RSSDI
TEXTBOOK OF
DIABETES MELLITUS

VOLUME 2

RSSDI TEXTBOOK OF
DIABETES MELLITUS

SECOND EDITION

Editor-in-Chief
BB Tripathy

Executive Editor
HB Chandalia

Editors
AK Das

PV Rao

SV Madhu

V Mohan

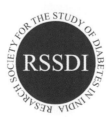

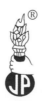

JAYPEE BROTHERS MEDICAL PUBLISHERS (P) LTD

New Delhi • Panama City • London

Jaypee Brothers Medical Publishers (P) Ltd.

Headquarter

Jaypee Brothers Medical Publishers (P) Ltd
4838/24, Ansari Road, Daryaganj
New Delhi 110 002, India
Phone: +91-11-43574357
Fax: +91-11-43574314
Email: jaypee@jaypeebrothers.com

Overseas Offices

J.P. Medical Ltd.
83 Victoria Street London
SW1H 0HW (UK)
Phone: +44-2031708910
Fax: +02-03-0086180
Email: info@jpmedpub.com

Jaypee-Highlights Medical Publishers Inc.
City of Knowledge, Bld. 237, Clayton
Panama City, Panama
Phone: +50-73-010496
Fax: +50-73-010499
Email: cservice@jphmedical.com

Cover illustration depicts the concept of expanded etiology of type 2 diabetes which includes pancreas, liver, kidney, intestinal tract and adipose tissue.

Website: www.jaypeebrothers.com
Website: www.jaypeedigital.com

Inquiries for bulk sales may be solicited at: jaypee@jaypeebrothers.com

This book has been published in good faith that the contents provided by the contributors contained herein are original, and is intended for educational purposes only. While every effort is made to ensure accuracy of information, the publisher and the editors specifically disclaim any damage, liability, or loss incurred, directly or indirectly, from the use or application of any of the contents of this work. Where appropriate, the readers should consult with a specialist or contact the manufacturer of the drug or device.

RSSDI Textbook of Diabetes Mellitus

Second Edition: 2008
Revised and Reprint: **2012**

ISBN: 978-93-5025-489-9

Printed at: Ajanta Offset & Packagings Ltd., New Delhi

MMS Ahuja: A TRIBUTE

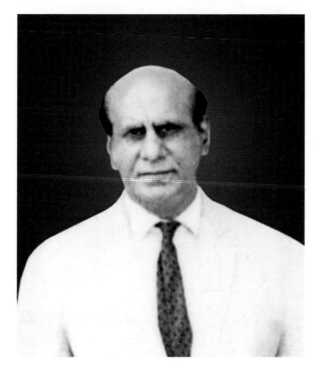

Professor MMS Ahuja was one of the major driving forces behind this textbook. It is unfortunate that he passed away on July 12, 1998, when this textbook was in its initial stages of preparation.

Professor Ahuja was Head of the Departments of Medicine and Endocrinology at the prestigious All India Institute of Medical Sciences (AIIMS) for several decades. He combined the qualities of a compassionate physician, an inspiring teacher and an inquisitive researcher—a combination difficult to find in modern times. He was a prolific writer and edited a highly popular series of review books entitled *Progress in Medicine*. In the areas of diabetology, his research work covered epidemiology, ketosis-resistant diabetes in young, cardiovascular complications, nutrition and patient education. He has left his distinctive stamp in these fields.

Professor Ahuja was one of the founders of Research Society for the Study of Diabetes in India (RSSDI) and the major working force behind this society's progress. He founded and edited the *International Journal of Diabetes in Developing Countries* from 1980 onwards, until the time of his collaboration with other editors. It took us a great deal of time to pick the threads of editorial process where he left them and ultimately put this book together. This textbook continues to bear the stamp of his excellence.

We, the editors of this textbook, owe a great deal of gratitude to our pioneering colleague, Professor Ahuja and pay him a respectful tribute.

Editors

CONTRIBUTORS

Subrat Kumar Acharya
Professor of Gastroenterology
All India Institute of Medical Sciences
New Delhi, India

Prashant Aggarwal
Senior Resident in Clinical Immunology
Sanjay Gandhi Postgraduate Institute of Medical
Sciences, Lucknow, Uttar Pradesh, India

SR Aravind
Consultant Diabetologist
Diacon Hospital
Bengaluru, Karnataka, India

Ashok Kumar Bajaj
Professor of Dermatology
MLN Medical College
Allahabad, Uttar Pradesh, India

JS Bajaj
Former Professor of Medicine
All India Institute of Medical Sciences
New Delhi, India

Sarita Bajaj
Professor of Endocrinology
MLN Medical College
Allahabad, Uttar Pradesh, India

V Balaji
Consultant Diabetologist
V Seshiah Diabetes Care and Research Institute
Chennai, Tamil Nadu, India

Samar Banerjee
Professor of Medicine
NRS Medical College
Kolkata, West Bengal, India

BC Bansal
Former Professor of Neurology Medical College
Rohtak, Haryana, India

Geetha K Bhat
Professor of Endocrinology and Metabolism
MS Ramaiah Medical College
Bengaluru
Karnataka, India

Eesh Bhatia
Professor of Endocrinology
Sanjay Gandhi Postgraduate Institute of Medical
Sciences, Lucknow, Uttar Pradesh, India

Vijayalakshmi Bhatia
Professor of Endocrinology
Sanjay Gandhi Postgraduate Institute of Medical
Sciences, Lucknow
Uttar Pradesh, India

Hemraj B Chandalia
Director
Dr Chandalia's Diabetes Endocrine Nutrition
Management and Research Centre
Mumbai, Maharashtra, India

Shaival H Chandalia
Consultant Endocrinologist
Jaslok Hospital and Research Centre
Mumbai, Maharashtra, India

PS Chatterjee
Head
School of Tropical Medicine
Kolkata, West Bengal, India

Swapna Chaturvedi
Dietician
All India Institute of Medical Sciences
New Delhi, India

Subhankar Chowdhury
Professor of Endocrinology
Institute of Postgraduate Medical Education and
Research, Kolkata, West Bengal, India

Paresh Dandona
Head, Division of Endocrinology
State University of New York at Buffalo, New York

Ashok Kumar Das
Director-Professor of Medicine
Jawaharlal Institute of Postgraduate Medical
Education and Research
Puducherry, India

BK Das
Associate Professor of Medicine
SCB Medical College, Cuttack, Orissa, India

PK Das
Professor of Medicine
SCB Medical College, Cuttack, Orissa, India

Sidhartha Das
Professor of Medicine
SCB Medical College,
Cuttack, Orissa, India

R Deepa
Research Biochemist
Dr Mohan's Diabetes Specialties Centre
Chennai, Tamil Nadu, India

Sandeep Dhindsa
Assistant Professor
State University of New York at Buffalo, New York

Ketan Goswami
Senior Fellow in Endocrinology
Southern Illinois University School of Medicine
Springfield IL

R Goswami
Associate Professor of Endocrinology
All India Institute of Medical Sciences
New Delhi, India

Leif Groop
Professor of Endocrinology
Lund University,
Malmö, Sweden

OP Gupta
Former Professor of Medicine
Civil Hospital
Ahmedabad, Gujarat, India

Sunil Gupta
Consultant Diabetologist
Diabetes Care n' Research Centre
Nagpur, Maharashtra, India

DK Hazra
ICMR Emeritus Medical Scientist
Sarojini Naidu Medical College
Agra, Uttar Pradesh, India

Aspi J Irani
Consultant Pediatrician
Dr B Nanavati Hospital
Mumbai, Maharashtra, India

RV Jayakumar
Professor of Endocrinology
Amritha Institute of Medical Sciences
Kochi, Kerala, India

Sushil Jindal
Associate Professor of Medicine
Peoples' College of Medical Sciences
Bhopal, Madhya Pradesh, India

Shashank R Joshi
Professor of Endocrinology
Seth GS Medical College
Mumbai, Maharashtra, India

Sandhya A Kamath
Professor of Medicine
Topiwala National Medical College
Mumbai, Maharashtra, India

Anil Kapur
Managing Director
World Diabetes Foundation, Lyngby, Denmark

A Kanungo
Chairman
Cuttack Diabetes Research Foundation
Bhubaneswar, Orissa, India

Romesh Khardori
Chief, Division of Endocrinology
Southern Illinois University School of Medicine
Springfield IL

AL Kirpalani
Professor of Nephrology
Bombay Hospital Institute of Medical Sciences
Mumbai, Maharashtra, India

Suman Kirti
Consultant Physician
Holy Family Hospital, New Delhi, India

N Kochupillai
Former Professor of Endocrinology
All India Institute of Medical Sciences
New Delhi, India

Venkata Ranga Rao Kodali
Department of Medicine
Jenny O' Neill Diabetes Centre
Derby, United Kingdom

Chandramohan Kolluru
Ophthalmologist
Aravind Eye Care System
Madurai, Tamil Nadu, India

Ajay Kumar
Consultant Physician
Diabetes Care and Research Center
Patna, Bihar, India

PS Lamba
Consultant Endocrinologist
Endocrine and Diabetes Management Centre
Mumbai, Maharashtra, India

RD Lele
Director
Jaslok Hospital and Research Centre
Mumbai, Maharashtra, India

SV Madhu
Professor of Endocrinology
University College of Medical Sciences,
Delhi, India

PC Manoria
Director
Heart Care Centre
Bhopal, Madhya Pradesh, India

Pankaj Manoria
Interventional Cardiologist
Escorts Heart Institute
New Delhi, India

AR Marita
Associate Director, Research and Development
Nicholas Piramal India Ltd
Mumbai, Maharashtra, India

Tiven Marwah
Assistant Professor of Endocrinology
VS General Hospital
Ahmedabad, Gujarat, India

Thomas Mathew
Assistant Professor of Medicine
St John's Medical College
Bengaluru, Karnataka, India

Suresh D Mehtalia
Consultant Physician
Sir HN Hospital
Mumbai, Maharashtra, India

PSN Menon
Head
Department of Pediatrics
Jaber Al-Ahmed Anned Forces Hospital, Kuwait

Anoop Misra
Consultant Physician
Fortis Hospital, New Delhi, India

Ramnath Misra
Professor of Immunology
Sanjay Gandhi Postgraduate Institute of Medical
Sciences, Lucknow
Uttar Pradesh, India

Sonal V Modi
Chief Nutritionist
Dr Chandalia's Diabetes Endocrine Nutrition
Management and Research Centre
Mumbai, Maharashtra, India

V Mohan
Chairman
Madras Diabetes Research Foundation
Chennai, Tamil Nadu, India

Susana A Moran
Emory School of Medicine,
Atlanta, GA, USA

C Munichoodappa
Director
The Bangalore Hospital
Bengaluru, Karnataka, India

MV Muraleedharan
Former Professor of Endocrinology
Medical College
Thrissur
Andhra Pradesh, India

Nutan Nabar
Research Associate
ICMR Advanced Centre of Reverse Pharmacology
Mumbai, Maharashtra, India

SJ Nagalotimath
Former Director
Karnataka Institute of Medical Sciences
Hubli, Karnataka, India

Dinesh K Nagi
Consultant Endocrinologist
Pinderfields Hospital
Wakefield, United Kingdom

Ramachandra G Naik
Consultant Endocrinologist
Bombay Hospital and Medical Research Centre
Mumbai, Maharashtra, India

M Balaraman Nair
Consultant Pathologist
Diagnostic and Research Centre
Thiruvanathapuram, Kerala, India

KM Venkat Narayan
Professor of Medicine
Emory School of Medicine
Atlanta GA

P Namperumalsamy
Chairman, Aravind Eye Care System
Postgraduate Institute of Ophthalmology
Madurai, Tamil Nadu, India

Anant Nigam
Consultant Diabetologist
Nigam Diabetes Centre
Jaipur, Rajasthan, India

Timothy O'Connor
Assistant Professor
Southern Illinois University School of Medicine
Springfield IL

Amy Olson
Instructor
Southern Illinois University School of Medicine
Springfield IL

MV Padma
Professor of Neurology
All India Institute of Medical Sciences
New Delhi, India

NC Panda
Former Professor of Biochemistry
SCB Medical College
Cuttack, Orissa, India

Kaushik Pandit
Research Scientist in Endocrinology
Institute of Postgraduate Medical Education and
Research, Kolkata
West Bengal, India

Vijay Panikar
Professor of Medicine
KG Somaiya Medical College
Mumbai, Maharashtra, India

SP Pendsey
Director
Diabetes Research Centre
Nagpur, Maharashtra, India

R Pradeepa
Research Nutritionist
Dr Mohan's Diabetes Specialties Centre
Chennai, Tamil Nadu, India

G Prasanth
Senior Resident in Medicine
Jawaharlal Institute of Postgraduate Medical
Education and Research
Puducherry, India

KM Prasanna Kumar
Senior Professor of Endocrinology and Diabetes
MS Ramaiah Medical College and Hospital
Bengaluru, Karnataka, India

G Premalatha
Consultant Diabetologist
Dr Mohan's Diabetes Specialties Centre
Chennai, Tamil Nadu, India

V Radha
Head, Molecular Genetics
Dr Mohan's Diabetes Specialties Centre
Chennai, Tamil Nadu, India

P Raghupathy
Former Professor of Pediatrics
Christian Medical College
Vellore, Tamil Nadu, India

A Ramachandran
President
India Diabetes Research Foundation
Chennai, Tamil Nadu, India

Pinjala Ramakrishna
Professor of Vascular Surgery
Nizam's Institute of Medical Sciences University
Hyderabad
Andhra Pradesh, India

PG Raman
Former Professor of Medicine
Gandhi Medical College
Bhopal, Madhya Pradesh, India

Kim Ramasamy
Chief Medical Officer
Aravind Eye Care System
Madurai, Tamil Nadu, India

D Sudhaker Rao
Director, Bone and Mineral Research Laboratory
Henry Ford Hospital
Detroit MI

Murlidhar S Rao
Professor of Cardiology
MR Medical College
Gulbarga
Karnataka, India

PV Rao
Professor of Endocrinology
Nizam's Institute of Medical Sciences University
Hyderabad, Andhra Pradesh, India

SS Rastogi
Consultant Endocrinologist
Research Centre for Diabetes and
Clinical Nutrition
Delhi, India

Radha Reddy
Consultant Endocrinologist
Chaparral Medical Group
Rancho Cucamonga CA

M Rema
Chief Ophthalmologist
Dr Mohan's Diabetes Specialties Centre
Chennai, Tamil Nadu, India

BK Sahay
Former Professor of Medicine
Osmania Medical College
Hyderabad, Andhra Pradesh, India

Rakesh K Sahay
Assistant Professor of Endocrinology
Gandhi Medical College
Hyderabad, Andhra Pradesh, India

GS Sainani
Physician
Jaslok Hospital and Research Centre
Mumbai, Maharashtra, India

Rajesh G Sainani
Consultant Gastroenterologist
Jaslok Hospital and Research Center
Mumbai, Maharashtra, India

KC Samal
Former Professor of Endocrinology
SCB Medical College
Cuttack, Orissa, India

Ami Ritesh Sanghvi
Fellow in Diabetology
Dr Mohan's Diabetes Specialties Centre
Chennai, Tamil Nadu, India

CB Sanjeevi
Associate Professor of Diabetes and Endocrinology
Karolinska Institute
Stockholm, Sweden

S Sarin
Insurance Services
New Delhi, India

Subrata Sarkar
Joint Research Director
Swami Prakashananda Ayurveda Research Centre
Mumbai, Maharashtra, India

V Seshiah
Medical Director
V Seshiah Diabetes Care and
Research Institute Chennai
Tamil Nadu, India

Nishit F Shah
Consultant Endocrinologist
PD Hinduja National Hospital
Mumbai
Maharashtra, India

Sanjiv Shah
Deputy Director
Swami Prakashananda Ayurveda Research Centre
Mumbai
Maharashtra, India

Siddharth N Shah
Consultant Diabetologist
SL Raheja Hospital
Mumbai
Maharashtra, India

Rekha Sharma
Chief Dietician
All India Institute of Medical Sciences
New Delhi, India

Dhananjay Shukla
Ophthalmologist
Aravind Eye Care System
Madurai, Tamil Nadu, India

C Snehalatha
Head of Laboratory
Dr A Ramachandran's Hospital
Chennai, Tamil Nadu, India

GR Sridhar
Consultant Endocrinologist
Endocrine and Diabetes Centre
Visakhapatnam, India

MC Srivastava
Physician
Diabetes Self-care Foundation
New Delhi, India

N Sudha
Consultant Pediatrician
Dr Mohan's Diabetes Specialties Centre
Chennai, Tamil Nadu, India

BB Tripathy
Former Professor of Medicine
SCB Medical College
Cuttack, Orissa, India

Devjit Tripathy
Assistant Professor
University of Texas Health Science Center
San Antonio TX

S Uthra
Fellow in Diabetology
Dr Mohan's Diabetes Specialties Centre
Chennai, Tamil Nadu, India

Ashok DB Vaidya
Principal Investigator
ICMR Advanced Centre of Reverse Pharmacology
Mumbai, Maharashtra, India

Rama Ashok Vaidya
Dean, Medical Research Centre
Kasturba Health Society
Mumbai, Maharashtra, India

Premlata K Varthakavi
Professor of Endocrinology
TN Medical College
Mumbai, Maharashtra, India

Vasumathy Vedantham
Retina-Vitreous Service
Aravind Eye Care System
Madurai, Tamil Nadu, India

Naval K Vikram
Department of Medicine
All India Institute of Medical Sciences
New Delhi, India

Stalin Viswanathan
Senior Resident in Medicine
Jawaharlal Institute of Postgraduate Medical
Education and Research
Puducherry, India

Vijay Viswanathan
Director
Diabetes Research Centre
Chennai, Tamil Nadu, India

Jasjeet S Wasir
Department of Medicine
All India Institute of Medical Sciences University
New Delhi, India

PREFACE TO REVISED SECOND EDITION

It gives me great pleasure to present the second revised edition of the *RSSDI Textbook of Diabetes Mellitus*. We were out of print of this book for the past one year because of a heavy demand for the book. While we were engaged in producing the Third Edition, we thought it appropriate to publish a Revised Second Edition. Jaypee Brothers Medical Publishers (P) Ltd, New Delhi, India, has undertaken the publishing of the revised edition. From our side, we have revised the book to make it virtually error-free.

I acknowledge assistance of all authors and my co-editors who served as section editors for this task. Professor V Mohan and Professor SV Madhu have undertaken this task earnestly. I have been ably assisted by my editorial staff, Dr Debanshu Roy, Dr Nishi Shah and Ms Patricia Sadri. I thank all my collaborators for their support.

HB Chandalia
Executive Editor

PREFACE TO THE SECOND EDITION

It is a matter of great pleasure and satisfaction for us that there has been a demand for second edition within two years of publication of the first. We are indeed grateful to our professional collegues in the country for their appreciation and encouraging remarks.

As already described in the last preface the first edition was compiled over a disorderly background following the sad demise of Professor MMS Ahuja who initiated the venture. As if that was not enough, at their first meeting, following release of the book, the editors decided to choose me (BB Tripathy) seven years his elder, as the Editor-in-Chief for the next edition of the book by over-ruling my objections, while Dr HB Chandalia was chosen as Executive Editor.

Following approval of the Society (RSSDI), the new list of editors was drawn up. The name of Professor Ahuja had to be dropped in any case. Most unfortunately, we also lost Professor Sam GP Moses, a buoyant personality with encyclopedic memory and remarkable for his coinage of apt phrases and epithets in course of his exceptionally eloquent delivery of addresses. As a replacement, the rest of us decided to invite a refreshingly young, resilient researcher and erudite scholar, Dr Viswanthan Mohan, Director of the celebrated Madras Diabetes Research Foundation and founder of Dr Mohan's Diabetes Specialities Center at Chennai, Tamil Nadu, India.

All policy decisions were taken by consensus arrived at a number of meetings convened at all the conference and gatherings held during the last three years or over.

The **second edition** presents a thoroughly revised, considerably expanded version of the first. While the chapters in the first edition numbered 62, it has escalated to 95 in the second.

Changes: Only Chapters 19, 56, 57 and 58 (in part) of the first edition have been reproduced as such in the second. All others have been rewritten, altered and supplemented as per requirement.

Some 23 new Chapters have been added, conspicuous among them, are Morphology of Pancreatic Islets (4), Biology of Insulin Action (6) Latent Autoimmune Diabetes in Adults (9), Role of Adipose Tissue (19), Anti-inflammatory Action of Insulin (7), Immunogenetics of Type 1 Diabetes (3) Nutrition Management in Special Situations (38), GI System, Bone Diseases and Rheumatological Manifestations (70, 72, 73 respectively) and Computers in Diabetes Management (86).

Furthermore "Epidemiology" has been split to 4 divisions in place of 2, in the first edition. Similarly, Oral Antidiabetic drugs from 1 to 3, Monitoring of controls from 1 to 3, Macrovascular Complication into 2, Peripheral Vascular Disease and Diabetic Foot split into two, Eye Disorders into two chapters, Role of Paramedical Personnel is presented in a separate chapter (89) while Prevention of Type 2 Diabetes has been dealt with in 3 chapters (91, 92, 93).

New contributors include some high profile international figures such as P Dandona, Leif Groop, KM Venkat Narayan, Romesh Khardori and D Sudhaker Rao. The name of Dinesh K Nagi needs a mention although he was kind enough to contribute the same topic to the last edition.

Equally important names from the national field are Balaraman Nair, Sunil Gupta, Sushil Jindal, RG Naik, P Raghupathy, Anoop Misra, Ajay Kumar, Ashok Vaidya, Sandhya Kamath, Samar Banerjee, Murlidhar S Rao, P Ramakrishna, P Namperumalsamy, Subrat Kumar Acharya, Ramnath Misra and Anant Nigam. Devjit Tripathy, an upcoming talent having worked wonders in collaboration of Leif Group and P Dandona is now a faculty member of the famous San Antonio Institute in Texas as a colleague of FM Heffner.

First authors have been altered in some 32 chapters for refreshing new contributions or occasionally for lack of positive response from the past ones. Naturally, these chapters have been fully revised and supplemented.

ACKNOWLEDGMENTS

I may be excused for writing this section in first person as tributes have to be paid to the rest of my editorial colleagues.

I am extremely fortunate to have the galaxy of editorial colleagues who have given me their utmost support in choosing the topics and their authors, in solving problems of all sorts as bound to crop up in course of this stupendous effort.

I have depended on Professor HB Chandalia and Professor AK Das for moral support for all my deeds and misdeeds. I had to look for their advice in most difficult circumstances. Professors SV Madhu and V Mohan have helped me most by undertaking to write chapters where assigned authors have failed to comply or the contributions did not appear to be adequate. In such circumstances, I send SOS messages to either of them for their help. This project would have failed to come through without their compliance in spite of their own personal/family problem or pressing preoccupations.

Professor PV Rao has undertaken the most onerous task of final verification of references, compilation of the index and implementation of printing and binding of the book at the final stage as he had done in case of the first edition. The next to follow, i.e. arrangement for circulation and marketing of the product have been entrusted entirely to the Executive Editor, Professor HB Chandalia of Mumbai, the commercial capital of the country.

In continuity, we have to express our heartfelt gratitude and eulogies to Mudrika Graphics, the printers of the Textbook. They managed to print the first edition initially under chaotic conditions. Thanks to their forbearance and sincere efforts, the book came out clear and sound with good get up and firm binding. We hope to have even a better product from them in case of the second edition. We are grateful to them for their best possible cooperation.

On my personal side, I am at a loss for ideas and words how to properly express my utmost gratitude to Sri Bidhu Bhusan Parija who has handled the papers we received, looked after the correction and retyping as well as the scrutiny of the final version to be dispatched for printing. He has executed volumes of correspondence with exceptional efficiency, sincerity, alacrity and hardwork inspite of advancing age beyond 75 years. I could never have ventured to undertake the task as Editor-in-Chief if he was not there with me. He was the one who has helped me through almost all of my other undertakings such as organizing conferences workshops and update sessions.

My wife, and my daughter-in-law Padmaja have provided me peace of mind as well as comforts for my physique during the trying periods so as to enable me to concentrate on my overwhelming task. Unfortunately, my wife cruelly left me high and dry on July 12, 2006 for her heavenly abode.

Dr SC Tej, my erstwhile clinical assistant, has helped me for nearly two years till he retired at age 86 years due to physical disability.

Lastly I have to state that I must have committed many errors and whimisical acts in course of my working for the book inspite of best of my intentions. These might have involved alterations, subtractions or additions in case of some of the chapters contributed by reputed scholars. All that I can do now is to very humbly solicit to be pardoned for all my faults partly in view of my age (5th year past 80) as well as for limitations in my knowledge and capacity.

Wishing the best to all those involved in preparing and marketing the *RSSDI Textbook of Diabetes Mellitus* Second Edition (2008), I solicit indulgent farewell from one and all.

BB Tripathy
HB Chandalia
AK Das
PV Rao
SV Madhu
V Mohan

PREFACE TO THE FIRST EDITION

With explosive increase in its prevalence, diabetes mellitus, as a chronic medical disorder, is to be reckoned on par with hypertension and atherosclerosis. A versatile disease, diabetes, in view of its frequent clinical and epidemiological link with the other two, constitutes a health problem of paramount concern for a very large proportion of the world population.

In the course of the last few decades, India has emerged as the country with the highest number of patients with diabetes. In keeping with this, in India, diabetology has emerged as a major specialty in the practice of both general medicine and endocrinology. Over the last thirty years, several centers have adopted diabetes as a single disease specialty for the state-of-the-art investigations and clinical care.

The idea of compiling a *Textbook on Diabetes Mellitus* was mooted with the above in view. Bearing in mind the fact that there already exist a number of exclusive books on diabetes on the global scene, this publication was planned keeping several special objectives in view. A large number of primary care physicians as well as an increasing number of specialists are in need of comprehensive knowledge on both basic and applied aspects of the disease. Publications from abroad are very expensive. Prices keep on rising steeply from edition to edition. Further, beginning from 1960s, it has been explicitly shown that problems associated with diabetes in India are in several respects distinct from those in the West, the major source of the available publications. Attempts to cover the special features of diabetes among diverse ethnic groups have been made in the two editions of the International Textbook of Diabetes Mellitus. Yet, it was felt that India needs a book of her own to cater to the needs of the burgeoning number of medical practitioners dealing with diabetes in this country as well as to those of its neighbors in South, Mid and South East Asia.

The Research Society for the Study of Diabetes in India (RSSDI) was founded in 1972 ostensibly for promoting academics and research on the intricate subject of diabetes mellitus. The Society has experienced phenomenal growth in membership and activities during the 90s of the last century. About four and half years back, Professor MMS Ahuja, a pioneer in establishing RSSDI, initiated a proposal for compiling a textbook on diabetes. Some of us quickly got together to process the basics and to set the program in motion. Unfortunately, the sad demise of Professor Ahuja in July 1998 left us high and dry. Records of the initial work were hard to trace out. It took us close to a year to recover from the shock and reorganize the undertaking right from the start.

As is evident from the list of editors, this is a collaborative work of several persons placed at long distances from each other. Professor PV Rao was assigned the pivotal role of keeping the records and looking after the printing, which he has done with great alacrity in the face of numerous difficulties in communication and coordination.

Although only a small body of basic research has originated from modern India, clinical and epidemiological studies have been numerous. These, for sure, are of considerable importance for medical practitioners and patients of this country. Only a small number of these works have been published or abstracted in the world literature and therefore most fail to hit books published in the West. The *RSSDI Textbook of Diabetes Mellitus* is purported to highlight data generated in India wherever relevant. Due scope has been provided for exposition of areas where Indian investigators have contributed valuable original ideas such as on planning of diet with higher carbohydrate content, use of insulin and sulfonylurea in combination, application of Yoga in the management of diabetes, an indigenous inexpensive method for the estimation of glycohemoglobin, identification and analysis of fibrocalculous pancreatic diabetes and malnutrition modulated diabetes mellitus, characterization of the quite common low weight type 2 diabetes as well as elaborate sequential study of epidemiology of diabetes in various social classes of ethnic Indians.

The scope of the textbook was proposed to be wide so as to be of service to general practitioners as well as to broaden their academic outlook. It was scrupulously designed to target the requirements of family physicians, academicians, clinical researchers and diabetes oriented health professionals at large. Diabetes along with its complications is a multiorgan disease covering all subspecialities of medicine as well as pediatrics, ophthalmology, obstetrics, surgery and orthopedics. While keeping all these in view, the contents have been designed and presented in a classic textbook style. Individual chapters are grouped into sections dealing with historical aspects, biochemical basis, pathogenesis, genetics, stages and classes, epidemiology, clinical details, management, complications and prevention. Each chapter is comprehensive and reasonably elaborate. Lists of references are adequate and appropriate. Contributions provided by experienced professors as well as senior and young clinical researchers from all parts of the country and some from abroad, have enriched the contents to the best possible extent. Many of the authors happen to be devoted members of the RSSDI.

Most notable shortcoming is the long delay of nearly three years of gestational period. Due to multiplicity of authors and editors, there is bound to be some overlap among the chapters. A few papers have been modified and even replaced after editorial scrutiny. Care has been taken to refer the papers back to the authors for updating, corrections and finally for reading of the proof copies prior to the final print.

The editors and the executives of the RSSDI are indeed thankful to various authors for devoting a lot of time and energy for preparing their contributions. Our thanks are due to Dr Rachel Thomas-Jacob for proofreading, the printers and numerous other persons who have helped individual editors and Professor PV Rao in the final lap of publication of our most cherished textbook on diabetes.

Publications on diabetes as well as CME and update sessions on the topic have been very popular during the recent decades. Our effort to bring out a comprehensive treatise on this popular subject, we earnestly hope, will receive fond acceptance from the readers. If this book addresses the questions they have in their minds or if it stimulates their thinking on this subject, our purpose would be served.

Sam GP Moses
BB Tripathy
HB Chandalia

CONTENTS

VOLUME 1

SECTION 1: PREAMBLE

SECTION 2: PHYSIOLOGY AND METABOLISM

SECTION 6: GENETICS AND IMMUNOLOGY

SECTION 7: CLINICAL PROFILE

SECTION 8: MANAGEMENT

VOLUME 2

SECTION 9: COMORBID CONDITIONS

SECTION 10: COMPLICATIONS

SECTION 11: DIABETES THROUGH LIFE AND EVENTS

SECTION 12: LIVING WITH DIABETES

SECTION 13: HEALTH CARE DELIVERY

SECTION 14: PREVENTION

Section 9

COMORBID CONDITIONS

Chapter 49

COMORBID CONDITIONS: OBESITY AND DYSMETABOLIC SYNDROME

Hemraj B Chandalia, PS Lamba

CHAPTER OUTLINE

DEFINITION AND SIGNIFICANCE OF COMORBID CONDITIONS

Over a period of time, diabetes takes serious toll of micro- and macrovasculature. Hence, those risk factors that are known to impact on the vascular system are extremely important to be recognized and addressed. There are a series of markers of vascular disease being studied aggressively at present. A study of these markers has a predictive value in the emergence of vascular disease. Hence, these are also viewed as comorbid conditions. In essence, study of these comorbid conditions lends additional depth to patient's clinical evaluation, making it truly comprehensive.

The importance of some comorbid conditions even supersedes the importance of metabolic control of diabetes. For example, looking from the viewpoint of coronary artery disease, management of hypertension, high LDL-cholesterol and tobacco abuse are considered class I interventions because the benefits of such interventions have been adequately documented. Control of diabetes, HDL-cholesterol, triglycerides, physical inactivity and obesity are considered class II interventions because they appear to have strong causal association with coronary heart disease (CHD), but the intervention data are limited.[1] Considering these facts, recognition of comorbid conditions become a very important strategy; more than even metabolic control of diabetes. Hypertension and high LDL-cholesterol are two risk factors, where the clinical outcome is so obvious, if poor control persists. In a situation like diabetic nephropathy, the pre-eminence of the control of hypertension over that of control of diabetes is well documented.[2]

Diabetes mellitus has been considered a multiorgan, multisystem disease. In older time, syphilis and now hepatitis B and AIDS have held similar status. Hence diabetology training without good training in internal medicine is considered a poor strategy. In-depth study and control of comorbid conditions, which is best done by an internist cum endocrinologist is an important strategy for a successful long-term outcome in diabetes.

TOBACCO ABUSE

It is a very important risk factor, which is often dutifully recorded in the patient history. However, a planned action to combat this menace is seldom initiated. In India, besides tobacco smoking, chewing tobacco and use of tobacco snuff and paste is rampant. In this form,

TABLE 49.1	Health hazards of tobacco abuse
Premature death	*Deaths in the year 2000*
Total number	4.8 million
• Deaths due to cardiovascular disease	1.7 million
• COPD	1.0 million
• Lung cancer	0.9 million
Risk as compared to nonsmokers	
• Fatal heart disease	2 times
• Lung cancer	10 times
• Strokes	2–3 times
• Acid peptic ulcer	2–3 times
• Cancer of mouth, esophagus, throat,	
• peripheral vascular disease	2 times
• Breast cancer, osteoporosis	Increased

COPD: Continuous obstructive pulmonary disease

the addiction also affects lot of females. Hence, a good diabetes center must also incorporate a good tobacco cessation program.

It is important to appreciate the morbidity and mortality associated with tobacco abuse, as this may need to be emphasized during the motivational phase of the cessation program. A few hazards of tobacco abuse are presented in **Table 49.1**.[3]

Tobacco Cessation Strategies

In order to help patients quit tobacco abuse, all tobacco users should be systematically identified at each visit and strongly urged to quit tobacco use. Those willing to quit should then be identified and systematic help offered to them. Literature related to cessation strategies should be available in the clinic.

At each follow-up visit, status of tobacco habit should be reviewed. Those patients who succeed should be congratulated. Those who fail in their attempts should be encouraged to learn the cause of failure and try again with a different strategy. Another tobacco user in the family reduces the chances of success, so also the alcohol habit, which is often associated with tobacco abuse. Use of inadequate dosage of nicotine replacement therapy is also associated with failure.[4,5] Benefits of cessation, even at an advanced age have been well documented and can serve as a motivational force.[6] Those having low consumption of tobacco or those suffering from acute vascular problem like acute coronary syndrome or peripheral vascular occlusion may decide to discontinue tobacco use abruptly, without any assistance. This method is called "cold turkey" and is quite successful, at least temporarily. It needs to be reinforced, in order to prevent relapse. Patients also need supportive treatment, like combating constipation or insomnia.

Nicotine replacement in de-escalating dosage is often the key to success and its use should be encouraged in all tobacco users except those with very low consumption. Contraindications to nicotine replacement are: pregnancy, ischemic heart disease and peripheral vascular disease. Nicotine patches can be used in low tobacco consumers while chewing gum or nasal spray should be used in heavy tobacco consumers. Patches are used in dosage of about 1 mg/hr initially and reduced every 1 to 2 weeks, over a period of 8 weeks to a dose of 5 to 8 mg/16 hr (waking hours). At this stage, total cessation is easy. Local skin reactions are common, but can be minimized by rotating application sites or using a steroid cream locally. Nicotine gum is available as 2 or 4 mg per piece preparation. Initially, a 2 or 4 mg piece per 2 hours maybe required. This should be reduced over the next eight weeks. The gum should be chewed till a "peppery" taste is experienced; thereafter it should be parked in the buccal cavity for about 30 minutes. Side effects like local soreness and dyspepsia can occur.

Another useful drug is an antidepressant—bupropion. It is used as a slow release preparation of 150 to 300 mg/day orally. It raises the intracerebral levels of dopamine and noradrenaline, much alike the action of nicotine. Usually the drug is administered for 1 to 6 months, with a decision to quit tobacco after 15 days. This drug is contraindicated with a history of seizures.

Weight gain is a common side effect of tobacco cessation strategies. Combined use of nicotine and bupropion minimizes weight gain. This is an important side effect in type 2 diabetics where obesity is a common comorbid condition. Hence, a simultaneous intensification of diet and exercise program should accompany a tobacco cessation program.

OBESITY

Epidemiology

Obesity is a highly prevalent disorder, commonly associated with type 2 diabetes. The prevalence of obesity is on the increase, mainly in the past two decades. Data from the National Health and Nutrition Examination Surveys (NHANES) reveal an increase in obesity (BMI >30) from 14.5 to 30.5% over a period of about 2 decades from 1980 to the year 2000.[7,8] Prevalence of overweight (BMI >25) was very high in the year 1999-2000, as 64% of adults in USA were overweight.[8] Commensurate with the rapid rise of obesity, a dramatic 30 to 40% increase in the prevalence of type 2 diabetes was observed between the years 1990 and 2000. Furthermore, a distressing rise in the prevalence of obesity has been reported in childhood, together with the advent of type 2 diabetes of childhood. In USA, more than 50% of children are either overweight or obese.[9] In the USA, prevalence of obesity in children 6 to 11 years of age doubled between the two NHANES studies in about two decades. In Japan, the situation is not as grim, but obesity doubled from 5 to 10% between 1974 and 1993.[10] In India, obesity has been described in 18.3% of school children especially from affluent communities[11] and emergence of type 2 diabetes of childhood is expected to occur rapidly in India.

The prevalence of obesity in Indian adults has been reported in the Second National Family Health Survey-2 (NFHS-2).[12] The prevalence varied in different states of India, from as low as 4 to 6% in Bihar and Orissa, to as high as 30 to 35% in Punjab and Delhi. Higher prevalence of obesity was associated with greater prosperity.

A series of studies from the years 1994-2004 from Rajasthan, India over a decade have demonstrated the rise in the prevalence of obesity and rural-urban differences.[13-16] The prevalence in urban areas was significantly high and over a decade, BMI in young adults (20–29 year age) increased from 21.1 ± 3.9 to 25.68 ± 11.1 and older people (50–59 year age) from 23.2 ± 5.7 to 27.8 ± 4.5 kg/m². At age of 50 to 59, 29.4% were overweight (BMI >25) and 7.6% obese (BMI >30) in 1995 while 82.3 were overweight and 32.4% were obese in the year 2004.

Definition and Diagnosis

Obesity is defined as an excess of adiposity. As it is difficult to determine the amount of body fat or body fat percent by simple clinical methods, various surrogate parameters have been utilized. BMI has been the most widely used parameter (**Table 49.2**). However, it does not reflect accurately the degree of adiposity, because body weight can be constituted by excess adipose tissue or muscle mass. To overcome this drawback, a simple waist measurement or waist/ hip ratio is used clinically. Normal values are presented in **Table 49.3**. It is obvious that if there is an increase in both the waist and hip circumferences, the W/H ratio may not be altered. Hence, an absolute waist circumference measurement or a sagittal diameter of waist (vertical

TABLE 49.2	Body mass index Wt (kg)/Ht (m²)	
	Normal	*Asian Indians*
Underweight	< 20	< 18
Normal	20–25	18–23
Overweight	> 25	> 23
Obese	> 30	> 28

distance between bed and top of abdomen in supine position) should be used. Abdominal fat, either intra-abdominal or extra-abdominal produces more insulin resistance and predisposes to cardiovascular disease as compared to the fat in the lower part (gluteofemoral) of the body. It has been demonstrated that Asian Indians have greater amount of body fat than Caucasians for a given BMI; thus the body fat percentage in Caucasians with BMI of 25 has been found to be equal to the percent body fat in Asian Indians with a BMI of 23.[17] Hence, the BMI of 23 is used as a cut-off point in Asian Indians.

The most accurate measurement of body fat is made by studying body composition by classic methods. For example, body water can be determined by underwater weighing and lean and fat body compartments estimated by using deuterium or tritiated water. The next accurate method to measure body fat is that by skin-fold measurements at suitable sites both on the body trunk and limbs. Determination of percent body fat by bioimpedance method is not very reliable, but used clinically because of the ease of its use. Body composition can be studied by using dual energy X-ray absorptiometry (DEXA), which gives estimates of body fat percent more accurately than bioimpedance method.

The measurements of truncal fat has been further partitioned into intra-abdominal and extra-abdominal compartments. These measurements are carried out by a single or multiple CT or MRI images of the truncal area and either a calculation of adipose tissue surface

TABLE 49.3	Assessment of truncal obesity	
	Males	*Females*
Waist (Indians)	≥ 102 cm ≥ 90 cm	≥ 88 cm ≥ 80 cm
W/H ratio	≥ 1	≥ 0.8
Sagittal diameter (Indians)	≥ 32 cm ≥ 29 cm	≥ 28 cm ≥ 25 cm

area by planimetry or a calculation of fat volume by a three-dimensional reconstruction of multiple images is made.

Some additional clinical parameters have been proposed to bring out the presence of truncal obesity. Total body weight divided by the abdominal girth is one such parameter. A summed value of skin-fold thickness over the trunk area (subscapular, suprailiac) gives some estimate of truncal obesity. The ratio of truncal skinfold thickness to limb skinfold (triceps, biceps, thigh) gives further insight into the distribution of body fat.

Etiology

The basic causes are genetic, environmental and hormonal.

Genetic Factors

The basic etiology of the common form of obesity is a complex interaction of multiple genes and environment. There are multiple susceptibility genes which either express directly through various hormones and enzymes to produce obesity or their expression is enhanced by the environmental influences. The environmental factors are too well described and continue to escalate in spite of being countered constantly in media headlines. These are high caloric intake mainly as fats, use of refined carbohydrates and low fiber foods, physical inactivity and mental stress.

Genetic factors are very obvious in rare cases of monogenic diseases due to gene mutations, like mutations of leptin or leptin receptor gene, prohormone convertase gene-1 (PC-1), pro-opiomelanocortin gene and melanocortin-4 receptor gene.

Environmental Factors

Nutritional: Overnutrition is part of an environmental problem leading to obesity. During certain phases of life, where nutrition is enhanced and physical activity declines, onset of obesity is precipitated. This can occur in children at the time of examination and women during pregnancy. The convalescent phase of any major illness can be associated with obesity, because physical activity may not commence while increased caloric intake occurs. Postenteric fever and posthepatitis obesity is still seen in the developing world. Physical inactivity increases with acculturation and urbanization. Although the calories expended in physical activity are not very large, the small energy imbalance so caused can result in slow weight gain (see under energy balance).

Medications: A variety of drugs can induce obesity. Corticosteroids uniformly cause weight gain, while oral contraceptive does so in some women. The treatment related weight gain in diabetics has been seriously discussed in the literature.[18-21] However, the weight gain connected with insulin, and sulfonylurea therapy is related to the weight loss occurring in the pretreatment period.[22] It occurs because the body weight moves towards its set point. The only drugs that can disturb the set point in diabetes and result in inordinate weight gain are thiazolidinediones. It is possible that this is determined genetically, as genetic polymorphism has been shown in animals exhibiting excessive weight gain with thiazolidinediones. However, most treated patients exhibit weight gain with these compounds, which is a major drawback of these drugs. The weight gain with thiazolidinediones has been ascribed to an accelerated recruitment of preadipocytes to adipocytes, a process likely to result in improved insulin sensitivity. The fat deposition is also described to be in the limbs and not truncal, but these facts need wider documentation.

Hormonal Factors

These are often invoked by the clinicians and patients alike in the causation of obesity, but are rarely responsible for moderate-to-severe obesity. Hypothyroidism is a common disease. It causes marginal weight gain, rarely exceeding five kilograms. Subclinical hypothyroidism can also cause weight gain and hence, forms an indication for treating subclinical disease. Hypercortisolism, induced by exogenous corticosteroids or endogenous secretion (Cushing's syndrome) also causes borderline weight gain of 2 to 5 kg due to excess adipose tissue and edema. Biochemical abnormalities in steroidal pathways, like an excess of 11-β-hydroxysteroid dehydrogenase type 1 (11-β-HSD) has recently been described as an important anomaly in obesity. This leads to increased conversion of cortisone to cortisol. Its significance remains to be established.

The most important endocrine obesity is seen in patients of insulinoma. The weight gain can be grossly excessive in this situation. However, insulinomas or similar disorders like nesidioblastosis are rare causes of obesity.

Energy Balance in Health and Disease

The basic equation of thermodynamics dictates that in a person in energy balance, the intake and expenditure are equal. Although this equation is inviolable, unknown and known alterations in metabolism can result in weight gain on a comparatively normal or moderately low calorie diet. This has always been enigmatic, but several possibilities are being explored to explain this phenomenon. It is possible that the intake is under-reported by obese subjects on a dietary recall.[23] The energy expenditure has a small component, called thermic effect of meal, which is described to be low in obese subjects.[24] Exercise also produces a thermic effect, which could be impaired in obese subjects.[25] In the metabolic pathways, there are certain wasteful pathways, which maybe hypoactive in obesity, thus allowing them to accumulate energy. The coupling and decoupling of oxidative phosphorylation is governed by certain enzymes. Polymorphism or impaired activity of uncoupling proteins has been shown in obese subjects.

The caloric equivalent of weight gain is 7000 kcal for each kilogram. Thus, a positive balance of 50 kcal/day will result in a slow and imperceptible weight gain of more than two kilograms in each year. Similarly, a small negative balance can result in substantial weight loss over the years.

Pathophysiology

Insulin Resistance

Excess of adipose tissue confers a state of insulin resistance in obesity. There has always been a debate whether insulin resistance or obesity, which of the two, is the primary event. In a group of 12 obese subjects, weight loss was induced by a hypocaloric diet. Serum insulin levels dropped on weight reduction, but when the subjects were refed for three days before post-weight loss testing, the insulin levels were similar to the pre-treatment levels.[26] The same phenomenon was observed in a group of 8 obese, impaired glucose tolerance subjects. This proves the point that insulin resistance is a primary abnormality. Recently, the relationship of obesity and insulin resistance was further dissected by studying insulin resistance in nonobese, nondiabetic individuals. The Asian Indians were shown to have insulin resistance even when nonobese.[27] This resistance is associated with polymorphism of ENPP1 (also known as PC-1) gene.[28] These seminal observations prove that insulin resistance is the primary event. In clinical practice, obesity and insulin resistance appear to coexist in most of the patients.

It is not only the quantity of adipose tissue, but dysfunction of adipose tissue that causes insulin resistance and cardiovascular disease.[29] Adipose tissue is an active endocrine organ. It gets inflamed in certain situations to produce more cytokines like interleukin-6 or tumor-necrosis factor-α. This process is also associated with a raised hypersensitive C-reactive protein level (HS-CRP), a marker now described to be associated with obesity, diabetes and cardiovascular disease. Leptin and resistin are increased and adiponectin is reduced in this situation. Increased leptin is probably caused by a state of leptin resistance while resistin is the main hormone responsible for insulin resistance. Adiponectin normally ameliorates insulin resistance.

Natural History and Clinical Course

Natural history of obesity gives an insight into the interventional strategies and treatment targets. Most obese subjects go through a familiar pattern of weight changes throughout their lives. They are usually obese in childhood and young adult life. Their body weight is distinctly above the ideal body weight. This weight is called desirable body weight for these individuals, as they maintain it at its set point for most part of their lives. With repeated pregnancies in females or a prolonged illness in both sexes, at times the weight settles down to a new set point, higher than the desirable body weight. This is called the settling point weight. Most obese subjects, when treated optimally, will reduce weight down to the settling point or rarely down to the desirable body weight, but almost never down to the ideal body weight.

On administration of hypocaloric diets the weight loss usually occurs in a stepladder pattern, the plateaus are usually due to water retention. At times, a plateau persists for a long time because with weight loss, the caloric expenditure is lowered.

In these situations, a further intensification of diet and exercise therapy is required. Very rapid weight loss can occur with starvation diets or very low calorie diets. Without dietary re-education, there is usually a relapse and weight gain. Such rapid changes in weight shatter the metabolic processes by causing rapid mobilization or accretion of fat and should be avoided. It must be added that the bariatric surgery has radically altered the course of the disease.

Complications

Obesity, unaccompanied by other cardiovascular risk factors, like hypertension or high LDL-cholesterol or tobacco abuse may not be responsible for any grave cardiovascular consequences. However, it is difficult to study obesity in its pure form. Extreme obesity obviously produces mechanical problems of weight-bearing joints, social unacceptability and psychological problems. Adipose tissue dysfunction may not be present, especially in young obese subjects. Such dysfunction maybe a function of senescent adipose tissue. These issues require further clarification in future. Most frequently, obesity is accompanied by other risk factors (metabolic syndrome) and hence a large number of complications are associated with obesity.

Cardiovascular Complications

In Framingham Heart Study,[30] the incidence of ischemic heart disease (IHD) increased by a factor of 2.4 in obese women and 2 in obese men. In Nurses Health Study, the increased risk of IHD as related to obesity was found to be present (RR 3.4) but low when adjusted for other risk factors (RR 1.9).[31] Obesity is associated with left ventricular hypertrophy and increased incidence of congestive heart failure and arrhythmia. Several types of lipoprotein abnormalities have been described in obesity. High triglycerides were emphasized by Albrink.[32] Additionally, dense LDL phenotype with low HDL-cholesterol is associated with obesity.[33]

Obesity is associated with an increased prevalence of hypertension. With the use of standard blood pressure cuffs, a spuriously high value is obtained. The distensible bladder in the cuff must cover the circumference of the arm as well as 75% of the length of the arm.

Increase in blood pressure has been described in the obese population in massive life insurance data. The Framingham study showed twice the prevalence of hypertension in obese as compared to nonobese subjects.[30] Obesity was described as the cause of hypertension in 30% of the individuals.[34] Weight gain is associated with raised blood pressure and weight loss has a salutary effect on the lowering of blood pressure. The mechanism of production of hypertension in obesity is probably via insulin resistance, which is associated with sodium retention, stimulation of the renin-angiotensin-aldosterone system and increased sympathetic activity.

Obesity and diabetes: Obesity and diabetes are closely interrelated, as both of them originate from a common pathogenetic mechanism; that is insulin resistance. High insulin levels and insulin resistance in obesity as well as early diabetes is well described.[26,35] In fact, the triad of obesity, insulin resistance and glucose intolerance or diabetes coexists in the metabolic syndrome.

In Nurses Health Study, where 1,14,824 women were followed for 14 years, it was demonstrated that risk of type 2 diabetes increases *pari passu* with an increase in BMI.[36] Distribution of body fat has independent influence on the development of diabetes.[37] Fasting blood glucose increased with increasing waist/hip ratio.[38] In USA, association of truncal obesity with diabetes has been particularly observed in Mexican Americans. Either measured as higher subscapular to triceps skinfolds or increased waist/hip ratio, the upper body obesity was associated with diabetes.[39] The mechanism of glucose intolerance in obesity is insulin resistance. This is induced mostly at the postreceptor levels; but at times at the receptor level, the receptor-kinase activity is decreased in obesity and diabetes.[40] In these situations, the glucose transporters are decreased in muscle and adipose tissue.[41] On the basis of insulin clamp studies, both the oxidative and nonoxidative glucose disposal have been shown to be impaired, the latter more than the former.[42] Impairment of glycogen synthase activity is one of the early abnormalities.[43]

Other Complications of Obesity

Cholelithiasis is found more commonly in the obese subjects. The risk of gallstones is two times more in women with a BMI over 30 kg/m^2 and seven times in those with BMI over 45 kg/m^2.[44] This is probably caused by a combination of cholesterol hypersecretion in the bile and reduced gallbladder motility. Rapid weight loss further renders the bile more lithogenic. The incidence of gallstones is markedly increased following bariatric surgery. Bile acid (ursodeoxycholic acid, UDCA) supplementation maybe indicated in these situations.

Obesity affects pulmonary function adversely. The lung compliance is lowered and work of breathing increased in obesity. There is alveolar hypoventilation with hypercarbia due to alterations in the respiratory drive. Obese subjects frequently suffer from sleep-disordered breathing or obstructive sleep apnea (OSA). Obstructive sleep apnea further aggravates insulin resistance due to increased sympathetic activity.[45] Medically as well as surgically induced weight loss improves a large number of respiratory abnormalities.[46]

Obesity increases osteoarthritis of knees and hip joints. The mechanism of production of osteoarthritis is direct weight-bearing trauma. Additionally, some systemic mechanisms like raised cholesterol, blood glucose or uric acid maybe operative through some unknown mechanism.

Obesity and hyperuricemia or gout have been associated in many studies. A cross-sectional study of

73,532 women aged 30-49 showed a significant association of obesity with gout.[47] In a Dutch study, serum uric acid levels were positively associated with body weight in men but not women.[48] In Fiji, both the Melanesian and Asian population showed a significant association of BMI with plasma uric acid levels in both diabetic and nondiabetic men and women.[49] More importantly, uric acid levels rise when obese subjects are on severely hypocaloric diets and this may, at times precipitate an attack of gout.

Obesity also affects endocrine function of several endocrine glands. Adrenocorticoid synthesis as well as degradation is increased, the cortisol levels and their diurnal variation remaining normal.[50] The total growth hormone secretion is lowered in obese subjects, with a blunting of periodic growth hormone spurts.[51] The insulin-like growth factor 1 (IGF-1) levels are, however normal, probably because of its stimulation by the hyperinsulinemic state.[51] Hyperinsulinemia and insulin resistance is present in obesity and has been described above.

Management of Obesity

Nutrition Therapy

(See Chapter 38)

Exercise Therapy

An inverse relationship between physical activity and body weight has been noted as early as in 1965 in the West Bengal population.[52] More importantly, exercise therapy prevents relapse; subjects with reportedly low physical activity have a three times possibility of relapse over a 10 year follow-up period as compared to those reportedly physically active.[53] Television viewing and lately, computer use has fostered physical inactivity.[54,55] Prolonged hours of television viewing can increase obesity 2 to 4 times in adults as well as adolescents.[54,55] The most evident mechanism of weight loss on exercise is quantitatively increased caloric expenditure. As the magnitude of this effect is not great, other explanations need to be invoked. These include thermic effect of exercise, increased cycling of substrates and elevated resting metabolic rate. Certain behavioral changes may occur with exercise, like decreased preference for fatty foods and psychological facilitation.[56] The resting metabolic rate increased by 10% in aerobic trained-individuals and 5% in resistance-trained individuals.[57] Several studies have shown a preferential fatty acid oxidation with slow and prolonged exercise as compared to brisk exercises, but these data have not been uniformly reproducible.[58,59]

In clinical practice, a combination of aerobic and resistance exercises should be prescribed. The precautions are same as in the case of diabetics undertaking exercises. The exercises should be brought to the target level gradually over 2 to 4 weeks time. In those who have never exercised before or in all subjects beyond 50 years age, a cardiovascular check-up is essential before instituting a full scale exercise program. Many obese subjects suffer from osteoarthritis of knees and hip joints, so that nonweight-bearing exercises may need to be prescribed. In urban centers in India, patients must have access to at least two types of exercise options, one indoor and other outdoor. In addition to a planned exercise program, incorporation of extra-activities in the daily schedule would give better results. For example, one can use stairs instead of an elevator or walk up to a colleague instead of using an intercom.

Behavioral Therapy

Behavioral approach is a powerful tool in the management of obesity. Eating pattern and exercise habits are learned behaviors and hence, can be modified. A large number of studies from 1970 to 1990 brought out the effect of behavioral therapy. In most of these studies, a weight loss of 3.8 to 8.5 kg occurred over 8 to 20 weeks of behavioral treatment.[60] A large number of subsequent studies have further established the role of behavioral therapy.[61-63] The most important components of behavioral therapy include self-monitoring, goal setting and stimulus or cue control. When applied to nutrition and exercise program, behavioral approaches improve the results substantially. Self-monitoring is an important component, so also is setting up of a realistic goal. Patient is guided to identify the cue or stimulus that is leading to excessive nutrient intake and strategies to eliminate the stimulus are undertaken. Some simple behavioral strategies are:

- Slow intake of food to allow time for experiencing satiation
- Fixing up time, place or crockery to be used for the meal to eliminate between meal intake
- Putting down fork and knife after each morsel
- Avoid eating while watching television.

Besides such nonspecific methods, specific strategies can be evolved after studying the eating behavior of the individual.

Pharmacotherapy

Although lifestyle interventions are useful in weight reduction, there are frequent failures and relapses.

Hence, search for medications has always been intensive in this area.

Noradrenergic serotonergic drugs: All of these compounds are in disuse at present except fluoxetine. The typical noradrenergic compounds were amphetamine, benzphetamine and diethylpropion. They have an abuse potential and are no longer used. The serotonergic drugs used earlier were fenfluramine and dexfenfluramine. On prolonged use, they were also shown to cause pulmonary hypertension and hence, their use is abandoned. Fluoxetine, a serotonergic compound has least side effects and is in use currently. Sibutramine is an inhibitor of reuptake of both serotonin and norepinephrine. It is the most widely used satiation-enhancing drug at present. In dosage of 5 to 20 mg/day, it produced significantly greater weight loss than placebo.[64] It is best used together with dietary re-education for the initial period of 2 to 3 months. However, long-term (up to 1 year) use of sibutramine has been reported with beneficial effects.[65] The side effects of sibutramine include headache, constipation, dry mouth, insomnia and a minimal rise in blood pressure.

Lipase inhibitor: Tetrahydrolipstatin (Orlistat, Xenical) is an inhibitor of pancreatic lipase. It prevents hydrolysis of dietary triglycerides and promotes its excretion through the fecal route.[66,67] More recently, in a study called XENDOS, orlistat has been used together with lifestyle changes in the prevention of type 2 diabetes.[68]

Orlistat is used in dosage of 180 mg twice a day with meals. The only unpleasant side effect is fecal soiling of clothes. On hypocaloric diets, it maybe possible to use the drug in dosage of 60–120 mg OD with the principal meal. This strategy avoids fecal soiling of clothes. In full dosage, the drug can cause malabsorption of fat-soluble vitamins. It should be given 2 hours before or after the ingestion of multivitamin or lipophilic drugs.

Pseudonutrients (See Chapter 38): These are extensively marketed by the food industry. Artificial sweeteners take place of sugar and many fat substitutes, which are either low caloric or calorie-free, take place of fat in the diet. The most eminent example of calorie free fat substitute is olestra.

Endocannabinoid receptor antagonists: This is a novel class of drugs, which antagonizes the cannabinoid type 1 receptor. Rimonabant is one such well-studied compound already in clinical use. In the Rio-Europe study, the drug was used in dosage of 5 or 20 mg per day in obese subjects with BMI >30 kg/m^2. It produced significant weight loss and improved HDL-cholesterol, triglycerides levels and insulin resistance.[69] In the Rio-lipid study, rimonabant was used in obese subjects with dyslipidemia.[70] In comparison to placebo, rimonabant at a dose of 20 mg produced significantly greater weight loss (6.7 ± 0.5 kg), reduced waist circumference (5.8 ± 0.5 cm), increased HDL-cholesterol (10 ± 1.6%) and reduced triglycerides (13 ± 3.5%). Rimonabant also increased adiponectin levels. The side effects of this drug include nausea, anxiety and depression.

Surgical Approach to Obesity

Of a variety of surgical approaches used in obesity, only two are currently in clinical use. Liposuction is recommended for removing localized bulges of fat, which do not respond to good medical management. It should not be used as a first line therapy to reduce body fat, as the procedure required will be extensive in such cases resulting in considerable blood loss and morbidity. Bariatric surgery of gastrointestinal tract has evolved through the past three decades. Earlier procedures like jejunoileal bypass produced considerable after-effects, including malnutrition and cirrhosis of liver. Two currently used procedures have produced good results with minimal morbidity. They are:
- Gastric Banding
- *Roux-en-Y bypass:* It is considered the method of choice whenever it is feasible.

The weight loss produced by bariatric surgery is massive. In morbidly, obese subjects (BMI > 40) or those with comorbidities like hypertension, diabetes and hyperlipidemia, bariatric surgery is the only effective method of weight control.

METABOLIC SYNDROME (Multimetabolic Syndrome, Syndrome X)

Definition and Diagnosis

The term syndrome X was coined by Gerald Reaven in the year 1988 to include four major components (The Deadly Quartet), obesity, insulin resistance, high triglycerides plus low HDL-cholesterol and hypertension. High insulin resistance can be present with or without impaired glucose tolerance or diabetes.[71] This concept emerged on the backdrop of several studies describing association of obesity, mainly abdominal obesity, hypertension, impaired glucose tolerance and hyperuricemia by Vague[72], Camus[73], Pyorala[74] and Modan.[75] Two important studies, one showing association of hyperinsulinemia and obesity and the other showing association of hyperinsulinemia and glucose intolerance.[26,35] and similar studies by Reaven—shaped the modern concept of syndrome X, later termed as multimetabolic syndrome. Later, this term has been used as an omnibus term to include all common metabolic diseases or markers of diseases or biochemical abnormalities described in these diseases.

In order to promote uniformity of data collection globally, serious efforts have been made by several organizations to define the syndrome. These include WHO, European Group for the study of Insulin Resistance (EGIR), National Cholesterol Education Program's panel on Detection, Evaluation and Treatment of High Blood Cholesterol in Adults (Adult Treatment Panel III), Association of Clinical Endocrinologists (AACE) and International Diabetes Federation.[76-80] The major differences between these classifications need to be resolved but notably WHO included patients of type 2 diabetes while EGIR excluded them. The ATP III criteria recognized three out of five abnormalities (abdominal obesity, elevated triglycerides, reduced HDL-C, elevated blood pressure and elevated fasting glucose) as diagnostic. The waist circumference cut-off points of the diagnosis of truncal obesity are better made specific to each ethnic group. Thus ATP III describes it as 102 cm in men and 88 cm in women and EGIR 94 cm in men and 80 cm in women. WHO has stipulated that waist circumference is made ethnic-specific. For Asian Indians, the cut-off point for waist circumference are 90 cm in men and 80 cm in women. **Table 49.4** gives WHO criteria.

Validity and Utility of Concept of Metabolic Syndrome

It is questionable whether metabolic syndrome (MS) represents an entity with common etiology. Insulin resistance has been described by Reaven to be central; however, etiology of the same remains to be settled. It is possible that various components of the metabolic syndrome arise from some susceptibility genes. Each of these components appears to be polygenic and it is quite possible that these components may share some of the susceptibility genes. As environmental influences are important in the expression of susceptibility genes, metabolic syndrome is manifest partly due to environmental influences.

The utility of the concept of metabolic syndrome stems from the fact that its components represent important cardiovascular risk factors.[81,82] It will always be advisable not to lose sight of these factors, once two or three components are found to coexist in the same individual. Thus, this concept serves the purpose of guiding the clinician to take a comprehensive approach. Metabolic syndrome increases lifetime risk of diabetes five-fold[82] and cardiovascular disease two-fold.[83] The list of abnormalities under the title of metabolic syndrome is being expanded continuously. From a clinical standpoint, the basic diseases under metabolic syndrome are obesity (general and truncal), dyslipidemia, dysglycemia and hypertension. Perhaps, hyperuricemia should be added to the list. The other features described are risk factors or markers of risk factors like hyperleptinemia, prothrombotic state (increased plasminogen activator inhibitor), proinflammatory state (increased C-reactive protein) and reduced adiponectin. The prevalence of metabolic syndrome is high in most communities, more so in Asian Indians. By NCEP criteria, 41.1% of Asian Indians were suffering from metabolic syndrome.[84] By using EGIR criteria, metabolic syndrome was present in 11.2% of Chennai (India) urban population.[85] In a multiethnic study in

TABLE 49.4	WHO criteria for the clinical diagnosis of metabolic syndrome
Clinical measure	IGT, IFG, T2DM
Insulin resistance	Lowered insulin sensitivity (Insulin sensitivity below lowest quartile for background population under investigation)
Plus any two of the following	
Body weight	Men: Waist-to-hip ratio > 0.90; Women: Waist-to-hip ratio > 0.85 and/or BMI > 30 kg/m^2
Lipid	TG $\geq$ 150 mg/dl and/or HDL-C < 35 mg/dl in men or < 39 mg/dl in women
Blood pressure	$\geq$ 140/90 mm Hg
Glucose	IGT, IFG or T2DM
Other	Microalbuminuria (urinary albumin excretion rate $\geq$ 20 µg/min or albumin-to-creatinine ratio $\geq$ 30 mg/g)

IGT: Impaired glucose tolerance; IFG: Impaired fasting glucose; T2DM: Type 2 diabetes mellitus; TG: Triglycerides; HDL-C: High-density lipoprotein cholesterol

Singapore, 28.8% of Indians, 24.2% of Malays and 14.8% of Chinese had metabolic syndrome.[86] As compared to these data, NHANES III showed a prevalence of 23.7% metabolic syndrome amongst the US population.[87]

Management of Metabolic Syndrome

It is in the context of metabolic syndrome, that one looks for a solution like polypill. A combination of statin, aspirin and β-blocker can reduce mortality by 83% and a combination of statin, aspirin, β-blocker and angiotensin converting enzyme (ACE) inhibitor can reduce mortality by 75%.[88] This issue has been critically reviewed.[89] Although the polypill may be effective, side effects from its individual components and fixed dose combination will restrict its efficient use. Any studies on the use of polypill are fraught with basic ethical and cost issues. Additionally, the components of polypill are controversial and a decision regarding the endpoints to be used in the study difficult.

Drugs like statins have pleiotropic effects and we would probably see more drugs that have effect both on PPAR-α and PPAR-γ receptors, thus incorporating the lipid and glucose lowering properties in one molecule. Presently, however, it must be appreciated that lifestyle interventions have all-pervasive effect on all the components of metabolic syndrome and should gain precedence over all drug therapies as they are almost devoid of side effects.

HYPERURICEMIA

Hyperuricemia is a common biochemical anomaly in the population at large. It is seen in 2 to 13% of non-hospitalized adults and 25% of hospitalized adults.

Etiology

Hyperuricemia can result either from decreased excretion (90% of the patients) or increased proportion of uric acid. Decreased excretion is usually idiopathic or due to renal insufficiency or metabolic acidosis. Diabetic nephropathy maybe accompanied by hyperuricemia.

Hyperuricemia can be a component of metabolic syndrome. More significantly, a weight reduction or starvation diet can lead to hyperuricemia, both due to increased production and decreased excretion of uric acid. A few commonly used drugs like thiazide or other diuretics, alcohol, pyrizinamide, nicotinic acid and cyclosporine cause hyperuricemia due to decreased excretion. Overproduction of uric acid is rare but should be considered in hemolytic states, alcohol abuse, obesity

and myeloproliferative or lymphoproliferative disorders.

Management

Asymptomatic hyperuricemia does not require treatment. It does not contribute to cardiovascular disease.[90] Hyperuricemia needs to be treated when symptomatic, producing either nephrolithiasis or uric acid nephropathy or gouty arthritis. Allopurinol, 100 mg TID is the key drug. Urine should be alkalinized in case of urolithiasis or uric acid nephropathy. In case of gouty arthritis, the immediate treatment consists of colchicine orally for 1 to 2 weeks in tapering dosage or indomethacin or other nonsteroidal anti-inflammatory drugs. This should be followed by long-term allopurinol, with an overlap therapy with colchicine and allopurinol for 1 to 2 weeks.

HYPERHOMOCYSTEINEMIA

Hyperhomocysteinemia has received increased attention as a cardiovascular risk factor in the past decade. Metabolism of homocysteine to methionine requires the presence of methionine synthetase and vitamin B_{12}, which in turn needs the presence of folic acid and methylenetetrahydrofolate reductase (MTHFR) (**Figure 49.1**). Homocysteine can alternatively be converted to cysteine in the presence of enzyme cystathione beta-synthetase, which is dependent upon the supply of pyridoxine (Vitamin B_6). Thus, normal homocysteine metabolism requires the presence of vitamin B_{12}, folic acid and pyridoxine.

Hyperhomocysteinemia in Asian Indians

The prevalence of hyperhomocysteinemia is high in India.[91-93] It has been ascribed to poor intake of B_{12} in vegetarians and destruction of folic acid because of prolonged cooking. Additionally, almost one-third of the Asian Indians have a polymorphism of the enzyme MTHFR.[94,95] Hyperhomocysteinemia has been described in obese insulin resistant children.[96] This has also been demonstrated in type 1 diabetes.[97] On the other hand, there are data to show that hyperhomocysteinemia and the common C677T variant of MTHFR gene are not associated with metabolic syndrome in type 2 diabetics.[98]

Significance of Hyperhomocysteinemia

Currently, a large number of studies have attempted to elucidate relationship of vascular complications in

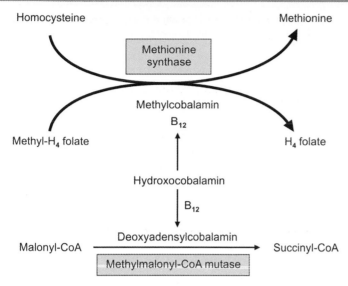

Figure 49.1 Role of vitamin B_{12} in homocysteine metabolism. Vitamin B_{12} deficiency leads to inhibition of both, methionine synthase and methyl malonyl CoA-mutase leading to hyperhomocysteinemia and methyl malonyl acidemia

diabetics and nondiabetics with hyperhomocysteinemia. The Hoorn study[99] failed to demonstrate any association between homocysteine levels and cardiovascular autonomic function in either diabetic or nondiabetic subjects. In HOPE-2 study, supplements of vitamins, folic acid, B_6 and B_{12} did not reduce the incidence of major cardiovascular events.[100] The homocysteine levels decreased by 2.4 micromol/liter in the active treatment group, while they rose by 0.8 micromol/liter in the placebo group. However, these data are vitiated by the fact that the placebo group also received folic acid from the fortified cereals. On the other hand, MTHFR gene polymorphism was associated with raised homocysteine levels and increased macroangiopathy (odd ratio 1.94, C1 95%: 1.31–2.89) in the Chinese population.[101] Raised homocysteine levels produced increased reactive oxygen species and platelet hyperactivity in type 2 diabetes mellitus.[102] A distinct effect of vitamin supplementation on the stroke mortality was observed in US and Canada.[103] After 1998, folate supplement was introduced in cereals, which showed a fall in stroke mortality rate from 2.9 to 0.3% per year.

Management

As hyperhomocysteinemia is highly prevalent in India in both diabetics and nondiabetics,[91] one would consider universal vitamin supplementation, especially if the link with vascular disease is unequivocally proven. If homocysteine levels are above 12 micromol/liter. It is recommended that a vitamin supplement containing methylcobalamin 500 mg, folic acid 5 mg and pyridoxine 10 mg is given. It is interesting to note that two commonly used drugs in diabetes—metformin and fenofibrate raise homocysteine levels. The clinical significance of this side effect needs further study.

SUMMARY

Recognition and optimal management of comorbid conditions is essential in diabetes. Certain comorbidities are more powerful determinants of the disease outcome than hyperglycemia. Two very well-recognized comorbidities, hypertension and dyslipidemias are discussed elsewhere. This chapter describes other comorbid conditions, tobacco abuse, obesity, metabolic syndrome, hyperuricemia and hyperhomocysteinemia.

REFERENCES

1. Gaziane MJ, Manson JE, et al. Primary and secondary prevention of coronary heart disease: Heart disease (6th edn). Braunwald E, Zipes DP, Libby P (Eds): Philadelphia: WB Saunders; 2001. pp. 1040-65.
2. Zatz R, Rehtz Dunn B, Mayer TW, et al. Prevention of diabetic glomerulopathy by pharmacologic amelioration of glomerular capillary hypertension. J Clin Invest. 1986;77:1925-30.
3. Parmet S, Lynm C, Glass RM. JAMA Patients page: Smoking and the heart. JAMA. 2003;290:146.
4. Murphy-Hoefer R, Griffith R, Peterson LL, Crossett L, Iyer SR, Huller MD. A review of interventions to reduce tobacco use in colleges and universities. Am J Preventive Medicine. 2005; 28:188.
5. Schroeder SA. What to do with a patient who smokes? JAMA. 2005;294:482.
6. Critchley JA. Mortality risk reduction associated with smoking cessation in patients with coronary heart disease: a systematic review. JAMA. 2003;290:88.
7. Flegal KM, Carroll MD, Kuczmarski RJ, Johnson CL. Overweight and obesity in United States: prevalence and trends, 1960-1994. Int J Obesity. 1998;22:39-47.
8. Flegal KM, Carroll MD, et al. Prevalence and trends in obesity among US Adults, 1999-2000. JAMA. 2002;288:1723-7.
9. Dietz WH, et al. Overweight in childhood and adolescence. N England J Med. 2004;350:855-7.
10. WHO Consultation. Obesity: preventing and managing the global epidemic. WHO Tech Rep. 2000;894:1-37.
11. Misra A, Vikram NK, Arya S, Pandey RM, et al. High prevalence of insulin resistance in postpubertal Asian Indian children is associated with adverse truncal body fat patterning, abdominal adiposity and excess body fat. Int J Obes Relat Metab Disord. 2004;28:1217-26.

12. International Institute for Population Sciences and ORG-MARG. National Family Health Survey (NFHS—2) 1999, India. Mumbai: International Institute for Population Sciences, 2000.

13. Gupta R, Gupta VP, Ahluwalia NS. Educational status, coronary heart disease and coronary risk factor prevalence in rural population of India. BMJ. 1994;309:1332-6.

14. Gupta R, Prakash H, et al. Prevalence of coronary heart disease and coronary risk factors in an urban population of Rajasthan. Indian Heart J. 1995;47:331-8.

15. Gupta R, Gupta VP, et al. Prevalence of coronary heart disease and risk factors in an urban Indian population, Jaipur Heart Watch-2. Indian Heart J. 2002;54:59-66.

16. Gupta R, Sarna M, et al. High prevalence of multiple coronary risk factors in *Punjabi Bhatia* community, Jaipur Heart Watch-3. Indian Heart J. 2004;57:646-52.

17. Banerji MA, Faridi N, et al. Body composition, visceral fat, leptin and insulin resistance in Asian Indian men. J Clin Endocrinol Metab. 1999;84:137-43.

18. United Kingdom Prospective Diabetes Study (UKPDS) Group. Intensive blood-glucose control with sulphonylureas or insulin compared with conventional treatment and risk of complications in patients with type 2 diabetes (UKPDS 33). Lancet. 1998;352:837-52.

19. The DCCT Research Group. Weight gain associated with intensive therapy in the diabetes control and complications trial. Diabetes Care. 1988;11:567-73.

20. Welle S, Nair KS. Effect of sulphonylurea and insulin on energy expenditure in type 2 diabetes mellitus. J Clin Endocrinol Metab. 1988;66:593-7.

21. Makimattila S, Nikkila K, et al. Causes of weight gain during insulin therapy with and without metformin in patients with non-insulin-dependant diabetes mellitus. Diabetologia. 1999;42:406-12.

22. Chandalia HB, Lamba PS, et al. Weight gain in type 2 diabetics with different treatment modalities. Metabolic syndrome and related disorders. 2005;3:130-6.

23. Lichtman SW, Pisarska K, et al. Discrepancy between self-reported and actual caloric intake and exercise in obsess subjects. N Engl J Med. 1992;327:1893-8.

24. Norgan NG, Durnin JVGA. The effect of 6 weeks of overfeeding on the bodyweight, body composition and energy metabolism of young men. Am J Clin Nutr. 1980;33:978-8.

25. Beilinski R, Schutz Y, et al. Energy metabolism during the postexercise recovery in man. Am J Clin Nutr. 1985;42:69-82.

26. Boshell BR, Chandalia HB, et al. Serum insulin in obesity and diabetes mellitus. Am J Clin Nutr. 1968;21:1419-28.

27. Chandalia M, Abate N, et al. Relationship between generalized and upper body obesity in insulin resistance in Asian Indian Men. J Clin Endocrinol Metab. 1999;84:2329-35.

28. Abate Nicola, Chandalia M. ENNP1/PC-1 K121Q polymorphism and genetic susceptibility to type 2 diabetes. Diabetes. 2005;54:1207-13.

29. Chandalia M, Abate N. Metabolic Complications of obesity: inflated or inflamed? Journal of Diabetes and its Complications. 2006;21:128-36.

30. Hubert HB, Feinlab M, Mcnamara OM, Castelli WP. Obesity as an independent risk factor for cardiovascular disease: a 26-year follow-up of participants in the Framingham Heart Study. Circulation. 1983;67:967-77.

31. Manson JE, Colditz GA, Stampfer MJ. A protective study of obesity and risk of heart disease in women. N Eng J Med. 1990;322:882-9.

32. Albrink MJ, Meigs JW. Interrelationship between skin-fold thickness, serum lipids and blood sugar in normal men. Am J Clin Nutr. 1964;15:255-61.

33. Austin MA, King MC, Vranizank M, Krauss BM. Atherogenic lipoprotein phenotype: a proposed genetic marker for coronary heart disease. Circulation. 1990;82:495-506.

34. Stamler R, Stamler J, Riedlinger WF, Algera G, Roberts RH. Weight and blood pressure. Findings in hypertension screening of 1 million Americans. JAMA. 1978;240:1607-9.

35. Kriesberg RA, Boshell BR, et al. Insulin secretion in obesity. N Engl J Med. 1967;27:314.

36. Colditz GA, Willet WC, Stampfer MJ, et al. Weight as a risk factor for clinical diabetes in women. Am J Epidemiol. 1990;132:501-13.

37. Ohlson LO, Larsson B, Svardsudd K, et al. Influence of body fat distribution on the incidence of diabetes mellitus. Diabetes. 1985;34:1055-8.

38. Lundgren H, Bengtsson C, Blohme G, Lapidus L, Sjostrom L. Adiposity and adipose tissue distribution in relation to incidence of diabetes in women: Results from a prospective population study in Gothenburg, Sweden. Int J Obes. 1989;13:413-23.

39. Haffner SM, Stern MP, Braxton DM, Hazuda HP, Patterson JK. Incidence of type 2 diabetes in Mexican Americans predicted by fasting insulin and glucose levels, obesity and body fat distribution. Diabetes. 1990;39:283-8.

40. Caro JF, Dohm LG, Pories WJ, Sinha MK. Cellular alterations in liver, skeletal muscle and adipose tissue responsible for insulin resistance in obesity and type 2 diabetes. Diabetes Metab Rev. 1989;5:665-89.

41. Hissin OJ, Foley JE, Wardzala LJ, et al. Mechanism of insulin-resistant glucose transport activity in enlarged adipose cell of the aged, obese rat. J Clin Invest. 1982;70:780-90.

42. Bogardus C, Lillioja S, Howard BV, Reaven G, Mott D. Relationships between insulin secretion, insulin action, and fasting glucose concentration in nondiabetic and non-insulin-dependant diabetic subjects. J Clin Invest. 1984;74:1238-46.

43. Eriksson J, Frassila-Kallunki A, Ekstrand A, et al. Early metabolic defects in persons at increased risk for non-insulin-dependant diabetes mellitus. N Eng J Med. 1989;321:337-43.

44. Stampfer MJ, Maclure CM, Colditz GA, Manson JE, Willen WC. Risk of symptomatic gallstones in women with severe obesity. Am J Clin Nutr. 1992;55:652-8.

45. Iyer S, Iyer R. Sleep and Obesity in the causation of metabolic syndrome. IJDDC. 2006;26:63-9.

46. Schwartz AR, Gold AR, Schubert N, et al. Effect of weight loss on upper airway collapsibility in obstructive sleep apnea. Am Rev Respir Dis. 1991;144:494-8.

47. Rimm AA, Werner LH, Yserloo BV, Bernstein RA. Relationship of obesity and disease in 73,532 weight conscious women. Public Health Rep. 1975;90:44-54.

48. Loenen HM, Eshuis H, Lowik MR, et al. Serum uric acid correlates in elderly men and women with special reference to body composition and dietary intake (Dutch Nutrition Surveillance System). J Clin Epidemiol. 1990;43:1297-303.

49. Tuomilehto J, Zimmet P, Wolf E, et al. Plasma uric level and its association with diabetes mellitus and some biologic para-

meters in a biracial population of Fiji. Am J Epidemiol. 1988;127:321-36.

50. Glass AR. Endocrine aspects of obesity. Med Clin North Am. 1989;73:139-60.

51. Veldhuis JD, Iranmanesh A, Ho KKY, et al. Dual defects in pulsatile growth hormone secretion and clearance subserve the hyposomatotropism of obesity in man. J Clin Endocrinol Metab. 1991;72:1224-8.

52. Mayer J, Purnima R, Mitra KP. Relation between caloric intake, body weight and physical work: studies in an industrial, male population in West Bengal. Am J Clin Nutr. 1956;4:169-75.

53. Williamson DF, Madans J, Anda RF, et al. Recreational physical activity and ten-year weight change in a US national cohort. Int J Obes. 1993;17:279-86.

54. Tucker LA, Bagwell M. Television viewing and obesity in adult females. Am J Public Health. 1991;81:908-11.

55. Gortmaker SL, Dietz WH, Cheung LWY. Inactivity, diet and fattening of America. J Am Diet Assoc. 1990;90:1247-52.

56. Poehlman ET, Melby CL, Badylak SF, Calles J. Aerobic fitness and resting energy expenditure in young adult males. Metabolism. 1989;38:85-90.

57. Poehlman ET, Gardner AW, Ades PA, et al. Resting energy metabolism and cardiovascular disease risk in resistance and aerobically trained males. Metabolism. 1992;56:968-74.

58. Ballor DL, Smith DB, et al. Neither high nor low intensity exercise promotes whole-body conservation of protein during severe dietary restrictions. Int J Obes. 1990;14:279-87.

59. Ballor DL, McCarthy JP, Wilterdink EJ. Exercise intensity does not affect the composition of diet and exercise-induced body mass loss. Am J Clin Nutr. 1990;51:142-6.

60. Wadden TA. The treatment of obesity: an overview. In Stunkard AJ, Wadden TA (Eds): Obesity Theory and therapy. New York: Raven Press; 1993. pp. 197-218.

61. Pascale RW, Wing RR, Butler BA, Mullen M, Bononi P. Effects of a behavioral weight loss program stressing calorie restriction versus calorie plus fat restriction in obese individuals with NIDDM or a family history of diabetes. Diabetes Care. 1995;18(9):1241-8.

62. Viegener BJ, Perri MG, Nezu AM, et al. Effects of an intermittent, low fat, low calorie diet in behavioural treatment of obesity. Behav Ther. 1990;21:499-509.

63. Agras WS, Taylor CB, Feldman DE, Losch M, Burrett KF, et al. Developing computer – assisted therapy for the treatment of obesity. Behav Ther. 1995;21:99-109.

64. Weintraub M., Rubio A, Golik A, Byrne L. Sibutramine dose ranging, efficacy study. Clin Pharm. 1991;50(3):330-7.

65. Smith IG, Goulder MA. Randomised Placebo-controlled trial of long-term treatment with sibutramine in mild or moderate obesity. J Fam Pract. 2001;50:505-12.

66. Hauptman JB, Jeunet FS, Hartmann D. Initial studies in humans with novel gastrointestinal lipase inhibitor Ro 18-0647 (tetrahydrolipstatin). Am J Clin Nutr. 1992;55:309-13S.

67. Tonstad S, Pometta D, Erkelens DW, et al. The effects of gastrointestinal lipase inhibitor, orlistat, on serum lipids and lipoproteins in patients with primary hyperlipidemia. Eur J Clin Pharmacol. 1994;46:405-10.

68. Torgenson JS, Hauptnaan J, Boldrin MN, et al. Xenid in the prevention of diabetes in obese subjects (XENDOS) study: a randomized study of orlistat as an adjunct to lifestyle changes for the prevention of type 2 diabetes in obese subjects. Diabetes Care. 2004;27:155-61.

69. Van Gaal LF, Rissanen AM, Scheen AJ, Zigler O, Rossner S for the RIO-Europe Study Group. Effects of the cannabinoids-1 receptor blocker rimonabant on weight reduction and cardiovascular risk factors in overweight patients: 1 year experience from the RIO-Europe Study. Lancet. 2005;365:1389-97.

70. Despres JP, Golay A, Sjostrom L. Rimonabant in obesity-Lipids (RIO-Lipids) Study Group. Effects of rimonabant on metabolic risk factors in overweight patients with dyslipidemia. N Engl J Med. 2005;353:2121-34.

71. Reaven G. Banting Lecture. Role of insulin resistance in human disease. Diabetes. 1988;37:1595-607.

72. Vague J. La differentiation sexeulle, facteu determinant des formes de l'obesite. Presse Medl. 1947;53:339-40.

73. Camus J, Goutte. Diabete, hyperlipemie, un trisyndrome metabolique. Rev Rheumatol. 1966;33:10-4.

74. Pyorala K. Relationship of glucose tolerance and plasma insulin to the incidence of coronary heart disease: results from two population studies in Finland. Diabetes Care. 1979;2:131-41.

75. Modan M, Halkin H, Almong S, et al. Hyperinsulinemia. A link between hypertension, obesity and glucose intolerance. J Clin Invest. 1985;75:809-17.

76. World Health Organisation. Definition, diagnosis and classification of diabetes mellitus and its complications. Report of a WHO consultation; 1999.

77. Balkau B, Charles M. Comment on the provisional report from WHO consultation. European Group for the study of Insulin Resistance (EGIR). Diabet Met. 1999;16:442-3.

78. Executive summary of the third Report of the National Cholesterol Education Program (NCEP) Expert Panel on Detection, Evaluation and Treatment of high Blood Cholesterol in Adults (Adult Treatment Panel III). JAMA. 2001;285:2486-97.

79. Einhorn D, Reaven G, Cobin R, et al. American College of Endocrinology Position Statement on the Insulin Resistance Syndrome. Endocr Pract. 2003;9:237-52.

80. International Diabetes Federation. The IDF consensus worldwide definition of metabolic syndrome. Available at http://www.idf.org/webdata/docs/IDF_Metasyndrome_definition.pdf (last accessed August 16,2006).

81. Stern MP, Williams K, Gonzalez-Villalpando, Hunt KJ, Haffner SM C, et al. Does metabolic syndrome improve identification of individuals at risk of type 2 diabetes and/or cardiovascular disease? Diabetes Care. 2004;27:2676-81.

82. Grundy SM. Metabolic syndrome: connecting and reconciling cardiovascular and diabetes Worlds. J Am Coll Cardio. 2006;47:1093-100.

83. Eckel R, Grundy S, Zimmet P. The metabolic syndrome. Lancet. 2005;365:1415-28.

84. Ramchandran A, Snehalata C, Satyavani K, et al. Metabolic syndrome in urban Asian Indian adults: a population study using modified ATP-III criteria. Diabetes Res Clin Pract. 2003;60:199-204.

85. Mohan V, Shanthirani S, Deepa R, et al. Intraurban differences in the prevalence of the metabolic syndrome in southern India: The Chennai Urban Population Study (CUPS No.4). Diabetic Med. 2001;18:280-7.

86. Tan CE, Ma S, Wai D, et al. Can we apply the National Cholesterol Education Program Adult Treatment Panel definition of the metabolic syndrome to Asians? Diabetes Care. 2004;27: 1182-6.

87. Ford ES, Giles WH, Dietz WH. Prevalence of the metabolic syndrome among US adults: findings from the Third National Health and Nutrition Examination Survey. JAMA. 2002;287: 356-9.

88. Gupta R, Prakash H, Gupta RR. Economic issues in coronary heart disease prevention in India. J Hum Hypertens. 2005;19: 655-7.

89. Combination Pharmacotherapy and Public Health Research Working Group. Combination pharmacotherapy for cardiovascular disease. Ann Intern Med. 2005;1443:593-9.

90. Culleton BF, et al. Serum uric acid risk for cardiovascular disease and death. The Franghimham Heart Study. Ann Intern Med. 1999;7:131.

91. Refsum H, et al. Hyperhomocysteinemia and elevated methylmalonic acid indicate a high prevalence of cobalamin deficiency in Asian Indians. Am J Clin Nutr. 2001;74:233-41.

92. Misra A, et al. Hyperhomocysteinemia and low intakes of folic acid and vitamin B in urban North India. Eur J Nutr. 2002;41:68-77.

93. Yajnik C, et al. Vitamin B_{12} deficiency and Hyperhomocysteinemia in rural and urban Indians. JAPI. 2006;54:775-81.

94. Mukherjee M, et al. A low prevalence of the C677T mutation in the methylenetetrahydrofolate reductase gene in Asian Indians. Clin Genet. 2002;61:155-9.

95. Kalita J, et al. Methylenetetrahydrofolate reductase gene polymorphism in Indian stoke patients. Neurology India, 2006;54:260-3.

96. Martos R, Valle M, et al. Hyperhomocysteinemia correlates with insulin resistance and low-grade systemic inflammation in obese prepubertal children. Metabolism. 2006;55(1): 72-7.

97. Dinleyici EC, Kirel B, et al. Plasma total homocysteine levels in children with type 1 diabetes: relationship with vitamin status, methylenetetrahydrofolate reductase genotype, disease parameters and coronary risk factors. J Trop Pediatr. 2006;52(4):260-6.

98. Russo Gt, DiBenedetto A, et al. Mild hyperhomocysteinemia and the common C677T polymorphism of methylene tetrahydrofolate reductase gene are not associated with the metabolic syndrome in type 2 diabetes. J Endocrinol Invest. 2006;29(3):201-7.

99. Spoelstra-De, Man AM, Smulders YM, et al. Homocysteine levels are not associated with cardiovascular autonomic function in elderly Caucasian subjects without or with type 2 diabetes mellitus: the Hoorn Study. J Intern Med. 2005; 258(6):536-43.

100. Lonn E, Yusuf S, et al. Homocysteine lowering with folic acid and B vitamins in vascular disease. Heart Outcomes Prevention Evaluation (HOPE) 2 Investigators. New Eng J Med. 2006;354: 1566-77

101. Sun J, Xu Y, Zhu Y, Lu H. Methylenetetrahydrofolate reductase gene polymorphism, homocysteine and risk of macroangiopathy in type 2 diabetes mellitus. J Endocrinol Invest. 2006; 29(9):814-20.

102. Signorello MG, Viviani GL, et al. Homocysteine, reactive oxygen species and nitric oxide in type 2 diabetes mellitus. Thromb Res. 2006 (E-pub ahead of print).

103. Yang Q, et al. Improvement in stroke mortality in Canada and United States, 1990 to 2002. Circulation. 2006;113:1335-43.

Chapter 50

HYPERTENSION IN DIABETES

Sandhya A Kamath

CHAPTER OUTLINE

- Introduction
- Etiology of Hypertension in Diabetes
- Pathophysiology
- Diabetic Nephropathy
- Complications
- Screening for Hypertension in Diabetes
- Management of Hypertension in Diabetes
- The Indian Scenario
- Summary

INTRODUCTION

Hypertension and diabetes mellitus are interrelated diseases, which, if untreated, strongly predispose to atherosclerotic cardiovascular disease. Lifestyle and genetic factors are important in the genesis of both conditions. Diabetes mellitus (DM) and hypertension coexist three times more commonly than predicted by chance. Hypertension is twice as prevalent among diabetic patients when compared to the general population.[1] Hypertension occurs more frequently in persons with type 1 or insulin-dependent diabetes mellitus (IDDM) than in those with type 2 or non-insulin-dependent diabetes mellitus (NIDDM). It is seen in almost all the patients who develop nephropathy. The prevalence of hypertension in type 2 diabetes increases with age, which is about 40 to 60% in the age range of 45 to 75 years.[2] The development of type 2 DM is 2.5 times more likely in hypertensive patients than in normotensive persons within 5 years.[3] In type 2 DM, hypertension antedates the diagnosis of diabetes by years and even decades, 8 times more frequently than the reverse. Hypertension is more prevalent in diabetic men than women before the age of 50 years, and reverse is true after the age of 50 years.[4] In obese diabetic patients, who account for 90% of patients with type 2 DM, hypertension is more common than obese persons without diabetes. This connection is even stronger in those who have truncal obesity along with the "dysmetabolic syndrome" of insulin resistance.

ETIOLOGY OF HYPERTENSION IN DIABETES

1. Essential hypertension accounts for the majority of hypertension in persons with diabetes, particularly in those with type 2 diabetes, who constitute more than 90 percent of those with a dual diagnosis of diabetes and hypertension.
2. Diabetic nephropathy, which commonly occurs after 15 years of diabetes in one of three persons with type 1 diabetes and one of five persons with type 2 diabetes, appears to be another important cause of hypertension.
3. Dysmetabolic syndrome X in which hypertension is associated with insulin resistance and glucose intolerance (including type 2 diabetes mellitus), a

characteristic dyslipidemia (hypertriglyceridemia, low HDL-cholesterol, high LDL, excess small, dense LDL particles), truncal obesity, procoagulant changes (elevated plasminogen activator inhibitor-I and fibrinogen) and hyperuricemia.

4. Secondary hypertension:
   a. Endocrine diseases causing both hypertension and diabetes, e.g. Cushing's syndrome, Conn's syndrome, pheochromocytoma, acromegaly.
   b. Hypertension due to diabetic complications, besides diabetic nephropathy, repeated pyelonephritis, can give rise to chronic pyelonephritis and end-stage renal disease.
   c. Drugs causing hypertension and diabetes, e.g. oral contraceptives, glucocorticoids.
   d. Antihypertensive drugs causing diabetes—potassium losing diuretics, e.g. thiazides (especially chlorthalidone), β-blockers, diazoxide.
5. Isolated systolic hypertension due to accelerated atherosclerosis is an important feature in diabetes mellitus.

PATHOPHYSIOLOGY

Hyperinsulinemia and hyperglycemia, both independently can raise the blood pressure.

Hyperinsulinemia is present in both type 1 DM and type 2 DM. Exogenous insulin is administered to patients with type 1 DM because of deficient endogenous insulin. Obesity-induced insulin resistance in type 2 DM results in increased insulin secretion in a futile attempt to maintain euglycemia. Hyperinsulinemia causes or aggravates hypertension in a number of ways[3] **(Figure 50.1)**. These include increased platelet adhesion and aggregation, and an imbalance between coagulation and fibrinolytic activities leading to a procoagulant state, endothelial dysfunction, lipoprotein abnormalities and vascular smooth muscle cell alterations.

Hyperglycemia *per se* inhibits endothelium-derived relaxation and stimulates transcription of the genes for growth factors acting on vascular smooth muscle cells.

Hypertension can exhibit several kinds of pathological features in patients with diabetes:[5]

1. Hypertension associated with diabetic nephropathy is a form of renal hypertension with sodium and fluid retention and volume expansion, increased peripheral vascular resistance, and increased cardiac output, especially if anemia is present.
2. Isolated systolic hypertension can occur at any age and is considerably more common in persons with diabetes than in those without. Accelerated

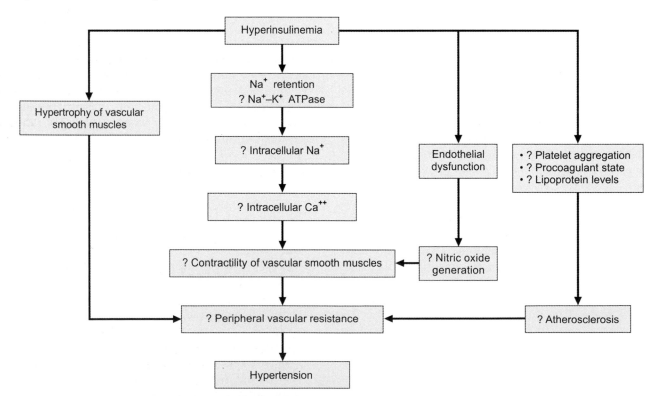

Figure 50.1 Mechanisms of hypertension in insulin resistance

atherosclerosis in patients with diabetes makes them lose their elasticity and become rigid. Blood ejected from the left ventricle enters the arterial tree with restricted capacity for expansion. This leads to undue increase in systolic blood pressure.

3. Supine hypertension with orthostatic hypotension sometimes occurs in patients with autonomic neuropathy and is difficult to treat in persons with diabetes. Maintenance of erect blood pressure involves several mechanisms. These include intact baroreceptor reflexes, cardiac output, blood volume and vasoactive hormones (catecholamines, renin-angiotensin-aldosterone system). In a normal individual, these mechanisms compensate for one another; and hence compromise in the function of one does not result in orthostatic hypotension. Autonomic neuropathy in diabetes blunts the above mechanisms. Compromise in any one of the mechanisms can give rise to orthostatic hypotension. Postural hypotension is also seen in the elderly and those treated with vasodilators and diuretics.

4. In most individuals with diabetes, increased peripheral vascular resistance related to accelerated atherosclerosis characterizes hypertension.

DIABETIC NEPHROPATHY

Only up to 30% of patients with type 1 DM develop nephropathy, but all patients who develop nephropathy develop hypertension.[6] About 20 to 40% of patients with type 2 DM may develop nephropathy in 20 years, but this nephropathy is not always accompanied by hypertension as in patients with type 1 DM.

Microalbuminuria is the earliest manifestation of nephropathy. This is a transitional phase when the blood pressure steadily and progressively starts rising. By the time gross albuminuria develops, almost all patients with type 1 DM and many patients with type 2 DM develop hypertension.

It is not yet clear whether hypertension initiates nephropathy or vice versa. But there is a definite etiological relationship between the two; the presence of nephropathy accelerates hypertension, and hypertension accelerates nephropathy. Systolic blood pressure (SBP) correlates better than diasystolic blood pressure (DBP) with renal disease progression in diabetes.[7] The rate of decline in renal function among patients with diabetic nephropathy has been reported to be a continuous function of arterial pressure down to approximately 125 to 130 mm Hg SBP and 70 to 75 mm Hg DBP.

Hypertension is present in many patients of type 2 DM at the time of diagnosis. This does not suggest that these patients have renal disease of any sort. It is more commonly essential hypertension. Similarly, micro-albuminuria/albuminuria in patients with type 2 DM does not always predict nephropathy. Albuminuria may be due to some other renal disease, especially in older persons.

COMPLICATIONS

An estimated 35 to 75 percent of diabetic complications can be attributed to hypertension.[5] The macrovascular and microvascular complications of diabetes are increased further when hypertension accompanies diabetes. Patients who have both diabetes and hypertension have more renal disease and atherogenic risk factors, including dyslipidemia, hyperuricemia, elevated fibrinogen, and left ventricular hypertrophy.[4] Hypertension contributes to the leading causes of morbidity and mortality in persons with diabetes, including coronary heart disease, stroke, peripheral vascular disease, lower extremity amputations, and end-stage renal disease. The United Kingdom Prospective Diabetes Study (UKPDS) demonstrated that each 10 mm Hg decrease in SBP was associated with average reduction in rates of diabetes-related mortality by 15%; myocardial infarction by 11%; and the microvascular complications of retinopathy or nephropathy by 13%.

The presence of microalbuminuria in type 1 DM precedes nephropathy and is also a marker for coronary artery disease. The progression to diabetic retinopathy is also hastened by hypertension. Therefore, simultaneous control of BP and blood glucose is very important in patients with diabetes and hypertension for decreasing cardiovascular events and other diabetic risk and outcomes.[2]

SCREENING FOR HYPERTENSION IN DIABETES

All diabetic patients must be regularly screened for hypertension and vice versa. Obese hypertensives or those receiving antihypertensives that can raise blood glucose should be screened for diabetes at least once every year. If blood glucose is raised, these potentially diabetogenic drugs should be changed, by which normoglycemia maybe restored.

All diabetic patients with other cardiovascular risk factors, such as nephropathy, obesity, dyslipidemia, smoking and poor glycemic control should also be checked frequently for hypertension.

Measurement of Blood Pressure

Blood pressure should be measured in the supine and standing position as recommended by JNC. Check should also be made for postural hypotension. If marked postural hypotension exists, the antihypertensive agent should be reduced or changed.

Investigations of Hypertension in Diabetes

The hypertensive diabetic patient should be investigated to exclude causes of secondary hypertension, to assess the extent of end-organ (heart, kidney, retina, peripheral vascular one) damages and to identify other potentially treatable factors, such as dyslipidemia and drug-induced hypertension. Investigations should include cardiac function tests, renal function tests, lipid profile and others to exclude secondary hypertension **(Table 50.1)**. It is imperative to note whether the patient has any other cardiovascular risk factors like smoking, alcoholism, dyslipidemia and family history of cardiovascular disease.

TABLE 50.1	Investigation for hypertension in diabetes

- History
  - Heart disease—cardiac failure, chest pain
  - Past history of renal disease
  - Smoking or alcohol abuse
  - Drug intake
  - Family history of hypertension, cardiovascular disease
- Physical examination
  - Pulse rate (tachycardia in pheochromocytoma)
  - Blood pressure in supine and erect positions
  - Peripheral pulsations
  - Renal bruit
  - Brachiofemoral delay
  - Cardiac size (especially left ventricular size)
  - Features of Cushing's syndrome, thyroid disease, acromegaly
  - Signs of renal disease
  - Fundus
- Blood biochemistry—glucose, urea nitrogen, creatinine, lipids
- Urine for microalbuminuria/albuminuria
- Chest X-ray—cardiac size, pulmonary edema
- Additional investigations when required
  - ECG—arrhythmias, left ventricular hypertrophy, ischemia
  - Echocardiography—chamber hypertrophy, ischemic dyskinesia
  - Ultrasonography for kidneys: shape and size
  - Carotid intimal medial thickness

TABLE 50.2	List of ACEI and ARB classes of drugs in common use

- ACEI   Dosase
  Enalapril   2.5–40 mg/day
  Ramipril   2.5–20 mg once day
  Perindopril   2–8 mg once day
- ARB
  Losartan   50–100 mg/day
  Ibresartan   150–300 mg/day
  Candesartan   8–12 mg/day
  Telmisartan   20–80 mg/day
- Combination
  Losartan 50 mg plus ramipril 2.5/5 mg
  Telmisartan 40 mg plus ramipril 2.5/5 mg

ACEI: Angiotensin converting enzyme inhibitor; ARB: Angiotensin-II receptor blocker

MANAGEMENT OF HYPERTENSION IN DIABETES

The NHLBI (National Heart, Lung and Blood Institute) clinical advisory committee has confirmed the benefit of therapy in patients with hypertension and diabetes that includes lifestyle modification (weight reduction, increased physical activity, moderation of salt and alcohol intake) and the appropriate use of antihypertensive therapy[8] **(Table 50.2)**.

Goal for Levels of Blood Pressure to be Achieved

The NHLBI (JNC) and American Diabetic Association (ADA) have recommended a goal for BP of less than 130/80 mm Hg in patients with diabetes and hypertension. Data supporting this are found in the following studies:[8]

1. The United Kingdom prospective diabetes study (UKPDS) observed that near optimal control of hypertension (144/82 mm Hg) led to 44 percent fewer diabetes-related strokes, 37 percent fewer cases of microvascular disorders due to diabetes (particularly diabetic retinopathy) and 32 percent fewer diabetes-related deaths.
2. The results of the hypertension optimal treatment (HOT) randomized trial showed that in patients with diabetes mellitus there was a 51% reduction (p = 0.005) in major cardiovascular events in target diastolic BP group less than 80 mm Hg compared with target group of less than 90 mm Hg.
3. A meta-analysis[9] of multiple prospective randomized studies of more than 12 months duration

reviewed the effect of drug treatment on morbidity and mortality in diabetic hypertensive persons. This analysis concluded that antihypertensive treatment to less than 130/85 mm Hg reduces the risk for cardiovascular events.[6]

4. Subanalysis of the diabetic cohort in the Sys-Eur trial suggests that further reduction in diastolic blood pressure below 85 mm Hg is beneficial. While systolic blood pressure was reduced by a comparable amount in each group (22 ± 16 mm Hg, nondiabetic vs 22.1 ± 14 mm Hg, diabetic group), the risk reduction in mortality from CVD was 13% for the nondiabetic and 76% for the diabetic patients. Thus, the benefit conferred per mm Hg blood pressure reduction appears to be greater in persons with type 2 diabetes than in those with hypertension but no coexistent diabetes mellitus.

Antihypertensive Pharmacological Therapy

JNC 7 has recommended that hypertensive persons with target organ damage/clinical cardiovascular disease and/or diabetes should be promptly initiated on pharmacotherapy in order to protect the heart, brain, kidney and the vascular tree against arteriosclerotic damage, which is the main cause of mortality in types 1 and 2 diabetes mellitus.

Antihypertensive Therapy and New-onset Diabetes Mellitus

Antihypertensive therapy has been suggested to potentially increase the risk for type 2 diabetes mellitus, specifically with diuretics and β-blockers. Many clinical trials have provided evidence on the contrary and favored the use of antihypertensive agents in the treatment of hypertension whenever indicated.

1. The atherosclerosis risk in community (ARIC)[1] study prospectively studied 12,550 hypertensives without diabetes to examine the independent relationship between the use of antihypertensive medicines and the risk for the subsequent development of type 2 diabetes mellitus. Thiazide diuretics, ACE inhibitors or calcium channel blockers (CCBs) did not incur a greater risk for subsequent diabetes than non-receipt of antihypertensive therapy. Patients taking β-blockers had a 28% higher risk of developing diabetes than those without medications.

2. The heart outcome prevention evaluation (HOPE) trial demonstrated a 30% decrease in new onset diabetes with ramipril. It clearly reinforces the fact that normotensive diabetic patients can be protected against cardiovascular complications by antihypertensive treatment with ACE inhibitors.

Evidence-based Medicine and Hypertension in Diabetes

Many other trials have demonstrated the benefit of antihypertensive pharmacotherapy in the treatment of hypertension and diabetes mellitus:

1. The UKPDS noted that BP lowering with captopril or β-blocker was effective in reducing microvascular and macrovascular complications of diabetes.

2. The captopril prevention project (CPP) also demonstrated equal benefits for BP reduction in terms of primary outcome with captopril or the diuretic and β-blocker based regimens.

3. The systolic hypertension in the elderly program (SHEP) study showed benefit using low-dose chlorthalidone alone or in combination with atenolol for reducing stroke and CAD in elderly patients.

4. The losartan intervention for end-point (LIFE) reduction in hypertension study and ALLHAT have demonstrated that adequate BP control improves CVD outcomes, especially stroke, when aggressive BP targets are achieved

Antihypertensive Drugs to be Used in Diabetes Mellitus

Based on clinical trial data four classes of drugs were noted to be effective as first line therapy: low-dose thiazide diuretics, β-blockers, CCBs and ACE inhibitors (ACEI).

Most diabetic patients would require more than one drug to achieve a therapeutic goal of less than 130/80 mm Hg. This is supported by the following evidence:

1. Multiple drugs were required in UKPDS to achieve tight control of 144/82 mm Hg versus less tight control of 154/87 mm Hg.

2. The HOT trial also confirms that multiple drug regimens are required to reach the goal for most hypertensive diabetic patients.

3. Meta-analysis of multiple prospective randomized studies also concluded that more than 60% of diabetic hypertensives will require more than one drug to control BP.[1] The combination drugs may actually be more beneficial than monotherapy with any individual agent or class.

RAS Blockade: The ACEIs and ARBs

Many patients with diabetes and hypertension may have albuminuria, which confers an increased cardiovascular risk. ACE inhibitors in this situation appear to afford unique benefit. They have a protective effect on the development of diabetes. Treatment with ACE inhibitors is now considered mandatory in diabetic nephropathy. ACE inhibitors exert beneficial effects by:

1. Improving blood flow through microcirculation in the skeletal muscle.
2. Improving insulin action in mediating glucose transport at cellular level.
3. Improved insulin sensitivity.
4. Decreased hepatic clearance of insulin.
5. Decrease intraglomerular pressure.
6. An anti-inflammatory effect.
7. Improved blood flow to the pancreas.
8. An effect on abdominal fat.
9. Do not adversely affect the metabolic status.

Therapy with an ACEI also is an important component of most regimens to control BP in diabetic patients.[7]ACEIs maybe used alone for BP lowering but are much more effective when combined with a thiazide-type diuretic or other antihypertensive drugs. The ADA has recommended ACEIs for diabetic patients over 55-year-old at high risk for CVD and β-blockers for those with known CAD. In the micro-hope sub-analysis of the HOPE study, which included both hypertensive and normotensive individuals, high-risk diabetic patients treated with ACEI added to conventional therapy showed a reduction in combined MI, stroke, and CVD death of about 25% and reduction in stroke by about 33% compared with placebo plus conventional therapy.

Secondly, RAS blockade for management of hypertension may also be achieved by use of angiotensin II receptor blocking (ARB) agents instead of or in addition to angiotensin converting enzyme inhibition (ACEI). Change over to ARB becomes necessary in a proportion of cases that develop untreatable cough on use of ACEI category of drugs. Furthermore, better blood pressure control and repression of LVH can be achieved by combining ARB with ACEI because of more complete blockage of RA system. Adding ARB maybe needed particularly in cases with escape of ACE activity in spite of full doses of ACEI agents. Although ARB drugs improve BP and microalbuminuria in patients with diabetes, an increased incidence of acute myocardial infarction (AMI) has been observed in some trials. Therefore, these should be used only in cases with clear cut indications. Commonly used ACEI and ARB agents are listed in **Table 50.2**.

Diuretics

On the basis of SHEP results, JNC 7 recommends low-dose diuretics for treatment of hypertensive patients with type 2 diabetes. If the dose is low (25 mg or less of hydrochlorothiazide), adverse effects on carbohydrate metabolism, worsening hypoglycemia, hypokalemia, and hypomagnesemia are uncommon. Furthermore, this class of agents is generally as effective as ACE inhibitors in lowering blood pressure in patients with diabetes. Indeed, long-term data (4 years) indicate that diuretics have the same effect as ACE inhibitors on reducing the progression of renal disease in patients with type 2 diabetes.[7] It is likely that volume expansion contributes to the elevated arterial pressure in these individuals. In the diabetic subgroup of ALLHAT, therapy with chlorthalidone reduced the primary end-point of fatal CAD and MI to the same degree as lisinopril or amlodipine. Thus, diuretics are effective antihypertensive agents in these patients but should be used in low doses.

Beta-blockers

Several concerns limit the usefulness of β-blockers in treating persons with diabetes:

1. These agents have adverse effects on glucose and lipid metabolism.
2. They can reduce awareness of hypoglycemia in patients with diabetes and prolong recovery from hypoglycemia.
3. They can reduce peripheral blood flow in patients who already have a compromised peripheral vascular system.
4. Thus, except under special circumstances (e.g. in the presence of angina pectoris and postmyocardial infarction), β-blockers should be used with caution in patients with diabetes and hypertension. β₁-selective agents are beneficial in diabetic patients as part of multidrug therapy, but their value as monotherapy is less clear.[7]

Calcium Channel Blockers

Some studies have raised concern about the safety of calcium channel blockers (CCBs) in diabetic hypertensives. The appropriate blood pressure control (ABPC) trial and the fosinopril amlodipine cardiovascular events trial (FACET) used antihypertensive treatment with ACE inhibitors (enalapril or fosinopril) and CCBs (nifidipine or amlodipine) in patients with type 2 diabetes. They found a favorable effect with ACE inhibitors (or an unfavorable effect with CCBs). In contrast, the

STOP-2 trial, HOT trial, and the SHEP trial produced indirect evidence regarding a protective role of CCBs in hypertensive diabetic patients. With these data, JNC 7 has recommended that CCBs are beneficial in diabetics as part of multidrug therapy, but their value as monotherapy is less clear. Calcium-channel blockers should not be used inpatients with diabetes who have had a recent coronary event.[10]

Angiotensin-II Receptor Blockers

They represent a potential alternative to ACE inhibitors in treating patients with diabetes or renal disease. With respect to microvascular complications, the ADA has recommended both ACEIs and ARBs for use in type 2 diabetic patients with chronic kidney disease because these agents delay the deterioration in glomerular filtration rate (GFR) and the worsening of albuminuria.

Inhibition of the Renin-Angiotensin System

There is an increased activation of the RAS cascade in conditions such as hypertension and diabetes.[11] Hence modulation of this system has become essential in treating hypertension and delaying the onset of diabetic nephropathy. ACEIs alone have not provided a satisfactory response. Either insufficient BP control or continued microalbuminuria may prevail in spite of high doses of ACEIs. This could be due to alternative pathways of converting angiotensin-I to angiotensin-II, 'ACE escape' phenomenon, or tissue ACE activity. ACEIs do not completely block the conversion of angiotensin-I (Ang-I) to Ang-II. Alternative pathways exist, and these pathways may produce 60 to 70% of Ang-II. 'ACE escape' develops during long-term treatment with ACEI resulting in rise to pretreatment levels of angiotensin-II and aldosterone levels. Tissue ACE activity is not always sufficiently blocked by regular dose of ACEI.

Combining an ACEI and angiotensin receptor blocker (ARB) counteract the above mechanisms.[11] Dual blockade simultaneously inhibits ACE and angiotensin-I receptors. This gives a more complete inhibition of the RAS, blocks the effects of both non-ACE pathways and tissue ACE activity and thus vastly enhances the desired therapeutic effect. Conditions characterized by an activated RAS cascade such as hypertension, heart failure and nephropathy in both diabetic and nondiabetic subjects will benefit from this treatment.

Special Considerations in Diabetic Patients with Hypertension

Kidney Disease

Diabetes mellitus is presently the leading cause of end-stage renal disease. The risk of diabetic renal disease increases with age and duration of diabetes. The development of nephropathy after 15 years of diabetes has been observed in more than 30 percent of persons with type 1 diabetes and in more than 20 percent of those with type 2 diabetes.[9] In type 1 diabetes, microalbuminuria, mesangial cell hypertrophy, and blood pressure are correlated and herald the development of diabetic nephropathy. An exaggerated blood pressure response to exercise may unmask incipient nephropathy in persons with diabetes. Hypertension accelerates the rate of progression of diabetic renal disease, and control of blood pressure as well as glucose may retard this progression rate.

Considerations for Therapy

1. Renal disease contributes to hypertension in patients with diabetes through several pathogenic mechanisms: sodium and water retention (extracellular fluid volume expansion) and increased vascular resistance.
2. Microalbuminuria that indicates the presence of diabetic nephropathy.
3. The progression of diabetic nephropathy appears to be correlated with a rise in blood pressure.
4. Compounding these renal abnormalities is the contribution of hyperglycemia *per se* to the volume expansion and consequent hypertension.

Thus, therapeutic approaches should include normalization of blood glucose in addition to the use of agents that will reduce both intravascular volume and intrarenal pressure.

ACE inhibitors are useful in this situation. In a recently reported randomized multicenter clinical trial, during a median follow-up of 3 years, treatment with an ACE inhibitor significantly decreased the rate of increase in creatinine and the rate of decline of creatinine clearance. The combined end-point of mortality, dialysis, and transplantation was reduced by 50 percent with ACE inhibitor therapy. These benefits appeared to occur independently of effects on blood pressure, and in both normotensive and hypertensive diabetic patients with nephropathy suggesting that ACE inhibitors may have special salutary effects in persons with type 1 diabetes and renal disease. It has not been determined whether these results pertain to persons with type 2 diabetes and renal disease.

Risks with ACE Inhibitors

1. A major risk of ACE inhibitors is an acceleration of renal insufficiency, particularly in those with bilateral renal artery stenosis a more common occurrence in the persons with diabetes mellitus. Close monitoring of renal function and serum potassium should be performed in the first few weeks after initiation of therapy if bilateral renal artery disease is suspected.
2. ACE inhibitors may cause hyperkalemia particularly in those individuals with renal failure or hyporeninemic hypoaldosteronism (type IV renal tubular acidosis).
3. Care must be exercised in initiating ACE inhibitor therapy in patients receiving diuretics because there maybe a profound drop in blood pressure and a decline in renal function.

Supine Hypertension with Orthostatic Hypotension

Supine hypertension with orthostatic hypotension in patients with diabetes mellitus is associated with autonomic neuropathy and is most difficult to treat. Occasionally, the upright blood pressure falls to such an extent that patients are unable to assume the upright posture, which maybe aggravated by many antihypertensive medications that cause orthostatic hypotension.[5]

Treatment

To reduce symptoms, the goal of therapy is to increase the upright pressure and to lower the supine pressure.

1. To increase the upright pressure, 9-alpha-fluoro-hydrocortisone, which produces sodium retention and can increase volume, is prescribed in small doses of 0.05 to 0.20 mg daily. Elevation of supine blood pressure and precipitation of heart failure are potential complications of this mineralocorticoid agent. Good elastic hose fitted to cover the legs and thighs and perhaps to waist level (such as Jobst stockings) maybe beneficial.
2. Both drugs and mechanical maneuvers can help in lowering supine pressure.
   - Short-acting vasodilators (i.e. ACE inhibitors, calcium antagonists, hydralazine) can be taken shortly before bedtime to reduce nocturnal supine blood pressures. Initial doses should be small and slowly titrated upward to prevent orthostatic hypotension in the morning hours.
   - Mechanically elevating the head end of the bed 10 inches will allow gravity to decrease the supine blood pressure.

Drugs for Managing Hypertensive Emergencies in Diabetic Patients

The pharmacologic treatment of hypertensive emergencies in patients with diabetes is not different from that for persons who do not have diabetes.[2] Treatment usually is administered with parenteral agents including sodium nitroprusside and various adrenergic blocking agents. However, the potential detrimental effects of several agents in producing uncontrolled drops in blood pressure or increased cardiac output should be considered carefully in patients with diabetes who may have concomitant CVD and cerebrovascular disease. Diazoxide may exacerbate hyperglycemia and therefore is contraindicated.

THE INDIAN SCENARIO

India today has the largest number of diabetic patients in any other country. Presently 35 million Indians have diabetes mellitus and it is estimated that by 2025 approximately 74 millions will have diabetes mellitus.[12] It has also been estimated that by 2025, one-third of the adult Indian population will have hypertension. This alarmingly high prevalence of diabetes and hypertension in the Indian population has been attributed to have dysmetabolic syndrome X. Several studies have shown a high incidence of this syndrome in Indians compared to the Eestern population.[13-15] The Chennai urban population study (CUPS) study has confirmed that subjects with glucose intolerance have a greater risk of hypertension.[4] Another latest epidemiological study, the Chennai urban rural epidemiology study (CURES) study,[16] has provided valuable data on diabetes, hypertension and obesity in India. It has reported a very high prevalence of diabetes mellitus (16%) and hypertension (23%). A higher socioeconomic status is associated with increased prevalence of both diabetes and hypertension, which is in contrast to the situation in some other developing countries. With increase in obesity particularly abdominal obesity, a sharp rise in both hypertension and diabetes has been observed.

CONCLUSION

Diabetes and hypertension frequently coexist and predispose to atherosclerotic cardiovascular disease and renal failure. There is a high prevalence of both diabetes and hypertension in the Indian population. This is attributed to the high prevalence of dysmetabolic syndrome X in Indians. Antihypertensive therapy must be promptly instituted in all diabetic patients with any degree of high blood pressure. The target BP for diabetic patients is lower than in the remaining population of hypertensive. All major classes of antihypertensive drugs are appropriate to treat hypertension in diabetic patients, but ACE inhibitors are special. They prevent CAD and protect the kidneys. A-II receptor antagonists have a potential role. Long-term clinical studies are still ongoing.

SUMMARY

The cutaneous manifestations in diabetes mellitus are due to multiple factors like metabolic disturbances, chronic degenerative changes and complications due to therapy. Diabetics are more prone to develop bacterial, fungal and viral infections. Patients with recurrent furuncles or carbuncle should always be investigated for diabetes. Monilial balanoposthitis and vulvo-vaginitis as well as extensive ring worm infections are common amongst diabetics. Pruritus vulvae are quite frequent in diabetic females.

Eruptive xanthomas are a characteristic, but uncommon complications of diabetes with associated hypertriglyceridemia. The lesions come in crops and regress when hyperlipidemia is controlled.

Necrobiosis lipoidica is the most specific, but very rare manifestation of diabetes. Majority of the patients either have diabetes or develop diabetes later or have first-degree relatives with diabetes. Diabetic dermopathy is the most common dermatosis associated with diabetes. Diabetic bullae are pathognomonic of diabetes. They are painless, noninflammatory bullae, and commonly appear spontaneously on the feet and hands. Granuloma annulare is another uncommon disorder and disseminated and diffuse granuloma annulare has strong association with diabetes.

Various dermatoses like acanthosis nigricans, generalized vitiligo, perforating dermatoses, skin tags, generalized pruritus and knuckle pebbles also need to be secreened for diabetes.

REFERENCES

1. Ferdinand Keith C. Update in pharmacologic treatment of hypertension. Cardiol Clin. 2001;19:279-94.
2. American Diabetes Association. Hypertension management in adults with diabetes. Diabetes Care. 2004; 27:565-7.
3. Gress TW, Nieto FJ, Shahar E, Wofford MR, Brancati FL. Hypertension and antihypertensive therapy as risk factors for type 2 diabetes mellitus. Atherosclerosis Risk in Communities Study. N Engl J Med. 2000;342:905-12.
4. Shantirani CS, Pradeepa R, Deepa R, Premlatha G, Saroja R, Mohan V. Prevalence and risk factors of hypertension in a selected South India population: the Chennai urban population study. JAPI. 2003;51:20-7.
5. National Blood Pressure Education Program Working Group. Report of hypertension in diabetes. NIH Publication No. 94-3530.
6. A Richard Christlieb, Andrez S Krolewski, James H Warram. Hypertension. In Joslin's Diabetes Mellitus, 13th edn. BI Waverly Pvt Ltd; 1996. pp. 817-35.
7. Seventh Report of the Joint National Committee on Prevention, Detection, Evaluation and Treatment of High Blood Pressure. Hypertension. 2003;42:1206.
8. Sowers JR, Reed J. Clinical advisory treatment of hypertension and diabetes. J Hypertension. 2000;2(2):132-3.
9. Chowdhary TA, Kumar S, Barnett AH, et al. Treatment of hypertension in patients with type 2 diabetes: a review of recent evidence. J Hum Hypertens. 1999;13:803-11.
10. Snow V, Weiss KB, Mottur-Pilson C. The evidence base for tight blood pressure control in the management of type 2 diabetes mellitus. Ann Intern Med. 2003;138:587-92.
11. Andersen NH, Mogensen CE. Inhibition of renin-angiotensin system, with particular reference to dual blockade treatment. J Renin-Ang-Aldo System. 2001;2:146-52.
12. Pradeepa R, Deepa, V Mohan. Epidemiology of diabetes in India—Current perspectives and future projections. JIMA. 2002;100.
13. Das UN. Metabolic syndrome is common in Indians: but why and how? JAPI. 2003;51:987-98.
14. Bhopal R. Epidemic of cardiovascular disease in South Asians. BMJ. 2002;324:625-6.
15. Arvind Gupta, Rajeev Gupta, Mukesh Sarna, et al. Prevalence of diabetes: impaired fasting glucose and insulin resistance syndrome in an urban India population. Diabet Resear Clinl Pract. 2003;61:69-76.
16. Mohan V. Prevalence of diabetes and hypertension in South Indian population—the Chennai urban rural epidemiology study (CURES). Asian J Diabetol. 2003;5:29-30.

FURTHER READING

1. Nilsson Peter M. Hypertension in diabetes mellitus. In John C Pickup, Pickup JC,G (Eds). 3rd edn. Blackwell Science Ltd; 2003. pp. 55.1-55.16.

Chapter 51

DYSLIPIDEMIA IN DIABETES

Subhankar Chowdhury, Kaushik Pandit

CHAPTER OUTLINE

- Introduction
- Lipoprotein Physiology
- Lipoproteins and Atherosclerosis
- Nature of Dyslipidemia in Diabetes
- Screening for Dyslipidemia in Diabetes
- Treatment of Dyslipidemia in Diabetes
- Conclusion

INTRODUCTION

Lipid disorders are not uncommon in diabetes. They may arise from a lack (in type 1 diabetes) or a defect in the action (in type 2 diabetes) of insulin; in type 2 diabetes part of the problem maybe a causally independent component of the 'metabolic/dysmetabolic syndrome'. Besides, an individual with diabetes may also have some form of familial/genetic dyslipidemia.

Whatever the mechanism, they contribute importantly to the considerable increase in the risk of atherosclerosis and consequent mortality in diabetes. In the Framingham study, it was documented that the incidence of cardiovascular disease in diabetic men was twice that among nondiabetic men, and in diabetic women it was about three times.[1] The absolute risk of cardiovascular death has been found to be much higher for diabetic than nondiabetic people in the large multiple risk factor intervention trial, irrespective of the presence of other risk factors.[2] However, apart from dyslipidemia, other factors also contribute towards the increased risk of coronary heart disease (CHD) in diabetes, e.g. hypertension, obesity, hyperglycemia, oxidative stress and smoking.[2-4]

LIPOPROTEIN PHYSIOLOGY

All the major lipids in our body, namely cholesterol, triglycerides and phospholipids have important physiological functions as follows:
1. Cholesterol
   - Structural constituent of cell membranes
   - Precursor of steroid hormones
   - Precursor of bile acids
2. Triglycerides
   - Major energy store of the body
3. Phospholipids
   - Structural constituent of cell membranes.

Structure

Lipoproteins are macromolecular complexes carrying hydrophobic lipids like triglycerides and cholesterol esters in plasma; these latter comprise the core of the lipoproteins and are enveloped by the amphiphilic (i.e. both hydrophobic and hydrophilic) monolayer of phospholipids, free cholesterol and proteins which solubilize the lipids for transport in plasma. The proteins, called apoproteins (or apolipoproteins), not only play a mechanical role in lipid transport, but also regulate lipoprotein metabolism.

Several major subclasses of lipoproteins have been defined by their physical-chemical characteristics, namely, chylomicrons, very low density lipoproteins (VLDL), intermediate density lipoproteins (IDL), low density lipoproteins (LDL) and high density lipoproteins (HDL). The size of the particles decreases (while density increases), continuously from the chylomicrons (diameter 75 to 1200 nm) to the HDL (diameter 5 to 12 nm). Roughly, there is a reciprocal relationship between the triglycerides and cholesterol contents of the lipoproteins, with chylomicrons and VLDL being high in triglycerides (80 to 90% and 50 to 80% respectively of triglycerides and 2 to 7% and 5 to 15% respectively of cholesterol) and LDL-C and HDL-C being relatively high in cholesterol (40 to 50% and 15 to 25% respectively of cholesterol and 5 to 15% and 5 to 10% respectively of triglycerides); the phospholipid content shows a gradual increase from 5 to 10% in chylomicrons to 20 to 30% in HDL-C.

Metabolism

For the sake of easy understanding this may be discussed under two broad groups, the metabolic handling of dietary lipids (exogenous) and that of endogenous lipids.

Dietary (Exogenous) Lipids

Dietary fats are absorbed into the intestinal mucosa as fatty acids, monoglycerides, glycerol and cholesterol; here they are re-esterified to triglyceride and cholesterol ester, which are incorporated in the lipid core of chylomicrons and enter the circulation via the thoracic duct. Medium-chain triglycerides can be absorbed directly into the portal circulation without the need for packaging into chylomicrons. Apolipoprotein B48 is necessary for formation and secretion of chylomicron from the intestinal cell. In the circulation, chylomicrons acquire additional apoproteins C and E from circulating HDL. Of these, apoprotein CII (apo CII) activates an enzyme, lipoprotein lipase (LPL) located on the endothelium of capillaries in skeletal muscle and adipose tissue, while apo CIII inhibits it. The net effect is hydrolysis of triglyceride component of chylomicrons in muscle and fat to yield fatty acids and glycerol; while both maybe used as fuel, some fatty acids may be re-esterified to triglycerides and stored in adipose tissue. In the process of catabolism of chylomicrons, triglycerides get depleted from the core while surface apo CII, CIII, free cholesterol and phospholipids are transferred to HDL-C. The chylomicron remnant (with a cholesterol-ester-rich core) is then taken up by the hepatocytes with the help of apo E following binding to hepatic LDL receptors. In effect, chylomicrons deliver dietary triglycerides to muscle and adipose tissue, while dietary cholesterol goes to the liver.

Endogenous Lipids

Endogenous lipid synthesis occurs primarily in the liver. Triglycerides are made from fatty acids that maybe synthesized locally or derived from the circulation. Cholesterol is synthesized in the liver (with hydroxymethylglutaryl coenzyme A reductase (HMG-CoA reductase) as the rate-limiting step), but some of the cholesterol transported out of the liver may actually be derived from the circulation, e.g. from chylomicron remnants. These lipids are secreted from the liver as VLDL with apo B100 being the major apoprotein. Once in circulation VLDL acquires apo C and E from HDL. In the plasma VLDL, like chylomicrons, loses triglycerides by the action of LPL in muscle and adipose tissue and gets converted to smaller and denser VLDL remnants. These remnants can have two fates: the larger (triglyceride rich) ones are likely to be taken up by the liver directly, with the help of apo E binding to LDL receptors; the smaller ones undergo progressive triglyceride (and redundant surface component) depletion to get converted to LDL through IDL; apo E and hepatic triglyceride lipase (HTGL) are actively involved in this process. Apo B100 is the only protein that remains on the surface of the LDL and cholesterol the predominant lipid in the core. Thus, the cholesterol-rich LDL particles are basically derived from VLDL.

LDL particles are further subclassified in terms of decreasing size from LDL 1 to 3. The small dense LDL3 is catabolized more slowly[5] and is more susceptible to oxidation.[6] About 60% of the LDL is taken up by the liver (through apo B100 attachment site on the LDL receptor), where cholesterol can be utilized for bile acid synthesis, while the remainder is delivered to peripheral tissues, including the adrenal cortex and gonads, where cholesterol is used for steroid hormone synthesis. The cholesterol content of the hepatocyte feeds back negatively on both *de novo* cholesterol synthesis and hepatic LDL receptor number.

Reverse Cholesterol Transport

HDL provides the means for reverse cholesterol transport from the peripheral cells to the liver. Nascent HDL particles containing the crucial apoprotein A1 and phospholipids are produced by the liver and intestine.

These particles accept free cholesterol from peripheral cells and other lipoproteins; this cholesterol thus aquired is esterified by the enzyme lecithin cholesterol acyltransferase (LCAT) to cholesterol ester, which moves to the hydrophobic core of HDL. LCAT is present in the HDL particle itself and is activated by apo A1. Nascent HDL, by acquiring more and more cholesterol (and also by receiving redundant surface components from other lipoproteins), is converted to larger and less dense HDL2. HDL2 can be taken up directly by the liver. More commonly, cholesterol esters from HDL2 are exchanged with triglycerides from triglyceride-rich apo B lipoproteins (chylomicrons and VLDL) with the help of cholesterol ester transport protein (CETP). The reverse cholesterol transport is complete when these apo B lipoproteins are taken up by the liver.

Thus, there are four important enzymes that control lipoprotein metabolism: LPL, HTGL, LCAT and CETP; defects in any of these enzymes can cause disturbances in plasma lipids, all of such disorders are rare clinical entities.

LIPOPROTEINS AND ATHEROSCLEROSIS

LDL-Cholesterol

Plasma cholesterol is well-recognized risk factor for atherosclerosis-related diseases, in particular coronary heart disease (CHD). This is well illustrated in the multiple risk factor intervention trial (MRFIT) where CHD death was positively correlated to plasma cholesterol level independent of hypertension and smoking.[2] It is believed that 80% of the worldwide variation in CHD incidence can be explained by differences in levels of plasma cholesterol.[7] It is the cholesterol carried in LDL that is primarily implicated in atherosclerosis.

A common, heritable phenotype characterized by the predominance of small, dense LDL3 particles (LDL subclass B) is associated with increased concentration of plasma triglycerides, reduced levels of HDL-C and increased risk of CHD in comparison with subjects with larger LDL (LDL subclass A).

LDL, modified by oxidation, is avidly taken up by 'scavenger' receptors on macrophages and endothelial cells in the arterial wall leading to the formation of cholesterol-laden foam cells; this sows the seed for atherosclerosis. These scavenger receptors differ from classical LDL receptors in that they are not down-regulated by increasing amounts of cholesterol inside the cell. Oxidized LDL may also stimulate secretion of cytokines and growth factors by endothelial cells,

smooth muscle cells and macrophages. This results in complex changes in the arterial wall involving further attraction of macrophages, proliferation of smooth muscle cells and laying down of extracellular matrix, altogether completing the process of atherosclerosis.

HDL-Cholesterol

HDL-cholesterol has a strong negative correlation with CHD risk.[8] HDL-cholesterol may protect against atherosclerosis by several hypothetical mechanisms:
1. Most attractively, by reverse cholesterol transport from foam cells in the arterial wall to the liver.
2. By protecting LDL from oxidation.
3. Indirectly, by lowering of apo B containing lipoproteins which deliver cholesterol to the endothelium.

Triglycerides and VLDL

The relationship between plasma triglyceride level and CHD risk is still not settled beyond doubt. Many studies have found a significant positive correlation between plasma triglyceride level and CHD risk on univariate analyses; however, quite often, this is lost on multivariate analyses where other factors like HDL-cholesterol are also included. The apparent risk of hypertriglyceridemia maybe secondary to other associated disorders like:
1. Low HDL-cholesterol.
2. Preponderance of small dense LDL3 subfraction (which is more atherogenic because of greater propensity to oxidation and slower catabolism).
3. Higher level of the coagulation factor VII (now recognized as an independent risk factor for CHD).
4. Higher level of plasminogen activator inhibitor-1 (PAI-1) (which can promote CHD by inhibiting fibrinolysis).

While it is true that atherosclerotic plaques do not contain triglycerides, we are to remember that triglyceride-rich lipoprotein particles like VLDL (more specifically VLDL remnants) also contain significant amounts of cholesterol ester and hence maybe atherogenic.

Moreover, in a recently published meta-analysis involving seventeen population-based prospective studies, TG was found to be an independent risk factor for CHD even after adjustment for HDL-cholesterol.[9,10]

Lipoprotein(a)

This is a LDL particle which has an additional apoprotein, designated apo(a), attached covalently to the apo B100. Apo(a) has striking structural similarity to plasminogen. The physiological role of lipoprotein (a) [Lp(a)] is not well understood. However, its plasma level is positively associated with CHD in nondiabetic population.[11]

Risk Factors versus Markers

A variable can be a predictor for CHD in an observational study, but not in clinical trials if the variable is a marker (or closely associated with other risk factors) rather than a true risk factor. Modification of a marker may or may not change the actual risk of CHD.

LDL-cholesterol is a recognized risk factor for CHD and its lowering has been unequivocally beneficial in clinical trials. It is possible that elevated triglyceride may be a better marker of CHD than elevated LDL-cholesterol in type 2 diabetics in an observational study, because triglyceride levels are more correlated with other components of the insulin resistance syndrome than is LDL-cholesterol. However, triglyceride lowering may not be so effective. Since clinical trials provide stronger data than observational studies, primary emphasis should be placed on LDL lowering, while interventions to lower the triglyceride levels and raise HDL-cholesterol levels may also be very useful.[12,13]

NATURE OF DYSLIPIDEMIA IN DIABETES

Lipid Disorders in Diabetes

The lipid abnormalities associated with diabetes are better termed as 'dyslipoproteinemia' or 'dyslipidemia', rather than 'hyperlipoproteinemia' or 'hyperlipidemia', because there maybe changes in both the quantity and quality of the lipoproteins. The two main determinants of these changes are the type of diabetes and the degree of glycemic control.

Dyslipidemia in Type 2 Diabetes

Dyslipidemia is more frequent in type 2 diabetes and is a major contributor to the high-risk of CHD seen in this condition.

Quantitative Changes

The most frequent form of quantitative dyslipidemia is increased triglycerides.[14-16] The United Kingdom prospective diabetes study (UKPDS) has shown that the hypertriglyceridemia of type 2 diabetes is already present at the time of diagnosis.[17] In fact, this has been noted in the prediabetic phase as well.[18] This is also influenced by the presence of other factors unrelated to hyperglycemia or insulin resistance, e.g. presence or absence of nephropathy, obesity, hypothyroidism, the frequent occurrence of genetically determined lipoprotein disorders (familial combined hyperlipidemia or familial hypertriglyceridemia), alcohol and estrogen usage.

The other quantitative dyslipidemia associated with type 2 diabetes is low HDL-cholesterol concentration. In the multivariate analysis, the male diabetic had lower HDL-cholesterol levels than corresponding nondiabetic subjects after adjusting for other variables.[19] UKPDS confirmed this; and found the abnormality more commonly in diabetic females.[20] The prospective cardiovascular Munster (PROCAM) study in the German population also noted the prevalence of low HDL-cholesterol in diabetic subjects.[21] The same feature was again noted in a Finnish population study. The future risk for CHD death in the study was found to be two-fold to four-fold higher in diabetic subjects with low HDL-cholesterol than in diabetic patients without it.[22] Other studies noted that it is the HDL2 subfraction which is specifically depressed in the high-risk population with CHD in diabetes.[23,24] The low HDL cholesterol may persist despite achievement of glycemic control.

Total and LDL-cholesterol concentrations in diabetics most often approach those in nondiabetic, especially on achievement of good metabolic control.

The similarity of plasma total cholesterol levels in type 2 diabetes and in those without diabetes should not lead one to conclude that cholesterol has no coronary risk effect in diabetics. The multiple risk factor intervention trial has shown that the incidence of coronary mortality increases in a curvilinear manner with increasing concentrations of serum cholesterol both in those with and in those without diabetes. The two curves were similar in shape but differed, with the curve for those with diabetes being higher than the curve for those without. At any given serum cholesterol concentration, those with diabetes had a risk of CHD mortality between two and four times greater than those without diabetes.[2] There maybe several reasons for this. First, the level of cholesterol in serum reflects the level of all lipoproteins, not just LDL. Thus, an elevation of serum cholesterol may, in part, indicate an increase in the triglyceride-rich lipoproteins as well. Second, there may be many nonlipoprotein atherogenic factors, e.g. advanced glycation end-products that might increase the risk in diabetes. Third, LDL maybe modified in a way that would make any given amount more atherogenic such as glycation and oxidation. Another aspect also needs mention. The LDL-cholesterol concentration is usually calculated by Friedewald formula [LDL-cholesterol = total cholesterol – {HDL-cholesterol + triglyceride/5} (all concentrations in mg/dl)]. However, in diabetes, the calculated LDL-cholesterol correlates poorly with that actually determined by ultracentrifugation, probably because of changes in cholesterol: triglyceride ratio in VLDL.[25]

LDL distribution is tilted towards smaller and denser LDL3 particles (LDL B phenotype) which have greater atherogenic potential.[26] Feingold et al found that normolipidemic men with diabetes have two-fold increase in the percentage of individuals with the LDL B phenotype compared with normolipidemic men without diabetes.[27] In the Kaiser Permanente Women Twins Study, prevalence of LDL phenotype B has been found to be an integral feature of insulin resistance syndrome.[28] Conversely, subjects with predominance of small LDL had a greater than two-fold increased risk of developing type 2 diabetes mellitus over a follow-up period of 3.5 years.[29]

HDL particles show enrichment in triglycerides, increased cholesterol to protein ratio and a selective reduction of apo AI. There is also increased glycosylation of apo AI and AII, which appears to accelerate HDL catabolism so that there is rapid clearance before they have circulated long enough to acquire sufficient cholesterol to become HDL2.[30] Glycosylation of HDL probably also impairs its ability to promote cholesterol efflux from cells *in vitro*.[31]

Lp(a) is of special interest in type 2 diabetes because of its known association with CHD. Studies have shown higher levels,[32] no difference[33] and even lower levels[34] in type 2 diabetic subjects. However, most of the studies on Lp(a) and type 2 diabetes are small and except for a few do not account for the apo(a) phenotype, which is a major determinant of Lp(a) concentration. The consensus appears to be that the diabetic state does not have any impact on Lp(a) concentration,[35] though diabetic patients with CHD have been found to have higher Lp(a) concentration than those without CHD.[36] A recent study from South India echoes the same conclusion that in diabetic population Lp(a) is an independent risk factor for CHD, though the level is not increased.[37]

Diabetic subjects have been found to have greater glycation of LDL particles, which are more susceptible to oxidation.[38] Increased oxidized LDL has also been found in diabetic subjects.[39]

Mechanism of Dyslipidemia in Type 2 Diabetes

Insulin resistance, which is important in the genesis of type 2 diabetes itself, can also cause hypertriglyceridemia and the preponderance of small dense LDL particles maybe explained in terms of hypertriglyceridemia.

Insulin normally inhibits hormone-sensitive lipase in adipose tissue; insulin resistance, therefore, causes unrestrained lipolysis leading to increased flux of fatty acids to the liver, which ends in higher hepatic triglyceride synthesis. On the other hand, activity of the endothelial insulin-dependent lipoprotein lipase will be less, resulting in diminished triglyceride clearance from triglyceride-rich lipoproteins. The direct effect of insulin on hepatic triglyceride and VLDL synthesis appears to depend on the duration of exposure. Short-term exposure inhibits,[40] while chronic hyperinsulinemia increases VLDL triglyceride secretion from the liver.[41] In type 2 diabetes, hyperinsulinemia does occur secondary to insulin resistance, but whether the liver remains sensitive to the VLDL secretory effects of chronic exposure to insulin is not clear. It may well be that in type 2 diabetes, both deficient (on adipose tissue lipase and endothelial LPL) and excessive (on hepatic VLDL secretion) insulin action may underlie the raised triglyceride. As a consequence of triglyceride enrichment of VLDL, there is increased transfer of triglycerides to LDL with the help of CETP; these triglyceride-rich LDL particles are substrates for hepatic lipase activity leading to the formation of small dense LDL.

Hyperinsulinemia, Dyslipidemia and CHD

It is common knowledge that insulin resistance and the compensatory hyperinsulinemia (if pancreatic β-cells are competent) are associated with an atherogenic plasma lipid profile, comprising elevated triglyceride and depressed HDL-cholesterol levels. A number of prospective studies, albeit in nondiabetic subjects, have also found plasma insulin to be an independent and statistically significant correlate of CHD. This naturally raises the important issue of the long-term safety of the use of insulin in type 2 diabetes, where hyperinsulinemia is already believed to exist. However, administration of insulin to both insulin-dependent (i.e. insulinopenic) and noninsulin-dependent (i.e. hyperinsulinemic) diabetics (to control hyperglycemia) or indeed to nondiabetic subjects produces a decrease in serum triglyceride levels.[42] Also, insulinoma is associated with low plasma concentrations of triglycerides.[43] Hence, direct role of hyperinsulinemia in the genesis of hypertriglyceridemia has been questioned. It is insulin resistance rather than consequent hyperinsulinemia that maybe consists as the cause of high triglyceridemia.

Moreover, in the UKPDS the intensive glycemic control group, many of whom were treated with insulin, far from showing increased CHD mortality actually showed a non-significant 16% decrease.[14]

Dyslipidemia in Type 1 Diabetes

It differs from that in type 2 diabetes in two important respects:
1. It is closely related to the degree of glycemic control.
2. Low HDL-cholesterol is not a feature (in the absence of renal involvement).

In poorly controlled type 1 diabetics, the characteristic lipid abnormality is increased triglycerides. This can be well explained by absolute deficiency of insulin. As expected, the level normalizes with adequate insulinization.

In the Wisconsin epidemiological study on diabetic retinopathy (WESDR), the mean levels of total and HDL-cholesterol were similar in type 1 diabetic subjects and age matched control population.[44] In the DCCT population (n = 1569), lipids and lipoproteins were similar to nondiabetic subjects participating in the lipid research clinics program.[45]

In fact, type 1 diabetic subjects who are in good control tend to have normal (and sometimes even better than normal) levels of lipoproteins (lower levels of triglyceride and cholesterol and higher levels of HDL-cholesterol).[46,47] Regarding qualitative changes in plasma lipids, it maybe noted that LDL size is not different in type 1 diabetes mellitus compared to controls. However, type 1 diabetic subjects have an increased cholesterol to triglyceride ratio in VLDL particles which may not resolve with intensive insulin therapy.[48] A lower lecithin (a phospholipid) content of VLDL and IDL has also been reported in type 1 diabetic patients.[49]

Lp(a) levels have been variously reported as high or normal in type 1 diabetes.

Presence of nephropathy (even at the stage of microalbuminuria) adversely affects practically all aspects of lipid profile leading to elevation of LDL-cholesterol, VLDL triglycerides and reduction of HDL-cholesterol, particularly HDL2.[50]

Dyslipidemia in 'Malnutrition-related Diabetes'

WHO recognized malnutrition-related diabetes mellitus as a separate type of diabetes in 1985. These patients tend to have rather low levels of cholesterol and triglycerides, which may partly explain their low rates of macrovascular disease. However, current view tends to be against identifying this as a separate class of diabetes.

Diabetic Dyslipidemia and Ethnicity

In an analysis in UKPDS cohort followed up for nine years, it was noted that the Asian Indian population cohort had lower total cholesterol, LDL-cholesterol and HDL-cholesterol, but higher triglyceride compared to the White Caucasian (WC) and Afro-Caribbean (AC) cohort. This probably signifies that the Asian Indians are more insulin resistant, a fact that has been proved in many other studies comprising multi-ethnic population.[51-54]

During the follow-up period of nine years, the Asian Indians showed a similar decrease of total and LDL-cholesterol as well as of triglyceride level compared to the WC and AC peer cohorts, but there was no significant change in HDL-cholesterol level, which showed an upward trudge in the other groups. This was seen despite a less significant increase in body weight and marginal worsening of blood pressure and glycemic parameters amongst the cohorts. The lipid changes were not related to the lipid lowering therapy because less than 2% of the population was receiving it.

SCREENING FOR DYSLIPIDEMIA IN DIABETES

Frequency

This should be done on an annual basis, especially in type 2 diabetics because of their higher risk of atherosclerosis-related diseases. Once an abnormality is detected, testing may need to be more frequent, e.g. to titrate the dose of lipid lowering agent.

Tests

Total cholesterol, HDL-cholesterol and triglycerides should be checked on fasting state (only triglyceride levels are significantly affected by meals within previous 12 hours). Unless there is urgency, lipid profile should be checked only after achieving good glycemic control; this can obviate some needless lipid lowering prescriptions.

Most clinical laboratories cannot measure LDL-cholesterol directly, but give a calculated value based on Freidewald formula; however, as we have already seen, this is liable to be fallacious in diabetics. On the other hand, many standard recommendations [e.g. the National Cholesterol Education Program (NCEP) in the USA)] on interventions in lipid control depend heavily on the LDL-cholesterol level.[55] As a rough substitute intervention maybe initiated at a total cholesterol level that is one-and-a-half times the recommended LDL-cholesterol value.

In diabetics, it maybe instructive to know the LDL and HDL subfractions (especially as the harmful small dense LDL maybe elevated despite a normal total LDL) as well.

If fasting lipids are normal, there is a scope for studying postprandial lipemia because of known defect in clearing chylomicrons in diabetics and which probably has influence on atherogenesis as chylomicron remnant particles are highly atherogenic.

TREATMENT OF DYSLIPIDEMIA IN DIABETES

Goals

The American Diabetes Association (ADA) recommendation [based on the NCEP adult treatment panel III (ATP III) guidelines] states that the first goal is to lower LDL-cholesterol, followed by HDL-cholesterol elevation and triglyceride lowering.[55,56]

The current recommendations of primary goal of therapy for LDL-C is to lower it to below 100 mg/dl. In people with diabetes over the age of 40 years with a total cholesterol of more than or equal to 135 mg/dl, statin therapy is recommended to achieve an LDL-C reduction of 30% irrespective of baseline LDL-C level.

Since the publication of ATP III, major clinical trials of statin therapy with clinical end-points have been published. These trials addressed issues that were not examined in previous clinical trials of cholesterol-lowering therapy. This necessitated a relook at the problem and issue new guidelines. In the recently published updated recommendation of NCEP ATP III, it was proposed that patients with diabetes and manifest cardiovascular disease it is reasonable to target a goal of less than 70 mg/dl; and in people with diabetes without manifest cardiovascular disease, a target of less than 100 mg/dl (which is equal to target of nondiabetic people with cardiovascular disease) is recommended.[57]

Raising HDL-cholesterol levels appears desirable, but pharmacologically difficult in type 2 diabetes. In the recent ADA recommendation, the goal for HDL-C has been set at more than 40 mg/dl. In women, an HDL-C goal 10 mg/dl higher maybe appropriate.

Though triglyceride lowering has been recommended there are no widely-accepted targets. However, the recent ADA recommendation suggests pharmacological intervention at triglyceride levels >400 mg/dl, with a target of 150 mg/dl even in the absence of other risk factors; in the case of severe hypertriglyceridemia (>1000 mg/dl), severe dietary fat restriction (<10% of calories), in addition to pharmacological therapy is necessary to reduce the risk of pancreatitis. Improved glycemic control is also very effective for reducing triglyceride levels and should be aggressively followed before the introduction of fibrates.[56]

Treatment Modalities

The options are lifestyle measures, glycemic control and specific lipid-modifying drugs. As a general principle, pharmacological therapy should be initiated only after behavioral interventions are used. However, in patients with clinical CHD or very high LDL-C levels (>200 mg/dl), pharmacological therapy should be initiated along with behavioral therapy. Studies conducted by the American Heart Association have found that medical nutrition therapy can reduce LDL-C only by up to 15 to 25 mg/dl; hence, if the LDL-C exceeds the goal by 25 mg/dl, the physician may decide to institute pharmacological therapy at the same time as behavioral therapy for high risk patients (e.g. diabetic patients with a prior myocardial infarction and/or other CHD risk factors).[58]

However, before implementing any therapy for dyslipidemia we must exclude other secondary causes like hypothyroidism (even if subclinical), renal disease (nephrotic syndrome and chronic renal failure causing separate types of dyslipidemia), alcoholism, liver disease (chronic obstructive liver disease as well as acute hepatitis) and drugs (nonspecific β-blockers, thiazides, glucocorticoids, anabolic steroids, estrogen, progesteron, sertraline, isotretinoin, cyclosporine, and HIV protease inhibitors). Correction of the underlying abnormality may cure dyslipidemia.

Lifestyle Measures

Diet

Dietary treatment is a necessary foundation of drug treatment. The NCEP of USA recommends a step I diet for practically all Americans, with a step II diet for greater cholesterol lowering (Table 51.1). In long-term studies, the Step II diet decreased serum LDL-C concentration by 8 to 15%. A diet more restricted in fat than in step II diet results in little additional reduction in LDL-C, rather it raises triglyceride and lowers HDL-cholesterol concentrations.[59]

The benefits of restriction of saturated fat with replacement by mono and polyunsaturated fats are believed to act in the following manner:

TABLE 51.1	Two-step approach to treatment of hypercholesterolemia	
Nutrients	Step I diet	Step II diet
Total calories	To achieve and maintain desirable body weight	To achieve and maintain desirable body weight
Total fat	<30% of total calories	<30% of total calories
Fatty acid		
Saturated	<10% of total calories	<7% of total calories
Monounsaturated	10–15% of total calories	10-15% of total calories
Polyunsaturated	≤10–15% of total calories	≤10% of total calories
Cholesterol	<300 mg/day	<200 mg/day
Carbohydrate	50–60% of total calories	50–60% of total calories
Protein	10–20% of total calories	10–20% of total calories

1. Upregulation of LDL receptors in the liver, allowing greater hepatic uptake of LDL-cholesterol.
2. Increased conversion of cholesterol to bile acids and increased bile acid secretion from the liver.
3. Secretion of bigger VLDL particles with diminished cholesterol content from the liver.

Diets low in fat are invariably rich in carbohydrates and carbohydrates tend to decrease not only LDL-cholesterol but also HDL-cholesterol; the beneficial effect may thereby be minimized or negated. It has been recognized that partial replacement of dietary carbohydrates by monounsaturated fats not only helps improve glycemic control, but also favorably impacts on the dyslipidemia in type 2 diabetes (by increase of HDL-cholesterol and decrease of triglycerides, with no difference in LDL-cholesterol).[59] A recent report suggests that not all carbohydrates lower HDL-cholesterol; carbohydrates with a low glycemic index may actually raise it.[60] While the concept of 'good' and 'bad' carbohydrates has been by now both intensively as extensively worked out, it is yet to catch the fancy of the Western population.

Special mention maybe made of the consumption of margarines and fish oils.

Margarine: This is derived by partial hydrogenation of vegetable oils and is therefore devoid of cholesterol. However, during this manufacturing process trans-isomers of polyunsaturated fatty acids are formed (in place of natural cis-isomers) which can raise LDL-cholesterol and Lp(a) and lower HDL-cholesterol.[61] At present, adverse effects of trans-fatty acids maybe considered as equivalent to saturated fatty acids. So margarine may not be a safer alternative to butter; in fact, unrestricted intake of margarine, in the mistaken belief of its safety, based on 'zero cholesterol' advertisements, maybe more harmful.

Fish oil: In nondiabetics marine fish oils, rich in w-3 (n-3) polyunsaturated fatty acids, have multiple salutary effects: (a) reduction of triglycerides, (b) reduction of platelet aggregation and (c) reduction of blood pressure. However, concern has been raised that in type 2 diabetes large doses (>7 gm/day) maybe harmful by causing (a) increase in LDL-cholesterol and (b) worsening of glycemic control.[62] A meta-analysis of 26 published trials on diabetics has shown that fish oils decrease triglyceride to a significant extent in type 2 diabetic subjects and do not increase glycated hemoglobin.[63] Hence, fish intake should be encouraged in the diet, even if fish oil supplementation is not indicated routinely in type 2 diabetes, except in the vegetarians.

In addition to reducing hypercholesterolemia, diet can also help to: (a) achieve weight loss (relevant for the obese) and thereby reduce hypertriglyceridemia, (b) improve insulin resistance and (c) reduce blood pressure.

However, it has to be remembered that up to 50% of Indian diabetes patients in (including type 2) maybe nonobese (some are actually underweight) and thus calorie restriction should not be indiscriminately advocated in the Indian context. Moreover, strict restriction of foods rich in saturated fats and cholesterol (e.g. butter, ghee, egg, mutton) will serve no useful purpose unless the individual has hypercholesterolemia (remembering, of course, that the cut-off levels are more stringent in presence of diabetes). The diet should be designed to maintain an optimum ratio (<10:1) between n-6 and n-3 polyunsaturated fats.

Exercise

It can be successfully incorporated in a weight-reducing program and thereby improve (a) insulin sensitivity and (b) glycemic control. The effects on lipid profile are also beneficial, with lowering of triglyceride and LDL-cholesterol and elevation of HDL-cholesterol.[64]

While it is well established that the benefits of lifestyle modification in a diabetic patient extend beyond improvement of dyslipidemia, the stark reality is that long-term compliance generally is poor. Hence, pharmacological intervention is called for quite frequently.

Glycemic Control

Both in type 1 and type 2 diabetes, plasma triglycerides falls almost parallel with blood glucose, whatever may be the modality of improving glycemic control. While tightening of glycemic control in type 1 diabetes changes the lipid profile to become normal (or, even super-normal), LDL and HDL-cholesterol stages usually do not show impressive changes in type 2 diabetes.

As mentioned earlier, there should be no hesitation in using insulin for achieving glycemic control, as this does not cause any worsening, in fact can only improve dyslipidemia. Among the oral hypoglycemic agents, biguanides and thiazolidinediones seem to have an edge over sulfonylureas because of insulin sensitizing property. Among thiazolidinediones, pioglitazone appears to be more lipid-friendly than rosiglitazone.

Finally, because of the influence of glycemic control on lipid levels, it will be cost-effective in most situations (especially in a developing country like India) to defer estimation of plasma lipids till reasonable glycemic control is achieved.

Specific Lipid-modifying Drugs

The major classes of lipid-modifying drugs are as follows:
1. Statins (HMG-CoA reductase inhibitors).
2. Fibrates (Fibric acid derivatives).
3. Cholesterol absorption inhibitors (Bile acid sequestrants and azetidinones).
4. Nicotinic acid.
5. Miscellaneous.

The first three are first-line therapy against hypercholesterolemia, while fibrates are most effective for lowering of triglycerides **(Table 51.2)**.

TABLE 51.2	Lipid-modifying drugs		
Type	*Mechanism*	*Effect on lipid profile*	*Dose*
HMG-CoA reductase inhibitors (Statins)	↓ Cholesterol synthesis; ↑ LDL receptor	↓ LDL cholesterol 25–40%; ↓ Triglycerides 10–30%	Lovastatin 10–80 mg/d Simvastatin 5–80 mg/d Atorvastatin 10–80 mg/d Pravastatin 10–40 mg/d Fluvastatin 10–40 mg/d Rosuvastatin 5–20 mg/d
Fibrates	↑ Fatty acid oxidation → Hepatic triglycerides synthesis ↑ LPL → ↑ Triglycerides hydrolysis	↓ Triglycerides 25–40% ↑ HDL cholesterol ↑ or ↓ LDL cholesterol	Gemfibrozil 600 mg BD Bezafibrate 200 mg TD (400 mg OD) Fenofibrate 67–200 mg, or 54–160 mg in micronized form Ciprofibrate 100 mg OD
Bile acid sequestrant	↓ Reabsorption of bile acids in intestine → ↑ Synthesis of new bile acids and ↑ LDL receptor	↓ LDL cholesterol 20–30% ↑ HDL cholesterol ↑ Triglycerides	Cholestyramine 8–12 g BD or TD Colestipol 10–15 g BD or TD
Azetidinone	↓ Absorption of cholesterol from intestinal micelles	↓ LDL-C by 15%	Ezetimibe 10 mg OD usually along with statins
Nicotinic acid	↓ Hepatic triglyceride synthesis; ↓ Secretion of apo B100 containing lipoprotein; ↓ VLDL → LDL conversion	↓ LDL cholesterol 15–25% ↓ VLDL cholesterol 25–35% ↓ Lp(a) 30% ↓ HDL cholesterol 25% ↓ Triglycerides 25–85%	50–100 mg TD; gradually increased to 1000–2500 mg TD

The most commonly used groups statins and the fibrates, will be discussed in some detail.

Statins

Mechanism of action: These drugs are structurally similar to hydroxymethylglutaryl-Coenzyme A (HMG-CoA), a precursor of cholesterol, and are competitive inhibitors of the rate-limiting enzyme in cholesterol biosynthesis, HMG-CoA reductase. These agents also upregulate hepatic LDL receptor activity. Because endogenous cholesterol synthesis is maximal at night, the statins are best administered in the evening.

Additionally, some statins may activate endothelial nitric oxide synthase[65] and diminish uptake of LDL by vascular smooth muscle cells,[66] thus may reduce CHD beyond that achieved by cholesterol lowering.

Efficacy: Statins are the most effective agents for lowering cholesterol, the maximal LDL-cholesterol reduction achieved with different statins range from 25 to 60%. Atorvastatin and simvastatin are the most efficacious. These drugs also lowers triglyceride levels, though by a lesser extent of 10 to 30%. Atorvastatin and simvastatin (along with pravastatin) being are relatively more efficacious than lovastatin, fluvastatin or cerivastatin. There can be a slight elevation of HDL-cholesterol by 5 to 10%.

The utility of the statins for both primary prevention (i.e. prevention in subjects who have not yet suffered from myocardial infarction) and secondary prevention (i.e. prevention of progression of CHD in those who have already sustained a myocardial infarction) of heart disease is by now established beyond doubt in the general population with reduction of coronary artery disease by 25 to 60% and the risk of death from any cause by about 30%[67,68] (Chapter 56).

There are few studies solely on diabetics. But the conclusions from diabetic subgroup analyses of the many big trials are that diabetics benefit equally, if not more, compared to nondiabetic counter parts from the use of statins.

Considering secondary prevention trials, we can refer to the diabetic subgroup analysis[69] of the Scandinavian simvastatin survival study (4S study) (5% of the 4444 subjects were diabetic) where LDL-cholesterol levels were rather high to start with, or the cholesterol and recurrent events (CARE) study (11% of the study subjects were diabetic, absolute number of diabetics being 586)[70] where mean LDL-cholesterol of 139 mg/dl was only modest. In the former, the reduction of risk of CHD among diabetic subjects was 55% (significantly higher than 32% observed in nondiabetics), while in the latter the risk reduction was less (around 25%) and similar in diabetics and nondiabetics. It appears that the benefit is greater, higher the initial LDL-cholesterol level.

Primary prevention trials on diabetic subjects with statins are scarce. In a recently conducted large clinical trial in Britain, heart protection study (HPS) with 40 mg of simvastatin (and antioxidants) in the age group of 40 to 75 years was carried out to assess the efficacy of primary prevention of CHD in diabetic and nondiabetic persons. The results of the study showed that with the usage of statin the rate of first major vascular events are reduced by about a quarter.[54]

In another recently published similar primary prevention study in 2,838 patients with type 2 diabetes with atorvastatin, collaborative atorvastatin diabetes study (CARDS) has shown use of atorvastatin in patients with type 2 diabetes causes significant reduction in mortality by 27%, acute coronary events by 36% and stroke by 48%.[71]

Adverse effects: The most common are gastrointestinal upset, muscle aches (not frank myopathy) and hepatitis. Rarer are myopathy, peripheral neuropathy and CNS side effects like insomnia, bad dreams and difficulty in concentrating. Atorvastatin or pravastatin, which do not penetrate the CNS, maybe tried when CNS side effects are prominent. The risk of myopathy is increased in the elderly, in presence of renal impairment and when co-prescribed with fibrates, nicotinic acid, erythromycin or cyclosporine. Cerivastatin has been withdrawn by its original manufacturer because of reports of fatal phethnyolysis.

Fibrates

Mechanism of action: These partly resemble short chain fatty acids and increase the oxidation of fatty acids, with diminished triglyceride synthesis and VLDL secretion from the liver. These also increase LPL activity in muscle and adipose tissue vasculature causing increased triglyceride clearance.

Some fibrates may also reduce fibrinogen levels.

Efficacy: Fibrates are effective triglyceride-lowering agents, reducing plasma levels by 25 to 60%; this is accompanied by a beneficial increase in HDL-cholesterol concentration by 10 to 20%. Depending on initial LDL-cholesterol level they can cause increase (if initial level is low) or decrease (if initial level is high) of LDL-cholesterol; fenofibrate appears to be the most effective in lowering LDL-cholesterol. Fibrates also tend to increase the proportion of favorable large and bouyant LDL particles.[72]

To determine the clinical benefit derived from the apparently favorable influence of fibrates on lipid profile in diabetics, one should look at the results of clinical trials, which are much smaller compared to those on statins.

For secondary prevention gemfibrozil and bezafibrate have been used more often than others. In the recently reported bezafibrate coronary angiographic intervention trial (BECAIT), bezafibrate reduced coronary events in 92 men over a 5 year period.[73] The diabetes atherosclerosis intervention study (DAIS) was a multicenter, double-blind, randomized, placebo-controlled trial in collaboration with the WHO which studied micronized fenofibrate versus placebo in 418 patients with type 2 diabetes for at least 3 years.[74] Half of the patients had a clinical history of CHD; it was thus a mixture of a primary and secondary intervention trial. It showed significantly less angiographic progression of coronary artery disease in the fenofibrate group.[75] Another large secondary prevention trial, the bezafibrate infarction prevention trial, is underway in Israel on 3000 diabetics.[76]

In a study from Finland, comparing the efficacy of simvastatin and gemfibrozil in diabetic patients, it was found that simvastatin was useful in both mixed and isolated hypercholesterolemia, whereas gemfibrozil was useful in patients with high triglyceride and low or normal LDL-cholesterol levels.[77]

Amongst the primary prevention trials, the best known is the Helsinki heart study; it showed that gemfibrozil caused a significant reduction of CHD events, especially in those with elevated triglyceride and lower HDL-cholesterol levels.[78] There was no effect on mortality. The diabetic subgroup comprised 135 subjects. In these subjects gemfibrozil reduced the risk of CHD by 60%, although the result was not statistically significant.

The SENDCAP study suggests that improving dyslipidemia in type 2 diabetic subjects with bezafibrate results in a reduction in the incidence of coronary heart disease, despite no effect on the progress of ultrasonically measured arterial disease (in the carotid and femoral arteries).[79]

Adverse effects: Most common are gastrointestinal upsets (more with gemfibrozil) and gallstones. Others include erectile dysfunction in men and myositis.

In one placebo-controlled study, clofibrate use was associated with higher mortality as a result of diseases of the biliary tract and cancer, though this has not been reproduced in other studies, nor with other fibrates.

Azetidinone

Ezetimibe belongs to a group of selective and very effective 2-azetidinone cholesterol absorption inhibitors which act on the level of cholesterol entry into enterocytes. Recent data indicated that the drug prevents the formation of a heterocomplex consisting of annexin-2 and caveolin-l and leads to specific inhibition of an NPClLI -dependent cholesterol uptake pathway required for uptake of micellar cholesterol into enterocytes.[80] Ezetimibe does not inhibit cholesterol synthesis in the liver, or increase bile acid excretion. Instead, ezetimibe localizes and appears to act at the brush border of the small intestine and inhibits the absorption of both biliary and disease cholesterol, leading to a decrease in the delivery of intestinal cholesterol to the liver. This causes a reduction of hepatic cholesterol stores and an increase in clearance of cholesterol from the blood; this distinct mechanism is complementary to that of HMG-CoA reductase inhibitors.[80]

Ezetimibe is not recommended as a monotherapy option till date. But in a clinical trial setting it has significantly reduced LDL cholesterol by a mean of 16.9%, compared with an increase of 0.4% with placebo in patients to primary hypercholesterolemia.[81]

In a double-blind, placebo-controlled study in patients with primary hypercholesterolemia, ezetimibe when coadministered with a statin significantly lowered total cholesterol, LDL-C and TG, and increased HDL-C compared to placebo (coadministration therapy with statin caused additional reduction of LDL-C by 34 to 41%, TG by 21 to 23%, and increased HDL-C by 7.8 to 8.4%, depending on the dose of statin.[82]

Nicotinic Acid or Niacin

Nicotinic acid or niacin is a very useful agent in the treatment of dyslipidemia. It decreases LDL-cholesterol and triglycerides, increases HDL-cholesterol to a significant extent and is the only agent known to reliably decrease Lp(a). The major adverse effect is flushing of skin and rarely hepatitis. It was believed to have the tendency to worsen glycemic control in patients with diabetes. But recent data from clinical trials on patients with diabetes have put to rest such unfounded fears, and niacin can be safely used in patients with diabetes and niacin therapy maybe considered as an alternative to statin drugs or fibrates for patients with diabetes in whom these agents are not tolerated or fail to sufficiently correct hypertriglyceridemia or low HDL levels.[83]

Bile Acid Sequestrants

Bile acid sequestrants are now used only as adjuncts to statins for further lowering of cholesterol. An important limitation is their tendency to raise triglyceride levels. Prominent gastrointestinal side effects often affect patient compliance.

Cholesteryl ester transfer protein (CETP) is a plasma protein that mediates the exchange of cholesteryl ester in HDL for triglyceride in VLDL. This process decreases the level of antiatherogenic HDL-cholesterol and increases proatherogenic VLDL and LDL-cholesterol, so CETP is believed to be potentially atherogenic. A CETP inhibitor thereby may increase the HDL concentration. A synthetic CETP inhibitor known as torcetrapib has been used in a randomized controlled trial in humans to test the efficacy of elevating HDL-cholesterol. The results of the trial suggest that torcetrapib increases HDL to a significant extent as monotherapy (46 to 106 percent), whereas in association with atorvastatin there is further elevation of HDL.[84]

Plant sterols and stanols, which are structurally related to cholesterol, decrease the incorporation of dietary and biliary cholesterol into micelles. This lowers cholesterol absorption. Furthermore, these components increase ABC-transporter expression, which may also contribute to the decreased cholesterol absorption. Consequently, cholesterol synthesis and LDL receptor activity increase, which ultimately leads to decreased serum LDL-cholesterol concentrations.

Plant sterols and stanols also lower plasma lipid-standardized concentrations of the hydrocarbon carotenoids, but not those of the oxygenated carotenoids and tocopherols. Also, vitamin A and D concentrations are not affected. Although absorption of plant sterols and stanols (0.02–3.5%) is low compared to cholesterol (35–70%), small amounts are found in the circulation and may influence other physiological functions.

A meta-analysis of 41 trials showed that intake of 2 gm per day of stanols or sterols reduced LDL by 10%. Effects are additive with diet or drug interventions: eating foods low in saturated fat and cholesterol and high in stanols or sterols can reduce LDL by 20%, adding sterols or stanols to statin medication is more effective than doubling the statin dose.[85]

In a randomized prospective trial with plant stanol esters on children with the aim of atherosclerosis prevention in childhood (STRIP study), the results showed that plant stanol esters reduce serum cholesterol concentration in healthy children irrespective of their gender or apoE4 phenotype.[86]

Miscellaneous

Orlistat, a pancreatic lipase inhibitor, was noted to cause significant reductions in total cholesterol, LDL-cholesterol, triglycerides and apolipoprotein B concentration in obese type 2 diabetics.[87]

Similar results have been reported with pramlintide, a synthetic amylin analog.[88]

Acipimox is a nicotinic acid congener that does not worsen glycemic control in diabetes. It causes significant triglyceride lowering along with decreasing total cholesterol and apolipoprotein B. But it has no significant effect in elevating HDL-cholesterol or apolipoprotein A1 level.[89]

Fish oils containing eicosapentaenoic acid and docosahexaenoic acid (n-3 polyunsaturated fatty acids) are known to decrease triglycerides. However, as already discussed, large doses increase LDL-cholesterol and may worsen glycemic control.

Dietary 'soluble' fibers like guar gum and pectin cause mild lowering of cholesterol.

Oral estrogen in postmenopausal women can lower LDL-cholesterol by 10% and raise HDL-cholesterol by 15%.

Finally, severe hypercholesterolemia can be treated by apheresis.

Newer Vistas in Lipid Modification

The newer statins in the pipeline are pitavastatin and nisvastatin which are currently undergoing clinical trials.[90] Pitavastatin showed a high potency in decreasing LDL and its catabolism is not mediated by the cytochrome P-450-3A4, thus reducing the potential for drug-drug interaction.[91]

The newer cholesterol absorption inhibitor which is undergoing trials is colesevelam and has shown a clinical efficacy similar to that of other resins, with minimal gastrointestinal side effects, improving tolerability and patient compliance.[92]

Other modalities are still at an experimental stage. Squalene synthase is the enzyme that converts farnesyl pyrophosphate to squalene in the cholesterol biosynthesis pathway, and inhibitors of squalene synthase enzyme, namely TAK-475 and 1,1-bisphosphonates inhibit hepatic cholesterol biosynthesis. They have shown significant lowering of LDL-C and triglyceride in animal studies but does not cause an elevation of HDL-C.[93,94] Microsomal triglyceride transfer protein (MTP) inhibitors are agents, which block the hepatic secretion of very low density lipoproteins (VLDL) and the intestinal secretion of chylomicrons. Hence, they are powerful agents to cause reduction of postprandial lipemia, but suffer from the drawback of potential adverse effects due to blockage of intestinal fat absorption and hepatic lipid secretion.[95] Implitapide, a new MTP inhibitor, reduces plasma cholesterol and triglyceride levels by 70% and 45%, and VLDL secretion rate by liver by 80%.[96] Naringenin, the principal flavonoid in grapefruit, reduces plasma lipids *in vivo* as well as inhibits apoB secretion and cholesterol esterification. The possible mechanism of action is by inhibition of hepatic MTP activity.[97] The acyl-CoA cholesterol acyltransferase (ACAT) is an important enzyme in the cholesterol transport pathway. Inhibitors of this enzyme namely avasimibe, KY-455 and MCC-147 have shown significant reduction of serum esterified and free LDL-cholesterol levels. ACAT inhibitors increase reversible binding of apoA-I to the cells and enhance apoA-I-mediated release of cellular cholesterol and phospholipid, but did not influence nonspecific cellular cholesterol efflux to lipid microemulsion. It was therefore concluded that the ACAT inhibitor increased the release of cholesterol from the cholesterol-loaded macrophages by increasing the expression of ABCA1, putatively through shifting cholesterol distribution from the esterified to the free compartments.[98,99] SC-435, a competitive inhibitor of ileal apical sodium-dependent bile acid cotransporter (ASBT) inhibits ileal bile acid absorption and the hepatic nuclear receptor FXR (farnesoid X receptor), which regulates cholesterol 7 alpha-hydroxylase. To keep the biliary bile acid output intact liver increases bile acid production from hepatic cholesterol. This leads to lowering of plasma cholesterol. This agent has shown promise in animal studies.[100] Upregulation of low-density lipoprotein receptor (LDLr) is a key mechanism to control elevated plasma LDL-cholesterol levels. A new class of compounds has been detected that directly binds to the sterol regulatory element-binding protein (SREBP) cleavage-activating protein (SCAP). SCAP ligands reduced both LDL-cholesterol and triglyceride levels by up to 80%.[101] Gemcabene, a new lipid-altering agent has undergone an efficacy and tolerability study in a double-blind, randomized controlled trial and has shown its efficacy in reducing LDL-cholesterol but lacks the property of elevating HDL-C or reducing triglycerides.[102] Lifibrol is a new hypocholesterolemic compound which effectively lowers LDL-cholesterol. Lifibrol causes a competitive inhibition of HMG-CoA synthase, an important enzyme in the cholesterol synthesis pathway. It, however, does not have the property of inhibiting the HMG-CoA reductase. A potential advantage of lifibrol is that therapeutic concentrations do not interfere with the production of mevalonate which is required not only to synthesize sterols but also as a precursor of electron transport moieties, glycoproteins and farnesylated proteins.[103] Peroxisome proliferator activated receptor alpha (PPAR-α) plays a significant role in lipid metabolism in addition to its activity in the glucose metabolism. Activation of PPAR-β leads to an elevation of HDL-C and reduction of triglycerides. A novel compound PD-72953, is found to have PPAR-α stimulating property. Animal studies have shown that PD-72953 causes an elevation of HDL-C and reduction of triglycerides.[104]

Rational Choice of Drugs

- This is guided primarily by the type of dyslipidemia. Comorbid conditions also need to be considered
- For isolated moderate hypercholesterolemia due to elevated LDL-cholesterol the first choice is a statin. While there is really not much of a difference between the different statins, for coexistent mild to moderate hypertriglyceridemia atorvastatin scores over the other agents
- For individuals developing CNS side effects with simvastatin, atorvastatin or pravastatin maybe tried
- For severe hypercholesterolemia a statin maybe combined with ezetimibe
- For moderate hypertriglyceridemia with low HDL-cholesterol and normal LDL-cholesterol, treatment is best initiated with a fibrate
- For severe hypertriglyceridemia fish oils maybe added to fibrates
- For moderate mixed dyslipidemia a statin or a fibrate maybe tried first; it maybe necessary to combine the two, of course with greater safety monitoring
- In presence of renal failure, statins are safer than fibrates because of predominant biliary excretion.

CONCLUSION

Cardiovascular complications in type 2 diabetics is pretty common, which has been documented in various large prospective trials. This is not decreased by strict glycemic control alone. Dyslipidemia in the form of increased triglyceride and decreased HDL-cholesterol has been noted to be a common occurrence in type 2 diabetics. Increased LDL-cholesterol has been implicated as the etiological agent in the causation of atherosclerotic vascular disease. In diabetics, apart from the genetic dyslipidemic phenotype, qualitative change in LDL-cholesterol (LDL B phenotype and oxidized LDL) has also been implicated as the cause of increased incidence of cardiovascular complications. The decreased HDL-cholesterol concentration also contributes to the increased incidence of cardiovascular disease. Insulin resistance and/or hyperinsulinemia has been implicated as the etiological phenomenon behind the increased triglyceride and decreased HDL-cholesterol concentration. In type 1 diabetics, HDL-cholesterol does not decrease and lipid disorder is closely related to degree of hyperglycemia. All type 2 diabetics should undergo annual lipid check up for cholesterol, triglyceride and HDL-cholesterol. The treatment goals for diabetic with or without CHD is stricter compared to people without diabetes. The ADA recommendation for treatment of dyslipidemia in diabetics harps on LDL lowering. Statins are the most common drugs used, followed by fibrates.

REFERENCES

1. Kannel WB, McGee DL. Diabetes and glucose tolerance as risk factors for cardiovascular disease: the Framingham study. Diabetes Care. 1979;2:120-6.
2. Stamler J, Vaccaro O, Neaton JD, Wentworth D. Diabetes, other risk factors, and 12-yr cardiovascular mortality for men screened in the multiple risk factor intervention trial. Diabetes Care. 1993;16:434-44.
3. Pyörälä K, Laakso M, Uusitupa M. Diabetes and atherosclerosis: an epidemiologic view (Review). Diabetes Metab Rev. 1987;3:463-524.
4. Bierman EL. Atherogenesis in diabetes (Review). Arterioscler Thromb. 1992;12:647-56.
5. Caslake MJ, Packard CJ, Series JJ, et al. Plasma triglyceride and low density lipoprotein metabolism. Eur J Clin Invest. 1992;22:96-104.
6. De Graaf J, Hak-Lemmers HLM, Hectors MPC, et al. Enhanced susceptibility to *in vitro* oxidation of the dense low density lipoprotein subfraction in healthy subjects. Arterioscler Thromb 1991;11:298-306.
7. Law MR, Wald NJ, Wu T, Hackshaw A, Bailey A. Systematic underestimation of association between serum cholesterol concentration and ischaemic heart disease in observational studies: data from the BUPA study. BMJ. 1994;308:893-6.
8. Gordon DJ, Probstfield JL, Garrison RJ, et al. High density lipoprotein cholesterol and cardiovascular disease: four prospective American studies. Circulation. 1989;79:8-15.
9. Hokanson JE, Austin MA. Plasma triglyceride level is a risk factor for cardiovascular disease independent of high-density lipoprotein cholesterol level: a meta-analysis of population-based prospective studies. J Cardiovasc Risk. 1996;3:213-9.
10. Austin MA, Hokanson JE, Edwards KL. Hypertriglyceridemia as a cardiovascular risk factor. Am J Cardiol. 1998; 81(4A):7B-12B.
11. Haffner SM, Morales PA, Stern MP, Gruber MK. Lp(a) concentrations in NIDDM. Diabetes. 1992;41:1267-72.
12. Haffner SM. Management of dyslipidemia in adults with diabetes (Technical review). Diabetes Care. 1998; 21:160-78.
13. American Diabetes Association. Management of dyslipidemia in adults with diabetes (Position statement). Diabetes Care. 1998; 21:179-82.
14. Wilson PW, Kannel WB, Anderson KM. Lipids, glucose tolerance and vascular disease: the Framingham study. Monogr Atheroscler. 1985;13:1-11.
15. Harris MI. Hypercholesterolemia in diabetes and glucose intolerance in the U.S. population. Diabetes Care. 1991;14:366-74.
16. Steiner G. The dyslipoproteinemias of diabetes. Atherosclerosis. 1994;110(Suppl):S27-S33.
17. UKPDS Group. UK prospective diabetes study XXVII: plasma lipids and lipoproteins at diagnosis of NIDDM by age and sex. Diabetes Care. 1997;20:1683-7.
18. Haffner SM, Stern MP, Hazuda HP, Mitchell BD, Patterson JK. Cardiovascular risk factors in confirmed prediabetic individuals. Does the clock for coronary heart disease start ticking before the onset of clinical diabetes? JAMA. 1990;263:2893-8.
19. Uusitupa M, Sitonen O, Voutilainen E, et al. Serum lipids and lipoproteins in newly diagnosed non-insulin dependent (type II) diabetic patients, with special reference to factors influencing HDL-cholesterol and triglyceride levels. Diabetes Care. 1986;9:17-22.
20. UKPDS Group. UK prospective diabetes study XI: biochemical risk factors in type 2 diabetic patients at diagnosis compared with age-matched normal subjects. Diabet Med. 1994;11:534-44.
21. Assmann G, Schulte H. The prospective cardiovascular Munster (PROCAM) study: prevalence of hyperlipidemia in persons with hypertension and/or diabetes mellitus and the relationship to coronary heart disease. Am Heart J. 1988;116:1713-24.
22. Laakso M, Lehto S, Penttila I, Pyorala K. Lipids and lipoproteins predicting coronary heart disease mortality and morbidity in patients with non-insulin-dependent diabetes. Circulation. 1993; 88:1421-30.
23. Laakso M, Voutilainen E, Pyorala K, Sarlund H. Association of low HDL and HDL2 cholesterol with coronary heart disease in noninsulin-dependent diabetics. Arteriosclerosis 1985;5:653-8.
24. Falko JM, Parr JH, Simpson RN, Wynn V. Lipoprotein analyses in varying degrees of glucose tolerance. Comparison between non-insulin-dependent diabetes, impaired glucose tolerant, and control populations. Am J Med. 1987;83:641-7.
25. Rubies-Prat J, Reverter JL, Senti M, et al. Calculated low-density lipoprotein cholesterol should not be used for management of lipoprotein abnormalities in patients with diabetes mellitus. Diabetes Care. 1993;16:1081-6.
26. Stewart MW, Laker MF, Dyer RG, et al. Lipoprotein compositional abnormalities and insulin resistance in type 2 diabetic patients with mild hyperlipidemia. Arterioscler Thromb. 1993;13:1046-52.
27. Feingold KR, Grunfeld C, Pong M, Doerrler W, Krauss RM. LDL subclass phenotypes and triglyceride metabolism in non-insulin-dependent diabetes. Arterioscler Thromb. 1992;12:1496-502.
28. Selby JV, Austin MA, Newman B, et al. LDL subclass phenotypes and insulin resistance syndrome in women. Circulation. 1993;88:381-7.

29. Austin MA, Mykkänen L, Kuusisto J, et al. Prospective study of small LDLs as a risk factor for non-insulin dependent diabetes mellitus in elderly men and women. Circulation. 1995;92:1770-8.

30. Witztum JL, Fisher M, Metro T, Steinbrecher V, Glam RI. Nonenzymatic glycosylation of high density lipoprotein accelerates its catabolism in guinea pigs. Diabetes. 1982;31:1029-34.

31. Duell PB, Oram JF, Beirman EL. Nonenzymatic glycosylation of HDL and impaired HDL-receptor mediated cholesterol efflux. Diabetes. 1991;40:377-84.

32. Ramirez LC, Arauz-Pacheco C, Lackner C, et al. Lipoprotein(a) levels in diabetes mellitus: relationship to metabolic control. Ann Intern Med. 1992;117:42-7.

33. Haffner SM, Morales PA, Stern MP, Gruber MK. Lp(a) concentrations in NIDDM. Diabetes. 1992;41:1267.

34. Rainwater DL, MacCleur JW, Stern MP, Vandeberg JL, Haffner SM. Effects of noninsulin dependent diabetes mellitus in Lp(a) concentrations and apolipoprotein(a) size. Diabetes. 1994;43:942-6.

35. Haffner SM. Lipoprotein(a) and diabetes. Diabetes Care. 1993;16:835-40.

36. Cömlekci A, Biberoglu S, Kozan Ö, et al. Correlation between serum lipoprotein(a) and angiographic coronary artery disease in non-insulin-dependent diabetes mellitus. J Intern Med. 1997;242:449-54.

37. Mohan V, Deepa R, Haranath SR, et al. Lipoprotein(a) is an independent risk factor for coronary artery disease in NIDDM patients in South India. Diabetes Care. 1998;21:1819-23.

38. Lyons TJ. Glycation and oxidation: a role in the pathogenesis of atherosclerosis. Am J Cardiol. 1993;71:26B-31B.

39. Berliner JA, Territo M, Navab M, et al. Minimally modified lipoproteins in diabetes. Diabetes. 1992;41(suppl 2):74-6.

40. Durrington PN, Newton RS, Weinstein DB, Steinberg D. Effects of insulin and glucose on very low density lipoprotein triglyceride secretion by cultured rat hepatocytes. J Clin Invest. 1982;70:63-73.

41. Wiggins D, Gibbons GF. The lipolysis/esterification cycle of hepatic triacylglycerol. Its role in the secretion of very low density lipoprotein and its response to hormones and sulphonylureas. Biochem J. 1992;284:457-62.

42. Pietri AO, Dunn FL, Grundy SM, Raskin P. The effect of continuous subcutaneous insulin infusion on very low-density triglyceride lipoprotein metabolism in type I diabetes mellitus. Diabetes. 1983;32:75-81.

43. Nikkila EA. Regulation of hepatic production of plasma triglycerides by glucose and insulin. In Lundquist F, Tygstrup N (Eds): Regulation of Hepatic Metabolism. Copenhagen: Munksgaard; 1974. pp 360-78.

44. Klein BE, Moss SE, Klein R, Surawicz TZ. Serum cholesterol in Wisconsin epidemiologic study of diabetic retinopathy. Diabetes Care. 1992;15:282-7.

45. The DCCT Research Group. Lipid and lipoprotein levels in patients with IDDM: diabetes control and complication trial experience. Diabetes Care. 1992;15:886-94.

46. Sosenko JM, Breslow JL, Miettinen OS, Gabbay KH. Hyperglycemia and plasma lipid levels: a prospective study of young insulin dependent diabetic patients. N Engl J Med. 1980;302:650-4.

47. Strobl W, Widhalm K, Schober E, Frisch H, Poliak A, Westphal G. Apolipoproteins and lipoproteins in children with type 1 diabetes: relation to glycosylated serum protein and HbA1. Acta Paediatr Scand. 1985;74:966-71.

48. Rivellese A, Riccardi G, Romano G, Giacco R, et al. Presence of very-low-density lipoprotein compositional abnormalities in type 1 (insulin-dependent) diabetic patients: effects of blood glucose optimisation. Diabetologia. 1988;31:884-8.

49. Bagdade JD, Subbaiah PV. Whole-plasma and high density lipoprotein subfraction surface lipid composition in IDDM men. Diabetes. 1989;38:1226-30.

50. Jensen T, Stender S, Deckert T. Abnormalities in plasma concentrations of lipoproteins and fibrinogen in type 1 (insulin dependent) diabetic patients with increased albumin excretion. Diabetologia. 1988;31:142-5.

51. McKeigue PM, Shah B, Marmot MG. Relation of central obesity and insulin resistance with high diabetes prevalence and cardiovascular risk in South Asians. Lancet. 1991;337:382-6.

52. Davis TME, Cull CA, Holman RR. Relationship between ethnicity and glycemic control, lipid profiles and blood pressure during the first 9 years of type 2 diabetes. UK prospective diabetes study (UKPDS 55). Diabetes Care. 2001;24:1167-74.

53. Stevens RJ, Kothari V, Adler AI, Stratton IM, Holman RR (UKPDS Group). The UKPDS risk engine: a model for the risk of coronary heart disease in type II diabetes (UKPDS 56). Clin Sci. 2001;101:671-9.

54. Heart Protection Study Collaborative Group. MRC/BHF heart protection study of cholesterol-lowering with simvastatin in 5,963 people with diabetes: a randomised placebo controlled trial. Lancet. 2003;361:2005-16.

55. NCEP Expert Panel on Detection, Evaluation and Treatment of High Blood Cholesterol in Adults. Executive summary of the third report of the national cholesterol education program (NCEP) expert panel on detection, evaluation and treatment of high blood cholesterol in adults (Adult treatment panel III). JAMA. 2001;285:2486-97.

56. American Diabetes Association. Dyslipidemia management in adults with diabetes (Position statement). Diabetes Care. 2004;27 (suppl 1):S68-S71.

57. Grundy SM, Cleeman J, Merz NB, et al for the Coordinating Committee of the National Cholesterol Education Program. implications of recent clinical trials for the National Cholesterol Education Program adult treatment panel III guidelines. Circulation. 2004;110:227-39.

58. Grundy SM, Balady GJ, Criqui MH, et al. When to start cholesterol-lowering therapy in patients with coronary heart disease: a statement for healthcare professional from the American Heart Association task force on risk reduction. Circulation. 1997;95:1683-5.

59. Garg A, Bonanome A, Grundy SM, Zhang Z-J, Unger RH. Comparison of a high-carbohydrate diet with a high monounsaturated-fat diet in patients with noninsulin dependent diabetes mellitus. N Engl J Med. 1988;319:829-34.

60. Frost G, Leeds AA, Dore CJ, Madeiros S, Brading S, Dornhorst A. Glycemic index as a determinant of serum HDL-cholesterol concentration. Lancet. 1999;353:1045-8.

61. Zock PL, Katan MB. Hydrogenation alternatives: effects of trans-fatty acids and stearic acid versus linoleic acid on serum lipids and lipoproteins in humans. J Lipid Res. 1992;33:399-410.

62. Schectman G, Kaul S, Kissebach AH. Effect of fish oil concentrate on lipoprotein composition in NIDDM. Diabetes. 1988;37:1567-73.

63. Friedberg CE, Janssen MJ, Heine RJ, Grobbee DE. Fish oil and glycemic control in diabetes: a meta-analysis. Diabetes Care. 1998;21:494-500.

64. Vanninen E, Uusitupa M, Siitonen O, Laitinen J, Lansimies E. Habitual physical activity, aerobic capacity and metabolic control in patients with newly diagnosed type 2 (noninsulin dependent) diabetes mellitus: effect of 1-year diet and exercise intervention. Diabetologia. 1992;35:340-6.

65. Kaesemeyer WH, Caldwell RB, Huang J, Caldwell RW. Pravastatin sodium activates endothelial nitric oxide synthase independent of its cholesterol-lowering actions. J Am Coll Cardiol. 1999;33:234-41.

66. Llorente-Cortes V, Martinez-Gonzalez J, Badimon L. Esterified cholesterol accumulation induced by aggregated LDL uptake in human vascular smooth muscle cells is reduced by HMG-CoA reductase inhibitors. Arterioscler Thromb Vasc Biol. 1998;18:738-46.

67. The Scandinavian Simvastatin Survival Study Group. Randomised trial of cholesterol lowering in 4,444 patients with coronary heart disease: the Scandinavian simvastatin survival study (4S). Lancet. 1994;344:1383-9.

68. Shepherd J, Cobbe SM, Ford I, et al. Prevention of coronary heart disease with pravastatin in men with hypercholesterolaemia. N Engl J Med. 1995;333:1301-7.

69. Pyorala K, Pedersen TR, Kjekshus J, et al. Cholesterol lowering with simvastatin improves prognosis of diabetic patients with coronary heart disease: a subgroup analysis of the Scandinavian Simvastatin Survival Study (4S). Diabetes Care. 1997;20:614-20.

70. Sacks FM, Pfeffer MA, Moye LA, et al. The effect of pravastatin on coronary events after myocardial infarction in patients with average cholesterol levels: cholesterol and recurrent Event Trial Investigators. N Engl J Med 1996;335:1001-9.

71. Colhoun HM, Betteridge DJ, Durrington PN, et al for CARDS investigators. Primary prevention of cardiovascular disease with atorvastatin in type 2 diabetes in the Collaborative Atorvastatin Diabetes Study (CARDS): multicentre randomised placebo-controlled trial. Lancet. 2004;364:685-96.

72. de Graaf J, Hendriks JC, Demacker PN, Stalenhoef AN. Identification of multiple dense LDL sub-fractions with enhanced susceptibility to in vitro oxidation among hyper-triglyceridaemic subjects: normalization after clofibrate treatment. Arterioscler Thromb. 1993;13:712-9.

73. Ericsson CG, Hamsten A, Nilsson J, et al. Angiographic assessment of effects of bezafibrate on progression of coronary artery disease in young male post infarction patients. Lancet. 1996;347:849-53.

74. Steiner G. The diabetes atherosclerosis intervention study (DAIS): a study conducted in cooperation with the World Health Organization. The DAIS Project Group. Diabetologia. 1996;39: 1655-61.

75. Goldbourt U, Behar S, Reicher-Reiss H, et al. Rationale and design of a secondary prevention trial of increasing serum high-density lipoprotein cholesterol and reducing triglycerides in patients with clinically manifest atherosclerotic disease (the bezafibrate infarction prevention trial). Am J Cardiol. 1993;71: 909-15.

76. Tikkanen MJ, Laakso M, Ilmonen M, et al. Treatment of hypercholesterolemia and combined hyperlipidemia with simvastatin and gemfibrozil with NIDDM. A multicenter study. Diabetes Care. 1998;21:477-81.

77. Manninen V, Tenkanen L, Koskinen P, et al. Joint effects of serum triglyceride and LDL cholesterol and HDL cholesterol concentrations on coronary heart disease risk in the Helsinki Heart Study: implications for treatment. Circulation. 1992;85:37-45.

78. Koskinen P, Mänttäri M, Manninen V, et al. Coronary heart disease incidence in NIDDM patients in the Helsinki heart study. Diabetes Care. 1992;820-5.

79. Elkeles RS, Diamond JR, Poulter C, et al. Cardiovascular outcomes in type 2 diabetes. A double-blind placebo-controlled study of bezafibrate: the St. Mary's, Ealing, Northwick Park Diabetes Cardiovascular Disease Prevention (SENDCAP) Study. Diabetes Care. 1998;21:641-8.

80. Seedorf U, Engel T, Lueken A, Bode G, Lorkowski S, Assmann G. Cholesterol absorption inhibitor Ezetimibe blocks uptake of oxidized LDL in human macrophages. Biochem Biophys Res Commun. 2004;320:1337-41.

81. Dujovne CA, Ettinger MP, McNeer JF, et al for Ezetimibe Study Group. Efficacy and safety of a potent new selective cholesterol absorption inhibitor, ezetimibe, in patients with primary hypercholesterolemia. Am J Cardiol. 2002;90:1092-7.

82. Melani L, Mills R, Hassman D, et al for Ezetimibe Study Group. Efficacy and safety of ezetimibe coadministered with pravastatin in patients with primary hypercholesterolemia: a prospective, randomized, double-blind trial. Eur Heart J. 2003;24:717-28.

83. Elam MB, Hunninghake DB, Davis KB, et al. Effect of niacin on lipid and lipoprotein levels and glycemic control in patients with diabetes and peripheral arterial disease: the ADMIT study: a randomized trial. Arterial Disease Multiple Intervention Trial. JAMA. 2000;284:1263-70.

84. Brousseau ME, Schaefer EJ, Wolfe ML, et al. Effects of an inhibitor of cholesteryl ester transfer protein on HDL cholesterol. N Engl J Med. 2004;350:1505-15.

85. Miettinen TA, Gylling H. Plant stanol and sterol esters in prevention of cardiovascular diseases. Ann Med. 2004;36:126-34.

86. Tammi A, Ronnemaa T, Miettinen TA, et al. Effects of gender, apolipoprotein E phenotype and cholesterol-lowering by plant stanol esters in children: the STRIP study. Special Turku Coronary Risk Factor Intervention Project. Acta Paediatr. 2002; 91:1155-62.

87. Hollander PA, Elbein SC, Hirsch IB, et al. Role of orlistat in the treatment of obese patients with type 2 diabetes. A 1-year randomized double-blind study. Diabetes Care 1998; 21: 1288-94.

88. Thompson RG, Pearson L, Schoenfeld Sl, Kolterman OG. Pramlintide, a synthetic analogue of human amylin, improves the metabolic profile of patients with type 2 diabetes using insulin. The Pramlintide in type 2 diabetes group. Diabetes Care. 1998; 21:987-93.

89. Fulcher GR, Catalano C, Walker M, et al. A double blind study of the effect of acipimox on serum lipids, blood glucose control and insulin action in non-obese patients with type 2 diabetes mellitus. Diabet Med 1992; 9:908-14.

90. Yamamoto A. New statins under clinical development: nisvastatin and rosuvastatin. Nippon Rinsho 2001;59(Suppl 3): 605-8.

91. Bolego C, Poli A, Cignarella A, Catapano AL, Paoletti R. Novel statins: pharmacological and clinical results. Cardiovasc Drugs Ther. 2002;16:251-7.

92. Bays H, Dujovne C. Colesevelam HCl: a non-systemic lipid-altering drug. Expert Opin Pharmacother. 2003;4:779-90.

93. Nishimoto T, Amano Y, Tozawa R, et al. Lipid-lowering properties of TAK-475, a squalene synthase inhibitor, *in vivo* and *in vitro*. Br J Pharmacol. 2003;139:911-8.

94. Ciosek CP Jr, Magnin DR, Harrity TW, et al. Lipophilic 1,1-bisphosphonates are potent squalene synthase inhibitors and orally active cholesterol lowering agents *in vivo*. Biol Chem. 1993; 268:24832-7.

95. Chang G, Ruggeri RB, Harwood HJ Jr. Microsomal triglyceride transfer protein (MTP) inhibitors: discovery of clinically active inhibitors using high-throughput screening and parallel synthesis paradigms. Curr Opin Drug Discov Devel. 2002;5:562-70.

96. Shiomi M, Ito T. MTP inhibitor decreases plasma cholesterol levels in LDL receptor-deficient WHHL rabbits by lowering the VLDL secretion. Eur J Pharmacol. 2001;431:127-31.

97. Borradaile NM, de Dreu LE, Barrett PH, Behrsin CD, Huff MW. Hepatocyte apoB-containing lipoprotein secretion is decreased by the grapefruit flavonoid, naringenin, via inhibition of MTP-mediated microsomal triglyceride accumulation. Biochemistry. 2003;42:1283-91.

98. Sugimoto K, Tsujita M, Wu CA, Suzuki K, Yokoyama S. An inhibitor of acylCoA: cholesterol acyltransferase increases expression of ATP-binding cassette transporter A1 and thereby enhances the ApoA-I-mediated release of cholesterol from macrophages. Biochim Biophys. Acta 2004;1636:69-76.

99. Raal FJ, Marais AD, Klepack E, Lovalvo J, McLain R, Heinonen T. Avasimibe, an ACAT inhibitor, enhances the lipid lowering effect of atorvastatin in subjects with homozygous familial hypercholesterolemia. Atherosclerosis. 2003;171(2):273-9.

100. Li H, Xu G, Shang Q, Pan L, et al. Inhibition of ileal bile acid transport lowers plasma cholesterol levels by inactivating hepatic farnesoid X receptor and stimulating cholesterol 7 alpha-hydroxylase. Metabolism. 2004;53:927-32.

101. Grand-Perret T, Bouillot A, Perrot A, Commans S, Walker M, Issandou M. SCAP ligands are potent new lipid-lowering drugs. Nat Med. 2001;7: 1332-8.

102. Bays HE, McKenney JM, Dujovne CA, et al. Effectiveness and tolerability of a new lipid-altering agent, gemcabene, in patients with low levels of high-density lipoprotein cholesterol. Am J Cardiol. 2003;92:538-43.

103. Scharnagl H, Schliack M, Loser R, et al. The effects of lifibrol (K12.148) on the cholesterol metabolism of cultured cells: evidence for sterol independent stimulation of the LDL receptor pathway. Atherosclerosis. 2000;153:69-80.

104. Bisgaier CL, Essenburg AD, Barnett BC, et al. A novel compound that elevates high density lipoprotein and activates the peroxisome proliferator activated receptor. J Lipid Res. 1998;39:17-30.

Section 10

COMPLICATIONS

Chapter 52

DIABETES COMPLICATIONS: OVERVIEW

SV Madhu

CHAPTER OUTLINE

- Introduction
- Diabetes Exposure and Risk of Complications
- Importance of Glycemic Control in Development of Chronic Complications
- Mechanisms of Diabetic Tissue Damage

- Cellular and Molecular Mechanisms of Hyperglycemia-induced Cellular Damage
- Role of Oxidative Stress in Development of Diabetic Complications
- Unifying Hypothesis for Diabetic Complications
- Summary

INTRODUCTION

The disease burden of diabetes mellitus is primarily due to the burden of its many complications. Diabetes exposure, which results from the level as well as duration of hyperglycemia, represents a metabolic state that favors the development of several long-term complications of the eye, kidney and heart. The question of whether control of glycemia leads to reduction in the risk of complications had been a matter of debate till recently. By now several carefully conducted, prospective, randomized clinical studies like diabetes control and complications trial (DCCT),[1] United Kingdom prospective diabetes study (UKPDS)[2] and the Kumamoto study[3] have clearly laid this debate to rest once and for all. Strict control of glycemia has now been shown in these studies to prevent complications considerably in both type 1 and type 2 diabetes. Also, there has been substantial progress in the past 2 to 3 decades in our understanding of the pathways that lead to the development of chronic complications in diabetes mellitus. Oxidative stress, protein kinase C (PKC) and advanced glycation end-products (AGEs) pathways

among others have been elucidated in great detail. This has not only contributed to our understanding of pathogenesis of diabetic complications but has also opened up novel areas of therapeutic potential which may help delay their development.

A wide spectrum of complications may develop in case of diabetes. These include the acute metabolic complications, the late complications and others as shown in **Table 52.1**. The late complications maybe microvascular, macrovascular or neuropathic.

DIABETES EXPOSURE AND RISK OF COMPLICATIONS

Retinopathy, particularly nonproliferative retinopathy is typically seen in patients with type 1 DM but is very rare in those without diabetes suggesting that it is diabetes exposure that drives its development.[4]

While the relationship between hyperglycemia and various stages of diabetic retinopathy was suggested by several earlier studies, it was in the DCCT that, for the first time, the dose-response relationship was established between hyperglycemia and the development

TABLE 52.1	Complications of diabetes mellitus

1. Acute metabolic complications
   a. Diabetic ketoacidosis (DKA)
   b. Hyperosmolar hyperglycemic nonketotic state (HHNS)
   c. Lactic acidosis

2. Chronic complications
   a. Microvascular
      i. Retinopathy
      ii. Nephropathy
      iii. Neuropathy
   b. Macrovascular
      i. Hypertension
      ii. Coronary heart disease (CHD)
      iii. Cerebrovascular disease (CVD)
      iv. Peripheral vascular disease (PVD)

3. Others
   a. Cardiac
      i. Diabetic cardiomyopathy
   b. Infection
      i. Bacterial
      ii. Fungal
      iii. Mycobacterial
   c. Ocular
      i. Infections
      ii. Cataract
      iii. Glaucoma
   d. Dermatological
      i. Necrobiosis lipoidica diabeticorum
      ii. Granuloma annulare
      iii. Diabetic bullae
      iv. Diabetic scleroderma
   e. Connective tissue
      i. Osteopenia, osteoarthritis
      ii. Scleroderma diabetic corum
      iii. Carpal tunnel syndrome
      iv. Dupuytren's disease
      v. Flexor tenosynovitis
      vi. Adhesive capsulitis of shoulder
      vii. Limited joint mobility (LJM)
   f. Oral
      i. Periodontal disease
      ii. Caries, xerostomia and candidiasis

and progression of diabetic retinopathy. A nonlinear threshold value of 8.5% HbA_{1c} above which there is a steep rise in incidence of retinopathy has been demonstrated, that imputes its implications for pathogenesis as well as care of diabetes.[1] Several other allied factors, such as hypertension, neuropathy, cardiac autonomic neuropathy, dyslipidemia and local ocular factors also increase the risk of retinopathy in the diabetic patient.[4]

The natural history of diabetic kidney disease, wherever it occurred is a relentless progression from normoalbuminuria to microalbuminuria and overt proteinuria and from there to end-stage renal diseases (ESRD).[5] Many studies have demonstrated that the level of diabetes exposure is the strongest risk factor for progression from normoalbuminuria to microalbuminuria,[6,7] the threshold value for HbA_{1c} being 8.1%.[8] However, the effect of hyperglycemia on the progression of microalbuminuria to overt proteinuria and then to ESRD is not so clear. A number of factors other than hyperglycemia have been shown to increase the risk of diabetic kidney disease—predisposition to hypertension, elevated blood pressure, cigarette smoking, high serum LDL-cholesterol levels and genetic predisposition to diabetic kidney disease may promote development of overt proteinuria.[4] While all the risk factors mentioned above have been clearly demonstrated in type 1 diabetes, data in patients with type 2 diabetes are less well documented. Available data suggest a similar relationship by and large. Studies in Asians, where type 1 DM is rare and type 2 DM occurs at a younger age, have shown that there is a higher risk of diabetic nephropathy. This maybe due to poorer glycemic control or due to a higher genetic or other environmental susceptibility among Asians.[8]

Diabetes is frequently associated with the development of premature atherosclerotic vascular disease.[9] This increased risk has been attributed to the high prevalence of multiple atherosclerotic risk factors among diabetic patients.[9,10] However, studies have also shown that the excess of coronary artery disease (CAD) in type 2 diabetics cannot be accounted for by the levels of four major risk factors identified for CAD, viz. hypertension, smoking, serum cholesterol and age; suggesting a role for other factors.[9,10] Diabetes specific exposure including hyperglycemia, diabetic dyslipidemia, treatment with insulin and diabetic nephropathy are all believed to contribute to this increase in risk[4] but still cannot explain the entire risk. Thus, there has been a search for nonconventional increase in risk factors like Lp(a), homocysteine and postprandial lipemia.

Lipid abnormalities in the postprandial state particularly hypertriglyceridemia may contribute significantly to the high macrovascular risk of diabetes. Postprandial hypertriglyceridemia has been shown to be present in type 2 diabetes in various studies[11] including those from our institution[12] **(Figure 52.1)** which appears to result from an interaction between the diabetic state and obesity. Postprandial hypertriglyceridemia has also been shown to be associated with carotid intimal medial thickness[13] and also with postprandial oxidative stress and endothelial dysfunction.[14]

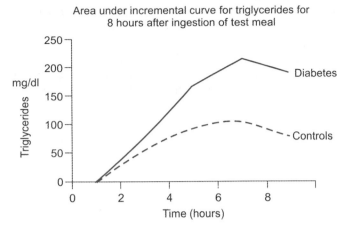

Figure 52.1 Postprandial lipid abnormalities in type 2 diabetes mellitus

All these recent observations suggest that postprandial lipemia particularly postprandial hypertriglyceridemia plays an important role in diabetes related atherosclerotic vascular disease and it would appear that the long recognized atherogenic potential of triglycerides especially in diabetes is attributable primarily to its altered metabolism in the postprandial state.

The risk of CAD in diabetes is seen much before the diagnoses of diabetes well into the prediabetes categories particularly impaired glucose tolerance (IGT). There is a wide variation in the prevalence of CAD among different diabetic populations. This has been attributed to the fact that prediabetic (insulin resistance and hyperinsulinemia) and diabetic exposure may affect the progression but not the frequency of atherosclerotic lesions so that populations with infrequent initial atherosclerosis like Pima Indians, Tokyo-Japanese, and Hong Kong-Chinese, may remain unaffected by diabetes exposure.[4]

IMPORTANCE OF GLYCEMIC CONTROL IN DEVELOPMENT OF CHRONIC COMPLICATIONS

Several clinical, observational and retrospective studies in the 1950s, 1960s and 1970s suggested a positive relationship between hyperglycemia and development of the late complications of diabetes. However, all these studies had limitations and remained inconclusive. Early observational studies in the late seventies, eighties and nineties that contributed significantly in supporting a relationship between glycemia and diabetic complica-

tions included the Brussels study[15] and the Wisconsin study.[16] In the former, Pirart[15] observed over 4000 patients in Brussels for up to 25 years and concluded that a longer duration of diabetes and cumulative glycemic control correlated significantly with the frequency and severity of diabetic complications, such as retinopathy, nephropathy and neuropathy. However, this study had some limitations and it was still not clear whether strict control of glycemia could reduce complications. The Wisconsin epidemiological study of diabetic retinopathy (WESDR) was a carefully conducted prospective epidemiological study in a large population cohort of diabetic subjects who were followed up for 10 years.[16]

WESDR data clearly demonstrated a strong and consistent relationship between glycemia (baseline glycated hemoglobin) and incidence and progression of microvascular (diabetic retinopathy, vision loss, nephropathy) and macrovascular (lower extremity amputation and cardiovascular disease mortality) complications in patients with either type of DM.

Several prospective intervention trials were conducted in the seventies and eighties particularly in type 1 DM. The Steno, Oslo and Kroc studies used continuous subcutaneous insulin infusion (CSII) and the Stockholm diabetes intervention study (SDIS) used multiple dose insulin injections (MDI), and the Dallas diabetes prospective trials (DDPT) were the most important of these. All the studies reported in varying degree a positive impact of glycemic control on development of various diabetic complications. However, all these studies were small and of short duration, and in none of them did the intervention start early enough in the course of diabetes to have major impact.[4]

Diabetes Control and Complications Trial[1]

Diabetes control and complications trial (DCCT) was the landmark study that for the first time unequivocally demonstrated that strict control of glycemia reduces the risk of several long-term complications in type 1 diabetes. This was a huge randomized, multicentric controlled clinical trial conducted in 1,441 subjects across 29 centers in USA. A 726 of these ("Primary prevention" cohort) had no incidence of diabetic complications and had duration of diabetes of less than 5 years. The remaining 715 ("secondary prevention" cohort) had mild-to-moderate background diabetic retinopathy and either macro- or microalbuminuria with disease duration of under 15 years. Subjects were randomly assigned to either intensive therapy (CSII/MDI) aimed at near normal glycemia or conventional therapy and followed up for a

TABLE 52.2	DCCT: Impact of intensive therapy on reduction of long-term complications

End-point risk reduction
- First appearance of retinopathy — 27%
- Progress of retinopathy — 60%
- New nephropathy — 34%
- Progress of nephropathy — 43%
- New neuropathy — 69%
- Progress of neuropathy — 57%
- Macrovascular disease — 44%

TABLE 52.3	UKPDS: Summary of results

End-point risk reduction of complications
- Any diabetes related end-point — 12%
- Microvascular end-points — 25%
- Myocardial infarction — 16%
- Cataract extraction — 24%
- Retinopathy at twelve years — 21%
- Albuminuria at twelve years — 33%

mean duration of 6.5 years. The intensively treated group achieved a median GHb throughout the study of 7.2% vs 9.1% in the conventional group and mean blood glucose of 155 mg/dl, vs 231 mg/dl. The results of the study are given in **Tables 52.2 and 52.3.** The most important adverse events in the intensive therapy group was a 3 times higher incidence of severe hypoglycemia, and an increased weight gain. The relationship of glycemic exposure and the risk for progression of diabetic complications was a curvilinear one with a steep relationship at higher levels of HbA$_{1c}$ **(Figure 52.2)**. This continuous relationship would suggest that any improvement in glycemic control is beneficial. Thus, DCCT showed unequivocally that intensive therapy that achieves near normoglycemia is associated with a significant delay in the onset and progression of diabetic retinopathy, nephropathy and neuropathy in type 1 DM.

The EDIC study,[17] a follow-up of to DCCT showed that the intensively treated group continued to have a lower incidence of complications after 4 years, despite comparable post-DCCT glycemic states with the control groups an exposition of glycemic memory and long-term effect normoglycemia.

Studies in Type 2 DM

The Kumamoto study[3] in Japan was a small study of 110 patients with type 2 DM who were followed up for 6 years following either intensive insulin therapy (MDI) or conventional insulin therapy.

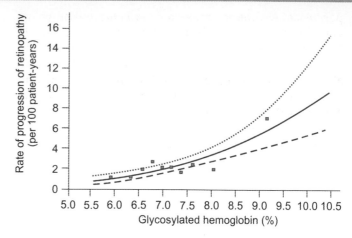

Figure 52.2 DCCT: Relationship of glycosylated hemoglobin and diabetes complications

Over 6 years, glycemic control in the 2 groups were similar to DCT (HbA$_{1c}$ 7.1 vs 9.4% and mean blood glucose 157 mg/dl vs 221 mg/dl). Progression of retinopathy was reduced by 69% and nephropathy by 70%. Risk of macrovascular complications were reduced by 54%.

The United Kingdom prospective diabetes study (UKPDS)[2] was another landmark study similar to DCCT but involving type 2 DM patients. This was a prospective study of over 5000 diabetic patients followed in 23 centers in UK for 20 years. In the main study, 3,867 newly diagnosed diabetic patients were randomly assigned to either intensive therapy (sulfonylureas or insulin) or conventional therapy (diet initially and later oral drugs or insulin). HbA$_{1c}$ decreased from 7.9 to 7.0% in the intensive treatment group with a 25% risk reduction in microvascular complications. UKPDS also showed clearly that in diabetes with hypertension additional tight control of blood pressure (mean BP over 9 years 144/82 vs 154/87 mm/dl) was associated with a reduction in microvascular end-points by 37%.

MECHANISMS OF DIABETIC TISSUE DAMAGE[4,18-20]

The major cause of tissue damage in diabetes is vascular disease affecting the micro- and macrocirculation. There is progressive narrowing and occlusion of lumen of the vessels that results in decreased perfusion, ischemia and tissue damage. There is increased permeability to plasma proteins that may get deposited in the vessel wall. Also, there occurs expansion of the extracellular matrix around perivascular cells such as the pericytes in the retina and the mesangial cells in the glomeruli leading to thickening of the basement membrane. In large vessels, there is increased deposition of collagen and lipids in atherosclerotic plaques. Endothelial mesangial and arterial smooth muscle hyperplasia and hypertrophy also result in vascular wall thickening. All these processes coupled with an increased coagulability in the vessel leads to vascular occlusion and diabetes tissue damage. Damage of diabetic tissues occurs in those tissues, which fail to downregulate their glucose uptake in the face of hyperglycemia with the resultant intracellular hyperglycemia.

CELLULAR AND MOLECULAR MECHANISMS OF HYPERGLYCEMIA-INDUCED CELLULAR DAMAGE

There are four major pathways that are thought to be activated in the causation of diabetic complications:[4]
1. Activation of polyol or (aldose reductase) pathway.
2. Increased formation of intracellular advanced glycation end-products (AGEs).
3. Activation of protein kinase C (PKC) isoforms.
4. Over activity of the hexosamine pathway.

Increased Activation of the Polyol Pathway[18-23]

Polyol pathway is inactive in the nondiabetic state **(Figure 52.3)**; most of the glucose being metabolized through the glycolytic pathway. In diabetes mellitus, hyperglycemia and the resultant increase in intracellular glucose and other glucose-derived substrates for aldose reductase like methylglyoxal lead to activation of the polyol pathway and increased glucose flux through this pathway **(Figure 52.4)**.

Aldose reductase is located in nerves, retina, lens, glomeruli and walls. Also in these tissues, glucose uptake is insulin independent, and hence, there is rise in intracellular glucose in direct proportion to blood glucose levels of blood levels. Thus, it is these tissues that are the primary targets of diabetic tissue damage

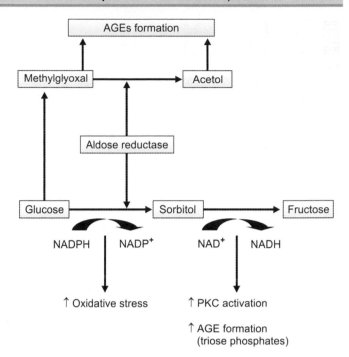

AGE: Advanced glycation end-products; PKC: Protein kinase C; NADPH: Nicotinamide adenine dinucleotide phosphate; NAD: Nicotinamide adenine dinucleotide

Figure 52.4 Polyol pathway in diabetes mellitus

resulting in neuropathy, retinopathy, cataract, nephropathy and vasculopathy.

Activation of the polyol pathway causes tissue damage by several mechanisms—osmotic damage secondary to sorbitol accumulation, increased oxidative stress secondary to decreased NADPH levels, PKC activation from increased NADH/NAD+ ratio, and increased AGE formation secondary to methylglyoxal and acetol and to raised NADH/NAD+ ratio.

Formation of Advanced Glycation End-products[4,18-20,24,25]

Glucose and the other glycating compounds such as decarbonyl-3 deoxy glucosone, methylglyoxal and glyoxal react with proteins and nucleic acids to form glycation products. These reactions are reversible to start with but later on they become less reversible to yield early glycation products and finally with the development of glucose-derived cross-links between protein molecules these become completely irreversible and lead to the formation of AGEs. The advanced glycation alters the structural and functional characteristics of these proteins and renders them nonfunctional in most cases. Hyperglycemia in diabetes mellitus induces

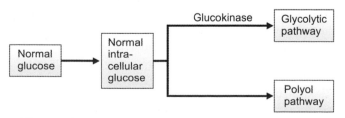

Figure 52.3 The polyol pathway in nondiabetic states

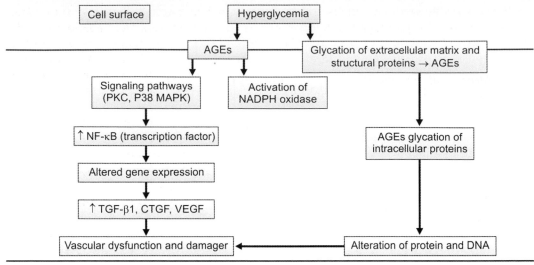

AGEs: Advanced glycation end-products
PKC: Protein kinase C
TGF-β1: Transforming growth factor beta 1
CTGF: Connective tissue growth factor
VEGF: Vascular endothelium-derived growth factor
NF-κB: Nuclear factor kappa B
P38 MAPK: P38 mitogen activated protein kinase

Figure 52.5 AGE and vascular complications

irreversible glycation of both intracellular and extra-cellular proteins. It is believed that increased intracellular glucose is the primary factor that drives both intracellular and extracellular AGE formation. The high intracellular glucose leads to increased formation of intracellular glucose derived decarbonyl precursors which readily react with the amino groups of intra- and extracellular proteins. These decarbonyl precursors of methylglyoxal and glyoxal generate AGEs at a much faster rate than glucose itself and are detoxified by the glyoxalase system.

Several animal and human studies support an important role for AGEs in the pathogenesis of diabetes complications **(Figure 52.5)**. AGE accumulation has been demonstrated in glomerular tissues of rats as well as humans[4,20,26] and retinal tissues[27,28] of diabetic animals. AGE infusion in animals resulted in pathological changes similar to those induced by hyperglycemia.[29]

We studied the serum AGE levels in controls and type 2 diabetic patients with and without microvascular complications.[30] Serum AGEs were significantly raised in type 2 DM as compared to controls. There was a progressive and significant increase in the levels of AGEs from healthy controls to diabetic patients without microvascular complications to those with microvascular complications. The study reinforces the importance of

AGEs in the development of microvascular complications in diabetes.

Aminoguanidine, an inhibitor of AGE, has been shown to prevent the pathological changes of experimental diabetic retinopathy[31] and nephropathy.[32] AGE-induced tissue damage results from both extracellular and intracellular effects.

Extracellular Effects of AGEs

The AGEs modify extracellular structure proteins including type 1 and type 2 collagen and laminin[33,34] by forming intermolecular covalent cross-linking bonds. These changes alter the function of various tissues particularly blood vessels and the glomerular basement membrane with a reduction in vascular wall elasticity and increased glomerular permeability to albumin.[26] Adhesion, proliferation and migration of endothelial cells are also impaired by AGEs. Binding of AGE to its receptors on endothelial cells (RAGE) affects expression of several genes thrombomodulin, tissue factor and VCAM-1 resulting in increased coagulability.[35-39] Vascular permeability is also increased. RAGE has also been shown to mediate generation of reactive oxygen species (ROS) and cause NF-κB activation, a pathway that has been well elucidated to lead to oxidative stress induced tissue damage.

AGE can also bind to specific receptors on monocytes and macrophages resulting in increased production of cytokines like interleukin-1, tumor necrosis factors-α (TNF-α), transforming growth factor-β (TGF-β), macrophage colony-stimulating factor (MCSF) and granulocyte colony stimulating factor (GCSF) which are known to mediate tissue damage and inflammation.[35-37]

Intracellular Effects of AGEs[40]

Glycation of intracellular proteins causes altered function leading to altered intracellular signaling and cell dysfunction. Altered extracellular matrix, secondary to advanced glycation results in abnormal binding with matrix receptors on cell surfaces and this leads to cellular dysfunction. Also, binding of glycated plasma proteins on macrophage receptors leads to increased ROS production and activation of the transcription factor NF-κB causing pathological gene expression of many genes that bring about tissue damage.

Increased Activation of Protein Kinase C[18-20,41-47]

Excessive and persistent activation of the diacylglycerol-protein kinase C (DAG-PKC) is also

believed to mediate hyperglycemia induced diabetic tissue damage. PKC activation can result from several mechanisms **(Figure 52.6)**. Hyperglycemia mainly activates PKC-β and PKC-δ isoforms as shown from animal studies in retina, glomeruli and vascular tissues.

PKC activation particularly the β isoform, has been shown in experimental studies to cause abnormalities of retinal blood flow, increased permeability of vessels, pathological angiogenesis especially in the retina through vascular endothelium-derived growth factor (VEGF).

Some of the structural and hemodynamic effects of PKC activation are secondary to inhibition of nitric oxide production and altered gene expression for vasoactive and growth factors such as ET-1 (endothelin-1), VEGF, TGF-β1 and connective tissue growth factor (CTGF). PKC also induces expression of adhesion molecules: platelet/endothelial cell adhesion molecule (PECAM) and intracellular adhesion molecule (ICAM). Furthermore, PKC activation is associated with increased expression of plasminogen activator inhibitor-1 (PAI-1) that promotes hypercoagulopathy. It thus appears that PKC activation has a central role to play in the development of diabetic vascular complications.

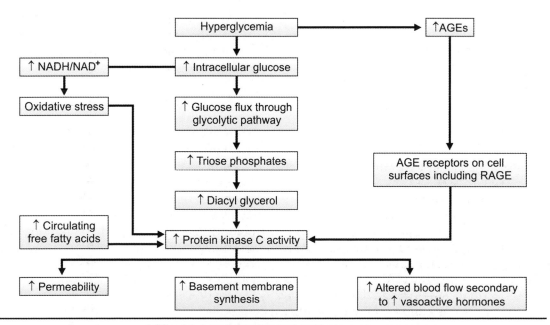

AGEs: Advanced glycation end-products
RAGEs: Receptor for advanced glycation end-products
NADPH: Nicotinamide adenine dinucleotide phosphate
NAD: Nicotinamide adenine dinucleotide

Figure 52.6 Activation of protein kinase C in diabetic vascular complications

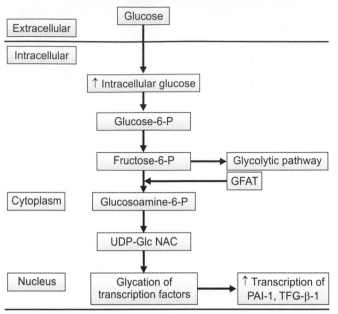

PAI-1: Plasminogen activator inhibitor-1;
TGF-β-1: Transforming growth factor-beta 1;
GFAT: Glutamine fructose-6-phosphate aminotransferase;
UDP-Glc NAC: UDP-N-acetyl glucosamine

Figure 52.7 Role of hexosamine pathway in diabetic complications

Increased Flux through the Hexosamine Pathway[48-53]

Shunting of glucose into the hexosamine pathway has recently been suggested as an important mechanism for hyperglycemia induced tissue damage **(Figure 52.7)**. Fructose-6-phosphate is diverted from the glycolytic pathway to increase production of glucosamine-6-phosphate, a substrate utilized to form UDP-N-acetyl glucosamine. This causes glycation of transcription factors for many genes in the nucleus particularly TGF-α, TGF-β and PAI-1. This altered gene expression as well as altered protein function together mediates the development of diabetes complications.

ROLE OF OXIDATIVE STRESS IN DEVELOPMENT OF DIABETIC COMPLICATIONS

Oxidative stress is defined as a condition where the overall generation of free radicals exceeds the total antioxidant levels in the body. Oxidative stress can result from overproduction of ROS and/or decreased efficiency of inhibitory and scavenging antioxidant systems. Targets of ROS can be direct such as peroxi-

dation of the lipids of cell membranes, oxidation, cross-linking and fragmentation of protein enzymes amino acids (enzymes) and single strand breaks and cross-linking of DNA or indirect such as activation of stress sensitive signaling pathways that regulate gene expression resulting in tissue damage. Antioxidant defense systems help to reduce the oxidative stress and keep oxidative damage in check by scavenging oxidative radicals. These include antioxidant enzymes like superoxide dismutase (SOD), catalase (CAT) and glutathione peroxides (GSH-Pox), chain breaking antioxidants like vit E, beta-carotene, GSH, vit C protein bound thiol groups, and transition metal binding proteins like ferritin, transferrin, lactoferrin and ceruloplasmin.[54,55]

Oxidative stress plays a crucial role in the development of the late complications of diabetes mellitus. In a study undertaken at our institution, we demonstrated that there is significantly enhanced oxidative stress in T2DM patients which is present early in the course of the disease, increases with increasing duration of DM, is present even in patients without evidence of significant micro- or macrovascular complications, predates the development of long-term complications and correlates best with postprandial glucose levels.[56]

Increased generation of ROS in diabetes mellitus reported from other studies includes increased lipid peroxidation,[57-59] decreased NO end-products along with increased malondialdehyde (MDA) levels[60] and elevated diene conjugates in T2DM with microvascular complications but not in those without.[61] On the other hand, lowered antioxidative defenses such as decrease in leukocyte vit C,[57] erythrocyte superoxide dismutase (SOD) activity,[62] total radical trapping capacity[63] and reduced glutathione (GSH)[64] have been recorded in some patients. However, normal SOD and GSH[57,65] have also been reported.

Antioxidant status, lipid peroxidation and nitric oxide end-products were estimated at our center in patients of type 2 diabetes mellitus with and without nephropathy. Patients with nephropathy were very carefully selected to avoid confounders. Serum MDA was higher in T2DM patients compared to controls and higher in T2DM with nephropathy compared to those without. Erythrocyte superoxide dismutase (SOD), catalase (CAT) activities were lower in T2DM and CAT activity and GSH levels in erythrocytes were lower in diabetes with nephropathy when compared with controls. The study clearly showed that oxidative stress is increased and antioxidant defenses are compromised in diabetic patients with nephropathy thus

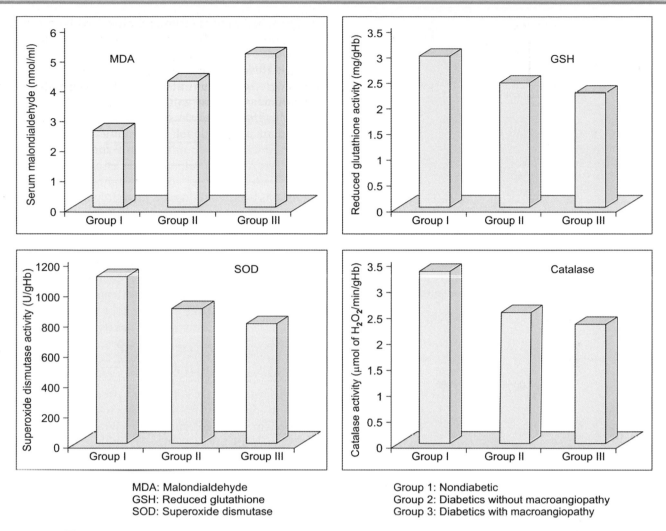

MDA: Malondialdehyde
GSH: Reduced glutathione
SOD: Superoxide dismutase

Group 1: Nondiabetic
Group 2: Diabetics without macroangiopathy
Group 3: Diabetics with macroangiopathy

Figure 52.8   Assessment of oxidative stress in type 2 patients with and without macroangiopathy

demonstrating a clear role for this pathway in the development of nephropathy.[66]

We assessed oxidative stress in type 2 diabetic patients with and without macroangiopathy.[67] There was a progressive increase in oxidative stress (MDH levels) and a progressive decrease of antioxidant defense systems (GSH, SOD and catalase) from control subjects, diabetic patients without macroangiopathy and diabetic patients with macroangiopathy suggesting that enhanced oxidative stress in diabetes with reduced antioxidative defense mechanism may play an important role in pathogenesis of macroangiopathy **(Figure 52.8)**. When parameters of oxidative stress were measured in the fasting state as well as 2, 4, 6 and 8 hours after a standardized high fat, low carbohydrate

(CHO) meal challenge in diabetic subjects with and without macroangiopathy it was found that there was a significant increase in TBARS, a measure of oxidative stress following a high fat meal challenge which peaked at 4 to 6 hours and declined at 8 hours in nondiabetics as well as both diabetic study groups **(Figure 52.9)**. Clearly, there was a significantly higher postprandial (PP) oxidative stress and a deficient antioxidant defense system observed in T2DM patients particularly those with macroangiopathy in addition to fasting abnormalities suggesting a specific role for PP oxidative stress in the development of diabetic macroangiopathy. The magnitude of PP hypertriglyceridemia was a major determinant of PP oxidative stress in this group **(Figure 52.10)**. It would appear from this study[68] and

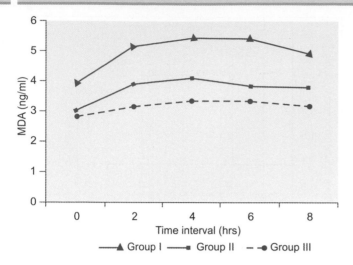

Figure 52.9 Postprandial MDA levels in patients of type 2 diabetes mellitus with and without macroangiopathy

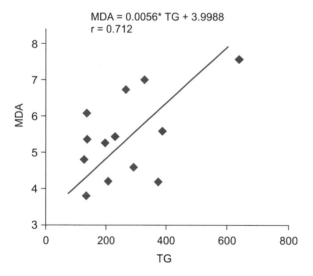

MDA: Malondialdehyde; TG: Triglyceride; PPTG: Postprandial triglyceride; PP MDA: Postprandial malondialdehyde

Figure 52.10 Correlation of PPTG levels at PP MDA levels in type 2 diabetes mellitus with macroangiopathy

from other studies[69] that the increased risk of macro-vascular disease in diabetic subjects conferred by PP hypertriglyceridemia and PP hyperglycemia is mediated by an increase in postprandial oxidative stress and thereby through activation of stress sensitive gene expression.[70]

Thus, oxidative stress resulting from increased production of ROS or their inadequate removal plays a key role in the pathogenesis of late diabetic complications. Hyperglycemia induced oxidative stress leads to tissue damage, the pathways for which have been well elucidated in recent years.

Hyperglycemia-induced late diabetic complications result from a cycle of self-perpetuating oxidative stress mediated cellular damage that is brought about by hyperglycemia dependent NF-κB activation in patients with diabetes mellitus. The importance of NF-κB in this regard has been well documented. In patients with DM, NF-κB activation correlates positively with HbA_{1c} and significantly with severity of albuminuria in those with nephropathy. Also, antioxidant lipoic acid treatment significantly suppresses NF-κB activation. Activation of NF-κB which is a transcription factor, triggers gene expression of a variety of genes that result in tissue damage **(Figure 52.11)**.[70-75]

UNIFYING HYPOTHESIS FOR DIABETIC COMPLICATIONS[76-79]

Recent studies suggest that overproduction of super-oxides in mitochondria secondary to excessive glucose metabolism is the common underlying initiating event that drives all other pathways including the polyol pathway, AGEs production, PKC activation and hexosamine pathway activation.[70] This is believed to be due to oxidative stress related pathways that are known to be operating in diabetes mellitus. Hyper-glycemia-induced increase in mitochondrial superoxide can also induce mitochondrial DNA mutations. It is hypothesized that this could sustain the elevated superoxide production long after euglycemia is restored and thereby result in continued activation of all major pathways that cause diabetic complications.

SUMMARY

Long-term complications of diabetes mellitus contribute a major health problem in addition to acute metabolic complications and infections. The atherosclerotic macrovascular complications like coronary artery disease, stroke and peripheral vascular disease are assuming high proportions. Diabetic tissue damage occurs primarily in tissues where glucose uptake is insulin independent and therefore the influx of glucose into the cells is unregulated and greatly increased in the face of hyperglycemia. Target organ damage in diabetes occurs

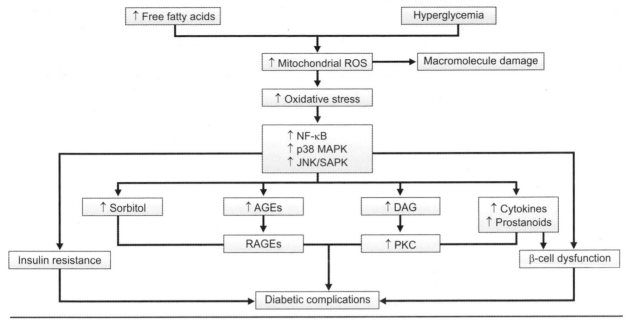

AGEs: Advanced glycation end-products
RAGEs: Receptor for advanced glycation end-products
DAG: Diacylglycerol
PKC: Protein kinase C
ROS: Reactive oxygen species
NF-κB: Nuclear factor kappa B
MAPK: Mitogen activated protein kinase
JNK: Janus kinase
SAPK: Serine activated protein kinase

Figure 52.11 Elevated FFA and hyperglycemia in the pathophysiology of diabetes complications via the generation of ROS

mainly in the eyes, kidneys, nerves, heart and blood vessels; although no organ of the body is spared. Overall, the vascular wall appears to be the primary target in diabetes-related complications regardless of the organs. Since little can be done after the development of overt complications, the emphasis has always been on preventing or delaying complications. The role of hyperglycemia in the development of diabetic complications and the beneficial effects of strict glycemic control have now been well established by well designed controlled clinical trials. There are four major pathways that are believed to mediate the development of complications—the polyol pathway, the advanced glycation end-product pathway, the protein kinase pathway and the hexosamine pathway. While the first two have for long been well elucidated, the role of the protein kinase pathway and the hexosamine pathway is being increasingly understood of late. Hyperglycemia is the initial trigger for most

steps of these pathways, which through a cascade of events specific to each pathway result in diabetic tissue damage. The role of oxidative stress is critical in this process and several studies including studies done at our institution support a very important role for reactive oxygen species (ROS) in oxidative stress. Major links in the oxidative stress pathway particularly the stress sensitive gene expression mechanisms and the events leading to NF-κB activation have now been fully elucidated, thereby greatly enhancing our understanding the basis of diabetic complications. Recently, a unifying concept for the development of diabetic complications has been proposed that links all the major pathways through a common trigger, i.e. oxidative stress. Recent understanding of the cellular and molecular mechanisms that mediate diabetic complications has opened up novel areas of potential therapeutic benefit in this regard.

REFERENCES

1. Diabetes Control and Complications Trial Research Group. The effect of intensive treatment of diabetes on the development and progression of long-term complications in insulin-dependent diabetes mellitus. N Engl J Med. 1993;329:683-89.

2. UKPDS Research Group. UK prospective diabetes study 16. Overview of 6 years' therapy of type II diabetes: a progressive disease. Diabetes. 1994;44:1249-58.

3. Okhubo Y, Kishikawa H, Araki E, et al. Intensive insulin therapy prevents the progression of diabetic microvascular complications in Japanese patients with noninsulin-dependent diabetes mellitus: a randomized prospective 6-year study. Diabetes Res Clin Pract. 1995;28:103-17.

4. Andrzej S, Krolewsk, James H, Warram, Maria Beatriz S, Freire. Epidemiology of late diabetic complications: a basis for the development and evaluation of preventive programs. Endocr Metab Clin North Am. 1996;25:217-42.

5. Mogensen CE, Christensen CK, Vittinghus E. The stages in diabetic renal disease with emphasis on the stage of incipient diabetic nephropathy. Diabetes 1983;32:64-78.

6. Chase PH, Jackson WE, Hoops SL, et al. Glucose control and the renal and retinal complications of insulin-dependent diabetes. JAMA. 198;261:1155-60.

7. Krolewski AS, Laffel LMB, Krolewski M, et al. Glycated hemoglobin and risk of microalbuminuria in patients with insulin-dependent diabetes mellitus. N Engl J Med. 1995; 332:1251-5.

8. Warram JH, Rich SS, Krolewski AS. Epidemiology and genetics of diabetes mellitus. In Kahn CR, Weir GC (Eds): Joslin's Diabetes Mellitus. Phaladephia: Lea and Febiger; 1994. pp. 201-15.

9. Haffner SM, Lehto S, Ronnemaa T, Pyorala K, Laakso M. Mortality from coronary heart disease in subjects with type 2 diabetes and in nondiabetic subjects. N Engl J Med. 1998;339: 229-34.

10. Fontbonne A. Relationship between diabetic dyslipo-proteinemia and coronary heart disease risk in noninsulin-dependent diabetes. Diabetes Metab Rev. 1991;7:179-89.

11. Lewis GF, O'Meara NM, Soltys PA. Fasting hyper-triglyceridemia in noninsulin-dependent diabetes mellitus is an important predictor of postprandial lipid and lipoprotein abnormalities. J Clin Endocr Metab. 1999;72:934-44.

12. Madhu SV, Mittal V, Krishna Ram B, Srivastava DK. Postprandial lipid abnormalities in type 2 diabetes mellitus. J Assoc Physic Ind. 2005;53:1043-46.

13. Shinichi Teno, Uto Y, Nagashima H, Endoh Y, IwamotoY, Omorin Y. Association of postprandial hypertriglyceridemia and carotid intima-media thickness in patients with type 2 diabetes. Diabetes Care. 2000;23:1401-6.

14. Anderson RA, Evans ML, Ellis GR, Graham J, Morris K, Jackson SK, et al. The relationships between postprandial lipemia, endothelial function and oxidative stress in healthy individuals and patients with type 2 diabetes. Atherosclerosis. 2001;154:475-83.

15. Pirart J. Diabetes mellitus and its degenerative complications. A prospective study of 4400 patients observed between 1947 and 1973. Diabetes Metab. 1977;3:97-107,173-82,245-56.

16. Klein R. Hyperglycemia and microvascular and macrovascular disease in diabetes. Diabetes Care. 1995;18:258-68.

17. Diabetes Control and Complications Trial/Epidemiology of Diabetes Interventions and Complications Research Group. Retinopathy and nephropathy in patients with type 1 diabetes four years after a trial of intensive therapy. N Eng J Med. 2000; 342:381-9.

18. Brownlee M. Biochemistry and molecular cell biology of diabetic complications. Nature. 2001;414:813-20.

19. King GL, Brownlee M. The cellular and molecular mechanisms of diabetic complications. Endocrinol Metab Clin North Am. 1996;25:255-70.

20. He Zhiheng, MR Christian, KL George. Pathogenesis of diabetes microvascular complications. Defronzo RA, Ferrannini E, Keen H, Zimmet P (Eds): International Textbook of Diabetes Mellitus. 3rd edn. Chichester: John Weley and Sons Ltd; 2004. pp. 1135-59.

21. Vader Jag DL, Robison B, Taylor KK, Hunsaker LA. Reduction of trioses by NADH-dependent aldo-keto-reductases: adose reductase, methylglyoxal and diabetic complications. K Biol Chem. 1992;267:4364-9.

22. Greene D, Lattimer SA, Sima AAF. Sorbitol, phosphoinositides and sodium-potassium-ATPase in the pathogenesis of diabetic complications. N Engl J Med. 1987;316:599-606.

23. Kinoshita JH, Nishimura C. The involvement of aldose redutase in diabetic complications. Diabetes Metab Rev. 1988;4:323.

24. Bownlee M, Cerami A, Vlassara. Advanced glycosylation end- products in tissue and the biochemical basis of diabetic complications. N Engl J Med. 1988;318:1315-21.

25. Vlassara H, Palae MR. Diabetes and advanced glycation end- products. J Intrim Med. 2002;251:87-101.

26. Tanji N, Markowitz GS, Fu C, Kishinger T, Taguchi A, Pischetsrieder M, Stern D, Schmidt AM, D' Agati VD. Expression of advanced glycation end-products and their cellular receptor RAGE in diabetic nephropathy and nondiabetic renal disease. J Am Soc Nephrol. 2000;11:656-66.

27. Stitt AW, Li YM, Gardiner TA, Bucala R, Archer DB, Vlassara H. Advanced glycation end-products (AGEs) co-localize with AGE receptors in the retinal vasculature of diabetic and of AGE-issued rats. Am J Pathol. 1971;50:523-31.

28. Stitt AW, Moore JE, Sharkey JA, et al. Advanced glycation end- products in viteous: structural and functional implications for diabetic vitreopathy. Invest Ophthalmol Vis Sci. 1998;39:2517-23.

29. Stit AAAW, Li YM, Gadiner TA, et al. Advanced glycation end-products (AGEs) co-localize with AGE receptors in the retinal vasculature of diabetic and of AGE-infused rats. Am J Pathol. 1997;150:523-31.

30. Gupta A, Tripathi AK, Madhu SV, Tripathi RL. Role of advanced glycosylated end-products on polymorphonuclear oxidative function leading to oxidative stress in type-2 diabetes mellitus. MD Thesis, University of Delhi; 2006.

31. Ammes HP, Martin S, Federlin K. Geisen K, Brownlee M. Aminoguanidine treatment inhibits the development of experimental diabetic retinopathy. Roc Natl Acad Sci USA. 1991;88:11555-8.

32. Soulis-Liparota T, Cooper M, Papazoglou D, Clarke B,

Jerums G. Retardation by aminoguanidine of development of albuminuria, mesangial expansion, and tissue fluorescence in streptozocin-induced diabetic rat. Diabetes. 1991;40:1328-34.

33. Tanak S, Abigad G, Brodsky B, Eikenbarry EF. Glycation induces expansion of the molecular packing of collagen. J Mol Biol. 1988;203:495-505.

34. Boyd-White J, Williams JC Jr. Effect of cross-linking on matrix permeability: a model for AGE-modified basement membranes. Diabetes. 1996;45:348-53.

35. Vlassara H. The AGE-receptor in the pathogenesis of diabetic complications. Diabetes Metab Res Rev. 2001;17:436-43.

36. Horiuchi S, Higashi T, Ikeda K, et al. Advanced glycation end- products and their recognition by macrophage and macrophage-derived cells. Diabetes. 1996;45:573-6.

37. Li J, Schmidt AM. Characterization and functional analysis of the promoter of RAGE (the receptor for advanced glycation end-products). J Biol Chem. 1997;277:16498-506.

38. Vlassara H, Fuh H, Donnell T, Cybulsky M. Advanced glycation end-products promote adhesion molecule (VCAM-1, ICAM-1) expression and atheroma formation in normal rabbits. Mol Med. 1995;1:447-56.

39. Schmidt AM, Hori O, Chen JX, et al. Advanced glycation end- products interacting with their endothelial receptor induce expression of vascular cell adhesion molecule-1 (VCAM-1) in cultured human endothelial cells and in mice: a potential, mechanism for the accelerated vasculopathy of diabetes. J Clin Invest. 1995;96:1395-403.

40. Giadino I, Edelstein D, Brownlee M. Nonenzymatic glycosylation *in vitro* and in bovine endothelial cells alters basic fibroblast growth factor activity: a model for intracellular glycosylation in diabetes. J Clin Invest. 1994;94:110-7.

41. Koya D, King Gl. Protein kinase C activation and the development of diabetic complications. Diabetes. 1998;47:859-66.

42. Xia P, Kramer RM, Kind GL. Identification of the mechanism or the inhibition of Na, K-adenosine triphosphatase by hyperglycemia involving activation of protein kinase C and cytosolic phospholipase A$_2$. J Clin Invest. 1995;96:733.

43. Ishi H, Koya D, King GL. Protein kinase C activation and its role in the development of vascular complications in diabetes mellitus. J Mol Med. 1998;76:21-31.

44. Aiello LP, Bursell SE, Clermont A, Duh E, Ishi H, Takagi C, Mori F, Ciulla TA, Ways K, Jirousek M Smith. Retinal permeability is mediated by protein kinase C *in vivo* and suppressed by an orally effective beta-isoform-selective inhibitor. Diabetes. 1997;46:1473-80.

45. Lynch JJ, Ferroo TJ, Blumenstock FA, Brockenauer AM, Malik AB. Increased endothelial albumin permeability mediated by protein kinase C activation. J Clin Invest. 1990;85:1991-8.

46. Derubertis FR, Craven PA. Activation of protein kinase C in glomerular cells in diabetes—mechanism and potential links to the pathogenesis of diabetic glomerulopathy. Diabetes. 1994;43:1-8.

47. Kim YS, Kim BC, Song CY, Hong HK, Moon KC, Lee HS, Advanced glycosylation end-products stimulate collagen mRNA synthesis in mesangial cells mediated by protein kinase C and transforming growth factor-beta. J Lab Clin Med. 2001;138:59-68.

48. Marshall S, Bacote V, Traxinger RR. Discovery of a metabolic pathway mediating glucose-induced desensitization of the glucose transport system: role of hexosamine biosynthesis in the induction of insulin resistance. J Bio Chem. 1991;266:4706-12.

49. Hawkins M, Barzilai N, Liu R, et al. Role of the glucosamine pathway in fat-induced insulin resistance. J Clin Invest. 1997; 99:2173-82.

50. Scheicher ED, Weigret C. Role of the hexosamine biosynthetic pathway in diabetic nephropathy. Kidney Int. 2000;77:S13-8.

51. MeClain DA, Paterson AH, Roos MD, Wei X, Kudlow JE. Glucose and glucosamine regulate growth factor gene expression in vascular smooth muscle cells. Proc Natl Acad Sci USA. 192;89:8150-4.

52. Daniels MC, McClain DA, Crook ED. Transcriptional regulation of transforming growth factor beta by glucose: investigation into the role of the hexosamine biosynthesis pathway. Am J Med Sci. 2000;319:138-42.

53. Goldberg HJ, Whteside CI, Fantus IG. The hexosamine pathway regulates the plasminogen activator inhibitor-I gene promoter and Sp 1 transcriptional activation through protein kinase C-beta I and delta. J Biol Chem. 2002;277:33833-41.

54. Baynes J. Role of oxidative stress in development of complications. Diabetes. 1991;40:405-12.

55. Irshad M, Chaudhary PS. Oxidant-antioxidant system: role and significance in human body. Ind J Exp Biol. 2002;40:1233-9.

56. Narang P, Singh S, Tondon OP, Madhu SV, Sharma SB, et al. Status of oxidative stress in early and late type 2 DM. MD Thesis, Delhi University; 2004.

57. Akkus I, Kalak S, Vural H, Caglayan O, et al. Leukocyte, lipid peroxidation, superoxide dismutase glutathione peroxidase and serum and leukocyte vitamine C level of patients with type 2 diabetes mellitus. Clin Chim Acta. 1996;244:221-7.

58. Nourooz-Zaden J, Rahimi A, Taj Addin Sarmadi J, Tritschleer H, et al. Relationships between plasma measures of oxidative stress and metabolic control in NIDDM. Diabetologia. 1997;40:647-53.

59. Nagasaka Y, Fujii S, Kaneko T. Effects of high glucose and sorbitol pathway on lipid peroxidation of erythrocytes. Horn Metab Res. 1989;21:275-6.

60. Vanizor B, Orem A, Karahan SC, et al. Decreased nitric oxide end-products and its relationship with high density lipoprotein and oxidative stress in people with type 2 diabetes without complications. Diabet Research Clin Pract. 2001;54:33-9.

61. Jennings PE, Jones AF, Florkoski CM, Lunec J, et al. Increased diene conjugates in diabetic subjects with microangiopathy. Diab Med. 1987;4:452-6.

62. Skrha J, Hodinar A, Kvasnicka J, Hilgertova J. Relationship of oxidative stress and fibrinolysis in diabetes mellitus. Diabet Med. 1996;13:800-5.

63. Ceriello A, Bortolotti N, Falleiti E, Taboga C, et al. Total radical trapping antioxidant parameter in NIDDM patients. Diabetes Care. 1997;20:197-7.

64. Yoshida, Hirokawa J, Tagami S, Kawakami Y, et al. Weakened cellular regulation of glutathione synthesis and efflux. Diabetologia. 1995;38:201-10.

65. Giri R, Kesavulu MM, Kameshwara RB, Ramana V, et al. Hyperlipidemia, increased lipid peroxidation and changes in antioxidant enzymes, Na$^+$-K$^+$ ATPase in erythrocytes of type 2 diabetic patients in Andhra Pradesh. Ind J Clin Biochem. 1999;14:168-75.

66. Bhatia S, Shukla R, Madhu SV, et al. Antioxidant status, lipid peroxidation and nitric oxide end-products in patients of type 2 diabetes mellitus with nephropathy. Clin Biochem. 2003;36:557-62.

67. Singhania N, Puri D, Sharma SB, Madhu SV. Assessment of oxidative stress in type 2 diabetic patients with and without macroangiopathy. MD Thesis, University of Delhi; 2004.

68. Saxena R, Madhu SV, Shukla R, Prabhu KM, Gambhir Jasvinder K. Postprandial hypertriglyceridemia and oxidative stress in patients of type 2 diabetes mellitus with macrovascular complications. Clin Chem Acta. 2005;359:101-8.

69. Ceriello A, Bortolotti N, Motz E, et al. Meal-generated oxidative stress in type 2 diabetic patients. Diabetes Care. 1998;21:1529-33.

70. Nishikawa T, et al. Elevated FFA and hyperglycemia in the pathophysiology of diabetes via the generation of ROS. Kidney Int. 2000;58:26-30.

71. Nishikawa T, et al. Hyperglycemia-induced ROS formation and inhibitory effects of mitochondrial uncoupling agents and manganese superoxide. Nature.

72. Mercurio F, et al. Exogenous and endogenous stimuli leading to ROS generation and activation of stress-sensitive gene expression. Oncogene. 1999;18:6163-71.

73. Barnes PJ, et al. Model of NF-κB activation by hyperglycemia, FFA, and cytokines. N Engl J Med. 1997;336:1066-71.

74. Pieper GM, Riaz-ul-Haq. Activation of nuclear factor-kappa B in cultured endothelial cells by increased glucose concentration prevention by calphostin C. J Cardiovasc Pharmacol. 1997;30:528-32.

75. Yereni KK, Bai W, Khan BV, Medford RM, Natarajan R. Hyperglycemia-induced activation of nuclear transcription factor kappa B in vascular smooth muscle cells. Diabetes. 1999;48:855-64.

76. Wallace DC. Disease of the mitochondrial DNA. Annu Rev Biochem. 1992;61:1175-212.

77. Wei YH. Oxidative stress and mitochondrial DNA mutations in human aging. Proc Soc Exp Bial Medical. 1998; 217:53-63.

78. Nishikawa T, Du Edelstein DXL, Yamagishi S, et al. Normalizing mitohondrial superoxide production blocks three pathways of hyperglycemic damage. Nature. 2000;404:787-90.

79. Scivttaro V, Ganz MB, Weiss MG. AGEs induced oxidative stress and activate protein kinase C-beta (II) in neonatal mesangial cells. Am J Physiol. 2000;278:F676-83.

Chapter 53

ACUTE METABOLIC COMPLICATIONS

Hemraj B Chandalia

Acute metabolic emergencies in diabetes are mostly preventable and eminently treatable. A good knowledge of their pathogenesis and management strategies is likely to produce a successful outcome. The emergencies to be considered in this chapter are Diabetic Ketoacidosis (DKA), Hyperglycemic Hyperosmolar Nonketotic State (HHNKS) and lactic acidosis. Hypoglycemia in diabetic patients is an important iatrogenic emergency and is discussed elsewhere.

DIABETIC KETOACIDOSIS

Definition

Three essential components of DKA are hyperglycemia, ketosis and resultant metabolic acidosis. A firm diagnosis of DKA requires these three criteria to be fulfilled. Usually, the blood glucose is more than 250 mg/dl, pH <7.3, urine ketones moderately positive, serum ketones positive in 1 : 4 dilution and bicarbonate <15 mEq/L.

Etiology and Precipitating Factors

The basic etiology is total or subtotal insulinopenia. How this leads to genesis of DKA is discussed in pathogenesis. However, the immediate clinical ante-cedents are important to identify, because it is possible to apply preventive approach at this level **(Table 53.1)**. In most patients, it is omission or reduction of insulin dosage in an insulin-dependent diabetic (IDDM or type 1). At times, DKA is the presenting feature of type 1 diabetics: it is estimated that 20% of DKA is accounted for by undiagnosed type 1 diabetics at times even from the elderly group. In type 1 diabetics on pump therapy, failure of pump can result in rapid advent of DKA. This is because pumps deliver regular insulin on minute-to-minute basis and their failure

TABLE 53.1		Etiology, clinical antecedents and prevention of DKA
Etiology	:	Insulinopenia
Clinical antecedents	:	Omission of insulin dose
		Undiagnosed type 1 DM
		Stress situations with resultant increase in contrainsulin hormones
Prevention or early diagnosis	:	Educate type 1 diabetics regarding sick-day routine
		Suspect type 1 DM in sick children with polyuria, polydipsia and weight loss

results in total nonavailability of insulin in a short period. At times, infection or an acute cardiovascular event places increased insulin demands on the patient. This is probably brought about by an increased secretion of contrainsulin hormones like catecholamines, cortisol, glucagon and growth hormone. Theoretically, in this situation, a type 2 diabetic, especially one with subtotal insulinopenia can develop DKA. In practice, however, most type 2 diabetics under such stressful situations with increased insulin demands develop a hyperglycemic, hyperosmolar state (HHNKS). They are usually nonketotic but at times have mild-to-moderate acetonuria and are often mistakenly diagnosed as having DKA (see HHNKS). Their blood pH is usually normal.

In some situations, so-called type 2 diabetic patients can develop a full-blown DKA. It is possible that these patients are truly type 1 diabetics having slow immune-destruction of their β-cells (Late onset autoimmune diabetes of adults) or suffer from other forms of type 1 diabetes. Thirty-nine percent of type 2 diabetics in India may have islet cell antibody 512 (ICA 512) positivity.[1] These patients are true type 1 diabetics, masquerading as type 2 diabetics. To confound this issue further, it is known that one-third of metabolic decompensations seen in diabetes are of mixed type, e.g. DKA coupled with a hyperosmolar state or starvation ketosis or alcoholic ketosis or lactic acidosis.

More recently, a number of psychotropic drugs (clozapine, olanzapine),[2,3] 'ecstasy' (3,4-methylenedi-oxymethamphetamine) ingestion[4] and treatment of kidney transplant patients with FK506/tacrolimus[5] have been shown to aggravate diabetes or precipitate an acute episode of DKA. An isolated example of DKA caused by growth hormone treatment in a patient of Prader-Willi syndrome has also been reported.[6] A fatal episode of DKA has been described with the combined use of ritonavir, stavudine and didanosine in a child suffering from HIV infection.[7]

Prevalence and Mortality

Prevalence of DKA is difficult to establish. Faich[8] reported a prevalence of 1.6% in Rhode Island. The annual rate was 0.46 per 100 patients with diabetes. At Diabetes, Endocrinology and Nutrition Management and Research Center, Mumbai, Maharashtra, India a group of 162 type 1 diabetics are on long-term follow-up. They make about 2% of the total clinic population of diabetics. There were 42 episodes of DKA in these patients requiring hospitalization. Of these 42 episodes of DKA,

15 occurred before the diagnosis was made and 24 before the patient presented to our center. Only three episodes occurred in two patients on regular follow-up at our center from 1988 to 1998. This brings out the importance of follow-up and patient education in specialized clinics.

Mortality in DKA is falling rapidly over the last six decades because of insulin therapy, better understanding of fluid, electrolytes and acid-base disturbances and finally, patient education and empowerment. Near 100% mortality of preinsulin era was brought down to 30% with the advent of insulin. Advent of antibiotic therapy and an improved understanding of fluid and electrolyte therapy brought down the mortality to about 10% in most centers around the world. Mortality is closely related to the severity of DKA at the time of presentation. It is also closely related to osmolarity and state of consciousness of the patient. In established diabetes centers, DKA as a primary disease has been associated with as low a mortality as 2.7%.[9] When coupled with acute vascular events and infections as primary diseases, mortality can still be high. In our patients with primary diagnosis of DKA, we have had no mortality in the past ten years.

Pathogenesis

Metabolic changes of DKA arise from absolute insulinopenia or subtotal insulinopenia with increased levels of counter-regulatory hormones like catecholamines, glucagon, cortisol and growth-hormone.[10] These hormonal changes result in increased glucose concentration because of (i) inadequate glucose utilization by insulin-sensitive tissues like muscles, adipose tissue and liver, (ii) increased glycogenolysis and most important, (iii) increased glucose production by the liver from amino acids **(Figure 53.1)**. Such hormonal milieu also leads to lipolysis, resulting in increased free fatty acid (FFA) and glycerol. The FFA undergo β-oxidation to generate ketone bodies and are also converted in the liver to very low-density lipoproteins (VLDL). Ketone bodies generated are acetone, acetoacetic acid and β-hydroxybutyric acid. β-hydroxybutyric acid is derived from acetoacetic acid by a process of reduction. In most patients of DKA, β-hydroxybutyrate to acetoacetate ratio is 4 : 1.[11] Furthermore, when reducing ions or substances like ascorbic acid are present in abundance, β-hydroxybutyrate may form the sole ketoanion. As the usual methods for testing ketone bodies (ketostix, ferricyanide test) detect only acetone and acetoacetic acid, these tests can be falsely-negative when the redox state is

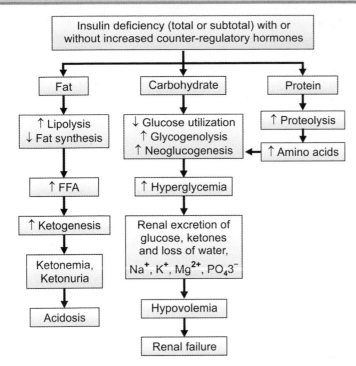

Figure 53.1 Pathophysiology of DKA

TABLE 53.2	Average deficits of water and electrolytes per kg of body weight in diabetic ketoacidosis
Water	100 ml
Na^+	7-10 mEq
Cl^-	3-5 mEq
K^+	3-5 mEq
Mg^{2+}	1-2 mEq
$PO_4{}^{3-}$	1-2 mEq

predominantly towards a more reduced state. Recently, a direct measurement of β-hydroxybutyrate has been introduced.[12] The amount of ketones is moderate to large in the urine (45–90 mg/dl, 3 to 4 + on ketostix) as compared to starvation ketosis where the amount of ketones is small (<30 mg/dl, 1 to 2 + on ketostix). Plasma ketones are positive in the undiluted state and 1 : 2 dilution, a finding not seen in starvation ketosis or HHNKS.

Overall, the metabolism in DKA simulates that in starvation, but the intensity of lipolysis, gluconeogenesis and ketogenesis is very high in DKA, resulting in profound acid-base and electrolyte disturbances **(Table 53.2).** Osmotic diuresis results in loss of large amounts of water, sodium, potassium, magnesium and phosphate. Overall, water loss is more than the loss of cations. In other words, the loss is hypo-osmolar and not iso-osmolar. The amount of water lost is 5 percent of body water in mild and 10 percent or more of body water in well developed DKA. Thus, the loss of water is 50 to 100 ml, sodium 7 to 10 mEq, potassium 3 to 5 mEq, chloride 5 to 7 mEq per kilogram of body weight. Hyperglycemia causes shift of water from intracellular to extracellular and intravascular compartment. This water is further lost by osmotic diuresis through kidneys. Serum sodium is modified by hyperglycemia

and hyperlipidemia. For every 100 mg of blood glucose rise above the baseline blood glucose of 100 mg/dl, serum sodium drops by 1.6 mEq.[13] Hyperlipidemia can be very severe at times; triglycerides of over 1000 mg/dl are not unusual. This can be easily seen in the fundus in the form of lipemia retinalis or at the bedside by looking at the serum, which is lipemic. The lipids reduce the aqueous compartment of the blood in which serum Na^+ is present and hence, cause spurious lowering of serum sodium. The net result of these various opposing events (water loss raising serum Na^+; hyperglycemia and hyperlipidemia decreasing serum Na^+) is such that serum Na^+ is almost normal or slightly low at the time of presentation. Total body potassium is negative by 3 to 5 mEq/kg of body weight, but the initial serum potassium could either be normal, high or low, depending upon the following factors:

i. Osmotic loss through kidneys decreasing serum K^+.
ii. Vomiting or acute gastric dilatation causes loss of potassium and decreases serum K^+.
iii. Decreased intravascular volume and diminished GFR decreases K^+ excretion and raises serum K^+.
iv. Metabolic acidosis causes migration of intracellular potassium into extracellular compartment and thus raises serum potassium. As acidosis is reversed by bicarbonate and insulin therapy, there is migration of potassium into the intracellular compartment resulting in severe and at times life-threatening hypokalemia.[14]

Metabolic acidosis is an important feature of DKA. The ketone bodies, except acetone which can be eliminated through lungs are fixed anions. They encroach on the alkali reserve and as acidosis progresses, result in low blood pH. In mild DKA, pH is about 7.3 but in severe acidosis it can be as low as 7.0 or 6.8. Metabolic acidosis is accompanied by respiratory alkalosis as a compensatory mechanism; this causes further lowering of peripheral bicarbonate, which cannot be used as an accurate guide to judge the degree of acidosis. This acidosis is reversible and hence with treatment, the ketone body generation stops, ketone utilization and excretion continues and bicarbonate is regenerated.

Management of DKA

General Guidelines

A patient with DKA needs urgent hospitalization. General nursing care and supportive measures are instituted immediately, depending upon the severity of DKA and state of consciousness. It is important to ask for laboratory investigations initially and periodically thereafter as indicated in **Table 53.3**. At the same time, two intravenous lines are secured, one for fluid, electrolyte and acid-base correction and the other for insulin therapy. A search is made for the possibility of an infection, notably of skin, lungs or urinary tract. Clinical examination and simple investigations will also reveal any vascular problem like a myocardial infarct, stroke or peripheral vascular occlusion. The treatment should preferably be initiated in emergency room, continued in intensive care for 1 to 3 days and thereafter be undertaken in the general ward. **Table 53.3** summarizes the treatment.

Fluid and Electrolyte Therapy

Fluid and electrolyte therapy is aimed at the replacement of previous losses, concurrent losses and daily requirements. As a general rule, the pace of replacement, especially of previous losses should be commensurated with the speed with which DKA has developed. As it takes about 48 to 72 hours to develop DKA, full replacement of previous losses and correction of acid-base disturbance is best undertaken with the same speed. This is true of any severe fluid and electrolyte problem as rapid correction is fraught with further disequilibrium, especially along the blood-brain barrier. Excessive and too rapid rate of fluid administration also increases the possibility of development of an adult respiratory distress syndrome. Thus, one-fourth previous losses can be replaced in first 4 to 6 hours, another one-fourth by 24 hours, the last one-half in 24 to 48 hours. Concurrent losses continue unabated till hyperglycemia is controlled.

Replacement of Water and Salt

This is the most important and urgent aspect of fluid therapy. As the water loss is in excess of salt loss, ideal repair fluid will be a half normal saline. However, in the initial period, half-normal saline is likely to cause a

TABLE 53.3	Protocol for the management of DKA (moderately severe)

On Admission: *Initial treatment*

Obtain complete blood count (CBC), blood glucose (BG), electrolytes, creatinine, urine glucose and ketone, plasma ketone, blood gases

Secure two intravenous (IV) lines:

Line 1: Give 10-20 units human regular insulin IV bolus

100 ml normal saline + 100 units regular human insulin: Infuse at the rate of 5-10 units/hr. Flush out first 10 ml fluid rapidly.

Line 2: Normal saline 1 liter over 1 hour; simultaneously infuse (through piggyback or bivalve) sodium bicarbonate 50-100 mEq in 250-500 ml of normal saline over 1 hour (optional)

0-4 hours: Monitor BG and K^+ hourly

Line 1: Continue insulin Infusion

Line 2: May infuse 500-1000 ml of ½ normal saline

Change to 5% dextrose when BG drops to about 200 mg/dl Start potassium chloride (KCl) 40 mEq per liter of IV fluids if serum K^+ <3.5 mEq/L or if urine output is good and BG is dropping

4-24 hours: Monitor BG and K^+ 2 hourly.

Line 1: Reduce insulin infusion rate to 2-5 units/hours IV when BG drops to 200 mg/dl

Line 2: 5% dextrose solution IV to correct half of calculated fluid requirement: KCl 40 mEq per liter of IV fluids

24-48 hours: Repeat CBC, electrolytes, and creatinine once a day

Line 1: IV insulin infusion at 1-5 units/hour; Give 10-20 U subcutaneous (SC) human regular insulin 2 hours before discontinuation of insulin infusion. Use basal (infusion) + bolus (IV 4-8 U regular insulin) regime when patient is on IV fluids + oral feeds

Line 2: 5% Dextrose infusion. Reduce IV fluids infused when able to retain fluids PO

After 48 hours: Shift to oral feeds
Start multiple dose insulin regime SC
Start KCl PO

further contraction of blood volume and cellular edema with the migration of water from the vascular bed to the intracellular compartment.

Hence, normal saline is considered an ideal initial replacement fluid. About a liter of normal saline must be infused in the first 1 to 2 hours of treatment; subsequently, the infusion pace is slowed as per general guidelines provided above. However, excess of saline infusion is fraught with danger: (i) because the previous losses are not iso-osmotic, water loss being in excess of NaCl loss and (ii) the chloride in normal saline is in excess of physiological requirement, so that large amount of saline produces a state of hyperchloremic acidosis. For these reasons, saline infusion should be replaced by 5% dextrose infusion after 4 to 6 hours of initial treatment. At this point usually the blood glucose has started a steady, linear decline and as such, supply of nutrients in the form of dextrose is called for. In practice, usually these events coincide, in exceptional cases half-normal saline can be used if blood glucose is still high and adequate saline has already been infused in the first 4 to 6 hours. Infusion of dextrose at the right time obviates several difficulties: (i) it provides the calories and prevents hypoglycemia, (ii) it provides free water once glucose is metabolized, and (iii) it forestalls possibility of excessive Na⁺ and Cl⁻ load.

Potassium Therapy[14]

As outlined in pathophysiology, initial serum potassium can be often normal, low or high. When very low initially, potassium infusion is started right away. In most cases, potassium drops after 4 to 6 hours of hydration and insulin therapy and at times drops to dangerously low levels. As glucose utilization proceeds intracellularly, potassium migrates from extracellular fluid to intracellular compartment. In case alkali is being administered, the potassium drop is aggravated, because alkalosis causes migration of potassium to intracellular sites. It is recommended that 20 to 30 mEq of potassium chloride be added to each liter of saline or other IV fluids. Theoretically, one-third of potassium replaced can be in the form of potassium phosphate (KPO_4), but in practice, the need of phosphate replacement in patients of DKA is rare (*vide infra*). Intravenous KCl should be continued to maintain the serum K⁺ at 4 to 5 mEq/liter. Potassium infusion should not ordinarily exceed 40 mEq/hr. It may be necessary to administer about 150 to 300 mEq of KCl in the first 24 hours. Monitoring of serum K⁺ is required at 1 to 2 hour intervals during this critical period **(Table 53.4)**.

Bicarbonate Therapy

This has been the most controversial aspect of therapy in DKA[15-17] **(Table 53.5)**. Theoretically, a metabolic acidosis can be best corrected by alkali therapy. However, the following features of metabolic acidosis in DKA call for a great caution in the use of alkali **(Figure 53.2)**:
1. Acidosis in DKA usually develops slowly over 2 to 3 days and hence needs correction at the same pace. As fluid and insulin therapy reverses the acidosis, a good amount of self-correction is possible.

TABLE 53.4	Potassium therapy in diabetic ketoacidosis

1. Do serum K⁺ initially, every one-hour for 6 hours, every 2 hours for next 6 hours and 12 hourly thereafter
2. Initial serum K⁺: Low, normal or high
3. If initial serum K⁺ is low, give 40 mEq KCl per liter of fluids to start with. Make sure urine output is adequate (>50 ml/ hour)
4. Potassium will drop precipitously after 2-4 hours of treatment and successful lowering of blood glucose. Continue 40 mEq KCl per liter of IV fluids administered
5. On institution of oral feed, 15-20 mEq KCl is recommended thrice a day p.o.

TABLE 53.5	Bicarbonate therapy in diabetic ketoacidosis

1. Give bicarbonate only if pH is < 7.2. Attempt correction only up to pH 7.2
2. Give half of the calculated dose. Do not repeat the dose
3. Give sodium bicarbonate diluted in normal saline or 5% dextrose in ratio of 1 : 4 (bicarbonate 1 part, saline 4 parts) over one hour

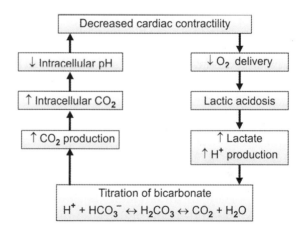

Figure 53.2 Mechanism of the deleterious effects of bicarbonate therapy

2. Rapid correction of peripheral acidosis can, for a period, aggravate intracerebral acidosis.
3. Lastly, oxygen dissociation and hence oxygen delivery to the tissues, is better in the acidotic state as compared to alkalotic state. Hence, sudden correction can jeopardize brain oxygenation and result is cerebral edema.
4. Elimination of ketone bodies through the kidneys is also better in the acidotic environment.
5. Alkali therapy also aggravates hypokalemia.
6. Use of sodabicarb also generates CO_2 resulting in aggravation of intracellular acidosis for some time.

Against all these arguments is the fact that a severe metabolic acidosis, especially when pH is less than 7.0, is likely to produce multiple organ dysfunction and must be corrected. Use of newer type of alkalinizing drugs, like carbicarb (a combination of sodium carbonate and sodabicarb) and THAM may be advantageous in this regard.

At present, the guidelines for alkali therapy have been fairly well established. Alkali therapy may be considered if pH is less than 7.2. If pH is less than 7.0, alkali therapy is considered essential. In any case, the dose of sodabicarb required is 50 percent of that calculated by the routine formula:

Soda bicarb (mEq) = (bicarb deficit) × (1/3 body water)

Recently, noninvasive monitoring of end-tidal CO_2 or transcutaneous CO_2 (TC–CO_2) has been shown to be a reliable guide to the bicarbonate concentration and hence acid-base status of the patient.[18,19] Usually a single dose of sodabicarb in slow infusion over half to one hour is considered adequate. The dose often works out to be 50 to 150 mEq and is hardly ever required to be repeated because the whole metabolic acidosis starts reversing in 4 to 6 hours of effective fluid and insulin therapy. If possible 7.5% soda bicarb solution (supplying 0.9 mEq/ml) should be diluted 1:4 by dextrose or saline solution, as concentrated soda bicarb is known to have caused severe thrombophlebitis of peripheral veins or even extensive tissue necrosis.

Magnesium and Phosphate Therapy[20-22]

Deficit of magnesium can be quite high. Profound, unexplained weakness, should suggest hypomagnesemia and if confirmed, treated.

It is important to understand the interaction of magnesium, parathormone, potassium and calcium ions. In hypomagnesemia, parathormone secretion is inhibited and concomitant hypocalcemia is resistant to correction. When required, a couple of doses of magnesium sulfate, 2 ml of 50% solution, intra muscular (IM) is sufficient to produce initial correction. In most patients, early institution of oral feeds takes care of magnesium deficit.

Phosphate therapy is also theoretically desirable. The erythrocyte concentration of 2,3-diphosphoglycerate is depleted in DKA. A normal concentration of (2,3-DPG) is required for optimum oxygen delivery to tissues. However, use of phosphate containing fluids is associated with hypocalcemic tetany and hence is not routinely recommended. Again, early institution of oral feeds, especially with milk replenishes phosphate quite

TABLE 53.6	Insulin therapy in diabetic ketoacidosis

1. IV insulin bolus 10-20 units
2. IV 5-10 units/hours till blood glucose is about 250-300 mg/dl
3. IV 2-5 units/hours till blood glucose is about 200 mg/dl
4. IV 1-2 units/hours plus 6-12 units IV bolus TDS, premeal, when on oral feed and IV fluids are being continued (Basal-bolus plan)
5. SC 6-12 units STAT one hour before stopping IV insulin infusion
6. SC multiple dose (usually 3 doses) regime when IV fluids are being discontinued

IV: Intravenous; SC: Subcutaneous
Note: Link all insulin doses to patient's previous insulin requirements. Always use human regular insulin. Switch patient to multiple SC dose regime when patient is on oral feed.

rapidly. Severe hypophosphatemia (serum level <1.5 mg/dl) is associated with skeletal muscle weakness, respiratory depression and hemolysis. In such situations, phosphate can be replaced conveniently by undertaking one-third of potassium replacement in the form of potassium phosphate.

Insulin Therapy in Diabetic Ketoacidosis[23,24] (Table 53.6)

Insulin therapy is obviously an important aspect of therapy in DKA. However, the blood glucose is known to drop considerably with hydration alone, if undertaken prior to insulin therapy. As DKA is a grave metabolic emergency and the initiating event is insulin deficiency, it will be unwise to withhold insulin either in the initial or subsequent part of its management.

The type of insulin to be used is regular human insulin. At present, these insulins are in extensive use. The immunological insulin resistance observed with conventional insulin is almost never seen with the use of human insulin. Keeping in mind such a possibility, it is advisable to use only human insulin in this emergency. The preferred route of administration of insulin is by continuous intravenous (IV) infusion. Although it is possible to administer insulin in mild DKA by subcutaneous (SC) or IM route, in moderately severe DKA with volume depletion and variable SC insulin absorption, it is better to resort to IV insulin. As insulin half-life is less than 8 minutes, repeated IV boluses are ineffective. On the other hand, if an IV infusion is set-up without a bolus, the desired concentration of plasma insulin (about 100 µU/ml) is achieved only after a lapse of 30 minutes to 2 hours. Considering these facts, the recommended method is to give a small bolus of 10 to 20 units human regular insulin IV and start a drip of insulin at the rate of 5 to 10 units/hour. Some authors have suggested a loading dose of 0.3 to 0.4 U/kg. Some investigations have shown that a loading dose is not required. The present author uses a loading dose and links it with the patients' previous insulin requirement, as this is a measure of patient's insulin sensitivity. About 20% of total daily requirement should be used as a loading dose. We usually link the continuous infusion rate to patient's previous requirements; 5 U/hour is initiated in those needing small insulin doses (<40 units/d) while higher infusion rate is used for those needing larger doses. This appears to be the most rational approach. Several studies have compared low dose insulin regimes with high dose regimes. Low dose regimes reduce the risk of hypokalemia and hypo-glycemia, but in the event of poor response, can be risky. The doses recommended here are somewhere inbetween and employed by most diabetologists. When using insulin by continuous infusion through a simple drip (with some flow regulator like dial-flo) or a syringe-pump (preferable mode), the problem of insulin adsorption is real. There are several methods to obviate this problem:

- Use larger doses (about 30 to 50% more) than required
- To flush about 50 ml of insulin containing fluid rapidly before connecting to patient
- Add human albumin or 5 ml of patient's blood or 2 ml of patient's serum to the IV fluid before adding insulin.

We routinely employ the second method in our patients of DKA or any emergency in diabetic patients calling for insulin infusion.

If fluid overload is the problem, as in DKA with left ventricular failure or renal failure, larger amount of insulin can be used IV, alternatively insulin can be given IM in doses of 5 to 10 units every hour.[25] We do not recommend SC insulin till all metabolic parameters are stabilized. At that point, and about an hour before the discontinuation of IV insulin infusion, a SC dose of 6 to 12 units of regular insulin is given. Thereafter, a multiple dose insulin regime is instituted.

General Management and Supportive Measures

Leukocytosis can occur in DKA and is not necessarily indicative of an infection. However, with a positive diagnosis of infection, appropriate antibiotics are required. In India, gastrointestinal infections, especially food poisoning of all varieties are common precipitating factors and would require treatment with appropriate antibiotics like ciprofloxacin or norfloxacin combined with tinidazole. In patients with vascular episodes or in gravely ill, elderly patients, heparinization has been considered but is not routinely recommended unless the complicating disease itself is a clear indication for heparinization (e.g. thromboembolism). Patients often have an acute gastric dilation; this may be treated by continuous aspiration, augmenting amount of fluids and electrolytes administered (water, Na^+, K^+) and probably using prokinetic drugs. Unconscious patients will require general nursing care. Urinary catheterization is often required in drowsy or unconscious patients with retention or to assess the hourly urinary output.

Metabolic Complications of DKA

Several complications are likely to develop in the course of treatment of DKA. A knowledge of the pathophysio-logy of these complications is essential so that they can be forestalled.

Hypokalemia

If blood glucose is lowered too rapidly and if soda-bicarb is used in large dose, lowering of serum potassium becomes precipitous and life-threatening. In situations where a timely and accurate potassium reading is not available, which may happen in remote areas of our country, it is good to note that whenever blood glucose starts dropping clearly, potassium supplement is called for. If urine output is good at this point, there is no contraindication to instituting a potassium chloride infusion in normal saline or 5% dextrose solution. In a good ICU setting, potassium should be estimated initially and thereafter 2 hourly for the first 12 hours and less frequently thereafter.

Hypoglycemia

This was a known complication until the insulin therapy was rationalized. If large doses of insulin are used in IV boluses, IM or subcutaneously, there is a possibility of hypoglycemia. At times, extra doses of insulin were recommended for continuing acetonuria. Fortunately, such approaches have been abandoned at the present time. Intravenous infusion of insulin is the preferred mode of treatment. When the response starts, the drop of blood glucose is linear and predictable. Once the blood glucose is lowered to 200 mg%, it is advisable to institute a 5% dextrose infusion.

Cerebral Edema

This complication can arise after 4 to 6 hours of successful therapy. The precipitating factors appear to include:[26 -28]

1. A rapid lowering of blood glucose. In well developed DKA, the brain generates some osmolar substances, so called idiogenic osmoles to hold intracellular water in place in the face of grave extracellular hyperosmolarity. With rapid lowering of blood glucose, extracellular osmolarity is reduced and water migrates intracerebrally.

2. Rapid alkalinization reduces oxygen delivery to the tissues including brain or aggravates intracerebral acidosis transiently (*vide supra*, soda-bicarb therapy). This results in cerebral edema. In order to prevent cerebral edema, soda-bicarb should be used judiciously and blood glucose should be lowered slowly. To reiterate a basic principle of metabolic corrections, the time taken to correct an anomaly should be about the same as that taken to develop the anomaly. As DKA usually develops over 24 to 72 hours time (pump withdrawal DKA and a few situations excepted), euglycemia should only be aimed at within 24 to 72 hours time. If a patient is doing well initially regarding the state of consciousness, but starts deteriorating after 4 to 6 hours of treatment, cerebral edema should be suspected. It can be confirmed by venous congestion or mild papilledema in the fundi or by a CT scan. In such a situation, the pace of metabolic corrections should be slowed down. It may be necessary to use mannitol or corticosteroids as anti-edema measures. Recently, hypertonic saline has been used.[29]

Adult Respiratory Distress Syndrome[30, 31]

Use of excessive fluids, especially crystalloids can result in adult respiratory distress syndrome (ARDS). At the time of presentation, a patient of DKA usually has an increased colloid osmotic pressure (COP) because of gross deficits of water and sodium. During the course of treatment the COP falls and creates a tendency towards edema formation. This results in pulmonary edema and a gradual decrease in PO_2, which can easily be monitored by pulse oximetry. It is advisable to recognize this complication early on as a reduction in the volume of crystalloids infused and use of a colloid solution like albumin for infusion can forestall the development of ARDS.

Relapse of DKA

As IV insulin infusions are usually employed in the treatment of DKA at present, a relapse is possible with the cessation of insulin infusion. It is, therefore, considered important to inject insulin SC or IM almost 1 to 2 hours prior to the time at which IV infusion is proposed to be discontinued. It is important to bear in mind that DKA is indicative of total endogenous insulinopenia; hence, assured delivery of insulin is essential at all phases of treatment.

Nonmetabolic Complications of DKA

Infections and vascular events dominate the scene in most elderly patients of DKA. Infections are often located in skin, lungs and urinary tract; e.g. carbuncle, pneumonia, urinary tract or foot infection and can be serious and lead to life-threatening septicemia. Mucormycosis is an interesting but rare type of infection in DKA and should be considered if clinical presentation indicates sinusitis, rhinitis or disturbance of external ocular movement or proptosis. Foot problems are often a combination of vascular occlusion and infection. Patient may present with a major vascular event like myocardial or cerebral infarction. The outcome is often dependent upon the severity of these nonmetabolic complications. Occasionally, a vascular event is precipitated during DKA, probably induced by hypotension, severe dehydration and profound hemobiological changes like sludging, hyperosmolarity, increased platelet aggregation and hyperviscosity.

Prevention and Early Intervention

The prognosis in DKA is strongly related to the severity of metabolic disturbance at the time of presentation. State of consciousness and degree of hyperosmolarity at presentation are important factors. Hence, early detection and intervention is important, which can be most effectively done by patient-education and empowerment and training of primary-care physicians.

Type 1 diabetic patients must know a sick-day routine and should have a rapid access to a knowledgeable physician. They should report to hospital early if they are unsuccessful in combating DKA with a few supplemental doses of insulin or especially if presence of vomiting precludes adequate fluid replacement orally. In the past 10 years, our center has not experienced a single death due to DKA mainly due to these precautions. In this period, all of our patients have been hospitalized in a conscious or drowsy state and have

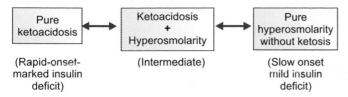

Figure 53.3 Clinical spectrum of DKA and hyperglycemic hyperosmolar nonketotic state

been either ambulatory or transported in a wheel-chair at the time of admission.

HYPERGLYCEMIC HYPEROSMOLAR NONKETOTIC STATE

Hyperglycemic Hyperosmolar Nonketotic State (HHNKS) along with DKA are increasingly being recognized as one of the most serious complications of diabetes mellitus and if misdiagnosed and either untreated or undertreated, it carries a high mortality.[32-39] Whereas DKA is associated predominantly with type 1 diabetes, HHNKS is associated with type 2. But, it is important to realize that any of these metabolic emergencies can occur in any type of diabetes mellitus, irrespective of the age or gender of the patient. It is important for the physician to realize that HHNKS and DKA represent a continuum with DKA at one end of the spectrum and HHNKS at the other **(Figure 53.3)**.

As discussed, DKA with significant hyperosmolarity typically indicates a total absence of insulin (type 1 diabetes), the onset tends to be acute, it is accompanied by modest degrees of hyperglycemia, usually less or around 300 mg/dL and there is invariably evidence of gross ketoacidosis. At the other extreme end of the spectrum, HHNKS typically occurs with lesser degree of insulin deficiency, usually in type 2 diabetes, patients tends to be older, onset is more gradual and there is either no ketoacidosis or mild insignificant ketonemia.[34,40] The most common clinical situation in a hospitalized patient is that of a type 2 diabetic who is ill with some concurrent illness like a stroke, myocardial infarction or acute infection and is found to have severe hyperglycemia and is diagnosed as DKA. Upon closer scrutiny, the patients are found to have only a mild ketonemia and near normal blood pH and are indeed suffering from HHNKS. Not so commonly recognized is the fact that the patient with DKA who has come in a comatose state to the emergency is inevitably suffering from a hyperosmolar state.[41] The estimated prevalence of the intermediate state is about 33%.[41] It is imperative

to recognize that the comatose patient must be treated for the hyperosmolar state and failure to do so is the major cause of mortality in the hyperosmolar-DKA syndrome.[40] Although rare, juvenile patients with type 1 diabetes may present with HHNKS.[42]

Definition

The essential components of HHNKS are:[40]
1. Blood glucose >700 mg/dl.
2. Serum osmolarity >320 mOsm/L or >340 mOsm/L (when patient comatose).
3. Serum bicarbonate >15 mEq/L.
4. Serum pH >7.3.
5. Urinary ketones negative or weak positive.
6. Serum ketones negative in 1 : 4 dilution.

The major criteria is a very high blood glucose associated with markedly elevated serum osmolarity (>340 mOsm/L, if the patient is comatose), with minimal or no ketoacidosis.

Pathogenesis

Partial or complete absence of insulin, initiates the hyperglycemia, which leads to the development of the hyperosmolar state. Insulin deficiency greatly enhances hepatic gluconeogenesis. The resulting excess of glucose is released into the extracellular space, where in the absence of adequate amounts of insulin, glucose can neither be normally transported into the cell, nor can the glucose that enters the cell be normally metabolized. The excess glucose is thereby restricted to the extracellular space. The combined hepatic overproduction and inadequate peripheral utilization of glucose therefore results in progressively increasing hyperglycemia. The amount of insulin needed to prevent lipolysis from the adipose tissue and ketogenesis in the liver is less than that needed to promote glucose utilization in all the sensitive tissues.

As shown in **Figure 53.4**, in HHNKS, there is enough insulin available, which prevents the activation of hormone sensitive lipase and thus prevents lipolysis in the adipose tissue. Similarly, in the liver, excess ketogenesis is prevented as enough insulin is available to counteract the effects of counter-regulatory hormones especially glucagon.[43-46]

Most critical to the understanding of the pathogenesis of HHNKS is the role of hyperglycemia, which on one hand causes osmotic shifts within the body, and on the other hand, causes severe osmotic diuresis with loss of free water and electrolytes from the body.[47,48] These changes are responsible for the hyperosmolar and hypovolemic state and death in the HHNKS.[43,49,50]

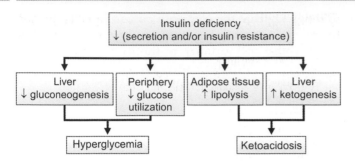

Figure 53.4 Pathophysiology of hyperglycemic hyperosmolar nonketotic state and diabetic ketoacidosis syndrome

As shown, in **Figures 53.4 and 53.5**, early in the course of the development of hyperosmolar state, hyperglycemia is responsible for the osmotic diuresis and for the hyperosmolarity of the extracellular fluid space (ECF). The increased glucose concentration in the ECF in turn causes an osmotic shift of water out of the cells into the smaller extracellular space. The result is a modest loss of extracellular fluid volume. The movement of fluid from the intracellular to the extracellular vascular space serves the important function of providing an "autotransfusion" that is by compensating for the water lost by osmotic diuresis, it initially preserves the vascular volume, thereby preventing hypovolemia and its serious consequences. This phenomena will be later discussed in the section detailing the treatment of HHNKS, since inappropriate therapy can cause reversal of autotransfusion into the vascular space, resulting in severe hypovolemia and death. With increasing hyperglycemia, the renal threshold for

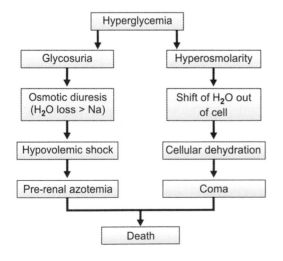

Figure 53.5 Osmotic effects of hyperglycemia

glucose (when further exceeded results in) massive osmotic diuresis with increasing loss of water and potassium in urine. As a result, both intracellular and extracellular dehydration results **(Figure 53.5)**. At this last stage of HHNKS, transfer of water from the intracellular to the extracellular space is no longer adequate to maintain the vascular volume. This results in cellular dehydration including brain dehydration and coma. An increasing loss of volume from the extracellular space leads to hypovolemic shock or vascular collapse. Either or both of these consequences may be responsible for a fatal outcome **(Figure 53.5)**.

The important point emphasized so far is that the coma in HHNKS or for that matter in DKA, is the result of hyperglycemia and the consequent hyperosmolarity and is not linked to acidosis.[43,49,50] Fulltop et al[42] and others[40,49,50] have demonstrated that there is no correlation between serum pH and either mental status or mortality in patients with HHNKS-DKA syndrome. By contrast, there is a very good correlation between depression of the sensorium and serum glucose levels. More significantly, plasma osmolarity is very closely related with degree of obtundation. In fact, various studies[40,43,49] demonstrate that coma does not occur until the plasma osmolarity exceeds approximately 340 mOsm/L. This means that if a patient with DKA presents in a coma and has a calculated serum osmolarity of 310 mOsm/L, the coma is not due to DKA or HHNKS and another cause, e.g. stroke or meningitis, must be sought for.

Osmolarity is readily calculated at the bedside by the formula shown in **Box 53.1**. Note that a value of 20 rather than the actual molecular weight of glucose (180/10), is used to convert glucose from milligrams per deciliter to milliequivalents per liter. In addition to making it easier to calculate, the value 20 more accurately reflects the osmotic activity of the glucose molecule.

In clinical situations, one should use the bedside calculation of effective osmolarity rather than the freezing point depression method to obtain the estimate of osmolarity.[47] **Figure 53.6** shows how that in a decompensated diabetic state, the lack of insulin aggravated

Box 53.1: Calculation of serum osmolarity
$2\,(Na + K)\,(mOsm/L) + \dfrac{Glucose\ (mg/dl)}{20}$
$=$ "Effective" Osmolarity (mOsm/L)

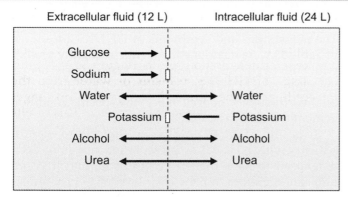

Figure 53.6 Compartmentalization of osmotically active molecules in insulin deficient states

TABLE 53.7	Precipitating factors in HHNKS-DKA syndrome

1. Too little insulin
2. Infection (even minor)
3. Severe stress (physical or emotional)
4. Hypokalemia (usually diuretic induced)
5. Renal failure
6. Inadequate fluid intake:
   - Old age (reduced sensitivity to thirst)
   - Infancy (poor access to water)
   - Incapacitation occurring at any age (poor access to water)

by severe insulin resistance, prevents glucose from entering the intracellular space, and the glucose is confined to the smaller extracellular space, resulting in more severe hyperglycemia. Sodium, even under normal conditions, does not enter the intracellular space to a significant extent. By contrast, urea, alcohol and a number of other compounds that are measured by freezing point depression method of determining osmolarity, pass freely back and forth between the extracellular and intracellular spaces. Thus, these molecules are not osmotically active and are thus clinically irrelevant. The "calculated" osmolarity includes only the osmotically effective molecules (glucose, sodium, and perhaps potassium), but the "measured" osmolarity includes many molecules that do not play a role in producing cellular dehydration.[40]

Thus, a patient of type 2 DM, aged 50 years who presents with fever and a measured osmolarity of 345 mOsm/L but a calculated osmolarity of 310 mOsm/L, is not comatose due to HHNKS, but is more likely to have meningitis or such other complications leading to coma.

Precipitating Factors

As already mentioned, inadequate insulin therapy, infection and an acute cardiovascular event can precipitate either DKA or HHNKS (**Table 53.7**). Special mention, however must be made of certain precipitating factors, which are more likely to precipitate HHNKS. Stress, usually physical, but occasionally emotional, can precipitate HHNKS by causing an increase in catecholamines and cortisol. Hypokalemia is an important cause. It aggravates the hyperglycemic state by reducing insulin secretion as well as by decreasing insulin sensitivity.[30] More often than not, hypokalemia is a consequence of osmotic diuresis and diuretic abuse.

A major and probably essential factor in producing HHNKS is the inability of the patient to sense the need for, or have access to water. The patient may either suppress or not recognize thirst, or the patient may be unable to obtain water because of a physical disability (e.g. in the very young or the very old). There is evidence that the thirst center may become less sensitive with age.[40] Additionally, once established, the hyperosmolar state may suppress the sensitivity to insulin, there by initiating a vicious cycle. Antidiuretic hormone secretion reaches a maximum at an osmolarity of about 295 mOsm/L, thereafter thirst and increased water intake, normally serve as the only protection against more severe hyperosmolarity. It is difficult, if not impossible, to produce hyperosmolar coma in the patient who can obtain and drink adequate amounts of water.[45]

In hospitalized, mentally obtunded patients or tube-fed patients, inadequate supply of water can occur, unless there are clear instructions to provide appropriate amounts of free water in the tube-feeding plan. This factor coupled with use of drugs listed in **Table 53.8** form the two commonest precipitating causes of HHNKS.

A large number of commonly used drugs can precipitate HHNKS (**Table 53.8**). Thiazide diuretic

TABLE 53.8	Drugs than can precipitate HHNKS	
Drugs	*Effects*	
1. Cortisone	Decreased insulin secretion, increased insulin resistance	
2. Thiazides	"	
3. Furosemide	Decreased insulin secretion, Increased water loss	
4. Dilantin sodium	"	
5. Beta blockers	"	
6. Calcium channel blockers	"	
7. Alcohol	Subclinical pancreatitis	

induces hypokalemia, which in turn causes hypergly-cemia by reducing insulin secretion and inducing hormone resistance. Propranolol and other β-blockers decrease insulin secretion, as does dilantin sodium. Calcium channel blockers also reduce insulin secretion. Alcohol may act by producing subclinical pancreatitis. On the other hand, given the large number of patients who simultaneously receive a thiazide diuretic, calcium channel blocker and β-blocker, HHNKS or DKA is rare. However, they can induce this condition, singly or in combination.

Corticosteroid use is probably the most common iatrogenic cause of HHNKS. Cortisol induces a marked peripheral resistance to insulin. Deaths have been reported due to HHNKS in patients not known to be diabetic at the time they receive cortisol.[52] In addition, to inducing peripheral resistance, cortisol may also be instrumental in the production of ketone bodies by the liver and it is unlikely that significant DKA-HHNKS occurs in hypoadrenal states (e.g. Schmidt's syndrome), wherein both insulin and cortisol are deficient. There is a case report of HHNKS being precipitated by lithium-induced diabetes insipidus.[53] HHNKS has also been reported in central diabetes insipidus.[54]

Mortality

Mortality rate in HHNKS approaches 20 to 40% as compared to 3 to 9% in DKA.[55,56] This is explained by severe concomitant complications and older age. Inappropriate therapy (inadequate fluid replacement) and associated vascular complications (myocardial infarction, strokes and thrombosis in lower extremities) contribute to both morbidity and mortality.

TABLE 53.9	Major signs and symptoms of HHNKS: Hyper-glycemic hyperosmolar nonketotic state; DKA: Diabetic ketoacidosis syndrome

- In 50–60% of HHNKS, hyperosmolar coma is the first sign of diabetes
- Dehydration can be manifested by thirst, decreased turgor, soft eyeballs and orthostasis (HHNKS)
- Temperature is usually normal or low, but if elevated, infection is usually present
- Stupor, coma and convulsions are more common in HHNKS, than in DKA
- Kussmaul breathing indicating pH <7.2 (DKA)
- Abdominal pain is present in at least 30% patients (DKA-HHNKS)
- Vomiting is seen in 50–60% of patients (DKA). Causes further dehydration. May precipitate hyperosmolar state

Clinical Features

The major signs and symptoms of HHNKS are shown in **Table 53.9**. As mentioned, patients frequently present with both hyperosmolar coma and ketoacidosis; hence, the symptoms of the two are combined, but depending on their frequency of occurrence, the specific condition is mentioned in parenthesis.

It is important to emphasize that, 50 to 60% of patients with HHNKS at presentation have not been diagnosed to have diabetes mellitus earlier. It is not unusual, therefore, for the diagnosis of hyperosmolar coma to be seriously delayed until the elevated plasma glucose suggests the correct diagnosis.[54-59]

The signs and symptoms of HHNKS linked to hyperosmolarity induced dehydration are thirst, decreased turgor, soft eyeballs, hypotension and orthostasis **(Table 53.9)**. It is worth emphasizing that hyperosmolar state or ketoacidosis do not cause an elevation of body temperature. Presence of fever in a comatose or acidotic diabetic patient is an indication of infection, which usually is the precipitating factor.

Obtundation, stupor, coma and generalized or partial seizures are characteristic of severe HHNKS and are rarely, if ever, observed in pure DKA.[50,57] Kussmaul respiration, abdominal pain and vomiting are more often linked to DKA.

The laboratory data observed in HHNKS is shown in **Table 53.10**. Marked hyperglycemia, usually greater than 800 mg/dl, is typical of hyperosmolar coma, and a total osmolarity above 340 mOsm/L is required for coma to be present. For all practical purposes, coma is never seen till this level of hyperosmolarity is attained. For the hyperosmolar state a serum osmolarity of

TABLE 53.10	Laboratory abnormalities in HHNKS
Plasma glucose	>700 mg/dl
Hyperosmolarity	340 mOsm/L
	(>320 mOsm/L-significant 280–295 mOsm/L-normal)
Sodium	Low, normal or high, but total body sodium always low
Potassium	Normal or high
Urine ketones	Nil or mild+
pH	>7.3
Bicarbonate	>15 mEq/L
Temperature	Normal or low
Leukocytosis	15,000–40,000 cells/mm^3 in DKA even without infection. Normal in pure HHNKS

320 mOsm/L is sufficient and this warrants a prompt therapeutic response to prevent onset of coma.

Serum sodium may be low, normal or high; however, total body sodium is always low. Potassium maybe normal or high, but again there is total body potassium deficit. Serum ketones, if measured, are below 7 mm/L and serum bicarbonate more that 15 mEq/L and pH is usually more or equal to 7.3. Contrary findings suggest an acidotic state, either DKA or the intermediate syndrome. As noted temperature is normal, unless an infection is present. Pure HHNKS does not affect the leukocyte count, however, DKA or acidosis can cause severe leukocytosis (15,000 to 40,000/cells/mm^3 with a marked shift to the left). Leukocytosis, therefore, *per se*, does not indicate infection.

Management of HHNKS

Fluid Replacement

The principle of treatment is to correct the hyperosmolar state and dehydration that is primarily responsible for coma and death in this syndrome. Hyperosmolarity is simply treated by rapidly correcting the water deficit. The electrolytes are replaced with saline containing potassium. The hyperglycemia is corrected primarily by fluid replacement,[58,59] as well as with insulin. Ketones and acidosis, if at all associated, are simultaneously corrected by the same measures.

The importance of adequate fluid replacement during insulin therapy cannot be over emphasized.[33,37,56-61] If insulin is administered to the hyperosmolar patient without simultaneously correcting the fluid deficit, glucose and water move from the vascular space into the cells and the "autotransfusion" described earlier is reversed.[40] The result is an acute loss of vascular volume, worsening of the hypernatremia, shock and increased mortality **(Figure 53.7)**.

Adequate fluid replacement is defined as replacing one-half of the water deficit in the first five hours. The average water deficit in the patient with hyperosmolar coma, with or without acidosis, is about 10% of the total body weight. A 50 kg patient with total body water would therefore have a deficit of about 5 liters and should receive a net intake of about 3 liters of water during the first five hours that is approximately 750 ml per hour. A recommended protocol for fluid replacement in HHNKS is shown in **Table 53.11**.

The choice between normal saline or one-half normal saline as the vehicle for fluid replacement is controversial.[16-18] It is reasonable to employ normal saline if the serum sodium is decreased or the patient is hypotensive. If serum sodium is elevated, initial fluid

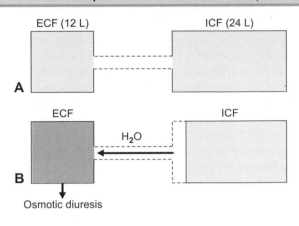

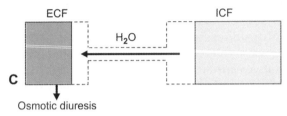

Figure 53.7 Fluid balance in hyperglycemic hyperosmolar state

A. Normal glycemia and hydration
B. Early: Extracellular fluid (ECF) is hyperosmolar, causing H$_2$O to shift from intracellular fluid (ICF) to ECF– an autotranfusion
C. Late: Continued osmotic diuresis cause dehydration, volume loss and hyperosmolarity in both ECF and ICF

TABLE 53.11	Fluid replacement in HHNKS

- Estimated H$_2$O deficit 10% of body weight
- Replace 50% of deficit in the first five hours
  A. Normal saline if:
     i. Hypotensive
     ii. Na <140 mEq/L
  B. One-half normal saline if:
     i. Na >145 mEq/L
     ii. Patient normotensive

Rate	Hours	Volume
	½–1	1L
	2	1 L
	3	500 ml-1L
	4	500 ml-1L
	5	500 ml-1L
	Total 1st 5 hours	3.5–5 L
	6th–12th hour	250–500 ml/hr

replacement should consist of one-half normal saline, followed by normal saline when the sodium returns to normal; or preferably dextrose solution when blood glucose is controlled or alternatively free water orally or through nasogastric tube. As vast majority of patients are conscious or in mentally obtunded patients where nasogastric tube is in place, it is possible to give water orally. This simplifies the fluid therapy considerably.

The rate of fluid replacement, as noted, is critical. There is almost unanimity in the literature that at least 1 to 2 liters of fluid should be administered in the first hour.[33,35,37,39,40,58,60] This is irrespective of age or associated disease. If physicians persist in correcting at the rate of 150 to 250 ml hour, the result is that 24 hours later, the serum osmolarity, far from being corrected, actually increases and the patient remains comatose. There are two major reasons why physicians are reluctant to infuse fluids rapidly in-patients with HHNKS; firstly, the fear of causing congestive heart failure and secondly the fear of causing cerebral edema. Literature does not support the concept that fluid replacement in the severely dehydrated patient causes congestive cardiac failure.[36,40,58,60] The one exception to this may be in the severely acidotic patient, since, it is well established that acidosis from any cause leads to segregation of fluid in the pulmonary bed. However, acidosis is usually never severe in HHNKS. Additionally, a large number of studies, reviewed by Rosenbloom[59] have documented that cerebral edema in HHNKS-DKA syndrome is unrelated to either the rate of fluid replacement or the rate of correction of hypernatremia or hyperglycemia. Finally, cerebral edema is not related to the tonicity of the hydrating solution. Assessment of the patient's hydration status during therapy is made by clinical evaluation. One has to judge hydration by evaluating turgor, blood pressure, degree of orthostasis, monitoring of central venous pressure and urinary output as well as reckoning of the fluid balance with meticulous care. Serum glucose and sodium, corrected or uncorrected are of much less value in determining the patient's state of hydration.

Insulin

While insulin therapy is less critical in the HHNKS, yet it should be instituted immediately after establishing the diagnosis. The principles and the dosage followed are the same as that for DKA and are shown in **Table 53.6.** When serum glucose levels decrease to about 250 to 300 mg/dl, 5% glucose in saline is to be infused at the rate of 250 to 500 ml/hour. Insulin drip must however continue at the rate of 1 to 2 U/hour to maintain a blood glucose of approximately 200 mg/dl. The same weaning of regimen from intravenous to subcutaneous should be followed as advised for DKA.

The replacement of potassium is as for DKA. Acidosis is never prominent in HHNKS, hence, bicarbo-

TABLE 53.12	Complications of HHNKS

1. Infections: Urinary tract, pneumonia (aspiration and linked to dehydration), pancreatitis
2. Disseminated intravascular coagulopathy
3. Venous and arterial thrombosis: (e.g. femoral arterial occlusion)
4. Myocardial infarction
5. Cerebrovascular accident
6. Hypoglycemia
7. Hypokalemia
8. Cerebral edema

nate therapy has no role to play. Phosphates and magnesium are rarely required except when phosphates level is less than 1.5 mEq/L, one can either give potassium phosphate (one-third of potassium replacement) or potassium hydrogen phosphate. There is, however, justifiable concern that intravenous phosphate will lower both serum calcium and cause metastatic calcium phosphate deposits in soft tissues. Early oral replacement of phosphate (in the form of milk) is preferred.

Complications

There are a number of complications that may accompany or follow the successful treatment of HHNKS. The metabolic complications are similar to those in DKA, except that in the absence of severe acidosis, pulmonary complications such as collection of fluid in the pulmonary vascular bed and ARDS are less common. However, few other complications tend to predominate **(Table 53.12).**

The extent of the complications is probably directly related to the duration of symptoms and inversely related to the rate at which the hyperosmolar state is reversed.[40,59] Urinary tract infections may occur due to poor flow and pneumonia may be due to dehydration or aspiration, the result of the obtunded state or hyperosmolar state induced convulsions. Obviously, infection can be a precipitating factor or a complication of the HHNKS.

Pancreatitis can likewise both precipitate and complicate the hyperosmolar state. There is very marked hypertriglyceridemia, which, may be a contributory to hyperosmolarity. Hyperosmolarity *per se*, perhaps due to impairment of blood flow to the pancreas may cause pancreatitis,[10] and this may be obvious a day or two after the patient has regained consciousness.

Disseminated intravascular coagulopathy has been reported following an episode of HHNKS. Arterial thrombosis, myocardial infarction, stroke, and femoral arterial thrombosis have been noted, following an episode of HHNKS. Cerebral edema is occasionally observed, but is not linked to the rate or amount of fluid administered.

There is good data demonstrating that the prompt recognition of the HHNKS and institution of adequate therapy has consistently reduced the mortality and complications of this potentially disastrous complication of diabetes mellitus.[33,40]

LACTIC ACIDOSIS

Explosive in onset and often unyielding to therapy, lactic acidosis usually reflects the presence of an underlying disorder that, if left untreated, leads to death. Lactic acidosis has the poorest prognosis amongst all of the acute metabolic complications of diabetes mellitus. Thus, it is extremely important to prevent this condition and we should also be able to detect it early, so that remediable measures can be instituted prior to the onset of irreversible damage.

Definition: For the sake of convenience, lactic acidosis is defined as a metabolic acidosis in which the arterial blood lactate equals or exceeds 5 mmol/L (45 mg/dl) and the arterial pH is below 7.35. Regardless of the specific biochemical criteria, it should be emphasized that lactic acidosis may not necessarily produce "acidemia", depending upon (i) the magnitude of hyperlactatemia, (ii) the buffering capacity of the body, and (iii) the coexistence of other conditions (e.g. liver disease, sepsis) that predispose to tachypnea and alkalosis. Thus hyper-lactatemia is synonymous with lactic acidosis and may be associated with acidemia, a normal pH, or alkalemia. The typical laboratory findings associated with lactic acidosis are shown in **Table 53.13**.[64,65]

Pathogenesis

The lactate ion arises from the reduction of pyruvate. Lactate dehydrogenase (LDH) catalyzes the reversible formation and removal of lactate in all cells.

$$\text{Pyruvate} + \text{NADH} + \text{H}^+ \leftrightarrow \text{Lactate} + \text{NAD}^-$$

TABLE 53.13	Laboratory findings typically associated with lactic acidosis

- Elevated anion gap
- Hyperuricemia
- Hyperphosphatemia
- Leukocytosis
- Normokalemia

In the healthy, rested, overnight-fasted adults, the basal lactate concentration usually ranges between 0.75 to 1 mmol/L (6.8 to 9.0 mg/dl). It has been estimated that under basal conditions, whole body lactate production by healthy adults averages 0.8 mmol per kg body weight per hour, or about 1400 mmol per 70 kg per human per 24 hours.[60] Major sources of lactate production include skin, erythrocytes, brain, skeletal muscles and intestinal mucosa.[61,63] Pyruvate, the basic metabolite for lactate production is derived mainly from oxidation of lactate via LDH, from proteolysis by a variety of dehydrogenation and transamination reactions and from glycolysis by the Embden-Meyerhof pathway. Six amino acids (alanine, cysteine, glycine, serine, threonine and tryptophan) provide the protein derived carbon backbones for pyruvate formation. In the basal state proteolysis contributes about 15% of the lactate generated intracellularly.[60,62] The largest and quantitatively the most important pathway for pyruvate genesis is from glycolysis. Glycolysis occurs in the cytoplasm at a rate largely determined by three unidirectional reactions catalyzed by hexokinase (HK), 6-phosphofructokinase (PFK) and pyruvate kinase (PK). Of these, PFK is the most important. Glycolysis *per se* does not produce lactic acid, but provides its conjugate base, lactate, ATP and water. Hydrolysis of ATP in turn generates protons in an amount stoichiometrically equivalent to that of lactate. The major source of lactate generation is anaerobic glycolysis when one mole of glucose generates 2 moles of ATP and 2 moles of lactate.[63]

Approximately 1400 mmol of lactic acid is produced endogenously and consumed daily by a typical human being. Diffusion of 1400 mmol of acid into the ECF destroys 1400 mmol of $NaHCO_3$, converting the alkali to sodium lactate. Hepatic oxidation of extracted sodium lactate regenerates lost bicarbonate in this cyclical process. In the healthy state, lactate production is balanced by lactate removal. When there is plentiful supply of oxygen to tissues, the metabolism of pyruvate is primarily oxidative rather than reductive. Pyruvate in the presence of PDH is converted to acetyl coenzyme A in the mitochondria. This is then further incorporated into the tricarboxylic acid (TCA) cycle and leads to generation of 38 moles of ATP, compared to 2 moles of ATP when only anaerobic glycolysis occurs and lactate is the end-product. Consumption of lactate by oxidative reactions occurs in all cells except erythrocytes, which lack mitochondria. The other major routes for lactate removal are via biosynthetic mechanisms, involving either the decarboxylation of pyruvate to acetyl-CoA or via net synthesis of glucose from pyruvate. Quantitatively the most important nonoxidative process of lactate removal is by gluconeogenesis by the liver and to a lesser extent, the kidney cortex. Here, it is either reduced to glucose or oxidized to carbon dioxide and water. The liver accounts for approximately 50% and the kidneys for about 30% of the whole body lactate uptake in the resting state.[62]

During fasting, neoglucogenesis assumes the major route of lactate use (at least in the liver), and the glucose released into the circulation becomes available for uptake and catabolism by peripheral tissues. Lactate released by these tissues then serves as a substrate for hepatic and renal glucose synthesis. This process of carbon shuttling between sites of a glucose synthesis and anaerobic glycolysis is called Cori's cycle. Lactate uptake by liver and kidney is concentration-dependent and is saturable and both organs can respond to hyperlactatemia by increasing lactate extraction by several folds above the basal rates. When the renal threshold for lactate is reached, excretion becomes another mechanism for lactate removal. The operation of the Cori's cycle also involves the continual production (via glycolysis) and removal (via oxidative phosphorylation) of hydrogen ions and thus is crucial for maintaining the acid-base equilibrium. Protons liberated in the cytoplasm by the hydrolysis of ATP during glycolysis are used by the mitochondrial respiratory chain for synthesis of new ATP, available to drive such undergoing processes such as gluconeogenesis. Thus, hepatic and renal functional adequacy is of paramount importance in lactate homeostasis. Failure of these two organs either singly or jointly associated with anaerobic conditions (hypoxia, septicemia, etc.) will definitely lead to life-threatening lactic acidosis.[63]

In summary, hyperlactatemia or lactic acidosis will result when its production exceeds its use or disposal. From the above discussion it is obvious that:
1. Mitochondrial oxygen supply determines the efficiency by which substrate fuels are oxidized and energy is generated.
2. The liver plays a pivotal role in both the production and use of lactate and hydrogen ions and in maintaining whole body acid-base balance.
3. Lactic acidosis results from a fundamental disorder of pyruvate metabolism, of which hyperlactatemia is an indicator, and from an imbalance between ATP hydrolysis and ATP production.

Considerable hyperuricemia is often associated with lactic acidosis because lactate competes with urate for secretion by the renal tubules, thereby competitively reducing urate excretion.[66] Hyperphosphatemia results from widespread cellular efflux due to persistent, unreplenished ATP hydrolysis and tissue hypoxia.[67] Acidemia-induced catecholamine release prompts demargination of white blood corpuscles, causing leukocytosis.[68] Lactic acidosis typically does not cause hyperkalemia. Unlike mineral acidic ions (e.g. HCl), the lactate ion more readily permeates the cell membranes. This cellular entry prevents the development of electrical gradients resulting from isolated H^+ entry into the cells, which would favor extrusion of cationic K^+ down the electrochemical gradient.[69]

Blood samples for lactate assays should be collected in tubes containing 10 mg of sodium fluoride and 2 mg of potassium oxalate, or rapidly precipitated with perchloric acid, to avoid *in vitro* lactate synthesis by red blood cells. Samples should be kept on ice until plasma is separated from unprecipitated specimen. This should be done within 15 minutes of collection.[70]

Most cases of lactic acidosis are considered to be acquired **(Table 53. 14)**. This is in contrast to congenital lactic acidosis which is caused by a wide array of inborn errors of metabolism that are due to genetic defects in gluconeogenesis, PDH, TCA cycle or the respiratory chain.[70]

Acquired lactic acidosis has been conventionally classified into type A (due to tissue hypoxia) and type B in which factors other than tissue hypoxia are the primary cause.[62,71] However, in a clinical setting, patients with lactic acidosis can rarely be classified as purely hypoxic (type A) or nonhypoxic (type B), as by the time lactic acidosis is diagnosed, multiple precipitating or exacerbating causes can be identified and these are inexorably linked. As a result, most cases of lactic acidosis, on diagnosis, are best classified as mixtures of type A and type B and reflect problems in both the production and removal of lactate and protons.[63]

Adverse Consequences of Lactic Acidemia

Severe acidosis is defined as pH <7.2. The adverse consequences of severe acidosis are listed in **Table 53.15**. These consequences are not linked to the cause of acidosis and can occur in metabolic, respiratory or mixed forms of acidoses. The effects on the cardiovascular system are especially life-threatening and include hypotension, decreased cardiac output, centralization or pooling of blood volume and reduced hepatic and renal blood flow. Of special note is the increased likelihood of re-entrant arrhythmias and a reduced threshold for ventricular fibrillation, while the defibrillation threshold remains unaltered. Acidosis triggers a

TABLE 53.14	Classification of acquired lactic acidosis

Type A: Due to tissue hypoxia
1. Tissue hypoperfusion
   - Abnormal vascular tone or permeability
   - Left ventricular failure
   - Decreased cardiac output
   - Massive catecholamine excess
2. Reduced arterial oxygen content
   - Asphyxia
   - Hypoxia (PaO_2 <35 mm of Hg)
   - Carbon monoxide poisoning
   - Life-threatening anemia

Type B: Not due to tissue hypoxia
1. Common disorders
   - Sepsis
   - Hepatic failure
   - Renal failure
   - Diabetes mellitus
   - Cancer
   - Malaria
   - Cholera
2. Drugs or toxins
   - Biguanides
   - Ethanol
   - Salicylates
   - Methanol
   - Ethylene glycol
   - Cyanide
   - Nitroprusside
   - Niacin
   - Catecholamines
   - Diethylether
   - Papavarine
   - Paracetamol
   - Nalidixic acid
   - Isoniazid
   - Streptozotocin
   - Sorbitol, xylitol, fructose
   - Parenteral nutrition
   - Lactulose
   - Theophylline
   - Cocaine
   - Vitamin deficiency
   - Paraldehyde
3. Other conditions
   - Strenuous muscular exercise
   - Grand mal seizures
   - D-lactic acidosis
   - Hypoglycemia

TABLE 53.15	Major adverse consequences of severe acidemia

1. *Cardiovascular*
   - Impairment of cardiac contractility
   - Arteriolar dilatation, venoconstriction and centralization of blood volume
   - Increased pulmonary vascular resistance
   - Reduction in cardiac output, arterial blood pressure, hepatic and renal blood flow
   - Sensitization to re-entrant arrhythmias and reduction in threshold of ventricular fibrillation
   - Attenuation of cardiovascular responses to catecholamines
2. *Respiratory*
   - Hyperventilation
   - Reduced strength of respiratory muscles and muscle fatigue
   - Dyspnea
3. *Metabolic*
   - Increased metabolic demands
   - Insulin resistance
   - Inhibition of anaerobic glycolysis
   - Reduction of ATP synthesis
   - Hyperkalemia
   - Increased protein degradation
4. *Cerebral*
   - Inhibition of metabolism and cell volume regulation
   - Obtundation and coma

Although metabolic demands may be augmented by the associated sympathetic surge, acidemia decreases the uptake of glucose in tissues by inducing insulin resistance and inhibits anaerobic glycolysis by depressing PFK activity. This has grave consequences on survival, as anaerobic glycolysis is the main source of energy during hypoxia. The uptake of lactate by the liver is curtailed and the liver can be converted from the premier consumer of lactate to a net producer. Acidemia promotes potassium egress from the cells leading to hyperkalemia. Brain metabolism and the regulation of its volume are impaired, resulting to progressive obtundation and coma.

Diabetes Mellitus and Lactic Acidosis

Diabetes mellitus sets the stage for lactate accumulation in several ways.[73] Insulin normally activates PDH, the rate-limiting enzyme for the oxidation of pyruvate. Insulinopenia causes a build up of pyruvate, which in turn is converted to lactate. Insulin deficiency also provokes muscle catabolism, providing more alanine to serve as additional substrate for pyruvate synthesis. About 10 to 15% of

sympathetic discharge but also progressively attenuates the effects of catecholamines on the heart and vasculature. Thus, at pH less than 7.2, the direct effects of acidemia predominate.[72]

Box 53.2: Normal anion gap
$Na^+ - (Cl^- + HCO_3^-) = 8\text{-}16$
$(Na^+ + K^+) - (Cl + HCO_3) = 12\text{-}20$

acutely ill diabetic patients have blood lactate levels greater than 5 mmol/L and the diabetic predisposition to lactic acidosis seems particularly more heightened during ketoacidotic episodes. This may be attributed to an inhibitory effect of ketones on hepatic lactate uptake.[56,65] Increase in $NAD/NADH^+$ ratio, hypoperfusion and an increase in H^+ concentration accompanying the volume depletion and the acidemia of DKA, all lead to lactate accumulation. Thus, it is not surprising that lactic acidosis can be observed in any acute metabolic emergency linked with any type of diabetes mellitus. In diabetic ketoacidosis (more often in type 1 diabetes), the presence of a high anion gap **(Box 53.2)** in the absence of significant ketonemia should make one suspect an associated lactic acidosis. Ideally, this should be confirmed by an arterial plasma lactate level, and active remedial measures must be taken.

Diabetic ketoacidosis is often linked with hypoxia (either as a complication of uncontrolled or prolonged ketoacidosis or as a precipitating cause such as fulminant pneumonia). Further acidosis *per se* induces insulin resistance, inhibits PFK activity, inhibits anaerobic glycolysis and leads to depressed cardiac output, central blood pooling, reduced hepatic plus renal blood flow and hypotension, all of which contribute to causation of lactic acidosis. In this situation, the hepatic extraction of lactate is markedly inhibited, rather the liver itself becomes a net lactate producer. Further, reduced renal blood flow impairs the excretion of lactate.

In hyperglycemic hyperosmolar nonketotic state (HHNKS), acidosis is usually not marked. If present, lactic acidosis needs exclusion. Often HHNKS is precipitated by myocardial infarction and renal failure, both conditions tending to favor lactic acidosis. Further, severe volume loss and hypotension also contribute to hyperlactatemia. Patients with type 2 diabetes frequently have very mild hyperlactatemia under basal conditions,[73] a condition which has been attributed to a defect in pyruvate oxidation. Hyperlactatemia during ketoacidosis may be due, in part, to an inhibitory effect of ketones on hepatic lactate uptake.[74] Biguanides, especially phenformin has been linked with membrane dysfunction of renal and hepatic mitochondria, which can lead to lactic acidosis. This is discussed further below.

Biguanides and Lactic Acidosis

Biguanides are guanidine derivatives of which three compounds, phenformin, buformin and metformin have glucose lowering activity. Of these, phenformin and metformin have found maximal clinical application.

Phenformin and Lactic Acidosis

Phenformin (phenethyl biguanide) was widely used in our country till recently. It has been clearly linked with lactic acidosis. Phenformin was withdrawn from several countries in the seventies because of the high-risk of lactic acidosis associated with it.[75,76] The frequently fatal side effect was a consequence of their capacity to bind to mitochondrial membranes and uncouple oxidative phosphorylation.[77] Metformin binds poorly to mitochondrial membranes and is therefore associated with a ten-fold reduced risk of lactic acidosis.[78] The blood glucose lowering potential of phenformin appears to be related, in part, to its ability to enhance the rate of glucose utilization in the peripheral tissues and increase the conversion of glucose to lactate. Phenformin may also inhibit pyruvate oxidation to acetyl-CoA.[79,80] Experimental models of phenformin induced lactic acidosis have demonstrated that extra- hepatic splanchnic lactate production was increased and hepatic uptake was reduced, due to a fall in the portal vein blood flow.[71,81] Although phenformin may increase blood lactate modestly in the basal state, most cases of phenformin-induced lactic acidosis were attributed to either high drug levels (due to overdose or failure of renal excretion) or the consequences of serious illnesses (renal failure, shock), that themselves predispose to acidosis.[82,83]

Raised pyruvate levels may be related to defective utilization of pyruvate caused by the partial inhibition of the TCA cycle. This in turn may be linked to phenformin-induced inhibition of certain essential enzymes such as succinic dehydrogenase and the cytochrome oxidases.[84,85] In order to maintain supply of ATP, enhanced glycolytic conversion of glucose to pyruvate occurs. Diminished gluconeogenesis may also contribute to the fall in blood glucose levels, since intermediates of TCA cycle are needed for gluconeogenesis. An alternate theory explains the elevation of blood pyruvate and lactate as a consequence of enhanced activity of the hexose monophosphate shunt. It has been further hypothesized that the liver is unable to utilize the excess lactate due to changes in its pH. The fall in the hepatic pH is probably brought about by the direct effect of the drug.[86]

Lactate Adaptation

Although phenformin induced lactic acidosis was widely reported from the West, reports from the Indian subcontinent reflected otherwise.[87] Hardly any or only a few cases were reported, while the drug was very widely used. This low incidence has been attributed to a high carbohydrate intake, suboptimal doses of phenformin and lesser prevalence of concurrent alcohol intake in the Indian population.[86] To elucidate this phenomena, a series of patients were studied on phenformin therapy. Lactate levels were estimated prior to and after four weeks of treatment with phenformin. In another group, lactate levels were estimated in patients who had been on phenformin for more than six months.[88,89] It was observed that a significant proportion of patients demonstrated hyperlactatemia on initiation of therapy. However, after six months of therapy, the blood lactate levels came back to normal. This implies that on prolonged therapy, the blood lactate levels drop because of a process of adaptation. The exact mechanism of this adaptive process is not known, but may be linked to altered drug pharmacokinetics. It is possible that under adverse circumstances like increasing the dose of phenformin, hypoxic insult, renal, cardiac or hepatic failure, this adaptation in a previously compensated patient breaks down leading to lactic acidosis. Genetically conferred defect in hepatic hydroxylation impedes the metabolism of phenformin.[88] This subset of patients develop brisk hyperlactatemia following phenformin and are especially prone to lactic acidosis. It is possible that such patients who have a brisk hyperlactatemia on initiation of phenformin therapy, may have adverse clinical reactions and may thus discontinue the medication. Therefore, these patients may have been inadvertently excluded from the study.[90]

Metformin and Lactic Acidosis

Metformin (N-1,6-dimethyl biguanide) is a bisubstituted guanidine with two polar methyl groups.[91,92]

Phospholipids are considered to be the primary and unspecific binding site for the nonpolar side chain of metformin and the drug may exert a variety of metabolic effects via alteration of biological membrane functions.[77,92] The bioavailability of ingested metformin is only 50 to 60% and peak plasma concentration of about 10 mmol/L are reached about two hours of ingestion of 500 to 1000 mg of the drug.[93,94] Very high concentrations of the drug accumulate in the intestinal wall.[95,96] Metformin does not bind to plasma proteins and is excreted unmetabolized in the urine and partially in the feces. The estimated elimination half-life is 2 to 5 hours.[96,97] As mentioned, metformin binds poorly to mitochondrial membranes in contrast to phenformin. Consequently, it improves insulin stimulated nonoxidative glucose metabolism, whereas glucose oxidation remains more or less unaffected.[98-100] Phenformin, on the other hand, has a clear inhibitory effect on glucose oxidation.[77] **Table 53.16** enlists the predominant differences between phenformin and metformin regarding their potential to cause lactic acidosis. between phenformin and metformin. This is linked with marked reduction in the incidence of hyperlactatemia, which is ten-fold lower than with phenformin.[78]

The prevalence of metformin-induced lactic acidosis is estimated to be about 0.24 cases per 10,000 patient-years[101] in contrast to phenformin, with which a rate of 1.5 cases per 10,000 patient-years was reported. In a recent study, Brown et al[102] found only 10 cases amongst 41,000 person-year usage; of these, four were confirmed, three were possible and three were borderline cases of lactic acidosis. All of them had at least one medical condition that could have caused lactic acidosis on its own. Berger and Campbell[103] estimated the prevalence at 0.01 to 0.067 per 1000 person-years and a mortality of 33%.

Can lactic acidosis occur with normal renal function? Extensive review of literature reveals an odd isolated case report, but most studies have shown that

TABLE 53.16	Phenformin and metformin: potential for causation of lactic acidosis	
	Phenformin	Metformin
Pharmacokinetics	Hydroxylation in liver (30%); Genetic polymorphism + Excreted in urine	Excreted in urine and feces unchanged
Mitochondrial membrane	Binds avidly	Binds poorly
Prevalence of Lactic acidosis:		
Ratio	10–20 times that of metformin	

TABLE 53.17	Metformin: Contraindications

- Impaired renal function
- Impaired hepatic function
- Cardiac failure
- Hypoxia of any origin, poor tissue perfusion, respiratory failure
- Proposed I.V. radiological contrast studies
- Acutely ill patients with dehydration, hypotension, perioperative period
- Type 1 diabetes mellitus (without insulin)
- Diabetes with complications, lean diabetic

lactic acidosis with metformin is inevitably linked with renal compromise. Lalau et al[104] studied 14 cases of metformin associated lactic acidosis and found clinical evidence of shock or hypoxia in 13 patients and the 14th had nonsteroid anti-inflammatory agent-induced anuria. Amongst these patients, significant metformin accumulation was documented only in 10 patients. In another study, Connaly et al[105] studied metformin levels in diabetics with moderately raised serum creatinine levels (120-160 µmol/L) and compared them with normal volunteers taking metformin and diabetics with normal serum creatinine (80-120 µmol/L). They found that plasma lactate levels are higher in diabetic subjects taking metformin compared to normal volunteers, but within the diabetic groups, the small elevation in serum creatinine was not associated with a higher lactate level.

Yet caution has to be exercised in the use of metformin. Common contraindications to metformin use are enlisted in **Table 53.17**. It must be avoided in the elderly, during any acute illness, perioperatively, and during IV contrast studies, in any condition linked to hypoxia, if there is evidence of impaired renal, hepatic or cardiac function.[77,93,106]

In conclusion, it must be stated that biguanide-induced lactic acidosis should be considered in the differential diagnosis of metabolic acidosis with an increased anion gap. Metformin is the preferred biguanide and phenformin use should be discouraged. Metformin should not be used in any diabetic with renal or hepatic impairment, congestive heart failure, alcohol abuse, proposed IV radiological contrast studies, poor tissue perfusion and hypoxia.

Clinical Presentation

As obvious from the preceding discussion, lactic acidosis arises most often in the presence of a life-threatening concomitant disease. In the diabetic, it usually presents as a result of severe sepsis, ketoacidosis, HHNKS, myocardial infarction, renal or hepatic failure, major trauma or surgery. Alcoholic binges, severe exercise in poorly controlled type 1 diabetes or poisoning (salicylates, ethylene glycol, methanol, cyanide, nitroprusside, theophylline), should be excluded.

Unexplained tachypnea associated with hypotension, and deteriorating mental status without significant ketonemia in a diabetic should point towards lactic acidosis.[61,72,80] Although an elevated anion gap and a low serum bicarbonate (in absence of significant ketonemia) point towards lactic acidosis, both these criteria may not be fulfilled in many cases with significant lactic acidosis. In conditions such as associated hepatic failure and sepsis, which induce metabolic alkalosis, these findings may be masked. Hyperventilation increases the likelihood of respiratory alkalosis. Hence, in any critical condition where lactic acidosis is a possibility, measurement of arterial or central venous blood lactate is essential to confirm the diagnosis. Various studies have demonstrated that lactate levels >10 mmol/L are associated with a very poor prognosis.[62,63,72] Significant hyperlactatemia should be considered at lactate levels >5 mol/L and treatment initiated at that stage.[70,72] Controversy still prevails as to whether levels between 3 to 5 mmol/L need energetic management in absence of significantly lower pH values.[63,70,107]

Management

The cornerstone of therapy for lactic acidosis is to treat the precipitating cause. Stoppage of biguanides, alcohol or other offending toxin is a prerequisite. In DKA or HHNKS, fluid replacement and insulin therapy must be given adequately. If there is an associated condition such as sepsis, hepatic, renal or myocardial compromise, it should be treated promptly. Patients may require ventilatory assistance. Cardiovascular collapse should be managed by fluid replacement (preferably normal or diluted saline preparations). Drugs that specifically increase myocardial contractility or reduce after load are preferable. Vasoconstrictive agents must not be used as they further aggravate the lactic acidosis (**Table 53.18**).

TABLE 53.18	Management of lactic acidosis

- Hydration
- Sodabicarbonate, dichloroacetate, carbicarb
- Forced diuresis or hemodialysis
- Insulin and thiamine

Severe lactic acidosis (pH <7.2) is an indication for alkali therapy. The use of alkali in moderate and mild acidosis has been and still is a subject of controversy. Potential ill effects of alkali administration are shown in **Figure 53.2**.[60] Intravenous alkali administration may increase lactate production, particularly in the splanchnic bed, decrease portal vein flow, lower intracellular pH in muscle and liver, raise circulating lactate levels, lower arterial pH and worsen cardiac output.[70]

Sodium bicarbonate is usually given diluted in normal saline in a dose of 1–2 mmol/kg (44 mmol = 50 ml in 500 ml normal saline) over a period of few hours. It should never be given as a bolus and used mainly as a temporary measure while controlling the major precipitating condition. It should only be given when arterial pH is <7.2.

Dichloracetate (DCA) has recently been proposed as a potential therapy in lactic acidosis. Theoretically, it has the following advantages:

1. It is the most potent known pharmacologic stimulus of PDH, the rate-limiting enzyme for the aerobic oxidation of glucose, pyruvate and lactate, PDH activation occurs within minutes and in virtually all tissues following parenteral DCA administration.
2. Under certain experimental conditions DCA may inhibit glycolysis and thereby lactate production.
3. DCA exerts a positive inotropic effect that has been attributed to improvement in myocardial glucose use and ATP production. This effect has been linked to increased cardiac output, and increased blood pressure in patients with heart failure or hypotension or both.[63,108]

However, the theoretical potential of DCA has not been proven in a controlled clinical trial.[109] Although various reports indicated that it was well tolerated and associated with increased pH and reduced lactate levels, the magnitude of change was small and it did not alter hemodynamics or survival.

Carbicarb: A buffering agent, which is an equimolar mixture of sodium bicarbonate and sodium carbonate ($Na_2 HCO_3$). Carbicarb has a buffering capacity similar to sodium bicarbonate, but does not generate carbon dioxide. Reports of controlled studies with carbicarb in patients with metabolic acidosis are still awaited.[110-112]

Thiamine and Insulin: Thiamine is a cofactor for PDH. For a patient with lactic acidosis who is vitamin deficient (e.g. alcoholism), thiamine is a safe and useful medication. It is also of benefit in beriberi induced lactic acidosis and congenital deficiency of either PDH or pyruvate carboxylase. Insulin stimulates the activity of PDH. Further its anabolic effect reduces the generation of alanine from the skeletal muscle, thus reducing the substrate for lactic acid formation. In most diabetic emergencies, insulin therapy as such is mandatory and achieving glycemic control must be an early target.[113]

Forced diuresis and hemodialysis has been advocated especially in the presence of fluid overload. Hemodialysis is the preferred modality in the presence of significant renal compromise. However, it is important to remember that the majority of diabetic emergencies are associated with hypovolemia.

In conclusion, it is emphasized that lactic acidosis is perhaps the most dangerous of the metabolic emergencies a diabetic may face. Prevention and continual awareness of the situations in which it can occur, can go a long way in its early detection and prompt management.

SUMMARY

A diabetic patient is prone to three acute metabolic complications, singly or in a mixed form: diabetic ketoacidosis, hyperglycemic hyperosmolar nonketotic state and lactic acidosis. Diabetic ketoacidosis is usually caused by the omission of insulin in a type 1 diabetic. Prevalence and mortality in DKA is rapidly changing with better understanding of its pathogenesis, patient-education and standardization of fluid, electrolyte and insulin therapy. Management of DKA illustrates some very basic principles of fluid-electrolyte and insulin therapy. Treatment requires replacement of water, saline, potassium and at times sodabicarb. Insulin is usually administered as intravenous infusion. Major metabolic complications are: hypokalemia, cerebral edema and hypoglycemia. Hyperglycemic hyperosmolar nonketotic state is usually found in type 2 diabetics, often elderly ones who have poor access to water due to mental obtundation. Water deficit is of colossal amounts, but there is minimal or no acidosis and insulin infusion is required in amounts smaller than that in DKA. Lactic acidosis can occur in any anoxic, hypoperfusion state. Though rare, it is an important complication of biguanide therapy. Acidosis is severe and management calls for large doses of sodabicarb intravenously. Administration of thiamine and insulin is also beneficial.

REFERENCES

1. Sanjeevi CB. Immune markers in insulin-dependent diabetes patients from India. In Das Ashok Kumar (Ed): Medicine Update. Mumbai: Assn Physicians India. 1998;641-8.
2. Torrey EF, Swalwell CI. Fatal olanzapine-induced ketoacidosis. Am J Psyciatry. 2003;160:2241.
3. Meatherall R, Younes J. Fatality from olanzapine-induced hyperglycemia. J Forensic Sci. 2002;47:893-6.
4. Seymore HR, Gilman D, Quin JD. Severe ketoacidosis complicated by 'ectasy' ingestion and prolonged exercise. Diabetic Med. 1996;10:908-9.
5. Toyonaga T, Kondo T, Miyamura N, Sekigami T, Sonoda K, Kodama S, Shirakami A, Shirotani T, Araki E. Sudden onset of diabetes with ketoacidosis in a patient treated with FK 506/tacrolimus. Diab Res Clin Pract. 2002;56:13-8.
6. Yigit S, Estrada E, Bucci K, Hyams J, Rosengren S. Diabetic ketoacidosis secondary to growth hormone treatment in a boy with Prader-Willi syndrome and steatohepatitis. J Pediatr Endocrinol Metab. 2004;17:361-4.
7. Cetin M, Yetgin S, Kara A , Turner AM, Gunay M, Gumru KF, Gurgey A. Hyperglycemia, ketoacidosis and other complications of L-asparaginase in children with acute lymphoblastic leukemia. J Med. 1994;25:219-29.
8. Faich GA, Fishbein HA, Ellis SE. The epidemiology of diabetic acidosis: a population-based study. Am J Epidemiol. 1983;117-551.
9. Kitabchi AE, Fisher JN, Murphy MB, Rumbal MJ. Diabetic ketoacidosis and hyperglycemic, hyperosmolar nonketotic state. In Kalin RC, Weir GC (Eds): Joslin Diabetes Mellitus, 13 edn. Philadelphia: Lea and Febiger;1994. pp.740.
10. Gelfand RA, Matthews DE, Bier DM, Sherwin RS. Role of counter-regulatory hormones in the catabolic responses to stress. J Clin Invest. 1984;74:2238-48.
11. Adrogue HJ, Wilson H, Boyd AE III, et al. Plasma acid-base patterns in diabetic ketoacidosis. N Engl J Med. 1982;307:1603-10.
12. Vanelli M, Chiari G, Capuano C, Iovane B, Bernardini A, Giacalone T. The direct measurement of 3-β-hydroxy butyrate enhances the management of diabetic ketoacidosis in children and reduces time and costs of treatment. Diabetes Nutr Metab. 2003;16:312-6.
13. Katz MA. Hyperglycemia-induced hyponatremia, calculation of expected serum sodium depression. N Engl J Med. 1973;289:843-4.
14. Beigelman PM. Potassium in severe diabetic ketoacidosis (editorial). Am J Med. 1973;54:419-20.
15. Cohen RD. Kitabchi AE, Murphy MB. When is bicarbonate appropriate in treating metabolic acidosis including diabetic ketoacidosis? In Gitnick G, Barnes HV, Duffy TP, et al (Eds): Debates in Medicine. Chicago: Year Book Medical Publishers; 1990. pp. 200-33.
16. Garella S, Dana CL, Chazan JA. Severity of metabolic acidosis as a determinant of bicarbonate requirements. N Engl J Med. 1973;289:121-6.
17. Narins RG, Cohen JJ. Bicarbonate therapy for organic acidosis: the case for its continued use. Ann Intern Med. 1987;106:615-8.
18. Garcia E, Abramo TJ, Okada P, Guzman DD, Reisch JS, Wiebe RA. Capnometry for noninvasive continuous monitoring of metabolic status in pediatric diabetic ketoacidosis. Crit Care Med. 2003;31:2539-43.
19. Joseph T. Noninvasive monitoring of the response to therapy during diabetic ketoacidosis: is end-tidal CO_2 useful? Crit Care Med. 2003;31:2562-3.
20. Zipf WB, Bacon GF, Spencer ML, et al. Hypocalcemia, hypomagnesemia and transient hypoparathyroidism during therapy with potassium phosphate in diabetic ketoacidosis. Diab Care. 1979;2655-68.
21. Ditzel J. Effect of plasma inorganic phosphate on tissue oxygenation during recovery from diabetic ketoacidosis. Adv Exp Med Biol. 1973;37A:163-72.
22. Fisher JN, kitabchi AE. A randomized study of phosphate therapy in the treatment of diabetic ketoacidosis. J Clin Endocrinol Metab. 1983;57:177-80.
23. Burghen GA, Ettledorf JN, Fisher JN, et al. Comparison of high dose and low dose insulin by continuous intravenous infusion in the treatment of diabetic ketoacidosis in children. Diab Care 1980;3:15-20.
24. Kitabchi AE, Ayyagari V, Guerra SMO, Medical House Staff. The efficacy of low dose versus conventional therapy of insulin for treatment of diabtic ketoacidosis. Ann Intern Med. 1976;84:633-8.
25. Alberti KGMM, Hockaday TDR, Turner RC. Small doses of intramuscular insulin in the treatment of diabetic "coma". Lancet. 1973;2:515-22.
26. Duck SC, Weldon VV, Pagliara AS, et al. Cerebral edema complicating therapy for diabetis ketoacidosis. Diabetes. 1976; 25:111-5.
27. Fein IA, Rackow EC, Sprung CI, et al. Relation of colloid osmotic pressure to arterial hypoxemia and cerebral edema during crystalloid volume loading of patients with diabetic ketoacidosis. Ann Intern Med. 1982;96:570-5.
28. Krane EJ, Rockoff MA, Wallman JK, et al. Subclinical brain swelling in children during treatment of diabetic ketoacidosis. N Engl J Med. 1985;312:1147-51.
29. Curtis JR, Bohn D, Daneman D. Use of hypertonic saline in the treatment of cerebral edema in diabetic ketoacidosis. Pediatr Diabetes 2001;4:191-4.
30. Carrol P, Matz R. Adult respiratory distress syndrome complicating severely uncontrolled diabetes mellitus. Report of nine cases and a review of the literature. Diab Care. 1982;5:574-80.
31. Sprung CL, Rackow EC, Fein IA. Pulmonary edema: a complication of diabetic ketoacidosis. Chest. 1980;77:687-8.
32. Alberti KGMM, Natrass M. Severe diabetic ketoacidosis. Med Clin North Am. 1978;62:799.
33. Barret EJ, Felig P. Diabetic ketoacidosis: pathogenesis and treatment. Medical Grand Rounds. 1983;2:321-34.
34. Clements RS, Vourgant B. Fatal diabetic ketoacidosis: major cause and approaches to their prevention. Diabetes Care. 1978; 1:314.
35. Fulltop M. The treatment of severely uncontrolled diabetes mellitus. Adv Intern Med. 1984;29:327.
36. Kriesberg RA. Diabetic ketoacidosis: new concepts and trends in pathogenesis and treatment. Ann Intern Med. 1978;88:681.
37. Schede D, Eaton RP, Alberti KGMM, et al. Diabetic coma—ketoacidotic and hyperosmolar. Alburque, NM: University of New Mexico Press; 1981.
38. Matz R. Hyperosmolar nonacidic diabetes (HNAD). In Rifkin H, Porte D Jr (Eds): Diabetes mellitus: Theory and Practice. New York: Elsevier Science; 1990. pp. 604-16.
39. Siperstein MD. Diabetes ketoacisosis and hyperosmolar coma. Endocrine and Metabolic. Clin North Am. 1992;21(2):415-32.

40. Carroll P, Matz R. Uncontrolled diabetes mellitus in adults: experience in treating diabetic ketoacidosis and hyperosmolar coma with low dose insulin and a uniform treatment regimen. Diabetes Care. 1983;6:579.

41. Basso A, Dalla Paola L, Erle G, Nacamulli D, Armanani D. Hyperosmolar coma at the onset of type 1 diabetes in a child. J Endocrinol Invest. 1997;20(4):234-9.

42. Fulltop M, Tannenbarm H, Dreyer N. Ketotic hyperosmolar coma. Lancet. 1976;2:635.

43. Miles JM. Effect of acute insulin deficiency on glucose and ketone body turnover in man: evidence for the primarily role of overproduction of glucose and ketone bodies in the genesis of diabetic ketoacidosis. Diabetes. 1980;29:2926.

44. Felts PW. Ketoacidosis. Med Clin North Am. 1983;67:831.

45. Foster DW, McGarry JD. The metabolic derangements and treatment. N Eng J Med. 1938;309:159.

46. Feig PV, McCurdy JD. The hypertonic state. N Eng J Med. 1977;56:38.

47. Gennaire J. Serum osmolarity, uses and limitations. N Eng J Med. 1984;310:102.

48. Areiff AI, Carroll HJ. Cerebral edema and depression of sensorium in nonketotic hyperosmolar coma. Diabetes. 1974;23:531-5.

49. Beigelman PM. Severe diabetic ketoacidosis (diabetic coma). Diabetes. 1971;20:490-500.

50. Wachtel TJ, Silliman RA, Lamberton P. Predisposing factors for diabetic hyperosmolar state. Arch Intern Med. 1987;147:499-501.

51. Umpierrez GE, Kelly JP, Navarrete JE, Casals MH, Kitabehi AE. Hyperglycemia crisis in urban blacks. Arch Intern Med. 1997;157(6):669-75.

52. Fujikawa LS, Meisler DM, Nozic RA. Hyperosmolar hyperglycemia nonketotic coma: a complication of short-term corticosteroid use. Ophthalmology. 1983;90:239-42.

53. Azam H, Neorton RW, Morris AD, Thompson CJ. Hyperosmolar nonketotic coma precipitated by lithium induced nephrogenic diabetes insipidus. Post Graduate Med J. 74(867):39-41.

54. Amundson CD, Olsen, Wade CD. Partial central diabetes insipidus complicating nonketotic hyperglycemic hyperosmolar coma. J Am Osteopathic Assoc. 1996;96(10):603-4.

55. Berger W. Diabetic emergencies. Schweizerisce Rundscharin fur Medzin Praxis. 1997;86(18):308-13.

56. Batista MS, Silva DF, Ferraz HB de Andrade LA. Complex partial seizures, aphasia as initial manifestation of nonketotic hyperglycemia: case reports. Arquivos de Neuro Psiquitria. 1998;56(2):296-9.

57. Waldhouse W, Klienberger G, Korn A, et al. Severe hyperglycemia: effects of rehydration on endocrine derangements and blood glucose concentration. Diabetes. 1979;28:557.

58. Gonsalez-Campay JM, Robertson RP. Diabetic ketoacidosis and hyperosmolar nonketotic state. Gaining control over extreme hyperglycemic complications. Post Graduate Med. 1996;9996:143-52.

59. Rosenbloom AC. Intracerebral crisis during treatment of diabetic ketoacidosis. Diabetes Carc. 1990;13.

60. Kriesberg RA. Lactic acidosis: an update. J Intensive Care Med. 1987;2:76-84.

61. Cohen RD, Woods HF. Clinical and biochemical aspects of lactic acidosis. London: Blackwell Scientific Publishing; 1976. p. 276.

62. Madias NE. Lactic acidosis. Kidney Int. 1986;28:252-74.

63. Stacpoole PW. Lactic acidosis. Endo Metab Clin North America. 1993;22(2):221-45.

64. Narins RG, Krishna GG, Yee J, Ikemiyashiro D, Schmidt RJ. The metabolic acidosis. In Narins RG (Ed): Clinical Disorders of Fluid and Electrolyte Metabolism. New York: McGraw-Hill Inc; 1994. pp. 769-825.

65. Narins RG, et al. Lactic acidosis and the elevated anion gap. Hosp Prac. 1980;125.

66. O'Connor LR, Klein KL, Bethune JE. Hyperphosphatemia in lactic acidosis. NEJM. 1977;277:707-9.

67. Relman AS. Lactic acidosis. Trans Am Clin Climatol Assoc.1971;82:70.

68. Goodkin DA, Narins RG. Quantitation of serum potassium changes during acute acid-base disturbances. In Whelyon A (Ed): Potassium in Cardiovascular and Renal Medicine. New York: Marcell Decker; 1986. p. 67.

69. Savoy J, Kaplan A. A gas chromatographic method for determination of lactic acid in blood. Clin Chem. 1966;12:559.

70. Wright EC, Stacpoole PW, The DCA-Lactic Acidosis Study Group. Causes, natural history and course of lactic acidosis in adults. Clin Res. 1991;38:1964.

71. Cohen RD, Woods HF. Lactic acidosis revisited. Diabetes. 1983; 32:181-91.

72. Adrogue JH, Madias NE. Management of life-threatening acid-base disorders. NEJM. 1988;338(1):26-34.

73. Reaven GM, Hollenbeck C, Geng CY, et al. Measurement of plasma glucose, free fatty acid, lactate and insulin for 24 hours in patients with NIDDM. Diabetes. 1988;37:1020-4.

74. Metcalfe HK, Monson JP, Welch SG, et al. Inhibition of lactate removal by ketone bodies in rat liver. Evidence for a quantitatively important role of the plasma membrane lactate transporter in lactate metabolism. J Clin Inves. 1986;78:743-7.

75. Luft D, Schmulling RM, Eggstein M. Lactic acidosis in biguanide treated diabetes: a review of 330 cases. Diabetologia. 1978;14:75-87.

76. Natrass M, Alberti KGMM. Biguanides. Diabetologia. 1978;14: 71-4.

77. Schaffer G. Biguanides: molecular mode of action. Res Clin Forums. 1979;1:21032.

78. Widen E, Groop L. Biguanides: metabolic effects and potential use in the treatment of insulin resistance syndromes. In Marshall SM, Home PD (Eds): The Diabetes Annual (8). Elsevier Science BV; 1994. pp. 227-41.

79. Dembo AJ, Marliss EB, Halpege ML. Insulin therapy in phenformin associated lactic acidosis. Diabetes. 1975;29:28-35.

80. Searle GL, Siperstein MD. Lactic acidosis associates with phenformin therapy. Diabetes. 1975;24:741-5.

81. Arieff AI, Park R, Leach W, et al. Pathophysiology of experimental lactic acidosis in dogs. Am J Physiol. 1980;239: 7135-42.

82. Misbin RI. Phenformin associated lactic acidosis: pathogenesis and treatment. Ann Intern Med. 1977;87:591-5.

83. Assan R, Heuelin C, Girard JR, et al. Phenformin induced lactic acidosis in diabetic patients. Diabetes. 1975;24(4):791-800.

84. Kruger FA, Skillman IG, Haniw GJ, et al. The mechanism of action of hypoglycemic guanidine derivatives. Diabetes. 1960; 9:170.

85. Altschild RA, Kruger FA. Inhibition of hepatic neoglucogenesis in guinea pig by phenformin. Ann New York Acad Sci.1968; 8:612.

86. Chandalia HB, Rangnath M. Biguanide induced lactic acidosis. J Assoc Physic Ind. 1990;38:(9):520-2.

87. Vishwanath M, Ramachandran A, Snehalata C. Phenformin induced lactic acidosis. Antiseptic. 1978;75:559-65.

88. Chandalia HB, Sadikot S. Blood lactic acid levels in diabetics treated with phenformin—for a process of adaptation. In Bajaj JS (Ed): Diabetes Mellitus in Developing Countries. Delhi: Interprint; 1984. pp. 337-9.

89. Chandalia HB. Metformin induced lactic acidosis. In Munichoodappa C (Ed): Proceeding of the Fourth National Congress on Diabetes, Bengaluru. Diabetes Care. 1980;215-9.

90. Chandalia HB. Metformin induced lactic acidosis. Bull Jaslok Hosp. 1980;5:45-6.

91. Sterne J. Pharmacology and mode of action of hypoglycemic agents. London: Academic Press;1969;11:193-245.

92. Herman LS, Melander A. Biguanides: basic aspects and clinical uses. In Alberti KGMM, Defronzo RA, Keen H, Zimmet P (Eds): International Textbook of Diabetes Mellitus. Chichester, UK: Wiley; 1992. pp. 773-95.

93. Schaffer G. Biguanides: a review of history, pharmacodynamics and therapy. Diabetes Metab Rev. 1983;9:148-63.

94. Pentikainen PJ, Neuvonen PJ, Penttib A. Pharmacokinetics of metformin after intravenous and oral administration to man. Eur J Clin Pharmacol. 1979;16:195-202.

95. Bailey C. Biguanides and NIDDM. Diabetes Care. 1992;15:755-72.

96. Herman LS. Metformin: a review of its pharmacologic properties and therapeutic use. Diabetes Metab. 1979;5:233-45.

97. Tucker CT, Casey C, Phillips PJ, Connor H, Ward JD, Wood HF. Metformin kinetics in healthy subjects and in patients with diabetes mellitus. Br J Clin Pharmacol. 1981;12:235-46.

98. Riccio A, Del Prato S, DeKreutzenberg W, Tiengo A. Glucose and lipid metabolism in noninsulin-dependent diabetes: effect of metformin. Diabetes Metab. 1991;17:180-4.

99. Groop L, Widen E, Franssila–Kallunki A, Ekstrand A, et al. Different effects of insulin and oral antidiabetic agents on glucose and energy metabolism in type 2 (noninsulin dependent) diabetes mellitus. Diabetologia. 1989;32:599-605.

100. Widen E, Eriksson J, Groop L. Metformin normalizes non oxidative glucose metabolism in normoglycemic individuals at increased risk of noninsulin-dependent diabetes. Diabetes. 1991;41:354-8.

101. Wilholm BE, Myrhed M. Metformin induced lactic acidosis in Sweden 1977 to 1991. Eur J Clin Pharmacol. 1993;44(6):589-91.

102. Brown JB, Pedula K, Barzilay J, Herson MK, Latare P. Lactic acidosis rates in type 2 diabetes. Diabetes Care. 1998;10(10):1659-63.

103. Berger A, Campbell DK. Biguanide induced lactic acidosis. Hoemone Metab Res; 1985.

104. Lalau JD, Lacroix C, Compagnon P, et al. Role of metformin accumulation in metformin associated lactic acidosis. Diabetes Care. 1995;18(6):779-84.

105. Connolly V, Keeson CM. Metformin treatment in NIDDM patients with mild renal impairment. Postgrad Med J. 1996;72 (848):352-4.

106. McCartney MM, Gilbert FJ, Murchison LE, et al. Metformin and contrast media: a dangerous combination. Clinical Radiol. 1999;54(1):29-33.

107. Cady LD Jr, Weil MH, Afifi AA, et al. Quantitation of severity of critical illness with special reference to blood lactate. Crit Care Med. 1973;1:75-80.

108. Hindman BT. Sodium bicarbonate in the treatment of subtypes of acute lactic acidosis: physiological considerations. Anesthesiology. 1990;72:1064-76.

109. Stacpoole PW, Wright EC, Baumgartner TG, et al. A controlled clinical trial of dichloracetate for treatment of lactic acidosis. N Eng J Med. 1992;327:1564-9.

110. Blecic S, DeBacker D, Deleuse M, et al. Correction of metabolic acidosis in experimental CPR: comparative study of sodium bicarbonate, carbicarb and dextrose. Am Emerg Med. 1991;20: 235-78.

111. Shapiro JI, Whalen M, Filey G, et al. Intracellular pH responses to sodium bicarbonate (B) and carcicarb (C) in ammonium chloride (AC) and hypercapnic (H) acidosis in the rat. Clin Res. 1998;36:374A (Abstract).

112. Filey GF, Kindig NB. Carbicarb: an alkalizing ion generating agent of possible clinical usefulness. Trans Am Clin Climatol Assn. 1984;96:141-53.

113. Guariglia A, Gonzi GL, Regoliski G, Vinci S. Treatment of biguanide induced lactic acidosis, reproposal of the "physiological" approach and review of literature. Ann Ital Med Int. 1994;9(1):35-9.

Chapter 54

HYPOGLYCEMIA

Siddharth N Shah, Shashank R Joshi

DEFINITIONS

For Adults

Hypoglycemia or low blood glucose is a clinical state associated with low (less than 50 mg/dl) or relatively low plasma glucose concentration usually associated with signs and symptoms of autonomic hyperactivity and neuroglycopenia.

The Diabetes Control and Complications Trial (DCCT) has defined hypoglycemias as: an event resulting in seizure, coma, confusion, irrational or other symptoms consistent with hypoglycemia (e.g. sweating, palpitation, hunger or blurred vision) in conjunction, with:

- A laboratory-determined or finger stick blood glucose less than 50 mg%
- Amelioration by treatment that raises blood glucose
- Prodromal symptoms of hypoglycemia (e.g. sweating, palpitations, hunger or blurred vision) remembered by the subject as occurring shortly before the event

- Severe hypoglycemia, coma or seizure or a reaction requiring hospitalization or intravenous glucose or glucagons.

For Neonates

The definition of hypoglycemia in newborn infants has been debated for decades, as there is no absolute consensus regarding threshold values for diagnosis or treatment. This is because there is no absolute correlation between plasma glucose values, clinical symptoms and long-term sequelae. In 1992, the majority of pediatricians defined a safe blood glucose concentration to be at least 2 mm (or plasma glucose >2.5 mm). They recognized an infant with symptoms of hypoglycemia has higher risk of neurological damage than an asymptomatic infant.

INTRODUCTION

Hypoglycemia occurring several hours after meals was described for the first time in 1922. In 1927, hyper-insulinism was recognized in a patient with malignant pancreatic islet cell tumor who has episodes of severe hypoglycemia. Prior to the discovery of insulin and oral hypoglycemic agents, many patients with different types of diabetes developed ketoacidosis which proved to be fatal. Today, with advances in the management of diabetes and its complications, cases of hypoglycemia progressing to coma and death are much more common instead.

Glycemic control makes a difference for people with types 1 and 2 diabetes mellitus (DM), but the barrier of hypoglycemia in reality does not allow the therapist to achieve the desired glycemic targets. Therefore, maintenance of euglycemia over a lifetime of diabetes, and thus full realization of its well-known potential macrovascular benefits, iatrogenic hypoglycemia is the major limiting factor in strict glycemic management in diabetes. Even early in the course of T2DM, when patients are responsive to oral agent and defenses against hypoglycemia are intact, true euglycemia maintained over time because of the fear of hypoglycemia.

Hypoglycemia is the major hazard of insulin treatment. Patients experience symptoms of hypoglycemia when the blood glucose concentration is less than 50 mg/dl, but individual susceptibility varies considerably. At its mildest, it is no more than a slight inconvenience yet it is both a hazard and unembarrass-

ment. Hypoglycemia occurs not uncommonly in patients on sulfonylureas especially elderly patients on long acting drugs like chlorpropamide and glibenclamide.

ETIOLOGY (TABLE 54.1)

The most common cause of hypoglycemia is iatrogenic, i.e. drug induced. Hypoglycemia secondary to alcohol, insulinoma, and liver disease and that associated with endocrine dysfunction and neonatal hypoglycemia are among the other causes of hypoglycemia.

Fed State Hypoglycemia (Table 54.2)

Nonspecific reactive functional hypoglycemia is the most frequent cause of hypoglycemia in the normal population and is associated with anxiety. These patients tolerate physical exercise and prolonged fasting very well.

In early diabetes, hypoglycemia is seen to occur 3 to 5 hours after a carbohydrate rich meal. It is absolved when pancreatic exhaustion occurs. There is a strong family history of diabetes. Fasting blood sugar is normal or elevated, prolonged fast is well tolerated.

In reactive hypoglycemia due to leucine sensitivity which measures release of insulin from the β-cells,

TABLE 54.1	Causes of fasting hypoglycemia	
Underproduction	*Overutilization*
a. Hormone deficiencies 1. Hypopituitarism 2. Adrenal insufficiency 3. Catecholamine deficiency 4. Glucagon deficiency	a. Hyperinsulinism 1. Insulinoma 2. Exogenous insulin overdose 3. Sulfonylurea overdose 4. Insulin autoimmunity
b. Enzyme defects 1. Glucose-6-phosphatase 2. Liver phosphorylase 3. Pyruvate carboxylase	b. Appropriate insulin level 1. Extrapancreatic tumors 2. Cachexia with fat depletion, e.g. advanced cancer
c. Substrate deficiency 1. Ketotic hypoglycemia of infancy 2. Severe malnutrition; muscle wasting (?) 3. Late pregnancy	
d. Acquired liver disease 1. Hepatic congestion 2. Cirrhosis 3. Severe hepatitis	
e. Drugs 1. Alcohol 2. Propranolol 3. Salicylates	

TABLE 54.2	Fed state (reactive) hypoglycemia

Early (Alimentary) within 2 to 3 hours after meals	*Late (occult diabetic) 3 to 5 hours after meals*
a. Alimentary hyperinsulinism	a. Delayed insulin release due to β cells dysfunction
b. Postgastrectomy (dumping syndrome)	b. Counter-regulatory deficiency of growth hormone, glucagon, cortisone, autonomic response, epinephrine
c. Functional fructose intolerance	
d. Hereditary fructose intolerance	
e. Galactosemia	
f. Leucine sensitivity	

hypoglycemic convulsions occur after an injection of leucine in infants and small children. There is a fall in blood glucose within 20 minutes with marked rise of serum insulin levels. It is a self-limiting disease occurring in infants up to 5 months of age and is rarely seen in adults.

Pseudohypoglycemia

Pseudohypoglycemia occurs in certain chronic leukemias when the leukocyte counts are markedly elevated. This artifactual low blood glucose reflects utilization of glucose by leukocytes after the blood sample has been drawn. Such a hypoglycemic finding is not associated with symptoms. Other artifactual hyoglycemias may be seen with improper sample collection or storage errors in analytic methodology, or confusion between whole blood and plasma glucose values. Plasma glucose is about 15% higher than corresponding whole-blood glucose values.

Normal Glucose Counter-regulation

Energy requirements are met from substrates derived from food and substrates stores as fat, protein, and glycogen. Insulin is the primary endocrine mediating the anabolic phase of metabolism while the counter-regulatory hormone levels are suppressed. The metabolic adjustment during the catabolic phase includes the activation of glycogenolysis and gluconeogenesis in the liver use of free fatty acid derived from triglyceride stored in adipose tissue

The first defense against falling plasma glucose concentration is decreased insulin secretion and activation of glucose of counter-regulatory hormones. Glucagon plays a primary role in the glucose counter-regulatory process. Epinephrine becomes important when glucagon is deficient. Other factors such as cortisol and growth hormone are involved in case of prolonged

TABLE 54.3	Glycemic threshold for physiologic and pathophysiologic responses
	Glycemic threshold
Decreased insulin secretion	83 ± 3
Increased counter-regulatory hormones section:	
Epinephrine	69 ± 2
Glucagon	68 ± 2
Growth hormone	66 ± 2
Cortisol	58 ± 2
Symptoms of hypoglycemia	53 ± 2
Cognitive dysfunction	49 ± 2

hypoglycemia in case of neurotransmitters and other metabolic substrates are also involved. The normal physiological response to falling blood glucose concentrations, the decline in insulin secretion and it occurs at a glycemic threshold of 83 mg/dl. The symptoms of hypoglycemia are seen on the average at blood glucose of 54 mg/dl and those of cognitive dysfunction at 49 mg/dl. The glycemic threshold of various counter-regulatory hormones is elaborated in **Table 54.3**.

PATHOGENESIS

Hypoglycemia is most commonly encountered due to overdosage with insulin or oral hypoglycemic drugs. This may be caused by any one or a combination of the following factors:

1. If more than the required dose of insulin or oral drug is administered.
2. If a meal is skipped, which is inadequate or is unduly delayed after insulin injection or oral drugs.
3. Unusual physical exertion such as swimming, cycling, running, and weight lifting, especially after taking insulin.

In early diabetes with partial decompensation there is islet inertia and insulin is not released till, blood glucose levels reaches 200 mg/dl. Blood sugar then falls fairly rapidly due to large release of insulin, leading to hypoglycemia (reactive hypoglycemia). Rapid gastric emptying in postgastrectomy patients with brisk absorption of glucose results in excessive insulin release, leading to fall of glucose concentration and hypoglycemic symptoms.

When the liver function is severely impaired, hypoglycemia occurs because glycogen storage and insulin are deficient in hepatic disease. Accumulation of serum insulin leads to fasting hypoglycemia, diabetic type of glucose tolerance test due to inability of the liver to store glucose as glycogen or epinephrine. Alcohol induces slowing of the Krebs' cycle with impairment of gluconeogenesis, giving rise to reduced glucose output and hypoglycemia. There is no rise of serum insulin during hypoglycemia.

Fasting hypoglycemia in an otherwise healthy adult is most commonly due to an adenoma of the islet of Langerhans. The cause of hypoglycemia due to extrapancreatic tumors is not clear but a high level of non-suppressible insulin like activity may play a role. In leucine sensitivity, leucine stimulates the release of insulin from the β cells like a sulfonylurea compound. In hereditary fructose intolerance, accumulation of fructose-1-phosphate by unknown mechanisms gives rise to hypoglycemia.

Drugs like salicylates, mono amino oxidase inhibitors, phenylbutazone, methotrexate, probenecid, clofibrate and dicoumarine potentiate the action of oral hypoglycemic drugs and hence care must be taken during their administration. When taken with oral hypoglycemic drugs, alcohol may produce hypoglycemia. Nonselective β-blockers mask the adrenergic symptoms of hypoglycemia and also delay recovery.

In patients without symptoms, one must be alert to diagnose artifactual hypoglycemia. Whole blood glucose values may be spuriously low in polycythemia vera, leukemia and hemolytic crisis.

Glucose Issues in Newborn

Glucose homeostasis has some unique features in a newborn compared to the adult. Throughout gestation, the fetus receives its entire supply of glucose and energy from the maternal circulation via the placenta. Thus, there is no need for fetal glucose production. Many workers have demonstrated that fetal new glucose production is nonexistent. The activity of important rate-limiting enzymes of gluconeogenesis such as pyruvate carboxylase, phosphoenolpyruvate carboxykinase (PEPCK), glucose-6-phosphatase and fructose-1,6-diphosphatase of gluconeogenesis is low. It does not increase until the perinatal period, and reaches adults levels only after several hours to days of extrauterine life. On the other hand, the enzymes active for glycogen synthesis and glycogenolysis are present before the accumulation of glycogen during the last 1 to 2 months of gestation. Glucose is the primary substrate for brain metabolism and the brain utilizes several time more glucose than muscle and fat. Infants have a large brain in relation to body weight ratio (12% in infants versus 2% in an adult), in reaction resulting in about three times higher glucose turnover rates on a per kg body weight basis in an infant compared to an adult, approximately 6 mg/kg/min (5-6 hours of fast) versus 2 mg/kg/min (overnight fast), respectively. Further, 90% of total glucose utilization in infants is by the brain.

Following cessation of the transplacental flow of nutrients, most healthy full-term newborns promptly initiate hepatic glucose production to meet their high glucose demands. After a decrease during the first two hours of life, blood glucose concentrations gradually increase and normoglycemia is established and maintained. Lipolysis and lipid oxidation increase immediately following birth, as indicated by a rapid postnatal increase in plasma concentrations of glycerol and free fatty acids, high glycerol turnover rates and decreasing respiratory quotient. Hepatic glycogen content is limited, and within a few hours of fasting, the neonate is dependent on gluconeogenesis as the primary mechanism to maintain euglycemia. Both glycerol and alanine have been demonstrated to contribute to glucose production within the first 6 to 8 hours after birth. Lipids are of substantial importance in the maintenance of glucose homeostasis in infants. Glycerol component is used directly for glucose production via gluconeogenesis; further free fatty acids (FFA) generated by lipopolysis are utilized for oxidative metabolism and production of ketone bodies (hydroxybutyric acid and acetoacetic acid). Both plasma FFA and ketone bodies can be used by a variety of body tissues, thus decreasing the demands of these tissues for glucose as an energy source. Ketone bodies, but not FFA, can cross the blood-brain barrier and partially supplant the need for glucose. Most healthy full-term infants adapt rapidly to the metabolic demands of extrauterine life. However, some infants, although born at term, have disturbed glucose metabolism and are at risk of hypoglycemia [e.g. infants with transient hyperinsulinemia, growth retarded infants with persistent hyperinsulinemia (PHHI) and infants with hormone and enzyme defects].

Hypoglycemia in newborn can have serious adverse effects and if untreated, hypoglycemia leads to neuroglycopenia with seizures, impaired neurological development, mental retardation and even death.

CLINICAL FEATURES

The signs and symptoms of hypoglycemia can be divided into those due to autonomic hyperactivity and those resulting from neuroglycopenia, as shown in **Table 54.4**. The manifestations are varied and will depend mainly on the rate of fall of blood glucose level and the ability of the patients' endocrine system to counteract. For example, some patients on insulin may complain of few symptoms despite very low blood glucose whereas a patient with Sheehan's syndrome may feel very uncomfortable even with moderately low blood glucose level.

Patients may present with weakness, palpitation, nervousness, sweating and mental confusion progressing to unconsciousness. History of insulin administration or history of having consumed oral hypoglycemic agent may be available. Short-acting insulin may produce hypoglycemia up to 4 to 6 hours after injection whereas intermediate-acting insulin may produce hypoglycemia in the evening past midnight. It is rare to find prolonged hypoglycemia with short-acting oral drugs to coma is more commonly encountered in elderly diabetics who are on chlorpropamide or glibenclamide. Whipple's triad consisting of symptoms of hypoglycemia with low blood glucose values and intermediate relief after ingestion of glucose is characteristic of β-cell tumor. Occasionally, the tumor is associated with severe diarrhea, muscle wasting and/or carcinoid syndrome. These patients get tired and do not tolerate prolonged exercise. It may also present as a part of multiple adenomatosis or neurofibromatosis. Even gastrin producing Zollinger-Ellison syndrome may be associated.

After a severe bout of alcohol, hypoglycemia can occur especially, if the patient takes very little food. Hypoglycemia may be intermittent and may not be reproduced by fasting. Patients who have undergone gastrectomy complain of nausea, abdominal discomfort, diarrhea, sweating, palpitation and giddiness (dumping syndrome).

After ingestion of sugar or fruit, severe vomiting and hypoglycemia occur in hereditary fructose intolerance. Liver enlargement, jaundice, cirrhosis, albuminuria, aminoaciduria and mental retardation due to chronic hypoglycemia have been observed in children. Older children show strong dislike for sugar and fruits.

INVESTIGATIONS

A. *Diagnosis of postprandial hypoglycemia:* The only unequivocal diagnostic test is the demonstration of low plasma glucose concentration (less than 50 mg/100 ml) during spontaneously developed symptoms. A 5-hour oral glucose tolerance examination showing a plasma glucose value of 50 mg/ml or less is suggestive.

B. *Diagnosis of β-cell adenomas (insulinoma)*
   1. Serum insulin level of 20 µU/ml or more in the presence of blood glucose values below 40 mg/dl.
   2. Elevated circulating proinsulin level; this is characteristic and does not occur in factitious hyperinsulinism.
   3. Demonstration of increasing ratio of insulin to glucose.
   4. Nonsuppression of C-peptides during hypoglycemia induced by 0.1 unit of insulin per kg body weight per hour. A normal person would suppress the peptide level to 50% or more during hypoglycemia.
   5. Glucose tolerance test is not helpful.
   6. Computerized tomography (CT) scan may not pick-up the tumor.
   7. Pancreatic arteriography can locate tumor preoperatively.

In normal persons, the insulin/glucose ratio is always less than 0.4; in insulinomas, the ratio is greater than 0.4 and often above 1.0. Multiple sampling is required

TABLE 54.4	Signs and symptoms of hypoglycemia
Autonomic hyperactivity	*Neuroglycopenia*
Adrenergic	Headache
Palpitation	Fatigue
Sweating	Mental dullness
Anxiety	Dizziness
Tremors	Blurring/clouding of vision
Tachycardia	Confusion
Parasympathetic	Abnormal behavior
Hyperactivity	Amnesia
Nausea	Seizure
Hunger	Unconsciousness

TABLE 54.5	Differential diagnosis of hypoglycemia
Fasting (Postabsorptive) hypoglycemia	*Reactive (Postprandial) hypoglycemia*

Fasting (Postabsorptive) hypoglycemia

- Iatrogenic
- Drugs
  - Insulin
  - Sulfonylureas
  - Alcohol
  - Pentamidine
  - Quinine
  - Quinidine
  - Salicylates
  - Sulfonamides
- Organ failure
  - Hepatic
  - Renal
  - Cardiac
- Non-β-cell tumors
- Endogenous hyperinsulinism
- Insulinoma microadenomatosis
- Autoimmune hypoglycemia
- Antibodies to insulin
- Insulin receptors
- Sepsis

Reactive (Postprandial) hypoglycemia

- Congenital enzyme deficiencies
- Galactosemia
- Hereditary fructose intolerance
- Alimentary hypoglycemia

- Idiopathic (functional)
- Reactive hypoglycemia

Hypoglycemia of infancy and childhood
  Neonatal hypoglycemia
  Congenital enzyme deficiency
  Ketotic hypoglycemia of childhood

because patients with insulinoma may secrete insulin episodically.

In islet cell tumors, provocative tests with tolbutamide, glycogen or leucine may be of help but the overlap between normal and insulinoma patients is so wide to render the tests of little value.

In factitious hypoglycemia, the triad of low blood sugar, high immunoreactive insulin and suppressed plasma C-peptide immunoreactivity is pathognomonic of exogenous insulin administration. When sulfonylureas are suspected as being responsible, a chemical test of the plasma to detect the drugs may be required.

DIFFERENTIAL DIAGNOSIS

Hypoglycemia should be differentiated mainly from hyperglycemia especially when a patient is in coma. Differential diagnostic features of hypoglycemia are given in **Table 54.5**. Differentiating features of hyper-

glycemia and hypoglycemia are mentioned in **Table 54.6**. Hypoglycemia may also present as transient ischemic attacks, giddiness, mental confusion, convulsion or coma and may be mistaken for a neurological illness.

Although food, especially free carbohydrates, will relieve symptoms regardless of the cause, persons without a hypoglycemic disorder may feel better after eating. A suspected patient has to undergo 5-hour oral glucose tolerance test with plasma sampling every half hour and at the time the symptoms occur. A good history will clinch the diagnosis of iatrogenic hypoglycemia.

COURSE AND PROGNOSIS

If detected early, hypoglycemia is reversible and can be prevented. Surgical removal of β-cell tumor alleviates all symptoms. If hypoglycemia occur only at night and

TABLE 54.6 Differential diagnosis of hypoglycemic and hyperglycemic coma

Symptoms, signs and laboratory findings	Hypoglycemic coma	Hyperglycemic coma
Physical findings		
Pulse rate	Increased	Increased
Pulse volume	Full	Weak
Temperature	May be decreased	May be decreased
Respiration	Shallow or normal	Rapid and deep (air hunger)
Blood pressure	Normal	May be increased
Skin	Clammy, sweating	Dry
Tongue	Moist	Dry
Tissue turgor	Normal	Decreased
Eyeball tension	Normal	Reduced
Breath	No acetone	Acetone present, fruity odor
Reflexed	Brisk reflexes	Diminished reflexes
Laboratory tests		
Urine glucose*	Negative to positive depending on timing of last voiding	Positive
Plasma glucose	Low	Raised ++++ 300 mg/dl or over
Plasma acetone**	Negative	Usually raised
Bicarbonate***	Normal	Low less than 200 mg/L
Blood pH	Normal	Diminished less than 7.3

*Sometimes urine is negative for sugar but positive for acetone in patients with hypoglycemic coma. This is due to starvation ketosis.

**In case of diabetic ketoacidosis with very severe complicating lactic acidosis, urine and plasma acetone may be negative. Rarely, uremic patients with diabetic ketoacidosis have positive plasma acetone but negative urine acetone.

***In patients with severe acute or chronic respiratory failure, plasma bicarbonate may be normal or increased despite concomitant presence of metabolic acidosis or diabetic ketoacidosis.

is not detected, it might lead to loss of memory and mental dullness.

COMPLICATIONS

Hypoglycemia may be misdiagnosed as hyperglycemia and if not treated promptly may lead to death. Chronic hypoglycemia may lead to loss of memory, clouding of vision, blunted mental activity, confusion, abnormal behavior, convulsions and coma.

Somogyi Effect

Insulin treated diabetic patients may show a rapid swing to hyperglycemia after episodes of hypoglycemia. The rebound hyperglycemia or Somogyi effect is thought to be caused by actions of hormonal antagonists or insulin secreted in response to hypoglycemia.

Hypoglycemia Unawareness

Some elderly, long-standing diabetic subjects on sulfonylurea do not get adrenergic symptoms and present with severe neuroglycopenic symptoms such as confusion, convulsions or coma during the hypoglycemic episodes. About a decade back, when patients taking porcine insulin were shifted on human insulin in UK. Some of the insulin-dependent diabetic patients also developed hypoglycemia unawareness. It is characterized by low sympathetic response with insignificant increase in circulating epinephrine and glucagons. Since the hypoglycemia-induced glucagons response is invariably reduced in patients with diabetes after 5 years, the main factor responsible for unawareness of hypoglycemia is inadequate response of epinephrine. Autonomic neuropathy was initially thought to be the main factor responsible for inadequate counter-regulation. However, many diabetic patients with established autonomic neuropathy have adequate counter-regulatory response, while many with inadequate response have no evidence of autonomic neuropathy. It is postulated that hypothalamus has specialized area, which detects hypoglycemia and triggers autonomic response. Exposure of this area to hypoglycemia might reset the trigger threshold at a lower level resulting in diminished counter-regulation.

MANAGEMENT

Hypoglycemia associated with unconsciousness or stupor should be treated on an emergency basis. The treatment of choice is to give 25 to 50 ml of 50% glucose solution over a period of 2 to 3 minutes. One milligram of glucagon injected IV is preferable in an emergency, the patient regaining consciousness within 15 minutes to permit ingestion of sugar. History of the precipitating cause of hypoglycemia must be ascertained and the future course of action chalked out to prevent further episodes.

The treatment of reactive hypoglycemia of fed state is alteration in dietary habits. Frequent small feeds are advised in nonspecific reactive hypoglycemia; the diet should contain some slowly absorbable carbohydrates and more protein. Anticholinergic drugs, such as probanthine 15 mg three times day, may be useful in reducing rapid gastric emptying. Tolbutamide in small doses may be given twice daily before meals in patients with early diabetes. Reactive hypoglycemia in leucine sensitivity can be treated by avoiding leucine containing protein such as milk. Diazoxide has also been tried. Propranolol in small doses may be useful in both situations.

Alcohol-induced hypoglycemia is prevented by reducing the intake of alcohol and increasing the ingestion of food.

Hereditary fructose intolerance requires avoiding foods containing sugar or fructose. Other carbohydrates and milk can be taken without fear.

Measures to avoid hypoglycemia in patients on insulin and/or sulfonylureas:

1. Do not delay, skip or reduce usual food intake.
2. Take a carbohydrate containing snack before physical exercise.
3. Avoid insulin injections in the limb which is actively involved in the exercise.
4. Avoid exercise during the peak time period of insulin action, i.e. 2 to 4 hours and 6 to 12 hours after injection for plain and intermediate-acting insulin, respectively.
5. When shifting to human insulin, the time gap between plain insulin injections and food intake should be reduced since human plain insulin is absorbed faster.
6. When changing over from conventional insulin highly purified insulins in those patients requiring more than 40 units of insulin per day true with reduced total insulin dosage by 205.
7. Do not use sulfonylureas in patients with hepatic and/or renal insufficiency.
8. Ask the patient to avoid alcohol.
9. In older patients, do not insist on a very tight control of blood glucose, and short-acting sulfonylureas should be preferred to long-acting in these patients.
10. Periodically monitor blood glucose (at least every 3 months).

Directions for Treatment

Severe Hypoglycemia

Severe hypoglycemia should be treated initially with intravenous glucose, whenever possible. If parenteral glucose cannot be used, dissolve the lyophilized glucagons using the accompanying diluting solution and use immediately. For adults and for pediatric patients weighing more than 44 lb (20 kg), give 1 mg (1 unit) by subcutaneous, intramuscular or intravenous injection. For pediatric patients weighing less than 44 lb (20 kg), give 1 mg (5 unit) or a dose equivalent to 20 to 30 mg/kg. Discard any unused portion. An unconscious patient will usually awaken within 15 minutes following the glucagons injection. If the response is delayed, there is no contraindication to the administration of an additional dose of glucagon; however, in view of the deleterious effects of cerebral hypoglycemia, emergency aid should be sought so that parenteral glucose can be given. After the patient responds, supplemental carbohydrate feeds should be given to restore liver glycogen and to prevent secondary hypoglycemia.

Glucagon is contraindicated in patients with known hypersensitivity to it or in patients with known pheochromocytoma. Glucagon should be administered cautiously to patients with a history suggestive of insulinoma, pheochromocytoma, or both. In patients with insulinoma, intravenous administration of glucagon may produce an initial increase in blood glucose; however, because of glucagon's hyperglycemic effects, the insulinoma may release insulin and cause subsequent hypoglycemia. A patient developing symptoms of hypoglycemia after a dose of glucagon should be given glucose orally or intravenously, whichever is most appropriate. Exogenous glucagons also stimulate the release of catecholamines. In the presence of pheochromocytoma, glucagons can cause the tumor to release catecholamines, which may result in a sudden and marked increase in blood pressure. If a patient develops a sudden increase in blood pressure, 5 to 10 mg of phentolamine mesylate may be administered intravenously in an attempt to control the blood pressure. Generalized allergic reactions, including urticaria, respiratory distress, and hypotension, have been reported in patients who received glucagon by injection.

Glucagon is effective in treating hypoglycemia only if sufficient liver glycogen is present. Because glucagon is of little or no help in states of starvation, adrenal insufficiency, or chronic hypoglycemia; hypoglycemia in these conditions should be treated with glucose.

Beta-Cell Tumors

Surgical removal, chemotherapy and irradiation help in eradication of the tumor. If hypoglycemia occurs it is treated symptomatically. Carbohydrate feeding every 2 to 3 hours is usually effective in preventing hypoglycemia. Glucagons should be available for emergency use. Diazoxide 300 to 600 mg daily orally has been useful along with a thiazide diuretic. Octreotide, somatostatin analogs have been used in metastatic tumors.

Neonatal Hypoglycemia

Hypoglycemia in the immediate postpartum period needs recognition, as the phenomenon is transient. Associated with hypoglycemia, there are hyperbilirubinemia, polycythemia and hyperviscosity, respiratory distress syndrome and necrotizing enterocolitis which must be recognized and treated. Every newborn of diabetic mothers must be given a 5% glucose infusion for the first six hours and subsequently blood glucose monitored to prevent fatal hypoglycemic convulsions.

Autoimmune Hypoglycemia

This may be associated with insulin antibodies or insulin receptor antibodies. The age of onset varies from a few days to an advanced age. Hypoglycemia occurs at any time and is often self limited.

Insulin receptor antibodies are observed in diabetic patients with type B insulin resistance associated with acanthosis nigricans. Most of these patients have pre-existing insulin resistant diabetes and evidence of autoimmune disease before the development of hypoglycemia.

Hypoglycemia due to Non-β-cell Tumor

A. Mesenchymal tumors constitute 45 to 64% of reported cases of β-cell tumor with hypoglycemia.
   Histologic types—fibrosarcoma, lymphosarcoma, liposarcoma, rhabdomyosarcoma, hemangiopericytomas, leiomyosarcoma, mesotheliomas.
   Clinical types—both sexes; around 5th decades; 1/3rd in chest, 2/3rd in abdomen, large and easily detectable.
B. Hepatomas (22% of cases), large adrenal tumors, Ca lung. These large tumors metabolize large amount of glucose. They may secrete insulin-like polypeptides.

Prophylactic Measures

Adequate education of diabetic patients and their relatives is necessary so that hypoglycemia can be avoided or treated effectively at an early state. Patients should carry a card stating that they have diabetes and are treated with insulin or oral hypoglycemic agents. Relatives, friends or colleagues at work or at school should be familiar with the signs of hypoglycemia and its emergency treatment. The importance of regular meals and snacks must be emphasized, and treatment should be adjusted appropriately for sporting activities or for special situations such as fasting before radiological procedures or minor surgery. If β-blocking drugs are used these should be cardioselective. Use of highly purified human insulins should reduce the problem of hypoglycemia associated with occasional release of insulin from high titers of insulin antibodies.

The therapeutic goal has to be modified in elderly diabetic patients with autonomic neuropathy, hypoglycemia unawareness or severe diabetic complications. Very strict glycemic control should be avoided where the risks of hypoglycemia outweighs any potential benefit, such as in long-standing IDDM patients who have impaired glucose counter-regulation, or in elderly or mentally subnormal patients. Intensive insulin therapy may also be impractical in treating infants or very young children. Moderate hyperglycemia may have to be accepted in these individuals to avoid the greater risk of low blood glucose concentrations. Although there is no evidence in humans that hypoglycemia causes fetal damage in early pregnancy, very tight glycemic control reduces the ability to perceive hypoglycemic symptoms and increases the risk of coma and convulsions, which are clearly undesirable for fetal development. Rapid tightening of glycemic control is now considered to have an initial potentially adverse effects on established microangiopathy and also increase vulnerability to hypoglycemia.

Social Implications

Because of the potential risk of hypoglycemia, with IDDM individuals are usually advised not to participate in high-risk sporting activities, such as hang-gliding, parachute jumping or scuba-diving. They may also be excluded from certain types of employment, e.g. steeple jacks, deep-sea divers and airline pilots. They are usually debarred from driving public-service vehicles and may not be permitted to operate some forms of machinery. Problematic hypoglycemia is a frequent reason for a patients driving license to be revoked, which may have medico-legal implications, e.g. repercussions on employment. The relationship of hypoglycemia to criminal responsibility has recently been reviewed.

BIBLIOGRAPHY

1. Agneta L Sunehag, Morey W Haymond. Glucose extremes in newborn infants. Clinics in Perinatology. 2002;29(2):245-60.
2. Archambeaud-Moaveraux F, Hac MC, Nadoion S, et al. Autoimmune-insulin syndrome. Biomed Pharmacother. 1989;43:581-6.
3. Ariky RA. Hypoglycemia associated with liver disease and ethanol. Endocrinol Metab Clin North Am. 1989;118:75-90.
4. Bolli G, De Feo P, Perrielto G, et al. Reactive hypoglycemia in humans. J Clin Invest. 1985;75:1023-31.
5. Cryer PE, Binder C, Bolli GB, et al. Hypoglycemia in IDDM. Diabetes. 1989;38:1193-9.
6. Cryer PE. Glucose counter-regulation. The prevention and correction of hypoglycemia in humans. Am J Physiol. 1993; 264:E149-55.
7. Cryer PE. Iatrogenic hypoglycemia in IDDM: Consequences, risk factors and prevention. In Marshall SM, Home PD, Alberti KGMM, Kralt LP (Eds): Diabetes Annual. Amsterdam: Elsevier; 1993; 7:317-31.
8. Davis M, Sharnoon H. Counter-regulatory adaptation to recurrent hypoglycemia in normal humans. J Clin Endocrinol Metab. 1991;73:995-1001.
9. EIrick H, Witten TA, Arai Y. Glucagon treatment of insulin reactions. N Eng J Med. 1958;258:476-80.
10. Fajans SS, Vinik AL. Insulin-producing islet cell tumors. Endocrinol Metab Clin North Am. 1989;18:45-74.
11. Field JB. Hypoglycemia: definitions, clinical presentation, classification and laboratory test. Endocrinol Metab Clin North Am. 1989;18:27-44.
12. Glucagon. Mosby's drug. Drug Consult; 2005.
13. Gold AE, Deary'IJ, Frier BM. Recurrent severe hypoglycemia and cognitive function in type 1 diabetes. Diabetic Med. 1993;10:503-8.
14. Horeldt F. Reactive hypoglycemia. Metabolism. 1956;24:1195.
15. Joshi SR. Hypoglycemia. Ind Pract. 1998;51(2):127-37.
16. Peitzman SJ, Agarwal BN. Spontaneous hypoglycemia in end-stage renal failure. Nephron. 1977;19:131-39.
17. Seltzer HS. Drug-induced hypoglycemia. Endocrinol Metab Clin North Am. 1989;18:163-83.
18. Service FJ, Mcmahon MM, O'Brien PC, et al. Functioning insulinoma: incidence, recurrence and long-term survival of patients. Mayo Clin Proc. 1991;66:711-19.
19. Shah SN. Insulin therapy in NIDDM. In Munjal YP (Ed): Medicine Update. 1997;7:220-9..
20. Talwalkar PG. Life-threatening hypoglycemia in elderly NIDDM patients on sulfonylurea: a comparative study. Ind J Int Med. 1993;3:146-8.
21. The Diabetes Control and Complications Trial Research Group. The effect of intensive treatment of diabetes on the development and progression of long-term complications in insulin-dependent diabetes mellitus. N Eng J Med. 1993;329:977-86.

Chapter 55

ACUTE INFECTIONS IN DIABETES MELLITUS

BK Das, PK Das

CHAPTER OUTLINE

- Introduction
- Common Microorganisms associated with Infections in Diabetic Patients
- Urinary Tract Infections
- Respiratory Tract Infections
- Abdominal and Gastrointestinal Infections
- Skin and Soft Tissue Infections
- Rhinocerebral Mucormycoses
- Malignant Otitis Externa
- Foot Infections
- Summary

INTRODUCTION

It is commonly believed that patients with diabetes are more susceptible to infection. However, there are reports which suggest lack of strong evidence for this association.[1] But at the same time, many observations allude to the fact that many infections are commonly seen in diabetic subjects, some occurring with increased frequency and severity, and a few exclusively associated with them. Recent findings support a causal relationship between high blood glucose and infection as evidenced by decrease in morbidity with improved glycemic control[2,3] and worsening of diabetes during infection.

Several factors contribute to increased predilection for infection which includes, importantly, an altered immunity. The innate immune system is predominantly affected manifesting as dysfunction of polymorpho-nuclear cells,[4] as well as, monocytes and macrophages.[5] There is limited T-lymphocyte dysfunction as evidenced by hyporesponsiveness to phytohemagglutinin but normal response to *Candida* antigen.[6] Humoral immune system is unaffected with B-lymphocytes showing normal antibody production when challenged by vaccines. There is evidence which suggests that good glycemic control corrects some of the immunological defects.[7] Therefore, it is imperative that blood glucose levels should be closely monitored in diabetic subjects with infection.

Other predisposing factors, as outlined in **Table 55.1**, which increase susceptibility to infection, are ketoacidosis, peripheral vascular disease, peripheral neuropathy, frequent catheterization and dialysis in patients of chronic renal failure.

Urinary tract, respiratory tract and deep soft tissue infections occur with increased frequency, and some of them can lead to complications and high mortality.[8] Some infections are exclusively associated in patients with diabetes, namely, rhinocerebral mucormycosis and invasive otitis externa **(Table 55.2)**.

Host Defense: Innate cellular immunity is more affected than adaptive immunity. Abnormalities in functions of

TABLE 55.1	Predisposing factors for infections in diabetes mellitus

Primary factors
- Altered innate immunity: PMNLs, monocyte/macrophage dysfunction
- Defective complement-mediated function
- Cytokine mediated (TNF-α and IL-1)

Secondary factors
- Peripheral vascular disease
- Peripheral neuropathy
- Gastroparesis
- Chronic renal failure and dialysis
- Ketoacidosis
- Urinary catheters and intravascular lines

PMNLs: Polymorphonuclear leukocytes;
TNF-α: Tumor necrosis factor alpha;
IL-1: Interleukin-1

TABLE 55.2	Common infections in diabetes mellitus

Infections-associated with increased incidence
- Genitourinary tract infections
  - Cystitis
  - Pyelonephritis
  - Renal and perinephric abscess
  - Balanoposthitis and vulvovaginitis
- Respiratory tract infections
  - *S. aureus* pneumonia
  - Gram-negative pneumonia
  - Tuberculosis
  - Lung abscess
- Skin and soft tissue infections
  - Surgical wound infection
  - Pyomyositis
  - Foot infection
- Abdominal infections
  - *Salmonella enteritidis*
  - *Campylobacter jejuni*

Infections predominantly associated with diabetes
- Malignant otitis externa
- Rhinocerebral mucormycosis
- Emphysematous cholecystitis
- Emphysematous pyelonephritis
- Emphysematous cystitis
- Necrotizing fasciitis
- Fournier's gangrene

polymorphonuclear leukocytes (PMNLs), monocytes and lymphocytes have been widely reported. PMNLs have abnormalities of chemotaxis, adherence, phagocytosis, oxidative bursts and intracellular killing.[4]

Despite increased expression of adhesion molecules and free radical activation, significantly lower neutrophilic chemotaxis has been observed in diabetic subjects.[4] Leukocyte dysfunction has been attributed to poor glycemic control.[7] There is a negative correlation between glycated hemoglobin and bactericidal activity of neutrophils.

Although several mechanisms have been postulated, it is currently believed that advanced glycation end products (AGEs) have a role in immune dysfunction. Hyperglycemia or presence of AGEs correlate with low level, persistent activation of PMNLs[5,8] characterized by spontaneous oxidative burst and release of enzymes like myeloperoxidase, elastase and neutrophil granule components. The end result is an exhausted PML incapable of adequate response to a challenge by an infectious pathogen.[8] Tolerance, as a result of spontaneous hyperexcitement, has also been reported in peripheral blood mononuclear cells in diabetic subjects.[4]

Besides, the activity of antibacterial proteins like lysozyme and lactoferrin gets affected after binding to AGE-modified proteins. The enzymatic and bactericidal function of lysozyme is inhibited along with bacterial agglutinating and killing activity of lactoferrin.[9] There is significant reduction in the number of phagocytic cells.[10] Abnormalities in monocyte/macrophage chemotaxis and phagocytic function have also been reported. Chemiluminescence studies have demonstrated improved function of these cells with regard to phagocytic activity on controlling blood glucose.[11]

Proinflammatory cytokines like TNF-α, IL-1 and IL-8 are increased in diabetic patients in basal state, but significantly less IL-2 and IL-6 are produced on stimulation of cells from these subjects.[8] IL-1 and TNF-α are known to increase glucose flux and oxidation.[12] Stress related to hyperglycemia causes release of these cytokines.

The complements an important arm of the innate immune system, is affected in hyperglycemic state. There is an abnormality of the opsonic binding site of C3 which increases susceptibility to *Candida* infection.[13]

Humoral immunity in diabetic subjects is unaffected as evidenced by normal levels of circulating immunoglobulins as compared to healthy controls, and good antibody response to vaccination challenge.[8]

Cell-mediated adaptive immunity is affected as evidenced by poor lymphoproliferative response to phytohemagglutin and *S. aureus*. But a dichotomy is revealed by normal response to *Candida albicans*.[6]

There are several studies which indicate that good glycemic control rectifies immune deficiencies resulting in reduced risk of infection.[2,3,14]

COMMON MICROORGANISMS ASSOCIATED WITH INFECTIONS IN DIABETIC PATIENTS

Organisms that cause pulmonary infections are similar to those found in nondiabetic population, however, gram-negative infections and *Mycobacterium tuberculosis* are more commonly observed. An increase in incidence of *Staphylococcus aureus* infection has been reported but a recent study failed to corroborate that evidence.[15] Mortality is also unaffected in diabetic patients with *Staphylococcus aureus* bacteremia.[16] A high incidence of group B Streptococcal bacteremia,[17] *Klebsiella* related infections,[18,19] certain enteric pathogens like *Salmonella enteritidis*[20] and *Campylobacter,*[21] Hepatitis C[22] and *Candida* infection[23] are commonly observed with increased frequency in patients with diabetes.

URINARY TRACT INFECTIONS

Symptomatic as well as asymptomatic urinary tract infection is commonly encountered in diabetic subjects,[24] with higher incidence of bacteriuria *seen in compared to* controls.[25] This observation is not reported in diabetic men. In an Indian series, symptomatic infection was reported to be 14% in mostly menopausal diabetic women.[26] In another study, the prevalence of urinary tract infection (UTI) in diabetes mellitus was found to be 9%.

Several factors have been implicated for increase in incidence of UTI like use of catheters, presence of autonomic neuropathy, diabetic cystopathy with resultant increased residual urine and vesicourethral reflux.[1,27] Other concomitant causes like vaginitis, cystocele and rectocele also contribute to higher incidence.[8] Interestingly, diabetic women with bacteriuria do not have higher glycosylated hemoglobin compared to nonbacteriuric diabetic women.[8]

Diabetes *predispose patients* to severe infections of upper urinary tract. Acute pyelonephritis is several times more common in diabetic subjects, commonly with bilateral involvement.[28] They are also at increased risks for complications like renal papillary necrosis, renal or perinephric abscess, and rarely, emphysematous pyelonephritis.[8] Emphysematous cystitis is another extremely rare complication that occurs predominantly in patients with diabetes.

E. coli is the most common pathogen isolated in UTI and complications associated with it. Other organisms isolated are *Klebsiella* and *Proteus* species. Presence of *Pseudomonas* and *Candida* in the isolate indicates a possibility of use of catheters and instrumentation of the urinary tract. Besides being a saprophytic colonizer, *Candida* sometimes causes invasive infection of lower as well as upper urinary tract in diabetes.[23]

Clinical presentations of UTI in diabetic subjects do not differ from nondiabetics. The general management also remains the same except when complications develop, which should be suspected when high temperature persists into fourth or fifth day despite adequate antimicrobial therapy.

Investigations like radiography, demonstrating air in the bladder wall or lumen in *case emphysematous cystitis,*[29] or gas in kidney in emphysematous pyelonephritis, ultrasonography, computerized or magnetic resonance imaging (MRI) scans for renal/perinephric abscess, and retrograde pyelography for renal papillary necrosis, assist in diagnosing complications.[8]

Treatment depends on the nature of complications. Appropriate antimicrobial therapy is supported by surgical intervention in case of abscess, and emphysematous pyelonephritis, where mortality is 60 to 80% with medical therapy alone.[29] In a study from North India, mortality related to UTI in diabetic patients was 2.4%.[30]

In case of fungal infection, resolution occurs in most cases without treatment, or on removal of urinary catheter. Antifungal like oral fluconazole is preferred in invasive cases.[31]

Asypmtomatic bacteriuria is not an indication for antimicrobial therapy. Since prevalence of upper tract involvement in diabetic women with bacteriuria is high, management of asymptomatic bacteriuria in diabetic patients has remained debatable.

RESPIRATORY TRACT INFECTIONS

The issue regarding increased susceptibility of diabetic patients to respiratory tract infection compared to nondiabetics has not been resolved.[32] The overall incidence of community acquired pneumonia is not higher in patients with diabetes.[33] However, diabetic subjects hospitalized with pneumonia have a higher risk of death than those without diabetes.[34] The incidence of bacteremia, delayed resolution of pneumonia, and recurrence of infection may also be higher in these patients.

Certain organisms like *Staphylococcus aureus*, gram-negative infections and *Mycobacterium tuberculosis* infect patients with diabetes more often, while some microorganisms like *Streptococcus pneumoniae*, *Legionella* and influenza virus cause increase in morbidity and mortality in patients with diabetes.[32] In the Indian series, 11.6% of diabetic patients presented with pneumonia, and *Klebsiella* was the commonest organism isolated.[26]

There is increased colonization of upper airway by *Staphylococcus aureus*[35] and gram-negative bacteria in diabetic patients, which may be responsible for increased incidence of bacterial pneumonias.[8] Colonization by *Staphylococcus aureus* make patients susceptible to lower respiratory tract infection following an attack by influenza virus which affects mucosal ciliary activity.[8] Increased incidence of bacterial pneumonia, ketoacidosis and mortality has also been reported among diabetic patients during epidemics of influenza and pneumonia.[32] Mortality due to bronchopneumonia in diabetes was 17.4% in an Indian study.[30] Diabetic patients have increased incidence of tuberculosis and most of them have advanced disease at the time of diagnosis.[40] Fungal infections like aspergillosis and *Cryptococcus neoformans* can also cause primary pneumonia.

It is recommended that diabetic patients receive pneumococcal and influenza vaccine annually[36] to reduce morbidity and mortality. This is a cost-effective preventive strategy.

ABDOMINAL AND GASTROINTESTINAL INFECTIONS

There is increased susceptibility to certain enteric pathogens in diabetes because of gastrointestinal dysmotility syndrome.[8] Normal motility is an important host defense mechanism against infection. *Salmonella enteritidis*[20] and *Campylobacter* infections[21] are reported with increased frequency. Diabetes is also a risk factor for infection with *Listeria monocytogenes*, in whom mortality is higher than in healthy individuals.[37] Emphysematous cholecystitis is a rare form of acalculous cholecystitis seen predominantly in male diabetics.[38] It results from ischemia of the gallbladder wall and infection with gas producing organisms. Frequently pathogens cultured include anaerobes such as *Clostridium* and aerobes like *E. coli*.[39] The natural course is marked by gangrene, perforation and higher mortality compared to patients with acute cholecystitis.[40] A plain radiograph is diagnostic, demonstrating a gaseous ring, 1 to 2 days after the attack. Prompt antibiotic therapy and early surgical intervention reduces mortality.

SKIN AND SOFT TISSUE INFECTIONS

There are no controlled studies to prove a higher association of skin and soft tissue infections like folliculitis,

furunculosis and subcutaneous abscess in patients with diabetes.[1] However, diabetic patients are more predisposed to postsurgical wound infection[14] in case of poor glycemic control. Both cutaneous fungal infections and pyomyositis caused by *S. aureus* occur with increased frequency.[39]

Several skin and soft tissue infections like diabetic foot, necrotizing fasciitis and Fournier's gangrene occur exclusively in these patients. Seventy five percent of patients with necrotizing fasciitis have diabetes.[1] The infection spreads along fascial planes and subsequently affects muscle and skin. The infection is usually polymicrobial and categorized as type I, if caused by an anaerobe in combination with facultative anaerobes like Streptococci or Enterobacteria, and type II, if caused by group A β-hemolytic streptococci alone or in combination with Staphylococci.[41] Common sites affected include abdominal wall, extremities, perineum and in obese diabetic women, the vulva. The infection is life-threatening and needs immediate surgical debridement along with broad-spectrum antibiotics. Despite appropriate therapy mortality is nearly 60%.[1]

Fournier's gangrene is a form of necrotizing fasciitis with predilection for the scrotum, penis and perineum. An estimated 40 to 60% of patients with this condition is associated with diabetes.[42] Predisposing genito-urinary or colorectal pathologies are found in most cases.[43] Infection is polymicrobial which includes *Clostridium*, gram-negative bacilli, bacteroides and anaerobic Streptococci. Mortality ranges between 20 to 35% despite adequate therapy.[44]

RHINOCEREBRAL MUCORMYCOSES

Around 50 to 75% of cases of rhinocerebral mucormycosis occur in diabetic patients[38] with ketoacidosis acting as an important predisposing factor.[45] This condition is caused by *Rhizopus* and *Mucor* species of fungi. Several reasons have been postulated for increased susceptibility of this infection among acidotic diabetics possibly because of increased availability of iron for the pathogen,[46] lack of serum inhibitory activity,[47] and defective pulmonary macrophage function due to hyperglycemic state.[48] It is an invasive disease involving the nasal cavity, sphenoidal sinus, cavernous sinus, orbit, frontal lobe, carotid artery and jugular vein. Early diagnosis and aggressive treatment is mandatory. Recently, lipid complex formulations of amphotericin B has allowed higher doses of the drug with lower systemic toxicity.[49] If untreated, the disease is universally fatal.

MALIGNANT OTITIS EXTERNA

Invasive otitis externa affects elderly subjects with diabetes[50] and can be life-threatening due to its intracranial extension. Predisposing factors like poor glycemic control, use of hearing aids, swimming in contaminated pools, and use of nonsterile water for ear irrigation[6] contribute to the development of this infection. Majority of cases are caused by *Pseudomonas*[51] and sometimes, secondary to colonization by *Aspergillus* of the external auditory canal.[52] Spread of infection leads to cranial osteomyelitis, facial nerve palsy,[6] lower cranial nerve palsies as well as involvement of sigmoid sinus and the meninges.[51] Mortality is close to 30% in patients with extensive intracranial involvement.[53]

Early diagnosis depends on demonstration of *Pseudomonas* by gram-stain and culture. Tissue biopsy is mandatory to exclude noninvasive otitis. MRI with gadollinium is the radiological examination of choice for its ability to delineate soft tissue and bone involvement.[38] Technetium and gallium scans are superior to CT or MRI in demonstrating early temporal bone osteomyelitis. Management includes surgical debridement of necrotic tissue and appropriate antipseudomonal therapy.

FOOT INFECTIONS

In patients with diabetes, foot infection is an extremely common problem. Clinically, manifest neuropathy is present in 25% of cases and close to 40% of patients with indecent foot ulcer will require amputation within three years. Several factors contribute to increased susceptibility to foot infection. Presence of neuropathy, vasculopathy, minor trauma, skin breakdown caused by dermatophytes and paronychia results in entrance of pathogens which progresses leading to life-threatening infection if not treated early.

Foot infection may be mild or severe. Mild infection is superficial when there is no evidence of ischemia, systemic toxicity or bone involvement. Severe infection is associated with manifestations mentioned above.[8] Mild infection can be controlled with appropriate antibiotic therapy while moderate to severe infection will require debridement, evaluation of osteomyelitis and necessary surgical intervention. Empiric coverage with antibiotics should include agents active against *Staphylococcus aureus*, *Pseudomonas*, enterococci and anaerobes.[8] Details regarding foot infection in diabetes is covered in Chapter 64.

SUMMARY

Many specific infections and some exclusive ones are commonly seen in patients with diabetes. Some of the infections are associated with dangerous complications which need early recognition. Defective innate immunity contributes to increased susceptibility to infection, and mostly immune deficiencies are linked to glycemic control. Blood glucose levels should be meticulously controlled in the presence of infection and appropriate antimicrobial therapy started early to reduce morbidity and mortality.

REFERENCES

1. Wheat LJ. Infection and diabetes mellitus. Diabetic Care. 1980;3:187-97.
2. Zerr K, Furnary A, Grunkmeier G, et al. Glucose control lowers risk of wound infection in diabetics after open heart operation. Ann Thoracic Surg. 1997;63:356.
3. Rassias A, Marrin C, Arruda J, et al. Insulin infusion improves neutrophil function in diabetic cardiac surgery. Anaesth Analg. 1999;88:1011.
4. Delamaire M, Maugendre D, Moreno M, et al. Impaired leucocyte function in diabetic patients. Diabetic Med. 1997;14:29.
5. Geerlings SE, Hoepelman A. Immune dysfunction in patients with diabetes mellitus. FEMS Immunol and Med Micro. 1999;26:259.
6. Deresinki S. Infections in diabetic patients: strategies for clinicians. Infectious Disease Reports. 1995;1:1.
7. Gallacher S, Thomson G, Fraser WD, et al. Neutrophil bactericidal function in diabetic mellitus: evidence for association of blood glucose control. Diabetic Med. 1995;12:916.
8. Calvet HM, Yoshikawa TT. Infections in diabetes. Infectious Disease Clinics of North America. 2001;15(2):407-19.
9. Li YM, Tan AX, Vlassara H. Antibacterial activity of lysozyme and lactoferrin is inhibited by binding of advanced glycation modified proteins to a conserved motif. Nat Med. 1995;1:1057-61.
10. Katz S, Klien B, Elian I, et al. Phagocytic activity of monocyte chemotactic responses in diabetes mellitus. Diabetic Care. 1983;6:479.
11. MacRury SM, Gemmel CG, Paterson KR, et al. Changes in phagocytic function with glycemic control in diabetic patients. J Clin Pathol. 1989;42:1143-57.
12. Ling P, Bistrian B, Mendez B, et al. Effects of systemic infusion of endotoxin, tumor necrosis factor and IL-1 on glucose metabolism in the rat: relationship to endogenous glucose metabolism and peripheral tissue glucose uptake. Metabolism. 1994;43:279-84.
13. Hosletter MK. Handicaps to host defenses: effects of hyperglycaemia on C3 and *Candida albicans*. Diabetes. 1990;39:271-5.
14. Pomposelli J, Baxter J, Babineari T, et al. Early postoperative glucose control predicts infection rate in diabetic patients. JPEN. 1998;22:77.
15. Breen JD, Karchmen AW. Staphylococcal infections in diabetic patients. Infect Dis Clin North Am. 1995;9:11-24.

16. Cooper G, Plat R. *Staphylococcus aureus* bacteremia in diabetic patients: endocarditis and mortality. N Eng J Med. 1982;73:658-62.

17. Farley MM, Harvey RC, Shell T, et al. A population based assessment of invasive disease due to *Group B Streptococcus* in nonpregnant adults. N Eng J Med. 1993;328:1807-11.

18. Leibovici L, Samra Z, Konisberger H, et al. Bacteremia in adult diabetic patients. Diab Care. 1991;14:89-94.

19. Wang JH, Liu YC, Lee SS, et al. Primary liver abscess due to *Klebsiella pneumoniae* in Taiwan. Clin Inf Dis. 1998;26:1434-8.

20. Telzak EE, Greenberg MSZ, Budnick LD, et al. Diabetes mellitus—a newly described risk factor for infection from *Salmonella enteritidis*. J Inf Dis. 1991;164:538-41.

21. Neil KR, Slack RC. Diabetes mellitus, antisecretory drugs and other risk factors for *Campylobacter* gastroenteritis in adults: a case control study. Epidemiol and Infect. 1997;119:307-11.

22. Fraser GM, Harman I, Meller N, et al. Diabetes mellitus is associated with chronic hepatitis C but not chronic hepatitis B infection. Israel J Med Sc. 1996;32:526.

23. Vazquez JA, Sobel JD. Fungal infection in diabetes. Infect Dis Clin North Am. 1995;9:97-116.

24. Sobel JD. Pathogenesis of urinary tract infection: role of host defenses. Infect Dis Clin North Am. 1997;11:531-49.

25. Vejlsgaard R. Studies on urinary tract infection in diabetes. I Bacteriuria in patients with diabetes mellitus and in control subjects. Acta Med Scand. 1964;179:173-82.

26. Sridhar CB, Anjana S, Thomas Mathew J. Acute infections, RSSDI Textbook of Diabetes Mellitus. 2002;Chapter 34:471-7.

27. Geerlings SE. Asymptomatic bacteriuria may be considered a complication in women in diabetes. Diabetes mellitus women ASB Utrecht study group. Diab Care. 2000;23:744-9.

28. Ellenbogen PH, Talner LB. Uroradiology of diabetes mellitus. Urology. 1976;8:413.

29. Patterson JE, Andriole VT. Bacterial urinary tract infections in diabetes. Inf Dis Clin North Am. 1997;11:735.

30. Bhansali A, Chattopadhya A, Dash RR. Mortality in diabetes—a retrospective analysis from a tertiary care hospital in North India. Diabetes Research and Clinical Practice. 2003;60:119-24.

31. Leu HS, Huang CT. Clearance of funguria with short course antifungal regimens: a prospective randomized controlled study. Clin Infect Dis. 1995;20:1152-7.

32. Koziel H, Koziel MJ. Pulmonary complications of diabetes mellitus: pneumonia. Infect Dis Clin North Am. 1995;9:65-96.

33. Woodhead MA, Macfarlane JT, McCracken JS, et al. Prospective study of the etiology and outcome of pneumonia in the community. Lancet. 1987;i:671-4.

34. Fine M, Smith M, Carson C, et al. Prognosis and outcome of patients with community acquired pneumonia. JAMA. 1996;275:134.

35. Lipsky BA, Pecoraro RE, Chen MS, et al. Factors affecting staphylococcal colonization among NIDDM patients. Diab Care. 1987;10:483.

36. ACP Task Force on Adult Immunization: immunization for immunocompromised adults. Guide for Adult Immunization. Philadelphia, ACP 1994. pp. 49.

37. Skokberg K, Syrjanen J, Jahkola M, et al. Clinical presentation and outcome of Listeriosis in patients with and without immunosuppressive therapy. Clin Infect Dis. 1992;17:143.

38. Nirmal J, Caputo J, Wietekamp M, et al. Infections in patients with diabetes mellitus. N Eng J Med. 1999;341:1906.

39. Nirmal J, Mahajan M. Infection and diabetes. Textbook of Diabetes, 3rd edn. John C Pickup, G Williams (Eds). Blackwell Publishers 2003;40:1.

40. Mentzer RM Jr, Golden GT, Chandler JG, Horsley JS III. A comparative appraisal of emphysematous cholecystitis. Am J Surg. 1975;129:10-5.

41. Giuliano A, Lewis F, Hadley K, et al. Bacteriology of necrotizing fascitis. Am J Surg. 1977;134:52-7.

42. Paty R, Smith AD. Gangrene and Fournier's gangrene. Urol Clin North Am. 1992;19:149.

43. Sentochnik DE. Deep soft tissue infections in diabetes patients. Infect Dis Clin North Am. 1995;9:53.

44. Bilton BD, Zibari GB, Mcmillan RW, et al. Aggressive surgical management of necrotizing fasciitis serves to decrease mortality: a retrospective study. Am Surg. 1998;64:397.

45. Artis WM, Fountain JA, Delcher HK, Jones HE. A mechanism of susceptibility to mucormycosis in diabetic ketoacidosis: transferrin and iron availability. Diabetes. 1982;31:1109-14.

46. Meyer BR, Wormser G, Hirschan SZ, et al. Rhinocerebral mucormycosis: premortem diagnosis and therapy. Arch Intern Med. 1979;139:557.

47. Gale GR, Welch AM. Studies of opportunistic fungi. I. Inhibition of *Rhizopus oryzae* by human serum. Am J Med Sci. 1961;241:604.

48. Waldorf AR, Ruderman N, Diamond RD. Specific susceptibility to mucormycosis in murine diabetes and bronchoalveolar macrophage defense against Rhizopus. J Clin Invest. 1984;74:150.

49. Walsh TJ, Heimenz JW, Seibel NL, et al. Amphotericin B lipid complex for invasive fungal infections: analysis of safety and efficacy in 556 cases. Clin Inf Disease. 1998;26:1383.

50. Sapico F, Bessman A. Infections in the diabetic patient. Infect Dis Clin Pract. 1995;1:339.

51. Tierney MR, Baker AS. Infections of the head and neck in diabetes mellitus. Inf Dis Clin North Am. 1995;9:195.

52. Philips P, Bryce G, Shepard J, et al. Invasive external otitis caused by *Aspergillus*. Rev Infect Dis. 1990;12:277-81.

53. Rubin J, Yu VL. Malignant external otitis: insights into pathogenesis, clinical manifestations, diagnosis and therapy. Am J Med. 1988;85:391.

Chapter 56

CHRONIC INFECTIONS IN DIABETES MELLITUS

Samar Banerjee

CHAPTER OUTLINE

INTRODUCTION

Infection in diabetes is one of the common and important terminal events. This complication by hampering glycemic control worsens the prognosis in a diabetic person. Diabetes Mellitus (DM) predisposes a person to infection and infection in turn overwhelms the metabolic control. Effective control of either affects the control of the other condition. Diabetes is considered as a secondary immune deficiency disorder by World Health Organization[1] as the disease is characterized by:

- Frequent, severe, prolonged and recurrent infections
- Alteration of at least one of the immune response mechanisms (e.g. polymorphonuclear leukocytes or lymphocyte response) determines the development of infection.

Chronic hyperglycemia impairs host defense. Some infections occur more in diabetic whereas some other infections occur equally both in diabetic and nondiabetic subjects.

- *Chemotaxis*: By this process polymorphonuclear cells migrate to the site of infection in response to chemotactic substances secreted by microorganisms. In diabetes, diminished chemotaxis has been noted and is well-correlated to metabolic control.[2]

- *Phagocytosis*: Adhesion and ingestion of foreign particles are the stages of phagocytosis and is triggered by serial mechanisms involving actin, myosin, immunoglobulin and complement system. Phagocytosis is impaired in long-standing uncontrolled diabetes, together with intrinsic defect of polymorphs from increase in sialidase enzyme secretion and reduction of cell membrane sialic acid. High level of blood glucose saturates lectin receptors which fail to initiate phagocytosis.[3]

- *Killing activity*: This activity is produced by lysosomal enzymes from polymorphs after phagosome and lysosome fusion and is dependent upon both oxidative and nonoxidative mechanisms. Decrease in this activity with high blood glucose and restoration by insulin therapy of this activity within 48 hours has been noted in diabetes.[4] Production of sorbitol also hampers the oxidative killing process.

- *Lymphocytic function*: In type 1 diabetes mellitus, reduction of total number of lymphocytes, especially of CD4 (helper cells) have been noted and this may be due to insulin deficiency.[5] Normalization of glycemic control reverses this effect. Because of this CD4 deficiency probably poor antibody response against hepatitis B vaccine is also observed reflecting poor cellular and humoral response.[6]
- *Immunoglobulins*: Lower level of immunoglobulins both IgG and IgA is reported in diabetic persons.[7]
- *Complement*: In diabetic patients often low C4 levels associated with C4A null gene has been seen in 25% of cases of type 1 diabetes mellitus.[8] Deficiency of C1q and C3 complement has also been observed.

Beyond these immune factors, local factors have also predisposing nature to infections as follows:

- Hyperglycemia predisposes to bacterial and fungal infection by altering the endothelial function and oxidative stress.
- Angiopathy both micro-and macrovascular produces anoxia and results in microbial proliferation impaired oxygen dependent polymorphonuclear function and improper perfusion of antibiotics.
- Sensory motor neuropathy produces pressure sores, ulcers, abnormal pressure points in the foot due to small joint arthropathy and small muscle myopathy of foot and microangiopathy predisposing to diabetic foot. Autonomic neuropathy is a predisposing cause of chronic urinary tract infection because of retention in the bladder. It also impairs the microvascular circulation and peripheral gangrene. Microvascular impairment also leads to reduced renal blood flow and frequent renal infection and eventual papillary necrosis.

SECONDARY FACTORS

The factors which render a diabetic more vulnerable to infection are as follows:

- Frequent hospitalizations
- Diabetic ketoacidosis
- Intravenous/intramuscular drug/fluid/blood administrations
- Inappropriate antibiotic usage
- Peripheral vascular diseases
- Neuropathy
- Gastroparesis, reflux and pulmonary aspiration
- Indwelling catheterization
- Frequent minor/major surgery
- Chronic renal failure requiring dialysis, blood transfusion.

CHRONIC INFECTIONS

Infections occurring commonly in diabetes are bacterial, fungal or viral.

Chronic infections more commonly seen in diabetes are as follows:

Bacterial
- Tuberculosis
- Pyelonephritis
- Cholecystitis
- Periodontal infection.

Fungal
- Candidiasis
- Rhinocerebral mucormycosis.

Viral
- Viral hepatitis particularly hepatitis C
- HIV infections.

Out of all these chronic infections, the most important are diabetic foot, cholecystitis, pyelonephritis, candidiasis, rhinocerebral mucormycosis, hepatitis C and HIV.

HEPATITIS C AND DIABETES

Both hepatitis C virus (HCV) infection and diabetes are spreading as epidemic worldwide. Both are slowly and silently developing, diagnosed very late and often with complications at diagnosis.

Allison et al first reported the incidence between these two diseases HCV and DM in 1994.[9] In a study of 100 patients, with cirrhosis, 50% of cases related to hepatitis had diabetes whereas HCV-ve cirrhosis group had diabetes in 9% of cases with an odds ratio of 10.0 (95% confidence interval, 3.4 to 20.3). Subsequent studies have also supported this association. Similarly, higher incidence of HCV infection is noted amongst diabetics than nondiabetics.

Amarapurkar et al (2002) from India[10] compared the etiology of chronic liver diseases with and without DM, and found higher evidence of HCV than hepatitis B virus (HBV) in diabetic than nondiabetic subjects **(Table 56.1)**

Wang et al studied 2327 consecutive subjects in the community and found anti-HCV positivity to be strongly associate with type 2 DM in subjects aged 35 to 49 years (odds ratio 3.3). Sonographic evidence of fatty liver and chronic liver disease in HCV+ve cases were also moderately associated with type 2 DM. No correlation with hepatitis B infection and alcohol

TABLE 56.1	Etiology of chronic liver disease in India				
	Nonalcoholic steato hepatitis with cirrhosis	NASH	Cryptogenic cirrhosis	HBV	HCV
Diabetic group	11.3%	18.9%	22.6%	17%	13.2%
Nondiabetic group	1.7%	13.0%	7.8%	30.43%	13%

consumption were noted.[11] Diabetes mellitus may also be significantly associated with hepatocarcinogenesis in chronic HCV patients as studied in 311 liver biopsies of HCV patients by Tajawa et al.[12]

Third National Health and Nutrition Examination Survey (NHANES III) published in 2000 proved unique association between HCV infection and DM,[13] where presence of HCV infection amongst persons above 40 years are statistically higher for the development of DM than HCV-ve person (odds ratio 3.77). But hepatitis B infection does not increase the risk of developing DM.[14] Incidence of DM amongst HCV chronic infection are higher than those with chronic HBV infection, alcoholic liver disease and biliary cirrhosis.[15] Petit et al (2001) observed that older age, obesity, severe liver fibrosis and family history of DM are related to potential risk or developing DM in HCV infected patients.[16] In patients with cirrhosis planned for hepatic transplantation development of type 2 DM is five times higher in those who were of HCV origin[17] **(Table 56.2)**.

This study has also shown that HCV-related liver failure, pretransplantation diabetes and male sex were independent predictors of developing DM, one year after transplantation.

Though majority of studies showed increased prevalence of DM amongst HCV chronic infection cases, Mangia et al reported negative correlation between these two.[18] They reported high rate of DM in patients suffering from cirrhosis irrespective of etiology.

A prospective nine-year study has shown persons with predisposing risk factors of DM are 11 times higher in coexistent HCV infection than those without.[19] Genotype 1a and 1b infections constitute 70% of HCV infection but whether particular genotype involves diabetic persons is not settled. Though some workers claim genotype 2a to be more often seen in diabetes with HCV infection, others claim DM in HCV does not have any special predilection for this genotype.[20,21] Moreover, alcohol does not exert any additive effect over HCV infection in development of DM.

Mode of Transmission of HCV

Conventionally, raised ALT in diabetes indicates fatty liver, but this is also seen frequently due to coexistent HCV infection as documented in United Kingdom prospective diabetes study trial. Though finger prick for blood sugar examination and insulin injection is a mode of transmission, different studies have ruled out the possibility.[22]

Pathogenesis of Diabetes in HCV Infection

Multiple mechanisms have been suggested for the association but none are clearly confirmed **(Table 56.3)**.[22]

Insulin Resistance

This is observed in all cases of cirrhosis regardless of etiology and is considered a key factor in the development of hepatogenous diabetes mellitus. HCV infection is reported to induce insulin resistance as observed in 250 cases of HCV-infected patients.[23] This may be possibly due to liberation of different cytokines like tumor necrosis factor alpha (TNF-α) which inhibits tyrosine kinase phosphorylase pathway. Insulin resistance is also an independent predictor of hepatic

TABLE 56.2	Incidence of diabetes mellitus in cirrhosis and after hepatic transplant		
	Before transplant	1st year transplant	5th year of transplant
HCV-related cases	29%	37%	41%
HBV-related cases	6%	10%	
Cholestatic liver disease	4%	10%	

TABLE 56.3	Pathogenesis of diabetes mellitus in HCV infection

- Hyperinsulinemia, insulin resistance
- Pancreatic infection by HCV
- Insulin deficiency or poor insulin secretion
- Autoimmune β-cell damage
- Nonalcoholic fatty liver disease
- Increased iron stores

fibrosis and is irrespective of degree of hepatic failure and lowest with genotype 3 HCV.

Caronia et al (1999) observed diabetes in 23.6% cases of HCV+ve cases and 9.4% cases of HBV-related cirrhosis. Fasting insulin level in 30 cases out of 127 HCV-related cirrhosis patients were significantly higher as consistent with insulin resistance. Reduced acute insulin response indicating β-cell dysfunction was observed in all these cases.[30]

Insulin Deficiency

Grimbert et al found lower value of serum insulin and C-peptide amongst 17 cases of HCV chronic infection and diabetes but when compared to 9 HCV-ve diabetes the result appeared not to be statistically significant probably because of low sample size.[15]

Pancreatic Infection by HCV

Whether like coxsackie, cytomegalo or mumps virus, HCV can infect pancreas and lead to diabetes has been thought of. But the viruses other than HCV, leads to type 1 DM and HCV is associated with type 2 DM.

Autoimmune β-cell Damage due to HCV

Though the genome of HCV has been identified within pancreas, evidence of β-cell damage by HCV directly or indirectly by immune response is questionable. Piquer et al studied this hypothesis and could not find higher incidence of GAD antibody, tyrosine phosphatase antibody or islet cell antibody in patients with HCV infection than normal population.[24] But increasing incidence of type 1 DM is seen after interferon therapy in HCV infection probably due to amplification of previously existing autoimmune response to β-cells.[25] Moreover, interferon therapy in healthy volunteer is reported to induce insulin resistance.[26]

Nonalcoholic Fatty Liver Disease

This entity is known for its association with diabetes mellitus and with HCV infection but obesity and dyslipidemia are determining risk between HCV infection and steatosis.[27] Metabolic steatosis and viral steatosis are both probably responsible for this condition.

Increased Iron Stores

Excess iron store is a known factor for development of secondary diabetes. Fourty percent cases of HCV infected persons have higher iron stores. Serum ferritin was studied by Hernandez in 123 patients infected with HCV (55 diabetic, 68 nondiabetic). Serum ferritin was four times in the diabetic group suggesting etiological correlation for diabetes in HCV infection.[28]

Effect of DM on HCV+ve Chronic Liver Disease

Retrospective cross-sectional study of 1195 patients with chronic HCV discloses a synergistic liver damaging effects of DM and HCV. The three-way interaction between the stages of chronic liver disease, diabetes and enzymatic cholestasis suggests that diabetes is a risk factor for the progression of viral liver disease at least in part by induction of cholestasis.[29]

High blood glucose in HCV-infected persons leads to advanced and higher fibrosis. These effects are mediated via receptors for advanced glycation end (AGE) products in hepatic stellate cells and increased oxidative stress through key inflammatory factors such as TNF-α and interleukin-6 (IL-6).[31]

DIABETES MELLITUS AND TUBERCULOSIS

Tuberculosis in diabetes is 2 to 5 times more frequent usually diagnosed late, asymptomatic and is usually due to reactivation of an old focus than fresh infection. The risk of acquiring tuberculosis was found to be 4.8 times higher compared to general population in a study of 1529 diabetic patients.[32] The risk was highest in type 1 DM patients. In a large cohort of 8793 patients, Patel in India reported tuberculosis to be the most commonly associated illness with DM.[33] Swai et al in a prospective seven-year follow-up of 1250 patients found that 5.4% cases developed pulmonary tuberculosis and 0.2% spinal tuberculosis. In 25.7% cases, tuberculosis was detected before DM, in 45.7% after DM and in 20.6% simultaneously.[34] They observed higher incidence of tuberculosis in younger age, with type 1 DM, poorly controlled group with low BMI.

Though chances of tuberculosis are higher in diabetes, infection rate by *Mycobacterium tuberculosis* and tuberculin sensitivity are not higher compared to those without diabetes.[35]

Higher sputum positivity, more extensive lung involvement particularly cavitations are noted. Though lower lobe involvement was claimed to be more in diabetes in earlier reports, recent observations suggest that distribution of lung affection is same as in nondiabetic subjects.[36]

Causes of Increased Susceptibility to Tuberculosis in Diabetes

- Neutrophilic dysfunction (discussed earlier).
- Lowered production of interleukin-1b from monocytes, more so in poorly controlled groups.
- Thickened alveolar epithelium and pulmonary basal lamina leading to reduction of diffusion capacity, lung capacity and elastic recoil.
- Reduced bronchial reactivity and dilation due to diabetic autonomic neuropathy.

Bacteriological conversion, relapse rate are same in diabetic and nondiabetic subjects. But relapse in diabetes mostly with resistant strains is associated with poor prognosis.[37] Correlation of relapse with diabetic control is still a conflicting issue.

Prevalence of Diabetes Mellitus in Tuberculosis

As diabetic subjects are well known to be prone to develop tuberculosis, tuberculosis affected patients have also higher prevalence of diabetes mellitus with prevalence rates varying from 1.9 to 41% in different studies.[32]

Jawad et al reported diabetes mellitus and impaired glucose tolerance (IGT) in 20% each of cases with tuberculosis,[38] 50% of them recovered on antituberculosis therapy.

Probable Causes of Higher Prevalence of Diabetes Mellitus in Tuberculosis

- Reciprocal worsening of the two process by each other
- Malnutrition and low body mass index (BMI)
- Pancreatic tuberculosis in rare cases
- Stress-induced diabetes mellitus due to tuberculosis
- Pituitary and adrenocortical hyper-reactivity
- Vitamin D deficiency.

Diabetic state usually improves on treatment with antituberculosis drugs. But rifampicin can produce alimentary glycosuria and early phase hyperglycemia due to possibly augmented glucose absorption from the intestine; intravenous glucose tolerance test (GTT) in normal.[39]

In active pulmonary tuberculosis, immunoreactive insulin, C-peptide and glucose levels before and after glucagon injection demonstrated insulin deficiency.[40] Antituberculous therapy is also detrimental to insulin secretion as reported by Egarova[41] who suggests insulin therapy at all times.[41] Purified protein derivative of *Mycobacterium tuberculosis* is also cytotoxic to islet cells.

F Bacakoglu et al (2000) studied 927 cases of culture positive tuberculosis and found DM in 12.3% persons.[42]

This study showed that DM does not alter the symptomatology, tuberculosis reactivity rate, or drug response, resistance or localization of the lesion in upper or lower zones of the lung. But in persons above 40 years and in female patients, lower lung field involvement is significantly high. Smear positive cases and radiologically reticulonodular appearance were less in tuberculosis with diabetes mellitus than opacity, cavitation, pleural involvement. Cavitary lesions were more common in type 1 diabetes mellitus than the type 2 variety.

Cavitary lesions though maintain high bacterial population, less smear positivity is noted in diabetes which may be related to muscle weakness and less effective expectoration. Higher frequency of lower lobe disease in elderly may be due to immunological alteration or higher frequency of primary tuberculosis, increased alveolar oxygen pressure in lower lobes.

Mona Bashar found 36% cases suffer from multiple drug resistance-TB (MDR-TB) amongst diabetics compared to 10% of nondiabetics controls (p <0.01).[43] Out of these 36% and 23% never received antitubercular drugs. Some 14% of diabetic group and 1% of nondiabetic group died of active TB, 20% of diabetic group had extrapulmonary tuberculosis compared to 5% of the nondiabetic group. The study strongly recommended directly observed therapy (DOT) therapy to avoid MDR-TB at least with four drugs while sensitivity report is awaited. If rifampicin and isoniazid (INH) resistance is detected, then two new drugs including the one injectable should be recommended.

Management strategy in tuberculosis with diabetes requires some special alterations:
- Requirement of high calorie and high protein diet (2000–2400 cal per day) in order to:
  - Compensate negative nitrogen balance
  - Prevent further infection or reactivation
  - Better insulin secretion.
- Problems with antitubercular drugs in diabetes mellitus:
  - Rifampicin
    - i. Accentuate destruction of sulfonylurea by drug interaction through P450 cytochrome oxidase enzyme
    - ii. Increase insulin requirement
    - iii. Augments intestinal glucose absorption.
  - Isoniazid
    - i. Antagonizes sulfonylurea action
    - ii. Rarely cause pancreatitis.
  - Biguanides
    - i. Loss of appetite and weight
    - ii. Malabsorption of glucose.

TABLE 56.4	Incidence of diabetes mellitus in tuberculosis patients	
Author	Total	Tuberculosis %
Himasworth 1938	230	6.8%
Bencot et al 1952	3106	4%
Neogi and Roy 1952	1862	3.3%
Turner and Warnick 1957	1851	1.8%
Deshmukh et al 1966	241	8.35%
Dehmkar et al 1975	400	7.8%

TABLE 56.5	Incidence of tuberculosis amongst diabetic subjects	
Author	% of diabetes	Total cases
Landis et al 1919	0.17 to 0.33	6.8%
Weiner and Karea	14.2%	305
Nichols 1957	11.0%	851
Deshmukh et al 1966	14.0%	200
Nanda and Tripathy 1968	12%	875
Lahiri and Sen 1974	8% Male, 5% Female	
Bhatia 1975	14%	150
Bahulkar 1975	4.5%	470

- Insulin is the only mode of treatment for lowering any degree of blood sugar within minimum time as few days of hyperglycemia may affect the anti-tuberculosis response. Insulin also helps in inflammatory response and healing process. Incidence of diabetes in tuberculosis patients and tuberculosis in diabetic patients studied before 1980 are presented in **Tables 56.4 and 56.5** respectively.[44]

Anorexia, weakness, sweating and weight loss are common both to tuberculosis and diabetes. So appearance of any one illness over another is detected very late.

Peculiarities of Tuberculosis in Diabetes

In diabetes, tuberculosis have the following characteristics:
- Relative paucity of physical signs and diagnosis made at far advanced stage
- Extensive caseation of lung tissue and cavitary lesions (bilateral or unilateral) is more in number
- Little pleural involvement
- Greater tendency of hemoptysis
- Less chance of endobronchial tuberculosis.

The severely of tuberculosis depends upon the duration of diabetes in uncontrolled stage. If diabetes is controlled judiciously, response of tuberculosis to drugs is same as in nondiabetic groups.

Preventive Management

- Diabetic persons who were Mantoux test (MT) negative and have recent conversion to tuberculin test should have INH prophylaxis, if they are in close contact with a infective case.
- All diabetic subjects at the initial diagnosis and every year, thereafter must have a X-ray chest done.
- All diabetic subjects with abnormal weight loss, unexplained cough or sudden increase of insulin requirement should have sputum examination and chest X-ray.

PERIODONTAL DISEASE AND DIABETES MELLITUS

Periodontitis or infection of the anchoring tissues surrounding the teeth is usually due to an anaerobic gram-negative organism. This has been claimed as sixth complication of diabetes mellitus by Loe in 1993. Poorly controlled diabetics are likely to develop this chronic infection as periodontal disease (PD) and in turn, this has the potential to alter blood sugar control.

Periodontal disease consists of six categories:
1. Gingival disease—the commonest form
2. Chronic periodontitis
3. Aggressive periodontitis
4. Periodontitis as a manifestation of systemic disease
5. Necrotizing periodontal disease
6. Periodontal abscess.

Chronic periodontal disease is a slowly progressing disease and remains undetected for long time. For these reasons, regular dental check-up is necessary for diabetic persons. It has been postulated that subgingival bacterial contents are higher in DM, leading to more severe disease. This is equally applicable for type 1 and type 2 disease but is dependent upon glycemic control. Regardless of the usual cases of higher infection rate in diabetes mellitus (DM), the effect of interaction between AGE monocytes and its receptor (RAGE) results in chronic release of proinflammatory cytokines like IL-1β, TNF-α and IL-6 from monotypes with matrix metalloproteinases leading to bone destruction.[45]

Alteration in both neutrophilic cellular and collagenase activity by degrading newly formed collagen, impair wound healing in diabetes. In type 1 DM, there is increased risk of PD with age and duration of DM and inadequate glycemic control.

Compared to nondiabetic controls, high incidence of periodontal disease is also seen amongst Pima Indians with type 2 DM.[46] Severe degree periodontal disease is also considered to be associated with higher risk of diabetic complications like proteinuria, stroke, angina, myocardial infarction and heart failure than in diabetic patients with mild periodontal disease.[47]

When treatment of periodontal disease with ultrasonic scaling alone or combined with doxycycline was given, significant reduction of HbA$_{1c}$ was noted after three months, more in the doxycycline treated group. The effects of doxycycline probably were due to altered host response by inhibition of protein kinase C and prevailing excess of IL-1β and TNF-α.[48] On the reverse, good diabetic control accelerates response to treatment for periodontal disease.

Finally, it can be accepted that periodontopathic bacteria increase cytokine release, which may amplify AGE-mediated adverse response and vice versa. Thus periodontal disease either precipitates or aggravates the diabetic process and its complications, and periodontal disease and diabetes mellitus enjoy a two-way relation. Proper dental health is another avenue to diabetic control.

HIV INFECTION AND DIABETES

Insulin resistance and its clinical associates like IGT, DM and dyslipidemia are increasing both in the general population and HIV-infected population in a similar scale. In June 1997, soon after introduction of protease inhibitors (PI), as part of highly active antiretroviral therapy (HAART), FDA issued a warning for increasing cases of hyperglycemia with HAART. The prevalence of Frank DM in people with HIV is rather low with study reports ranging from 0.5 to 15%. But IGT is much higher as estimated to be 15 to 25%. Some degrees of insulin resistance are also noted up to 50% cases on protease inhibitor therapy.[49] Coinfection with HCV is found in 40% cases of HIV+ve persons and is more likely to develop diabetes mellitus insulin resistance (IR). Mehta et al observed that HCV+ve people are four times more likely to develop type 2 DM than HCV-ve persons but no association with hepatitis B was found. If HCV infection occurs in HIV+ve cases, the risk of developing hyperglycemia becomes five times higher.[50] Elevated level of ALT liver enzyme is an indicator for liver inflammations and predicts insulin resistance (IR) in HIV cases with lipodystrophy in presence or absence

of hepatitis B or C. Whether HIV-related hyperglycemia will have the negative health sequences like complications of diabetes mellitus are not yet settled but probably will have the same fate as in HIV-ve cases with hyperglycemia.

One interesting fact is that HAART therapy in children rarely promotes IR, as in adults but develop elevated serum lipid levels equally. Living long with HAART therapy, a HIV person can acquire DM as age-related problems.[51] Common causes of IR in HIV infection are described in **Table 56.6**.

Protease Inhibitor Therapy

Protease inhibitor (PI) therapy directly affects blood glucose metabolism than due to alteration of body fat gain or loss.

Kathelien Mulligan et al compared treatment of 21 HIV+ve cases with protease inhibitor, 9 cases with nucleoside reverse transcriptase inhibitors (NRTI) and 12 cases with no antiretroviral therapy and observed as follows:[52]

Protease Inhibitor-treated Cases

- Elevated fasting insulin and blood glucose, increased triglycerides and LDL.
- Signs of insulin resistance after 3.4 months on average without body shape change at the time.

Nucleoside Reverse Transcriptase Inhibitors treated Cases

No change with blood glucose and lipid is observed with NRTI therapy.

The observations with PI therapy are shown in **Table 56.7**.[51]

Among the protease inhibitors, indinavir is strongly related to glucose intolerance and insulin resistance has been detected within 2 to 8 weeks of treatment even in

TABLE 56.6	Common causes of insulin resistance in HIV infection

- PI therapy
- Lipodystrophy
- Increased local or systemic inflammatory mediators
- Hepatic lipid accumulation
- Muscle lipid accumulation
- Hepatitis C infection
- Reduced systemic adiponectin, leptin and increased resistin
- Low testosterone

TABLE 56.7	Other observations with HIV therapy		
Investigators	Impaired glucose tolerance (IGT)	Diabetes mellitus	Altered insulin sensitivity
George Behren Rabi Walli et al	46%	13%	61%
Frank Goefel et al			55% with PI, 27% with NRTI
WIHS report		2.8 cases per 100 persons years on PI	1.4 cases per 100 persons years on NRTI developed DM

HIV-ve persons. Regarding other protease inhibitors, atazanavir has lowest effect and amprenavir (after 48 weeks of therapy) and saquinavir have got moderate effect on insulin and glucose. The probable mechanisms for PI-induced blood glucose abnormalities are:[51]

- Reduced peripheral uptake by interfering with GLUT-4 activity in the fat and muscle cells up to 26 to 45% in pharmacologic dose, within minutes and reversed after withdrawal which may lead to fat loss in limbs and face.
- Diminished β-cell secretion due to failure to recognize hyperglycemia as GLUT-2, which transports glucose inside β-cell are suppressed by PIs.
- Increased hepatic glucose output up to 47% within 4 weeks of indinavir therapy, due to increase in both glycogenolysis and gluconeogenesis.
- Suppression of adipocyte differentiation, defective expression of PPAR-δ receptors.

Blood Glucose and Lipodystrophy

Loss of peripheral fat and gain in visceral or abdominal fat is known to be associated with IR. This lipodystrophic changes like loss of fat from face and limbs are also present in HIV+ve cases, more so on PI treatment. IR amongst PI therapy are more prevalent in cases with buffalo hump (with fat accumulation at the back of neck). Hadigan et al in a series of 101 HIV+ve cases in the Framingham offspring study have observed several cases with body fat changes.[53] They have also reported insulin resistance in men with AIDS-related wasting syndrome treated with NRTI. Out of them in 52 cases with low testosterone level hypogonadic males, testosterone administration improved IR as body shape and body mass were only minimally altered.[51]

Fatty Acid Metabolism

High blood level of free fatty acids related to visceral fat accumulation and peripheral fat loss interfere with glucose metabolism and produce IR. Hadigan et al

found that HIV+ve cases receiving antiretroviral therapy had heightened fasting lipolysis which was aggravated after glucose administration (opposite in normal persons). This indicates presence of higher free fatty acids and IR but does not exclude role of other factors.

Other Causes for Diabetes Mellitus

HIV-induced β-cell damage has been thought of but not supported by reasonable experiments. Higher level of cortisol, a hormone seen during stress and chronic illness was thought to be a contributing factor but ruled out in recent experiments. HAART therapy produces immune recovery and increased number of TNF receptors have been observed in HIV+ve cases. Mynarcik et al demonstrated elevated TNF receptors to be associated with IR in HIV+ve cases.[54] Imbalance in other cytokines like interleukin IL-1, IL-6, IL-10 may also contribute to blood glucose abnormality.[52] He also observed changes with adipocyte hormones, high level of resistin and low levels of leptin and adiponectin in cases of lipodystrophy in HIV+ve cases.

Recently, Natasha et al reported resolution of DM after initiation of antiretroviral therapy in two HIV-infected patients, the one treated with PIs and another with NRTI.[55] Probably HIV may directly damage β-cell or produce IR by cytokines, hormonal disturbances or unknown mechanisms.

Diagnosis and Monitoring of Diabetes Mellitus in HIV+ve Cases

Fasting blood glucose two hours after 75 g glucose test and fasting serum insulin level are utilized to assess the abnormality in most of the cases. International AIDS Society recommends (2002 Guidelines) fasting blood glucose before HAART, 3 to 6 months after drugs and at least annually thereafter. For persons with high-risk for IR, only oral glucose tolerance test (OGTT) may be performed. They do not recommend insulin estimation.

Management of Blood Glucose Changes

Options

- Lifestyle changes
- Substitution of PIs by other antiretroviral drugs such as nevirapine or efavirenz or abacavir, if possible
- Antidiabetic drugs same as used in HIV-ve cases, do not usually require some insulin therapy.

Oral Hypoglycemic Agents

If lifestyle modification is not adequate or substitution of PIs are not possible, oral hypoglycemic agents (OHA's), e.g. metformin and thiazolidinediones particularly rosiglitazones are of choice to control the glycemic state. Both of these drugs alone or in combination have its effect on improvement in insulin resistance, body fat distribution, free fatty acids and lipid profile in HIV+ve cases also. Sulfonylureas which worsen hyperinsulinemia and produce drug interaction with HAART should better be avoided. Insulin can be used according to the need of the situation.

Drug Interactions between HAART and OHA

- Avoid metformin in patients with NRTI (especially d4T and ddI) as both precipitate lactic acidosis and more so in HIV+ve patients with gross weight loss.
- Avoid thiazolidinediones in cases with liver damage due to associated hepatitis B or C. But rosiglitazone has less impact in liver and fewer interactions with PI. Fluid overload with rosiglitazone and pioglitazone should be kept in mind in cases of AIDS patients with compromised cardiac and renal functions. Insulin is reserved for severe cases of type 2 DM or adverse effects of OHA.

Conclusion

Diabetic patients are at higher risk for acquiring HIV infection because of multiple needle prick, if improperly sterilized or recycled needles are used. Diabetic subjects can also contract HIV from multiple surgical interventions or dialysis and blood transfusion when chronic renal failure develops.

Whether HIV infections alone, like HCV, can produce DM or IGT is not yet clear but it is proved beyond doubt that HAART regimen particularly indinavir is definitely correlated. Between lipodystrophy associated IR and PI-associated IR, the former is more contributory and irreversible than the latter. The risk of acquiring DM in HIV+ve cases are more with HCV infections, obesity and genetic background. Screening for DM should be done with PI therapy and more frequently in high-risk cases. Lifestyle modification is of choice, metformin or glitazones can be added subsequently.

RHINOCEREBRAL MUCORMYCOSIS

Fifty percent of these cases occur in diabetic persons and may present with a life-threatening flare in a person chronically infected with the fungus, *Rhizopus oryzae*. During diabetic ketoacidosis, the inhibitory effect of serum wanes and the disease flares up. But this inhibitory effect is restored after correcting acidosis.[56] Early manifestations are facial, ocular or nasal pain with nasal stuffiness and discharge. Subsequent manifestations are proptosis, chemosis, necrotic black lesions on palate or nasal mucosa, fever, headache, ophthalmoplegia and visual loss from cavernous sinus thrombosis. Hemiparesis may be seen due to thrombosis of cerebral vessels.

Diagnosis is confirmed by demonstration of blood and nonseptate haphazardly branching hyphae from biopsy of necrotic tissue. MRI is essential to identify extent of involvement. Surgical debridement of infected tissue, drainage of the sinuses along with amphotericin B injection is the choice of therapy.

CHOLECYSTITIS

Chronic cholecystitis with or without cholelithiasis is very common in diabetes, probably because of supersaturation of bile, chronic infection, impaired gallbladder motility, decreased cholecystokinin release and hepatic impairment. Emphysematous cholecystitis, an uncommon gas producing virulent infection, is similar to acute cholecystitis, but more frequent in males, with higher mortality due to gangrene or perforation. Some 35% of cases occur in diabetes and 50% contain gallstones. Crepitus on abdominal palpation, demonstration of gas in X-ray or CT scan helps in diagnosis. Prompt cholecystectomy with broad-spectrum antibiotics like ampicillin-sulbactam 3 gm intravenously every 6 hours are the choice of treatment.[56]Agarwal et al (2004) from India studied 91 cases of diabetes for gallbladder function by USG. Both increased fasting gallbladder volume and decreased ejection function of gallbladder were correlated with autonomic neuropathy. Gallbladder volume showed positive correlation with BMI, age and LDL cholesterol.[57]

CHRONIC PYELONEPHRITIS AND CYSTITIS

Chronic urinary tract infection (UTI) is 2 to 4 times more common in diabetes, particularly in women and in presence of autonomic neuropathy with retention in bladder. Bilateral infection is also more often seen with diabetes. Acute manifestations are emphysematous pyelonephritis presenting with fever, loin pain, hematuria, pneumaturia, abdominal mass is a life-threatening situation and in 90% cases occurs in diabetes only.

Failure of remission of fever with therapy for UTI for 3 to 4 days in a diabetic patient possibility of emphysematous pyelonephritis and perinephric abscess should be thought of. Chronic fungal urinary tract infection particularly due to candidiasis is also common in diabetes. It can involve both upper and lower urinary tracts. Infection localized to the bladder may be also due to colonization than infection but pyuria supports the latter. Indwelling catheter if any, should be removed. Bladder irrigation with amphotericin B, single dose of amphotericin B or oral fluconazole for 4 days are the treatment of choice.[57]

CHRONIC INFECTIONS IN DIABETIC FOOT

This is a frequent complication and most neglected issue by both the patient and treating physician. This is discussed in a separate chapter.

FUNGAL INFECTIONS IN DIABETES

These are very common but most neglected situations presenting as oropharyngeal candidiasis and candidal vulvovaginitis (a common mode of presentation in type 2 DM), intertriginous candidiasis (which may lead to gangrene of foot) and paronychia.

Infections Strongly Associated with DM

- Group B streptococcal bacteremia
- *Klebsiella* infections
- Lung abscess
- Endophthalmitis
- Thyroid abscess
- *Salmonella enteritidis*
- Tuberculosis
- Hepatitis C
- Candidiasis.

Measures for Prevention of Infections in Diabetes

- Maintenance of good hygiene
- Standard immunization
- Frequent check-up
- Foot care
- Antibiotics usage, catheterization, IV lines with proper care and above all good metabolic control.

SUMMARY

- Diabetes mellitus (DM) is often complicated by acute or chronic infections, as it is a secondary immune deficiency disorder. DM produces alterations of both cellular and humoral immunity.
- Common chronic infections in diabetes are tuberculosis, pyelonephritis, staphylococcal infections, cholecystitis, candidiasis, viral hepatitis and HIV.
- Hepatitis C and diabetes are very commonly associated. Hepatitis C may be an etiological agent for diabetes mellitus. Hyperglycemia also leads to advanced fibrosis due to hepatitis C.
- Incidence of tuberculosis in DM is 2 to 5 times higher, recurrence with multidrug resistant bacteria is more common. More cavitary lesions, less sputum positivity and with relative paucity of symptoms and signs are the notable features. Treatment for DM should be done preferentially with insulin.
- Periodontitis is a complication of DM and DM may develop from periodontitis also. Proper dental care should be a part of diabetic control.
- Protease inhibitor therapy in HIV infection can lead to development of insulin resistance. But whether HIV produces β-cell damage is not known. HIV and DM may be complicated by HCV infection.
- Rhinocerebral mucormycosis, cholecystitis, chronic urinary tract infection and candidiasis are other common chronic infections in DM.

REFERENCES

1. WHO. Immunodeficiency: report of a scientific group. Technical report series 630. Geneva: World Health Organization, 1978.
2. Moutschen MP, Scheen AJ, Lefebvre PJ. Impaired immune responses in diabetes mellitus: analysis of the factors involved. Relevance to the increased susceptibility of diabetic patients to specific infections. Diabetes Metab. 1992;18:187-201.
3. Pozzilli P, Signore A, Leslie RDG. Infections, immunity and diabetes. International Textbook of Diabetes Mellitus, 2nd edn. KGMM Alberti et al (Eds). John Wiley and Sons 1997;2:1231-41.
4. Gin h, Brottier E, Aubertin J. Influence of glycemic normalization by an artificial pancreas on phagocytic and bacterial functions of granulocytes in insulin-dependent diabetic patients. J Clin Pathol. 1984;37:1029-31.

5. Drell DW, Notkins AL. Multiple immunological abnormalities in patients with type 1 (insulin-dependent) diabetes mellitus. Diabetologia. 1987;30:132-43.

6. Pozzilli P, Arduini P, Visalli N, Sutherland J, Pezzella M, Galli C, et al. Reduced protection against hepatitis B virus following vaccination in patients with type 1 (insulin-dependent) diabetes. Diabetologia. 1987;30:817-9.

7. Hoddinott S, Dornan J, Bear JC, Farid NR. Immunoglobulin levels, immunodeficiency and HLA in type 1 (insulin-dependent) diabetes mellitus. Diabetologia. 1982;23:326-9.

8. Vergani D, Johnston C, B-Abdullah N, Barnett AH. Low serum C4 concentrations: an inherited predisposition to insulin-dependent diabetes? Br Med J. 1983;286:943-8.

9. Allison ME, Wreghitt T, Palmer CR, Alexander GH. Evidence for a link between hepatitis C infection and diabetes mellitus in a cirrhotic population. J Hepatol. 1994;21:1135-9.

10. Amarapurkar D, Das HS. Chronic liver disease in diabetes mellitus. Trop Gastroenterol. 2002;23(1):3-5.

11. Wang CS, Wang ST, Yao WJ, Change TT, Chou P. Community-based study of hepatitis C virus infection and type 2 diabetes: an association affected by age and hepatitis severity status. Am J Epidemiol. 2003;158(12):1154-60.

12. Tazawa J, Maeda M, Nakagawa M, Ohbayashi H, Kusano F, Yamane M, et al. Diabetes mellitus may be associated with hepatocarcinogenesis in patients with chronic hepatitis C. Dig Dis Sci. 2002;47(4):710-5.

13. Mehta SH, Brancati FL, Sulkowski MS, Strathdee SA, Szklo M, Thomas DL. Prevalence of type 2 diabetes mellitus among persons with hepatitis C virus infection in the United States. Ann Intern Med 2000;133:529-99.

14. Fraser GM, Harman I, Meller N, Niv Y, Porath A. Diabetes mellitus is associated with chronic hepatitis C but not chronic hepatitis B infection. Isr J Med Sci. 1996;32:526-30.

15. Grimbert S, Valensi P, Levy-Marchal C, Perret G, Richardet JP, Raffoux C, et al. High prevalence of diabetes mellitus in patients with chronic hepatitis: a case-control study. Gastroenterol Clin Biol. 1996;20:544-8.

16. Petit JM, Bour JB, Galland-Jos C, Minello A, Verges B, Guiguet M, et al. Risk factors for diabetes mellitus and early insulin resistance in chronic hepatitis C. J Hepatol. 2001;35(2):279-83.

17. Bigam DL, Pennington JJ, Carpentier Awanless IR, Hemming AW, Croxford R, Creig PD, et al. Hepatitis C related cirrhosis: a predictor of diabetes after liver transplantation. Hepatology. 2000;32:87-90.

18. Mangia A, Schiavone G, Lezzi G, Marmo R, Bruno F, Villani MR, et al. HCV and diabetes mellitus: evidence for a negative association. Am J Gastroenterol. 1998;93:2363-7.

19. Mehta SH, Brancati FL, Strathdee SA, Pankow JS, Netski D, Coresh J, et al. Hepatitis virus infection and incident of type 2 diabetes. Hepatology. 2003,38:50-6.

20. Mason AL, Lau JY, Hoang J, Qian K, Alexander GJ, Xu L, et al. Association of diabetes mellitus and chronic hepatitis C virus infection. Hepatology. 1999;29:328-33.

21. Zein NN, Abdulkarim AS, Wiesner RH, Egan KS, Persing DH. Prevalence of diabetes mellitus in patients with end-stage liver cirrhosis due to hepatitis C, alcohol, or cholestatic disease. J Hepatol. 2000;32:209-17.

22. Gul Bahtiyar, John J Shin, Ayse Aytaman, James R Sowers, Samy I McFarlane. Association of Diabetes and Hepatitis C Infection: epidemiologic evidence and pathophysiologic insights. Curr Diab Reports. 2004;2:51-5.

23. Hui JM, Sud A, Farrell GC, Bandara P, Byth K, Kench JG, et al. Insulin resistance is associated with chronic hepatitis C virus infection and fibrosis progression. Gastroenterology. 2003;125:1695-704.

24. Piquer S, Hernandez C, Enriquez J, Ross A, Esteban JI, Genesca J, et al. Islet cell and thyroid antibody in patients with hepatitis C virus infection: effect of treatment with interferon. J Lab Clin Med. 2001;137(1):38-42.

25. Fabris P, Floreani A, Tositi G, Vergani D, DeLala F Betterle C. Type 1 diabetes mellitus in patients with chronic hepatitis C before and after interferon therapy. Aliment Pharmacol Ther. 2003;18(6):549-58.

26. Koivisto VA, Pelkonen R, Cantell K. Effect of interferon on glucose tolerance and insulin sensitivity. Diabetes. 1989;38:641-7.

27. Fiore G, Fera G, Nepoli N, Vella F, Schiraldi O. Liver steatosis and chronic hepatitis C virus infection: a spurious association? Eur J Gastroenterol Hepatol. 1996;8(2):125-9.

28. Hernandez C, Genesca J, Ignasi Esteban J, Garcia L, Simo R. Relationship between iron stores and diabetes mellitus in patients infected by hepatitis C virus: a case-control study [in Spanish]. Med Clin (Barc). 2000;115(1):21-2.

29. Cimino L, Oriani G, D'Arienzo A, Manguso F, Loguercio C, Ascione A, et al. Interactions between metabolic disorders (diabetes, gallstones and dyslipidemia) and the progression of chronic hepatitis C virus infection to cirrhosis and hepatocellular carcinoma: a cross-sectional multicentre survey. Dig Liver Dis. 2001;33(3):240-6.

30. Caronia S, Taylor K, Pagliaro L, Carr C, Palazzo U, Pertik J, et al. Further evidence for an association between noninsulin-dependent diabetes mellitus and chronic hepatitis C virus infection. Hepatology. 1999;30(4):1059-63.

31. Vlad Ratziu, Mona Munteanu, Frederic Charlotte, Luminita Bonyhay, Thierry Poynard. Fibrogenic impact of high serum glucose in chronic hepatitis C. J Hepatology. 2003;39:1049-55.

32. Olmos P, Donoso J, Rojas N, Landeros P, Schurmann R, Retamal G, et al. Tuberculosis and diabetes: a longitudinal-retrospective study in a teaching hospital. Rev Med Chil. 1989;117:979-83.

33. Patel JC. Complications in 8793 cases of diabetes mellitus 14 years study in Bombay Hospital, Mumbai, India. India J Med Sci. 1989;43:177-83.

34. Swai AB, Mclarty DG, Nugusi F. Tuberculosis in diabetic patients in Tanzania. Trop Doct. 1990;20:147-50.

35. Garcia PH, Cruz MF, Martines CT. PPD and chemoprophylaxis in diabetes mellitus. Aten Primaria. 1992;9:106-8.

36. Morris JT, Seaworth BJ, McAllister CK. Pulmonary tuberculosis in diabetes. Chest. 1992;102:539-41.

37. Kameda K, Kawabata S, Masuda N. Follow-up study of short-course chemotherapy of pulmonary tuberculosis complicated with diabetes mellitus. Kekkaku. 1990;65:791-803.

38. Jawad F, Shera AS, Memon R, Ansari G. Glucose intolerance in pulmonary tuberculosis. JPMA. 1995;45:237-8.

39. R Goswami, N Kochupillai. Endocrine Implications of Tuberculosis. SK Sharma (Ed). New Delhi: Jaypee Brothers Medical Publishers. 386-95.

40. Karachunskii MA, Balabolkin MI, Beglarian NR. Izmeneniia uglevodnogo obmena ubol'nykh thberkulezom {Changes in carbohydrate metabolism in patients with tuberculosis} Vestn Ross Akad Med Nauk. 1995;7:18-21.

41. Egorova IL. Inkretornia funksiia podzheludochnio zhelezy ubol'nykh tuberkulezom legkikh I sakharnym diabetom. The

incretory function of the pancreas in patients with pulmonary tuberculosis and diabetes mellitus. Probl Tuberk. 1991;9:36-8.

42. Feza Bacakoglu, Ozen Kacmaz Basoglu, Gursel Cok, Abdullah Saymer, Mahmut Ates. Pulmonary Tuberculosis in Patients with Diabetes mellitus. Respiration. 2001;68:595-600.

43. Mona Bashar. Increased incidence of multidrug-resistant tuberculosis in diabetic patients on the Bellevue chest service, 1987-1997: clinical investigations. Chest. 2001;120:1514-9.

44. Banerjee Samar (Ed). Endocrine and metabolic aspects in tuberculosis. Update on Tuberculosis. WB Branch: API, 25-9.

45. Lalla E, Lamster IB, Schmidt AM. Enhanced interaction of advanced glycation end products with their cellular receptor RAGE: implications for the pathogenesis of accelerated periodontal disease in diabetes. Ann Periodontol. 1998;3:13-9.

46. Jeffery Pucher, James Stewart. Periodontal disease and diabetes mellitus. Current Diabetes Report. 2004;4:46-50.

47. Thorstensson H, Kuylenstierna J, Hugoson A. Medical status and complications in relation to periodontal disease experience in insulin-dependent diabetics. J Clin Periodontal. 1996;23:194-202.

48. Grossi SG, Skrepcinski FH. Treatment of periodontal disease in diabetics reduces glycated hemoglobin. J Periodontal. 1997;68:713-9.

49. Dube M. Disorder of glucose metabolism in patients infected with human immunodeficiency virus. Clinical Infectious Diseases. 2000;31(6):1467-75.

50. Mehta S, et al. The effect of HAART and HCV infection on the development of hyperglycemia among HIV-infected persons. J Acquir Immune Defici Syndr. 2003;33(5):577-84

51. Liz Highleyman. Insulin Resistance and Diabetes. Bulletin of Experimental Treatments for AIDS. Winter 2003/2004. A Publication of the San Francisco AIDS Foundation.

52. Mulligan K, Grunfeld C, Tai VW, Algren, Pang M, Chernoff DN, et al. Hyperlipidemia and insulin resistance are reduced by protease inhibitors independent of changes in body composition in patients with HIV infection. J Acquir Immune Defic Syndr. 2000;23(1):35-43.

53. Hadigan C, Meigs JB, Corcoran C, Rietschel P, Piecuch S, Basgoz N, et al. Metabolic abnormalities and cardiovascular disease risk factors in adults with human immunodeficiency virus infection and lipodystrophy. Clin Infect Dis. 2001;32(1):130-9.

54. Mynarcik DC, McNurlan MA, Steigbigel RG, Fuhrer J, Gelato MC. Association of severe insulin resistance with both loss of limb fat and elevated serum tumor necrosis factor receptor levels in HIV lipodystrophy. J Acquir Immune Defic Syndr. 2000;25:312-21.

55. Natasha M, Julio SG Montaner, Gregory Bondy. Resolution of diabetes after initiation of antiretroviral therapy in two human immunodeficiency virus-infected patients. Endocrine Practice. 2004;10(3):199-201.

56. Joshi Nirmal, Caputo Gregory M, Weitekamp Michael R, Karchmer AW. Infections in patients with diabetes mellitus. NEJM. 1999;341(25):1906-12.

57. Agarwal AK, Miglani S, Singla S, Garg U, Dudeja RK, Goel A. Ultrasonographic evaluation of gallbladder volume in Diabetics. JAPI. 2004;52:962-5.

Chapter 57

MACROVASCULAR DISORDERS IN DIABETES: DETERMINANTS AND RISK FACTORS

Sidhartha Das

CHAPTER OUTLINE

- Introduction
- Burden of macrovascular disease in Diabetes with Special Reference to Indian
- Distribution and Profile of Atherosclerosis in Diabetic versus Nondiabetic Persons
- Likely Determinants/Risk Factors for the Development of Macrovascular Disease

---

INTRODUCTION

Macrovascular disease (MVD) is the most prevalent complication amongst diabetic subjects in the West. Almost two-thirds of deaths in diabetics is due to coronary artery disease (CAD), cerebrovascular disease (CVD) or peripheral vascular disease (PVD). The situation has worsened in the postinsulin era due to control over acute complications and infections in diabetes. The problem although more marked in those with type 2 diabetes is also a major cause of morbidity and mortality in type 1 diabetes. Therefore, the American Heart Association has designated diabetes mellitus (DM) as a major risk factor for cardiovascular disease.[1]

BURDEN OF MACROVASCULAR DISEASE IN DIABETES WITH SPECIAL REFERENCE TO INDIAN

Atherosclerosis (AS) is more prevalent in subjects with diabetes mellitus (DM) and quantum of involvement of vascular channels is more profound as compared to those without diabetes. Such association suggest the role of chronic hyperglycemia to be the common determi-nant as most other genetic, hormonal and metabolic parameters, thought to be risk factors (RF) or determi-nants for arteriosclerosis, are dissimilar in these two major types of diabetes mellitus. Prospective study and retrospective analysis in families with type 2 diabetes had revealed that MVD foreruns the development of overt hyperglycemia by decades, suggesting a likelihood of AS and DM sharing a "common soil" for growth and development in the individual.

Studies from USA and other Western countries reveal that CAD, acute myocardial infarction, congestive heart failure and PVD are common morbidities associated with DM. The situation in Indians is different as compared to the West as the four major risk factors for CAD, viz. hypercholesterolemia, hypertension and cigarette smoking are not very prominent among Indians with CAD as compared to the Framingham cohorts.[2]

However, MVD is one of the most established complications of diabetes in India with steady rise in the incidence of CAD amongst the urban population as well as amongst diabetic subjects **(Tables 57.1 and 57.2)**. The prevalence of PVD is much less amongst Indians as compared to diabetic subjects in the West **(Table 57.3)**. Although there has been substantial increase in the prevalence of PVD in Indians where it varies from 0.8%

TABLE 57.1	Prevalence of CAD in urban and rural India[3]		
Author	Year	Place	CD (%±SD)
Urban Population			
Mathur KS	1960	Agra	1.05 ± 0.3
Padmavathi	1962	Delhi	1.04 ± 0.3
Sarvotham SG	1968	Chandigarh	6.60 ± 0.6
Gupta SP	1975	Rohtak	3.63 ± 0.5
Chaddha SL	1990	Delhi	9.67 ± 0.3
Shety KS	1994	New Delhi	10.9
Gupta R	1995	Jaipur	7.59 ± 0.6
Singh RB	1995	Morabadad	8.55 ± 2.3
Begom TR	1995	Trivandrum	12.65 ± 1.5
Ramachandran	2001	Chennai	3.9
Mohan V	2001	Chennai	11
Gupta R	2002	Jaipur	7.30
Rural Population			
Dewan BD	1974	Haryana	2.06 ± 0.4
Jajoo UN	1988	Vidarbha	1.69 ± 0.3
Kutty VR	1993	Kerala	7.43 ± 0.8
Wander GS	1994	Punjab	3.09 ± 0.5
Gupta R	1994	Rajasthan	3.53 ± 0.3
Singh RB	1995	UP	3.09 ± 1.4

TABLE 57.2	Prevalence of CAD amongst diabetic subjects in India[3]			
Author	Year	Place	Prevalence of CAD (%)	
ICMR	1984-87	Multicentric	8.1%	Males
			4.7%	Females
Mohan V	2001	Chennai	21.4%	
Gupta PB	2001	Surat	19%	
Gupta S	2001	Nagpur	33.5%	Males
			21.5%	Females
Phatak SR	2002	Ahmedabad	20.2%	Males
			26.1%	Females

TABLE 57.3	Prevalence of PVD in diabetes[4]		
Author	Country	Year	Prevalence
ICMR (Multicentric-9 centres)	India	1984-87	0.8%
Mohan V, Premalatha G et al	India	1995	3.9%
Pendsey SP	India	1998	3.8%
Premalatha G et al	India	2000	6.3%
Ali SS, Das S et al	India	2005	10% (Foot in DM)
Janka HU, Standl E et al	Germany	1980	16%
Migdalis IN, Kourti A et al	Greece	1992	44%
Walters DP, Gatting W et al	UK	1992	23.5%
Marinelli MR, Beach KW et al	USA	1997	33%

(Foot in DM = those presenting with foot problems, 10% had PVD)

TABLE 57.4	Incidence of CVD in diabetics as compared to nondiabetic subjects[6]	
Place	Incidence	
• Alabama (USA)	3 times higher in DM	
• Norway	2 times higher in DM	
• Whitehall Study (UK)	2 times in DM	
• Finland	2 times in DM	
• Asia and Africa	15.8 (non-DM) : 54.7 (DM)	

TABLE 57.5	Prevalence of CVD among diabetic patients (%)[6]	
Place	Prevalence	
• Overall in India (1960 to 1970)	0.5–9.2	
• Cuttack, Tripathy BB, 1976	3.4	
• Madras, Shanti P, 1991	4.66	
• Madras, V Viswanathan, 1992	1.2	
• Hong Kong, 1970	5.6	
• Hong Kong, 1976	14.6	

TABLE 57.6	Incidence of DM amongst patients with CVD (%)[6]	
		In Percent
•	Study from 11 countries	2–28
•	West KM, North Carolina (USA)	13.9
•	West KM, Michigan (USA)	18.3
•	West KM, Africa	4–8
•	Lam KSL et al, Hong Kong	33.5
•	Das S, Cuttack, Orissa, India	8.0
•	Saroop KS et al, Mumbai, Maharashtra, India	32.0
•	Saroop KS et al, Pondicherry (Pudicherry)	32.0
•	Toole, Janway and Choi	28.0
•	Sabharwal, Anjaneyula and Mehndiratta	20.0

in epidemiological study to 10% in hospital-based publications, it is substantially low as compared to data published from Germany, Greece, USA and UK, where almost 80 to 90% of foot lesions in diabetics are due to atherosclerosis.[3-5]

The prevalence of CVD varies from 3.4 to 9.2% amongst diabetic subjects in India **(Tables 57.4 and 57.5)**.[6] However, the prevalence of DM amongst patient with CVD is much higher as compared to CAD or PVD **(Table 57.6)**. DM is more common (22.1%) cause for cerebral infarction than cerebral hemorrhage (6.35%) as shown by studies from India.[7]

DISTRIBUTION AND PROFILE OF ATHEROSCLEROSIS IN DIABETIC VERSUS NONDIABETIC PERSONS

Atherosclerosis tends to occur in patches with predilection for particular regions in the vascular channels. In the coronary circulation, the proximal left anterior descending artery (LAD), the carotid artery at the bifurcation and abdominal aorta at the origin of renal arteries are more susceptible to develop AS than the other parts of arterial tree. The growth of AS plaques do not occur in smooth linear pattern, but rather discontinuously with periods of waxing and waning of the process.[8] The process of AS is more widespread and extensive with rapid progress in patients with DM as compared to those without.[9] Besides coexistence of the other three risk factors (RF) like dyslipidemia, hypertension and smoking can increase the prevalence of AS in a multiple progressive manner. Studies on coronary angiography had shown higher prevalence of multivessel disease along with more extensive involvement in patients with diabetes as compared to nondiabetic subjects.[10] Further studies from South India had shown

that at any given age diabetic subjects had higher values of intima-medial thickness than those without diabetes and that the difference reached statistical significance over the age of 50 years.[11]

LIKELY DETERMINANTS/RISK FACTORS FOR THE DEVELOPMENT OF MACROVASCULAR DISEASE

Hyperglycemia

The contribution of hyperglycemia as an independent determinant or RF for developing MVD, coronary artery disease (CAD) in particular, has become apparent from the United Kingdom Prospective Diabetes Study (UKPDS). Several biochemical mechanisms consequent to metabolites of glucose can affect numerous cellular pathways both intra-and extracellularly, that can have adverse effect on cells of the vascular walls. These mechanisms can be summarized as:

a. *Increase in nonenzymatic glycation of proteins:* Besides excess glycation of intracellular proteins and plasma membranes; glucose forms glycated compounds and oxidants by causing glycation of primary amines of amino acids in extracellular matrix and fluid. These glycated products can act on inflammatory agents to release cytokines or directly cause vascular dysfunction. The ketoamine can undergo further modification and degradation to form insoluble complexes referred to as advanced glycation end products (AGE). Collagen, present all over to body, are rich in lysine, have long biological half-life and thus most susceptible to glycation and AGE formation. Such changes in the collagen of the vascular wall lead to excess LDL trapping and oxidation. Interestingly, there may be a threshold for these glycation effects in patients with DM, i.e. there is correlation between the degree of glycemia and MVD, whereas among people without DM, there is no such correlation as they fall below the glycemic threshold.

b. *Activation of polyol pathway:* Excess amount of glucose enters the intracellular compartment vascular endothelial cells independent of insulin for glucose transport and get metabolized through the sorbitol pathway. Excess of sorbitol cause change in the redox potential or alter signal transudation pathways, viz. activation of diacylglycerol and protein kinase C. All these adversely affect permeability, contractility, extracellular matrix, cell growth, angiogenesis, cytokine action and leukocyte adhesion processes the tissues of the vascular wall.

c. *Activation of diacylglycerol (DAG)-protein kinase C (PKC) cascade:* Intracellular DAG is the physiological activator of PKC. DAG is derived from multiple sources including hydrolysis of phosphatidylinositides, metabolism of phosphatidylcholine or *de novo* synthesis. PKC consists of a family of 11 isomers representing the major targets for lipid second messengers. Persistent hyperglycemia causes rise in DAG-PKC levels intracellularly in many tissues including aorta, heart, retina, glomeruli and even insulin sensitive tissues like liver and skeletal muscle but not in brain or peripheral nerves. However, transient rise in blood glucose does not cause this and such increase in intracellular DAG-PKC may require 3 to 5 days of persistent hyperglycemia. Increased activation of DAG-PKC cascade leads to multiple cellular and functional abnormalities in vascular cells. There occurs increased release of arachidonic acid and prostaglandin E2 production vis-a-vis decreased Na^+, K^+ ATPase activity which in turn affects cellular integrity as well as function like contractility, growth and differentiation. PKC activation can increase expression of transforming growth factor-β (TGF-β) which increases type IV and type VI collagens and fibronectins which suppress proteoglycans in extracellular matrix. Less production of proteoglycans like glucosaminoglycans in capillary endothelial surface leads to defect in lipoprotein lipase (LPL) binding and consequent poor clearance of VLDL. These metabolic defects lead to the typical dyslipidemia of DM (discussed below). Further, increase in collagen, particularly type-IV, leads to expansion of the basement membrane with vascular dysfunction.

d. *Oxidative stress:* Nonenzymatic glycation is a process that affects protein at any situation whether structural protein, coagulation protein, lipoprotein or carrier proteins in circulation. Hyperglycemia is an important generator of oxygen-free radicals (OFR) production and contributes to glucose auto-oxidation and increased AGE formation. All these combinedly increased the oxidative stress in the diabetic individual. The oxidative stress manifests as increase in NADH/NAD ratio in various cells and tissue with less of nitric oxide (NO) production in vessel wall. The biological activities of such cells are altered. In the vascular channel, the effect can be depressed activity of LPL, decreased insulin action with increased effector cell resistance, attenuated fibrinolysis, increased production of von Willebrand factor (vWF) and endothelin, defective production of endothelial derived relaxation factor (EDRF) and

increase in oxidized LDL. Oxidation, which is enhanced in diabetic state, not only modifies the phospholipid content of LDL but also the amino acid side chains of apoprotein B100 (Apo B100). Such oxidized Apo B100 mediates excess of receptor uptake of LDL by endothelial cell. The oxidized LDL molecule is:
- More recognized by macrophage scavenger receptors and readily taken up to form foam cells: fat-ladened scavenger cells/smooth muscle cells (SMC) in atheromatous lesions. Within the foam cells the degradation of oxidized LDL is impaired leading to further accumulation of lipids in these cells.
- Oxidized LDL increases the adhesion of circulating monocytes to damaged endothelium, enhancing their migration into the vascular intima.
- Oxidized LDL is more immunogenic forming antibody-lipoprotein complex which stimulate foam-cell formation and platelet aggregation as compared to nonoxidized LDL.
- Oxidized LDL has an increased affinity for getting bound to glucose-mediated crosslinks present in the matrix of the vascular intima. These are various hitherto known mechanisms by which increased oxidative stress can lead to enhanced AS and MVD in DM.

e. The enhanced flux of glucose into the cells via hexamine formation has been discussed above under (c) and (d). In general, the Na^+- K^+ pump is defective in diabetic subjects with uncontrolled hyperglycemia. This allows the excess flux and the likely explanation is through DAG-PKC activation.

Hyperinsulinemia–Insulin Resistance[12]

Insulin in physiological levels has antiatherogenic actions whereas in insulin resistance (IR), hyperinsulinemic (HI) situations, it promotes AS. At physiological levels, as insulin increases NO production, retards migration and growth of SMC from the subendothelial layer of vascular wall. The vascular cells are capable of responding to insulin with a wide variety of action. Insulin in situation of HI exerts its adverse effects on the vessel wall through other mediators and mechanisms rather than having a direct effect like enhancing mitogenicity.

In conditions of HI/IR as seen in obese type 2 diabetes, insulin may partly lose its metabolic effect but retains its growth-stimulating effect on vascular wall cells. In patients with HI, insulin exerts its atherogenic effect on SMC by enhancing the mitogenic action of more potential growth factors like platelet-derived growth factor (PDGF) and insulin-like growth factor (IGF). IR and HI can trigger various coagulation abnormalities that act as important factors for development of MVD in diabetes more so with type 2 diabetes. Generation of NO is suppressed in patients with HI. In brief, the mechanisms of enhanced atherosclerosis are:

- Insulin, proinsulin and oxidized LDL can induce increased expression and secretion of plasminogen activator inhibitor-l (PAl-l) by endothelial cell lines and hepatocytes. As PAl-l is a fast-acting inhibitor of fibrinolysis, it helps in thrombogenesis and vascular occlusion. PAl-l is now considered as a part of insulin resistance syndrome (IRS).
- A concentration of endothelial cell protein, vWF is elevated in IRS. This is a marker of endothelial cell dysfunction/damage and raised levels in plasma suggest endothelial cell injury and activation of atherogenesis. Further, secretion of vWF and other procoagulants as well as adhesive molecules indicate the existing procoagulant state.
- Levels of fibrinogen are elevated in IRS. This being an acute phase protein synthesized by liver in response to circulating interleukin-6 (IL-6) suggest role of acute phase cytokines in the abnormalities of coagulation and endothelial function. This is more so in obese diabetics where the adipose tissue secretes IL-6 and adipose tissue-expressed tumor necrosis factor-alpha (TNF-α). Both are proinflammatory cytokines and enhance atherogenesis.

Evidences from studies published in 1979 and 1980 from various parts of Europe and Australia had shown that HI is a predictor of future development of AS in men while the atherosclerosis risk in communities (ARIC) study revealed the reverse phenomenon, i.e. HI was RF for MVD in women. There are reports suggesting that HI did not correlate with AS in non-caucasians. Moreover, the major controversy was raised regarding the estimation of insulin in plasma since most assays also estimated proinsulin along with insulin. It was then thought that the proinsulin was the main culprit for increased prevalence of MVD in type 2 DM with HI which was spurious due to nonspecific assay.

However, two prospective studies, the Quebec Cardiovascular Study and the British Regional Heart Study that used specific immunoassay for insulin have revealed that, there is a threshold for the MVD enhancing effect of insulin and an increase of one standard deviation in specific insulin levels conferred a 70 percent increase in cardiovascular risk.

Dyslipidemia

Dyslipidemia is one of the well-known determinants of MVD. There have been great changes in the profile of lipid abnormalities in the population over the decades. Reports revealing normal values of pre-β-lipoproteins vis-a-vis hypercholesterolemia as RF for increased incidence of CAD in the 1950 have gradually been replaced by volumes of publications suggesting hypertriglyceridemia and abnormalities in LDL fraction with regards to size of the molecule and glycation of its apoproteins as the underlying dyslipidemia in diabetes for development of MVC.[13]

Our own findings of raised triglyceride (TG) levels in DM was originally attributed to the inherent high carbohydrate diet in our population. By early 1980s, we had enough published data to emphasize that raised levels of triglycerides (TG) and VLDL cholesterol (VLDL-C) were more characteristic lipid abnormalities in DM irrespective of nutritional status or body mass index (BMI). Current knowledge from the West corroborates that the major abnormality in diabetics is hypertriglyceridemia with level of cholesterol and LDL being nearly similar to that found in the general population.

Hypertriglyceridemia is one of the main markers of IR, even in diabetic subjects who are lean or low body weight. It is needless to re-emphasize today that most studies have endorsed the view that hypertriglyceridemia confers an increased risk for MVD, CAD in particular, in the general population. This risk of TG is independent of HDL. Hypertriglyceridemia refers to a situation of increased TG-rich lipoproteins. On ultra centrifugation of plasma from such patients, it is found that three-fourth of TG-rich lipoprotein molecules are smaller dense particles and float at a density range of 12 to 60 Sf. All these particles contain one molecule of Apo B 100 and so called intermediate density lipoprotein (IDL). The small dense IDL level is positively correlated with MVD in men with or without DM and is independent of LDL and HDL. Raised TG levels are also associated with increased levels of PAl-1.[13]

Prospective studies have shown that hypertriglyceridemia may antedate development of MVD in type 2 diabetes. Plethora of recent data on insulin sensitivity and CAD suggest that there could be a genetic predisposition for hypertriglyceridemia in patients with type 2 DM. Such genetic abnormality is not monogenic in origin and appears to be determined by genes that cluster in a particular region of one chromosome so as to express concurrently and produce the complex situation of hypertriglyceridemia in type 2 diabetes with increased propensity for MVD. Mutations have been detected in LPL gene locus present in chromosome 8 which can produce impaired clearance of VLDL from circulation. The apoproteins AI, CIII and AIV are known to modulate TG transport and metabolism where AI and AIV stimulate while C-III suppresses LPL activity. The genes for these apoproteins have been found to be located on the long arm of chromosome 11 and at least 14 mutations have been detected in patients with type 2 DM. These mutations can produce apoproteins and LPL that are defective in function and can slow VLDL clearance with consequent persistent hypertriglyceridemia.[13]

The near normal levels of plasma cholesterol in diabetics may be in reality misguiding since at any given concentration of cholesterol, diabetics are two to four times more prone to develop CAD as compared to nondiabetics. This could be due to the reason that the mere quantitative value of cholesterol or LDL may not be important as LDL may be modified, viz. nonenzymatically glycated, undergone oxidation, changed sized to smaller and denser particles. Over and above their interaction with coexistent nonlipid risk factors like AGE, hypertensions, changes in the coagulation cascade make them more atherogenic in diabetes. Further, plasma levels of HDL and its composition have been observed to be altered while efficacy with regard to reverse cholesterol transport subdued. The HDL cholesterol levels have been variably reported to be either low, normal or even raised in diabetes depending on the mode of treatment or state of metabolic control. The role of lipoprotein (a) [Lp(a)] as a determinate for MVD has been widely studied in nondiabetic population. It is genetically determined lipoprotein which varies in distribution and concentration from one ethnic group to the other and is supposed to be a RF for CAD. Certain studies suggest that Lp(a) has a reduced capacity to suppress cellular cholesterol synthesis and thus higher quantities of Lp(a) can get internalized into the endothelial cells through Apo B 100 receptors and cause excess intracellular cholesterol deposition. The plasma level of Lp(a) is more or less uniform in both types 1 and 2 DM but are higher in insulin treated subjects and subjects with IR. Levels of Lp(a) are not well-correlated with incidence of CAD but has a positive correlation with circulating insulin levels. Moreover, level of Lp(a) has been found to be raised in diabetic subjects with either macro-or microvascular disease indicating that it is associated with generalized vasculopathy in patients with DM.

Obesity and Hypertension

These two abnormalities have been well known to be part and parcel if IR and HI syndrome. Both of these make the individual more susceptible to MVD as established from population studies as well as clinical observations. Obesity confers more risk for CAD while hypertension has even greater bearing for development of stroke. Central obesity with increased visceral fat is a major determinant of IR and HI, since these are major promoters of cytokines as well as other products like non-esterified fatty acids responsible for insulin resistance associated with obesity. Besides, the visceral fat contains more receptors for cortisol and for insulin which further aggravates the state of insulin resistance. Both obesity and hypertension are well-established risk factors irrespective of diabetic state.

Rheology

As already discussed increased PAI-1, vWF and fibrinogen can enhance MVD. Levels of factor VII and VIII are elevated along with thrombin, antithrombin complexes, while antithrombin III, protein C and S are reduced. Platelet abnormalities are also observed in both type 1 and type 2 DM leading to increased aggregation and adhesion.

Smoking

Smoking enhances risk of PVD in diabetic subjects more than hundred times as compared to nondiabetic non-smokers. Cessation of smoking is associated with decrease in progression of atherosclerosis. There is strong evidence that smoking markedly increases the risk of both myocardial infarction and complication of peripheral vascular disease in those with diabetes, especially women. Smoking is believed to be associated with adverse changes in plasma lipids and lipoproteins, especially with low levels of HDL.

Homocysteine

Raised plasma levels of homocysteine (He) have been established as an independent determinant for MVD. Homocysteine (He) is an important branch point (intermediary metabolite) in the conversion of methionine to cysteine. In reality, the levels of *He* refer to a family of metabolites in plasma. The clearance plasma level depends on the metabolic efficiency of the individual and depended on the availability of vitamin B_6, B_{12} and folic acid. Nutritional deficiency of these vitamins are known to cause raised plasma levels of *He* because of poor conversion to cysteine. Levels above 16.2 mM/L have been found to be very strongly correlated with MVD. The levels are due to accentuated coagulability state, endothelial cell dysfunction and thrombosis. Studies on diabetic subjects have shown rise in prevalence of CAD and PVD in those with elevated *He* levels irrespective of the type of DM. However, studies on Indian type 2 diabetes patients have revealed linear relationship of plasma *He* levels with BMI and plasma insulin levels. The levels of *He* in healthy controls was about 9 mM/L.[14]

REFERENCES

1. Powers AC. Diabetes mellitus. In Harrison's Principle of Internal Medicine 16th edn; 2004. pp. 2152-90.
2. Enas EA, Mehta JL. Malignant atherosclerosis in young Indians: thoughts on pathogenesis, prevention and treatment. Clinical Cardiology. 1995;18:131-5.
3. Das S, Misra TK. Diabetes, lipids and coronary artery disease in Indians. In Gupta SB (Ed): Medicine Update Vol. 15. The Association of Physicians of India, Mumbai, Maharashtra, India; 2005. pp. 227-33.
4. Das S, Goenka RK. Diabetic dyslipidemia. In Bhattacharya PK (Ed): Medicine Update, Assam Chapter Vol 13. The Association of Physicians of India, Assam Chapter, Dibrugarh, Assam, India; 2003. pp. 559-63.
5. Ali SS, Das SK, Begum T. Foot involvement in diabetes mellitus. The Asian J of Diabetology. 2005;7:15-20.
6. Das S. Cerebrovascular complications in NIDDM. Jr Assn Phys India. 1993;41(Suppl 1):57-65.
7. Padma MV, Bajaj JS. Diabetes and Stroke. In Bansal BC (Ed): Recent Concepts in Stroke. The Association of Physicians of India, Mumbai, Maharashtra, India; 1999. pp. 79-95.
8. Peter Libby. The pathogenesis of atherosclerosis. Harrison's Principles of Internal Medicine, 16th edn; 2004. pp. 1425..
9. Fuster V, Corti R. Evolving concepts of atherothrombosis. In Fuster V (Ed): Assesing and Modifying the Vulnerable Atherosclerotic Plaques. American Heart Association. New York: Futura Publishing Company Inc; 2002. pp. 1-27.
10. Mishra TK, Das S, Patnaik UK, et al. Relationship of metabolic syndrome with quantum of coronary artery disease (CAD) in Indian patients with chronic stable angina. Metabolic Syndrome and Related Disorders, 2005 (in press).
11. Mohan V, Ravi Kumar R, Shanthi Rani S, et al. Intimal medical thickness of the carotid artery in South Indian diabetic and nondiabetic subjects: the Chennai Urban Population Study (CUPS). Diabetiologia. 2000;43:494-9.
12. Das S, Baliarsinha AK. Insulin resistance and dyslipidemia two-way relationship. In Venkatraman S (Ed): Medicine Update Vol 14. The Association of Physician of India, Mumbai, Maharashtra, India; 2004. pp. 100-5.
13. Misra A, Vikram NK. Insulin resistance syndrome (Metabolic syndrome) and Asian Indians. Current Science. 2002;83:1483-96.
14. Das S, Reynolds T, Patnaik A, et al. Plasma homocysteine concentration in type 2 diabetes patients in India relationship to body mass index. J Diabetes and its Complications. 1999;13:200-3.

Chapter 58

ATHEROSCLEROSIS IN DIABETES: PATHOGENESIS

V Mohan

INTRODUCTION

Atherosclerosis, a complicated multifactorial pathological process, affects mainly large and medium-sized arteries resulting in macrovascular disease. Virtually, all large vessels are involved and clinical manifestations result from the narrowing and thrombosis of coronary, cerebral and some peripheral arteries. Though the consequential end points of atherosclerosis are well defined, there is no clear explanation for the pathophysiology leading to atherosclerosis. Further the pathophysiology in diabetic subjects is even more complicated, as several cardiovascular risk factors are triggered due to metabolic alterations resulting in increased risk for atherosclerosis **(Figure 58.1)**. In the past few decades, accelerated development of atherosclerosis in diabetes, both causative factors and pathophysiology has been the subject of intense study.[1] These studies have improved the knowledge on the pathogenic mechanisms of atherosclerosis and the triggering factors that lead to acute clinical events.

ARTERIAL VESSEL WALL STRUCTURE

Endothelial cells, smooth muscle cells and extracellular matrix like elastic elements, collagen and proteoglycans are the basic constituents of the walls of arterial blood vessels. The vessel wall has three layers: the innermost layer—the tunica intima, middle layer—the tunica media and the outer layer—the tunica adventitia.

PATHOLOGY OF ATHEROSCLEROSIS

The pathological sequence of atherosclerosis involves macrophages that develop into foam cells and get

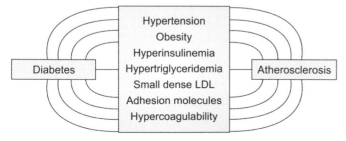

Figure 58.1 Link between diabetes and atherosclerosis

deposited at the junction of the tunica intima and tunica media layers of the artery and later progress into a fibrous atheroma.[2]

Important factors in the initiation and growth of plaques are:
- Endothelial dysfunction and injury
- Subendothelial, monocyte/macrophage accumulation
- Lipoprotein infiltration
- Smooth muscle cell proliferation
- Influx of T-lymphocytes and other inflammatory cells and progressive lipid accumulation in foam cells, finally leading to plaque formation, erosion, platelet aggregation and adhesion thrombosis.

FIBRINOLYSIS AND COAGULATION

Endothelium helps to regulate homeostasis of the cardiovascular system by releasing antithrombotic, fibrinolytic factors, and vasodilators. Diabetes is associated with several disorders of coagulation and fibrinolysis. Patients with diabetes mellitus tend to have increased plasminogen activator inhibitor (PAI-1) levels, decreased fibrinolysis, increased tissue plasminogen activator (tPA) and increased fibrinogen levels in common with metabolic syndrome.[3] Recent studies from Chennai, Tamil Nadu, India have shown levels of fibrinogen and PAI-1 to be associated with angiographi-

cally proven coronary artery disease (CAD)[4] that the relative odds ratios for CAD increased with increase in quartiles of fibrinogen and plasminogen activator inhibitor.[4] These imbalances in fibrinolysis and coagulation increase atherosclerotic progression in diabetic subjects.

LOW DENSITY LIPOPROTEIN

Increase in plasma cholesterol and its main transporter low density lipoprotein (LDL) is an important risk factor in atherosclerosis. In diabetic subjects, LDL tends to get modified due to hyperglycemia, oxidative stress and other metabolic abnormalities. Small dense LDL is considered to be more prone to oxidation and conformational changes,[5] which results in the lowering of LDL clearance by its receptors, triggering immunological changes **(Figure 58.2)**.[6] Some studies have shown the oxidizability of LDL to be associated with early structural changes.[7] Studies have shown that diabetic subjects had higher small dense LDL compared to normals.[8] Modified LDL stimulates endothelial cells to release adhesion molecules.

ADHESION MOLECULES AND CHEMOTACTIC PROTEINS

There is enhanced endothelial production of vascular cell adhesion molecules-1 (VCAM-1) and monocyte

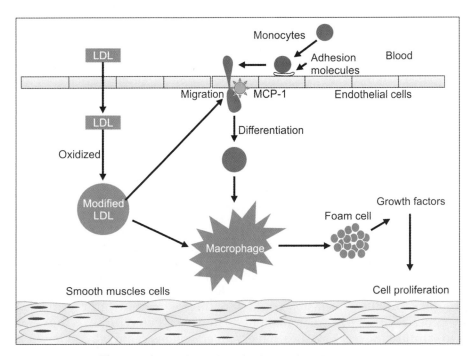

Figure 58.2 LDL induced atherosclerotic process

chemotactic protein-1 (MCP-1) in diabetic subjects, all of which are known to enhance the atherosclerotic process. The chemokine MCP-1 recruits and activates monocytes from the circulation to inflammatory site and this activation is stimulated by VCAM-1.[9]

Damage to the endothelium triggers adherence and aggregation of platelets at the site of damage. This enhances monocytes to further enter the tunica intima and proliferate within the tunica media junction of the artery. This combination of biochemical and anatomical alterations contributes to oxidative stress and increased vascular damage and the vicious cycle continues.

EARLY ATHEROSCLEROTIC CHANGES IN DIABETIC SUBJECTS

Basically the atherosclerotic process could be categorized into functional and structural changes in the artery. The first to occur would be functional changes in the arteries leading to the loss of elasticity. This is followed by structural changes like lipid infiltration and foam cell formation, leading to intimal thickening, plaque formation and finally narrowing of the lumen of the artery interfering with blood flow. The plaque eventually ruptures with consequent intraluminal thrombosis with blockage.

Functional changes can be studied by looking at flow-mediated dilatation or arterial stiffness. These preclinical atherosclerotic markers have gained wide recognition as they are useful surrogate markers for CAD and can also be used in studies on prevention and intervention of CAD.[10,11] In a population-based study, the mean IMT values among diabetic subjects were found to be higher compared to normal subjects.[12] More recently, IMT values were reported to increase progressively with increasing glucose intolerance. In subjects with normal glucose tolerance, the mean IMT values were lowest followed by those with impaired glucose tolerance and highest among the diabetic subjects.[13] Endothelial dysfunction measured as flow-mediated dilatation (FMD) of the brachial artery using high-resolution B mode ultrasonography was also found to be reduced in diabetic patients compared to age and sex-matched nondiabetic subjects.[14]

INFLAMMATION

Recent work suggests that coronary occlusion could be an inflammatory process, in which inflammation causes the plaque to rupture. Several studies have shown an association between inflammatory markers with diabetes. Inflammatory changes could take place near the rupture of the plaque, leading to instability of the fibrous tissue in the plaque, thus facilitating thrombosis. Studies on proinflammatory makers have revealed that cytokines like tumor necrosis factor-α (TNF-α), C-reactive protein (CRP) and interleukin-6 (IL-6) are strongly associated with CAD. Recent studies suggest that raised CRP plays a key role in mediating insulin resistance and coronary artery disease.[15,16] In a study on 150 South Indians, CRP levels were found to be higher among diabetic subjects with and without CAD compared to nondiabetic subjects without CAD.[17]

PLAQUE RUPTURE

The artery responds to the intimal hyperplasia with efforts for a protective action such as an enlargement, thereby increasing the lumen area. This protective process continues until the atheromatous material leads to 40% stenosis. Thereafter, compromise in the lumen area causes hemodynamically significant obstructions.

Acute manifestations of coronary atherosclerosis, viz. unstable angina, acute myocardial infarction, or sudden cardiac death are considered to share a common pathophysiologic phenomenon: thrombosis or a plaque rupture. Plaques need not necessarily block the arteries, rather, much like an abscess; they are ingrained within the arterial wall and may remain asymptomatic. Some plaques called "vulnerable plaques" could be eroded or may rupture. Such plaques are more dangerous than those that cause anginal pain. Several postmortem, retrospective studies have shown that plaque disruption plays a key role in the pathophysiology of acute coronary syndromes.[18,19] The fragility of atheromatous plaques has been related to their irregular formation and high lipid content with propensity to rupture. Unstable atheromatous plaques have an increased tendency to rupture. Studies have documented that diabetic subjects have more vulnerable plaques than nondiabetic subjects.[20]

CONCLUSION

Numerous factors and pathways are involved in the development of diabetes and atherosclerosis. The major pathways are intriguing and challenging to alter. However, behavioral changes or pharmacological interventions can modify many of them.

REFERENCES

1. Shwartz SM, Bornfeldt KE. How does diabetes accelerate atherosclerotic plaque rupture and arterial occlusion? Front Biosci. 2003;8:1371-83.
2. Ross R. Cellular and molecular studies of atherogenesis. Atherosclerosis. 1997;131 Suppl:S3-4.
3. Matsuo T, Kadowaki S, Okada K, Matsuo O. Activity of tissue plasminogen activator and plasminogen activator inhibitor in noninsulin-dependent diabetes mellitus. J Diabet Complications. 1990;4:119-121.
4. Deepa R, Velmurugan K, Saravanan G, Dwarakanath V, Agarwal S, Mohan V. Relationship of tissue plasminogen activator, plasminogen activator inhibitor-1 (PAI-1) and fibrinogen with coronary artery disease in South Indian male subjects. J Assoc Physicians India. 2002;50:901-6.
5. Tan KC, Ai VH, Chow WS, Chau MT, Leong L, Lam KS. Influence of low density lipoprotein (LDL) subfraction profile and LDL oxidation on endothelium-dependent and independent vasodilation in patients with type 2 diabetes. J Clin Endocrinol Metab. 1999;84:3212-6.
6. Packard CJ. Triacylglycerol-rich lipoproteins and the generation of small, dense low-density lipoprotein. Biochem Soc Trans. 2003;31:1066-9.
7. Uusitupa MI, Niskanen L, Luoma J, Vilja P, Mercuri M, Rauramaa R, Yla-Herttuala S. Autoantibodies against oxidized LDL do not predict atherosclerotic vascular disease in noninsulin-dependent diabetes mellitus. Arterioscler Thromb Vasc Biol. 1996;16:1236-42.
8. Mohan V, Deepa R, Velmurugan K, Gokulakrishnan K. Association of small dense LDL with coronary artery disease and diabetes in Urban Asian Indians. The Chennai Urban Rural Epidemiology Study (CURES 8). J Assoc Physicians India. 2005;53:95-100.
9. Lukacs NW, Strieter RM, Elner V, Evanoff HL, Burdick MD, Kunkel SL. Production of chemokines, interleukin-8 and monocyte chemoattractant protein-1, during monocyte: endothelial cell interactions. Blood. 1995;86:2767-73.
10. Yamasaki Y, Kawamori R, Matsushima H, et al. Atherosclerosis in carotid artery of young IDDM patients monitored by ultrasound high resolution B-mode imaging. Diabetes. 1994;43:634-9.
11. Celermajer D, Sorenson K, Bull C, Robinson J, Deanfield JE. Endothelium-dependent dilation in the systemic arteries of asymptomatic subjects related to coronary risk factors and their interaction. J Am Coll Cardiol. 1994;24:1468-74.
12. Mohan V, Ravikumar R, Shanthi Rani S, Deepa R. Intimal medial thickness of the carotid artery in South Indian diabetic and nondiabetic subjects. The Chennai Urban Population Study (CUPS). Diabetologia. 2000;43:494-9.
13. Mohan V, Gokulakrishnan K, Sandeep S, Srivastava BK, Ravikumar R, Deepa R. Carotid intimal medial thickness, glucose intolerance and metabolic syndrome in Asian Indians. The Chennai Urban Rural Epidemiology Study (CURES-22) Diabetic Medicine. 2006;23:845-50.
14. Ravikumar R, Deepa R, Shanthi Rani CS, Mohan V. Comparision of carotid intima-media thickness, arterial stiffness and brachial artery flow medicated dilatation in diabetic and nondiabetic subjects. The Chennai Urban Population Study (CUPS No 9). Am J Cardiol. 2002;90:702-7.
15. Festa A, D'Agostino R Jr, Howard G, Mykkanen L, Tracy RP, Haffner SM. Chronic subclinical inflammation as part of the insulin resistance syndrome: the Insulin Resistance Atherosclerosis Study (IRAS). Circulation. 2000;102:42-7.
16. Ridker PM, Hennekens CH, Buring JE, Rifai N. C-reactive protein and other markers of inflammation in the prediction of cardiovascular disease in women. N Engl J Med. 2000;342:836-43.
17. Mohan V, Deepa R, Velmurugan K, Premalatha G. Association of C-reactive protein with body fat, diabetes and coronary artery disease in Asian Indians. The Chennai Urban Rural Epidemiology Study (CURES-6). Diabet Med. 2005; 22:863-70.
18. Libby P, Theroux P. Pathophysiology of coronary artery disease. Circulation. 2005;111:3481-8.
19. Kullo IJ, Edwards WD, Schwartz RS. Vulnerable plaque: pathobiology and clinical implications. Ann Intern Med. 1998;129:1050-60.
20. Gyongyosi M, Yang P, Hassan A, Weidinger F, Domanovits H, Laggner A, Glogar D. Coronary risk factors influence plaque morphology in patients with unstable angina. Coron Artery Dis. 1999;10:211-9.

Chapter 59

CORONARY HEART DISEASE IN DIABETES

PC Manoria, Pankaj Manoria

CHAPTER OUTLINE

- Introduction
- Coronary Heart Disease in Diabetes: Epidemiology and Role of Risk Factors
- Metabolic Syndrome and Cardiovascular Disease
- Clinical Presentation, Complications and Mortality
- Prediabetes and Coronary Heart Disease
- Primary Prevention of CHD in Prediabetes
- Primary Prevention of CHD in Diabetes
- Management of CHD in Diabetes
- Summary

INTRODUCTION

The last few years have witnessed spectacular advances in the field of diabetes with coronary heart disease (CHD), both in terms of enhanced understanding and in the availability of a rich panoply of therapeutic options in terms of:

- Better control of dysglycemia with advanced pharmacotherapy coupled with nonpharmacological interventions
- Cardiovascular risk reduction with powerful antiatherosclerotic drugs like statins and angiotensin converting enzyme (ACE) inhibitors
- Refinements in percutaneous coronary interventions (PCI) coupled with increasing use of glycoprotein IIb/IIIa receptor antagonists and drug eluting stents (DES) to optimize not only the immediate results but also to minimize distressingly high restenosis rates in diabetics following PCI
- Advances in coronary artery bypass surgery (CABS) with better results and also making with the procedure more patient friendly.

But despite these advances, cardiovascular disease (CVD) is rampant in diabetics throughout the globe including India. With better control of infective and metabolic complications, diabetes has predominantly become a disease of the cardiovascular system.

About 80% of diabetic subjects succumb to a cardiovascular disease and out of this, a major chunk almost to the tune of 75% is contributed by CHD and the remaining 25% by cerebrovascular disease and peripheral vascular disease. CHD is therefore the leading cause of morbidity and mortality in diabetics and demands special focus and attention.

The growing epidemic of diabetes in India estimated at 35 millions by 2003, the rampant cardiovascular disease in them and the horrifying statistical projections for the next 20 years mounting up to 75 is a matter of serious concern and there is an urgent necessity to initiate a national program for prevention of diabetes and cardiovascular risk reduction (CVRR).

Keeping this in mind, a new subspecialty of diabetes, cardiodiabetology has emerged on the scenario and cardiologists and diabetologists are

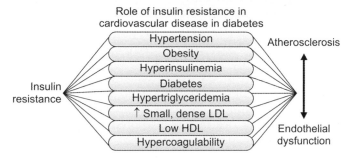

Figure 59.1 Multiple abnormalities that are frequently associated with insulin resistance and eventually lead to endothelial dysfunction and atherosclerosis

joining hands to target and minimize cardiovascular disease in diabetics.

Unlike microvascular disease which gets clicked with onset of diabetes, the macrovascular disease, predates the development of diabetes by several years and by the time the diagnosis of diabetes is made, the macrovascular territory is already studded with athero-occlusive disease.

Why athero-occlusive disease predates the onset of diabetes is a matter of active interest and research? The potential factors responsible for increased risk of athero-occlusive disease in diabetes include hyperinsulinemia and associated cluster of conventional risk factors coupled with genetic and environmental factors. Hyper-insulinemia predates the development of diabetes and is perhaps responsible for promoting athero-occlusive disease in prediabetic state. The strongest evidence to support association between hyperinsulinemia and CHD comes from Quebec Heart Watch Study.[1] The multifaceted mechanisms by which hyperinsulinemia cause insulin resistance and consequent hyper-insulinemia promotes CHD is outlined in **Figure 59.1**.

Besides this, the diabetic vessels are assaulted by a panoply of metabolic, hemostatic and other factors **(Table 59.1)**.

Most distressing is the fact that the risk of development of acute myocardial infarction (AMI) in a diabetic patient over a seven-year period is same as than a nondiabetic one who had already sustained myocardial infarction (MI) as was shown in the East West Study.[2] Thus diabetes has emerged as a cardiovascular disease. Interestingly, the American Diabetes Association (ADA) has identified diabetes as a cardiovascular disease and the National Cholesterol Education Programme (NCEP) Expert Panel on detection, evaluation and treatment of high blood cholesterol in adults (Adult Treatment Panel III) recognizes diabetes as a coronary heart disease risk equivalent thereby implying that the 10 years CHD risk in diabetics is >20%. Targeting CHD in diabetics at the time of diagnosis is too late. Attempts therefore should be made to target cardiovascular disease in prediabetic stage (infra).

CORONARY HEART DISEASE IN DIABETES: EPIDEMIOLOGY AND ROLE OF RISK FACTORS

Diabetes is categorically a cardiac risk factor for CHD and is independent of other known cardiac risks factors.[3,4] Men with diabetes are up to 3 times more likely to die of cardiovascular causes than men without diabetes; the relative risk for women with diabetes is even higher.[3,5-9] The risk of development of AMI in future in diabetics is like a nondiabetic patient with prior myocardial infarction.[2] People with diabetes also have twice the risk of death in the wake of AMI compared to people without diabetes.[10-14]

The pathogenesis of CHD in diabetes is multifaceted and is contributed by several risk factors like hypertension, dyslipidemia, microalbuminuria, smoking, central obesity, etc. Whether or not plasma glucose level is a risk factor for CVD has remained controversial. However, in a recent analysis of data United Kingdom Prospective Diabetes Study (UKPDS)[15] after adjustment

TABLE 59.1	Frequently observed metabolic, hemostatic and other abnormalities in patients with diabetes that may lead to risk of cardiovascular disease
• Hyperglycemia	• ↑ Small dense LDL cholesterol
• Hyperinsulinemia	• ↑ Apo B lipoprotein
• ↑ Levels of insulin growth factor (IGF-1)	• ↑ Tissue angiotensin II levels
• ↑ Intra-abdominal fat	• ↑ Serum fibrinogen
• ↑ Fatty acids	• ↑ Plasminogen activator inhibitor-1 (PAI-1)
• ↑ Triglycerides	• ↑ Oxidative stress
• ↓ HDL cholesterol	• ↓ Synthesis of EDRF (NO)

of other risk factors, a rise in glycated Hb of 1% was associated with a 14% rise in the risk of myocardial infarction.

Patients with diabetes often have clustering of risk factors such as hypertension, dyslipidemia and obesity and the summation of risk factors leads to a much steeper rise in the risk of CV mortality in diabetics compared to nondiabetic population.

Blood pressure: In people with diabetes, large epidemiological studies have clearly demonstrated a progressive continuous relationship between both systolic and diastolic blood pressure and risk of cardiovascular death or myocardial infarction.[3,16-21] In an epidemiological analysis of data from the UKPDS, a 10 mm rise in systolic blood pressure was associated with a 19% rise in stroke, a 12% rise in heart failure and a 17% rise in diabetes related death.[22]

Dyslipidemia: LDL-cholesterol is a progressive continuous CV risk factor in people with diabetes. Similar observations has been reported for relationship between low HDL-cholesterol and high triglyceride levels (a lipid profile characteristics of diabetes) and CV events. In the UKPD study, the risk of angina pectoris or prior MI increased 1.6-fold for every mmol increase LDL-cholesterol.[17] The severity of dyslipidemia is only modest in patients with diabetes but there is evidence in favor of a positive relationship between LDL cholesterol and CV risk even at relatively low range of LDL-cholesterol values.[22] In addition, there seems to be qualitative changes which make even these relatively low cholesterol levels dangerous in patients with diabetes. These factors include an increased rate of glycosylation of apolipoprotein B which in turn leads to increased incorporation of LDL-cholesterol into macrophages. In addition, LDL particles are smaller and more dense, facilitating oxidation and accumulation in the vessel wall. High HDL levels are also protective in diabetics[23] but HDL concentration tends to be low, partly caused by changes in the metabolism of triglyceride rich lipoproteins.

Albuminuria: A meta-analysis of prospective studies[24] and a recent epidemiological analysis of data from the Heart Outcome Preventive Evaluation (HOPE) study[25] have clearly shown that microalbuminuria is an independent risk factor for cardiovascular events as well as heart failure and stroke. Studies of patient with macroalbuminuria have documented an even higher relative risk of CV events.[16] Of considerable interest, however, is a recent evidence showing that the degree of albumin excretion is a continuous risk factor that extends right down into the normal albuminuric range.[25] Studies have also shown that renal insufficiency is also a risk factor for CV events. In the HOPE study, individuals with a serum creatinine ≥ 1.24 μmol/liter had 22% risk of MI stroke or CV death that exceeded the 15.1% incidence in people with better renal function (P <0.001).[26]

Several other risk factors also predict a high-risk of heart disease in people with diabetes. These include abdominal obesity, insulin resistance, proliferative, retinopathy, smoking and a cluster of features together known as the metabolic syndrome (MS).

METABOLIC SYNDROME AND CARDIOVASCULAR DISEASE

A number of recent studies have demonstrated that the presence of MS is associated with significant increase in the risk of CV events and cardiac mortality.[27-34] Large population based Italian study (22256 men and 18495 women) reported that the risk of death from all causes including cardiovascular diseases was increased with the number of metabolic abnormalities (high blood glucose, high blood pressure, low HDL-cholesterol and high triglyceride) in both men and women.[29] In the Framingham Offspring Study (2406 men and 2569 women aged 19 to 74 years), the participants with at least three risk factors related to metabolic syndrome had significantly increased risk for cardiovascular disease, up to 2.4-fold for men and 5.9-fold for women.[30]

Perhaps the most important data emphasizing the importance of CVD in patients with MS are those from a study by Lakka et al in which the investigators prospectively examined the relationship between MS and CVD and overall mortality in middle-aged men participating in the population-based Kuopio Ischemic Heart Disease Risk Factor Study who were followed for 11.4 years.[27] Utilizing both the ATP III and World Health Organization (WHO) definitions, Lakka et al demonstrated that even in the absence of diabetes or prior CVD, the presence of MS was associated with significant increased in the risk of CVD and all cause mortality **(Figure 59.2)**.

Another population-based study recently examined the relationship between the components of MS and the risk of CVD and diabetes. During the five-year observational period, the risk of incident CVD was found to increase with the number of components of MS and increased by more than five-fold in those with four or more components compared to those with only one component.[28]

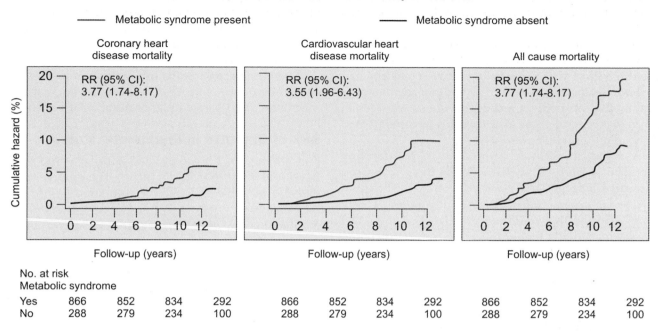

Figure 59.2 Adverse prognostic implication of cardiovascular metabolic syndrome

Recently published data from 11 prospective European cohort studies which included 6156 men and 5356 women also confirmed that nondiabetic subjects with metabolic syndrome have an increased risk from cardiovascular mortality.[31] In another study, the risk of cardiovascular disease was found to be markedly increased in patients with metabolic syndrome, and it was especially very high in patients who had both diabetes and features of metabolic syndrome.[32] The recent study by Ninomiya et al on the subjects participating in the NHANES III survey confirmed the strong and consistent relationship between incidence of myocardial infarction, stroke, and metabolic syndrome.[33]

Metabolic syndrome has also been shown to be a major predictor of cardiovascular risk in women as evidenced in the recent publication from the Women's Ischemia Syndrome Evaluations Study.[34]

The above evidence highlights not only the importance of increasing awareness among clinicians regarding the strong relationship between metabolic syndrome and cardiovascular disease but also the urgency of intervening and modifying the fatal cascade of events in these patients, leading to tremendous increase in mortality and morbidity which would have significant impact on society.

CLINICAL PRESENTATION, COMPLICATIONS AND MORTALITY

Ischemic chest pain is blunted in diabetes mellitus and myocardial ischemia or infarction may be associated with milder symptoms or may be totally silent. In the Framingham study,[35] 25% of myocardial infarctions were unrecognized. Silent infarctions are more common in diabetic (39%) as compared to nondiabetic subjects (22%). Healed scars on the myocardium in the absence of antemortem history of infarction are three times more common in autopsy studies on diabetics compared to nondiabetic patients.[11]

Similarly, during treadmill exercise test, angina is absent during ischemic episodes (painless ST depression) almost twice as commonly in subjects with diabetes than without diabetes. This is due to severe autonomic neuropathy in the former.[36-39] History therefore is not of much help in the diagnosis of myocardial infarction in diabetic patients.

The patient may present with atypical symptoms, such as dyspnea, fatigue, nausea, vomiting or confusion, leading to delay in the diagnosis. Solar et al[40] reported that 35% of diabetic patients with acute myocardial infarction were admitted initially to the medical wards and not to the coronary care unit.

Asymptomatic MI is associated with increased cardiac morbidity and mortality related to delay in seeking medical care.[37] Uretsky et al[41] compared diabetic and nondiabetic patients in whom AMI was associated with atypical symptoms. These patients were older than those with classic symptoms. A majority had no history of prior angina and so did not seek medical help for 12 to 24 hours. Cardiogenic shock was seen in 35% patients with atypical presenting symptoms and the hospital mortality was 50%.

In diabetes mellitus, immediate peri-infarction mortality is high. Diabetic women have increased morbidity and mortality (nearly twice in-hospital mortality in women when compared to men)[37] Czyzk et al[42] reported that middle-aged diabetics with AMI have a substantially higher mortality rate compared to nondiabetics of the same age.

Diabetic subjects develop complications of myocardial infarctions more often than without diabetes. These include cardiogenic shock, CHF and conduction disturbances,[36-42] etc. Anterior infarction is more common in diabetes. CHF was seen in 44% of diabetic women and 25% of diabetic men. The increased incidence of CHF in DM despite similar size of infarct could be due to more extensive CAD,[38] coronary microcirculatory disease, cardiomyopathy antecedent hypertension and autonomic neuropathy. On occasion, left ventricular free wall ruptures may be the presenting feature[43] and this may produce high mortality. High blood glucose on admission in DM with AMI is bad prognostic sign[44] and also contributes to mortality. Reinfarction, fatal and nonfatal are higher in the long-run.

Tanaka et al[45] examined the effects of DM and its treatment on the circadian variation of AMI. They studied 336 patients of AMI and found that peak onset occurred hours between 6 am and 12 noon in nondiabetic while such late morning peak was less prominent in diabetic patients. In diabetic patients receiving adequate treatment, however, the circadian pattern was well preserved, whereas in untreated diabetic patients, there were no peaks in the distribution of onset of AMI. These findings suggest that autonomic disturbances in DM may blunt the late morning peak in the frequency of onset of AMI.

PREDIABETES AND CORONARY HEART DISEASE

Prediabetes is an intermediate stage between normal and overt diabetes. Prediabetes includes impaired glucose tolerance (IGT) and impaired fasting glucose (IFG).

According to WHO, IGT is diagnosed when fasting plasma glucose is <126 mg/dl and 2 hours postprandial glucose is between 144 to 199 mg/dl.[46] According to ADA, IFG stage is diagnosed if fasting plasma glucose is 100 mg/dl to 125 mg/dl.[47]

The prediabetic state not only has high-risk of conversion into diabetes but also harbors ongoing macrovascular disease in large number of patients.

Risk of Diabetes in Prediabetic State

Both IFG and IGT are associated with increased risk for development of diabetes in future. The relative risk for diabetes in subjects with IGT compared to normal is 2.150. However, ethnic differences have been documented by Dowse[48] with Pima Indians having the highest incidence rate of 15 per 100 cases followed by rural Wanigelas, Nauruans, urban Samoans and Mauritius Indians. Both IFG and IGT have more or less similar risk for developing diabetes,[49,50] but they identify different set of individuals. A prospective study on six different populations revealed the incidence rate of diabetes in subjects with IGT to be 57.2/1000 persons years with range from 35.8/1000 to 87.3/1000 persons years in different populations.[51] A longitudinal study in Baltimore is followed up by natural history of diabetes and observed that subjects with NGT progress to the prediabetes, either IFG or IGT and then to diabetes.[52] 22% of subjects with IFG and 17% of subjects with IGT progressed to diabetes during 10 years follow-up. In contrast, a study in Taiwan demonstrated that 17.6% of IGT progressed to diabetes compared to 7.4% with impaired fasting glycemia.[53] Thus, there could be ethnic differences in conversion rates to diabetes in individuals with IFG or IGT in different populations. Given these high rates of conversion to diabetes among prediabetic subjects, it is alarming to observe that the overall prevalence of IGT in urban areas in India is 14.0% with a range from 5.9% to 30.1[54,55] Several studies on the natural history of diabetes have shown that IGT and IFG are prediabetes stages that precede diabetes[49-53,56] and these subjects are therefore an important target group for primary prevention.

Cardiovascular Disease in Prediabetes

Subjects with prediabetes not only have a high-risk for diabetes but are potentially at high-risk for cardiovascular disease.[57] Earlier studies have demonstrated that cardiovascular disease increased in a graded manner with deterioration of glucose intolerance.[58-60] There is indeed a consistent relationship of plasma

TABLE 59.2	Observation on relations between plasma glucose levels and cardiovascular disease	
Study	Study subjects	Incidence of cardiovascular disease mortality
Holsinki Policemen Study 1979[64]	Policemen aged 35-64 years	Higher in the upper 20% of plasma glucose and insulin distribution
Paris Prospective Study 1985[65]	Policemen aged 43-54 years	Higher in the upper 20% of plasma glucose
Whitehall Study 1983[66]	Men aged 40-64 years	In the 95th percentile of 2 hour postload plasma glucose
Chicago Heart Study 1986[66]	10789 men and 7919 women	Higher in subjects with 200 mg/dl one hour oral glucose load plasma levels
Da Qing Study 1993[67]	577 subjects with IGT	9.5 fold higher prevalence of electrocardiographically diagnosed heart disease compared to subjects with normoglycemia
MONICA Study 2003[68]	617 subjects who had oral glucose tolerance test	Odds ratio for unknown myocardial infarction was 4.1 in women with IGT compared to normal

glucose with cardiovascular disease without any threshold.[61] This has led to the introduction of the term 'dysglycemia' which is considered to be a risk factor for cardiovascular diseases.[62,63]

The relationship between plasma glucose levels and cardiovascular disease is shown in **Table 59.2**.

Prediabetes and Cardiovascular Disease— The Chennai Urban Population Study

The Chennai Urban Population Study (CUPS) is a population-based study involving two residential areas representing the lower and middle-income group in Chennai and Southern India. All individuals aged 20 years living in these two colonies were requested to participate in the study, which had an overall response rate of 90.2%. All study subsets underwent an oral glucose tolerance test excluding diabetes and were categorized as normal glucose tolerance (NGT), impaired glucose tolerance (IGT) or diabetes.

The prevalence of diabetes in this study population was 12% and 11% had coronary artery disease (CAD).[55,57,69] Prevalence of IGT in this population was 5.9%. CAD was diagnosed using medical history and Minnesota coding of 12 lead ECG. The prevalence of CAD among subjects with diabetes was 21.4% which is two times higher than that seen in normal glucose tolerance, while the prevalence of CAD in IGT was 14.9%. The prevalence of all cardiovascular risk factors was higher in IGT compared to normal **(Table 59.3)**. The risk for CAD thus seems to increase even at the stage of impaired glucose tolerance.

TABLE 59.3	Prevalence of coronary artery disease and cardiovascular risk factors in subjects with IGT compared to normal—The Chennai Urban Population Study (CUPS)[55]	
Parameters	Normal glucose tolerance	Impaired glucose tolerance (IGT)
Coronary artery disease (%)	9.1	14.9
Obesity (%) Body mass index 25 kg/m^2	23.6	54.1
Abdominal obesity (%) (Waist circumference) Male 90 cm Female 80 cm	23.5	62.2
Hypertension (%) SBP 140 mm Hg and/or DBP 90 mm Hg and/or Known hypertension	16.7	47.2
Hypercholesterolemia (%) Total cholesterol: 200 mg/dl	19.0	43.2
Hypertriglyceridemia (%) Serum triglycerides: 150 mg/dl	17.6	31.1
Low HDL levels (%) (HDL cholesterol) Males <40 mg/dl Females <50 mg/dl	36.5	35.1

Strategies for Prevention of Diabetes in Prediabetes State

Various attempts have been made to prevent diabetes by utilizing nonpharmacological measures as well as pharmacotherapy. The various diabetes prevention trials are exhibited in **Table 59.4**.

TABLE 59.4	Diabetes prevention trials		
Completed trials			
Study	Participants	Mean duration of follow-up	Intervention and risk reduction
Da Qing IGT and diabetes study[70]	577	6 years	Diet: 33% reduction Exercise: 47% reduction Diet plus exercise: 38% reduction
Diabetes prevention program[71]	3234	2.8 years	Lifestyle: 58% reduction Metformin: 31% reduction
Finnish study[72]	522	3.2 years	Lifestyle: 58% reduction
STOP NIDDM Acarbose study[73]	1429	3.3 years	Acarbose: 25% reduction
Ongoing trials			
Study	Participants	Intervention	Study start and end
NANSY	2224 M+F with IFG	Glimepiride	2000-2007
DREAM	4500 M+F with IGT	Ramipril and rosiglitazone	2002-2008

PRIMARY PREVENTION OF CORONARY HEART DISEASE IN PREDIABETES

Attempts have been made to prevent cardiovascular disease by lifestyle modification and pharmacotherapy.

Lifestyle Modification

Physical activity has been shown to have a strong relation with coronary artery disease.[74]

In the Malmo prevention study,[75] the intervention arm constituted 288 IGT subjects who were compared to 135 subjects on routine treatment. Intervention included dietary therapy and physical activity with annual check-up. The IGT routine group had two times greater risk for overall mortality compared to subjects with normal glucose tolerance while mortality rates in the IGT intervention group were similar to that seen in the normal group. This observation indicates that long-term intervention program and exercise help in weight reduction and also to reduce cholesterol levels, which could ameliorate vascular complications. Emphasis on lifestyle changes including dietary counseling and physical activity could reduce mortality in subjects with prediabetes.[75]

A randomized controlled trial utilizing behavioral intervention in 67 adults with IGT by Oldroyd et al[76] demonstrated that intervention in the form of regular diet and physical activity counseling with an adherence to recommendations over a six months period showed favorable effects in weight reduction and reducing blood pressure.

Pharmacological Approaches

Antihyperglycemic Therapy

The STOP NIDDM trial[77] published its report on cardiovascular disease mortality in subjects with IGT in 2003. According to this report, acarbose therapy decreased cardiovascular disease risk by 50% in subjects with IGT, the maximum risk reduction was observed for myocardial infarction with a hazard ratio of 0.09. Multivariate analysis revealed that fasting glucose and systolic blood pressure to be associated with cardiovascular disease apart from treatment with acarbose.[77]

Postprandial hyperglycemia has been associated with cardiovascular disease in many studies.[78,79] However, the benefit of glycemic control in reducing the risk for cardiovascular disease is still not clear in diabetic subjects as UKPDS showed that reduction in myocardial infarction in the intensive group compared to conventional therapy.[80] More recent studies (EDLC) reveal long-term beneficial effects of rigid glycemic control (in DCCT) on incidence of CVD.[81] Interventions to decrease glycemia, in the prediabetes stage may be beneficial as this not only decreases the risk for diabetes but would indirectly reduce cardiovascular disease risk as well.

Blood Pressure Control

The United Kingdom Prospective Diabetes Study (UKPDS) demonstrated that blood pressure reduction helps in preventing cardiovascular outcome.[80] Several substudies from major trials have documented the favorable effects of blood pressure reduction in reducing mortality in diabetic subjects.[82-84] Though these studies were performed in diabetic subjects, they support the notion that blood pressure reduction even among prediabetes stage would decrease CVD risk.

Angiotensin Converting Enzyme Inhibitors

The HOPE study showed that angiotensin converting enzyme inhibitors (ACEIs) inhibitors reduce cardiovascular disease events in subjects with IGT and also prevent diabetes.[85] This chance finding led to the DREAM trial, which will assess the effectiveness of ramipril and rosiglitazone in reducing the risk for both diabetes and cardiovascular disease outcomes in subjects with prediabetes using a factorial design.

Statins

There is no trial available with statins in prediabetic state. However, the substudies of 4S and CARE have shown beneficial effects of cholesterol lowering by statin in subjects with IFG.[86,87]

The 4S study compared the effect of simvastatin in reducing cardiovascular disease events in 3237 subjects with normal fasting glucose, 3237 subjects with IFG and 753 subjects with diabetes. After an average of 5.4 years of follow-up, subjects treated with simvastatin and IFG had significantly reduced coronary events, revascularizations and coronary mortality.[87] In the LIPID trial, pravastatin reduced cardiovascular disease events from 45.7 to 37.1% in subjects with IFG.[88] Another study on IFG from Spain showed that atorvastatin had potentially beneficial actions in addition to their cholesterol lowering effects on lowering the postprandial levels of triglycerides and increasing insulin sensitivity compared to placebo.[89]

Fibrate Therapy

There is no available fibrate trial dedicated to prediabetes.

In the BIP trial, it was observed that subjects with diabetes and IFG had significantly higher rate of cardiovascular disease end-points compared to normal. However, a clinically nonsignificant decrease in clinical outcome was observed in subjects with IFG on bezafibrate compared to placebo.[90]

Aspirin and Beta-blockers

There is no data with aspirin and beta-blockers in prediabetic state.

Although, there is no large data available on prevention of cardiovascular disease in prediabetes, subgroup analysis does show beneficial effects. Thus, besides lifestyle modification, pharmacotherapy may also be utilized for future prevention strategies to reduce the twin epidemics of diabetes and cardiovascular disease in our country.

PRIMARY PREVENTION OF CORONARY HEART DISEASE IN DIABETES

Antiplatelet Agents

In T2DM, aspirin therapy (75-162 mg/day) is recommended for all patients above 40 years or those who have additional risk factors (family history of CVD, hypertension, smoking, dyslipidemia or albuminuria). The same strategy is applicable for type 1 diabetes. Clopidogrel as an alternate for aspirin intolerant patients and an adjunctive in very high-risk patients must be considered.

Angiotensin Converting Enzyme Inhibitors and Angiotensin Receptor Blockers

Diabetic patients >55 years of age with history of CVD, hypertension, dyslipidemia, smoking or albuminuria should be offered ACEI to reduce the risk of CV events as was shown in the HOPE trial.[91]

In the HOPE trial, the primary composite end-point of MI, stroke and CV death was reduced to 22%, CV death by 25%, MI by 20% and stroke by 31% **(Table 59.5)**. In subjects, put on ACEI patients with diabetes also benefited immensely **(Tables 59.6 and 59.7)**. Both the macrovascular as well as microvascular outcome was better. Interestingly, the rate of new onset diabetes was reduced by 34%.[86]

The result of various trials of ACEI showing reduction of new onset diabetes is outlined in **Table 59.8**. The use of angiotensin receptor blockers (ARBs) is also associated with reduction of new onset diabetes **(Table 59.9)**.

The exact mechanism is not known but several mechanisms have been postulated like increase in pancreatic blood flow, anti-inflammatory action and mobilization of fat from anterior abdominal wall which is metabolically active.

TABLE 59.5 Hope trial: Primary adjudicated events—Ramipril vs Placebo

	Ramipril (%)	Placebo (%)	RR	95% CI	P
No. randomized	4645	4652			
Primary outcome MI, stroke, CV death	14.1	17.7	0.78	0.70-0.86	< 0.001
CV death	6.1	8.1	0.75	0.64-0.87	< 0.001
MI	9.9	12.2	0.80	0.71-0.91	<0.001
Stroke	3.4	4.9	0.69	0.56-0.84	< 0.001
Non-CV death	4.3	4.1	1.03	0.84-1.25	0.78
Death from any cause	10.4	12.2	0.84	0.75-0.95	0.006

TABLE 59.6 Hope trial: Diabetes adjudicated events—Ramipril vs Placebo

	Ramipril (%)	Placebo (%)	RR	95% CI	P
No. randomized	1808	1770			
Primary outcome MI, stroke, CV death	15.3	19.6	0.76	0.65-0.89	0.0007
CV death	6.0	9.6	0.62	0.49-0.79	0.00009
MI	10.1	12.7	0.79	0.65-0.96	0.015
Stroke	4.3	6.1	0.68	0.51-0.91	0.0097
Non-CV Death	4.5	4.4	1.03	0.75-1.40	0.87
Mortality	10.6	13.9	0.75	0.62-0.90	0.0024

TABLE 59.7 Hope trial: Other diabetes related events in follow-up—Ramipril vs Placebo

	Ramiptol	Overall Placebo	RR	Ramipril	Diabetics Placebo	RR
Randomized	4645	4652		1808	1770	
Diabetic complications	6.2	7.4	0.84	14.9	17.6	08.3
Overt nephropathy/renal dialysis	3.2	4.2	0.74	6.9	8.6	0.78
Laser therapy	3.7	4.0	0.92	9.4	10.5	0.88
New microalbuminuria	20.2	22.5	0.90	33.0	37.0	0.90
New diagnosis of diabetes	3.7	5.3	0.68	–	–	–

TABLE 59.8 Trials showing prevention of diabetes with an ACE inhibitor

Study	Comparison	Hazard ratio	Result
HOPE[92]	Ramipril vs placebo	0.66 (0.51-0.85)	Ramipril reduced the risk of diabetes by 34% vs placebo
CAPPP[93]	Captopril vs beta-blockers/diuretics	0.79 (0.67-0.94)	Captopril was associated with a low risk of diabetes vs beta-blockers/diuretics
SOLVD substudy[94]	Enalapril vs placebo	0.22 (0.10-0.46)	Enalapril significantly reduced incidence of diabetes in patients with LVD
ALLHAT[95]	Lisinopril vs amlodipine Lisinopril vs diuretics	8.1% vs 9.8% 8.1% vs 11.6%	Lisinopril was associated with a lower rate of diabetes vs CCB or diuretics
ASCOT-BPLA[96]	Amlodipine + Perindopril vs beta-blocker + Thiazide	0.70 (0.63-0.78)	Perindopril was associated with a lower incidence of new onset diabetes

TABLE 59.9	Trials showing prevention of diabetes with an ARB	
Study	*Comparison*	*Hazard ratio*
LIFE[97]	Losartan vs atenolol	0.75 (0.63-0.88)
SCOPE[98]	Candesartan vs control	0.80 (0.62-1.03)
ALPINE[99]	Candesartan/felodipine vs beta-blockers/diuretics	1 vs 8 patients

TABLE 59.10	Management strategies for CHD in diabetes

- Myocardial reperfusion in ST elevation MI (STEMI)
  - i. Thrombolytic therapy
  - ii. Primary angioplasty
- Glucose insulin potassium therapy
- Antiplatelet drugs
- Beta-blocker
- Angiotensin converting enzyme inhibitors
- Statins
- Management of unstable angina (UA) and Non-ST elevation MI (NSTEMI)
- Revascularization in multivessel CAD

The ACEIs also enhances glucose uptake in skeletal muscle by a bradykinin mediated mechanism and blunts serum accumulation of AGEs.

Statins

The CARDs trials[100] have revolutionized the use of statins in diabetes. Prior to this trial, there was no diabetes dedicated statin trial. The subgroup analysis of diabetics in primary prevention trials showed benefits. The CARDs study tested atorvastatin (10 mg) for primary prevention of CVD in 2838 patients of type 2 diabetes without any history of heart disease but having at least one of the following risk factors like hypertension, retinopathy, albuminuria.

The trial was halted two years earlier because of 37% relative risk reduction in CV events, 48% reduction in stroke and 27% reduction in overall mortality rate. What was very striking was that a very low dose of 10 mg atorvastatin has produced CV benefits. Most of the other trials of statins have utilized very high dose of statins which is usually not the practice in India.

Thus, all type 2 diabetic patients with risk factors for CVD should be offered statin.

Beta-blockers

There is no data with these agents on primary prevention of CHD in diabetic patients.

MANAGEMENT OF CORONARY HEART DISEASE IN DIABETES

This can be discussed under following heads (Table 59.10):

Myocardial Reperfusion in STEMI

Thrombolytic Therapy

This should be administered at the earliest, preferably at home or during transportation to a hospital. It is contraindicated in unstable angina (UA) and non-ST elevation MI (NSTEMI). There is no diabetic dedicated

thrombolytic trial but most of the trials have included diabetic patients also. It is seen that if the thrombolysis is completed in the first 2 hours, then the results of thrombolysis are same as primary angioplasty but after this window period primary angioplasty definitely scores over lytic therapy in all aspects.

The important aspects of thrombolytic therapy in diabetic with STEMI are outlined below:

- Diabetic patients are less likely to receive thrombolytic therapy. This is because they may not have chest pain because of associated neuropathy.
- Fear of diminished efficacy. This may happen because diabetics have enhanced platelet activity, elevated procoagulant activity and impaired intrinsic fibrinolysis.
- Patency rates of infarct related artery and mortality benefit.

Despite achieving similar patency rates as nondiabetics, the mortality is higher in diabetic patients (17.3% vs 10.2%) probably because of impaired endothelial dysfunction and diminished myocardial flow reserve.[101] However, in spite of several factors unfavorable to thrombolysis, they still derive substantial benefit from it. The fibrinolytic therapy trialists (FTTs) collaborative group[101] in an overview of 58,600 patients including 1529 diabetics showed that the absolute reduction in the 35 day mortality after thrombolysis in patients with DM was 3.7% compared with 1.5% in nondiabetic counterparts.

In diabetic patients, the mortality fell to 13.6% following thrombolysis as compared to 17.3% in the control group while in the nondiabetic group, the mortality was reduced to 8.7% vs 10.2% in the control group. The reocclusion with recurrent ischemia is also higher in diabetes 9.2% vs 5.3% in the GUSTO study.[102]

There is unnecessary fear of hemorrhagic strokes and ocular complications following thrombolytic therapy in diabetics as this has not been demonstrated in major studies, the FTT collaborative group and GUSTO study.

Primary Angioplasty

The primary angioplasty is more effective than thrombolytic therapy in diabetic too, like nondiabetic patients. The GUSTO IIb angioplasty substudy[103] in the diabetic subgroup showed that despite worse baseline clinical and angiographic profile, more severe stenosis and poor flow in the culprit artery, the procedural success was similar for diabetics and nondiabetics. However, restenosis is more common in diabetics in the long-run.

Glucose-insulin Infusion

The long-term results of diabetes and insulin-glucose infusion in the acute myocardial infarction (DIGAMI) study from Sweden showed that the mortality in diabetic patients with AMI can be reduced by 29% with an insulin-glucose infusion followed by multidose insulin therapy. At one year, 18.6% patients in the intervention group had died compared to 26.1% in the control group. The mortality reduction was particularly evident in patients who had a low cardiovascular risk profile and no previous insulin treatment.[103] These observed benefits from glucose-insulin infusions may be due to suppression of free oxidation of fatty acids. Free fatty acids potentiate ischemic injury by direct toxicity and by inhibition of glucose oxidation and increased oxygen demand. Some of these innovative treatments may be useful in reducing mortality in patients with DM after AMI.

Antiplatelet Drugs

All diabetic patients with CAD must be administered aspirin 75 to 160 mg/day indefinitely. Diabetic subjects have increased platelet activation and accelerated turnover of platelets. Thus, theoretically they may need higher doses or higher frequency of aspirin administration, or need additional antiplatelet agents like ticlopidine or clopidogrel. The subset analysis of the second International Study in Infarct Survival (ISIS-2) found no benefit of 160 mg per day of aspirin in diabetic patients.[104] Since this was a subgroup analysis, it could be a chance finding but it did put a question mark on the efficacy of low dose aspirin in diabetic patients. However, a meta-analysis of the Antiplatelet Trialists Collaborative Group[105] was done to determine the effect of antiplatelet therapy on vascular events. It showed a significant benefit of aspirin therapy in DM with or without vascular disease, for the combined end-point of stroke MI or vascular death. In diabetic patients, the vascular event rate with aspirin fell to 18.5% as compared to 22.3% in controls.[105] The magnitude of this benefit was similar in diabetics and nondiabetic subjects. Doses throughout this range seemed to have a similar effect. There was no appreciable evidence that either a higher aspirin dose or any other anitplatelet regimen was more effective than medium-dose aspirin in preventing vascular events.

Clopidogrel therapy as an alternative therapy in aspirin intolerant patients and adjunctive therapy in very high-risk patients must be considered. With aspirin resistance being increasingly recognized, the use of clopidogrel is likely to increase in future. But after the favorable results of recent trials like CLARITY and COMMIT/CCS2, aspirin plus clopidogrel has become mandatory therapy for STEMI. Distressingly enough, the reports of clopidogrel resistance are also coming. The use of glycoprotein IIb/IIIa receptor antagonists in diabetic patients undergoing PCI improves the results comparable to a nondiabetic state as was shown in the Epistent study.[106] The utility of this agent is not established in patients not being treated with PCI.

Beta-blockers

These are very useful in diabetic patients with coronary artery disease particularly AMI and post-MI state. The results of trials indicate that beta-blockers dramatically improve survival in patients following MI. A meta-analysis of randomized post-MI studies demonstrated that chronic beta-blockade is more effective in diabetic patients and is associated with a 48% reduction of mortality compared to 33% in nondiabetics. Clinicians are often reluctant to use beta-blockers in diabetes counterparts as it may interfere with glucose metabolism, worsen dyslipidemia and may mask symptoms of hypoglycemia. These are unnecessary concerns with use of beta-blockers in diabetes and their benefits outweigh the theoretical adverse risk. Moreover studies have not confirmed that use of beta-blocker leads to higher rates of hospitalization for low blood sugar spells. Prior beta-blocker use is also associated with significantly lower mortality in diabetics undergoing PCI. Beta-blocker remain significantly underutilized in post-MI patients and hypertensive diabetic patients and attempts must be made to widen the net of beta-blockers in diabetic patients. Of late, beta-blocker metoprolol CR/XL has demonstrated antiatherosclerotic effects on carotid IMT in BCAPS[107] and ELVA trial,[108] although these trials were not done exclusively in diabetic patients.

Angiotensin Converting Enzyme Inhibitors

All diabetic subjects with CAD should be put on ACEI. Patients with LVD as well as those with preserved LV function benefit from it. The macrovascular as well as microvascular outcomes are improved by ACEI in diabetics. The benefits of ACE inhibitors in diabetic subjects with athero-occlusive disease including CAD were shown in HOPE trial.[40] The Europa trial carried out in nearly 12000 patients with stable CAD (12% with diabetes) over a period of 4.2 years showed a 20% risk reduction in the composite end-point of death, MI and cardiac arrest.[109]

A retrospective analysis of the data of the GISSI-3 study[110] revealed a decreased 6-week mortality in diabetic patients with lisinopril (8.7% vs 12.4%), an effect that was significantly (p <0.025) higher than that observed in nondiabetic patients (5.6% vs 5.9%). An analysis from the MI collaborative group comprising the pooled data of consensus II, CCS-1 and GISSI-3 trials showed a trend towards higher benefit of ACE inhibition in diabetic patients (17.3 lives saved per 1000 with diabetes treated vs 3.5 lives saved per 1000 without). Even in the consensus II trial, which showed no overall improvement in mortality by intravenous enalapril, a 22% reduction in mortality was seen at 6 months in the diabetic subgroup.[111] The survival of myocardial infarction long-term evaluation (SMILE) study revealed 34% cumulative reduction in the risk of death or severe congestive heart failure (CHF) with zonfenopril at 6 weeks (risk reduction of 61% in diabetes and 23% in nondiabetic subject).[112] The trandolapril cardiac evaluation (TRACE) study also showed the benefit of ACE inhibition following AMI in diabetic patients with severe left ventricular dysfunction (ejection fraction < 35%).[113] One life was projected to be saved in 26 months by treating only 6 diabetic compared to 17 nondiabetic patients. Thus, the efficacy of ACE inhibitors in CAD patients with DM is overwhelming. ACE inhibitors in AMI improves left ventricular remodeling, the fibrinolytic balance, endothelial function and sympathovagal balance. It delays renal dysfunction and improves glycemic control.

Statins

There is no dedicated statin trial in diabetic subjects with CAD. However, the subgroup analysis of various secondary prevention trials have shown significant benefits in terms of CHD risk reduction, the benefits being more in diabetic subsets compared to the nondiabetic section **(Table 59.11)**. Statin should be used in all diabetic patients with CAD.

Management of Unstable Angina and NSTEMI

Thrombolytic therapy is contraindicated in unstable angina and NSTEMI as the clot in culprit artery in this subset is rich in platelets. Aspirin plus clopidogrel is used in all patients as shown in PCI[117] and PCI cure[118] trials. Low molecular weight heparin is also used in all patients and is preferable over unfractionated heparin.

The majority of recent trials of low molecular-weight heparins (LMWH) in ACS have shown their superiority over unfractionated heparin (UFH) in the 30-day incidence of a composite end-point of death, MI or recurrent angina.[119,120] They have been shown to be especially useful in the high-risk subgroups, i.e. patients with electrocardiographic changes, positive troponin, etc. The diabetic patients (n = 2175) in the randomized GUSTO IIb study[121] (n=12142) showed a tendency towards a lower risk of death or reinfarction with

| TABLE 59.11 | CHD prevention trials with statins in diabetic subjects |

Study	Drug	No.	Baseline LDL-C mg/dl (mmol/L)	LDL-C lowering	CHD risk reduction (overall)	CHD risk reduction (diabetes)
			Primary prevention			
AFCAPS/ TexCAPS[114]	Lovastatin	239	150 (3.9)	25%	37%	43%
			Secondary prevention			
Care[115]	Pravastatin	586	136 (3.6)	28%	23%	25% (p = 0.05)
4S[87]	Simvastatin	202	186 (4.8)	36%	32%	55% (p = 0.002)
LIPID[116]	Pravastatin	782	150 (3.9)	25%	25%	19%
4S extended	Simvastatin	483			32%	42% (P = 0.001)

hirudin as compared to heparin at 30 days (12.2% vs 13.9%) and 6 months (17.8% vs 20.2%).

In high-risk patients, an early invasive strategy with PCI is preferred over conservative strategies and this results in reduction in morbidity and mortality. The policy of using ACEI, statins and beta-blockers is same as in STEMI.

Revascularization in Multivessel Coronary Artery Disease

One-third of patients undergoing revascularization have diabetes and a poorer prognosis compared to nondiabetic subjects mainly due to adverse baseline variables. The National Heart Lung and Blood Institute (NHBLI) PTCA registry data showed that diabetic patients were older, had more comorbid conditions and triple vessel disease.

Trials after trials like RITA (1993),[122,123] ERACI (1993),[124] GABI (1994),[125] EAST (1994),[126] CABRI (1995),[127-130] BARI (1996),[131,132] ERACI-2 (2001),[133] ARTS (2001),[134,135] SOS (2001),[136,137] have shown that angina relief is better with CABG compared to PTCA and repeat revascularization is less with CABG. However, with use of glycoprotein IIb/IIIa receptor antagonists and drug-eluting stent (DES), the results of PTCA have improved. The preliminary data from ARTS-II trial has shown comparable data with both revascularization modalities.

Currently, new strategies are being tested in an ongoing bypass angioplasty revascularization investigation 2 diabetes (BARI 2D) trial.

The primary aim of the BARI 2D trial is to test the following two hypotheses of treatment efficacy in patients with type 2 diabetes and documented stable coronary artery disease in a setting of uniform glycemic control, and intensive management of all other risk factors, including dyslipidemia, hypertension, smoking and obesity.

- *Coronary revascularization hypothesis*: A strategy of initial elective revascularization of choice (surgical or catheter-based) combined with aggressive medical therapy results in lower five-year mortality compared with a strategy of aggressive medical therapy alone.
- *Method of glycemic control hypothesis* with a target HbA$_{1C}$ level of less than 7.0%, a strategy of hyperglycemic management directed at insulin sensitization results in lower five-year mortality compared with a strategy of insulin provision.

The BARI 2D trial will use a 2 × 2 factorial design with 2600 patients being randomized. The patients will be divided into four treatment groups: Revascularization with insulin sensitizing, revascularization with insulin providing, medical with insulin providing, and medical with insulin sensitizing.

The future revascularization evaluation in patients with diabetes mellitus—optimal management of multivessel disease (FREEDOM) trial is also ongoing to compare surgical revascularization vs PCI and after this trial, we will be able to know which strategy is better for diabetics with multivessel CAD.

SUMMARY

With better control of infective and metabolic complications, diabetes has emerged as a cardiovascular disorder and 70% of diabetic patients succumb to coronary artery disease particularly acute myocardial infarction.

Unlike microvascular disease which gets clicked with onset of diabetes, macrovascular disease predates the diagnosis of T2DM by several years. Therefore acceleration of targeting cardiovascular disease at the time of diagnosis of diabetes is too late. Attempts must be made to pick-up patients in prediabetic stage and those with metabolic syndrome. Lifestyle modification must be strictly implemented at this stage. There is no big trial of drugs in the prediabetic stage. Subgroup analysis from statin trials favor their use in them. The diabetes reduction assessment with ramipril and rosiglitazone medication (DREAM) trial is ongoing to assess the role of ACEI ramipril in prediabetic stage.

For primary prevention of CHD in diabetes, aspirin (after the age of 40 years), statins and ACEI are recommended in patients with risk factors. There is no trial available with beta-blockers.

For treatment of CHD in diabetes, aspirin, ACEIs and statins are mandatory. Beta-blockers are particularly useful in post-MI patients.

The treatment of ACS in diabetics is same as in nondiabetic subjects. The success rate of primary angioplasty is same in those with diabetes compared to nondiabetic patients. The restenosis rates after PTCA in diabetics is higher than CABG. In diabetic person with multivessel coronary artery disease, CABG is superior but rapid advances in PCI like glycoprotein IIB/IIIa receptor antagonist and DES, this modality is fast encroaching over CABG. The FREEDOM trial is in progress to decide the superiority or inferiority of one modality over another.

In view of the enormous increase in the incidence and prevalence of diabetes throughout the globe, particularly in this country, there is an urgent necessity to initiate a national program for prevention of diabetes, otherwise the disease will slowly engulf our population and we will not be able to control it with our limited resources.

REFERENCES

1. Despres JP, Lamarche B, Mauriege P, et al. Hyperinsulinemia as an independent risk factor for ischemic heart disease. N Engl J Med. 1996;334:952-7.
2. Haffner SM, Lehto S, Ronnemaa T, Pyroala K, Laakso M. Mortality from coronary heart disease in subjects with type 2 diabetes and in nondiabetic subjects with and without prior myocardial infarction. N Engl J Med. 1998;339:229-34.
3. Stamler J, Vaccaro O, Neaton JD, Wentworth D. Diabetes, other risk factors, and 12-year cardiovascular mortality for men screened in the multiple risk factor intervention trial. Diabetes Care. 1993;16:434-44.
4. Chen YT, Vaccarino V, Williams CS, Butler, J, Berkman LF, Krumholz HM. Risk factors for heart failure in the elderly: a prospective community- based study. Am J Med. 1999;106(6) 605-12.
5. Kannel WB, McGee DL. Diabetes and cardiovascular disease. The Framingham Study. JAMA 1979;241(19):2035-8.
6. Fuller JH, Shipley MJ, Rose G, Jarrett RJ, Keen H. Mortality from coronary heart disease and stroke in relation to degree of glycemia. The Whitehall Study. Br Med J (Clin Research Ed) 1983;287(6396):867-70.
7. Goldbourt U, Yaari S, Medalie JH. Factors predictive of long-term coronary heart disease mortality among 10059 male Israeli civil servants and municipal employees. A 23 years mortality follow-up in the Israeli Ischemic Heart Disease Study. Cardiology. 1993;82:100-21.
8. Barett-Connor E, Cohn BA, Wingard DL, Edelstein SL. Why is diabetes mellitus a stronger risk factor for fatal ischemic heart disease in women than in men? The Rancho Bernardo Study. JAMA. 1991;265:627-31.
9. Manson JE, Coldlitz GA, Stampfer MJ, Willett WC, Krolewski AS, Rosner B, et al. A prospective study of maturity-onset diabetes mellitus and risk of coronary heart disease and stroke in women. Arch Int Med. 1991;151:1141-7.
10. Malmberg K, Yusuf S, Gerstein HC, Brown J, Zhao F, Hunt D, et al. Impact of diabetes on long-term prognosis in patients with unstable angina and non-Q-wave myocardial infarction. Result of the OASIS (Organization in Assess strategies for ischemic syndromes) registry. Circulation. 2000;102:1014-9.
11. Behar S, Boyko EJ, Reicher-Reiss H, Goldbourt U. Ten-year survival after acute myocardial infarction: comparison of patients with and without diabetes. Am Heart J. 1997;133(3):290-6.
12. Make KH, Moliterno DJ, Granger CB, Miller DP, White HD, Wilcox RG, et al. Influence of diabetes mellitus on clinical outcome in the thrombolytic era of acute myocardial infarction. GUSTO-1 investigators. Global utilization of streptokinase and tissue plasminogen activator for occluded coronary arteries. J Am Coll Cardiol. 1997;30(1):171-9.
13. Miettinen H, Lehto S, Salomaa V, Mahonen M, Niemela M, Haffner SM, et al. Impact of diabetes on mortality after the first myocardial infarction. Diabetes Care. 1998;21(1):69-75.
14. Melchior T, Kober L, Madsen CR, Seibaek M, Jensen GV, Hildebrandt P, et al. Accelerating impact of diabetes mellitus on mortality in the year following an acute myocardial infarction. Eur Heart J. 1999;20(13):973-8.
15. Stratton IM, Adler AI, Neil HA, Matthews DR, Manley SE, Cull CA, et al. Association of glycemia with macrovascular and microvascular complications of type 2 diabetes (UKPDS 35); prospective observational study. BMJ. 2000;321(7258): 405-12.
16. Gall M-A, Borch-Johnsen K, Hougaard P, Nielsen FS, Parving H-H. Albuminuria and poor glycemic control predict mortality in NIDDM. Diabetes. 1995;44:1303-9.
17. Turner RC, Millns H, Neil HAW, Stratton IM, Manley SE, Mathews DR, et al. Risk factors for coronary artery disease in noninsulin-dependent diabetes mellitus. United Kingdom prospective diabetes study (UKPDS 23). Br Med J. 1998;316:823-8.
18. Wei M, Gaskill SP, Haffner SM, Stern MP. Effects of diabetes and level of glycemia on all-cause and cardiovascular mortality. The San Antonio Heart Study. Diabetes Care. 1998;21(7):1167-72.
19. Mehler PS, Jeffers BW, Estacio R, Schrier RW. Associations of hypertension and complications in noninsulin-dependent diabetes mellitus. AM J Hypertens. 1997;10(2):152-61.
20. Lehto S, Ronnemaa T, Pyorala K, Laakso M. Predictors of stroke in middle-aged patients with noninsulin-dependent diabetes. Storke. 1996;27(1):63-8.
21. Hadden DR, Patterson CC, Atkinson AB, Kennedy L, Bell PM, McCance DR, et al. Macrovascular disease and hyper-glycemia: 10-years survival analysis in Type 2 diabetes mellitus. The Belfast Diet Study. Diabet Med. 1997;14(8):663-72.
22. Adler AI, Stratton IM, Neil HA, Yudkin JS, Matthews DR, Cull CA, et al. Association of systolic blood pressure with macrovascular and microvascular complications of type 2 diabetes (UKPDS 36); prospective observational study. BMJ. 2000;321(7258):412-9.
23. Howard BV, Robbins DC, Sievers Ml, et al. LDL-cholesterol as a strong predictor of coronary heart disease in diabetic individuals with insulin resistance and low LDL. The Strong Heart Study. Arterioscler Thromb Vasc Biol. 2000;20:830-5.
24. Dinneen SF, Gerstein HC. The association of microalbuminuria and mortality in noninsulin-dependent diabetes mellitus. Arch Int Med. 1997;157:1413-8.
25. Gerstein HC, Mann JF, Yi Q, Zinman B, Dinneen SF, Hoogwerf B, et al. Albuminuria and risk of cardiovascular events, death, and heart failure in diabetic and nondiabetic individuals. JAMA. 2001;286(4):421-6.
26. Mann JF, Gerstein HC, Pogue J, Bosch J, Yusuf S. Renal insufficiency as a predictor of cardiovascular outcomes and the impact of ramipril. The HOPE randomized trial. Ann Intern Med. 2001;134(8):629-36.
27. Lakka HM, Laaksonen DE, Lakka TA, Niskanen LK, Kumpusalo E, Tuomilehto J, Salonen JT. The metabolic syndrome and total and cardiovascular disease mortality in middle aged men. JAMA. 2002;288:2709-16.
28. Klein BE, Klein R, Lee KE. Components of the metabolic syndrome and risk of cardiovascular disease and diabetes in Beaver Dam. Diabetes Care. 2002;25:1790-4.

29. Trevisan M, Liu J, Bahsas FB, et al. Syndrome X and mortality; a population based study: risk factor and life expectancy research group. Am J Epidemiol. 1998;148:958-66.

30. Wilson PW, Kannel WB, Silbershatz H, et al. Clustering of metabolic factors and coronary heart disease. Arch Intern Med. 1999;159:1104-9.

31. Hu G, Qias Q, Tuomilehto J, et al. Prevalence of the metabolic syndrome and its relation to all cause and cardiovascular mortality in nondiabetic European men and women. Arch intern Med. 2004;164:1066-76.

32. Alexander CM, Landsman PB, Teutsch S, et al. NCEP defined metabolic syndrome, diabetes, and prevalence of coronary heart disease among NHANES III participants, age 50 or older. Diabetes. 2003;52:1210-4.

33. Nonomiya JK, L'Itaien G, Criqui MH, et al. Association of the metabolic syndrome with history of myocardial infarction and stroke in the Third National Health and Nutrition Examination Survey. Circulation. 2004;109:42-6.

34. Kip KE, Marroquin OC, Keeley DE, et al. Clinical importance of obesity versus metabolic syndrome in cardiovascular risk in women. A report from the women's ischemia syndrome study evaluation (WISE) study. Circulation. 2004;109:706-13.

35. Kannel WB, Hjortlant M, Castelli WP. Role of diabetes in congestive heart failure: the Framingham study. AM J Cardiol. 1974;34:29-43.

36. Sainani GS, Sainani Rajesh. Diabetes mellitus and cardiovascular diseases: current concepts in diabetes mellitus. GS Sainani (Ed) 1993;73-87.

37. Jacoby RM, Nesto RW. Acute myocardial infarction in the diabetic patient—Pathophysiology, clinical course and prognosis. J Am Coll Cardiol. 1992;20:736-44.

38. Serrano-Rios M, Perez A, Saban Ruiz J. Cardiac complications in diabetes. In World Book of Diabetes in Practice: Princeton NJ (Ed). Elsevier. 1986;2:169-78.

39. Bhatia SG, Sainani GS, Nayak NN, et al. Valsalva maneuvers a test for autonomic neuropathy in diabetes mellitus. J Assoc Physician India. 1976;24:89-94.

40. Solar N, Bennet M, Pentecost B, et al. Myocardial infarction in diabetes. QJ Med. 1975;173:125-32.

41. Uretsky BF, Farquhar D, Berezin A, et al. Symptomatic myocardial infarction without chest pain: prevalence and clinical course. Am J Cardiol. 1977;40:498-503.

42. Czyzk A, Krolewski A, Szablowskas, et al. Clinical course of myocardial infarction among diabetic patients. Diabetic Care. 1980;4:526-9.

43. Zahger D, Miligalter E, Pollak A, et al. Left ventricular free wall rupture as the presenting manifestation of acute myocardial infarction in diabetic patients. Am J Cardiol. 1996;78:981-2.

44. Fava S, Aqulina Q, Azzopardi J, et al. The prognostic value of blood glucose in diabetic patients with acute myocardial infarction. Diabetic Medicine. 1996;13:803.

45. Tanka T, Fujita M, Fudo T, et al. Modification of the circadian variation of symptom onset of acute myocardial infarction in diabetes mellitus. Coronary Artery Disease. 1995;6:241-4.

46. Alberti KG, Zimmet PZ. Definition, diagnosis and classification of diabetes mellitus and its complications. Part 1: Diagnosis and classification of diabetes mellitus provisional report of a WHO Consultation. Diabet Med. 1998;15:539-53.

47. American Diabetes Association Clinical Practice Recommendations 2004. Diagnosis and classification of diabetes mellitus. Diabetes Care. 2004;27:S5-10.

48. Dowse GK. Incidence of NIDDM and the natural history of IGT in Pacific and Indian ocean populations. Diabetes Res Clin Pract. 1996;34 (Suppl):S45-50.

49. Keen H, Jarrett RJ, McCartney P. The ten year follow-up of the Bedford survey (1962-1972): glucose tolerance and diabetes. Diabetologia. 1982;22:73-8.

50. De Vegt F, Dekker JM, Jager A, Hienkens E, Kostense PJ, Stehouwer CD, Nijpels G, Bouter LM, Heine RK. Relation of impaired fasting and postload glucose with incident type 2 diabetes in a Dutch population: the Hoorn Study. JAMA. 2001;285:2109-13.

51. Edelstein SL, Knowler WC, Bain RP, et al. Predictors of progression from impaired glucose tolerance to NIDDM: an analysis of six prospective studies. Diabetes. 1997;46:701-10.

52. Meigs JB, Muller DC, Nathan DM, Blake DR, Andres R. Baltimore Longitudinal Study of Aging. The natural history of progression from normal glucose tolerance to type 2 diabetes in the Baltimore longitudinal study of aging. Diabetes. 2003;52:1475-84.

53. Chou P, Li CL, Wu GS, Tsai ST. Progression to type 2 diabetes among high-risk group in Kin-Chen, Kinmen. Exploring the natural history of type 2 diabetes. Diabetes care. 1998;21:1183-7.

54. Ramachandran A, Snehalatha C, Kapur A, et al. For the Diabetes Epidemiology Study Group in India (DESI). High prevalence of diabetes and impaired glucose tolerance in India: National Urban Diabetes Survey. Diabetologia. 2001;44:1094-101.

55. Mohan V, Shanthirani CS, Deepa R. Glucose intolerance (diabetes and IGT) in a selected South Indian population with special reference to family history, obesity and lifestyle factors. The Chennai Urban Population Study (CUPS 14). Journal of Association of Physicians of India. 2003;51:771-7.

56. Hiltunen L, Kivela SL, Laara E, Keinanen-Kiukanniemi S. Progression of normal glucose tolerance to impaired glucose tolerance or diabetes in the elderly. Diabetes Res Clin Pract. 1997;35:99-106.

57. Rennert NJ, Charney P. Preventing cardiovascular disease in diabetes and glucose intolerance; evidence and implications for care. Prim Care. 2003;30:569-92.

58. Rodriguez BL, Lau N, Burchfiel CM, et al. Glucose intolerance and 23 years risk of coronary heart disease and total mortality: the Honolulu Heart Program. Diabetes Care. 1999;22:1262-5.

59. Lowe LP, Liu K, Greenland P, Metzger BE, Dyer AR, Stamler J. Diabetes, asymptomatic hyperglycemia, and 22-year mortality in black and white men. The Chicago Heart Association Detection Project in Industry Study. Diabetes Care. 1997;20:163-9.

60. Jackson CA, Yudkin JS, Forrest RD. A comparison of the relationships of the glucose tolerance test and the glycated haemoglobin assay with diabetic vascular disease in the community. The Islington Diabetes Survey. Diabetes Res Clin Pract. 1932;17:111-23.

61. Balkau B, Shipley M, Jarrett RJ, et al. High blood glucose concentration is a risk factor for mortality in middle-aged nondiabetic men: 20-year follow-up in the Whitehall Study, the Paris Prospective Study, and the Helsinki Policemen Study. Diabetes Res Clin Pract. 1997;36:121-5.

62. Gerstein HC, Anand S, Yi QL, et al. DHARE investigators. The relationship between dysglycemia and atherosclerosis in South Asian, Chineses and European individuals in Canada: a randomly sampled cross-sectional study. Diabetes Care. 2003;26:144-9.

63. Gerstein HC, Pais P, Pogue J, Yusuf S. Relationship of glucose and insulin levels to the risk of myocardial infarction: a case-control study. J Am Coll Cardiol. 1999;33:612-9.

64. Pyorala K. Relationship of glucose tolerance and plasma insulin to the incidence of coronary heart disease: results from two population studies in Finland. Diabetes Care. 1979;2:131-41.

65. Eschwege E, Richard JL, Thibault N, et al. Coronary heart disease mortality in relation with diabetes, blood glucose and plasma insulin levels. The Paris Prospective Study, ten years late. Horm Metab Res. 1985; Suppl 15:41-6.

66. Pan WH, Cedres LB, Liu K, et al. Relationship of clinical diabetes and asymptomatic hyperglycemia to risk of coronary heart disease mortality in men and women. Am J Epidemiol. 1986;123:504-16.

67. Pan XR, Hu YH, Li GW, Liu PA, Bennett PH, Howard BV. Impaired glucose tolerance and its relationship to ECG-indicated coronary heart disease and risk factors among Chinese. Da Qing IGT and Diabetes Study. Diabetes Care. 1993;16:150-6.

68. Lundblad D, Eliasson M. Silent myocardial infarction in women with impaired glucose tolerance: the Northern Sweden MONICA study. Cardiovasc Diabetol. 2003;2:9.

69. Arvind K, Pradeepa R, Deepa R, Mohan V. Diabetes and Coronary artery disease. Indian J Med Res. 2002;116:163-76.

70. Li G, Hu Y, Yang W, et al. Effects of insulin resistance and insulin secretion of the efficacy of interventions to retard development of type 2 diabetes mellitus: the Da Qing IGT and Diabetes study. Diabetes Res Clin Pract. 2002;58:193-200.

71. Knowler WC, Barrett-Connor E, Folwer SE, et al. Diabetes Prevention Program Research Group. Reduction in the incidence of type 2 diabetes with lifestyle intervention or metformin. N Engl J Med. 2002;346:393-403.

72. Tuomilehto J, Lindstrom J, Eriksson JG, et al. Finnish Diabetes Prevention Study Group. Prevention of type 2 diabetes mellitus by changes in lifestyle among subjects with impaired glucose tolerance. N Engl J Med. 2001;344:1343-50.

73. Chiasson JL, Josse RG, Gomis R, Hanefeld M, karasik A, Laakso M. STOP-NIDDM Trial Research Group. Acarbose for prevention of type 2 diabetes mellitus: the STOP-NIDDM randomized trial. Lancet. 2002;359:2072-7.

74. Sesso HD, Paffenbarger RS Jr, Lee IM. Physical activity and coronary heart disease in men: the Harvard Alumni Health Study. Circulation 2000;102:975-980.

75. Eriksson KF, Lindgarde F. No. excess 12 years morality in men with impaired glucose tolerance who participated in the Malmo Preventive Trial with diet and exercise. Diabetologia. 1998;41:1010-16.

76. Oldroyd JC, Unwin NC, White M, Imrie K, Mathers JC, Alberti KG. Randomized controlled trial evaluating the effectiveness of behavioral interventions to modify cardiovascular risk factors in men and women with impaired glucose tolerance: outcomes at 6 months. Diabetes Res. Clin Pract. 2001;52:29-43.

77. Chiasson JL, Josse RG, Gomis R, Hanefeld M, Karasik A, Laakso M. STOP-NIDDM Trial Research Group. Acarbose treatment and the risk of cardiovascular disease and hypertension in patients with impaired glucose tolerance: the STOP-NIDDM trial. JAMA. 2003;290:486-94.

78. Bonora E. Postprandial peaks as a risk factor for cardiovascular disease: epidemiological perspectives. Int J Clin Pract Suppl. 2002;129:5-11.

79. Hanefeld M. Postprandial hyperglycemia: noxious effects on the vessel wall. Int J Clin Pract Suppl. 2002;129:45-50.

80. UK Prospective Diabetes Study (UKPDS) Group. Intensive blood glucose control with sulfonylureas or insulin compared with conventional treatment and risk of complications in patients with type 2 diabetes (UKPDS 33). Lancet. 1998;352:837-53.

81. DCCT/EDIC Study Research Group. Intensive diabetes treatment and cardiovascular disease in patients with type 1 diabetes. N Engl J Med. 2005;353:2643-53.

82. The Systolic Hypertension in the Elderly Program Cooperative Research Group. Implications of the systolic hypertension in the elderly program. Hypertension. 1993;21:335-43.

83. Hansson L, Zanchetti A, Carruthers SG, et al. Effects of intensive blood pressure lowering and low-dose aspirin in patients with hypertension; principal results of the hypertension optimal treatment (HOT) randomized trial. HOT Study Group. Lancet. 1988;351:1755-62.

84. Heart Outcomes Prevention Evaluation Study Investigators. Effects of ramipril on cardiovascular and microvascular outcomes in people with diabetes mellitus: results of the HOPE study and Micro-HOPE substudy. Lancet. 2000;355:253-9.

85. Yusuf S, Sleight P, Pogue J, Bosch J, Davies R, Dagenais G. Effects of an angiotensin converting-enzyme inhibitor, ramipril, on cardiovascular events in high-risk patients. The Heart Outcome Prevention Evaluation Study Investigators. N Engl J Med. 2000;342:145-53.

86. Goldberg RB. The benefits of lowering cholesterol in subjects with mild hyperglycemia. Arch Intern Med. 1999;159:2627-8.

87. Haffner SM, Alexander CM, Cook TJ, et al. Reduced coronary events in simvastatin treated patients with coronary heart disease and diabetes or impaired fasting glucose levels: subgroup analyses in the Scandinavian Simvastatin Survival Study. Arch Intern Med. 1999;159:2661-2667.

88. Keech A. Colquhoun D, Best J. Secondary prevention of cardiovascular events with long-term pravastatin in patients with diabetes or impaired fasting glucose: results from the LIPID trial. Diabetes Care. 2003;26:2713-21.

89. Costa A, Casmitjana R, Casls E. Effect of atorvastation on glucose homeostasis. Postprandial triglyceride response and C-reactive protein in subsets with impaired fasting glucose. Diabetic Med. 2003;20:713-45.

90. Arcavi L, Behar S, Casp A, Reshef N, Boyko V, Knobler H. High fasting glucose levels as a predictor of worse clinical outcome in patients with coronary artery disease: results from the bezafibrate infarction prevention (BIP) study. Am Heart J. 2004;147:239-15.

91. Yusuf S, Gerstein J, Hoogwer B, et al. Ramipril and the development of diabetes. JAMA. 2001;286:1882-5.

92. Hansson L, Lindholm LH, Niskanen L, et al. Effects of angiotensin-converting enzyme inhibition compared with conventional therapy on cardiovascular morbidity and mortality in hypertension: the Captopril Prevention Project (CAPPP) randomized trial. Lancet. 1999;353:611-6.

93. Vermes E, Ducharme A, Bourassa MG, et al. Enalapril reduces the incidence of diabetes in patients with chronic heart failure: insight from the studies of left ventricular dysfunction (SOLVD). Circulation. 2003;107:1291-6.

94. The ALLHAT Officers and Coordinators for the ALLHAT Collaborative Research Group. Major outcomes in high-risk hypertensive patients randomized to angiotensin-converting enzyme inhibitor or calcium channel blocker vs diuretic. The Antihypertensive and Lipid-lowering Treatment to Prevent Heart Attack Trial (ALLHAT). JAMA. 2002;288:2981-97.

95. Dahlof B, Sever PS, Pulter NR, Wedel H, Beevers DG, Caulfied M, Collins R, Kjeldsen SE, Kristinsson A, McInnes GT, Mehlsen J, Nieminen M, O'Brien E, Ostergren J. Prevention of cardiovascular events with an antihypertensive regimen of amlodipine adding perindopril as required versus atenolol adding bendroflumethiazide as required, in the Anglo-Scandinavian Randomized controlled trial. Lancet. 2005;366:895-906.

96. Lindholm LH, Ibsen H, Borch-Johnsen K, et al. LIFE study group. Risk of new-onset diabetes in the Losartan intervention for end-point reduction in hypertension study. J Hypertens. 2002;20:1879-86.

97. Lithell H, Hansson L, Skoog I, et al. SCOPE study group. The Study on Cognition and Prognosis in the Elderly (SCOPE): principal results of a randomized double-blind interventional trial. J Hypertens. 2003;21:875-86.

98. Lindholm LH, Persson M. Alaupovic P, et al. Metabolic outcome during 1 year in newly detected hypertensive: results of the antihypertensive treatment and lipid profile in a north of Sweden efficacy evaluation (ALPINE study). J Hypertens. 2003;21:1563-74.

99. Coltou HM, Betteridge DJ, et al. Collaborative Atorvastatin Diabetes Study (CARDS): effectiveness of lipid lowering for the primary prevention of major cardiovascular events in diabetes. Lancet. 2004;364:685-696.

100. Fibrinolytic Therapy Trialists (FTT) Collaborative Group: indications for fibrinolytic therapy in suspected acute myocardial infraction. Collaborative overview of early mortality and major morbidity result from all randomized trails of more than 1000 patients. Lancet. 1994;343:311-22.

101. Woodfield SI, Lundergan CE, Reiner JS, Green-house SW, Thompson MA, Rohbeck SC, et al. Angiographic findings and outcome in diabetic patients treated with thrombolytic therapy for acute myocardial infarction: the GUSTO-I experience. J Am Coll Cardiol. 1996;28:1661-9.

102. Hasdai D, Granger CB, Srivatsa SS, Criger DA, Ellis SG, Califf RM, et al. Diabetes mellitus and outcome after primary coronary angioplasty for acute myocardial infarction: lessons from the GUSTO-Ib is angioplasty substudy. Global use of strategies to open occluded arteries in acute coronary syndromes. J Am Coll Cardiol. 2000:35:1502-12.

103. Malmberg K, Ryden L, Hamsten A, Herlitz J, Waldenstrom A, Wedel H. Effects on insulin treatment on cause specific one-year mortality and morbidity in diabetic patients with acute myocardial infarction. DIGAMI Study Group. Eur Heart J. 1996;17:1337-44.

104. Second International Study of Infarct Survival (ISIS-2) Collaborative Group. Randomized trial of intravenous streptokinase, oral aspirin, both or neither among 17187 cases of suspected myocardial infarction: ISISI-2. Lancet. 1988;2:349-60.

105. Antiplatelet Trialists' Collaboration. Collaborative overview of randomized trials of antiplatelet therapy-I; prevention of death. Myocardial infarction and stroke by prolonged antiplatelet therapy in various categories of patients: BMJ. 1994;308:81-106.

106. Marso SP, Lincoff AM, Ellis SG, Bhatt DL, et al. Optimizing the percutaneous interventional outcomes for patients with diabetes mellitus. Results of the EPISTENT diabetic substudy. Circulation. 1999;100:2477-84.

107. Hedblad B, Wikstrand J, Janzon L, Wedel H, Berglund G. Low-dose metoprolol CR/XL and fluvastatin slow progression of carotid intima-media thickness: main results from the beta-blocker cholesterol-lowering asymptomatic plaque study (BCAPS). Circulation. 2001;103:1721-6.

108. Wiklund O, Hulthe J, Wikstrand J, Schmidt C, Olofsson SO, Bondjers G. Effect of controlled release/extended release metoprolol on cartotid intima-media thickness in patients with hypercholesterolemia: a 3-year randomized study. Stroke. 2002;33:572-7.

109. Efficacy of perindopril in reduction of cardiovascular events among patients with stable coronary artery disease: randomized, double blind, placebo controlled, multicentric trial (the EUROPA study). Lancet. 2003;362:782-8.

110. Zuanetti G, Latini R, Maggioni AP, Franzolsi M, Santoro L, Tognoni G, et al. Effect of the ACE inhibitor lisinopril on mortality in diabetic patients with acute myocardial infarction: data from the GISSI-3 study. Circulation. 1997;96:4239-45.

111. Swedberg K, Hed P, Kjekshus J, Rasmussen K, Rydeat L, Wedel H. Effects of early administration of enalapril on mortality in patients with acute myocardial infarction. Results of CONSENSUS-II. N Engl J Med. 1992;327:678.

112. Ambrosioni E, Borghi C, Magnani B. The effect of the angiotensin converting enzyme inhibitor zofenopril on mortality and morbidity after anterior myocardial infarction. The survival of myocardial infarction long-term evaluation (SMILE) study investigators. N Engl J Med. 1995;332:80-5.

113. Gustafson I, Hildebrandt P, Seibaek M, Melchior T, Torp-Pedersen C, Kober L, et al. Long-term prognosis of diabetic patients with myocardial infarction: relation to antidiabetic treatment regimen. The TRACE Study Group. Eur Heart J. 2000;21:1937-43.

114. Downs JR, Clearfield M, Weis S, Whitney E, Shapiro DR, Beere PA, Langendorfer A, Stein EA, Kruyer W, Gotto AM Jr, for the AFCAPS/TexCAPS Research Group. Primary prevention of acute coronary events with lovastatin in men and women with average cholesterol levels: results of AFCAPS/TexCAPS. JAMA. 1998;279:1615-22.

115. Goldberg RB, Mellies MJ, Sacks FM, Moyel LA, Howard BV, Howard WJ, Davis BR, Cole TG, Pfeffer MA, Braunwald E. Cardiovascular events and their reduction with pravastatin in diabetic and glucose intolerant myocardial infarction survivors with average cholesterol levels: subgroup analyses in the cholesterol and recurrent events (CARE) trial. Circulation. 1998;98:2513-9.

116. Long-term effectiveness and safety of pravastatin in 9014 patients with coronary heart disease and average cholesterol concentrations: the LIPID trial follow-up. Lancet. 2002; 359(9315):1379-87.

117. The CURE investigators. Effects of clopidogrel in addition to aspirin in patients with acute coronary syndromes without ST segment elevation. N Engl J Med. 2001;345:494-502.

118. Mehta Sr, Yusuf S, Peters RJG, et al. Effects of pretreatment with clopidogrel and aspirin followed by long-term therapy in patients undergoing percutaneous coronary intervention: the PCI-CURE study. Lancet. 2001;358:527-33.

119. Cohen M, Demers C, Gurfinkel EP, Turpie AG, Fromell GJ, Goodman S, et al. Low molecular weight heparins in non ST-segment elevation ischemia the ESSENCE trial. Am J Cardiol. 1998;82:19-24L.

120. Bernink PJLM, Antman EM, McCabe CH, Horacek T, Papuchis G, Mautrer B. Treatment benefit with enoxaparin in unstable angina is greatest in patients at highest risk: a multivariate analysis from TIMI IIB (Abstr). J Am Coll Cardiol. 1999;33(Suppl A):352A.

121. Angioplasty Substudy Investigators. The global use of strategies to open occluded coronary arteries in acute coronary syndromes (GUSTO IIb): a clinical trial comparing primary coronary angioplasty with tissue plasminogen activator for acute myocardial infarction N Engl J Med. 1997;366:1621-8.

122. RITA Trial Participants. Coronary angioplasty vs coronary artery bypass surgery. The randomized intervention treatment of angina (RITA) trial. Lancet. 1993;341:573.

123. Henderson RA. The randomized intervention treatment of angina (RITA) trial protocol: A long-term study of coronary angioplasty and coronary artery bypass surgery in patients with angina. Br Hert J. 1979;62:411.

124. Rodriguez A, Boullon F, Perez-Balino N, et al. Argentine Randomized Trial of Percutaneous Transluminal Coronary Angioplasty versus Coronary Artery Bypass Surgery in Multivessel Disease (ERACI). In: hospital results and 1 year follow-up. J Am Coll Cardiol. 1993;22:1060.

125. Hamm CW, Reimbers J, Ischinger T, et al for the German Angioplasty Bypass Surgery Investigation: A randomized study of coronary angioplasty compared with bypass surgery in patients with symptomatic multivessel coronary disease. N Engl J Med. 1994;331:1037.

126. King SB III, Lembo NJ, Wintraub WS, et al. Emory Angioplasty versus Surgery Trial (EAST): Design, recruitment and baseline description of patients. Am J Cardiol. 1995;75:42C.

127. CABRI Trial Participants. First-year results of coronary angioplasty versus bypass revascularization investigation (CABRI). Lancet. 1995;346:1179.

128. Kurbaan AS, Bowker TJ, Rickards AF. Differential restenosis rate of individual coronary artery sites after multivessel angioplasty: implications for revascularization strategy. CABRI Investigators. Coronary Angioplasty versus Bypass Revascularization Investigation. Am Heart J. 1998;135:703-8.

129. Kurbaan AS, Bowker TJ , Illsley CD, et al on behalf of the CABRI (Coronary Angioplasty versus Bypass Revascularization Investigation) Investigators: difference in the mortality of the CABRI diabetic and nondiabetic populations and its relation to coronary artery disease and the revascularization mode. Am J Cardiol. 2001;87:947-50.

130. Wahrborg P. Quality of life after coronary angioplasty or bypass surgery: 1-year follow-up in the coronary angioplasty versus bypass revascularization investigation (CABRI) trial. Eur Heart J. 1999;20:653-8.

131. Rogers WJ, Alderman EL, Chaitman BR, et al. Bypass angioplasty revascularization investigation (BARI): baseline clinical and angiographic data. Am J Cardiol. 1995;75:9C.

132. Schaff HV, Rosen AD, Shemin RJ, et al. Clinical and operative characteristics of patients randomized to coronary artery bypass surgery in the bypass angioplasty revascularization investigation (BARI). Am J Cardiol. 1995;75:18C.

133. Rodriguez A, Bernardi V, Navia J, et al. Argentine Randomized Study: Coronary Angioplasty with Stenting Versus Coronary Bypass surgery in Patients with Multiple-Vessel Disease (ERACI II): 30 days and one-year follow-up results. ERACI II Investigators. J Am Coll Cardiol. 2001;37:51-8.

134. Serruys PW, Unger F, Sousa JE, et al for the Arterial Revascularization Therapies Study Group: comparison of coronary artery bypass surgery and stenting for the treatment of multivessel disease. N Engl J Med. 2001;344:1117-24.

135. Serruys P. Three year results form the Arterial Revascularization Therapies Study (ARTS). Presented at the XXIII Congress of the European Society of Cardiology, Stockholm, Sweden, 2001.

136. Stables RH. Design of the Stent or Surgery Trial (SOS): a randomized controlled trial to compared coronary artery bypass grafting with percutaneous transluminal coronary angioplasty and primary stent implantation in patients with multivessel coronary artery disease. Semin Intervent Cardiol. 1999;4:201-7.

137. Stables R. SOS trial (Stent or Surgery trial). Presented at the 50th Scientific Session of the American College of Cardiol. Orlando, FL, March 2001.

Chapter 60

EPIDEMIOLOGY OF CORONARY ARTERY DISEASE IN DIABETES

OP Gupta, Tiven Marwah

CHAPTER OUTLINE

- Introduction
- Epidemiology of Coronary Artery Disease—Global, Indian and in Immigrant Indians
- Epidemiology of CAD in Type 1 Diabetes Mellitus
- Epidemiology of CAD in Type 2 DM—Special Features
- Impact of Diabetes on CAD in Women
- Impact of Diabetes on CAD Mortality
- CAD in Type 2 DM having Diabetic Nephropathy
- CAD in Diabetes—Indian Studies
- CAD in Prediabetes
- Prevalence of Pre-CAD Markers in DM
- Summary

INTRODUCTION

In the last 25 years, there has been a pandemic trend of occurrence of coronary artery disease (CAD) in India, particularly in urban areas.[1-3] This is also true for the rising magnitude of diabetes mellitus (DM) in the country.[3-5] Further, the prevalence of CAD in diabetics has now acquired a vicious form, which has become a major health problem in the region.[1,6-8] Many studies have consistently shown that people with diabetes are 2 to 4 times more prone to develop CAD as compared to nondiabetics.[3,4,9,10]

Several special features have been attributed to the occurrence of CAD in diabetics. It tends to occur at an early age, is usually more extensive and severe or is found in virulent form which is rapidly progressive. The relative risk of CAD in women with diabetes is higher than in men.[11-15] Further, the patients of CAD with diabetes have worse prognosis.[10,16,17,19-21] An excessive CAD mortality among diabetic individuals has been reported in a number of prospective studies encompassing a variety of ethnic and racial groups.[20-23] But currently as a population, Indians are most susceptible to all the three diseases namely CAD, diabetes and occurrence of CAD in diabetes.[2-4,24,25]

EPIDEMIOLOGY OF CORONARY ARTERY DISEASE—GLOBAL, INDIAN AND IN IMMIGRANT INDIANS

Global Studies

Early in the last century, there was a rapid rise in the global prevalence of CAD. Several reports indicate that during the past three decades, there has been a substantial increase of CAD in developing countries, particularly in India, while during the same time, there has been a significant decline in CAD mortality in developed countries.[1] The estimates from the Global Burden of Disease Study show that India faces the greatest burden of CAD.[2] The current estimate of 25 million CAD patients in India is projected to increase to 40 million by the year 2020 as shown in **Figure 60.1.**

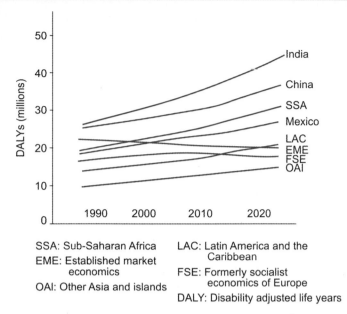

SSA: Sub-Saharan Africa
EME: Established market economics
OAI: Other Asia and islands
LAC: Latin America and the Caribbean
FSE: Formerly socialist economics of Europe
DALY: Disability adjusted life years

Figure 60.1 Burden of CAD 1990–2020[2]

Burden of CAD 1990-2020[2]

The coronary artery disease (CAD) is associated with high mortality rate and it is projected that mortality rates in India will increase by approximately 100% from the year 1985 to 2015.[24] The total number of CAD deaths from India and China equals that of the CAD deaths contributed by all developed countries put together. Moreover, Indians have a higher prevalence of premature CAD in comparison to other ethnic populations as reflected in epidemiological studies in India and on migrant Indians in the UK, Trinidad, Singapore and other countries.[6-8,25]

Indian Studies

Since 1960, several studies on the prevalence of CAD in urban and rural populations in India have been published **(Table 60.1)**.

At that period of time, the prevalence of DM in India was not considered to be high, moreover these reports are about prevalence of CAD in general or selected populations and not in subjects of diabetes.

As seen in **Table 60.1**,[2] the prevalence of CAD in urban population in India has progressively increased from 1.05% in 1960 (Agra, Uttar Pradesh, India) to 11.0% in 2001(Chennai, Tamil Nadu, India). In the Jaipur Heart Watch (JHW) studies, the prevalence of CAD was 7.59% in 1995 (JHW-1) and 7.30% in 2002 (JHW-2), indicating that there has not been significant difference in the prevalence of CAD in a comparatively short period of seven years in the same population.[3,4] However, in rural population there has been an increase in CAD

TABLE 60.1	Prevalence of CAD in urban and rural populations of India[5]				
Urban Population					
Author	*Year*	*Age group*	*Place (India)*	*Sample size*	*CHD (%+/-SD)*
Mathur KS	1960	30-70	Agra	1046	1.05+/-0.3
Padmavathi	1962	30-70	Delhi	1642	1.04+/-0.3
Sarvotham SG	1968	30-70	Chandigarh	2030	6.6+/-0.6
Guptra SP	1975	30-70	Rohtak	1407	3.63+/-0.5
Chaddha SL	1990	25-64	Delhi	13723	9.67+/-0.3
Reddy KS	1994	35-64	New Delhi		10.9
Gupta R	1995	20-80	Jaipur	2212	7.59+/-0.6
Singh RB	1995	20-70	Moradabad	152	8.55+/-2.3
Begom TR	1995	20-70	Trivandrum	506	12.65+/-1.5
Mohan V	2001	>20	Chennai	1262	11
Gupta R	2002	>=20	Jaipur	1123	7.3
Rural Population					
Author	Year	Age group	Place (India)	Sample size	CHD (%+/-SD)
Dewan BD	1974	30-70	Haryana	1506	2.06+/-0.4
Jajoo UN	1988	30-70	Vidarbha	2433	1.69+/-0.3
Kutty VR	1993	25-65	Kerala	1130	7.43+/-0.8
Wander GS	1994	30-70	Punjab	1100	3.09+/-0.5
Gupta R	1994	20-80	Rajasthan	8148	3.53+/-0.3
Singh RB	1995	20-80	UP	162	3.09+/-1.4

prevalence from 1.69%(1988) to 3.53%(1995) except for high prevalence reported in Kerala, India (7.43%) in 1993 **(Table 60.1)**.

Coronary Artery Disease in Immigrant Indians

In course of time, people of Indian origin have migrated to different countries of the world and they, in common, share the genetic predisposition to higher prevalence of CAD. Autopsy reports of Indian and Chinese done in Singapore in 1959 revealed that Indians have seven times higher prevalence of CAD than Chinese males.[26] Several other studies from Singapore,[27] Uganda,[28] South Africa,[29] and Fiji,[30] have also indicated that in Indians the prevalence of CAD was three times higher as compared to respective native populations. Between 1975 and 1985, the relative risk of death from CAD was found 2.6 in Indians compared to people of African origin.[31] Further, the St James Survey from Trinidad reported that ECG changes of CAD were seen in 14% Indian men under the age of 55 years.[32]

In the CAD mortality data for England and Wales for the period 1970-72 and 1979-83, the standard mortality ratio (SMR) for male Indians between 20 and 69 years of age was the highest at 136. Similarly, the SMR for Indian females was even higher at 146. In the Southall Study,[33] the prevalence of CAD was 4% in India-born men as compared to 2.3% in Europeans. Amongst the first generation immigrant Indian physicians in USA, it was found that CAD was 3 times more in Indian men (mean age 46.4 years) as compared to the men in Framingham offspring study (7.6% vs 2.5%).[7] Thus, it can be concluded that the prevalence of CAD among immigrant Indians is about 3 times higher than in indigenous populations. Further, the mortality due to CAD is quite high among Indian immigrants in all age groups particularly in young persons.

EPIDEMIOLOGY OF CORONARY ARTERY DISEASE IN TYPE 1 DIABETES MELLITUS

The long-term follow-up of patients with type 1 DM has demonstrated that the first indications of clinically manifested CAD appear late in the third or fourth decade of life, regardless of whether diabetes developed early in childhood or in late adolescence. The CAD risk increases rapidly after the age of 40 years. By 55 years of age, 35% of diabetic men and women are likely to die from a coronary event as compared to 8% of men and only 4% of women in general population.[34] Like in type 2 DM, women with type 1 DM lose most of their inherent protection from CAD observed in nondiabetic women.[34,35] The occurrence of severe coronary atherosclerosis in a subset of type 1 DM patients before the age of 55 years, irrespective of the duration of diabetes suggests that diabetes mainly accelerates the progression of early atherosclerotic lesions that commonly occur youth in the general population.[34]

Type 1 DM having Diabetic Nephropathy

Diabetic nephropathy develops in about 30 to 40% of type 1 DM patients.[36] Similarly, the prevalence of CAD rises sharply in presence of diabetic nephropathy.[34,37] It has been reported that kidney, involvement even in the earliest stages increases the risk of CAD. The patients with type 1 DM followed from the onset of micro-albuminuria developed CAD eight times more frequently than patients without microalbuminuria.[38] Microalbuminuria, therefore, is not only an indicator of renal disease but is also a strong risk factor for CAD. Krolewski[34] reported that the risk of development of CAD in patients with persistent proteinuria was 15 times higher as compared to those without proteinuria. The coronary angiographic studies have revealed that nearly all patients with diabetic nephropathy over the age of 45 years have one or more clinically significant stenosis in them.[39] A long-term follow-up study conducted at Steno Memorial Hospital, Denmark showed that patients with persistent proteinuria had a 37-fold increase in mortality from CAD relative to the general population, whereas patients without proteinuria had a cardiovascular mortality only 4.2 times higher.[37]

Several biochemical and metabolic abnormalities like hypertension, lipid abnormalities, fibrinolysis and coagulation alterations contribute to the atherosclerotic process in presence of diabetic nephropathy.[40] The risk for the development of diabetic nephropathy is only partially determined by glycemic control and is highly influenced by genetic susceptibility.[37,41,42] Further CAD is twice as common a cause of death among parents of diabetic patients with nephropathy than among parents of diabetic patients without nephropathy. The diabetic nephropathy subjects with CAD are six times more likely to have a family history of CAD than those who did not have a CAD. A history of cardiovascular disease in the father or both parents of a type 1 DM patient increases the risk of nephropathy in the offspring by three-and ten-folds, respectively.[43]

EPIDEMIOLOGY OF CORONARY ARTERY DISEASE IN TYPE 2 DM—SPECIAL FEATURES

The literature on the association between diabetes and CAD has increased exponentially in recent years. The interpretation of epidemiologic studies on the association between diabetes and CAD are often difficult because both conditions are common and may occur together also by chance.

Prevalence

Several studies have shown that people with diabetes are more likely to develop CAD as compared to people who do not have diabetes. Recent North American studies have reported on the prevalence of CAD in impaired standard oral glucose tolerance test (OGTT)[9,45-49] which estimate that the CAD prevalence rates vary between 29 to 43% which are significantly higher than those with normal OGTT. Each subset of diabetic population, like Americans (European-white), Mexicans (Hispanic) and of Japanese ancestry, nearly always had significantly more clinically manifested CAD than those without diabetes **(Figure 60.2)**.[15,46]

Further, the Strong Heart Study conducted in 13 American Indian Communities in Arizona, Oklahoma and Dakotas, similarly showed two to three fold increase in prevalence of CAD in diabetic than in nondiabetic subjects in all groups and both sexes.[50]

Moreover, the results of three well-planned Finnish studies in three regions of Finland[9,51-53] indicate that the rate of myocardial infarction (MI) was two to four times higher in diabetic subjects in comparison to the nondiabetic subjects. Similarly, angina pectoris was also

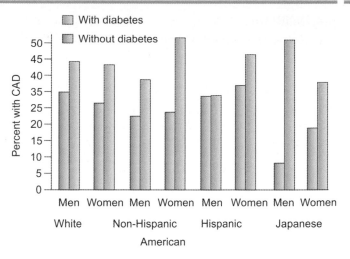

Figure 60.2 Age-adjusted prevalence of CAD in adults with and without diabetes[15,46]

found twice common in diabetic than in nondiabetic subjects.

Incidence Studies

In six prospective North American population and occupation based studies, the incidence of fatal CAD in persons with and without diabetes is shown in **Table 60.2**.[9,11-15,44]

In every study, the risk of fatal CAD was significantly greater among diabetics than nondiabetic subjects. The Wisconsin Study[54] and the Nurses' Health Study[12] are two large prospective studies of CAD in diabetes which separately reported CAD incidence in persons with type 1 diabetes or type 2 diabetes. Wisconsin study showed

TABLE 60.2	Risk of fatal CAD in diabetic vs nondiabetic white adults—US Studies[9]						
Population	Age year	Years follow-up	Sex	Number		Adjusted risk ratio	
				Diabetic	Nondiabetic	Duration	Multiple
Alameda County, CA[13]	>40	9	M	51	1648	—	1.5
			F	70	1982	3.5	3.1
Chicago, IL[14]	35-64	9	M	377	10843	4.0	3.8
			F	170	7860	5.9	4.7
NHANES I[44]	40-77	9	M	189	3151	2.3	2.4
			F	218	3823	2.8	2.6
Rancho Bernardo, CA[15]	40-79	14	M	207	893	1.8	3.3
			F	127	1224	3.3	3.3
Nurses' Health Study[12]	30-55	8	F	1483	114694	6.9	—
New Haven, CT[11]	>65	6	M	156	994	—	1.6
			F	230	1388	—	4.5

| TABLE 60.3 | Risk of fatal CAD or major CAD events (CAD fatal or nonfatal MI) in diabetic patients vs nondiabetic subjects—European population/occupation based study[9] | | | | | | | |

Population	Age years	Years follow-up	Sex	Type of diabetes	Number Diabetic	Number Nondiabetic	Adjusted risk ratio fatal major event Age	Adjusted risk ratio fatal major event Multiple
Population sample Finland	40-69	10	M	Previously diagnosed (unspecified)	273	12299	2.7	2.5
			F	Previously diagnosed (unspecified)	292	12008	3.4	9.4
Population sample, Gothenburg, Sweden	51-59	7	M	Previously diagnosed (unspecified)	232	6665	4.1	3.4
London civil servants	40-64	18-20	M	Known and New T2DM	191	17966	2.8	2.6
Paris policemen	44-55	17	M	Known T2DM	125	6055	3.5	2.3
				New T2DM	158		2	0.8

M—Male, F—Female

that CAD relative risk estimates in men with type 1 diabetes or type 2 diabetes were 9.1 and 2.4 respectively while in women, the same were 13.5 and 2.2. Among the nurses, the age-adjusted relative risks of CAD for diabetic vs nondiabetic women were 12.2 for type 1 diabetes and 6.9 for type 2 diabetes. While comparing the incidence of CAD in patients with type 1 and type 2 diabetes, Elizabeth Barret-Connor et al[9] concluded that the higher relative risks associated with type 1 diabetes than with type 2 diabetes may reflect the greater duration of diabetes, more severe metabolic disturbances and the relatively low CAD rates in young persons without diabetes.

The Prospective Studies in European Population

Table 60.3 shows that the risk of fatal CAD was markedly increased in diabetic than in nondiabetic subjects. Collins et al[16] published a prospective population-based study of diabetes and fatal cardiovascular disease from Fiji in which it is reported that death from all causes was significantly increased in Asian Indian men but not in Melanesian men with diabetes.

Epidemiological Variations According to Age, Sex and Duration of Diabetes Mellitus

The incidence and prevalence of CAD in diabetes mellitus vary according to age, sex, race and duration of DM and the presence of other risk factors.

In Framingham study, **Table 60.4**[17] (referred later) the average annual incidence of cardiovascular disease per 1000 persons at risk was calculated in three age groups, i.e. 45-54 years, 55-64 years and 65-74 years. Both in males and females the highest relative risk for CAD in diabetics was in the younger age group of 45-54 years. The overall prevalence of CAD in males diabetics is two-fold higher than in the nondiabetic whereas it is three-fold higher in the females diabetics than nondiabetics. The effect of duration of diabetes mellitus on the development of CAD was assessed in a 24-year follow-up study of patients in Joslin Center. The cause of death was CAD in 38% of men and in 39% of women.[55] The long-term effect of duration of diabetes mellitus on mortality rate due to CAD was compared with the subjects of Framingham Heart Study (Nondiabetic population) **(Figures 60.3A and B)**.[55]

| TABLE 60.4 | Average annual incidence of cardiovascular disease per 1000 persons at risk (Adopted from Framingham study)[17] | | | |

Age	Men Diabetics	Men Nondiabetics	Women Diabetics	Women Nondiabetics
45–54	31.7	12.3	24.8	4.3
55–64	48.1	25.1	37.9	12.6
65–74	57.1	28.4	40.4	22.4
Total	39.1	19.1	27.2	10.2

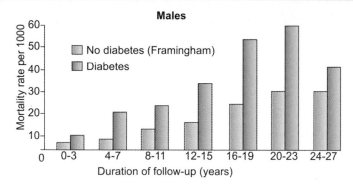

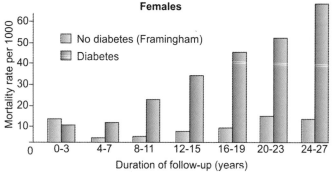

Figures 60.3A and B Age-adjusted mortality rate from CAD at Joslin Diabetes Center and in the Framingham Cohort[55]

Figure 60.4 shows CAD mortality according to 4-year intervals of duration of diabetes mellitus. As reported from the Joslin Center in the Framingham sample, the increasing risk of CAD with duration of follow-up reflects the effect of aging process, whereas in patients with diabetes, the increased risk reflects the combined effect of aging together with cumulative diabetes exposure. Diabetic patients had higher CAD-related mortality than did the nondiabetic patients

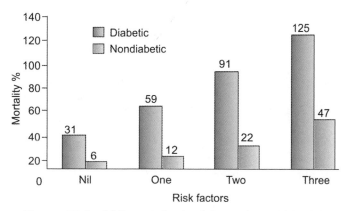

Figure 60.4 CAD mortality in diabetes in multiple risk factor intervention trial (MRFIT)[10]

during the first 3 years of follow-up. The magnitude of this excess mortality was increased in subsequent intervals of observation, indicating the cumulative effect of diabetes exposure on cardiac vasculature. The effect of diabetes duration on CAD risk is more prominent in women than in men.

The multiple risk factor intervention trial (MRFIT) study[10] demonstrated that the mortality increased markedly among diabetic compared to nondiabetic subjects due to the coexistence of multiple risk factors. The three classical major CAD risk factors, namely total cholesterol, high blood pressure and cigarette smoking carry a similar increased risk in persons with and without diabetes. These risk factors appear to have an additive effect. In the 12-year follow-up of the MRFIT trial, it was shown that patients with diabetes in presence of any patients in the presence of any of the risk factors, have two-fold higher mortality due to cardiovascular disease than those without diabetes.

Geographical and Ethnic Variations

There are considerable ethnic and geographical variations in the cardiovascular risk associated with diabetes. As reported by Peter Grant and Andrew Davies, the risk of myocardial infarction increases northwards through Europe, with the highest rates in parts of Finland and the UK.[56]

South Indians living in England have a relative risk of 1.4 for those suffering from myocardial infarction as compared with the English (Caucasians) while a relative risk is 3.8 as compared with their Chinese co-inhabitants in Singapore.[57] Similar variation is found in the USA, where prevalence of myocardial infarction is highest in non-Hispanic whites and blacks, and lowest in Hispanic whites, native Americans (including the Pimas)[58] and the Japanese.[59] The reasons for this variation are still unknown.

IMPACT OF DIABETES ON CORONARY ARTERY DISEASE IN WOMEN

In the general population, women are considered to be at a much lower risk of CAD mortality than men. Many studies have shown that diabetes erases this female advantage and increases the risk of heart disease much more in women than in men. Warren Lee et al[18] carried out a meta-analysis of ten prospective cohort studies and reported the impact of the risk of CAD in diabetic men and women. Their analysis suggests that the relative risk of CAD death from diabetes is indeed greater for women than men. Depending upon the

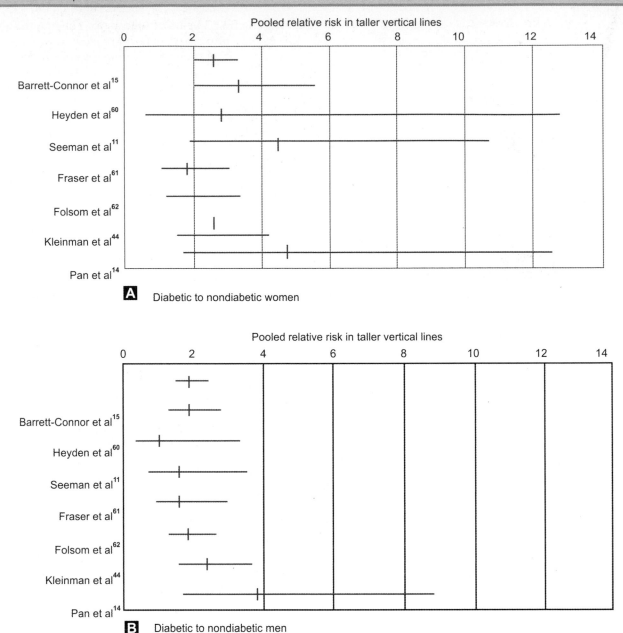

Figures 60.5A and B Risk factor adjusted relative risk of CAD death, diabetic to nondiabetic women and men (95% CI)[18]

analysis, the relative for women is 2.5 vs a relative risk[1,62] for men[18] **(Figures 60.5A and B)**.

The greater impact of diabetes mellitus on CAD mortality was also confirmed by two large profession-based studies done in USA—The Nurses' Health Study[63] and US Male Physicians study.[19] Hu et al examined mortality from all causes and from CAD among 12,1046 women-aged 30 to 55 years with type 2 diabetes in the Nurses' Health Study who were

followed up for two years. Compared with women with no diabetes or CAD at baseline, age-adjusted relative risks or fatal CAD were 8.7 for women with a history of diabetes and no CAD at baseline, 10.6 for women with a history of CAD and no diabetes at baseline, and 25.8 for women with both conditions at baseline.[63] Corresponding relative risks were substantially lower in a five-year follow-up of 91,285 US male physicians aged 40 to 84 years.[19]

IMPACT OF DIABETES ON CORONARY ARTERY DISEASE MORTALITY[64-66]

Various studies have shown that there is higher mortality from CAD in diabetic in comparison to nondiabetic people. A Finnish study by Haffner in 1998 compared the risk of myocardial infarction (MI) over a 7-year period in 1373 nondiabetic and 1059 diabetic subjects.[20] The patients with DM and no prior MI had a 20.2% incidence of MI during the seven-year follow-up, similar to that of nondiabetic subjects with prior MI (18.8%) **(Figure 60.6)**.

It also compared the probability of death from CAD in diabetics vs nondiabetic subjects and showed that the probability of mortality due to CAD is similar in diabetic subjects without prior MI as in nondiabetic subjects with prior MI **(Figure 60.7)**.[20]

Similarly, in the Organization to Assess Strategies for Ischemic Syndromes (OASIS) registry,[21] diabetic patients without prior cardiovascular disease had the same event rates for all outcomes, as did nondiabetic patients with prior cardiovascular disease. These results led the Adult Treatment Panel III of the National Cholesterol Education Programme to establish diabetes as a CAD equivalent requiring aggressive therapy.[67]

Gu et al utilized data from the first National Health and Nutrition Examination Survey (NHANES-1) and the NHANES-1 epidemiologic follow-up survey to analyze the mortality rates from CAD in diabetic and nondiabetic populations.[68] They found that overall mortality rates have declined significantly in the general population due to better medical care over the 22-year period of the survey (1971–1993). However, these improvements were

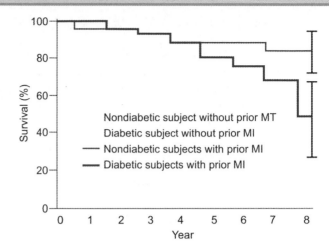

Figure 60.7 Comparison of Kaplan-Meier estimates of the probability of death from CAD in diabetic and nondiabetic subjects with and without prior MI[20]

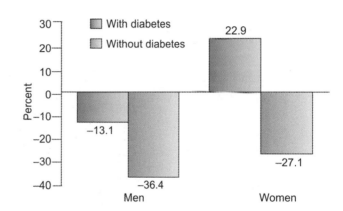

Figure 60.8 Nine-year rates of decline in heart disease mortality among adults aged 35 to 75 years, by sex and diabetes status[68]

not reflected in the diabetic population over the same period. In nondiabetic men and women, the mortality was reduced by 36.4 and 27.1%, respectively. By contrast, mortality fell by only 13.1% in diabetic men and has actually risen by 23% in diabetic women since the 1970s and 1980s[68] **(Figure 60.8)**.

CORONARY ARTERY DISEASE IN TYPE 2 DM HAVING DIABETIC NEPHROPATHY

In type 2 diabetes, the diabetic nephropathy in all the three stages namely microalbuminuria, macroalbuminuria and end-stage renal disease (ESRD) serves as a

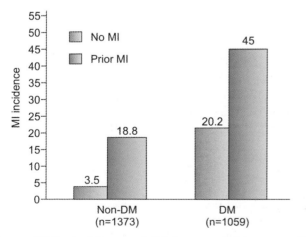

Figure 60.6 Incidence of fatal or nonfatal myocardial infarction (MI) in diabetic and nondiabetic subjects with or without prior MI[20]

fertile soil in the occurrence of ischemic heart disease and cardiomyopathy. Macroalbuminuria usually heralds the development of both microvascular (retinopathy) and macrovascular diseases.[39,69] Recent data suggest that microalbuminuria is a surrogate marker not only for glomerular injury but also for diffusely increased endothelial permeability which correlates with cardiovascular morbidity and mortality.[70,71] Moreover, microalbuminuria is thought to reflect widespread vascular and endothelial damage consequent to which the endothelial dependent vasorelaxation is impaired. This translates into increased damage to arteries leading to increased risk of cardiovascular death. The existence of diabetic nephropathy in any form increases the risk of cardiovascular death[37,72] **(Figures 60.9A and B)**.

Several mechanisms are implicated in development of atherosclerotic process in the presence of diabetic nephropathy. The onset of microalbuminuria is associated with the development of hypertension and with numerous prothrombotic and atherogenic changes, including raised triglycerides, low HDL-cholesterol and increased circulating levels of factor VII, PAI-1 and fibrinogen.[73,74]

Further in diabetic patients reaching ESRD, the overall mortality is reported to be greater than in nondiabetic patients. A study showed that in 35 to 44 years of age group, the three years survival rate of diabetic patients is 44% in men and 66% in women compared with 75 and 87% for nondiabetic patients with ESRD.[75] Most of the excess deaths are from CAD.[76] The commonest cause of deaths in diabetic patients who have undergone renal transplantation is also CAD which accounts for 40% of deaths in these patients.[77]

Prognosis of CAD in Diabetes Mellitus

Moreover, the prognosis after a CAD event is poorer among diabetic patients than among their nondiabetic counterparts. A high proportion of patients with type 2 diabetes die within one year of an acute myocardial infarction (MI) (44.2% of diabetic men, 36.9% of diabetic women) and a considerable number of patients die even before they reach hospital.[22] A recent study suggests that diabetes decreases the life-expectancy of an individual by eight years.[23] Survival rates in diabetic subjects with angiographically proven coronary artery disease are decreased by 30% as compared to their nondiabetic counterparts.[72]

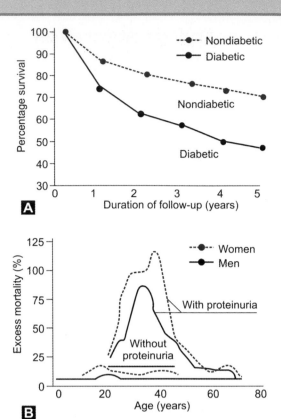

Figures 60.9A and B Cardiovascular mortality in diabetes and with and without proteinuria[37,72]

CORONARY ARTERY DISEASE IN DIABETES—INDIAN STUDIES

The first report to contrast the difference between the prevalence of CAD in general population and in diabetics was published in Framingham study[17] **(Table 60.4)**.

This indicates higher prevalence of CAD in male diabetic (39.1 per 1000) as compared to nondiabetic subjects (19.1) while in female diabetic subjects, it was 27.2 as compared to 10.2 respectively.[17]

Similar studies of prevalence of CAD in diabetics have been conducted in India, which are summarized in **Table 60.5**.[5]

The Indian Council of Medical Research (ICMR) multicentric study was carried out in different hospitals in 1984 to 1987. Hence, the figures are comparatively lower than the figures published in the recent studies in similar set of patients. The reports of Prevalence of

TABLE 60.5	Prevalence of CAD in diabetes in India[5]		
Author	Year	Place	Prevalence of CAD (%)
ICMR	1984-87	Multicentric	Male 8.1%, Female 4.7%
A Ramachandran	1998	Chennai (Tamil Nadu, India)	Male 3.9%, Female 10.3%
V Mohan	2001	Chennai (Tamil Nadu, India)	21.40%
PODIS	2001	Multicentric	4.50%
Gupta PB	2001	Surat (Gujarat, India)	19%
Phatak SR	2002	Ahmedabad (Gujarat, India)	Male 20.2%, Female 26.1%
Agrawal RP	2004	Bikaner, (Rajasthan, India)	19.2%, > 40 years

TABLE 60.6	Prevalence of CAD in migrant diabetic Indians[6,7]			
State	Country	Sample size (age cut-off in years)	Year	Prevalence of CAD (%)
London[6]	UK	1421 (40–69)	1993	17
Illinois[7]	USA	1688 (≥20)	1996	10

Diabetes Indian Study (PODIS) show comparatively low figures of prevalence of CAD as 4.5% because the study was conducted only in newly detected diabetics (Sadikot et al, personal communication). Ramachandran (1998)[78] has reported prevalence of CAD in diabetics as 14.2% in the population-based study in Chennai, South India, while Mohan et al[79] from the same city in 2001 observed prevalence of 21.4%. Similarly in other studies, Gupta et al have reported prevalence of CAD in diabetic subjects as 19%[80] and Phatak as 23.2%, which are comparable to the reports of Mohan et al.

Agrawal et al in their very recent study have reported the prevalence of CAD in diabetic subjects as 19.2% from western part of India.[81] They also observed increasing prevalence of CAD with increase in age from 40 years (2.9%) to more than 70 years (45%). Similarly, there was higher prevalence of CAD with increasing duration of diabetes, systolic and diastolic blood pressure and higher values of GHb%.[81] Deepa et al have made similar observations where they found prevalence of CAD increasing with age and duration of diabetes where prevalence of CAD reached 40% with diabetes of more than 20 years duration in clinic-based study. They found that 21.4% of diabetic subjects and 14.9% of the subjects with impaired glucose tolerance (IGT) had CAD as compared to 9.1% among subjects with normal glucose tolerance (NGT).

Some revealed higher incidence of diabetes and CAD in persons who had low birth weight but became obese in adulthood.[82] Children born small but grown heavy/tall were the most insulin resistant and had the highest levels of cardiovascular risk factors.[83]

Various epidemiological studies have reportedly mentioned that there is a higher prevalence rate of CAD among migrant Indians with diabetes compared to the native population[6,7] **(Table 60.6)**.

CORONARY ARTERY DISEASE IN PREDIABETES

Clinically evident type 2 diabetes is a well-established cause of CAD and its increased mortality. Many studies[84-89] have shown that even the subclinical states of glucose intolerance (comprising of undiagnosed diabetes and IGT) increase the risk of CAD and related mortality. Saydah et al[90] conducted a prospective study to compare the all cause mortality among individuals with diagnosed type 2 diabetes, undiagnosed diabetes and IGT with individuals having NGT in the general US population. They found that in comparison to those with NGT the multivariate adjusted relative risk (RR) of all cause mortality was greatest for adults with diagnosed diabetes (RR-2.11), followed by those with undiagnosed diabetes (RR-1.77) and those with IGT (RR-1.42). A similar pattern of risk was observed for CAD mortality[90] **(Figure 60.10)**.

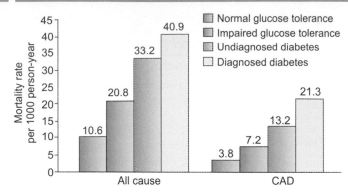

Figure 60.10 All cause and CAD mortality in the NHANES II mortality survey in different groups[90]

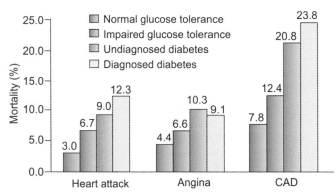

Figure 60.11 Correlation of mortality with history of CAD among NHANES II participants aged 30 to 74 years in different groups[90]

It was concluded that there was a gradient of mortality associated with abnormal glucose tolerance ranging from a 40% greater risk in adults with IGT to a 110% greater risk in adults with clinically evident diabetes.[90] There was also a significant gradient in incidence of angina, MI and all cardiovascular disease **(Figure 60.11)**.

Further, Haffner et al[91] examined the risk factors in confirmed prediabetic individuals and showed that the risk for CAD starts from the stage of IGT itself, i.e. even before overt diabetes sets in. He concluded that the clock for CAD starts ticking before the onset of clinical diabetes. Similar results were shown in South Indian population in CUPS study by Mohan and coworkers in Chennai.[92] In this study, the prevalence of CAD was higher among diabetic and subclinical diabetic subjects in comparison to controls. The prevalence rate of CAD was 9.1% in NGT subjects compared to 14.9% in IGT, 13.1% in newly diagnosed and 25.3% in those with known diabetes. Interestingly, the prevalence rate of

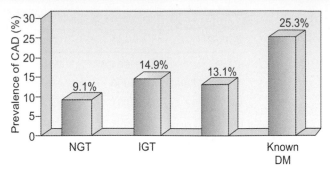

Figure 60.12 Prevalence of CAD in subjects with different degrees of glucose intolerance CUPS data[92]

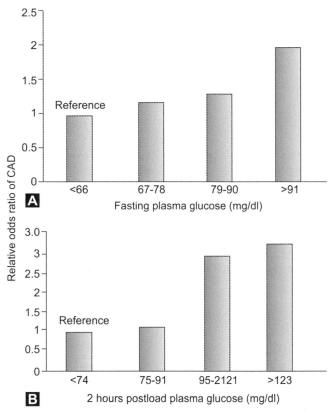

Figures 60.13A and B Relative odds ratio for CAD by quartiles of fasting and 2 hours postload plasma-glucose[92]

CAD was similar in subjects with IGT and newly detected diabetics **(Figure 60.12)**.

The odds ratio for CAD increased with increase in quartiles of fasting plasma glucose and 2 hours postglucose load plasma-glucose indicating a strong association of glycemia with CAD **(Figures 60.13A and B)**.

PREVALENCE OF PRE-CORONARY ARTERY DISEASE MARKERS IN DIABETES MELLITUS

The CAD is one of the end-points of atherosclerotic disease. With the advances in technology, it is possible to study atherosclerosis in its early stage and to predict clinical events of CAD.

Electron-beam computed tomography (EBCT) is a noninvasive technology for evaluating the extent of coronary artery atherosclerosis that relies on the detection of coronary artery calcium (CAC). Recent studies based on EBCT have demonstrated that diabetic patients have a substantially higher prevalence of CAC. The amount of calcium deposited in the coronary arteries correlates with the pathological extent of atherosclerosis and the presence of stenosis evaluated by coronary angiography which predicts future CAD events. A study by Sunita Schurgin demonstrated that patients with diabetes had a significant increase in the prevalence of CAC scores which were more than or equal to 400 (25.9%) as compared to the randomly selected (7.2%) and matched (14.4%) nondiabetic control groups[93] **(Figure 60.14)**.

Structural changes like carotid intimal medial thickness (IMT) and functional changes like endothelial dysfunction and arterial stiffness are the other methods to detect early atherosclerotic changes. These atherosclerotic markers are found to be higher in diabetic subjects in comparison to nondiabetic controls. In CUPS study, Shanti Rani et al[94] and Mohan et al[95] reported that the IMT values among diabetic subjects were significantly higher (0.95 mm) compared to normal subjects (0.74 mm).[95] Moreover, carotid atherosclerosis defined as IMT >1.1 mm was significantly higher in diabetic subjects (20%) compared to nondiabetic subjects (1%).[96] Similarly, endothelial function, which was assessed by flow-mediated dilatation decreased significantly in diabetic subjects compared to nondiabetic subjects.[96] Arterial stiffness was studied using pulse wave analysis and was markedly increased in diabetic subjects.[96] Thus, subclinical and preclinical CAD and its markers are significantly increased in diabetics in comparison to nondiabetic subjects.

SUMMARY

The epidemiological studies conducted in India in the past couple of decades on CAD in diabetics indicate that there has been several fold increase in their co-prevalence. This increase is significantly higher in urban population mainly after the age of 40 years. Asian Indian diabetic patients are particularly vulnerable to develop higher rates of CAD around the world. Alarming signal is that raised prevalence of CAD is quite significant even in IGT, which further aggravates, the morbidity and mortality from CAD in overt diabetes. Looking at the present magnitude of the problem and its tremendous potential of increase in future, an active public health policy and program are urgently needed to reduce the impact of the twin pandemics of CAD and DM in India.

ACKNOWLEDGMENTS

We deeply appreciate the enormous help rendered by Mr Ravi S Iyer and Deepak Keswani in the preparation of this chapter up to its final stage.

REFERENCES

1. Enas EA, Jacob S. Coronary artery disease in Indians in the USA. In Sethi KK (Ed): Coronary artery disease in Indians: a global perspective. Mumbai: Cardiological Society of India 1998. pp. 32-43.
2. Murray CJ, Lopez AD. Alternative projections of mortality and disability by cause 1990-2020: Global Burden of Disease Study. Lancet. 1997;349:1498-504.
3. Gupta R, Gupta VP, Sarna M, Bhatnagar S, Thanvi J, Sharma V, et al. Prevalence of coronary heart disease and coronary risk factors in urban Indian population: Jaipur Heart Watch-2. Indian Heart J. 2002;54:59-66.
4. Gupta R, Prakash H, Mazumdar S, Sharma S, Gupta VP. Prevalence of coronary heart disease and coronary risk factors in urban population of Rajasthan. Indian Heart J. 1995;47:331-8.
5. Gupta OP, Phatak S. Pandemic trends in prevalence of diabetes mellitus and associated coronary heart disease in India—their causes and prevention. Int J Diab Dev Countries. 2003;23:37-50.

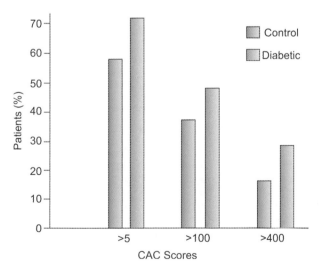

Figure 60.14 The distribution of coronary artery calcium (CAC) scores in diabetic patients compared with matched nondiabetic subjects[81]

6. Bahl VK, Prabhakaran D, Karthikeyan G. Coronary artery disease in Indians. Indian Heart J. 2001;53:707-13.

7. Enas EA, Garg A, Davidson MA, Nair VM, Huet BA, Yusuf S. Coronary heart disease and its risk factors in first-generation immigrant Asian Indians to the United States of America. Indian Heart J. 1996;48:343-53.

8. McKeigue PM. Coronary heart disease in Indians, Pakistanis, and Bangladeshis: etiology and possibilities for prevention. Br Heart J. 1992;67:341-2.

9. Elizabeth Barrett-Connor, Kalevi Pyorala. Long-term complications: diabetes and coronary heart disease. Jean-Marie Ekoe, Paul Zimmet, Rhys Williams(Eds). The epidemiology of diabetes mellitus: an International Perspective. John Wiley and Sons 2001;21A:301-17.

10. Stamler J, Vaccaro O, Neaton JD, Wentworth D. For the multiple risk factor Intervention Trial Research Group. Diabetes, other risk factors, and 12 year cardiovascular mortality for men screened in the MRFIT. Diabetes Care. 1993;16:434-44.

11. Seaman T, deLeon CM, Berkman L, Ostfeld A. Risk factors for coronary heart disease among older men and women: a prospective study of elderly community dwelling. Am J Epidemiol. 1993;138:1037-49.

12. Manson JE, Colditz GA, Stampfer MJ, et al. A prospective study of maturity onset diabetes and risk of coronary heart disease and stroke in women. Arch Intern Med. 1991;151:1141-7.

13. Wingard DL, Cohn BA. Coronary heart disease among women in Alameda county, 1965-73. In coronary heart disease in women: Proceedings of an NIH workshop. New York: Haymarket Doyma. 1987:Ch 11.

14. Pan W, Cedres LB, Liu K, et al. Relationship of clinical diabetes and asymptomatic hyperglycemia to risk of coronary heart disease mortality in men and women. Am J Epidemiol. 1996;123:504-16.

15. Barrett-Connor E, Cohn BA, Wingard DL, Edelstein SL. Why is diabetes mellitus a stronger risk factor for fatal ischemic heart disease in women than in men? The Rancho Bernardo Study. J Am Med Assoc. 1991;265:627-31.

16. Collins VR, Dowse GK, Cabealawa S, Ram P, Zimmet PZ. High mortality from cardiovascular disease and analysis of risk factors in Indian and Melanesians Fijians. Int J Epidemiol. 1996;25:59-69.

17. Kennel WB, McGee DI. Diabetes and glucose tolerance as risk factor for cardiovascular disease: the Framingham study. Diabetes Care. 1997; pp.120-31.

18. Warren Lee, et al. Impact of diabetes on CHD in women and men. Diabetes Care. 2000;123:964-7.

19. Lotufu PA, Gaziano JM, Chae CU, et al. Diabetes all cause and coronary heart disease mortality among US male physicians. Arch Intern Med. 2001;161:242-7.

20. Haffner SM, Lehto S, Ronnemaa T, et al. Mortality from coronary heart disease in subjects with type 2 diabetes and in nondiabetic subjects with and without prior myocardial infarction. N Engl J Med. 1998;339:229-34.

21. Malmberg K, Yusuf S, Gerstein HC, et al. Impact of diabetes on long-term prognosis in patients with unstable angina and non-Q wave myocardial infarction: results of the Organization to Assess Strategies for Ischemic Syndromes (OASIS) registry. Circulation. 2000;102:1014-9.

22. Miettinen H, Lehto S, Salomaa V, et al. Impact of diabetes on mortality after the first myocardial infarction: the FINMONICA Myocardial Infarction Register Study Group. Diabetes Care. 1998;21:69-75.

23. Roper NA, Bilous RW, Kelly WF, Unwin NC, Connolly VM. Excess mortality in a population with diabetes and the impact of material deprivation: longitudinal, population based study. BMJ. 2001;322:1389-93.

24. Reddy KS, Yusuf S. Emerging epidemic of cardiovascular disease in developing countries. Circulation. 1998;97:596-601.

25. Balarajan R. Ethnic differences in mortality from IHD and CVD in England and Wales. British Medical Journal. 1991;302:560-4.

26. Danaraj TJ, Acker MS, Danaraj W. Ong WH, Yam TB. Ethnic group differences in coronary heart disease in Singapore: an analysis of necropsy records. Am Heart J. 1959;58:516-26.

27. Chen AJ. Recent trends in the mortality and morbidity of cardiovascular diseases. Am Acad Med Singapore. 1980;9:411-15.

28. Shaper AG, Jones KW. Serum cholesterol, diet and coronary heart disease in Africans and Asians in Uganda. Lancet. 1959;2:534-7.

29. Wyndham CH. Trends with time of cardiovascular mortality in the populations of the RSA for the period 1968-1977. S Afr Med J. 1982;61:987-93.

30. Tuomilehto J, Ram P, Eseroma R, Taylor R, Zimmet P. Cardiovascular diseases in Fiji; analysis of mortality, morbidity and risk factor. Bull World Health Organ. 1984;62:133-43.

31. Miller GJ, Beckles GLA, Alexis SD, Byam NT, Price SG. Serum lipoproteins and susceptibility of men of Indian descent to coronary heart disease. The St James Survey. Trinidad: Lancet. 1982;2:200-3.

32. Beckles GL. Miller GJ, Kirkwood BR, Alexis SD, Carson DC, Byam NT. High total and cardiovascular disease mortality in adults of Indian descent in Trinidad, unexplained by major coronary risk factors. Lancet. 1986;1:1298-301.

33. McKeigue PM, Shah B, Marmot MG. Relation of central obesity and insulin resistance with high diabetes prevalence and cardiovascular risk in South Asians. Lancet. 1991;337:382-6.

34. Krolewski AS, Kosinski EJ, Warren JH, et al. Magnitude and determinants of coronary artery disease in juvenile-onset, insulin-dependent diabetes mellitus. Am J Cardiol. 1987;59:750-5.

35. Donahue RP, Orchard TJ. Diabetes mellitus and macrovascular complications: an epidemiological perspective. Diabetes Care. 1992;15:1141-55.

36. Earle K, Viberti GC. Familial, hemodynamic and metabolic factors in the predisposition to diabetic kidney disease. Kidney Int. 1994;45:434-7.

37. Borch-Johnsen K, Norgard K, Hommel E, et al. Is diabetic nephropathy an inherited complication? Kidney Int. 1992;41:719-22.

38. Jensen T, Borch-Johnsen K, Kofoed-Enevoldsen A, Deckert T. Coronary heart disease in young type 1 (insulin dependent) diabetic patients with and without diabetic nephropathy: incidence and risk factors. Diabetologia. 1987;30:144-8.

39. Manske CL, Wilson RF, Wang Y, Thomas W. Prevalence of and risk factors for angiographically determined coronary artery disease in type 1 diabetic patients with nephropathy. Arch Intern Med. 1992;152:2450-5.

40. Deckert T, Kofoed-Enevoldsen A, Norgaard K, Borch-Johnsen K, Feldt-Rsmussen B, Jensen T. Microalbuminuria, Implications for micro- and macrovascular disease. Diabetes Care. 1992;15:1181-91.

41. Seaquist ER, Goetz FC, Rich S, Barbosa J. Familial clustering of diabetic kidney disease. Evidence for genetic susceptibility to diabetic nephropathy. N Engl J Med. 1989;320:1161-5.

42. Marre M, Jeunemaitre X, Gallois Y, et al. Contribution of genetic polymorphism in the renin-angiotensin system to the development of renal complications in insulin-dependent diabetes: Genetique de la Nephropathie Diabetique (GENEDIAB) Study Group. J Clin Invest. 1997;99:1585-95.

43. Earle K, Walker J, Hill C, Viberti G. Familial clustering of cardiovascular disease in patients with insulin-dependant diabetes and nephropathy. N Engl J Med. 1992;326:673-7.

44. Kleinman JC, Donahue RP, Harris MI, Finucane FF, Madans JH, Brock DB. Mortality among diabetes in a national sample. Am J Epidemiol. 1998;128:389-401.

45. Scheidt-Nave C, Barrett-Connor E, Wingard DL. Resting electrocardiographic abnormalities suggestive of asymptomatic ischemic heart disease associated with noninsulin-dependent diabetes mellitus in a defined population. Circ. 1990;81:899-906.

46. Rewers M, Shetterly SM, Baxter J, Marshall JA, Hamman RF. Prevalence of coronary artery disease in subjects with normal and impaired glucose tolerance and noninsulin-dependent diabetes mellitus in a biethnic Colorado population. The San Luis Valley Diabetes Study. Am J Epidemiol. 1992;12:1321-30.

47. Mitchell BD, Hazuda HP, Haffner SM, Patterson JK, Stern MP. Myocardial infarction in Mexican Americans and non Hispanic Whites: The San Antonio Heart Study. Circ. 1991;83:45-51.

48. Fujimoto WY, Leonetti DL, Kinyoun JL, Shuman WP, Stolov WC, Wahl PW. Prevalence of complication among second generation Japanese American men with diabetes, impaired glucose tolerance or normal glucose tolerance. Diabetes. 1987;36:730-9.

49. Fujimoto WY, Leonetti DL, Bergstrom RW, Kinyoun JL, Stolov WC, Wahl PW. Glucose intolerance and diabetic complications among Japanese-American women. Diabetes Res Clin Pac. 1991;13:119-30.

50. Howard BV, Lee ET, Cowan LD, et al. Coronary heart disease prevalence and its relation to risk factors in American Indians. The Strong Heart Study. Am J Epidemiol. 1995;142:254-68.

51. Uusiyupa M, Siitonen O, Aro A, Pyorala K. Prevalence of coronary heart disease, left ventricular failure and hypertension in middle-aged newly diagnosed type 2 (noninsulin-dependent) diabetic subjects. Diabetologia. 1985;28:22-7.

52. Laakso M, Ronnemaa T, Pyorala K, Kallio V, Puukka P, Penttila I. Atherosclerotic vascular disease and its risk factors in noninsulin dependent diabetic and nondiabetic subjects in Finland. Diabetes Care. 1998;11:449-63.

53. Mykkanen L, Laakso M, Pyorala K. Asymptomatic hyperglycemia and atherosclerotic vascular disease. Diabetes Care. 1992;15:1020-30.

54. Moss SE, Klein R, Klein BE. Cause specific mortality in a population based study of diabetes. J Public Health. 1991;81:1158-62.

55. Andrzej S Krolewski, James H Warram. Epidemiology of late complication of diabetes in Joslin's diabetes mellitus (13th edn). Lea and Febiger; 1994. pp. 605-19.

56. Peter J Grant, Andrews Davies. Cardiovascular diseases and diabetes (3rd edn). In Textbook of Diabetes: Pickup Johnsons, Williams G (Eds). New York; 2003. pp. 56.1-56.24.

57. McKeigue PM, Ferrie JE, Pierpoint T, Marmot MG. Association of early onset coronary heart disease in south Asian men with glucose intolerance and hyperinsulinemia. Circulation. 1993;87:152-61.

58. Howard BV, Welty TK, Fabsitz RR, et al. Risk factors for coronary heart disease in diabetic and nondiabetic native Americans. Diabetes.1992;41(Suppl 2):4-11.

59. Cooper R, Cutler J, Desvigne-Nickens P, et al. Trends and disparities in coronary heart disease, stroke and other cardiovascular diseases in the United States. Circ. 2000;102:3137-47.

60. Heyden S, Heiss G, Bartel AG, Hames CG. Sex differences in coronary mortality among diabetics in Evans County. Georgia: J Chronic Dis. 1980;33:265-73.

61. Fraser GE, Strahan TM, Sabate J, Beeson WL, Kissinger D. Effects of traditional coronary risk factors on rates of incident coronary events in a low risk population. The Adventist Health Study. Circ. 1992;86:406-13.

62. Folsom AR, Szklo M, Stevens J, Liao E, Smith R, Eckfeldt JH. A prospective study of coronary heart disease in relation to fasting insulin, glucose and diabetes. The Atherosclerosis Risk in Communities (ARIC) study. Diabetes Care. 1997;20:935-42.

63. Hu FB, Stampfer MJ, Solomon CG, et al. The impact of diabetes mellitus on mortality from all cause and coronary heart disease in women. Arch of Intern Med. 2001;161:1717-23.

64. Simons LA, McCallum J, Friedlander Y, Simons J. Diabetes, mortality and coronary heart disease in the prospective Dubbo study of Australian elderly. Aust NZ J Med. 1996;26:66-74.

65. Kannel WB, Wilson PW. Risk factors that attenuate the female coronary disease advantage. Arch Intern Med. 1995;155:224-33.

66. Butler WJ, Ostrander LD Jr, Carman WJ, Lamphiear DE. Mortality from coronary heart disease in the Tecumseh study: long-term effect of diabetes mellitus, glucose tolerance and other risk factors. Am J Epidemiol. 1985;121:541-7.

67. Executive summary of the third Report of the National Cholesterol Education Program (NCEP), Expert panel on Detection, Evaluation and Treatment of High Blood Cholesterol in Adults (Adult Treatment Panel III). J Am Med Assoc. 2001;285:2486-97.

68. Gu K, Cowie CC, Harris MI. Diabetes and decline in heart disease mortality in US adults. JAMA. 1999;281:1291-7.

69. Mogersen CE. Microalbuminuria predicts clinical proteinuria and early mortality in maturity onset diabetes. N Eng J Med. 1984;310;356-60

70. Tuttle KR, Puhlman ME, Cooney SK, Short R. Urinary albumin and insulin as predictors of coronary artery disease: an angiographic study. Am J Kidney Dis 1999;34:918-25.

71. Valmadrid CT, Klein R, Moss SE, Klein BE. The risk of cardiovascular disease mortality associated with micro-albuminuria and gross proteinuria in persons with older onset diabetes mellitus. Arch Intern Med. 2000;160:1093-100.

72. Barzilay JI, Kronmal RA, Bittner V, et al. Coronary artery disease and coronary artery bypass grafting in diabetic patients aged 365 years. Am J Cardiol. 1994;74:334-9.

73. Gruden G, Cavallo-Perin P, Bazzan M, et al. PAI-1 and factor VII activity are higher in IDDM patients with microalbuminuria. Diabetes. 1994;43:426-9.

74. Bruno G, Cavallo-Perin P, Bargero G, et al. Association of fibrinogen with glycemic control and albumin excretion rate in patients with noninsulin- dependent diabetes mellitus. Ann Intern Med. 1996;125:653-7.

75. Geerlings W, Tufveson G, Brunner FP, et al. Combined Report on Regular Dialysis and Transplantation in Europe XXI (1990). Nephrol Dial Transplant. 1991;6(suppl 4):5-29.

76. Renal failure in diabetics in the UK: deficient provision of care in 1985. Joint Working Party on Diabetic Renal Failure of the British Diabetic Association, the Renal Association, and the Research Unit of the Royal College of Physicians. Diabetes Med. 1988;5:79-84.

77. Lemmers MJ, Barry JM. Major role for arterial disease in morbidity and mortality after kidney transplantation in diabetic recipients. Diabetes Care. 1991;14:295-301.

78. Ramachandran A. Epidemiology of vascular complications in type 2 diabetes in Indians. NNDU proceedings. 1999;101-5.

79. Mohan V, Deepa R, Shantirani S, Premlatha G. Prevalence of coronary artery disease and its relationship to lipids in a selected population in South India (CUPS No 5). Am J Coll Cardiol. 2001;38:687-97.

80. Gupta PB, Bhatt P, Thakker K. Vascular complications of type 2 diabetes mellitus. Guj Med J. 2002;59:9-12.

81. Agrawal RP, Ranka M, Beniwal R, Sharma S, Purohit VP, Kochar DK, Kothari RP. Prevalence of micro- and macro-vascular complications in type 2 diabetes and their risk factors. Int J Diab Dev Countries. 2004;24:11-8.

82. Fall CHD, Yagnik CS, Rao S, Coyaji KI. The effect of maternal body composition before pregnancy on fetal growth: the Pune Maternal Nutrition Study. In fetal programming: influences on development and disease in later life. Shaugan PM, O'Brien, Wheeler T, Barker DJP (Eds). RCOG: London. 1999; 21:231-45.

83. Yagnik CS. The origin of metabolic syndrome in Indians. In the metabolic syndrome; Sood OP, Ratan A(Eds). Ranbaxy Science Foundation 2000; pp. 17-29.

84. The DECODE study group. Glucose tolerance and mortality: comparison of WHO and American Diabetes Association—diagnostic criteria. Lancet. 1999;354:617-21.

85. Balkau B, Shipley M, Jarrett RJ, Pyorala K, Pyorala M, Forhan A, Eschwege E. High blood glucose concentration is a risk factor for mortality in middle-aged nondiabetic men: 20 year follow-up in the Whitehall study. The Paris Prospective Study, and the Helsinki Policemen Study. Diabetes Care. 1998;21:360-7.

86. Lowe LP, Liu K, Greenland P, Metzger BE, Dyer AR, Stamler J. Diabetes, asymptomatic hyperglycemia and 22 year mortality in black and white men: The Chicago Heart Association Detection Project in Industry Study. Diabetes Care.1997; 20:163-9.

87. Shaw JE, Hodge AM, deCourten M, Chitson P, Zimmet PZ. Isolated postchallenge hyperglycemia confirmed as a risk factor for mortality. Diabetologia. 1999;42:1050-4.

88. Stengard JH, Tuomilehto J, Pekkanen J, Kivinen P, Kaarsalo E, Nissinen A, Karvonen MJ. Diabetes mellitus, impaired glucose tolerance and mortality among elderly men: the Finnish cohorts of the seven countries study. Diabetologia. 1992; 35(8):760-5.

89. Wei M, Gaskill SP, Haffner SM, Stern MP. Effects of diabetes and level of glycemia on all cause and cardiovascular mortality. The San Antonio Heart Study. Diabetes Care. 1998;21:1167-72.

90. Saydah HS, Catherine M Loria, Eberhardt MS, Brancati FL. Subclinical states of glucose intolerance and risk of death in the US. Diabetes Care. 2001;24:447-53.

91. Haffner SM, Stern MP, Hazuda HP, Mitchell BD, Patterson JK. Cardiovsacular risk factors in confirmed prediabetic indivi-duals. Does the clock for coronary heart disease start ticking before the onset of clinical diabetes? JAMA. 1990;263:2893-8.

92. Arvind K, Pradeepa R, Deepa R, Mohan V. Diabetes and coronary artery disease. Indian J Med Res. 2002;116:163-76.

93. Schurgin Sunita, Rich Stuart, Mazzone Theodore. Increased prevalence of significant coronary artery calcification in patients with diabetes. Diabetes Care. 2001;24(2):335-8.

94. Shanthirani CS, Rema M, Deepa R, et al. The Chennai Urban Population Study (CUPS)—Methodological details (CUPS paper No 1). Int J Diab in Dev Countries. 1999;19:149-57.

95. Mohan V, Ravikumar R, Shanthirani CS, Deepa R. Intimal medial thickness of the carotid artery in South Indian diabetic and nondiabetic subjects. The Chennai Urban Population Study (CUPS). Diabetologia. 2000;43:494-9.

96. Ravikumar R, Deepa R, Shanthirani CS, Mohan V. Comparison of carotid intima-media thickness, arterial stiffness and brachial artery flow mediated dilatation in diabetic and nondiabetic subjects (CUPS No 9). Am J Cardiol. 2002;90: 702-7.

Chapter 61

NONCORONARY CARDIAC COMPLICATIONS IN DIABETES

Murlidhar S Rao

INTRODUCTION

Cardiovascular disorders accounts for over 70% of mortality among patients of diabetes mellitus. Diseases of the heart itself have been identified as the cause of mortality in 52 to 56% during 1965-68.[1] Ever since the observations of extensive atherosclerosis in coronary arteries at autopsy[2] and higher incidence of ischemic heart disease (IHD) in patients with diabetes (Levine 1922).[3] Coronary heart disease (CHD) was reckoned as the sole category of heart disease promoted by diabetes mellitus.

In 1967, Tripathy et al[4] presented their observation on *paroxysmal cardiogenic dyspnea {left ventricular (LV) failure}* in the absence of hypertension and any clinical or electrocardiographic evidence of ischemic heart disease (IHD) in five patients with poorly controlled diabetes mellitus. Diabetic cardiomyopathy was suggested as the possible cause of left ventricular insufficiency in these subjects.[4] The idea received little international cognizance until Rubler et al (1972)[5] and Hamby et al (1974)[6] documented pathological charges in the heart and clinical heart failure in diabetic patients which could not be ascribed to coronary artery disease, hypertension, valvular lesions or alcoholism. The cardiac conditions in these situations were specified as diabetic cardiomyopathy.

In addition Wheeler and Watkin[7] as well as Ewing et al[8] in 1973 ascribed certain clinical cardiovascular manifestations and altered responses to a number of evocative tests to cardiac autonomic neuropathy (CAN) in patients with diabetes mellitus.

Furthermore documentations of much higher incidence of symptomatic heart failure and sudden cardiac deaths in diabetic patients in the Framingham Study (Kannel et al, 1974)[9] needed explanations and exploration for other diabetes related factors that may operate over and above accelerated and excessive coronary atherosclerosis.

Over this background, the presently acknowledged noncoronary cardiac complications of diabetes can be discussed under the following three headings:
1. Diabetic cardiomyopathy and heart failure in diabetes
2. Cardiac autonomic neuropathy in diabetes
3. Sudden cardiac death in diabetes.

DIABETIC CARDIOMYOPATHY AND HEART FAILURE IN DIABETES

Epidemiology

The existence of a specific diabetic cardiomyopathy was first established by Rubler et al in 1972[5] based on their study of four adult diabetic patients with both Kimmelstiel-Wilson disease and congestive cardiac failure (CCF). None of patients had evidence neither of valvular, congenital, hypertensive or alcohol-related heart disease nor of significant coronary atherosclerosis. These patients had DM for 5 to 20 years. The Framingham workers also found that cardiac failure was more common among diabetic subjects and that this could not be explained by coronary artery disease.[9] Diabetes was shown to be an independent risk factor of CCF in the elderly population and 1% increase in the HbA$_{1c}$ increased the risk of CCF by 15%.[10]

The frequency of diabetes mellitus (DM) in patients among the patients suffering from cardiomyopathy with CCF is significantly greater than anticipated (Hamby et al, 1976).[6] In India, Tripathy (1973)[11] and Dutta et al (1976)[12] reported the existence of cardiac enlargement and failure in diabetes mellitus without obvious coronary artery or hypertensive disease suggesting a specific diabetic cardiomyopathy. Thus, there are evidences to suggest that diabetes mellitus may predispose to the development of a specific diabetic heart muscle disease which may lead to CCF.

Pathogenetic Mechanisms

The exact mechanisms by which diabetes mellitus may induce CCF independent of epicardial coronary artery disease (CAD) are unkown but several hypotheses based on scientific data have been put forward.

Intramyocardial Microangiopathy

This has been observed in diabetic heart.[13] Autopsy studies on 116 diabetic subjects have shown that the intramural arterioles and capillaries had hyaline thickening with PAS positive material in the vessel wall. Further studies demonstrated the capillary basement membrane thickening, increased degree of myocardial fibrin and even the capillary microaneurysms.[14,15] As such diabetic microangiopathy to some extent is likely to be responsible for diabetic cardiomyopathy.

Metabolic Factors

Hyperglycemia, impaired myocardial glucose uptake and increased turnover of free fatty acids (FFA) may all contribute to diabetes mellitus-related myocardial dysfunction. Oxidation of glucose in diabetic heart is impaired by lack of lactate utilization and decreased pyruvate dehydrogenase activity resulting in oxidative decarboxylation within the Kreb's cycle.

Endothelial Dysfunction

Uncontrolled diabetes mellitus (DM) results in impaired endothelium dependent vasodilatation seen in both T1 and T2DM and is responsible for reduced myocardial flow reserve in the absence of CAD.

Myocardial Fibrosis

Experimental and clinical data point to a potential role for myocardial fibrosis in diabetic cardiomyopathy. Intramyocardial accumulation of collagen is a well-demonstrated consequence of DM. Moreover, the deposition of advanced glycation end products (AGEs) may result in left ventricular hypertrophy and stiffness which may lead to left ventricular diastolic dysfunction. Abnormal accumulation of calcium ions in the myocardial cells, a significant depression of epinephrine-stimulated adenylate cyclase activity and a defective oxidative metabolism of heart mitochondria have been observed experimentally in diabetic rats.[16]

In summary, various mechanisms may induce a specific diabetic ++ myocardial disorder, i.e. cardiomyopathy. Whether diabetic cardiomyopathy alone is a common cause of CCF is, however not clear. Another possibility is that these myocardial alternations related to DM, may predispose to the development of CCF association with disorders such as CAD or hypertension.

Two-fold higher incidence of heart failure following myocardial infarction (MI) in patients with diabetes[17] may be attributed to coexisting cardiomyopathy. Further cardiac mortality is 1.6 to 2 times higher in diabetic subjects following advent of heart failure. Doubling of 4-year cardiac mortality rate (25.9 vs 14.5) has been observed in diabetic patients with MI compared to nondiabetic subjects despite smaller size of infarcts in the former. This has been attributed to poor compensatory hyperkinetic response of noninfarcted myocardium[18] on account of myocardium in the cardiac muscles.

It has been estimated that diabetes increase incidence of heart failure by 1.8-fold in hypertensive men and 3.7-fold in hypertensive women[19] because of associated cardiomyopathy. This may be attributed to adverse myocardial effect of DM in patients with both diabetes and hypertension.

Pathological Aspects

Cardiac histopathology has been described in diabetic patients with or without CCF. Accumulation of periodic acid Schiff (PAS) positive material in the myocardial

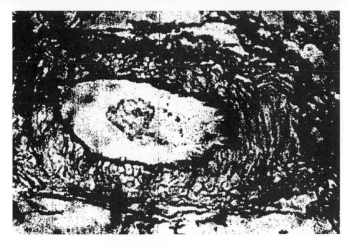

Figure 61.1 Endomyocardial biopsy showing excess of interstitial collagen

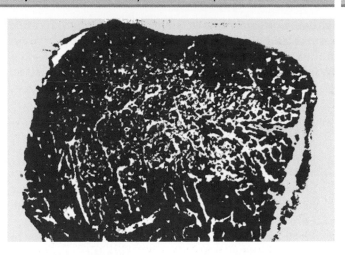

Figure 61.3 Endomyocardial biopsy showing thickening of wall of a small arteriole X 400

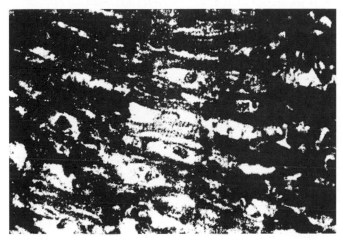

Figure 61.2 Endomyocardial biopsy showing periodic acid Schiff (PAS) positive material in the interstitium

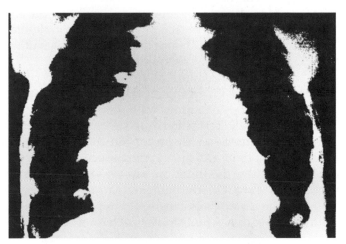

Figure 61.4 X-ray chest PA view of case no. 25 (Group II) showing cardiomegaly

interstitium, increased collagen deposits and interstitial fibrosis have all been documented **(Figures 61.1 and 61.2)**.[19] Hypertrophy is seen in some myocytes. Perivascular, interstitial and replacement fibrosis with fragmentation or degeneration of myocytes is commonly seen. Myocardial concentrations of triglycerides and cholesterol were diffusely increased in the autopsy studies by Regan et al.[20] Intramyocardial arteriolar and capillary basement membrane thickening **(Figure 61.3)**,[19] accumulation of neutral mucopolysaccharides in the intramural arterioles with endothelial proliferation with focal protuberances and development of microaneurysms in the capillaries of diabetic myocardium are other features that have been demonstrated in diabetic hearts.[14]

Clinical Profile

Specific diabetic cardiomyopathy is basically a chronic progressive state with myocardial diastolic dysfunction/ failure to begin with. Later on the systolic abnormalities supervene by the time the classical features of CCF are clinically observed. Effort intolerance of various grades and paroxysmal (nocturnal) dyspnea with cough, are the most common presenting features. Cardiomegaly **(Figure 61.4)**,[19] atrial and ventricular gallops and signs of pulmonary congestion are present. Studies linking DM with CCF have estimated the prevalence of DM in people with CCF to be around 20% compared to 4 to 6% in the control population.[21] Epidemiological studies have shown that there is increased risk of heart failure in diabetic subjects, especially those with poor glycemic control and also longer duration of diabetes.[22]

Noninvasive Studies

- *Electrocardiography (ECG)*: ECG changes mainly consist of diffuse T-wave abnormalities which are likely to be related to the underlying diabetic myocardial disease. ECG signs of left ventricular hypertrophy may be present without hypertension as was seen in the four original cases of Rubler et al.[5] If there is associated hypertension or coronary heart disease, then the corresponding ECG signs will be present.

  In addition, electrocardiographic evidences of conduction blocks such as right bundle branch block (RBBB) has been observed to be more frequent in subjects with diabetes than in controls.[19]

- Doppler echocardiography has emerged as an excellent noninvasive technique to demonstrate the various LV function abnormalities at any given time and also in the serial follow-up of patients.

  Earliest abnormality is LV diastolic dysfunction which can be shown on pulsed wave (PW) Doppler tracing of the LV inflow with sample volume at mitral valve cusps. Increased "A" wave velocity compared to 'E' wave, prolonged 'E' deceleration time, E/A ratio less than 1 all characteristic of the LV diastolic dysfunction are recorded **(Figure 61.5)**.[23] Many elderly persons (above 65 years of age) who are neither diabetic nor hypertension may also show this echo-Doppler pattern. The pattern, as seen in younger persons with diabetes of 5 to 20 years' duration without hypertension or coronary heart disease is suggestive of diabetic cardiomyopathy. Asymmetrical septal hypertrophy or even the concentric LVH may be seen on M-mode and 2-D echo. The LV dilatation may not be seen in a diabetic heart with LV diastolic dysfunction and normal systolic function but may occur when LV systolic dysfunction supervenes over the pre-existing diastolic abnormalities. This is consistent with the fact that a diabetic heart has a stiff and less compliant myocardium to start with (diastolic dysfunction) but later LV becomes dilated with poor ejection fraction (EF) (systolic failure) resulting in CCF[4] **(Figure 61.6)**. Functional mitral and tricuspid regurgitations (due to dilated LV and RV) can be demonstrated on CW Doppler. Left ventricular (LV) is dilated and shows global hypokinesia with poor EF. Newer Doppler echo

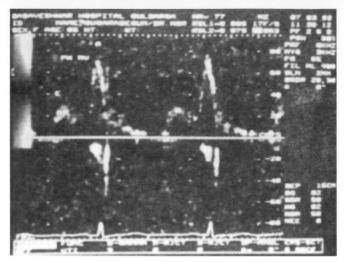

Figure 61.5 Pulse wave Doppler at the mitral valve showing the 'A' wave taller than 'E' (E/A ratio <1) and E-deceleration time, suggestive of LV diastolic dysfunction in one of our cases 14

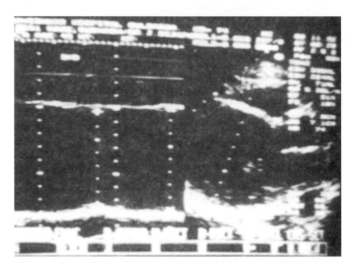

Figure 61.6 Dilated heart with poor LV function (EF < 40%) in another case of diabetic heart disease with chronic CCF. Functional mitral and tricuspid regurgitation was present in this case

imaging modalities like tissue Doppler imaging and myocardial contrast echo may throw more light on these abnormalities.

- Systolic time intervals (STIs) and apex cardiographic (ACG) tracing are other noninvasive techniques which are now not routinely done with the present advances in an echocardiography. For STIs, simultaneous (3 channel) recording of the ECG, phonocardiography and the carotid pulse tracings at 100 mm speed is done. Diabetic patients

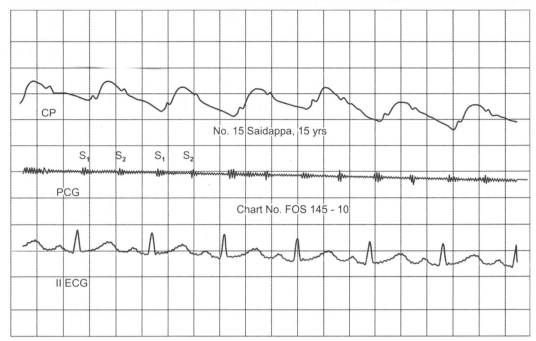

Figure 61.7 STI in a young diabetic showing prolonged PEP (PEPI: 136.8 m sec.) and increased PEPI/LVETI ratio (0.332) suggestive of reduced LV function. This boy aged 15 years had T1DM for >5 years, very poorly controlled[16]

have a shorter LV ejection time (LVET) and a longer pre-ejection period (PEP). Therefore, the ratio PEP/LVET is prolonged suggesting a reduction in LV function in diabetic patients **(Figure 61.7)**[19,24,25] even in the younger age group.

ACG technique is a mechanical displacement record with the transducer kept snugly at the LV apex on chest wall in the left lateral position (best palpable apical thrust position). This recording, once described as an external ventriculogram is done at 100 mm speed. Both systolic (systolic bulge) and diastolic abnormalities (rapid filling wave abbreviated) can be made out. Furthermore, 'a' wave of the ACG in the diabetic heart disease is abnormally tall, a sign of decreased compliance. This technique although a useful noninvasive method, is obsolete now and rarely done.

- Radionucleotide ventriculography has also been occasionally used to study ventricular function in diabetic patients. Most studies have shown normal resting ejection fraction but a lower EF in response to dynamic exercise in the diabetic patients compared to nondiabetic subjects.

Grossly, altered myocardial functions has been documented experimentally in diabetic dogs (Regan, 1974).[26]

Hence, the conclusion is that in diabetes left ventricle both contracts and relaxes in an abnormal way and many times this cannot be explained by occult or manifest coronary artery disease.

Invasive Studies

Cardiac catheterization, necessary to define the state of the coronary arteries, typically reveals:
- Elevated left ventricular end-diastolic pressure ($\uparrow$ LVEDP)
- Lower left ventricular end-diastolic volume ($\downarrow$ LVEDV)
- Normal coronary angiogram
- Normal lactate response to atrial pacing. Suggestive of absence of ischemia.

These observations suggest decreased compliance of the left ventricle without any coronary artery disease.[17] Besides, there is a low stroke volume index but normal ejection fraction (EF). Diminished LV filling is probably responsible for diminished stroke volume. When there is CCF in these patients, LVEF is decreased. In some diabetic patients, functional abnormalities of the coronary microvasculature (diminished coronary vasodilator reserve) might be visualized to explain the symptoms since their coronary angiograms may be normal.

Management

This is no different from treating failure due to other causes. ACE inhibitors (if not tolerated, angiotensin receptor blockers), β-blockers especially carvedilol or bisoprolol, diuretics preferably loop diuretics (furosemide), aldosterone antagonist spironolactone and in some instances, digoxin in this order are the drugs to be used apart from salt and fluid-restriction.

- *Angiotensin-converting enzyme inhibitors (ACEIs):* ACEIs are the preferred drugs to treat CCF in diabetics. In studies of left ventricular dysfunction (SOLVD),[27] for instance, the efficacy of enalapril was more marked in diabetic than in nondiabetic patients. In assessment of treatment with lisinopril and survival (ATLAS) trial[28] also, a longer risk reduction in diabetic patients with CCF was seen compared to the rest when treated with high dose of lisinopril.

  ACEIs are renoprotective as well as cardioprotective besides reducing the insulin resistance.
- *β-blockers:* Since these are known to have some hyperglycemic effects, their use in diabetes has been disputed. However, in diabetic patients with specific cardiomyopathy and CCF, carvedilol in appropriate doses results in symptomatic improvement and survival benefit.[29] Bisoprolol and metoprolol have also been found useful in diabetic patients with CCF.
- *Diuretics:* Loop diuretics (Furosemide) and spironolactone have been found to be beneficial in managing CCF in diabetic as well as nondiabetic subjects. Thiazides have hyperglycemic effects which may worsen the glycemic control in a diabetic and hence may not be preferred. Spironolactone has been shown to reduce the mortality in patients of heart failure {Rationale for the randomized aldactone evaluation study (RALES)}.[30]
- *Glycemic control:* Intensive glycemic control reduces the incidence of heart failure in patients with T2DM as shown in United Kingdom Prospective Diabetes Study (UKPDS).[31] Strict diabetic diet apart from salt and water restriction, glycemic control by insulin given in 3 to 5 small doses per day before each snack or meal are needed. HbA_{1c} should be kept within 65%. Tight glycemic control may itself ameliorate specific diabetic cardiomyopathy to some extent.

  Other risk factors in diabetic patients with or without CCF have also to be taken care of. Coexisting HTN and dyslipidemia/hyperlipidemia have to be treated with appropriate antihypertensive drugs as well as statins and/or fibrates.

Prognosis

The important determinants in the progression of specific diabetic heart muscle disease into clinical heart failure are poor glycemic control, coexisting CAD and HTN as well as the existence of microvascular disease. Intensive control of blood glucose and HTN will go a long way in preventing clinical heart failure.

A peculiar form of hypertrophic cardiomyopathy is seen among the 50% of the neonates born to diabetic mothers. High levels of fetal insulin which in turn is related to inadequate control of DM in the mother, is probably responsible for this neonatal cardiac hypertrophy. Strict control of blood glucose during pregnancy can reduce the chances of CCF in these infants although the echo appearance of LVH may persist.

CARDIOVASCULAR AUTONOMIC NEUROPATHY IN DIABETES

Prevalence

Autonomic neuropathy was generally recognized as a part of the spectrum of nerve damage in DM by Jordan in 1936 and Rundles in 1945.[32]

Cardiovascular autonomic neuropathy (CAN) is fairly common and a troublesome complication of both type 1 and type 2 DM. During 1970s, a series of tests were developed for the assessment of that part of the autonomic nervous system that innervates the circulatory systems. Ewing and Clarke[33] summarized in detail these methods and the limits of normality which are utilized to find out the objective evidence of existence of CAN in a diabetic. A multicenter study group[34] has shown that although the symptoms of CAN are present in 14 to 23% patients, the CAN on the basis of objective tests is present in 51% of T2DM. Indian studies also reveal the existence of CAN, on an objective basis in the range of 50 to 77% of diabetic subjects[35] with long-term diabetes.

Clinical Profile

Cardiovascular reflexes are important in maintaining the homeostasis during stress situations through both parasympathetic and sympathetic pathways of the autonomic nervous system. Cardiovascular autonomic neuropathy (CAN) in the diabetic patients with or without peripheral neuropathy, sometimes induce disabling situations such as severe postural hypotension and silent (painless) myocardial ischemia or infarction occasionally leading to sudden cardiac death. Sudden syncope, lightheadedness, transient visual loss, pallor, extreme weakness and diaphoresis are other symptoms. Postprandial hypotension, reduced exercise tolerance and ischemic pattern on ECG observed on treadmill testing or Holter monitoring are other manifestations of CAN in diabetic patient. In the Framingham study, 23% of all myocardial infarctions were detected only at routine ECG follow-up, about half of these were symptomatic (but had not been recognized) and about half were truly silent.[36] Neuropathy of the sympathetic afferent nerve fibers may be responsible for the painless infarctions.

Second major effect of CAN is to impair the response for various circulatory adjustments. On exercise, the diabetic patients are less able to increase their heart rate, blood pressure or cardiac output compared to the nondiabetic controls. Postural hypotension in CAN may often be exacerbated by administration of insulin to such subjects.[37]

Assessment

On testing for sympathetic and parasympathetic divisions of CAN, it has been seen that the parasympathetic fibers are affected earlier than sympathetic. CAN is usually not reversible with rare exceptions. Lastly, diabetic CAN subjects are at an increased risk of sudden death.

Tests Reflecting Cardiac Parasympathetic Damage

- *Heart rate response to deep breathing:* Continuous ECG is taken in deep inspiration and expiration (6 breaths/minute). The maximum and minimum R-R intervals are calculated. These are converted into beats/minute. The result is noted as the difference between maximum and minimum heart rate per minute (6 breathing cycles). Normally, this difference is 15 beats/minute, below this is abnormal. Less than 10 beats/minute are grossly abnormal.
- *Immediate heart rate response to standing:* Continuous ECG is recorded when the patient is lying down comfortably and then standing on position for up to 30th beat. The result is expressed as 30 : 15 ratio which is normal if greater than and equal to 1.04, borderline 1.01 and abnormal if less than and equal to 1.00.
- *Valsalva ratio:* Patient lying comfortably on a bed is asked to blow into a mouthpiece connected to a mercurial sphygmomanometer and holding it on a pressure of 40 mm Hg for 15 seconds, while ECG is

being continuously recorded. ECG taken after this Valsalva maneuver in lead II and V1 is looked into and the ratio of longest R-R interval to shortest R-R interval is calculated. This ratio is called Valsalva ratio.

Normal Valsalva ratio is 1.2, values between to 1.2 borderlines and 1.0 or less is abnormal.

Tests of Cardiac Sympathetic Damage

- *BP response to sudden standing (Postural hypotension):* The BP of the patient is recorded first in a quiet lying down position and then immediately on standing. Fall of BP on standing is normally less than 10 mm Hg. Fall of 30 mm Hg or more is definitely abnormal. Between 11 and 29 mm Hg is borderline.
- *BP response to sustained handgrip:* An inflated BP cuff is given to the patient for squeezing it continuously. The BP is recorded before, during and after the procedure. The maximum DBP during the procedure minus the resting DBP (before the test) is normally higher by 16 mm Hg. If it is less than 10 mm Hg, then the test is definitely abnormal. If it is 11 to 15 mm Hg, then it is borderline.
- *BP response to cold pressor test:* After rinsing the hand in ice-cold water, BP is recorded. Normally, the DBP rises by more than 8 mm Hg. Any value below this is considered as abnormal.

There are likely to be some pitfalls resulting in misdiagnosis while assessing the CAN tests in diabetes mellitus. The assessment is likely to be more accurate if the combination of tests is taken into consideration. It is also important to keep in mind of the various drugs worsening the autonomic neuropathy. Commonly used such drugs are ACE inhibitors, α-blockers, methyldopa, clonidine, phenothiazines, barbiturates and tricyclic antidepressants.

Lastly, an invariant pulse rate of 80 to 90 beats/min unresponsive to stress, exercise or sleep indicates near complete cardiac denervation. All the above tests are grossly abnormal and carotid sinus pressure has no effect on heart rate. This is similar to the denervated heart following cardiac transplantation.[38]

Management

Strict glycemic control may reverse early CAN and at least prevent its progression. Drugs found beneficial in some cases are antioxidants (alpha-lipoic acid), ACE inhibitors, aldose-reductase inhibitor and L-carnitine. Exercise prescription to diabetic subjects with CAN has to be specifically tailored on individual basis.

SUDDEN CARDIAC DEATH IN DIABETES

Definition and its Association

Sudden cardiac death (SCD) implies unexpected natural death, i.e. occurring within an hour of onset of symptoms in an individual with or without recognized cardiac disease. SCD in DM could occur in association with:

- Coronary artery disease (more than one previous myocardial infarction)
- Ischemic cardiomyopathy/chronic CCF
- Noncoronary heart disease like diabetic cardiomyopathy {with or without left ventricular hypertrophy (LVH)} or severe cardiac autonomic neuropathy
- Complex ventricular ectopy
- Positive family history of SCD
- Heavy smoking.

Cause of Sudden Cardiac Death

The SCD is more often due to ventricular tachycardia and ventricular fibrillation and less often due to bradycardia and cardiac asystole. The vast majority of patients who are victims of SCD have cardiac structural abnormalities which provide the substrate for ventricular tachyarrhythmias that are the causes for SCD in most cases. Electrolyte imbalance or proarrhythmic effect of some drugs may have triggering effect on fatal ventricular arrhythmias. Long standing, uncontrolled diabetes often associated with CAN, structural changes in the myocardium and small intramural vasculopathy, often with chronic CCF, render the heart vulnerable for malignant arrhythmias which result in SCD. Twenty-four hour ECG (Holter monitoring) monitoring often discloses various arrhythmias (like ventricular ectopics) or ischemic changes in ECG occurring silently is a useful technique to pick-up the diabetic patients at risk of SCD even those with normal autonomic function.[39] So also the tests of CAN, Doppler echocardiography and the presence of late potentials on signal-averaged ECG definitely help in identification of the susceptibility for SCD. Nuclear techniques such as thallium scan which shows perfusion defects (ischemic areas) and the metaiodobenzyl guanidine (MIBG) (an analog of the well-known antiadrenergic therapeutic agent guanethidine) scintigraphy that reveals accumulation defects (denervation areas) are very useful. The latter technique is used for cardiac sympathetic imaging.[40]

Moreover, in diabetic patients it has been shown that the circadian rhythm is disturbed and this probably plays an important role in the onset of acute cardiovascular syndromes including acute ventricular arrhythmias and SCD.[41] Acute cardiac events occur at the time with highest sympathetic and lowest parasympathetic activity, usually during the late morning peak in nondiabetic subjects. In patients with diabetes, this rhythm is lost and the acute episodes may occur in late night during sleep which may be fatal.

Management of Patients at Risk

Apart from glycemic control and BP control, some of the drugs like β-blockers in the background of CHD, ACEIs in the backdrop of CCF, antiarrhythmic drugs like amiodarone and sotalol have been found to be useful to some extent in preventing SCD. Devices like automatic implantable cardioverter defibrillator (AICD) are quite effective in detecting and terminating ventricular tachyarrhythmias and prevent SCD.[42]

SUMMARY

Noncoronary cardiac disease in diabetes mellitus could be in the form of specific diabetic cardiomyopathy, cardiac autonomic neuropathy or silently occurring potentially lethal ventricular arrhythmias often resulting in sudden cardiac death. Methods of identification of these syndromes on clinical and investigational basis have been described along with current thinking about the pathogenetic mechanisms and the management strategies to be adopted.

REFERENCES

1. Marks HH, Karll LP. Onset, course prognosis and mortality in diabetes mellitus. In Marbles A, White P, Krall LP (Eds): Joslin's diabetes mellitus. Philadelphia: Lea and Feabiger; 1971.p.209.
2. Brunt NL. On the heart in relation to diabetes. Practitioner. 1907;79:42-6.
3. Levine SA. Angina Pectoris: some clinical considerations. JAMA. 1922;39:928-33.
4. Tripathy BB, Panda NC, Tej SC. Paroxysmal cardiogenic dyspnea in diabetes mellitus (Abstract). Assoc Phys India. 1967;15:61.
5. Rubler S, Dulgash J, Yuceoglu YZ, et al. New type of cardiomyopathy associated with diabetic glomerulosclerosis. Amer J Cardiology. 1972;30:595-602.
6. Hamby RI, Sherman L, Mehta J, et al. Diabetic cardiomyopathy. JAMA. 1974;229:1749.
7. Wheeler T, Watkins J. Cardiac denervation in diabetes. Br Med J. 1973;4:584-6.

8. Ewing DJ, Campbell IW, Butt AA, et al. Vascular reflexes in diabetic autonomic neuropathy. Lancet. 1973;2:1354-6.

9. Kannel WB, et al. Role of diabetes in congestive heart failure: the Framingham study. Amer J Cardiology. 1978;34:29.

10. Chae CU, Glynn RJ, et al. Diabetes predicts congestive heart failure risk in the elderly. Circulation. 1998;98(Suppl 1):721.

11. Tripathy BB. Cardiac enlargement and failure in diabetes. J Indian Med Assoc. 1973;61:45.

12. Dutta AL, Das S, Panja M, et al. Profile of cardiac involvement in diabetes. J Diabetic Assoc India. 1976;16:43.

13. Blumethal HT, Alex M, Goldenberg S. A study of lesions of the intramural coronary branches in diabetes mellitus. Arch Pathol. 1960;70:27.

14. Factor SM, Okun EM, Minase T. Capillary microaneurysms in the human diabetic heart. N Engl J Med. 1980;302:384.

15. Panja M, Pal NC, Majumdar G, et al. Report of small vessel changes in the diabetic heart. J Assoc Phys India. 1976;24:637.

16. Saratchandra K. Noncoronary heart disease in diabetes: Diabetic cardiomyopathy in postgraduate medicine. Cardio diabetology (API). 1998;XII(Part I):139-42.

17. Stone PH, Muller JE, Hartwell T, et al. The effect of diabetes mellitus on prognosis and serial left ventricular functions after both coronary disease and diastolic left ventricular dysfunction to the adverse prognosis. The MILIS Study Group. J Am Coll Cardiol. 1989;14:49-57.

18. Hypertension in Diabetes Study (HDS) II. Increased risk of cardiovascular complications in hypertension type 2 diabetic patients. J Hyperens. 1993;II:319-25.

19. Misra R, Das JP, Tripathy BB, Samal KC, Didyadhar S. Studies on noncoronary cardic complications of diabetes mellitus. In Bajaj JS (Ed): Diabetes mellitus in developing countries. New Delhi: Inter print. 1984; pp. 271-7.

20. Regan TJ, et al. Evidence of cardiomyopathy in familial diabetes mellitus. J Clin Invest. 1977;60:885. Quoted in: Progress in Cardiology 2/1. Zipes DP, Rowlands DJ (Eds). Lea and Febriger 1989; pp. 107-25.

21. Banters C, Lamblin N, et al. Influence of diabetes on heart failure risk and outcome: a review. Cardio Diab. 2003;2:1-19.

22. Iribaren C, Karter AJ, Go AS, et al. Glycemic control and heart failure in adult patients with diabetes. Circulation. 2001;103:2668-73.

23. Rao MS, Natraj LB, Bijapure JB, et al. Echocardiographic evaluation of LV function in NIDDM. J Diab Assoc India. 1996;36:106-11.

24. Ahmed SS, Jaferi GA, Narang RM, Regan TJ. Preclinical abnormality of left ventricular function in diabetes mellitus. Am Heart J. 1975;89:153-8.

25. Rao MS, Mulimani M, et al. Left ventricular function studies in young diabetics by systolic time intervals (STIs). J Diab Assoc India. 1996;36:118-25.

26. Regan TJ, et al. Altered myocardial function and metabolism in chronic diabetes mellitus without ischemia in dogs. Circulation Research. 1974;35:222.

27. Shindler DM, Kostis JB, Yusuf S, et al. Diabetes mellitus: a predictor of morbidity and mortality in the studies of left ventricular dysfunction (SOLVD) trial and registry. Amer J Cardiol. 1996;77:1017-26.

28. Ryden L, Armostrong PW, Cleveland JG, et al. Efficacy and safety of high dose lisinopril in chronic heart failure patients at high CV risk including those with DM: results of ATLAS trial. European Heart J. 2000;21:967-78.

29. Packar M, Bristow MR, Cohn JN, et al. The effect of carvedilol on morbidity and mortality in patients with chronic heart failure. US carvedilol HF study group. NEJM. 1996;334:1349-55.

30. Pitt B, Zinnad F, Ramme W, et al. Randomized aldactone evaluation study (RALES): the effect of spironolactone on the morbidity and mortality in patients with severe HF. NEJM. 1999;341:709-17.

31. Stratton IM, Adler AI, Neil HA, et al. Association of glycemia with macro- and microvascular complications of T2DM (UKPDS 35): Prospective Observational Study. 2000;321:405-12.

32. Rundles RW. Diabetic autonomic neuropathy. Medicine (Baltimore). 1945;24:111-60.

33. Ewing DJ, Clarke BF. Diagnosis and management of diabetic autonomic neuropathy. BMJ. 1982;285:916-8.

34. Zeigler D, Gries FA, Spuler M, et al. The epidemiology of diabetic neuropathy: Diabetic Cardiovascular Autonomic Neuropathy Multicenter Study Group. J Diab and its Complications. 1992;6:49-57.

35. Mukhopadhyaya J, Ray S. Cardiac autonomic neuropathy in diabetes. Medicine Update (API). 2004;14:35-8.

36. Margolis JR, Kannel WB, Feinleib M, et al. Clinical features of unrecognized myocardial infarction silent and symptomatic (Framingham study). Amer J Cardiology. 1973;32:1-7.

37. Page MM, Watkins PJ. Provocation of postural hypotension by insulin in diabetic autonomic neuropathy. Diabetes. 1976;29:90-5.

38. Das AK, Balachandar J, Chandrasekhar S. Autonomic neuropathy of heart in diabetes. Int J Diab Dev Countries. 1995;15:146-8.

39. Ahluwalia G, Jain P, Chugh SK, et al. Silent myocardial ischemia in diabetics with normal autonomic function. Int J Cardiology. 1995;48:147-53.

40. Koistinen MJ. Airaksinen KE, Huikuri HV, et al. No difference in cardiac innervation of diabetic patients with painful and asymptomatic coronary artery disease. Diabetes Care. 1996;19:231-3.

41. Zarich Stuart, Waxman S, et al. Effect of autonomic nervous system on the circadian pattern of myocardial ischemia in DM. J Amer Coll Card. 1994;24:956.

42. Connolly SJ, Gent M, Roberts RS, et al. Canadian implantable defibrillator study (CIDS): a randomized trial of the implantable cardioverter defibrillator against amiodarone. Circulation. 2000;101:1297-302.

Chapter 62

DIABETES AND CEREBROVASCULAR DISEASE

BC Bansal, MV Padma, JS Bajaj

CHAPTER OUTLINE

- Introduction
- Diabetes as a Risk Factor for Stroke: The Evidence-based Studies
- Diabetes associated other Risk Factors for Stroke
- Pathogenesis of Stroke and Cerebrovascular Disease in Diabetes
- Stroke Subtypes and Pattern of Vascular Disease in Diabetes
- Summary

INTRODUCTION

Diabetes has long been a major health problem and has held for many years the dubious distinction of being the number one cause of adult blindness, kidney failure and nontraumatic limb amputation, besides being a recognized risk factor of considerable importance for coronary and cerebrovascular diseases. The turn of the millennium is witnessing several changing paradigms and newer perspectives in diabetes mellitus. One of these relates to the improved understanding of the relationship between metabolic profile of diabetes mellitus and cerebrovascular disease.

DIABETES AS A RISK FACTOR FOR STROKE: THE EVIDENCE-BASED STUDIES

Although medical and surgical therapies for impending or recent-onset stroke must be pursued, prevention is likely to be the most effective strategy in reducing the ravages of cerebrovascular disease (CVD). The development of atherosclerotic disease and stroke has been related to a number of host and environmental factors delineated in recent years, chiefly through prospective epidemiologic studies. The relative impact of each of these risk factors is becoming clearer, and controlled clinical trials have demonstrated the efficacy of risk factor modification in stroke prevention.

Sufficient data exists to implicate diabetes as an independent risk factor for stroke.[1] Large population studies have shown stroke to be more frequent and have a higher mortality in patients with diabetes,[2,3] with a predilection for women when compared to men. In a Swedish cohort, the highest rate was 6-fold in diabetic males but 13-fold in diabetic females. In the Framingham study,[4,5] peripheral arterial disease was significantly more in diabetics when compared to cerebral or coronary artery disease. However, incidence of cardiovascular disease was again more common in female counterparts with diabetes when compared to males. Among the 3776 patients in the United Kingdom Prospective Diabetes Study (UKPDS),[6,7] 2.6% developed stroke on a follow-up of 7.9 years. The prevalence of recognized diabetes in patients with acute stroke approximates between 8 and 24%. However, undiagnosed diabetes mellitus is estimated to be between 6 and 42%. In a recently published study by Gray et al,[8] it was concluded that one-third of all stroke patients may have diabetes mellitus. For patients presenting with poststroke hyperglycemia, impaired glucose tolerance or diabetes mellitus is present in two-thirds of all survivors at 12 weeks. Admission plasma glucose[3] 6.1 mmol, if combined with HbA_{1c} >6.2% were good predictors of the presence of diabetes mellitus following stroke.

Stress has been laid on assessment of diabetes before discharge of a stroke patient.[9] In a study to establish relationship between asymptomatic hyperglycemia, diabetes and stroke,[10] 7649 men aged 40-59 years were followed for a mean period of 16.8 years. Of these, 347 patients developed stroke. Men who developed diabetes during follow-up (N = 320) and men with established diabetes at initial recruitment (N = 98) showed significantly increased risk of stroke, even after adjustment of all associated risk factors. Higher levels of nonfasting glucose concentration were independently associated with a significantly increased risk of developing stroke.

Diabetics are known to have an increased susceptibility to coronary, femoral and cerebral artery atherosclerosis. Surveys of stroke patients and prospective studies have confirmed the increased risk of stroke in diabetes. In the United States, in the period 1976 to 1980, a medical history of stroke was 2.5 to 4 times more common in diabetics than in persons with normal glucose tolerance.[11] In the Framingham cohort, peripheral arterial disease with intermittent claudication occurs more than 4 times as often in diabetics.[5] The coronary and cerebral arteries are also affected but to a lesser extent. For atherothrombotic brain infarction, the impact of glucose intolerance, i.e. physician-diagnosed diabetes, glycosuria or a blood sugar greater than 150 mg% is greater in women than in men and is significant as well as an independent contributor to stroke.

The association of glucose intolerance and diabetes with subsequent incidence of stroke was examined prospectively in a cohort of middle-aged Japanese-American men from Honolulu Heart Program who were followed for approximately 22 years.[12] Incidence rates and risk estimates were compared for thromboembolic and hemorrhagic strokes. Adjustments for potential, confounding and mediating factors were used to determine whether observed relations were independent of other cardiovascular risk factors. The study showed that subjects with diabetes and elevated glucose appeared to be at an increased risk of thromboembolic but not hemorrhagic stroke. These associations were largely independent of other cardiovascular disease risk

factors. Excess risk was apparent in older as well as younger diabetic individuals and in hypertensive and nonhypertensive subjects with diabetes.

Although recurrence after ischemic stroke is frequent, with an annual incidence of 4 to 14%, the risk factors for stroke recurrence have not been firmly established. The risk for an initial cerebral infarction are well studied and include increasing age, hypertension, diabetes mellitus, cardiac disease, atrial fibrillation, coronary heart disease, congestive heart failure and cigarette smoking. Hier et al[13] studied stroke recurrence within two years after ischemic infarction. They prospectively studied stroke recurrence in 1,273 patients with ischemic stroke who were entered into the stroke data bank, with a median follow-up of 13 months. The two-year cumulative recurrence rate among these patients was 14.1%. Age, sex, history of hypertension, atrial fibrillation, or transient ischemic attacks and stroke location were not associated with a higher risk of stroke recurrence. Patients with an elevated blood pressure, an abnormal initial computed program, or a history of diabetes mellitus were at a higher risk of stroke recurrence. A multivariate model suggests that patients at the lowest risk for stroke recurrence have a low diastolic blood pressure, no history of stroke, no history of diabetes mellitus and an infarct of unknown cause.

Similar to two-year recurrence, Sacco et al[14] reported that the determinants of a 30-day stroke recurrence were a history of hypertension, admission diastolic blood pressure of >100 mm Hg, history of diabetes, and admission blood glucose level of >140 mg/dl. The risk of early recurrence was slightly but not significantly higher in patients with history of stroke and an abnormal admission ECG. The independent predictors of early recurrence were history of hypertension (odds ratio = 3.7) and initial blood glucose level (odds ratio = 1.8 for 100 mg/dl increment). In the Northern Manhattan Stroke Study,[15] admission glucose was a predictor of both stroke recurrence and mortality. For mortality, the effect was greater for 30-day outcome, while for recurrence; the effect was observed even among 30-day survivors. Admission glucose was a determinant of 30-day stroke recurrence in the NINDS Stroke Data Bank, while diabetes was a significant predictor of 2-year recurrence.

The European BIOMED stroke project[16] looked at *survival* and *functional* outcomes of stroke patients with and without diabetes mellitus. A total of 4,537 patients from seven countries with first time ever stroke were evaluated for demographics, risk factors, clinical presentation and outcome. It was observed that stroke

TABLE 62.1	Distribution of risk factors in stroke			
Risk factor	Infarct (n = 140)		Intracranial hemorrhage (n = 63)	
	No.	%	No.	%
Hypertension	79	56.4	57	90.5
Diabetes mellitus	31	22.1	4	6.35
Hyperlipidemia	7/80	8.8	1/32	3.12
Tobacco-chewing	11	7.8	5	7.9
Smoking	54	38.6	18	28.6
Alcohol	21	15	8	12.7
Previous history of stroke	16	11.4	7	11.1
Cardiac disease	32	22.9	10	15.9
Family history of stroke	38	27	16	25.4

patients with diabetes did poorly in terms of motor function, although case fatality rates, are not significantly higher among diabetics when compared to normoglycemics. Their study emphasized the need for early diagnosis and treatment of every case of diabetes.

Data from our country is inconsistent, sparse and generally derived from hospital admissions and many of the stroke patients are likely to be treated domestically in villages or would be admitted or seen by local medical practitioners. The incidence of stroke varies from 0.9 to 1% of all admissions in hospital from India,[1] rising to 4% when all emergencies are included. Stroke amongst diabetes has an incidence of 0.5 to 9.2%. Mortality data in diabetes with stroke range from 12 to 32.5%. In an ongoing project, 203 stroke patients, male and female, of all ages who attended the stroke clinic at the Neurosciences Center, All India Institute of Medical Sciences (AIIMS), New Delhi, India have been studied. The risk factor profile was analyzed in the above patients with special relevance to the population profile in urban northern India. The distribution of risk factors is given in **Table 62.1**. A number of patients had multiple risk factors, the constellation including hypertension, CAD, diabetes mellitus and hyperlipidemia as a part of dysmetabolism and smoking as a lifestyle acquisition.

DIABETES ASSOCIATED OTHER RISK FACTORS FOR STROKE

Although diabetes is an independent risk factor for stroke with its many underlying pathophysiological mechanisms, it has long been believed that hypertension

may be the main risk factor for strokes in diabetic patients, which also applies to patients with transient ischemic attacks (TIAs). Treatment of hypertension found at the time of diagnosis of diabetes reduces subsequent risk of both strokes and TIAs. In the recently published *Progress* study, use of perindopril and indapamide produced significant proportional stroke risk reduction in both diabetics (38%) and nondiabetics (28%). Therefore, the relationship between diabetes and hypertension seems much more complex. Since hypertension is a common, important and modifiable risk factor for both micro- and macrovascular complications of diabetes, a synergistic effect probably exists between the two leading to a final common pathway for vasculopathy causing stroke. Proteinuria has also been identified as an independent risk factor for stroke in one study.[17] However, among the Framingham cohort, no such correlation was found. In the UKPDS study, obesity or lack of exercise, poor glycemic control, hyperinsulinemia and dyslipidemia were not significantly associated with stroke. However, even though statistics may show nonsignificant events, presence of these risk factors is likely to worsen the underlying pathophysiological mechanisms responsible for stroke in diabetics and control of these potentially modifiable risk factors becomes essential.

PATHOGENESIS OF STROKE AND CEREBROVASCULAR DISEASE IN DIABETES[1,18]

Lists of the factors contributing to the pathogenesis of stroke are presented in **Table 62.2**.

Stroke in a diabetic patient may be related to the vasculopathy with its many underlying pathophysiological mechanisms or indirectly due to complications of diabetes and involvement of other organ systems. Both macrovascular and microvascular diseases have been thought to be having their own determinants and pathogenetic mechanisms, leading to enhanced atherogenesis or thrombosis. Since, no single factor can be alone responsible for such a chronic process to occur, it is likely that many recognized and not so recognized factors may work in unison. Complications of atherosclerosis are responsible for 50% of deaths in patients with type 2 diabetes, 27% of deaths in patients with type 1 diabetes of duration 35 years or less, and 67% of deaths in patients with type 1 diabetes of duration 40 years or more. CVD is a cause of death in about 10% of these patients. Since, multitude of pathogenic mechanisms may result in a final pathway of athero-

TABLE 62.2	Pathogenesis of stroke

VASCULOPATHY
- **Macrovascular disease (Enhanced atherosclerosis and others)**
  - *Hyperglycemia*
    - i. Increase in nonenzymatic glycation of proteins
    - ii. Activation of polyol pathway
    - iii. Activation of diacylglycerol (DAG) protein kinase C (PKC) cascades
    - iv. Increase of flux via the hexosamine metabolism
    - v. Enhanced flux of glucose
  - *Hyperinsulinemia—Insulin resistance*
  - *Dyslipidemia*
  - *Rheulogy*
    - i. *Procoagulant state*
      1. Decrease in PAI-1
      2. Increase in vWF
      3. Increase in fibrinogen
      4. Increase in factor VII
      5. Decrease in antithrombin III, protein C and S
    - ii. *Platelet abnormalities*
  - Homocysteine dysfunction
  - Endothelial dysfunction
    - i. Structural and functional changes
    - ii. Enhanced atherogenesis
    - iii. Impaired NO production
  - Microalbuminuria
  - Obesity and hypertension
- **Microvascular disease (Genetic theory, biochemical theory and hemodynamic theory)**
  - Basement membrane morphology and dysfunction
  - Endothelial cell dysfunction
  - Coagulation factors changes
  - Vascular permeability and blood flow

CARDIAC DYSFUNCTION AND EMBOLISM
- Myocardial infarction
- Cardiomyopathy

thrombosis, discussion of each factor would be beyond the scope of this chapter.

- *Hyperglycemia* may affect many cellular pathways both intracellularly and extracellularly and thereby lead to abnormality of vessel cell walls. Glucose forms glycated compounds or oxidants, which can act on inflammatory cells to release cytokines or directly act on vascular cells to cause vascular dysfunction. Further modifications leads to formation of advanced glycation end products (AGEs). Since collagen is highly susceptible to this changes, its presence in vessel wall leads to excess low density lipoprotein (LDL) trapping and oxidation. Activation of diacylglycerol (DAG), protein kinase C (PKC) cascade, leads to poor

clearance of very low density lipoprotein (VLDL) due to defects in lipoproteins lipase binding in capillary endothelial surface.

- *A procoagulant* state often exists in patients with diabetes as discussed here under. Insulin resistance and hyperinsulinemia, modulate effects on PA-I, von Willebrand factor (vWF) and fibrinogen. Platelet abnormalities are also observed in diabetics. These are:
  - Increased intercellular Ca^{++} mobilization
  - Reduced fluidity of cell membrane
  - Glycation related change in membrane adhesion and aggregation
  - Dyslipidemia-enhanced platelet aggregation.

Factors potentiating thrombosis: Patients with diabetes have increased concentrations of prothrombotic factors, fibrinogen and vWF. Elevated circulating levels of fibrinopeptide A in patients with diabetes mellitus reflect increased thrombin activity and hence increased fibrin generation in such patients. Platelets from patients with diabetes mellitus are prothrombotic, and exhibit increased adhesiveness, a decreased threshold for aggregation in response to agonists and an increased incidence of spontaneous aggregation *in vitro.* In addition, platelets from subjects with diabetes show an impaired ability to mediate vasodilatation. This impaired vasodilatation is secondary to the release of a short-acting platelet-derived substance that interferes with the ADP-induced dilatory response seen in normal vessels with intact endothelium.

Insulin modulates the reactivity of platelets. The exposure of platelets to insulin decreases aggregation of platelets by increasing synthesis of nitric oxide, which in turn increases the intraplatelet concentrations of the nucleotides cyclic GMP and cyclic AMP. Accordingly, insulin deficiency seen in type 1 diabetes and in the later stages of type 2 diabetes may contribute to increased platelet reactivity by decreasing the tonic inhibition of platelet reactivity induced by insulin.

Mechanisms of impaired fibrinolysis: Decreased fibrinolytic capacity is observed consistently in the blood from patients with diabetes, particularly those with type 2 diabetes. The decreased fibrinolytic capacity is secondary to increased concentrations of plasminogen activator inhibitor type 1 (PAI-1) without change in the concentration of tissue-type plasminogen activator. The mechanism responsible for the overexpression of PAI-1 as seen in subjects with diabetes and in other insulin-resistant states is likely to be multifactorial. The combination of hyperglycemia-insulinemia, hypertriglyceridemia and hyperglycemia increases the concentration of PAI-1 in human subjects. The hormonal (hyperinsulinemia) and metabolic (particularly hypertriglyceridemia) abnormalities of diabetes mellitus are critical determinants of the concentration of PAI-1 in blood. Increased production of PAI-1 from liver, adipose tissue and blood vessels, in subjects with diabetes mellitus (particularly obese subjects with type 2 diabetes) is well recognized. Therapies aimed at reduction of insulin resistance lead to reduction in hyperinsulinemia as well as PAI-1. Improved fibrinolytic capacity afforded by therapy that decreases hyperinsulinemia may retard progression of atherosclerosis.

- *Endothelial dysfunction* is common in diabetes and is generally caused by hyperglycemia and dyslipidemia. Impairment of NO leads to poor vasodilatation, and other factors which cause increased vasomotor tone, vascular permeability and vascular remodeling. There is enhanced disappearance of endothelium, weakening of tight junctions and changes in expressions of adhesion molecules. This is associated with basement membrane thickening and increase in enzymes mediating type 5 collagen synthesis and fibrinonectin predisposing to enhanced atherogenesis and obliteration of vessel caliber. Endothelial replication may be defective and apoptotic cell deaths may increase. Increased vascular permeability is most commonly seen in retina and glomerulus, and is not a major phenomena in cerebral blood vessels. However, raised vascular tone is related to vascular permeability increase and loss of antithrombotic activity of endothelium leads to thrombosis and occlusion of blood vessels.
- *Pathogenic role of hyperlipidemia*: Coronary artery disease (CAD) is a common cause of death in diabetes mellitus. The incidence of peripheral vascular disease and cerebrovascular disease is also considerably increased in these patients. The increased risk of vascular disease in diabetes cannot be completely explained by the presence of conventional risk factors. The increased risk, however, is due in part to lipid abnormalities.

Lipid abnormalities are twice as common in patients with type 2 diabetes as in the nondiabetic population and are more complex than in patients with type I (IDDM) owing to the interaction between obesity, insulin resistance and hyperinsulinemia commonly observed with this condition. In type 2 diabetes, the most common lipid abnormality seen is hypertriglyceridemia and reduced HDL-cholesterol levels. An

TABLE 62.3	Lipid abnormalities in diabetes mellitus

- Hypertriglyceridemia
- Low HDL-cholesterol
- Triglyceride-enriched HDL
- Dense LDL
- Abnormal LDL kinetics
- Elevated IDL
- Glycosylation of lipoproteins
- Oxidation of lipoproteins
- Increased Lp(a)

atherogenic constellation of lipid abnormalities including small dense LDL, hypertriglyceridemia, elevated IDL and apo-B levels, and reduced HDL and apo-A I levels occur more commonly in type II diabetes mellitus. The lipid abnormalities found in diabetes mellitus are listed in **Table 62.3**.

Triglycerides may be a risk factor for coronary artery disease because they are carried on atherogenic triglyceride-rich lipoprotein particles (direct role) or because they may be a marker for the presence of other atherogenic lipoprotein particles (indirect role) **(Table 62.4)**.

Although no direct studies have been done to correlate cerebrovascular atherogenesis with metabolic alterations in diabetes, mechanisms similar to those underlying CAD may be active or contributory. Few autopsy studies have reported on diabetes and degree of cerebral atherosclerosis. An increased frequency and severity of atherosclerosis in the circle of Willis, as well as in the middle cerebral, basilar and carotid arteries was observed in the diabetic compared with the nondiabetic subjects. In a recent study, prevalence of diabetes was significantly higher among Japanese subjects with atherothrombotic occlusion of the internal carotid and basilar arteries than in control subjects. Serum glucose was also weakly associated with large-

TABLE 62.4	Methods by which triglycerides may be atherogenic in diabetes

Direct
- Foam cell induction by remnant particles

Indirect
- Association with other atherogenic risk factors
- Decreased HDL-cholesterol
- Dense LDL phenotype
- Postprandial hypertriglyceridemia
- Insulin resistance
- Clotting abnormalities

vessel (circle of Willis) but not intracerebral small-vessel atherosclerosis after adjusting for other risk factors.

Other Possible Mechanisms to Explain Hyperglycemia-induced Worsening of Cerebral Ischemia

Plasma Glucose and Spreading Depression[19]

Spreading depression (SD) is a wave of ionic transients involving release of K^+ and uptake of Ca^{2+}, Na^+ and Cl^- through respective membrane channels and is most likely initiated and propagated by massive presynaptic release of large amounts of glutamate and resultant activation of N-methyl-D-aspartate (NMDA) receptors following local brain injury, including focal brain ischemia. In normal brain tissue, SDs repeatedly elicited over a 5-hour period do not lead to neuronal death. However, when such SDs repeatedly collapse ionic gradients, activation of NMDA receptors and gap junctions propagates SDs and possibly triggers a massive Ca^{2+} influx, which in energy-compromised neurons is adequate to trigger a cell death cascade. This hypothesis finds support in the finding that in focal brain ischemia SD increases the ischemic volume, probably by 23% per SD wave. Another determinant of brain injury in cerebral ischemia is plasma glucose. Cerebral ischemia triggers a massive genomic response that leads to induction of nearly 100 genes normally not transcribed, as well as modulation of the expression of constitutive genes. The role that these genes and their products play in the mechanisms of ischemic brain injury remains one of the challenges facing investigators in the field. Koistinaho and colleagues in a very recent elegant study, examined whether variations in plasma glucose modulate the pattern of gene expression following cortical SD. These investigators observed that changes in plasma glucose produce profound effects on the mRNA expression of the early gene c-fos, of the inflammatory early gene cyclooxygenase 2 (COX-2) involved in the inflammatory response, the heme oxygenase I (HO-I) also known as the heat-shock protein (HSP) and of protein kinase C (PKC)—an injury-inducible kinase. The findings of the study referred to raise the possibility that plasma glucose may have a profound effect on the molecular events triggered cortical SD, and possibly on postischemic gene expression. Thus, the deleterious effect of hyperglycemia may be mediated through alterations in gene expression. Future studies would indicate whether such deleterious effects ascribed to hypoglycemia with

respect of injury-induced early gene (s) expression are transcriptional, translational or post-translational.

Plasma Glucose and Regulation of Na⁺/Myo-inositol Cotransporter Gene Expression in Hippocampus[20]

Myo-inositol is accumulated into cells by means of the Na⁺/myo-inositol cotransporter (SMIT). In a recent study, the effects of hyperglycemia on the expression of SMIT-mRNA were examined in rat hippocampus. In normal control rats, SMIT-mRNA signals were predominantly located in the hippocampus, cerebellum and choroid plexus. A massive induction in the hippocampus was observed in the acute stage of induced hyperglycemia in the CA3/CA4, the molecular layer of the dentate gyrus and the hippocampal fissure. These changes returned to normal after normalization of glucose levels. These results suggest regional specificity of permeability of the blood-brain barrier and/or cellular differences in sensitivity to hyperglycemic stress would exist in the brain.

Plasma Glucose and Na-K ATPase in the Brain[21]

In a recent experimental study, Na-K ATPase activity in the brain decreased significantly after diabetes was induced with streptozotocin in rats. Largest decreases were observed in the hippocampus (−30%) and the cerebral cortex (−26%).

Insulin's Vascular Action[22]

In addition to its metabolic properties, insulin appears to exert physiologically significant effects on blood vessels via a number of mechanisms; insulin-mediated vasodilatation has both endothelium-dependent and independent components and may be coupled with intercellular glucose metabolism, thus providing a mechanism for targeting substrate delivery to tissues with specific metabolic requirements. The pathophysiologic significance of defects insulin's vascular action remains uncertain, but further elucidation of the underlying mechanisms may help to explain the observed epidemiologic associations between metabolic cardiovascular and perhaps cerebrovascular disorders. From a public health perspective, identification of individuals with elevated glucose levels provides an opportunity for intervention. Lifestyle changes including increased physical activity, reduction of body weight in the obese, and stress reduction may prove to be effective measures. The evidence appears strong in the case of those with known diabetes, in whom efforts to improve the modifiable risk factors for thrombo-embolic strokes may provide considerable benefit. In a recent review of Stroke Clinic Data by Joseph and colleagues,[23] the risk factor profile showed little improvement despite stroke clinic attendance over a second year follow-up. The finding that more than two-thirds of the diabetics had a serum glucose >137 mg/dl was indicative of an unsatisfactory control of blood sugar. Despite distinctly identified vascular risk factors, and possible attempts to achieve their control, these factors are often not adequately modified. A more aggressive dual focus on not only identification but also control of these factors, the introduction of strong incentives to improve both patient and physician behavior, and a team approach, perhaps widening the patient-doctor circle to include all members of the health care team including nurses, physicians assistants, and other ancillary staff, through multiprofessional education, may result in better compliance, and frequent follow-up, and enhanced metabolic control of diabetic state. A successful model such as multiprofessional education for diabetes integrated care (MEDIC) can be adopted for this purpose.[24]

STROKE SUBTYPES AND PATTERN OF VASCULAR DISEASE IN DIABETES

Ischemic stroke is by far common in diabetics than hemorrhagic stroke. Although diabetes with patho-physiologic mechanisms described are above respon-sible for the local thrombosis and atherosclerosis, worsening infection and inflammatory of the vessel will be responsible for the attendant stroke. Cerebral small vessel disease is far more common than large artery disease in diabetic population. In a Japanese population, lacunar infarction is the most common subtype of cerebral infarction compared to atherothrombotic or cardioembolic infarction. Carotid artery disease with significant stenosis does not seem to be the major cause of cerebral ischemia in diabetes. The frequency of transient ischemic attacks (TIAs) is increased by nearly 3-fold but diabetics may present with full-blown stroke without warning compared to the nondiabetic population. Stroke-like syndromes caused by hypogly-cemia and metabolic hypomotor coma or precoma are rare but well documented and may be confused with TIAs, or stroke. Seizures may also be triggered by metabolic derangements in susceptible patients.

Diabetes Mellitus and Acute Ischemic Stroke

Magnetic resonance spectroscopy (MRS) has contri-buted significant information on ischemic brain metabolism in the clinical patient.[3] In general, the clinical data substantiate the observations made when anoxia and ischemia are induced *in vitro* and in experimental stroke models. The potential of spectroscopy now extends to the diagnostic monitoring of metabolic change, in identifying markers of therapeutic window, in establishing prognosis and in determining stroke outcome. Further, important questions concerning ischemic cellular mechanisms may be pursued using MRS. Welch et al studied MRS in 66 patients with acute ischemic stroke in which acute clinical deficits signaled the first episodes of cerebral ischemia.[25] The findings confirm that high-energy phosphates deterioration and severe acidosis can be detected in an ischemic brain. The large variability in measures reflects the extreme heterogeneity of the metabolic response to ischemia. This is almost certainly due to the diversity of the time course, degree and extent of ischemia and the clinical status of the patient. Also, although metabolic deficits persist for days in some patients, in others energy recovery is apparent much earlier. Furthermore, recovery of energy metabolism takes place without commensurate clinical recovery. This is consistent with the concept that although high-energy phosphate metabolism is initially responsible for the neurologic dysfunction, other factors probably play a more important role in the persistence of the dysfunction and eventually in the causation of infarction. Disturbances of brain acid-base status are important in the mecha-nisms of ischemic neuronal damage. pH has a role in controlling local cerebral blood flow (CBF) and tissue oxygen delivery.[26] There is a pH dependence of membrane transfer mechanisms,[27,28] intracellular hydrogen ion concentration controls, and cytoplasmic enzyme activity (particularly the constellation of enzymes involved in glycolysis). Electron-chain transport in mitochondria culminating in ATP synthesis is pH linked, as is the chelation of ATP by Mg^{2+} for phosphoryl transfer reactions. The critical acid-base event in ischemic brain is a resultant of progressive deterioration of energy status and the ensuing stimulation of anaerobic glycolysis aimed at preserving ATP synthesis at the cost of lactic acid accumulation and CO-entrapment; these sequential changes, with a relatively minor contribution from ATP hydrolysis, seem primarily responsible for tissue acidosis.[28]

Glycemia and Acid-Base Status

Proposedly, the severity of acidosis is dependent on blood glucose concentration and brain glucose and glycogen stores, which in-turn, based on experimental evidence, may determine neurologic outcome.[29,30] When glucose delivery to the brain is continued as a result of incomplete ischemia or during reperfusion, there is apparent further stimulation of glycolytic activity, which further adds to the pool of metabolic acids at a time when the cell is already stressed to compensate for decreased pH. Pretreatment of animals with glucose prior to complete ischemia dramatically impairs the restitution of cerebral blood flow (CBF) and energy metabolism during the postischemic period; this is attributed in part to tissue lactic acidosis.[31] On the other hand, fasting and hypoglycemia markedly attenuate ischemic brain acidosis, reduce infarction size, and decrease ischemic neurologic deficit.[29,32] Neurologic outcome is worsened by high systemic blood glucose levels at the time of hospital admission for stroke.[33-35] Positron emission tomography (PET) studies have provided metabolic data to support the adverse influence of glucose.

Hyperglycemia and Acute Stroke

In a prospective study by Pulsinelli,[36] neurologic outcome in diabetic patients with stroke was significantly worse than in the nondiabetic with a significantly higher stroke-related mortality in the former. The neurologic outcome also was worse with high blood glucose levels; only 43% of patients with blood glucose levels above 120 mg/dl (6.6 mmol/L) returned to work, whereas 76% of those with lower levels of blood glucose regained employment. These findings are consistent with those of Asplund et al who also found that the presence of diabetes mellitus adversely affected the short- and long-term neurologic outcome in patients with ischemic and hemorrhagic strokes.[37] There exists a large data-set of experimental evidence affirming that transient ischemia is associated with a higher risk of permanent infarction in hyperglycemic animals. It is clearly documented that hyperglycemia adversely affects the recovery after global ischemia. Myers et al observed that the preischemic nutritional state of monkeys significantly affected the recovery following ischemia or hypoxia.[38] Siemkowicz and Hansen showed that after 10 minutes of complete brain ischemia in rats, all hyperglycemic animals died within 12 hours, while normoglycemic rats survived with either complete recovery or with minor

persistence of neurological deficits.[39] Further, the metabolic and neurophysiological recovery are depressed in hyperglycemic rats after global ischemia.[40] On histopathological examination, marked clumping of nuclear chromatin and cell sap was clearly observed after 30 minutes of incomplete ischemia in hyperglycemia animals; in contrast, the changes were either minimal or strikingly discrete in normoglycemic animals.[41] Myers et al[42] observed that hyperglycemia enlarges infarct size in cerebrovascular occlusion in cats. Hyperglycemic cats developed infarcts that were three times larger than those in the normoglycemic cats. Additionally, 25% of cats with hyperglycemia for one hour prior to, and six hours after. Middle cerebral artery (MCA) occlusion died of massive hemispheric edema and brainstem compression, an outcome strikingly absent in normoglycemic animals. Adequate reperfusion is of critical importance for recovery following global ischemia. It is postulated that transient ischemic attacks in patients with raised blood glucose might result in complete infarction due to impaired reperfusion of the ischemic area.[43]

Coexistence of several known systemic complications of diabetes could have contributed to the poorer neurologic outcome, following ischemic stroke. The presence of proliferative angiopathy of small cerebral blood vessels,[44,45] with or without severe cerebral arteriosclerosis in diabetic patients,[46] represents changes that potentially could interfere with the establishment of collateral blood flow to the ischemic zone, thereby enlarging the size of cerebral infarct. Other factors that might exacerbate ongoing cerebral ischemia in a patient with diabetes include, an impaired autoregulation of cerebral blood flow,[47] an increase in whole blood or plasma viscosity,[48] a reduced deformability of erythrocytes[28] and an increased adhesion of erythrocytes-to-endothelial cells.[49] The impaired synthesis of prostacyclin, a potent vasodilator and antiplatelet aggregating substance, in patients with diabetes, may also augment cerebral infarction.[50]

In view of the profound adverse effect of hyperglycemia on brain ischemia in otherwise normal animals, it logically follows that hyperglycemia *per se* may also affect adversely the outcome of an ischemic patient who is otherwise euglycemic. Animal models have demonstrated an important association between hyperglycemia and ischemic injury. Both increased[51,52] and reduced injury[53,54] patterns have been demonstrated with hyperglycemia in permanent focal ischemia models. Initially hyperglycemia may be neuroprotective[55] by reducing ischemic depolarizations through delayed breakdown of transmembrane ion gradients with extended anaerobic glycolysis.[56,57] With persistent ischemia, however, hyperglycemia produces a profound cellular acidosis due to the excessive substrate for the predominant anaerobic glycolysis occurring in hypoxemic/ischemic tissue.[58] Once a critical threshold of acidosis is reached, hyperglycemia becomes detrimental.[59] Proposed mechanisms for the deleterious effects of hyperglycemia and the resultant cellular acidosis include enzymatic dysfunction, enhanced free radical production[60] (lipid peroxidation) through increased iron-catalyzed hydroxyl radical production, depressed mitochondrial function by inhibited ADP-stimulated respiratory activity,[61] induction of endo-nucleases that may lead to programmed cell death[62] (apoptosis), increased intracellular Ca^{2+} accumulation,[63] and cellular edema.[64] The above mechanisms may also cause a worse outcome in hyperglycemic primary intracerebral hemorrhage (the excess lactate production occurring in the area of ischemia around the site of the hemorrhage). Melamed[34] reported a higher short-term mortality from ischemic cerebral infarction in patients who were hyperglycemic regardless of whether they were diabetic or nondiabetic. Although Melamed interpreted the findings as showing that increased hyperglycemia developed in patients with more extensive brain damage through a stress response, the findings could have been as easily interpreted the other way round. Feibel et al examined the stress response in stroke and demonstrated a greater mortality in patients who excreted more than 200 µg/day of urinary norepinephrine in the acute phase of the illness. Such observations are compatible with the inference that hyperglycemia augments cerebral infarction. Indeed, they imply a possible cyclic process in which stroke-induced stress causes hyperglycemia, which in-turn further extends the cerebral infarct thereby inducing further stress. Weir et al[65] studied whether hyper-glycemia can be an independent predictor of poor outcome after acute stroke. Plasma glucose concentration above 8 mmol/L after acute stroke predicted a poor prognosis after correcting for age, stroke severity, and stroke subtype. The effect of hyperglycemia on mortality was large. The estimated relative hazard of 1.87 was greater than that for hemorrhagic versus ischemic stroke and equivalent to adding more than 20 years to a patient's age. They concluded that raised glucose concentration is therefore unlikely to be solely a stress response and should arguably be treated actively. Hyperglycemia is also associated with an increase in cerebral edema following acute ischemia.

Berger et al[66] reported a larger cerebral edema either on autopsy or as evidenced by shift of the midline or ventricular compression on CT scan in hyperglycemic patients. It is suggested that increased cerebral edema is related to an initial phase of vasodilatation followed by worsened microvascular perfusion. It is possible that the small vessel disease known to occur in the brains of diabetic patients may be more "permissive" of fluid transduction across the blood-brain barrier leading to cerebral edema.

Retrospective analysis of 100 patients with acute hemorrhagic stroke admitted in the Neurosciences Center, All India Institute of Medical Sciences (AIIMS), New Delhi, India between January 1998 to January 1999, showed 12% to be known diabetics. The average blood glucose at admission was 191 mg% (110–460 mg%), of which 6 patients (50%) had a blood glucose of >140 mg%. Eight out of these 12 patients did not survive the stroke in the first 14 days (mortality—66.7%). Three patients who survived had average blood glucose of 120 mg%. Four patients who were not known diabetic were found to have an admitting blood glucose of >140 mg%. The average blood glucose in them was 276 mg%. All the 4 patients died during admission. The univariate correlation between baseline varieties and mortality of 14 days after major acute hemorrhagic stroke in these 100 patients is given in **Table 62.5**.

Although the above study had a limited number of patients, certain trends can be seen emerging. As against an overall mortality of 45%, the mortality in the group with diabetes 66.6%, suggesting a higher mortality in diabetics as against nondiabetics with stroke. The group of diabetics with an admitting blood glucose level of <120 mg% had survived stroke. This suggests that a better metabolic control in diabetes probably improves the prognosis in acute stroke. The group of four patients who were not known diabetic, but showed hyper-glycemia at the onset of stroke probably represents those who were undetected patients of type 2 diabetes, presenting with a catastrophic cerebrovascular event.

Retrospective analysis of 50 consecutive patients with acute ischemic stroke admitted to the Neurosciences Center, All India Institute of Medical Sciences, New Delhi, India between the months of June 1998 to January 1999 showed five patients to be known diabetics (10%). The average admitting blood glucose was 118 mg% (56–303 mg%). Twelve (24%) of the subjects in this group had an admitting blood glucose of >140 mg%. Nine patients who were not previously known to be diabetic, had blood glucose of >140 mg% (18%). Of these, only three (33.3%) had persistently high blood

| TABLE 62.5 | Univariate correlation between baseline varieties and mortality of 14 days after intracerebral hemorrhage in 100 patients |

Variable	Dead (n = 45) No. %	Alive (n = 55) No. %	X^2	P-value
Gender				
Male	27 (60)	35 (63.6)	0.161	0.6886
Female	15 (33.3)	23 (41.8)		
First BP systolic				
<139	7 (15.5)	6 (10.9)	1.25	0.53
139-200	20 (44)	32 (58)		
>200	15 (33)	17 (31)		
Diastolic				
<85	6 (13)	6 (11)	1.38	0.5
85-95	12 (26.7)	10 (18)		
>95	27 (60)	39 (70.9)		
Hemorrhagic volume				
<40 cm^3	8 (17.7)	34 (62)	30.6	0.0000
40-60 cm^3	8 (17.7)	2 (3.6)		
>60 cm^3	11 (24.4)	0		
Intraventricular hemorrhage				
Present	30 (66.6)	19 (34.5)	14.57	0.0001
Absent	12 (26.6)	39 (70.9)		
Level of consciousness				
0-Normal	0	8 (14.5)		
1-Drowsy	9 (20)	26 (47)	20.5	0.0001
2-Responding to pain	15 (33)	18 (32.7)		
3-Comatose	18 (40)	6 (10.9)		
Blood glucose				
>140 mg	12 (26.6)	4 (7.3)	5.42	0.199
<140 mg	31 (68.8)	53 (96.4)		

glucose levels requiring insulin or oral hypoglycemic agents at the time of discharge. There was no mortality in the first 14 days.

Serum Glucose and Cerebral Ischemia— Reperfusion Injury

Recent advances in the development of thrombolytic therapy in ischemic stroke and the PET demonstration of spontaneous reperfusion in early cerebral infarction have enhanced the significance of reperfusion-induced brain injury. Reperfusion following ischemia may exacerbate tissue injury by producing free radicals. Iron-catalyzed free radical formation is enhanced by lactic acidosis, which is aggravated by hyperglycemia, is also implicated in the pathogenesis of ischemic brain injury. As a mechanism for the adverse effect of hyperglycemia, most attention has focused on the neuronal effects of increased tissue lactate production and lowered tissue pH. An alternate or supplementary hypothesis to a direct neuronal effect is that hyperglycemia could enhance ischemic injury via an effect on the vasculature. In reversible focal ischemia, hyperglycemia consistently aggravates ischemic damage. Restoration of blood flow after 8 hours of occlusion is associated with a higher mortality than permanent occlusion.[52] Hyperglycemia increases damage to the blood-brain interface,[67] resulting in increased edema, and hemorrhagic transformation. Following MCA occlusion in cats, deCourten-Myers et al[68] found that the incidence and extent of hemorrhagic infarction on reperfusion were much greater in hyperglycemic compared with normo-glycemic animals. In another study, a glucose infusion resulted in a 75% hemorrhagic transformation rate compared with 9% in the noninfused group,

Hyperglycemia may increase hemorrhagic transformation by accelerating microvascular injury. Neuropathological studies have demonstrated reduced flow in the microcirculation,[61] which may be due to increased capillary endothelial cell swelling that reduces luminal diameter. A severe perfusion deficit has been demonstrated with hyperglycemia, which may further aggravate injury. Paljarvi et al[69] found that reperfusion after global ischemia caused excessive endothelial cell swelling and decreased luminal diameter in hyperglycemic rats while having little effect in normoglycemic rats. The occurrence of hemorrhage on reperfusion is of particular importance because it is the major complication in the use of thrombolytic drugs to restore CBF after an ischemic event. The most critical complication of intravenous recombinant tissue plasminogen activator (RTPA) therapy for acute ischemic stroke is intracerebral hemorrhage (ICH). In the National Institute of Neurological Disorders and Stroke (NINDS) RTPA trial,[70] 6.4% of rtPA-treated patients developed neurological deterioration due to ICH compared with only 0.6% in the placebo-treated group. In the European Cooperative Acute Stroke Study (ECASS-I) trial,[71] 20% of rtPA-treated patients developed parenchymal hematomas compared with 7% in the placebo arm.[72] Identifying patients who are at a high-risk of hemorrhagic complications may lead to improved patient selection and enhanced safety of this treatment. Nevertheless, few factors have been identified as predictors of symptomatic hemorrhage. In the NINDS rtPA trial, only stroke severity as defined by the National Institute of Health Stroke Scale (NIHSS)[73] and CT changes of mass effect, edema or hypodensity, were independent predictors of symptomatic hemorrhage. A statistical trend ($P >0.05$) was seen for age and the dichotomous variable blood glucose >300 mg/dl as baseline predictors of symptomatic hemorrhage. Recent human clinical study by Demechuk et al[74] closely examined the role of hyperglycemia in the setting of thrombolysis. Baseline serum glucose was the only independent predictor of hemorrhage. Serum glucose >1.1 mmol/L was associated with a 25% symptomatic hemorrhage rate. This study demonstrated a definite relationship between baseline serum glucose/diabetes history and intracerebral hemorrhage after rtPA treatment.

Further clinical studies, although academically desirable, are unlikely to be more informative than the present literature, given the uncontrollable nature of pre-existing microvascular disease in diabetes and stress-induced hyperglycemia in nondiabetic patients.

Accordingly, it seems wise to maintain blood glucose levels in the near-normal range in diabetic patients with a high-risk of stroke or with any symptoms suggesting impending or evolving cerebral ischemia. Similarly, glucose-containing infusions should be avoided in the immediate treatment of patients with acute or progressive stroke, in patients undergoing surgery that could affect cerebral blood flow (carotid endarterectomy) or in those who have had cardiac arrest. In stroke-prone patients scheduled for surgery of any kind, anesthetic agents without a tendency to raise the blood-brain glucose concentration should be used. Therapeutic interventions aimed at lowering glucose levels or neutralizing the effects of the acidosis have recently been studied. Insulin therapy,[75] tirilazad[76,77] (a free radical scavenger), deferoxamine,[59] and hypothermia[67] have all shown promising neuroprotection in hyperglycemic animal models.[78]

SUMMARY

Diabetes has long been a major health problem and is recognized as a leading cause of adult blindness, kidney failure and nontraumatic limb amputation, besides being a recognized risk factor of considerable importance for coronary and cerebrovascular diseases. Sufficient data exist to implicate diabetes as an independent risk factor for stroke.[79] Admission glucose was a determinant of 30-day stroke recurrence in the NINDS Stroke Data Bank, while diabetes was a significant predictor of 2-year recurrence.

Data from India are inconsistent and generally derived from hospital admissions and many of the stroke patients are likely to be treated domestically in villages or would be admitted or seen by local medical practitioners or RMPs. The relationship between diabetes and hypertension seems much more complex. Since hypertension is a common, important and modifiable risk factor for both micro- and macrovascular complications of diabetes—a synergistic effect probably exists between the two leadings to a final common pathway for vasculopathy causing stroke. Stroke in a diabetic patient may be related to the vasculopathy with its many underlying pathophysiological mechanisms or indirectly due to complications of diabetes and involvement of other organ systems. Both macro- and microvascular diseases have been thought to be having their own determinants and pathogenetic mechanisms, leading to enhanced atherogenesis or thrombosis. Complications of atherosclerosis are responsible for 50% of deaths in patients with type II diabetes, 27% of deaths in patients with type 1 diabetes of duration 35 years or less, and 67% of deaths in patients with type 1 diabetes of duration 40 years or more. Although no direct studies have been done to correlate cerebrovascular atherogenesis with metabolic alterations in diabetes, mechanisms similar to those underlying CAD may be active or contributory.

Ischemic stroke is by far common in diabetics than hemorrhagic stroke; as has been observed in previous studies. Although vascular diabetes with pathophysiologic mechanisms for local thrombolysis and atherosclerosis are the ones responsible, worsening infection and inflammation of the vessel will be responsible for the attendant stroke. Cerebral small vessel disease is by far more common than large artery disease in diabetic population. The severity of acidosis is dependent on blood glucose concentration and brain glucose and glycogen stores, which in turn, based on experimental evidence, may determine neurologic outcome. High systemic blood glucose levels worsen neurologic outcome at the time of hospital admission for stroke. Positron emission tomography (PET) studies have provided metabolic data to support the adverse influence of glucose.

Coexistence of several known systemic complications of diabetes could contribute to poorer neurologic outcome following ischemic stroke. The presence of proliferative angiopathy of small cerebral blood vessels, with or without severe cerebral arteriosclerosis in diabetic patients, represent changes that potentially could interfere with the establishment of collateral blood flow to the perischemic zone, thereby enlarging the size of cerebral infarct. Other factors that might exacerbate ongoing cerebral ischemia in a patient with diabetes include, an impaired autoregulation of cerebral blood flow, an increase in whole blood or plasma viscosity, a reduced deformability of erythrocytes and an increased adhesion of erythrocytes-to-endothelial cells. The impaired synthesis of prostacyclin, a potent vasodilator and antiplatelet aggregating substance, in patients with diabetes, may also augment cerebral infarction.[80]

At the present stage of our knowledge, it seems wise to maintain blood glucose levels in the near-normal range in diabetic patients with a high-risk of stroke or with any symptoms suggesting impending or evolving cerebral ischemia.

REFERENCES

1. Bansal BC, Yadav P, Tripathi BK, Agarwal AK. Diabetes and cerebrovascular disease. In Ahuja MMS, Tripathy BB, Moses Sam GP, Chandalia HB, Das AK, Rao PV, Madhu SV (Eds): RSSDI textbook of diabetes mellitus. Hyderabad: RSSDI; 2002. pp. 549-58.
2. Tuomilento J, Rastenyte D, Jousilahti D, et al. Diabetes mellitus as a risk factor for death from stroke. Prospective study of the middle aged Finnish population. Stroke. 1996;27:210-5.
3. Kuusisto J, Mykkanen L, Pyorala, et al. NIDDM and its metabolic control are important prediction of stroke in elderly subjects. Stroke. 1994;25:1157-64.
4. Lindegard B, Hillborn M. Associations between brain infarction, diabetes and alcoholism: observations from the Gothenberg population cohort study. Acta Neurol Scand. 1987;75:125-200.
5. Kannel WB, McGee DL. Diabetes and cardiovascular risk factor: the Famingham study. Circulation. 1979;59(1):8-13.
6. Dalal PM. Cerebrovascular disease (CVD) in type 2 diabetes mellitus. In Dash RJ (Ed): New Visas in Type 2 diabetes Vol 1. 229-45.
7. Davis TM, Millns H, Stratton IM, et al. Risk factors for stroke in type 2 diabetes mellitus. United Kingdom Prospective Diabetes Study (UKPDS 29). Arch Int Med. 1999;159:1097-103.
8. Gray CS, Scott JF, French JM, et al. Prevalence and prediction of unrecognized diabetes mellitus and impaired glucose tolerance following acute stoke. Aging. 2004;33:71-7.
9. Barata DM, Kim N, Concato J, et al. Hyperglycemia in patients with acute ischemic stroke: whether do we screen for unrecognized diabetes. QJM. 2003;491-7.
10. Wannamethee SG, Perry IJ, Shaper AG. Nonfasting serum glucose and insulin concentrations and the risk of stroke. Stroke. 1999;30:1780-6.
11. Davis ND, Hachinski V. Epidemiology of cerebrovascular disease. In Anderson D (Ed): Neuroepidemiology. A tribute to Bruce Schoenberg. Boca Raton: CRC Press; 1991. pp. 27-53.
12. Sacco RL, Wolf PA, Kennel WB, et al. Survival and recurrence: the Framingham Study. Stroke. 1982;13:290-5.
13. Radder GK. The use of NMR spectroscopy for the understanding of disease. Science. 1986;233:640-5.
14. Welch KMA, Levine SR, Martin G, et al. Magnetic resonance spectroscopy in cerebral ischemia. Neurologic Clinics. 1992;10(1):1-29.
15. Kuschinsky W, Whal M. Local chemical and neurogenic regulation of cerebral vascular resistance. Physiol Rev. 1978;58:656.
16. Meghberbi SE, Milan C, Minier D, Couvreur G, et al. Association between diabetes and stroke subtype on survival and functional outcome 3 months after stroke. Data from the European BIOMED stroke project. Stroke. 2003; 34:688-94.
17. Lund Anderson H. Transport of glucose from blood to brain. Physiol Rev. 1979;59:305.
18. Siesjo BK. Acidosis and brain damage: possible molecular mechanisms. J Cereb Blood Row Metab. 1985;5:S225-6.
19. Myers RE, Yamaguchi M. Tissue lactate accumulation as a cause of cerebral edema. In Neuroscience Abstracts, Vol 2. Bethesda, MD, Society for Neuroscience 1976;1042.
20. Welch KMA, Barkley GL. Biochemistry and pharmacology of cerebral ischemia. In Bamett JM, Mohr JP, Stein BM et al (Eds). Stroke: pathophysiology, diagnosis and management. New York: Churchill Livingstone. 1986;1:75-99.
21. Welsh FA, Ginsberg MD, Rieder W, et al. Deleterious effect of glucose pretreatment on recovery from diffuse cerebral ischemia in the cat. Stroke. 1980;11:355.

22. Chopp M, Welch KMA, Tidwell C, et al. Global cerebral ischemia and intracellular pH during hyperglycemia and hypoglycemia in the cat. Stroke. 1988;19:1383-7.

23. Melamed E. Reactive hyperglycemia in patients with acute stroke. J Neural Sci. 1976;29:269.

24. Pulsinelli WA, Sigsbee B, Rawlinson O, et al. Experimental hyperglycemia and diabetes mellitus worsen stroke outcome. Ann Neurol. 1980;8:91.

25. Pulsinelli WA, Levy DE, Sigsbee B, et al. Increased damage after ischemic stroke in patients with hyperglycemia with or without established diabetes mellitus. The Arner J Med. 1983;74:540.

26. Asplund K, Hagg E, Helmers C, et al. The natural history of stroke in diabetic patients. Acta Med Scand. 1980;207:417-24.

27. Myers RE, Yamaguchi S. Nervous system effects of cardiac arrest in monkeys. Arch Neurol. 1977;34:65-74.

28. Siemkowicz E, Hansen A. Clinical restitution following cerebral ischemia in hypo, normo and hyperglycemic rats. Acta Neural Scand. 1978;58:1-8.

29. Plum F. What causes infarction in ischemic brain? The Robert Wartenberg Lecture. Neurology. 1983;33:222-33.

30. Kalimo H, Rehnerona S, Soderfield B, Olsson Y, Siesjo BK. Brain lactic acidosis and ischemic cell damage histopathology. J Cereb Blood Flow Metab. 1981;1:313-27.

31. de Courten-Myers G, Myers RE, Schoolfield L. Hyperglycemia enlarges infarct size in cerebrovascular occlusion in cats. Stroke. 1988;19:623-30.

32. Nedergaard M, Diemer NH. Focal ischemia in the rat brain: with special reference to the influence of glucose concentration. Acta Neuropathol (Berl). 1987;73:131-7.

33. Ajex M, Baron EK, Goldenberg S, Blumenthal HT. An autopsy study of cerebrovascular accident in diabetes mellitus. Circulation. 1962;25:663-73.

34. Aronson SM. Intracranial vascular lesions in patients with diabetes mellitus. J Neuropathol Ex-Neurol. 1973;32:183-96.

35. Grunnet ML. Cerebrovascular disease: diabetes and cerebral atherosclerosis. Neurology. 1963;13:486-91.

36. Bentsen N, Larsen B, Larsen NA. Chronically impaired autoregulation of cerebral blood flow in long-term diabetics. Stroke. 1975;6:497-502.

37. Barnes AJ, Locke R, Scudder PR, et al. Is hyperviscosity a treatable component of diabetic microcirculatory disease? Lancet. 1977;11:789-91.

38. McMillan DE, Utterback NG, LaPuma J. Reduced erythrocyte deformability in diabetes. Diabetes. 1978;27:895-901.

39. Wautier JL, Paton C, Wautier MP, et al. Increased adhesion of erythrocytes to endothelial cells in diabetes mellitus and its relation to vascular complications. N Engl J Med. 1981;305:237-42.

40. Siberbauer KF, Schemthaner G, Sinzinger H, et al. Decreased vascular prostacyclin in juvenile on set diabetes. N Engl J Med. 1979;300:366-7.

41. Nedergaard M. Transient focal ischemia in hyperglycemic rats is associated with increased cerebral infarction. Brain Research. 1987;408:79-85.

42. de Courten-Myers GM, Kleinholz M, Wagner KR, Myers RE. Normoglycemia (not hypoglycemia) optimizes outcome from middle cerebral artery occlusion. J Cereb Blood Flow Metab. 1994;14:227-36.

43. Ginsberg MD, Prade R, Dietrich WD, et al. Hyperglycemia reduces the extent of cerebral infarction in rats. Stroke. 1987;18:570-4.

44. Kraft SA, Larson CP Jr, Shuer LM, et al. Effect of hyperglycemia on neuronal changes in a rabbit model of focal cerebral ischemia. Stroke. 1990;21:447-50.

45. Zasslow MA, Pearl RG, Shuer LM, et al. Hyperglycemia decreases acute neuronal ischemic changes after middle cerebral artery occlusion in cats. Stroke. 1989;20:519-23.

46. Huang NC, Yongbi MN, Helpem JA. The influence of preischemic hyperglycemia on acute changes in brain water ADCw following focal ischemia in rats. Brain Res. 1998;788:137-43.

47. Nedergaard M, Astrup J. Infarct rim: effect of hyperglycemia on direct current potential and (14C) 2-deoxyglucose phosphorylation. J Cereb Blood Flow Metab. 1986;6:607-15.

48. Els T, Rother J, Beaulieu C de Crispigny A, Moseley ME. Hyperglycemia delays terminal depolarization and enhances repolarization after peri-infarct spreading depression as measured by serial diffusion MR mapping. J Cereb Blood Flow Metab. 1997;17:591-5.

49. Wagner KR, Kleinholz M, de Courten-Myers GM, Myers RE. Hyperglycemia versus normoglycemic stroke: topography of brain metabolites, intracellular pH and infarct size. J Cereb Blood Flow Metab. 1992;12:213-22.

50. Siesjo BK, Ekholm A, Katsura K, Theander S. Acid base changes during complete brain ischemia. Stroke. 1990;21:194-8.

51. Siesjo BK, Bendek G, Kwide T. Influence of acidosis on lipid peroxidation in brain tissues in vitro. J Cereb Blood Flow Metab. 1985;5:253-8.

52. Hillerad L, Emster L, Siesjo BK. Influence of in vitro lactic acidosis and hypercapnia on repiratory activity of isolated rat brain mitochondria. J Cereb Blood Flow Metab. 1984;4:430-7.

53. OuYang YB, Mellergard P, Kristian T, et al. Influence of acid-base changes on intracellular calcium concentration of neurons in primary culture. Exp Brain Res. 1994;101:265-71.

54. Kraig RP, Petito CK, Plum F, Pulsinelli WA. Hydrogen ions kill brain at concentrations reached in ischemia. J Cereb Blood Flow Metab. 1987;7:379-86.

55. Weir CJ, Murray GD, Dyker AG, Lees KR. Is hyperglycemia an independent predictor of poor outcome after acute stroke? Results of a long-term follow-up study. BMJ. 1997;314:1303-6.

56. Berger L, Hakim AM. The association of hyperglycemia with cerebral edema in stroke. Stroke. 1986;17(5):865-71.

57. Dietrich WD, Alonso O, Busto R. Moderate hyperglycemia worsens acute blood-brain barrier. Injury after forebrain ischemia in rats. Stroke. 1993;24: 111-6.

58. de Courten-Myers GM, Kleinholz M, Wagner KR, Myers RE. Fatal strokes in hyperglycemic cats. Stroke. 1989;20:1707-15.

59. Paljarvi L, Rehncrona S, Soderfeldt B, Olsson Y, Kalimo H. Brain lactic acidosis and ischemic cell damage quantitative ultrastructural changes in capillaries of rat cerebral cortex. Acta Neuropathol (Berl). 1983;60:232-40.

60. The National Institute of Neurological Disorders and Stroke rtPA Stroke Study Group. Tissue plasminogen activator for acute ischaemic stroke. N Engl J Med. 1995;333:1581-7.

61. Hacke W, Kaste M, Fieschi C, et al. For the ECASS study group. Intravenous thrombolysis with recombinant tissue plaminogen activator for acute hemispheric stroke: the European Cooperative Acute Stroke Study (ECASS). JAMA. 1995;274:1017-25.

62. The NINDS rtPA Stroke Study Group. Intracerebral hemorrhage after intravenous t-PA therapy for ischemic stroke. Stroke. 1997;28:2109-18.

63. Larrue V, von Kummer R, del Zoppo G, Bluhmki E. Hemorrhagic transformation in acute ischemic stroke: potential contributing factors in the European Cooperative Acute Stroke Study. Stroke. 1997;38:957-60.

64. Demchuk AM, Morgenstern LB, Krieger DW, et al. Serum glucose level and diabetes predict tissue plasminogen active-for-related intracerebral hemorrhage in acute ischemic stroke. Stroke. 1999;30:34-9.

65. Auer RN. Insulin, blood glucose levels and ischemic brain damage. Neurology. 1999;51(Suppl 3):S39-43.

66. Maruki Y, Koehler RC, Kirsch JR, et al. Tirilazad pretreatment improves early cerebral metabolic and blood flow recovery from hyperglycemic ischemia. J Cereb Blood Flow Metab. 1995;15:88-96.

67. Kim H, Koehler RC, Hurn PD, et al. Amelioration of impaired cerebral metabolism after severe acidotic ischemia by tirilazad post-treatment in dogs. Stroke. 1996;27:114-21.

68. Hurn PD, Koehler RC, Blizzard KK, Traystman RJ. Deferoxamine reduces early metabolic failure associated with severe cerebral ischemic acidosis in dogs. Stroke. 1995;26:688-94.

69. Kuller LH, Dorman JS, Wolf PA. Cerebrovascular disease and diabetes. In Diabetes in America, Diabetes Data compiled for 1984. National Diabetes Data Group, Department of Health and Human Services. NIH Publication (No.85-1468) 1985;1-18.

70. Kannel WB, McGee DL. Diabetes and cardiovascular disease: the Framingham Study. JAMA. 1979;241:2035-38.

71. Burchfiel CM, Curb D, Rodriguez BL, et al. Glucose intolerance and 22-year stroke incidence. The Honolulu Heart Program. Stroke. 1994;25:951-7.

72. Hier DB, Foulkes MA, Suriontoniowski M, et al. Stroke recurrence within 2 years after ischemic infarction. Stroke. 1991;22:151-61.

73. Sacco RL, Shi T, Zamanillo MC, Kargman DE. Predictors of mortality and recurrence after hospitalized cerebral infarction in an urban community: the Northern Manhattan Stroke Study. Neurology. 1994;44:626-34.

74. Schneider DJ. Acceleration of atherosclerosis by abnormalities in thrombosis and fibrinolysis associated with diabetes mellitus. Current Opinion in Endocrinology and Diabetes. 1998;5:75-9.

75. Koistinaho J, Parsonen S, Yrjanheikki J, Chan PK. Spreading depression induced gene expression is regulated by plasma glucose. Stroke. 1999;30:114-9.

76. Leong SF, Leung TK. Diabetes induced by streptozotocin causes reduced Na-K ATPase in the brain. Neurochem Res. 1991;16:1161-5.

77. Yamashita T, Tamatani M, Taniguchi M, et al. Regulation of Na$^+$ myo-inositol cotransporter gene expression in hyperglycemic rat hippocampus. Brain Res Mol Brain Res. 1998;57:167-72.

78. Cleland SJ, Petric JR, Veda S, et al. Mechanisms and pathophysiologic significance of insulin vascular action. Current Opinion in Endocrinology and Diabetes. 1998;5:217-22.

79. Joseph LN, Babikian VL, Allen NC, Winter MR. Risk factor modification in stroke prevention: the experience of a stroke clinic. Stroke. 1999;30:16-20.

80. Bajaj JS. Diabetes care for the millions: a challenge for the next millennium. In: Diabetes (1994). Baba S, Kaneko T (Eds). Amsterdam: Excerpta Medica. 1995;95-102.

Chapter 63

PERIPHERAL ARTERIAL DISEASE IN DIABETES

Pinjala Ramakrishna

CHAPTER OUTLINE

- Introduction
- Incidence and Comorbidity
- Diagnosis of Peripheral Vascular Disease in Diabetes—Noninvasive Studies
- Clinical Problems and Management
- Medical Management
- Surgical Management

INTRODUCTION

Incidence, Pathophysiology and Diagnosis

Peripheral arterial disease is a condition characterized by atherosclerotic stenosis and occlusion of the lower extremity blood vessels. Peripheral arterial disease is a major risk factor for lower extremity amputation. The presentation of peripheral arterial disease in general population and smokers is well known and much studied in past few years but the management of peripheral arterial disease in diabetics is less clear and it is under diagnosed and under treated in many countries including India. Clear guidelines are yet to be established for the management of peripheral arterial disease in diabetes and many special issues are to be considered in the process. It has been estimated that 20% of symptomatic peripheral arterial disease patients have diabetes (Framingham Heart Study).[1] But it is not known what happens to this relation in the asymptomatic peripheral arterial disease. In diabetes, the pain is blunted due to neuropathy and classical claudication pain may not be perceived in some.[2,3]

INCIDENCE AND COMORBIDITY

Diabetes can affect any vascular bed in the body to variable degrees, but the effect of diabetes on peripheral vascular bed seems to be unique. The dysmetabolic state in diabetes affects arterial structure and function. These changes in arteries start even before the detection of diabetes. Peripheral arterial disease is four times more prevalent in diabetics than in nondiabetics. The arterial disorder typically involves the tibial and popliteal arteries but may spare the dorsalis pedis artery in the foot. Smoking, hypertension and hyperlipidemia contribute to increased prevalence of peripheral arterial disease in diabetes **(Figure 63.1)**.

It is observed that more than half of the peripheral arterial disease patients are asymptomatic or have atypical symptoms, one-third may have claudication and remaining have different expressions forms of the disease.[4] Melton found that the incidence of symptomatic occlusive arterial disease in diabetes was as high as 21.3 and 17.6 per 1000 person years for men and women.[5] Gangrene was noted in 20% of the patients with occlusive arterial disease. The cumulative

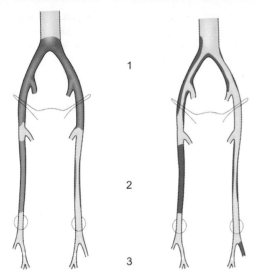

Peripheral vascular disease in diabetes

Figure 63.1 Distribution patterns of peripheral vascular disease are variable in diabetic patients with and without history of smoking. Involvement of the tibial arteries, popliteal artery and femoral artery is common. Now vascular surgeons feel vascular bypasses possible from the proximal arteries to the foot as it was found that dorsalis pedis and posterior tibial arteries are patent in the foot

incidence of vascular disease in diabetics has been estimated to be 15% at 10 years after the initial diagnosis of diabetes and 45% at 20 years.[6] The presence of lower extremity ischemia is detected by the clinical signs, symptoms and abnormal findings in noninvasive vascular tests. The common symptoms are claudication (pain during walking), pain occurring in the arch of the foot or forefoot at rest or during the night, with absent popliteal or posterior tibial pulses, thinned or shiny skin, loss of hair on the lower leg and foot, thickened nails. When legs are kept down the affected area becomes red and turns pale when the foot is elevated. The color changes are usually less prominent in case of excessive skin pigmentation. It was observed that 15 to 17% of patients with intermittent claudication were diabetics, 30 to 50% of patients undergoing lower extremity vascular surgery were found to be diabetic and 50 to 60% of patients undergoing lower extremity major amputation were found to have diabetes. The symptoms of ischemia were noted in relatively younger people suffering from diabetes. Type 2 diabetes patients with peripheral vascular disease have also shown a high incidence of mortality (22%) compared with those without peripheral vascular disease (4%) in a study.[7]

Smoking and hypertension are associated with proximal vessel disease (iliac, femoral arteries) but diabetes is typically associated with popliteal and tibial arterial disease. The estimations of prevalence of peripheral arterial disease in diabetes also depend on the type of method used for its diagnosis. Presence of claudication and absent pulses is not suitable enough to be used for studying the prevalence of peripheral arterial disease in people with diabetes. Ankle brachial index may be a better alternative to study prevalence of peripheral vascular disease in epidemiological studies. Approximately 27% of the diabetes patients with peripheral arterial disease show progression of symptoms over period of 5 years. Loss of a limb can be as high as 4 to 5% in them. In India and many other countries, peripheral vascular disease in diabetes is less often diagnosed and hence under treated. The prevalence of peripheral arterial disease in Europe and North America is estimated to be as high as 27 million. Yet peripheral arterial disease remains a largely under diagnosed and under treated disease. In epidemiologic studies, peripheral arterial disease detection rates were 20 to 30% when specific at-risk populations were screened. In an effort to guide diagnostic and treatment protocols, prevention of atherothrombotic disease network has recommended 5 actions. Initiate a screening protocol for patients at high-risk, improve treatment rates among patients who have been diagnosed with symptomatic peripheral arterial disease and increase the rates of early detection among the asymptomatic population.[6] When ABI alone was used over 40 years of age, Elhadd TA et al detected 20% incidence of peripheral arterial disease.[7] In diabetes patients above 50 years of age, prevalence of peripheral arterial disease was 29%, which was much more than the incidence shown based on the absent pulses and symptoms of peripheral arterial disease **(Figure 63.2)**.[8]

The deleterious nature of peripheral arterial disease is increased due to under diagnosis and under treatment. So, the recent developments suggest re-examination of traditional methods used to diagnose and manage peripheral arterial disease. These developments included data from community surveys of prevalence, treatment and outcomes, which have shed new light on the magnitude of the burden of peripheral arterial disease and its under treatment. The epidemiologic evidence shows that Ankle-Brachial Index (ABI—also known as the Ankle-Brachial Pulse Index or the Ankle/Arm Index) is an effective risk-assessment tool. Significant risk reduction can be achieved with pharmacological intervention in peripheral arterial disease.

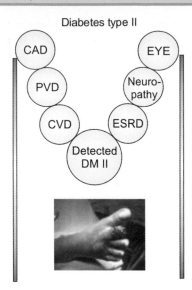

Diabetes type II

CAD — EYE — PVD — Neuro-pathy — CVD — ESRD — Detected DM II

Figure 63.2 Peripheral vascular disease in the diabetic patients should be always considered in association with the other macrovascular complications. It may be asymptomatic or symptomatic but certainly affects the quality of life and increases the risk of limb loss in the follow-up

Peripheral arterial disease is a progressive (slowly or rapidly) condition and it is anatomically characterized by thickening and stiffening of the arteries, arterial stenosis and occlusions in the peripheral arterial bed. It can lead to nonhealing wounds, gangrene, and eventual amputation. In those patients older than 55 years, peripheral arterial disease is an indicator of systemic arterial disease. In diabetic patients, tibial and plantar vessel calcification can be seen in the plain X-rays of leg and foot suggestive of peripheral arterial disease. Once peripheral arterial disease is diagnosed on the basis of claudication (symptomatology) and followed for five years—27% progress to leg ischemia, 4% require amputation, 20% develop nonfatal myocardial infarction and 30% would be the all-cause mortality in them. When critical limb ischemia is the initial diagnosis, then long-term prognosis is worse with 30% amputations and 20% mortality within 6 months.[9]

Fortunately most cases of peripheral arterial disease are asymptomatic. Data suggest that risk of systemic complication in asymptomatic peripheral arterial disease patients is same as the symptomatic. That means the incidence of atherothrombotic events, myocardial infarction (MI), stroke, impaired lower extremity functioning and internal carotid artery stenosis is similar in symptomatic and asymptomatic patients with peripheral arterial disease. This point was observed in the Limburg peripheral arterial occlusive disease (PAOD) study. A cross-sectional survey of 3650 patients aged 40 to 78 years showed that those with asymptomatic peripheral arterial disease had a risk factor and comorbidity profile comparable with that in symptomatic patients.[10]

In India, there are statistical data from individual large hospitals but national epidemiological studies are yet to be conducted. There is enough data from other countries in the world to suggest that the peripheral arterial disease significantly affects the quality of life. Three recent programs, the Prevention of Progression of Arterial Disease and Diabetes (POPADAD), the Minnesota Regional Peripheral Arterial Disease Screening Program and the Peripheral Arterial Disease Awareness, Risk and Treatment, New Resources for Survival (PARTNERS) Program have demonstrated high peripheral arterial disease detection rates of 20.1%, 26.5%, and 29%, respectively, when specific populations at risk were screened. The ongoing POPADAD study evaluates 8000 patients who are 40 years and older and had type 1 or type 2 diabetes mellitus but no clinical symptoms of arterial disease. In the preliminary recruitment phase, patients were enrolled from 227 primary care facilities and 27 major hospitals throughout Scotland. In these patients, 20.1% had an ABI value less than 0.95 suggestive of peripheral arterial disease.

Peripheral arterial disease is a powerful indicator of systemic atherothrombotic disorder, with or without evidence of symptoms. It was also observed that patients with peripheral arterial disease have an increased risk of MI and stroke and are 6 times more likely to die within 10 years than patients without peripheral arterial disease. In addition, the degree of symptom severity has been found to correlate with poor outcome. Patients with symptomatic peripheral arterial disease have a 15-year accrued survival rate of approximately 22%, compared with—a survival rate of 78% in patients without peripheral arterial disease symptoms. The patient survival rate for peripheral arterial disease is worse than the outcome for breast cancer and Hodgkin's disease.[11] Advanced age, smoking and diabetes are strongly associated with peripheral arterial disease. Other peripheral arterial disease risk factors are hypertension, hyperlipidemia, male sex, homocysteine-mia, elevated plasma fibrinogen levels, elevated glucose level, prior MI, heart failure, history of stroke, and history of transient ischemic attack. Despite the marked increase in risk of lower extremity atherosclerosis, we have inadequate information regarding the role of medical therapies in diabetic patients with PAD. In the beginning, doubts were raised about the role of tight glycemic control, aggressive blood pressure management, or the use of antiplatelet agents' effect on decreasing the incidence of intermittent claudication or critical limb ischemia. Although simvastatin decreased the rates of reported claudication in patients with CAD in Scandinavian Simvastatin Survival Study (4S), but the trial did not report data specific to patients with diabetes. Based on the recent studies, it is recommended that patients with diabetes should receive therapies of proven benefit because cardiovascular events remain the principal cause of death in patients with peripheral arterial disease.

DIAGNOSIS OF PERIPHERAL VASCULAR DISEASE IN DIABETES— NONINVASIVE STUDIES

Noninvasive vascular studies used for assessing peripheral vascular disease are transcutaneous oxygen (tcPO$_2$) measurement, ankle-brachial index (ABI) and absolute toe systolic pressure (ATSP). ABI is a non-invasive test, it can be easily done in the outpatients clinics with a handheld Doppler device. A blood pressure cuff is placed on the upper arm and inflated until no brachial pulse is detected by the Doppler device. The cuff is then slowly deflated until a Doppler detects return of pulse and pressure at that point is recognized as systolic pressure. This same test can be repeated on the legs, with the cuff wrapped around the distal calf with Doppler probe placed over dorsalis pedis or posterior tibial artery. The ankle systolic pressure divided by brachial systolic pressure gives ankle-brachial index (ABI). The sensitivity (95%) and specificity (100%) values are considered as satisfactory.[12] Solely with noninvasive tests, there is also a possibility that one may underestimate the severity of arterial insufficiency. So, if lower extremity ischemia is strongly suspected on clinical grounds, peripheral angiography or other imaging study should be performed to confirm or rule out suspected significant ischemia. We know that adequate tissue perfusion is needed for proper wound healing and arterial insufficiency should be suspected when an ulcer fails to heal with all the usual measures. ABI is a noninvasive, simple, inexpensive measurement to assess the patency of the lower extremity arterial system.[13] ABI is measured when the patient is lying in the supine position, with subsequent ankle and brachial blood pressure measurements using a 5 to 7 MHz handheld Doppler device. Ideally, the posterior tibial and dorsalis pedis artery systolic

pressures are both measured and compared with the arm pressure. An ABI measurement usually takes 10 minutes to perform. An ABI measurement is the most effective, accurate and practical method of PVD detection in our practice, it can be performed by technologists and nurses. Usually diagnosis of PVD is based on the presence of limb symptoms or an ABI less than 0.9. An ABI of 1.0 is generally considered normal. When the ABI value is less than 0.9, it has 95% sensitivity in predicting angiogram-positive vascular disease. Which means it is associated with 50% or greater stenosis in one or more major vessels. It is almost 100% specific in excluding healthy individuals. ABI value is less than 0.9 highly predictive of morbidity and mortality from cardiovascular events linked with PAD, when compared ABI is more sensitive and specific than several standard screening tests. POPADAD and aspirin for asymptomatic atherosclerosis (AAA) studies are evaluating the potential benefits of antiplatelet therapy in patients with a low ABI value. ABI can stratify the severity of both asymptomatic and symptomatic diseases with a numerical value. In a study to determine the relationship between ABI and morbidity, mortality in patients with PAD, the 5-year cumulative survival rate was 63% for patients with ABI value less than 0.50, 71% for patients with ABI value between 0.50 and 0.69, and 91% for patients with an ABI value between 0.70 and 0.89. Those with ABI value less than 0.90 are twice as likely to have coronary heart disease (CHD) than those with a normal ABI and have an increased risk of fatal and nonfatal MI, stroke, and death from cardiovascular causes, as well as all-cause death. ABI is a useful tool because it not only identifies PAD, but also detects the severity of PAD and helps in planning treatment (ABI >0.90, normal; 0.71–0.90, mild PAD; 0.41–0.70, moderate PAD; ≤ 0.40, severe PAD). But there are also some limitations for the ABI in the management of peripheral arterial disease. ABI does not measure the effectiveness of preventive treatment. Some elderly and diabetic patients have calcified arteries which prevent compression of blood vessels and flow by the blood pressure cuff. So that may result in falsely high ABI reading (>1.50). Patients with high grade aortoiliac arterial stenosis or occlusions may also occasionally present with a normal ABI at rest due to the presence of a rich collateral arterial network. These patients must be referred for other tests, such as toe pressure measurement, Doppler waveform analysis, pulse volume recording, duplex arterial ultrasound study, or exercise Doppler stress testing.

CLINICAL PROBLEMS AND MANAGEMENT

Gangrene of the Toes

Gangrene of the toes can result from four possible causes:

1. Atherosclerosis with thrombus formation.
2. Microthrombi formation secondary to infection. This can convert small vessels in the toes to endarteries resulting in gangrene.
3. Cholesterol emboli that break off from ulcerated plaques in the proximal larger vessels. This causes cyanosis and gangrene of the toes and the blue or purple toe syndrome. It is characterized by sudden onset of pain in the toes and a deep purplish discoloration of the involved toes. A sharp demarcation frequently occurs between normally perfused skin and ischemic areas. However, the dorsalis pedis and posterior tibial pulses are usually present. Cholesterol emboli to the foot can also result in painful petechiae, a livedo-reticularis pattern of the skin and myalgias because the emboli go both to the skin and muscle arteries. This constellation of signs and symptoms strongly suggests micro emboli. If the changes are bilateral, the source of the emboli is in the aorta. If it is unilateral, the source is in the iliac artery or below. Many patients who receive anticoagulation therapy with warfarin, thrombolytic therapy with streptokinase and tissue plasminogen activator can also develop blue toe syndrome. It is therefore extremely important to periodically check the toes and feet of patients receiving anticoagulants or thrombolytic therapy. The usual treatment of cholesterol emboli is removal of the ulcerated plaques, to prevent further embolization. Recently intra-arterial injections of prostaglandin E was suggested for the treatment of the blue toe syndrome.
4. The fourth cause of gangrene of the toes involves drugs that can affect the peripheral circulation, causing gangrenous changes in the toes. Vasopressors, such as dopamine (Inotropin), are frequently used to treat shock. Because of the norepinephrine-like vasoconstrictive effects of these agents, ischemic gangrene can develop in the toes and feet, particularly in diabetic patients who have peripheral arterial insufficiency. Dopamine exerts positive inotropic effects by direct action on the adrenergic receptors. When sufficiently large doses of inotropic drugs are administered, the predominant effect is vasoconstriction in all vascular beds. In patients with PAD, dopamine should be used with caution in as low a dose as possible. If a patient is in shock, the risk-benefit ratio would dictate the use of inotropic drugs despite the peripheral arterial risks. However, the feet of these patients must be inspected daily. Peripheral circulation can also be impaired by β-blockers commonly used for treatment of angina and hypertension.

Management of heel lesions continues to be a difficult problem, such that patients with severe heel ulcerations are often treated with primary amputation. The combination of distal neuropathy, repeated local trauma, prolonged periods of vessels. This causes cyanosis and gangrene of the toes and the blue or purple toe syndrome. It is characterized by sudden onset of pain in the toes and a deep purplish discoloration of the involved toes. A sharp demarcation frequently occurs between normally perfused skin and ischemic areas. However, the dorsalis pedis and posterior tibial pulses are usually present. Prolonged periods of decubitus pressure, and peripheral arterial disease make these lesions particularly problematic in the diabetic population. Although many reconstructive options are available for the treatment of heel ulcers, cornerstone to their management is the restoration of adequate arterial blood flow to the affected region. Although direct revascularization of the hindfoot by means of the posterior tibial artery is often an attractive option, its use is frequently limited, especially in the diabetic population with significant tibial atherosclerosis. Alternatively, blood flow to the foot may be restored by means of the dorsal circulation, with perfusion of the hindfoot provided through collateral pathways. Inframalleolar revascularization by dorsalis pedis artery bypass in the treatment of ischemic feet lesions has been found to be useful. One and five-year patency rates for grafts placed to the dorsalis pedis artery were satisfactory independent of the location of the lesion. With primary 5-year patency rates ranging between 55% and 60% and secondary patency rates between 60% and 70%. Although these grafts are now widely recognized as providing adequate and durable treatment for limb-threatening forefoot ischemia, their efficacy in the treatment of hindfoot ischemia also has shown by healing rates approaching 90% for heel lesions. Dorsalis pedis bypass effectively reverses local hindfoot ischemia to promote tissue healing. This finding is supported by a greater than 85% 5-year limb salvage rate for both forefoot and heel lesions.

Clinical presentation of ischemic heel lesions can extend over a wide-spectrum of pathology, ranging from localized skin fissures extending into the dermis to extensive necrosis of subcutaneous tissues and Achilles tendon with underlying calcaneal osteomyelitis. Of the patients with heel lesions reviewed in a series, the relative early nature of the lesions is illustrated by the need for operative debridement or reconstruction in only 23%. Those patients not requiring local heel procedures were treated with local wound care, packing of open wounds with normal saline or one-quarter strength povidone-iodine solution, and systemic antibiotics as indicated. Of patients with limited tissue loss, 88% demonstrated complete healing of their lesion. In patients with more extensive tissue loss requiring operative intervention, initial treatment consisted of prompt drainage of deep space infections with local wound care as described above. After revascularization in these patients, soft tissue coverage was obtained by means of a variety of procedures. If the lesions demonstrated a healthy granulation bed overlying the calcaneum, split thickness skin grafting over the defect is performed. With lesions demonstrating evidence of calcaneal exposure and presumed osteomyelitis, primary therapy consisted of partial calcanectomy with primary closure of the wound. If the extent of skin loss is too extensive for primary closure, skin edges were approximated with retention sutures, and the remaining defect was allowed to heal by secondary intention. Direct skin grafting to an exposed calcaneum or use of radiologic testing for the diagnosis of osteomyelitis was not used in these patients. Soft tissue defects too large for approximation after calcanectomy were treated with myocutaneous grafts. Patients who underwent operative debridement and reconstruction, complete healing of their lesions was accomplished in 81%. In reviewing 191 infrainguinal bypasses, Carsten et al determined that 5 of 17 major amputations that were performed despite a patent graft resulted from chronic neuropathic heel ulcers. But in another series of 432 with dorsalis pedis bypasses only two patients with nonhealing heel lesions and patent grafts ultimately required amputation. Smith et al showed that 13 of 23 (57%) patients required an average of 33 weeks after arterial bypass to completely heal their lesions. Six patients (26%) in their study lived with some wound areas remaining open, and two patients (9%) required amputation. Although 90% healing rate, with an average time to healing of 20 weeks, was shown in study with 0% major amputation rate.

The status of the pedal arch and its contribution to outflow resistance (and secondarily pedal graft patency) remains an area of controversy. Less well studied is the influence of an intact pedal arch on heel lesion healing,

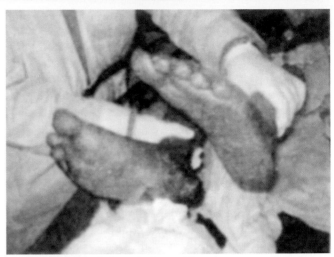

Figure 63.3 Ischemic foot with gangrenous changes noted after debridement of the heel ulcer

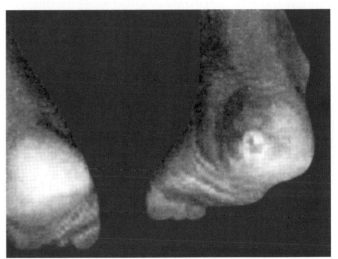

Figure 63.4 Nonhealing ischemic ulcer in the heel of foot secondary to diffuse atherosclerotic tibioperoneal vascular disease (multisegmental)

notably after placement of a dorsalis pedis bypass graft **(Figures 63.3 and 63.4)**. Our data demonstrate that both graft patency and lesion healing are not dependent on the angiographic presence of a complete arch. As such, one would argue that in the absence of an intact pedal arch, sufficient collateral pathways are present to revascularize the heel after restoration of pulsatile flow to the forefoot circulation.

Hypertension, Complicating Diabetes with Peripheral Arterial Disease

Adequate management of hypertension is equally important to improve the outcome of peripheral vascular disease patients with diabetes. Type 2 diabetes and hypertension are often seen together and this association increases risk of cardiovascular and renal disease. The prevalence of hypertension in type 2 diabetes is higher than that in the general population and they are also younger. At the age of 45 years, 40% of patients with type 2 diabetes are hypertensive and this can increase up to 60% by the age of 75. Hypertension increases the already existing high-risk of cardiovascular disease in type 2 diabetes. Hypertension is also a risk factor for the development of micro-albuminuria and possibly retinopathy. The treatment to achieve the target blood pressure reduces the incidence of stroke and myocardial infarction particularly in the elderly with peripheral vascular disease. Such patients are also at increased risk of peripheral limb edema after vascular surgical reconstruction. Patients with hypertension and type 2 diabetes assigned to tight control of blood pressure achieved a significant risk reduction— 24% for any end-points related to diabetes, 32% for death related to diabetes, 44% for stroke and 37% for microvascular disease. In addition, there was a 56% reduction in risk of heart failure. It is difficult to give tight blood pressure in our population when the upper limb blood vessels are affected by the peripheral vascular disease. The blood pressure in them can be falsely low. The United Kingdom Prospective Diabetes Study 38 (UKPDS 38) trial did not show any decrease in the amputation rates with tight blood pressure control.[14] ACE inhibitors improve endothelial function in cases with peripheral artery disease. A total of 3577 patients in the Heart Outcomes Prevention Evaluation (HOPE) study had diabetes, 1135 of whom had no clinical manifestations of cardiovascular disease, and the event rate in this group was about half that in the other patients (10.2 vs 18.7 percent). 4051 patients out of 9297 had peripheral arterial disease. Ramipril has shown to reduce the cardiovascular points equally in both the groups of this study, with and without peripheral arterial disease. This shows that the ramipril is effective in reducing the fatal and nonfatal ischemic events in the peripheral arterial disease patients but we do not have prospective randomized controlled trials to show the benefits of ACE inhibitors in peripheral arterial disease *per se*.[15,16]

The diagnosis of diabetes was found to be related to the level of an ABI in peripheral arterial disease as were the fasting blood glucose and fasting insulin levels. This relation appears to be independent of obesity as measured by body mass index.

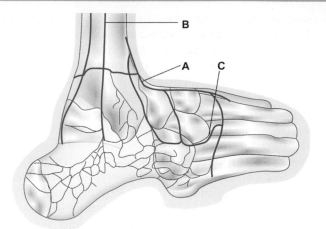

Figure 63.5 Arterial anastomosis around the ankle joint. The foot is supplied by the dorsalis pedis, posterior tibial and peroneal arteries. There is good communication between these important vessels through the collateral arteries: (A) Dorsalis pedis artery (B) Posterior tibial artery (C) Peroneal artery

Foot Ulcers and Peripheral Vascular Disease in Diabetes—Role of Noninvasive Studies and Angiograms for Predicting the Amputation

Various factors may influence the outcome of foot ulcers in diabetic subjects, but the severity of lower extremity arterial disease is the main independent risk factor for major amputation. Many studies have used noninvasive methods to assess peripheral arterial disease, but few have used angiography exclusively in diabetic subjects with foot ulcers. Available angiographic data have mostly been acquired from heterogeneous groups of diabetic subjects with critical limb ischemia with or without foot ulcers or subjects selected for vascular procedures **(Figure 63.5)**. The prognostic value for major amputation has also been investigated for the results of noninvasive vascular laboratory procedures but not for those of angiographic evaluation.

Can One Exclude Peripheral Arterial Disease in the Absence of Symptoms?

The absence of symptoms of ischemia does not exclude its diagnosis. Diabetic neuropathy can impair the sensations. This may result in inability to perceive claudication pain after exercise or ischemic rest pain in the legs. In one study on 103 subjects, in whom DSA detected hemodynamically significant stenosis, only 27 subjects (26.2%) showed ischemic pain while in 76 subjects (73.8%) this pain was completely absent.

Stenosis more than or equal to 50% of vessel lumen diameter were also detected in subjects with normal ABIs or normal values of $tcPO_2$. These results are not surprising. It is known that Doppler-derived ABI can be falsely high due to arterial media calcification and that the transcutaneous oximetry values may be influenced by various systemic and local factors (e.g. blood oxygenation, thickness of the skin, and the presence of inflammation or local edema). These conditions are particularly frequent in diabetic subjects with foot ulcers. Duplex scanning is considered be as effective as angiography. However, the arterial media calcification can also affect the findings of duplex scanning. The accuracy of duplex scanning is very high in the aortofemoral segment but lower in the distal arteries. This seems to be a particularly important limiting factor in the diabetic subjects with foot ulcers, in whom stenosis is prevalently distal tibial arteries.

Can Peripheral Arterial Disease be Excluded in Case of Palpable Foot Pulses?

The presence of palpable pulse cannot exclude the peripheral arterial disease. There can be good pulse in some patients due to adequate collateral circulation in spite of stenotic lesion (>50%). Just the absence of intermittent claudication or ischemic pain, a normal ABI, and a reassuring $tcPO_2$ value do not exclude the presence of an arterial occlusive disease similarly a palpable pulse cannot always exclude the peripheral arterial disease. Angiography draws attention to occlusive arterial disease that is not detectable with noninvasive laboratory procedures. In such cases, if the angiography had not been carried out, these could be considered as "neuropathic foot". But with the positive findings on angiography, these can be treated as "neuroischemic foot". This classification may not be important when the patients are prepared for major amputation. We can administer medication for arterial disease and improve the blood flow and thereby improve the quality of life in patients with subclinical ischemia in neuroischemic foot problems. These methods are useful for slowing down the progression of arterial disease and this is particularly meaningful in diabetic subjects with foot ulcers. But there is always concern about the adverse reactions to contrast material used in angiography when renal function may be compromised. So, there is obvious limitation to the use of angiograms. Few studies also demonstrated that adequate precautions before diagnostic angiogram can protect the renal function. Wagner grade 2 ulcer with defective healing over a month of outpatient treatment and Wagner grade >2 can be an indication for angiographic study in diabetic patients with foot ulcers. The angiographic evaluation can also provide prognostic information. By assigning to the stenosis found through angiography a score that takes into consideration their extent (percentage of vessel lumen reduction) and diffusion (involved segments of vascular tree), it is possible to obtain a numerical index, our angiographic score that evaluates the severity of the peripheral occlusive arterial disease and its prognostic value. Multivariate analysis has indicated the angiographic score to be an independent variable associated with major amputation. In clinical practice, this score could give a useful indication of whether the ulcer can be managed with or without major amputation. No patient with a score <10 underwent a major amputation, and all patients with a score >14 underwent a major amputation. There is also a statistically significant difference in angiographic score between subjects healed with or without a minor amputation. Nevertheless, the overlapping between the two groups does not allow the indication of precise cut-offs. The evaluation of the stenosis in popliteal and infrapopliteal arteries is particularly important: When there is a total occlusion of >2 of each of the arteries, the probability of major amputation is very high. Type 2 diabetes is more common than type 1 diabetes throughout the world. In a country like United States, type 2 diabetes accounts for 90% of the estimated 17 million people, or 6.2% of the US population, who currently suffer from diabetes.[16] C-reactive protein (CRP) for risk assessment in peripheral arterial disease with diabetes CRP is a strong independent predictor of death in type 2 diabetes. Patients with peripheral vascular disease are also known to show increased levels of CRP. Atherosclerotic vascular disease of the coronary or peripheral arteries is a chronic inflammatory process.[17] Vu JD et al noted that the likelihood of peripheral arterial disease is enhanced by the elevated CRP levels.[18]

Linnemann et al[19] examined in Germany 592 patients, aged 55 to 74 years (311 men, 281 women), with signs and symptoms of circulation deficits by duplex ultrasound for suspected cerebrovascular and peripheral vascular disease and followed over a period of 5 years. At baseline, 292 patients of the total group had type 2 diabetes (49.3%). Ischemic heart disease was present in 40.2%, internal carotid stenosis in 21.9% and peripheral arterial disease in 39.7% of the subjects. During the observation period, 104 patients had died, 72 (69.2%) due to cardiovascular causes. Nonfatal myocardial infarction occurred in 39 patients (7.4%), nonfatal stroke in 70 patients (13.3%) and amputations because of gangrene were unavoidable in 24 patients (4.6%), CRP was the strongest predictor of cardiovascular death in type 2 diabetic subgroup when compared to the traditional cardiovascular risk factors and the data of diabetic metabolic control.

CRP was correlated positively with plasma levels of triglycerides, C-peptide, postprandial glucose, albuminuria, and inversely with HDL-cholesterol in type 2 diabetic patients. CRP can be used a better predictor of death and cardiovascular events than traditional risk factors or parameters of metabolic control in type 2 diabetic patients at high-risk for cardiovascular end points. This will be a useful parameter in peripheral arterial disease patients to predict the outcome during the course of treatment.

MEDICAL MANAGEMENT

Two noninvasive modes of therapy have demonstrated benefit in improving walking distance in patients with PAD: Exercise and cilostazol. Exercise rehabilitation is currently suggested as the cornerstone of management. Supervised exercise therapy produces impressive increases in walking distance. Since 1966 many randomized controlled trials have shown benefit of supervised exercise therapies in individuals with peripheral arterial disease.[20] Meta-analysis showed that, supervised exercise programs increased walking distance by 122%. The mechanism underlying the benefit could be due to improved cardiovascular fitness, increased production of nitric oxide or modification of cardiovascular risk factors. Many advocate and feel that supervised exercise walking program, which can increase the walking distance, modify the risk factors and improve the insulin sensitivity. These programs call for at least three months of intermittent treadmill walking three times per week.

Cilostazol, a type III phosphodiesterase inhibitor, acts as antiplatelet drug and exerts favorable effects on improvement of walking distance through mechanism as yet unclear. Cilostazol increases walking distance by 35 to 50% above placebo in patients with claudication; however, we lack specific information for diabetic patients. It is remembered that this drug is contraindicated, if there is suspicion of cardiac failure. Pentoxifylline, a xanthine derivative, may affect blood rheology and decrease blood viscosity. Pentoxifylline improves claudication in some studies but not in others, and outcomes specific to patients with diabetes remain unknown.

Percutaneous Interventions and Thrombolytic Therapies for PAD in Diabetes

The outcomes of lower extremity revascularization through the percutaneous methods are dependent on many variables, including the arterial lesion location, length, degree of stenosis, distensibility, occlusion and the nature of distal runoff through the collateral arteries. In diabetes, distribution of atherosclerotic plaques is oriented more towards the distal arterial tree. So, they tend to have severe arterial occlusive disease below the knee and also in the runoff vessels. As the distal runoff declines, the results of percutaneous interventions worsen. The success of iliac artery stenting in diabetic patients varies among studies, but several groups have shown better than 90% patency at the end of one year. Femoral artery interventions have 1-year patency rates ranging from 29 to 80%. Diabetes adversely affects success rate in this type of medium and small vessels angioplasty. This finding may result in part from poor runoff in patients with diabetes. In diabetes patients with good distal runoff, patency rates were comparable to those of nondiabetic patients. The results of angioplasty are poor as we go down to the leg and foot level arteries. The outcomes of surgical revascularization in diabetes resemble those in patients without diabetes in terms of limb salvage, albeit more distal than that of nondiabetic patients. Combining the procedures is known as 'Hybrid' procedures. The iliac artery lesions are dilated and stented, while the femoral popliteal occlusions are bypassed. These patients will be requiring bypass operations to the tibial vessels either from the popliteal artery or femoral artery. The role of stents for the lower limb arteries in thigh and knee are still under evaluation. The restenosis rate is high as the reocclusion of the angioplasty segment is common. Antiplatelet drugs and anticoagulants as low molecular weight heparin and oral anticoagulant drugs have been used with a view to improve the patency of the treated segments of the arteries. Thrombolytic therapies are used to dissolve the fresh thrombus when it is detected during the angiography. The ability to pass the guidewire through the soft thrombus gives us a clue that it can be dissolved with thrombolytics. After giving the thrombolytic agent for 1 to 2 days, there can be either complete or partial recanalization of the affected arterial segment. It is also possible to see a residual lesion (stenosis) which can be dilated with suitable angioplasty balloon. The newer stents which are now used in the coronaries (drug eluting stents) are giving better hopes because they may inhibit the early restenosis in the peripheral arteries. But we need to wait for more studies to prove the same. The prevalence of type 2 diabetes is expected to increase dramatically in the coming decades, primarily due to the increasing prevalence of obesity.[21] Furthermore, the burden of prediabetes is already substantial with impaired glucose tolerance (IGT) affecting an estimated 16 million and impaired fasting glucose (IFG) affecting 10 million of US adults aged 40 to 74 years. Patients with type 2 diabetes, metabolic syndrome X, and prediabetes are often treated with antihypertensive medications because of concomitant hypertension or cardiovascular disease.[22,23] Revascularization should be considered when there are clinical signs of ischemia with positive noninvasive tests and vascular imaging confirming peripheral arterial occlusive disease. Adequate control of concomitant hypertension and hyperlipidemia can reduce the risk of peripheral arterial occlusive disease and its complications in diabetic people. Smoking is well-established risk factor for peripheral vascular disease in diabetic and nondiabetic population. So, smoking cessation is crucial for preventing the progression of occlusive arterial disease.[24]

Moderate and intense lipid lowering therapy in patients with peripheral arterial disease and diabetes patients with type 2 diabetes mellitus showing increased concentrations of low density lipoprotein cholesterol, decreased concentrations of high density lipoprotein cholesterol, hyperglycemia, hypertension, and smoking are at risk for coronary artery disease, defined as fatal and nonfatal myocardial infarction or angina. So, it is important to give attention to all these factors for patency of the reconstructed blood vessels and survival of the patients. Increased concentrations of low density lipoprotein cholesterol may be more pathogenic in patients with type 2 diabetes mellitus than in nondiabetic subjects because of the presence of small dense low density lipoprotein cholesterol particles and oxidation of glycated low density lipoprotein cholesterol. The 1.57 increased risk for an increment of 1 mmol/L in low density lipoprotein cholesterol concentration equates to a 36% risk reduction for a decrement of 1 mmol/L, similar to the 31% risk reduction achieved with a 3-hydroxy-3-methylglutaryl coenzyme A reductase inhibitor in men with hypercholesterolemia. The subgroup analysis of the simvastatin study showed that the diabetic patients had similar protection to that of nondiabetic patients. At the same time 4S study has shown 38% reduction in the risk of new or worsening symptoms of intermittent claudication.[25] A decreased concentration of high density lipoprotein cholesterol was an independent risk factor for coronary artery disease. The 15% decrease in the risk of coronary artery disease associated with a 0.1 mmol/L increment in high density lipoprotein cholesterol concentration is compatible with the 8 to 12% reduction reported from prospective American studies. Triglyceride concentration was a risk factor for coronary artery disease after adjustment for age and sex, but it was not an independent risk factor when the other variables were included in the model. This is in accord with other studies, possibly because of the greater biological variability of triglyceride than high density lipoprotein cholesterol measurements. However, it was also found over 6 months that the concentration of high density lipoprotein cholesterol was more variable than that of triglyceride, possibly because of low precision with the assay (coefficient of variation 6% vs 2%) and because patients were receiving dietary advice and had a more uniform dietary intake than in the general population. As control of plasma triglyceride and high density lipoprotein cholesterol concentrations is interlinked through lipoprotein lipase and hepatic lipase activities, it may not be feasible to separate the contributions of triglyceride and high density lipoprotein cholesterol to coronary artery disease. Postprandial triglyceride values may have an additional atherogenic role to the fasting values that were measured.

SURGICAL MANAGEMENT

Usually in patients presenting with severe claudication or critical limb ischemia, surgery is slightly superior to percutaneous transluminal angioplasty for revascularization in the femoral, popliteal, and infrapopliteal vessels, but this comes at a price of increased periprocedural cardiovascular morbidity and mortality. Many of the clinical complications of diabetes are ascribed to alterations in the vascular structure and function with subsequent end organ damage and death. These are nonocclusive microcirculatory dysfunction involving the basement of the capillaries and macrovasculopathy due to atherosclerosis affecting the coronary and peripheral vascular circulation.[26] Vascular surgical reconstruction or bypass improves blood flow to ischemic tissues affected by the macrovascular disease. Some 50% of these diabetic patients with foot ischemia will also have infection and most of these patients have neuropathy in addition.[27] Based on the initial observations of Goldenberg on amputated diabetic limbs in 1959, for very long time people were under the impression that the small arterioles are occluded in diabetes by a material which is positive for periodic-acid-Schiff stain. But that concept was refuted later by many.[28] It is a common misconception that patients with diabetes mellitus have an occlusive lesion in the microcirculation of the foot. The belief can be traced to an early study that described material that stained positive with periodic acid-Schiff stain in the arterioles of retrospectively examined amputation specimens from diabetic patients. Subsequent prospective studies with the use of standard histology and a delicate arterial casting technique failed to confirm the presence of an arteriolar occlusive lesion characteristic of diabetes mellitus. The casting studies demonstrated foci of small artery occlusion but the number of such foci was greater in nondiabetics than in diabetic subjects. These foci probably explain the propensity to localized gangrene in both groups. In patients undergoing femoropopliteal bypass, the physiological response to papaverine vasodilation was similar in diabetic and nondiabetic patients. This demonstrated the absence of any fixed resistance in the diabetic microcirculation.

The concept of small vessel disease has certainly given rise to pessimistic attitude of many but now that is refuted. Rejection of small vessel disease concept in itself has decreased the risk of major amputation in those with diabetes significantly.

Indications and Type of Surgical Treatment

Surgical procedures for ischemic limb salvage are well defined and based on the severity of symptoms and hemodynamic data. Primary indications for the surgical therapies both on hemodynamic data and clinical symptomatology. All the surgical procedures are aimed at relieving the symptoms of limb-threatening ischemia, such as rest pain, ulcers and gangrene of the toes. Chronic critical limb ischemia is defined not only by the clinical presentation but also by an objective measurement of impaired blood flow. Criteria for diagnosis includes one of the following:
- More than two weeks of recurrent foot pain at rest that requires regular use of analgesics and is associated with an ankle systolic pressure of 50 mm Hg or less, or a toe systolic pressure of 30 mm Hg or less, or
- A nonhealing wound or gangrene of the foot or toes, with similar hemodynamic measurements.[2]

The hemodynamic parameters are less reliable in diabetes patients because of calcification in arterial wall which can impair blood vessel compression by a blood pressure cuff. This can result in falsely high systolic pressure measurements that are greater than the actual pressure. Surgery is advised in the form of bypass or removal of the occlusions (atherothrombectomy/endarterectomy). Intermittent claudication is still a relative indication for surgical therapy. Surgery for the intermittent claudication is considered only when adequate trials of drugs and supervised exercise have failed to give the desired benefits to the patients. The results of surgery are conventionally measured in terms of vessel patency (graft patency), limb salvage and patients survival. All the patients may not have palpable pulses at the ankle level after a successful vascular bypass due to distal disease in the smaller arteries. A sustained increase of 15% in the ankle brachial index (ABI) is considered as improvement due to treatment. Postoperative duplex scanning or angiography are definitive in establishing the patency of the graft or treated segment but these are time-consuming and expensive to be considered at regular intervals in India. The results of bypass are measured as primary limb salvage and limb salvages. In the primary limb salvage, we are measuring the success of the initial procedure itself but in the secondary limb salvage, we measure the success of the procedure, its postoperative follow-up in terms of detection and treatment of the complications or restenosis.

In addition to the improvement in these objective parameters, we are looking at the changes in the quality of life of these patients before and after the intervention. The improvement in the quality of life may be a better measure and a more appropriate tool to assess successful outcome than patency of the graft, limb salvage and patient survival. Adequate relief of symptoms including pain, healing of ulcers, return to normal ambulation, independent living and general level of patient satisfaction are all considered to be valid parameters for comparing results of lower extremity surgical revascularization and nonsurgical methods for the treatment of peripheral arterial disease. Very few studies in the current practice are focusing on these issues and in the coming years more instruments for quality of life measurement are used to study and quantify the results of the surgical and nonsurgical treatments for lower limb ischemia.

It is difficult to carry out double blind randomized controlled trials in acute limb-threatening ischemia to compare surgery with other modes of therapy and obtain level one evidence in current practice. At the same time, it may not be acceptable to randomly assign patients with acute limb-threatening ischemia to surgical or nonsurgical procedures for this type of study. Results from the studies conducted on induction of claudication were not very different from each other. In study conducted by Lundgren and coauthors in 1989, 75 patients with intermittent claudication verified by laboratory testing were randomly assigned to either: (1) Surgery alone, (2) Surgery combined with exercise training, or (3) Exercise training alone. All the comparable patients were taken into these three groups: *ABI, toe blood pressure and calf blood flow*, and *walking performance* were examined as the endpoints of study. ABI and toe blood pressures significantly increased in the group with surgery and not with the exercise training alone. All the three groups have shown significant improvement in the calf blood flow and walking performance. The improvement was significantly greater in the surgery and exercise group but at the same time, complications were also more in the surgical group.

Advances in angiographic technology, surgical skills, and anesthesia/critical care contributed to the improved outcomes with infrapopliteal reconstruction/bypass for limb-threatening ischemia in general. Distal bypass operations have become important in diabetic patients whose pattern of occlusive disease frequently involves the tibial and popliteal vessels. The number of diabetic patients (greater than 90%) getting referred to the tertiary care hospitals with ischemic limb-threatening lesions is steadily increasing. This will also increase the demand for the peripheral vascular surgical services in India too. The current use of intra-arterial digital subtraction angiography (IADSA) improved the ability to visualize the distal arterial tree suitable for placement of the bypass grafts. A subset of individuals is identified where the tibial vessels are also extensively diseased but the dorsal pedal artery was spared. Vein bypass grafting to the dorsalis pedis artery was found to be useful in this subset of patients. The standard proximal operations such as aortoiliac and femoropopliteal bypass around the knee joint are same in the diabetic and nondiabetic subjects. In the proximal vessels, synthetic grafts are preferred because the veins cannot match the size of the large vessels. The inflow vessel (Iliac) lesions are more often subjected to the angioplasty with or without femoropopliteal bypass. The results of angioplasty are encouraging. The long stenotic lesions or occlusions of the femoropopliteal artery above the knee are bypassed with saphenous vein and simulta-neously the blocked tibial vessel is also bypassed if there is critical ischemia distally in the foot or toes. An ideal graft for bypass in the legs is an autogenous vein.

Graft Material for the Bypass Operations

The superiority of the autologous vein graft has been repeatedly documented in the vascular surgical literature.[29] Great saphenous vein is the longest vein in the body. The typical saphenous vein anatomy is seen only in 38.2% of patients in a venography study done by Shah and his group from Albany, USA.[30] The saphenous vein can be absent (4%), may be duplicated with other anomalies. The valves in the saphenous vein are usually bicuspid. Usually, there are six valves but there can be as many 13 valves in the great saphenous vein. The harvested saphenous vein is reversed and used as the bypass conduit. The diameter of the vein should be at least 4 mm to be considered for the femoropopliteal arterial bypass. *In-situ* saphenous bypass is found to be more suitable for the distal bypass as the smaller distal diameter of the vein matches diameter of the artery to which it is going be anastomosed. The results of *in-situ* saphenous vein bypass are as good as reversed saphenous vein. If the ipsilateral saphenous vein is not available contralateral vein graft is harvested for the bypass. If the veins are not available due to their utilization in coronary artery bypass grafting arm veins (cephalic/basilic veins) can be used as the alternative conduits for the bypass. Short saphenous veins can also be used for bypass. Early vein graft thrombosis is prevented by good anastomosis, preparation of vein graft with minimal trauma and irrigating it with substances such as heparin, papaverine and sodium nitroprusside. In the long-term follow-up, the veins used for the bypass also show atherosclerotic plaque formation, aneurysmal dilatation and discrete stenosis.[31] Long-term patency of the vein grafts is better than the synthetic in above or below the knee bypass operations. In few studies, the outcome with the ePTFE grafts and vein grafts were compared. In Indian practice whenever a suitable vein graft is available, it is first considered as it is cost-effective to the patient as well. Infrapopliteal arterial reconstructions for limb salvage are no longer regarded as controversial procedures. The overall functional results seem to be superior to those attained with lumbar sympathectomy or major amputations. Moreover recent data demonstrated that bypasses to infrapopliteal arteries when performed with short vein grafts can generate acceptable limb salvage despite the presence of poor angiographic runoff, high outflow resistance, or both.

Women with Diabetes and Peripheral Arterial Disease

The Framingham study has showed that the diabetes is powerful risk factor for atherosclerotic coronary and peripheral arterial disease independent of other risk factors and this risk seems to be slightly more in women.[32] Ischemic foot problems in diabetic women due to peripheral arterial disease need special attention because they are at high-risk of amputation. Type 2 diabetes mellitus is a well-established risk factor for coronary heart disease (CHD) in men. It is now well known that diabetic women are also at high-risk of cardiovascular disease.

The hyperglycemic status in diabetes eliminates the usual female (hormonal) advantage for coronary vascular mortality. The incidence of peripheral vascular events in women with diabetes and coronary heart disease is also higher than that in the nondiabetic women. The annual age and sex adjusted rate of lower extremity procedures such as peripheral angioplasty, bypass surgery, and amputation was 119 per 100,000 (in the state of Maryland).[33] Thus, individuals with coronary atherosclerosis appear to have a roughly 10-fold increased risk of lower extremity arterial disease requiring revascularization or amputation.[34]

Amputations and Survival in Patients with Peripheral Vascular Disease and Diabetes

Patients with nonreconstructable vascular disease are treated with supervised exercise therapy and anti-platelet drugs/anticoagulants. If there is no response to medication or when there is progression of the symptoms such as rest pain, ulcerations or gangrene, we need to consider amputation. Diabetic men and women have a 10.3 and 13.8 fold higher risk for the lower limb amputation (Siitonen et al, 1993).[33] They studied the Finnish population and noted men 349/100,000 and women 239.4/100,000 are undergoing lower limb amputations due to diabetes and peripheral vascular disease after excluding the other causes for amputations.[33]

Mean survival of the patients with peripheral arterial disease and diabetes after amputation also depends on many factors. The level of amputation is one of the important indicators of long-term survival after amputation. The survival is expected to be worse for higher level amputations. Nicholas T et al[34] have noted that mean survival time after first amputation is not different among the men and women with diabetes. When the analysis was done after adjustment for the level of an amputation (major and minor), the survivals were not different between the diabetic and nondiabetic people and the same was valid for indication of amputation, i.e. infection/ischemia. In the nondiabetic, the postamputation survivals were dependent on the age. The younger nondiabetic patients had better survivals but such a better survival is not particularly observed in the younger patients with diabetes. Ischemia and infection are both important causes for amputation in diabetes but ischemia is more important in the nondiabetic subjects. Redo procedures for avoiding an amputation is often required in diabetic patients. One or more limb revascularization procedures may be needed in peripheral arterial disease patients with diabetes for limb salvage. It was observed that only 14 to 15% of the diabetic and nondiabetic subjects may require multiple vascular procedures for limb salvage.

Therapeutic Footwear in Peripheral Arterial Disease and Diabetes (Figures 63.6 to 63.12)

Nonhealing foot ulcers are usually known to precede the amputations in many diabetic patients. In a study, Pecoraro et al[35] found that 84% of the patients gave history of an ulcer prior to amputation in their practice. So, it was proposed that prevention of ulcerations can lower rate of amputations in these patients. Depending on the clinical findings (Neuropathy, deformity, vasculopathy and past history of ulceration) and the risk of ulceration different categories of patients were identified. They are grouped as 0, 1, 2, 3. Based on the risk of ulceration, corrective footwear is recommended to the individual patients as per the need with the help of a Pedorthist. The initial observations made by Chantefau et al[36] from Germany were encouraging

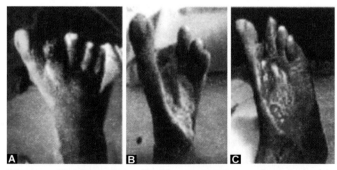

Figures 63.6A and B (A) The appearance of an ischemic wound after debridement of septic focus and amputation of the 2nd toe (B) The appearance of the same wound after bypass to the dorsalis pedis artery in the foot with a saphenous graft from the popliteal artery

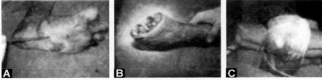

Figures 63.7A to C (A) Neuroischemic—septic foot in a diabetic person free flap (B) Amputation of the forefoot and healthy stump (C) Reconstruction/closure of the stump with a free flap (muscle and skin)

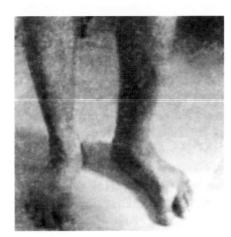

Figure 63.8 Postoperative photograph showing the course of the saphenous vein graft which is function well after femorodistal bypass to the anterior tibial artery in diabetic person for limb. The great toe ulcer after this bypass operation and the rest pain subsided. Patient is able to walk well but there is difficulty in getting suitable footwear for him due to deformity of the foot

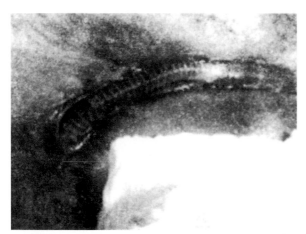

Figure 63.9 Infected synthetic vascular graft (Ringed graft) used the femorofemoral arterial bypass in suprapubic region. Wound cultures showed MRSA infection. The wound healed with after removal of exposed graft under the cover of injection (Vancomycin therapy)

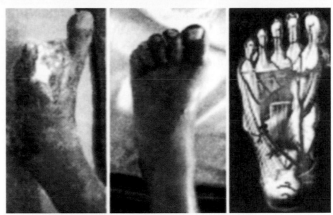

Figure 63.10 Septic foot in a diabetic person

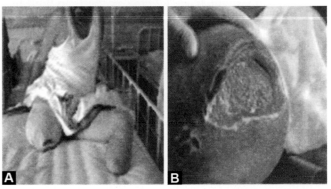

Figures 63.11A and B (A) Bilateral lower limb amputations secondary to nonreconstructable peripheral vascular disease in a diabetic person with ischemic gangrene. Right side above knee amputation and on left side below knee amputation was done. This patient also has non end-stage renal disease with raised creatinine level (2 mg%). (B) Nonhealing above knee stump after amputation with necrotic margins

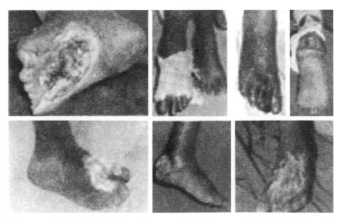

Figure 63.12 Peripheral vascular disease limbs in diabetic patients presenting with the septic complications. Peripheral vascular disease is an important component of the diabetic foot disease and increases morbidity and amputation risk

though some reviews raised their concerns about the results as groups of patients studied belonged to different categories. Edmonds et al followed their patients using the therapeutic footwear for 2.2 years (the compliant and noncompliant) patients with neuropathy and ischemia. The incidence of ulceration was significant in both groups of patients who have not used the prescribed shoes. Twenty-eight patients developed ulcers in special footwear group and 83 patients from the noncompliant group developed ulcerations in this study. Later similar findings were also note in the Dargis et al, (1999).[37] Uccioli et al[38] had similar findings in their studies with the use of the footwear in diabetic population. Ill-fitting shoes are known to precipitate the ulcerations. It was found that 88% women in USA wear chappals/shoes which are 1.2 cm smaller than their feet (Frey et al, 1993).[39] On the contrary in some countries, we see that many people do not wear chappals regularly or are using only Hawai slippers. Most of the middle-aged Indian women do not go for shoes. The tight-fitting small shoes can increase the foot pressures above 120 N/cm^2 and increased the risk of ulcerations. Young et al found that when the foot pressures are less than

112 N/cm^2. Ulceration was not seen in their patients. Similarly, patients wearing the shoes with heels are also at great risk of ulceration due to misdistribution of foot pressure. If the height of the shoe heel is more than 1.9 cm, then foot pressures will increase by 22%, 5 cm heel can produce 57% increase in the foot pressure and when the heel is above 8.3 cm, then the foot pressures increase by 76%. It is probably better for the diabetic patients with neuropathy and vasculopathy not to choose the fancy shoes with high heels.

Peripheral vascular disease in association with the other factors in diabetic person as shown in **Flow Chart 63.1**.

The risk of macrovascular disease in persons with diabetes is greater for any given risk factor, alone or in combination, then it is in persons without diabetes, and the therapeutic benefit of treating macrovascular risk factors in persons with diabetes appears to be at least equal to that seen in persons without diabetes. Given that the incidence of this disease is higher in those with diabetes, the absolute benefit will be greater. The high incidence of macrovascular disease in persons with diabetes makes it more likely that vascular specialists

Flow Chart 63.1 Peripheral vascular disease in association with the other factors in diabetic person

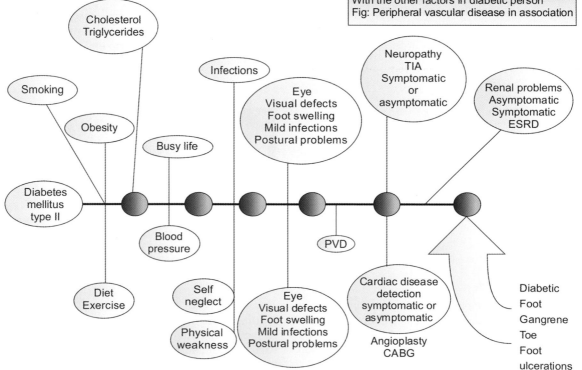

(cardiologist, vascular surgeon and angiologist) will often see a patient with diabetes. Thus, from a public health point of view they should have the opportunity to provide benefit to people with diabetes both by intervening in the development of cardiovascular disease by treating diabetes and other risk factors. The data provided here suggest that diabetes has similar proportional effects on disease risk in Eastern and Western populations and in men and women but is more strongly related to disease risk in younger than older individuals. This is of particular relevance to some developing countries, since the average age at which people suffer major cardiovascular events in such countries is much lower than that in higher-income countries.[40] Taken together with the evidence of rapidly increasing numbers of people with diabetes in countries such as India and China, the findings from this project suggest that unless preventive action is taken, the absolute impact of diabetes on the health of the populations of Asia will be enormous.

REFERENCES

1. Murabito JM, D'Agostino RB, Silbershatz H, Wilson WF. Intermittent claudication: a risk profile from the Framingham Heart Study. Circulation. 1997;96:44-9.
2. Hiatt WR. Medical treatment of peripheral arterial disease and claudication. N Engl J Med. 2001;344:1608-21.
3. Melton LJ, Macken KM, Palumbo PJ, Elveback LR. Incidence and prevalence of clinical peripheral vascular disease in a population-based cohort of diabetic patients. Diabetes care. 1980;3(6):650-4.
4. National diabetes fact sheet. National estimates and general information on diabetes in the United States. Atlanta GA: US Department of Health and Human Services, Centers for Disease Control and Prevention, 1997.
5. Beach KW, Bedford GR, Bergelin RO, Martin DC, Vandenberghe N, Zaccardi M, Strandness DE Jr. Progression of lower- extremity arterial occlusive disease in type II diabetes mellitus. Diabetes care. 1988;11:464-72.
6. Belch JJ, Topol EJ, Agnelli G, Bertrand M, Califf RM, Clement DL, Creager MA, Easton JD, Gavin JR 3rd, Greenland P, Hankey G, Hanrath P, Hirsch AT, Meyer J, Smith SC, Sullivan F, Weber MA. Critical issues in peripheral arterial disease and Management: a call to action. Arch Intern Med. 2003;163(8):884-92.
7. Elhadd TA, Robb R, Jung RT, et al. Pilot study of prevalence asymptomatic peripheral arterial occlusive disease in patients with diabetes attending a hospital clinic. Practical Diabetes Int. 1999;16:163-6.
8. Hirsch AT, Criqui MH, Treat-Jacobson D, Regensteiner JG, Creager MA, Olin JW, Krook SH, Hunninghake DB, Comerota AJ, Walsh ME, McDermott MM, Hiatt WR. PAD detection, awareness and treatment in the primary care. JAMA. 2001;286:1317-24.
9. Weitz JL, Byrne J, Clagett GP, Farkouh ME, Porter JM, Sackett DL, Strandness DE Jr, Taylor LM. Diagnosis and treatment of chronic arterial insufficiency of lower extremities: a critical review. Circulation. 1996;94:3026-49.
10. Hooi JD, stoffers HE, Kester AD, Rinkens PE, Kaiser V, van Ree JW, Knottnerus JA Risk factors and cardiovascular diseases associated with asymptomatic peripheral arterial occlusive disease: the Limburg peripheral arterial occlusive disease (PAOD) study. Scan J Prim Health Care. 1998;16:177-82.
11. Dormandy JA, Rutherford RB for the Transatlantic Inter Society Consensus (TASC) working group. Management of peripheral arterial diseases (PADs). J Vase Surg. 2000;31:S1-296.
12. Bernstein EF, Fronek A. Current status of noninvasive tests in the peripheral arterial disease. Surg Clin North Am. 1982;62:473-87.
13. Newman AB, Sisovick DS, Manolio TA, Polak J, Fried LP, Borhani NO, Wolfson SK. Ankle-arm index as a marker of atherosclerosis in the Cardiovascular Health Study. Circulation. 1993;88:837-45.
14. United Kingdom Prospective Diabetes Study (UKPDS) group. Tight blood pressure control and risk of macrovascular and microvascular complications type 2 diabetes (UKPDS 38). BMJ. 1998;317:703-13.
15. Yusuf S, Sleight P, Pogue J, Bosch J, Davies R, Dagenais G. Effects of an angiotensin converting enzyme inhibitor, ramipril on cardiovascular events in high-risk patients: the Heart Outcomes Prevention Evaluation Study Investigators. N Engl J Med. 2000;342:11553.
16. Centers for Disease Control and Prevention. National Diabetes Fact Sheet: General Information and National Estimates on Diabetes in the United States, 2000. Atlanta, GA: US Department of Health and Human Services, Centers for Disease Control and Prevention, 2002.
17. Ridker PM, Cushman M, Stampfer MJ, Tracy RP, Hennekens CH. Plasma concentration of C-reactive protein and risk of developing peripheral vascular disease. Circulation. 1988;97:425-28.
18. Vu JD, Vu JB, Pio JR, Malik S, Franklin SS, Chen RS, Wong ND. Impact of C-reactive protein on the likelihood of peripheral arterial disease in United States adults with the metabolic syndrome, diabetes mellitus and preexisting cardiovascular disease. Am J Cardiol. 2005;96(5):655-8.
19. Linneman B, Viogt W, Nobel W, Janka HU. C-reactive protein is a strong independent predictor of death in type 2 diabetes: association with multiple facets of metabolic syndrome. Exp Clin Endocrinol Diabetes. 2006;114:127-34.
20. Larsen OA, Lassen NA. Effect of daily muscular exercise in patients with intermittent claudication. Lancet. 1966;2:1093-96.
21. Boyie JP, Honeycutt AA, Narayan KM, Hoerger TJ, Geiss LS, Chen H, Thompson TJ. Projection of diabetes burden through 2050: impact of changing demography and disease prevalence in the US. Diabetes Care. 2001;24:1936-40.
22. Beckman JA, Creager MA, Libby P. Diabetes and athero-sclerosis: epidemiology, pathophysiology and management. JAMA. 2002;287:2570-81.
23. The Joint National Committee on Detection, Evaluation, and Treatment of High Blood Pressure: the sixth Report of the Joint National Committee on Detection, Evaluation, and Treatment of High Blood Pressure. Arch Intern Med. 1997;157:2413-46.

24. Lassile R, lepartalo M. Cigarette smoking and the outcome after lower limb arterial surgery. Acta Chir Scand. 1988;154:635-40.

25. Randomized trial of cholesterol lowering in 4444 patients with coronary heart disease: the Scandinavian simvastatin survival study (4S). Lancet. 1994;344:1383-9.

26. Williamson JR, Tilton RG, Chang K, Kilo C. Basement membrane abnormalities in diabetes mellitus: relationship to clinical microangiopathy. Diabetes Metab Rev. 1988;4:339-70.

27. Tannenbaum GA, Pompselli FB Jr, Marcacdo EJ, Gibbons GW, Campbell DR, Freeman DV, Miller A, LoGerfo FW. Safety of vein bypass grafting to the dorsal pedal artery in diabetic patients with foot infections. J Vase Surg. 1992;15:982-88.

28. LoGerfo FW, Coffman JD. Current concepts. Vascular and microvascular disease of the foot in diabetes. Implications for foot care. N Engl J Med. 1984;311:1615-9.

29. Taylor LM Jr, Edwards JM, Porter JM. Present status of reversed vein bypass grafting: five-year results of modern series. J Vase Surg. 1990;11:193-206.

30. Shah DM, Chang BB, Leopold PW, Corson JD, Leather RP, Karmody AM. The anatomy of the greater saphenous venous vein. J Vase Surg. 1986;3:273-83.

31. Szilagyi DE, Elliott JP, Hageman JH, Smith RF, Dall"Olmo CA. Biological fate of autogenous vein implants as arterial substitutes. Ann Surg. 1973;178:232-44.

32. Ruderman N, Haudenschild C. Diabetes an atherogenic factor. Prog Cardiovasc Dis. 1984;26:373-412.

33. Siitonen OI, Niskanen LK, Laakso M, Siitonen JT, Pyorala K. Lower extremity amputations in diabetic and nondiabetic patients. Diabetes Care. 1993;16(1):16-20.

34. Nicholas T, Sameer ALS, Michael GW, Boulton AJM, Edward BJ. Mortality in diabetic and nondiabetic patients after amputations performed from 1990 to 1995. A 5-year follow-up study. Diabetes Care. 2004;27:1598-604.

35. Pecoraro RE, Reiber GE, Burgess EM. Pathways to diabetic limb amputation: basis for prevention. Diabetes Care. 1990;13:513-21.

36. Chantelau E, Haage P. An audit of cushioned diabetic footwear: relation to patient compliance. Diabet Med. 1994;11:14-6.

37. Dargis V, Pantelejeva O, Jonushaite A, Vileikyte L, Boulton AJ. Benefits of a multidisciplinary approach in the management of recurrent diabetic foot ulceration in Lithuania: a prospective study. Diabetes Care. 1999;22(9):1428-31.

38. Uccioli L, Faglia E, Monticone G, Favales F, Durola L, Afdeghi A, et al. Manufactured shoes in the prevention of diabetic foot ulcers. Diabetes Care. 1995;18(10):1376-8.

39. Frey C, Thompson F, Smith J, et al. American orthopedic foot and ankle society women's shoe survey. Foot Ankle. 1993;14:78.

40. Yusuf S, Reddy S, Ounpuu S, Anand S. Global burden of cardiovascular diseases. Part I: general considerations, the epidemiologic transition, risk factors, and impact of urbanisation. Circulation. 2001;104:2746-53.

Chapter 64

DIABETIC FOOT SYNDROME

SP Pendsey

INTRODUCTION

The diabetic foot is often an inching painless surprise that holds in its dark portals a soon raising flood of complications. It is a quiet dread of disability, long stretches of hospitalization, mounting expenses, with the dangling end result of an amputated limb. The phantom limb plays its own cruel joke on the already demoralized psyche. The diabetic foot no wonder is one of the most feared complications of diabetes.

Diabetic foot is one of the commonest complications of diabetes. It is the leading indication for hospital admissions and is associated with prolonged stay. Major limb amputation is the endpoint of foot lesions in diabetics and is therefore the most feared complication of diabetes. It is interesting to note that many of the principles of etiology, treatment and prevention of diabetic foot problems were established by the pioneer work of Paul Brand. He developed his approach while treating plantar wounds in patients with Hansen's disease while working in India.[1]

A classical triad of neuropathy, ischemia, and infection characterizes the diabetic foot. The presence of infection and altered host response because of chronic hyperglycemia rapidly worsens the clinical picture from what appeared trivial just the other day, to one that now is suddenly limb or even life-threatening. Diabetic foot is seldom seen in isolation; it usually accompanies other macro- and microvascular complications of diabetes. It is hence essential to pay due attention to the other systems, renal and cardiovascular in particular, while managing the diabetic foot. Advanced diabetic foot is like a prothrombotic state and it is not uncommon to see a fresh cardiovascular or cerebrovascular event, while managing the diabetic foot.

Quantitative plantar pressure measurements have remarkably changed the understanding of the patho-genesis of foot ulcer. It has also refined the footwear prescription, which is so essential for high-risk feet. Newer antibiotics, recent therapies, and better dressing materials, have improved the clinical course of diabetic foot lesions to some extent. Inconceivably and equally painfully, it is the ignorance, whether on part of the patient or the primary care physician, which has remained the stumbling block in improving the outcome of diabetic foot lesions. Diabetic subjects need to be managed under the care of a multidisciplinary team with expertise in the many facets of care. In some centers in the developed world, it has been possible to reduce the amputation rate by 50%. The intensive application of patient education, prescribing appropriate footwear, multidisciplinary team approach, and the increasing use of infrapopliteal bypass by the vascular surgeons have been the major factors responsible for these improvements. The message concerning the team approach needs to be heard around the world.

In Western world, patient education and use of multidisciplinary team approach for the management and prevention of diabetic foot has resulted in successful reduction of the number of major amputations by 50% as the St Vincent Declaration had stated. In India, the scenario is quite demoralizing mainly because of lack of education, ignorance on the part of primary physicians and diabetic patients, barefoot walking, late reporting after the initial trauma and continued use of tobacco. Considering the current estimate of 35 million diabetics in India, it would not be an exaggeration to state that India might emerge as the country with highest amputations in diabetics in the coming years unless urgent preventive measures are taken.[2]

A well-structured organization with facilities for providing diabetic foot care is essential. For such an approach to be successful, concentrated efforts by all those working with diabetic patients are required. In addition, it is our responsibility to inform national health department of seriousness of the diabetic foot problem. Improvement in outcome is possible, if proper strategies are executed at national level.

EPIDEMIOLOGY

Foot Ulcers

Diabetic foot ulcers are common and estimated to affect 15% of all diabetic individuals during their lifetime.[3] An estimated 85% of amputations are preceded by diabetic foot ulcers.[4] Numerous risk factors for the development of foot ulcers have been suggested, the most important being peripheral sensory neuropathy followed by peripheral vascular disease. The proportion of neuropathic, neuroischemic and purely ischemic lesions in diabetics is 54%, 34% and 10%, respectively.

In India, prevalence of foot ulcers in diabetic patients in clinic population is 3%,[5] which is much lower than reported in the Western world.[6] A possible reasoning for the low prevalence in Indians is younger age and shorter duration of diabetes.

Peripheral Vascular Disease

Peripheral vascular disease (PVD) has been reported to be low among Asians[7-9] ranging between 3 to 6% as against 25 to 45% in Western patients.[10-12] The prevalence of PVD increases with advancing age and is 3.2% below 50 years of age and rises to 55% in those above 80 years of age.[13] Similarly, it also increases with increased duration of diabetes, 15% at 10 years and 45% after 20 years.[3] In India, the number of diabetic patients above the age of 80 years or with the duration of diabetes of more than 30 years is extremely low, thus explaining the low prevalence of PVD in Indian diabetics. In the coming years, with better diabetes care, the longevity of our diabetic patients would significantly increase and it would not be surprising to see an increasing prevalence of PVD in the Indian scene by the next 2 to 3 decades.[9]

Lower Extremity Amputations

Amputation rates in diabetics increase with advancing age and are generally higher in males than females. Racial and ethnic differences in amputation rates have been reported, highest in Pima Indians 24.1 per 100,000 person years and lowest in the diabetics of Asian ethnic origin 3.4 per 100,000 person years while in Caucasians, it is 14.2 per 100,000 person years.[14,15] Various studies have reported that approximately 50% of amputees will undergo second or contralateral amputation (leg)[16,17] within 1 to 3 years. At our center, this has been reported to be 8.92%.[5] Most of the Western studies have reported a high mortality after lower limb amputations ranging between 11 to 41% at 1 year, 20 to 50% at 3 years and 39 to 68% at 5 years.[16,18,19] At our center, it has been observed to be 14.28% at 2 years.[5]

Table 64.1 shows the differences among Western and Indian studies as far as major limb amputation is concerned. The increased mortality, contralateral limb amputation and the frequency of above knee amputations are higher in Western patients mainly because of older age, generalized atherosclerosis, and multisystem

TABLE 64.1	Limb amputation in diabetes—Differences among Western vs Indian experience[5]	
Limb amputation	*Western*	*Indian*
Mean age at amputation	75 years	61.25 years
Mortality at 2 years	50%	14.28%
Contralateral limb amputation at 2 years	30–50%	8.92%
AK: BK amputation	1 : 2	1 : 6
Indications Neuropathic	10%	76.78%
Ischemic	90%	23.21%

TABLE 64.2	Economics of treatment of diabetic foot: Cost of treatment for complete healing (in India)[16]	
Type of lesion	Treatment	Direct cost (US $)
Neuropathic ulcer	Ambulatory	56
Infected neuropathic foot	Ambulatory	165
Advanced diabetic foot	Salvage	1080
Advanced diabetic foot	Limb amputation	960
Advanced diabetic foot	Salvage then amputation	2650
Neuroischemic foot	Bypass	1960

involvement. In Western patients, the commonest indication for major limb amputations is neuroischemic foot. Unfortunately, in Indians the commonest indication, for major limb amputation, is invariably a neuropathic foot with secondary infection mainly because of incorrect or delayed treatment. Majority of the amputations in Indians are avoidable, provided early recognition and prompt and aggressive treatment is executed.

SOCIOECONOMICS

The cost associated with foot ulcers and lower extremity amputations is exorbitant. The mean cost of treatment of diabetic foot ulcers, from diagnosis until healing, in Sweden, in 1990 was US $14,527 including the cost of rehabilitation while that for major amputations was US $73,627.[20]

In India where majority of the patients are not medically insured, the cost involved in the management of diabetic foot is beyond their capacity, although, the cost involved is much less than reported from the Western world **(Table 64.2)**.

CLASSIFICATION

Diabetic foot is mainly classified into two types:

The neuropathic foot, in which neuropathy dominates and the neuroischemic foot, in which occlusive vascular disease is the main factor while neuropathy is present.

Neuropathy leads to fissures, bullae, neuropathic (Charcot) joint, neuropathic edema, and digital necrosis **(Figure 64.1)**. Ischemia leads to pain at rest, ulceration on foot margins **(Figure 64.2)** digital necrosis and gangrene. Differentiating between these entities is essential because their complications are different and

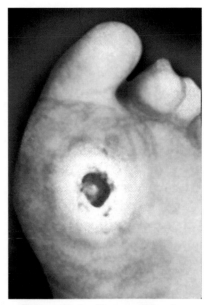

Figure 64.1   Neuropathic ulcer

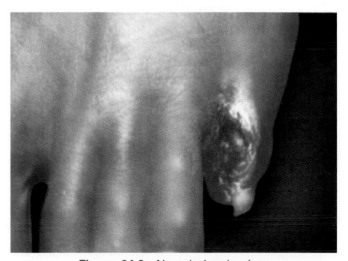

Figure 64.2   Neuroischemic ulcer

TABLE 64.3	Wagner's classification[21]
Grade 0	No ulceration in a high-risk foot
Grade 1	Superficial ulceration
Grade 2	Deep ulceration that penetrates up to tendon, bone or joint
Grade 3	Osteomyelitis or deep abscess
Grade 4	Localized gangrene
Grade 5	Extensive gangrene requiring major amputation

they require different therapeutic strategies. Purely ischemic foot, with no concomitant neuropathy, is rarely seen in diabetic patients and hence the management is same as for the neuroischemic foot. One also sees foot lesions in diabetics without any significant neuropathy or ischemia (Non-neuroischemic foot). Such foot lesions are secondary to trauma and are invariably infected because of underlying, uncontrolled and often undetected diabetes. Another classification (grading) of diabetic foot is known as Wagner's classification[21] is given in **Table 64.3**. It is more specific for neuropathic foot and secondary infection.

PATHOGENESIS

Biomechanics

The majority of foot ulcers in diabetics occurs as a consequence of mechanical trauma unnoticed by the patient due to neuropathy. Commonest sites of ulcerations are in the forefoot. Ulcers occur at sites of high pressure on either plantar or dorsal surfaces and are caused by undue bony prominences, ill-fitting footwear and toe deformities.

Chronic hyperglycemia and polyneuropathy causing damage to sensory, motor and autonomic nerve fibers lead to certain functional and structural changes in the foot. Chronic hyperglycemia leads to nonenzymatic glycosylation of proteins causing limited joint mobility, alteration in the elastic tissues of the plantar skin, and underlying collagen tissue. Foot deformities occur as a result of atrophy of intrinsic muscles of the foot. Further previous scars and toe amputations alter the architecture of the foot. Loss of elasticity, resilience, flexibility and free joint movements lead to a relatively rigid and unstable foot with altered weight-bearing pressure areas. Bony prominences develop underneath the foot pushing the fibro-fatty shock absorbing tissue forward, exposing the condyles of the metatarsal heads. The combination of various risk factors in the presence of

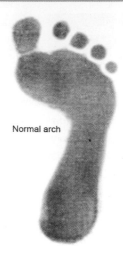

Figure 64.3 Foot impression of a normal weight-bearing foot

neuropathy increases the plantar pressures on the forefoot and hallux significantly thereby increasing the risk of foot ulceration.

Semiquantitative estimation of plantar pressures can be carried out using the inkpad **(Figure 64.3)** on which the patient's foot leaves an impression in different shades. Although, this method is quite specific, it is not very sensitive. Quantitative measurement of plantar pressures is now possible with many devices commercially available. All these require the use of a computer and special software.

For barefoot measurement, the patient walks onto the platform. In this situation, information from a single foot contact is collected. For in-shoe measurement, the matrix of transducers is manufactured into a thin pliable *insole*, which is placed in the shoe in direct contact with the foot. In this case, information from multiple steps can be obtained.

Healthy individuals remain ulcer free not necessarily because they have lower plantar pressures, vulnerable party but because they can feel pain. Studies carried out to measure peak plantar pressures in normal individuals reveal that peak pressure ranges from 50 to 300 kilopascals (kPa) with the lowest measures being on the midfoot region and the highest pressures being on the heel, and on the heads of the first three metatarsals and the hallux. Various studies in patients with diabetic neuropathy have revealed that peak plantar pressures are increased two to three folds. Elevated plantar pressure is now accepted as a major factor in the pathogenesis of plantar ulcers in diabetic subjects. Plantar pressure can identify areas of high pressure unsuspected on clinical examination and in-shoe measurement can refine the process of footwear prescription by defining the exact degree of pressure relief at high-risk areas.[22]

Neuropathic Foot

Neuropathic foot ulcerations result from two or more risk factors occurring together. In diabetic polyneuropathy (sensory, motor and autonomic), which leaves the foot with loss of protective sensations (LOPS), any damaging feelers or external injury is either less perceived or is not at all, resulting in an ulcer. Sensory neuropathy is the most important pre-requisite for foot ulcerations. All the other factors contribute to foot ulceration only in the presence of sensory neuropathy. Motor neuropathy results in atrophy and weakness of the intrinsic muscles of the foot (intrinsic minus foot), leads in clawed toes and abnormal walking pattern. The fibrofatty tissues which act like cushions for metatarsal heads (metatarsal cushions), are pushed forward due to deformities, leading to an increased pressure on the metatarsal heads. Autonomic neuropathy results in reduced or absent sweating causing plantar xerosis with cracks and fissures. Limited joint mobility, foot deformities and abnormal gait result in an altered biomechanical loading of the foot with elevated plantar pressures and probably increased shear forces. Loss of protective sensations coupled with the repetitive trauma on walking, in presence of raised plantar pressures, results in formation of plantar callus. Growth of plantar callus further increases the local skin pressure as it works as a foreign body on the skin surface. Neuropathic foot ulceration results from factors extrinsic the insensitive foot such as an external trauma, often together with intrinsic factors such as an increased plantar pressure. Plantar ulcers do not occur overnight but are a result of repetitive stress of walking and abnormal weight-bearing, resulting in chronic tissue damage.

Sensory, autonomic and motor neuropathy, contribute to the pathogenesis of neuropathic foot. Motor neuropathy leads to atrophy of the small muscles of the foot, with an imbalance between flexors and extensors. These changes result in clawing of the toes, prominent metatarsal heads and forward migration of the fibrofatty pads. As a result, high pressure develops under the metatarsal heads, both during standing and walking. High foot pressure combined with dry, brittle skin (a result of autonomic neuropathy) leads to callus formation, which acts as a foreign body and can cause tissue damage and foot ulceration **(Flow chart 64.1)**.[23]

TABLE 64.4	Factors contributing to foot ulceration[6]
Intrinsic factors	*Extrinsic factors*
Bony prominences	Inappropriate footwear
Limited joint mobility	Walking barefoot
Joint deformity	Falls and accidents
Callus	Objects inside shoes
Altered tissue properties	Activity level
Previous foot surgery	
Neuro-osteoarthropathic joint	

The nonenzymatic glycosylation of collagen leads to stiffness of the ligaments and is associated with restrictions in the range of motions of the joints of foot and ankle (limited joint mobility; LJM) leading to increased plantar pressures.[24] The development of sensory neuropathy with reduced or absent pain leads to susceptibility to trauma and development of ulcer. **Table 64.4** shows the extrinsic and intrinsic factors contributing to foot ulceration.

Charcot Foot

A Charcot joint or neuroarthropathy is defined as a relatively painless progressive arthropathy of single or multiple joints caused by an underlying neuropathy. The most frequent location of the neuropathic joint is the tarsometatarsal region followed by the metatarsophalangeal joints and the ankle and the subtalar joints.[25] The initial presentation is often a hot swollen foot, the precipitating event usually being a minor trauma.

The process of destruction takes place over a few months and leads to two classic deformities, the rocker-bottom deformity in which there is displacement and subluxation of the tarsus downwards and the medial convexity, which results from displacement of the talonavicular joint or from tarsometatarsal dislocation. If these deformities are not accommodated in properly fitting footwear, ulceration at vulnerable pressure points often develops. The pathophysiology of the Charcot foot is not well understood. Increased blood flow, possibly associated with autonomic neuropathy and increased osteoclastic activity are the two possible mechanisms responsible for the bony resorption in early phase.[26]

Pathogenesis

Multiple factors appear to contribute to the development of the Charcot foot. A peripheral neuropathy with loss of protective sensation, an autonomic neuropathy with increased blood flow to the bone, and mechanical trauma, has emerged as the most important

Flow chart 64.1 Schematic presentation of pathogenesis of diabetic foot ulcer

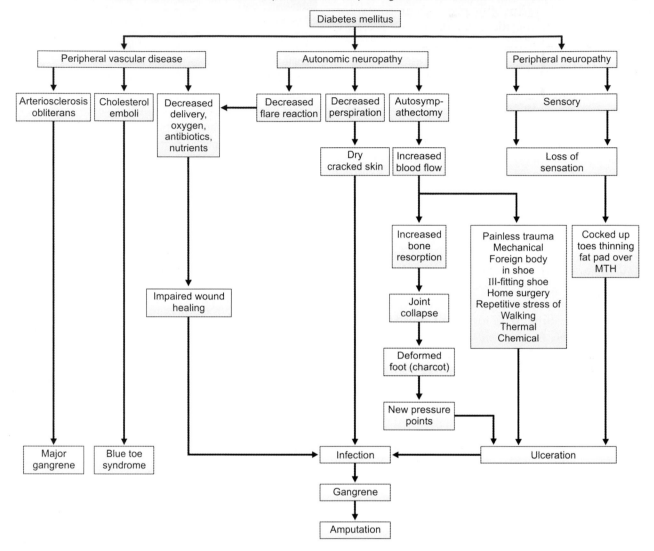

determinants. Basically, there is an increase in osteo-clastic (bone resorption) activity over an osteoblastic (bone deposition) activity. The autonomic neuropathy leads to an arterial dilatation (sympathetic denervation) and arteriovenous shunting, increasing blood flow which in turn causes bone resorption. The loss of protective pain sensation and presence of uninterrupted physical activity finally make these osteopenic bones susceptible to stress fractures, bone destruction, and collapse of the foot architecture.

Joint involvement: Although any point of the joint of the foot can be involved, the most frequent location of neuroarthropathy is the tarsometatarsal region, followed by metatarsophalangeal joint, the ankle, subtalar, and then the interphalangeal joints.

Radiologically, metatarsals show an atrophy or osteo-lysis of bone, often described as a *sucked candy* and *mortar and pestle* appearance of the metatarsophalangeal (MTP) or interphalangeal (IP) joint. An X-ray foot may reveal fragmentation, fracture, new bone formation, subluxation and dislocation of the joints.

Clinical Presentation

The clinical presentation of Charcot foot can be divided into three phases:
1. Acute onset
2. Bony destruction/deformity
3. Stabilization.

Acute onset: Classically, the Charcot foot at acute onset is hot, erythematous, and swollen with bounding pulses

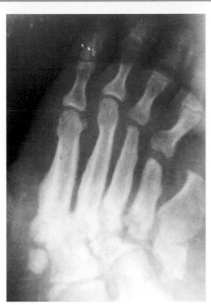

Figure 64.4 X-ray showing fragmentation of bone and dislocation of joints in Charcot foot

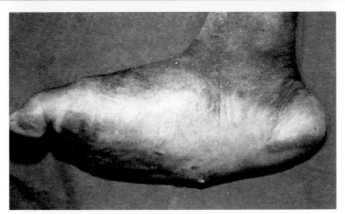

Figure 64.5 Rocker-bottom deformity of Charcot foot

and prominent veins. Usually, the pain or discomfort is minimal due to underlying neuropathy. A history of recent injury often precedes onset of the swelling. It is important to differentiate the acute stage of Charcot foot from cellulitis, as both have a red, hot, and swollen foot. Few differentiating features are: cellulitis is more likely in the presence of an ulcer which may show signs of infection, it is usually associated with fever, raised total leukocyte counts and raised erythrocyte sedimentation rate. An X-ray of the foot may be normal in the acute stage of Charcot. However, technetium diphosphonate bone scan may detect early bone damage.

Bone destruction/deformity: Clinically, the foot is swollen, warm and the medial arch of the foot is usually collapsed. An X-ray reveals fragmentation, fracture, new bone formation, subluxation and dislocation **(Figure 64.4)**. These damages develop very rapidly, within a few weeks of the onset. Classical deformities of the Charcot foot are a rocker-bottom foot **(Figure 64.5)**, with a medial convexity and ankle deformities. Involvement of tarsometatarsal joints leads to altered shape of the foot. The midfoot appears broad with the medial arch collapsed. Involvement of MTP and IP joint lead to deformities of the toes and the ankle joint involvement leads to a swollen hindfoot and deformities of the ankle.

Foot Infection

Infection in diabetic foot is a limb-threatening condition because the consequences of deep infection in a diabetic foot are more disastrous than elsewhere mainly because of certain anatomical peculiarities. Foot has several compartments which are inter communicating and the infection can spread from one into another, lack of pain allows the patient to continue ambulation further facilitating the spread. The foot also has soft tissues that cannot resist infection, like plantar aponeurosis, tendons, muscle sheaths and fascia. A combination of neuropathy, ischemia and hyperglycemia worsens the situation by reducing the defense mechanism.

Nonulcer Pathologies

Bone deformities, nail pathologies and dermatological infections are some of the nonulcer problems. Even a minor lesion can provide a portal of entry for infection and should never be underestimated. Foot deformities may be corrected nonsurgically (orthoses) or by proper footwear. Common bone deformities are hallux valgus, hammer toe, clawing of toes and pes cavus.

Fungal infections can provide a portal of entry for more serious infections. Tinea pedis is seen as macerated lesions with fissuring interdigitally. It should be promptly treated with local as well as systemic antifungal drugs. Infection of the nails (onychomycosis) is also common in diabetics and requires prolonged antifungal treatment.

Nail Deformities

Ingrowing toe-nails, thickening and other deformities of the nails are common in neuropathic and neuro-ischemic feet. Thickened nails can lead to subungual ulcers and deformed nails can traumatize the adjacent soft tissues. All these need to be cared for by regular nail clipping and attended by a podiatrist. Neglected nails may eventually cause damaging trauma to the adjacent parts.

DIAGNOSIS

Neuropathic Foot

It is the chronic sensorimotor and peripheral sympathetic neuropathies that can be assessed by detecting sensation to pinprick and cotton-wool and vibration using 128 Hz tuning forks. Knee and ankle jerks should be examined. It is difficult to examine autonomic nerves, except to note a dry skin with marked fissuring as indicative of a sweating deficit. Arteriovenous shunting which leads to the warm foot with distended dorsal foot veins is also an evidence of autonomic dysfunction. Using a handheld biothesiometer, one can assess vibration threshold. The vibration threshold increases with age and values must be compared with age-adjusted normograms.[21] Using the monofilament, one can assess the protective pain sensation. The filament is applied to the foot until it buckles. Buckling of the 5.07 monofilament occurs at 10 g of linear pressure and is the limit used to detect protective pain sensation.[24]

Sensations should be tested under the 1st, 3rd and 5th metatarsal heads, as well as the dorsal aspects. If the patient does not detect the filament, then protective pain sensation is assumed to be lost. The feet should also be examined for limited joint mobility, clawing of toes, callus formation, bunions, and callosities on the dorsum of foot. Nail changes onychauxis, onychomycoses and interdigital mycoses should be looked for.

Osteomyelitis

Osteomyelitis generally results from contiguous spread from deep soft tissue infection through the cortex to the bone marrow. Majority of the deep long-standing foot infections are associated with osteomyelitis. Diagnosing osteomyelitis in a patient with diabetic foot is often difficult. Major problems include differentiating soft tissue infection from bone infection and infections from noninfectious disorders (Charcot foot). Plain radiography usually shows focal osteopenia, cortical erosions or periosteal reaction in early stage and sequestration in the late stage. Radiographic changes take at least 2 weeks to be evident. Newer techniques like bone scan, computerized tomography (CT) scan, positron emission tomography (PET), magnetic resonance imaging (MRI) are being evaluated of which MRI is said to be more sensitive and specific.[27] A simple clinical test is probing to bone. A sterile metal probe is inserted into the ulcer if it penetrates to the bone it almost confirms the diagnosis of osteomyelitis. Chronic discharging sinus and sausage-like appearance of the toe are the clinical markers of osteomyelitis. Definitive diagnosis requires obtaining bone biopsy for microbial culture and histopathology.

MANAGEMENT

Diabetic foot should be managed using a multidisciplinary team approach. We at our center, involve several members in the team-like:

Podiatrist	Orthotist
Diabetologist	Surgeon
Educator	Nurse
Patient's relative	Primary physician

It is the diabetologist who should be the captain of the team. The motto of this team approach is to save the limb and not amputate it.

Neuropathic Foot

Management principles: It is now well recognized that the primary factor in the cause of diabetic plantar ulcer is the presence of an insensate foot due to neuropathy. This insensitivity allows excessive and prolonged stress and pressures to occur in the diabetic foot, which ultimately results in tissue breakdown. If the tissue breakdown (ulcer) goes unnoticed or untreated, an infection is imminent and major amputation is likely. If the ulceration is the result of an increased plantar pressure, the treatment should focus on reducing this pressure at the ulcer site. This relief of pressure can be achieved mainly by mechanical control (offloading), and by resting the affected foot.

The treatment of neuropathic ulcers involves callus removal, eradication and redistribution of the weight-bearing forces. Callus contributes to high plantar pressure and must be looked for and proper measures taken to prevent, limit and remove it. The removal of callus permits wound drainage and is best achieved using a scalpel. Callus should be removed carefully and evenly. Failure to remove the callus may lead to increased compression of the soft tissues, abscess formation.[28] Ulcers need rest to heal. Immobilization, nonweight-bearing and treatment of infection can achieve this.

Offloading: Ideally, the plantar ulcers must be managed with rest and avoidance of pressure. Total nonweight-bearing (bed rest) is neither practical nor acceptable to most of the patients. Various other methods of offloading are discussed below, in brief:
- *Wheelchair:* A light-weight, folding wheelchair can be of great help in achieving maximal offloading. It

is especially useful, if the ulcers are bilateral or infected.

- *Crutches:* This is an inexpensive and one of the most practical methods of offloading. The greatest advantage is ability to attend work. However, elderly patients and patients with amyotrophy find it difficult to walk with handheld crutches.
- *Walker:* A light-weight metallic, folding walker provides stability and is a good alternative for patients who cannot cope with crutches.
- *Total Contact Cast (TCC):* It is the *gold standard* among various methods used to aid the healing of plantar foot ulcers. The principle of TCC is to equalize loading of the plantar surface by a uniform *total contact* of the plantar surface with the cast material thereby increasing the weight-bearing area and minimizing the pressure at the ulcer site. Plantar pressure studies have shown a reduction in the pressure at the ulcer site with TCC by over 80%. Most of the ulcers heal in approximately 6 weeks.

The ideal indication for TCC is longstanding, nonhealing and noninfected plantar ulcer. The contraindications are infected plantar ulcer, noncompliant patient, ulcer depth greater than its width, swelling of the foot and ABI is 0.5 or less.

Infected Foot

Infection in a diabetic foot is limb-threatening and at times life-threatening and therefore, must be treated aggressively. Superficial infections should be treated with debridement, oral antibiotics and regular dressings. Deep infections are considered, when the signs of infection are combined with an evidence of involvement of deeper tissue structures such as bones, tendons or muscles. Although superficial infections are usually caused by gram-positive bacteria, the deep foot infections are invariably polymicrobial and caused by gram-positive, gram-negative bacteria and anaerobes. All patients with deep infections should be hospitalized and started on broad-spectrum antibiotics. The choice of antibiotics initially should be empirical but once the culture reports are known, it should be specific and narrowed down. Multiple injections of insulin or continuous insulin infusion should be instituted to achieve metabolic control. Patients should be posted for surgical debridement as early as possible (24–36 hours) and necessary medical work-up should be done preoperatively.

Surgical debridement should be carried out in an operation theater. The incision is made over the site of maximum fluctuation or webspace and deepened up to the second layer of the sole, cutting the plantar fascia along the line of flexor tendons till either pus or edema fluid is seen. All the devitalized tissue, sloughed tendons and infected bones should be debrided. If the infection is spreading proximally, an additional incision behind the medial malleolus should be given for better decompression.[29-31] After initial bold decompression, debridement is carried out regularly. Although the objective is to salvage the limb, the decision should be revised in favor of limb amputation, if the patient continues to show signs of worsening of infection and septicemia.

A multidisciplinary approach providing debridement, meticulous wound care, adequate vascular supply, metabolic control, improvement of nutritional status, empirical antimicrobial treatment and nonweight-bearing are the cardinal features in the treatment of infected diabetic foot.

Amputation

Amputation is the endpoint of diabetic foot lesions. Surgeons hate to perform amputation surgery and patients do not like it either. Major amputations result in considerable morbidity and at times even mortality. It leads to permanent disability to the patient. However, in diabetic foot lesions this unfortunate decision has to be taken in order to save the life.

Amputations are divided into minor (up to midtarsal level) and major amputations (above midtarsal level).

Various amputations carried out are toe disarticulation, ray amputation, transmetatarsal amputation, tarsometatarsal disarticulation, mid-tarsal disarticulation, ankle disarticulation, transtibial amputation (BK, below knee), knee disarticulation (TK, through knee), transfemoral amputation (AK, above knee) and hip disarticulation.[6,22]

Minor Amputations

Aggressive treatment of foot infection, better diabetes management and vascular reconstruction procedures have helped in salvaging many limbs, but the number of minor amputations have increased. In an infected foot, it is often necessary to carry out open amputations. To close the amputation wounds primarily, the tissue must be free of infection and well perfused. Skin grafts and reconstructive plastic surgery are often necessary for such open amputations.[22]

Minor amputations are indicated to remove gangrene, e.g. after revascularization for ischemia as part of debridement for foot infection or in the correction of foot deformities.[32]

Although healing may take several months, minor amputations do not compromise significantly the capability of walking except more proximal ones like midtarsal.

Once minor amputation has been performed, the risk for further ulceration is greatly enhanced and a lifelong close surveillance is indicated, with special attention to footwear, which must be modified or custom made in many cases.

Major Amputations

Major amputations are associated with considerable morbidity such as reamputation, and capability of walking as well as a high postoperative mortality. Long-term results show a high-risk of contralateral amputation and increased mortality.[14,18]

Major amputations are indicated in patients with neuroischemic feet where revascularization is not feasible, in advanced infections, in medically compromised patients and occasionally in cases with severe Charcot deformities.

Whenever a major amputation is planned the option of revascularization should be considered first. Glycemic control and nutritional status should be optimized. All the patients who have undergone a major amputation have a high-risk of subsequent contralateral amputation and therefore a surveillance program, for the remaining foot is crucial. Patients, after major amputation, should be referred to prostheses center for appropriate limb prosthesis.

PREVENTION

Preventing the diabetic foot ought to be the first priority. This can be achieved by identifying the high-risk individuals, like those with peripheral neuropathy, peripheral vascular disease, foot deformities, and presence of callus. They should receive intensive foot care education, regular attention by a podiatrist and should be advised proper footwear and insoles. Patients should be reviewed frequently, assessed for neuropathic and neuroischemic lesions and treated as necessary **(Table 64.5)**.

Preventing diabetic foot disease using the multidisciplinary team approach is a noble step in the right direction. However, the concept of a podiatrist and orthotist are as yet not well mooted. These specialties need to be developed urgently. Intensified education of high-risk patients, education of primary physicians and prescribing proper footwear, are essential components of this program.

Preventive Footwear (Characteristics)[22]

The footwear should be light in weight (up to 700 g/pair), nontraumatic and esthetically acceptable to patients.

Outsole: Shoes with a soft outsole bend easily and are not able to stabilize the foot while walking. Rigid soles absorb shock and reduce vertical pressure. The outsole should be tough to prevent penetrating injuries from sharp objects. It should be serrated as smooth outsoles are slippery. The heel should not be higher than 2 inches (5 cm). High heels increase pressure over forefoot.

Shoe size: It is extremely important to have a proper sized shoe. Patients with insensate feet tend to wear tight shoes, as they do not feel any discomfort. In loose shoes the foot slides, increasing the shear stress. Length of a shoe should allow ½ inch (1.25 cm) between the end of the shoe and the longest toe and can be measured using an appropriate device. The foot is widest at the first metatarsophalangeal joint and should match with the widest part of the shoe. Shoe size mentioned on the shoe varies among brands and styles.

Counter: The counter controls the heel and determines its fitting inside the shoe.

Shoes with laces or Velcro: Shoes should be fastened with laces or Velcro, to allow adjustability needed for edema

TABLE 64.5	Risk categorization system[6]	
Category	*Risk profile*	*Check-up frequency*
0	No sensory neuropathy	Once a year
1	Sensory neuropathy	Once every 6 months
2	Sensory neuropathy with signs of peripheral vascular disease and/or foot deformities	Once every 3 months
3	Previous ulcer/amputation	Once every 1–3 months

or deformities and allow the shoe to fit properly without the danger of it slipping off. Slip-on shoes may better be avoided.

Depth of the shoe: Footwear should have an extra depth to accommodate dorsal deformities and removable insoles.

Toe box: A rounded and high toe box is essential to accommodate dorsal deformities (clawed toes, hammer toes). A shoe with a narrow or tapered toe box aggravates friction and deformities like hallux valgus and rigid toecap causes toe compression.

Uppers: The uppers should have a soft inner lining to prevent friction injuries, like bunions. Uppers can also be made of elastic or a soft and flexible material instead of leather.

Insoles: Insoles give cushioning to the feet and allow distribution of plantar pressure; they also act like a shock absorber. They should be inserted inside the shoe without making the shoe too tight. They are made of microcellular rubber, ethyl-vinyl-acetate or polyethylene foam (Plastazote). Insoles wear out (bottoming out) and therefore need to be replaced periodically (3 to 6 months).

Dressing Material

Conventional dressings, such as gauze, impregnated gauze, gauze and cotton, packing strips have been in use for fifty years. Moist wound environment that these dressings provide are best for wound regeneration and repair and increasing the velocity of healing. Effective wound management aims to strike a balance, i.e. a moist environment to promote healing, but not so wet as to cause maceration and excoriation.

Two factors are important for natural wound healing. One is wound exudates, which is the generic term given to the liquid produced from wounds. Exudate keeps the wound moist, supplies nutrients and provides the medium for migration and mitosis of epithelial cells. This in-turn, keeps the wound supplied with leukocytes, helping to control microorganisms. Second factor is the presence of white cells in the wound. White cells play a major role in wound healing by cleaning the wound, removing potentially pathogenic microorganisms and producing collagen, the building block of new tissue. Excessive exudates can cause maceration and hence the dressing should be able to absorb excessive exudates from the wound. The characteristics of an ideal dressing are:

- To remove excess exudates and toxic components
- To maintain high humidity in the wound
- To allow gaseous exchange
- To provide thermal insulation
- To provide protection from secondary infection
- To allow removal without trauma at dressing change
- To be free from particulate and toxic components.

Newer Dressings

A wide variety of new dressing materials have been developed. However, none of the newer dressings fulfill all the characteristics of an ideal dressing.

Some of the newer dressings are film dressing, foam dressing, nonadherent dressings, hydrogels, hydrocolloids and alginates.

The treating foot care team has to make appropriate choice of dressing for a particular type of wound. It is important to note that there is a wide range of performance parameters within and between various types of newer dressings. Although no dressing fulfills all the characteristics of an ideal dressing, important factors to consider include user friendliness, cost effectiveness and ability to maintain a moist wound environment.

Newer Therapies

Wound healing is the process by which tissues respond to an injury. The process of wound healing is controlled by growth factors that initiate cell growth and proliferation by binding to specific high-affinity receptors on the cell surface. Growth factors (GF) have the ability to stimulate the mitosis of quiescent cells. Platelets, macrophages, epithelial cells, fibroblasts and endothelial cells produce GF. The growth factors most commonly involved in wound healing include platelet-derived growth factor (PDGF), fibroblast growth factor (FGF), epidermal growth factor (EGF) and insulin-like growth factor (IGF). Newer therapies provide various growth factors topically to promote and hasten wound healing.

Platelet-derived Growth Factors

The only topical growth factor that has shown convincing results to stimulate healing of chronic neuropathic diabetic ulcers is platelet-derived growth factor (PDGF-BB; becaplermin). Recombinant human PDGF-BB gel preparation is used for noninfected neuropathic ulcers. The gel preparation is spread over the wound and covered with nonadherent saline-soaked gauze dressing. The dressing changes once or twice every day. It has to be realized that this gel therapy is effective only, if other modalities like recurrent surgical debridement of ulcer and offloading are adhered to. The limitation of its generous use is prohibitive cost. However, recently, it has been made available in India, at one-tenth cost (Plermin).

Dermagraft

It is bioengineered human dermis designed to replace a patient's own damaged or destroyed dermis. It consists of neonatal dermal fibroblasts cultured *in vitro* on a bioabsorbable polyglactin mesh. Fibroblasts are screened extensively for infectious agents before they are cultured. As the fibroblasts proliferate within the mesh, they secrete human dermal collagen, fibronectin, growth factors and other proteins, embedding themselves into a self-produced dermal matrix. This results in a living, metabolically active dermal tissue with the structure of a papillary dermis of newborn skin.

Apligraf

Like human skin, Apligraf consists of living skin cells and structural protein. The lower dermal layer combines bovine type 1 collagen and human fibroblasts (dermal cells), which produce additional matrix proteins. The upper epidermal layer is formed by prompting human keratinocytes (epidermal cells), first to multiply and then to differentiate and replicate the architecture of the human epidermis.

Granulocyte Colony-Stimulating Factor

It is an endogenous hemopoietic growth factor that induces terminal differentiation and release of neutrophils from the bone marrow. Endogenous concentrations of granulocyte colony-stimulating factor (G-CSF) rise during bacterial sepsis, suggesting its role in the neutrophil response to infection. G-CSF improves function in both normal and dysfunctional neutrophils. Since, diabetes represents an immunocompromised state secondary to neutrophil dysfunction, the effect of recombinant human G-CSF (filgrastim) has been tried in diabetic foot infections. It is administered as a daily subcutaneous injection for one week.

G-CSF therapy has been shown to be associated with earlier eradication of pathogens from infected ulcers, quicker resolution of cellulitis, shorter hospital stay and shorter duration of intravenous antibiotic treatment. G-CSF therapy was seen to be associated with leukocytosis, due almost entirely to an increase in neutrophil count. Thus, G-CSF may be an important adjunct to conventional therapy.

Hyaff

It is an ester of hyaluronic acid, which is a major component of the extracellular matrix. It facilitates growth and movement of fibroblasts and in contact with wound exudates, produces a hyaluronic gel, which covers the wound and promotes granulation and healing. It has been found to be effective in neuropathic foot ulcers, especially with sinuses.

Although newer therapies have shown some promising results in promoting and hastening wound healing of noninfected plantar neuropathic ulcers, they are no substitute to the fundamental principles of management of plantar ulcers like offloading, pressure relief and callus removal.

The management of foot problem in diabetes has been updated by Michael et al.[33,34]

SUMMARY

A classical triad of neuropathy, ischemia, and infection characterizes the diabetic foot. The presence of infection and altered host response because of chronic hyperglycemia rapidly worsens the clinical picture from what appeared trivial just the other day, to be one that is suddenly limb or even life-threatening.

In Western world, patient education and use of multidisciplinary team approach for the management and prevention of diabetic foot has resulted in successful reduction of the number of major amputations by 50% as per the mandate of the St Vincent Declaration. In India, the scenario is quite demoralizing mainly because of lack of patient education, ignorance on the part of primary physicians, barefoot walking, late reporting after the initial trauma and continued use of tobacco. Considering the current estimate of 35 million diabetics in India, it would not be an exaggeration to state that India might emerge as the country with highest amputations in diabetic subjects in the coming years unless extensive preventive measures are taken.

Preventing diabetic foot should be managed using a multidisciplinary team approach. The motto of this team approach is to save the limb and amputate it in case of dire necessity.

Preventing diabetic foot should be the first priority. This can be achieved by identifying the high-risk individuals, like those with peripheral neuropathy, peripheral vascular disease, foot deformities and the presence of callus.

Although newer therapies have shown some promising results in promoting and hastening wound healing of noninfected plantar neuropathic ulcers, they are no substitute to the fundamental principles of management of plantar ulcers like offloading, pressure relief and callus removal.

REFERENCES

1. Brand PW. Insensate feet: a practical handbook on foot problems in leprosy. London: The Leprosy Mission, 1981.
2. Pendsey SP. Editorial. Int J Diab Dev Countries. 1994;14:35-6.
3. Palumbo PJ, Melton LJ. Peripheral vascular disease and diabetes. In Harris MI, Hamman RF (Eds): Diabetes in America. NIH Pub No 85-1468. Washington: US Government Printing Office; 1985:XVI-21.
4. Pecoraro RE, Reiber GE, Burgess EM. Pathways to diabetic limb amputation: basis for prevention. Diabetes Care. 1990;13:513-21.
5. Pendsey SP. Epidemiological aspects of diabetes foot. Int J Diab Dev Countries. 1994; 14:37-8
6. International Consensus on the Diabetic Foot by the International Working Group on the Diabetic Foot, 1999.
7. Mohan V, Premlatha G, Sastry NG. Peripheral vascular disease in noninsulin-dependent diabetes mellitus in South India. Diab Res Clin Pract. 1995;27:235-40.
8. DeSilva D. The prevalence of macrovascular disease and lipid abnormalities amongst diabetic patients in Sri Lanka. Postgrad Med J. 1993;69:557-61.
9. Pendsey SP. Peripheral vascular disease (PVD): an Indian Scenario. Dibetologia Croatia. 1998;27(4):153-6.
10. Migdalis IN, Kourti A, Zachariadis D, Samartzis M. Peripheral vascular disease in newly diagnosed noninsulin-dependent diabetes. Int Angiol. 1992;11:230-2.
11. Marinelli MR, Beach KW, Glass MJ, et al. Non-invasive testing vs clinical evaluation of arterial disease: a prospective study. J Am Med Assoc. 1979;241:2031-4.
12. Walters DP, Gatling W, Mullee MA, Hill RD. The prevalence, detection and epidemiological correlates of peripheral vascular disease: a comparison of diabetic and nondiabetic subjects in an English Community. Diab Med. 1992;9:710-5.
13. Janka HU, Standl E, Mehnert H. Peripheral vascular disease in diabetes mellitus and its relation to cardiovascular risk factors: screening with Doppler ultrasonic technique. Diabetes Care. 1980;3:207.
14. Nelson RG. Lower extremity amputations in NIDDM: 12-year follow-up study in Pima Indians. Diabetes Care. 1988;11:8-16.
15. Gujral JS, McNally PB, Burden AC. Ethnic differences in the incidence of lower extremity amputation secondary to diabetes mellitus. Diabetic Med. 1993;10:271-4.
16. Pendsey SP. Indian Scenario: the diabetic foot in complications of diabetes in Indian Scenario; Nidus 99 Diabetology Initiative in Diabetology: Proceedings; 1, 3.
17. Ebskov B, Josephson P. Incidence of reamputation and death after gangrene of the lower extremity. Prosthetics and Orthotics International. 1980;4:77-80.
18. Silbert S. Amputation of the lower extremity in diabetes mellitus. Diabetes. 1952;1:297-9.
19. Lee JS, Lu M, Lee VS, Russel D, Bahr C, Lee ET. Lower extremity amputation: incidence, risk factors and mortality in the Oklahoma Indian Diabetes Study. Diabetes. Study. Diabetes. 1993;42:876-82.
20. Apelqvist J, Ragnarson-Tennall G, Persson U, Larsson J. Diabetic foot ulcers in a multidisciplinary setting: an economic analysis of primary healing and healing with amputation. J Int Med. 1994;235:463-71.
21. Wagner EW. The dysvascular foot: a system for diagnosis and treatment. Foot Ankle. 1981;2:64-7.
22. Pendsey SP. Diabetic foot: a clinical atlas. New Delhi: Jaypee Brothers Medical Publishers, 2003.
23. Levin ME. Pathogenesis and management of diabetic foot lesions. In Levin ME, O'Neal LW, Bowker JH (Eds): The diabetic foot, 5th edn. St Louis: Mosby Year Book; 1993.
24. Boulton AJM. The pathogenesis of diabetic foot problems: an overview. Diabetic Med. 1996;13(suppl 1):512-6.
25. Sanders LJ, Frykberg RG. Diabetic neuropathic osteoarthropathy: the Charcot foot. In Frykberg RG (Ed): The high-risk foot in diabetes. New York: Churchill Livingstone 1991; pp. 227-38.
26. Klenerman L. The Charcot joint in diabetes. Diabetes Medicine 1996;13:S52-4.
27. Yuh WTC, Corson JD, Baraniewski HM, et al. Osteomyelitis of the foot in diabetic patients: evaluation with plain film, Tc-MDP bone scintigraphy and MR imaging. AJR. 1989;152:795-800.
28. Young MJ, Cavanagh PR, Thomas G, et al. The effect of callus removal on dynamic plantar foot pressures in diabetic patients. Diabetic Medicine. 1992;9:55-7.
29. Pendsey SP. Preventing the diabetic foot. In Kapur A, Thakur S (Eds): Proceedings of the Sixth Novo Nordisk Diabetes Update. 1997;27:55-61.
30. Pendsey SP. The diabetic foot and gangrene, in practical management of diabetes. Pendsey SP (Ed). New Delhi: Jaypee Brothers Medical Publishers. 1997;21:119-29.
31. Murali NS. Limb conservation in severe diabetic foot infection: a new technique. Int J Diab Dev Countries. 1994;14:55-9.
32. Albrechtsen SB, Henriksen BM, Holstein P. Minor amputations after revascularization for gangrene. Acta Orthop Scand. 1997;68(3):291-3.
33. Michael E Edmonds, Alethea VM Foster (Eds). Managing the Diabetic Foot. Blackwell Science 2000; pp.123-5.
34. Michael E Edmonds. New Treatments for Diabetic Foot Ulcers. In Andrew JM Boulton, Henry Connor, Peter R Cavanagh (Eds): the Foot in Diabetes. Wiley and Sons 2000; pp.179-84.

Chapter 65

PATHOGENESIS OF DIABETIC MICROVASCULAR COMPLICATIONS

Vijay Viswanathan

CHAPTER OUTLINE

- Introduction
- Morphologic Features
- Mechanisms of Hyperglycemia-induced Damage
- Summary

INTRODUCTION

Diabetes mellitus is associated with numerous long-term clinical complications that contribute to the increased morbidity and mortality from the disease despite the available measures for metabolic control.[1, 2] These complications may be divided into macrovascular complications, which include coronary artery, cerebral vascular and peripheral vascular disease; and microvascular complications that include retinopathy, nephropathy, and neurovascular defects along with autonomic neuropathy. Such complications may be manifested clinically as myocardial infarction, angina, stroke blindness, end-stage renal failure, congestive heart failure, defective nerve conduction and impaired wound healing. Evidence indicates a causal link between the degree of blood glucose control in diabetes and the development and progression of clinical complications.

The Diabetes Control and Complications Trial (DCCT)[1] and United Kingdom Prospective Diabetes Study (UKPDS)[2] have emphasized the role of tight glucose control as being important in reducing diabetic microvascular disease in type 1 diabetes mellitus (DCCT) and type 2 diabetes mellitus (UKPDS). The relation between tight glucose control and macrovascular complications is not as clear.[3] The importance of blood pressure control in reducing diabetic microvascular complications has been shown.[4] Apart from these factors, damage induced by hyperglycemia involves a complex interaction between many influences including genetic predisposition, smoking, body mass index, dyslipidemia and alterations in coagulation factors.[3]

This chapter will highlight on the pathophysiology of diabetic microvascular complications with respect to the morphological and biochemical changes.

MORPHOLOGIC FEATURES

Basement Membrane

The classic morphologic finding in diabetic microangiopathy is the thickening of basement membranes in capillaries.[5-7] This is a generalized phenomenon that affects basement membranes of both vascular and nonvascular tissues. The basement membranes of mammary ducts, testes and sweat glands also are thickened, as are sarcoplasmic and perineural basement membranes and alveolar epithelium[8–12] **(Table 65.1)**.

In most tissues, the basement membrane separates cells from the interstitial space. The exceptions are the glomerulus of kidney, in which the basement membrane is between endothelial cells of the capillary and epithelial cells of the Bowman's capsule, and in the

TABLE 65.1	Biochemical alterations of the basement membrane in diabetes mellitus
Composition	• Increased collagen content (type IV and VI) • Switch—(nodular sclerosis) type IV collagen reduces; type VI collagen increases • Reduction in heparin sulfate proteoglycan • Laminin—increased or decreased
Synthesis	• Increased synthesis of collagen • Increased glucosyltransferase activity (enzymatic glycosylation) • Increased nonenzymatic glycosylation of basement membrane collagen and albumin
Degradation	• Reduced degradation due to reduced activity of enzymes involved in glycoprotein degradations • Advanced glycation endproducts increase collagen crosslinking and prevent degradation

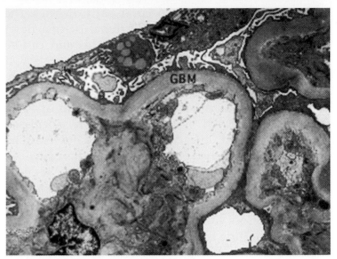

Figure 65.1 The glomerulus in diabetic nephropathy. The glomerular basement membranes are diffusely thickened in a uniform fashion. Mesangial regions are also expanded by excess mesangial matrix-like material

membrane is between the endothelial cell and the glial cell.[13] The glomerular basement membrane is continuous with the tubular basement membrane via the Bowman's capsule. In the retina, thickening of the basement membrane also is found between endothelial cells and pericytes (mural cells).[7, 14–16]

The chemical components of the basement membrane are now well recognized and include collagens (mainly type IV), chondroitin, heparin sulfate proteoglycans and various glycoproteins such as lamina.[17–20] Basement membranes in normal tissues form boundaries between similar cells and different cell types. They provide structural support, maintain architecture, modify cellular functions such as proliferation, and provide a filtration barrier. Thus, these alterations in basement membrane morphology can easily be envisaged as having functional consequences.

The initial description of diabetic renal glomeruli by Kimmelstiel and Wilson[21] thickening of the glomerular basement membrane has been recognized as a prominent morphologic feature of diabetic nephropathy. This thickening of the basement membrane in diabetes has classically been described as a slow process that occurs over many years.

The expansion of the mesangium is the other major lesion observed in diabetic glomerulopathy **(Figure 65.1)**. This expansion is thought to be the main factor leading to impaired renal function.[22] With the progressive increase in the mesangial matrix, there is a loss in capillary surface area (filtration area). Increase in mesangial volume fraction (mesangial volume/glomerular volume) also has a strong clinical correlation with declining glomerular filtration rate (GFR) and

albuminuria. Such a functional correlation is not exhibited for increases in the thickness of the glomerular basement membrane.[23] Along with changes in the composition of the basement membrane. Changes in the mesangium lead to altered permeability and eventually to glomerular occlusion, fibrosis and decreased filtering capacity **(Flow chart 65.1)**.

Flow chart 65.1 Schematic presentation of the pathway in the development of diabetic nephropathy

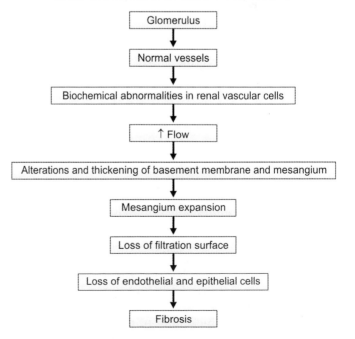

Functional changes also occur in early diabetes. The GFR and filtration fraction (GFR/renal plasma flow) increase early in the course of diabetes and can be corrected by intensive insulin treatment.[24–26] On account of the changes in the basement membrane permeability of the capillaries is altered such that the excretion of proteins with molecular weights of 44000 to 150000 is increased.[27] Albumin excretion is increased in diabetes and, like an elevated GFR, can be normalized by intensive insulin treatment or islet-cell transplantation.[24–26] Similar changes are seen in diabetic rats. This initial alteration in permeability seems to be due primarily to increased filtration pressures across the glomerulus. Later selectivity of the permeability barrier changes, that permits an increase in the leakage of plasma proteins. Fibrin accumulation, possibly related to decreases in fibrinolysis, may contribute to the precapillary occlusion seen in diabetes.[28–31]

Alterations in growth factor expression are also associated with diabetic nephropathy. In particular, transforming growth factor-β (TGF-β) expression was increased in mesangial cells exposed to high glucose for 48 hour,[32] in glomeruli from diabetic rats[33-37] and in glomeruli from patients with diabetic nephropathy.[38] TGF-β is a known regulator of extracellular matrix (ECM) accumulation, and has been shown to increase expression of collagen I, IV and fibronectin in mesangial and glomerular epithelial cells.[39–42] Evidence suggests protein kinase C (PKC) activation may be involved in the glucose-induced increase in TGF-β expression leading to ECM synthesis.

In a cross-sectional study from South India,[43] it was noted that the levels of TGF-β_1 was elevated in type 2 diabetic subjects. Treatment with insulin and angiotensin converting enzyme inhibitors (ACEIs) reduced the levels of TGF-β_1 in these subjects.

Changes in Vascular Cells

Beside the generalized changes in the basement membrane, specific changes in vascular cells have been documented. These changes in vascular cells vary depending on the tissue involving pericytes in diabetic retinopathy and glomerular endothelial cells, mesangial cells, and epithelial cells in diabetic nephropathy.[44– 48]

The earliest histologic change in diabetic retinopathy is the loss of retinal pericytes.[44–48] Normally, the ratio of endothelial cells to pericytes in the retinal capillaries is 1:1.[44,45] In parallel with loss of pericytes, several other histologic changes are observed, including increased capillary diameter, thickening of the basement memb-

rane, changes in retinal blood flow, increased vascular permeability, and formation of microaneurysms. It has been postulated that many of these changes are the consequence of the loss of pericytes.

In the glomeruli, at least three different types of vascular cells are involved in microvascular changes:[49–51] Glomerular endothelial cells, mesangial cells and epithelial cells. Mesangial cells, like pericytes, have contractile properties but react differently to diabetes, increasing their size and possibly their number as well.[5,6,13,49–51] The loss of glomerular filtration function is directly related to the expansion of the mesangium and the loss of the filtration surface formed by the endothelial and epithelial cells. In early stages of diabetes, there appears to be an expansion of the mesangium and mesangial cells. The basement membrane is also thickened, and the combination of this thickening and the expansion of the mesangium results in a gradual loss of the endothelial and epithelial cells. At the later stage of nephropathy, general fibrosis of the glomeruli leads to end-stage kidney disease similar to other glomerulosclerotic diseases.[5,6,13, 21,22]

Vascular Abnormalities

The abnormalities found in the endothelial and vascular supporting cells from diabetic patients or animals can be separated into four general categories:
1. Coagulation
2. Permeability
3. Flow and contractility
4. Regeneration

Coagulation

Multiple alterations in coagulation have been reported. In the endothelium, abnormalities have been found in the levels of activity of factor VIII, prostaglandins, fibrinolysis and other functions.[51,52] The levels of tissue plasminogen activator (TPA) are decreased the levels of tissue plasminogen activator inhibitor (PAI) are increased.

Another parameter used in assessing the coagulation state is von Willebrand factor antigen (vWF), which complexes with factor VIII to form factor VIII Ag: vWF.[53,54] This complex is produced by endothelial cells and is involved in formation of thrombi and in adhesion of platelets to the subendothelium.[55,56] Most studies have reported that levels of vWF are increased in both insulin-dependent and non-insulin dependent diabetic patients. Most studies have indicated that glycemic control, whether achieved by diet, sulfonylureas or insulin, normalizes vWF levels in patients.[57,58] The duration of the diabetic state seems to correlate with the level of vWF.[59,60]

Diabetes and hyperglycemia have been reported to affect the metabolism of prostaglandins, which are potent metabolites of endothelial cells that affect platelet aggregation and vascular thrombosis.[61,62] Prostaglandin I₂ (PGI₂) production in endothelial cells has been evaluated extensively because it is an inhibitor of platelet aggregation and adhesion. It is also a strong vasodilator.[62] These properties suggest that a reduction in the level of PGI₂ may lead to an increase in thrombosis and contractility.

Permeability

In retinal vessels, the vascular barrier is formed by tight junctions between capillary endothelial cells. Increases in permeability are probably due to abnormalities in the endothelial cells. The pericytes also may play a major role, since the normal ratio of pericytes to endothelial cells is one.

One of the earliest manifestations of diabetic vascular dysfunction, particularly in the retinal vessels and kidney, is an increase in vascular permeability to circulating macromolecules. Marked increases in albumin permeation have been reported in the eye, sciatic nerve, aorta and kidney obtained from three week diabetes rats.[63]

It has been suggested that activation of PKC stimulates the endothelial cell contractile apparatus to enhance vascular permeability via the phosphorylation of specific cytoskeletal proteins. PKC activation is reported to lead to the phosphorylation of the cytoskeletal proteins caldesmon, vimentin, talin and vinculin.[64–66]

Vascular endothelial growth factor (VEGF) stimulates both cell growth and permeability, and is the main factor responsible for regulation of hypoxia stimulated angiogenesis. Activation of the PKCβ isoforms is essential for VEGF-mediated cell growth.

Flow and Contractility

Atrial natriuretic peptide (ANP) has been shown to increase renal blood flow and filtration rate.[67] Infusion of antibodies to ANP normalizes renal blood flow, suggesting that ANP may have a role in increasing renal blood flow in the diabetic state. Other growth factors, such as growth hormone and insulin-like growth factor-I (IGF-I), have been implicated, since they can cause renal enlargement and increase the GFR[68-69] **(Table 65.2)**.

During the first 2 to 5 years of diabetes, retinal blood flow appears to be decreased. Blood flow has been reported to be increased when background retinopathy is present.[70] However, with advanced proliferative retinopathy, retinal blood flow appears to decrease again.[71,72] This decrease could increase hypoxia and further induce neovascularization.

Loss of capillary pericytes is one of the earliest and most specific features associated with clinical retinopathy in diabetes. As pericytes have a vital role in

TABLE 65.2	Growth factors involved in microangiopathic changes in the kidney and retina and the effect of diabetes on their production		

S No.	Growth factor	Relevant function	Effect of diabetes
1.	GHBP	Cellular proliferation Increased GFR	Long-term diabetes sustained increase in GHBP and increased GHBP mRNA
2.	IGF-1 GFBP-1, IGFBP-5	Cell proliferation	Early increase in IGF-1 mRNA and then normalization. IGFBP-1 and 5 normal in early but sustained increase later on Increase in renal receptor mRNA
3.	IGF-II	Cell proliferation	Increase in renal receptor mRNA
4.	Fibroblast growth factors (acidic and basic)	Cell proliferation Angiogenesis	Increased in patients with proliferative retinopathy (PR)
5.	Epidermal growth factor	Organogenesis, wound healing	Decreased urinary excretion
6.	Transforming growth factor-β	Cell growth and hypertrophy Extracellular matrix synthesis	Increased level in vitreous in patients with proliferative retinopathy Increased glomerular expression of mRNA
7.	Platelet derived growth factor	Cellular proliferation Extracellular matrix synthesis	Increased glomerular expression of mRNA

maintenance of capillary integrity, their loss in diabetes contributes to vessel dysfunction via altered ECM composition, increased vascular permeability, enlarged capillary diameter, impaired regulation of vascular tone, endothelial cell proliferation and microaneurysm formation. Each of these changes may contribute to abnormalities in retinal blood flow and the development of retinal ischemia. The ischemic retina is able to stimulate angiogenesis via the release of angiogenic growth factors such as VEGF. This factor contributes to increased endothelial cell proliferation and permeability and has been implicated in mediating intraocular neovascularization in patients with diabetic retinopathy.[73] These newly formed vessels in the retina tend to be fragile and prone to hemorrhage and leakage, which may induce further neovascularization and fibrosis of the retina, and lead to more severe proliferative form of retinopathy **(Flow chart 65.2)**.

The impairment in retinal blood flow in the early stages of diabetes may be a consequence of an increase in resistance to flow; diabetes-induced alterations in vasoactive factors in conjunction with changes in the PKC signal transduction pathway are suggested to be involved. One suggested mechanism by which diabetes-induced activation of PKC could alter vasoreactivity within the retina by altering the expression of endothelium-derived vasoactive factors such as the potent vasoconstrictor peptide endothelin-1 (ET-1), which has been identified in many retinal cells including the

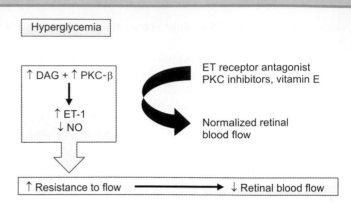

Figure 65.2 Schematic presentation demonstrating the proposed mechanism for the decrease in retinal blood flow in early diabetes

capillary endothelial cells and pericytes; or by the endothelium-derived vasodilator nitric oxide (NO) **(Figure 65.2)**.

In a study from Southern India, it was noted that the levels of ET-1 were elevated in patients with normo-albuminuria without any complications.[74] Similarly, in another study, it was noted that the endothelium dependent vasodilatation was impaired in normo-albuminuric subjects.[75] This study signifies the fact that the process of pathogenesis starts at a very early stage.

Alterations in the function of several vasoactive factors within the kidney have been suggested to contribute to the development of diabetes-induced hyperfiltration. Furthermore, each of these factors may be linked with activation of the diacylglycerol (DAG)-PKC pathway. Increased synthesis of the glomerular prostaglandins PGE_2, PGI_2 and $PGF_2\alpha$ has been reported to occur in glomeruli from two weeks diabetic rats.[76,77] Similarly, in cultured mesangial cells, exposure to high glucose increased PGE_2 and PGI_2, and increased release of arachidonic acid.[78] Such increases in vasodilatory prostaglandins (PGs) could lead to hyperfiltration **(Flow chart 65.3)**.

The potent vasodilator NO, may also contribute to increases in blood flow and in turn, glomerular hyperfiltration. However, it is important to note that a variety of changes have been reported to occur in diabetes, therefore the exact role for NO in the kidney is not clear.[79]

Changes to Endoneural Blood Flow

Experimental diabetic neuropathy has been characterized by decreased axonal transport, decreased nerve conduction velocity and impaired axon regeneration.

Flow chart 65.2 Schematic presentation of the progression of diabetic retinopathy

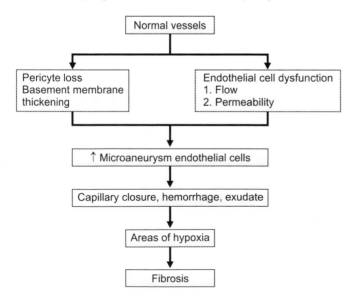

Flow chart 65.3 Effect of hyperglycemia on various pathogenic mechanisms

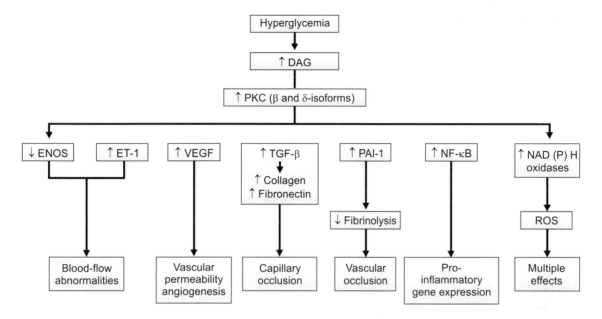

MECHANISMS OF HYPERGLYCEMIA-INDUCED DAMAGE

Hyperglycemia-induced nerve ischemia may contribute to the development of diabetic neuropathy, as vasodilator agents, which improve reductions in nerve blood flow, have been found to improve nerve defects.[80]

Hyperglycemia is suggested to cause diminished phosphoinositol (PI) turnover, which in turn leads to reduced availability of DAG, and in turn, a decrease in neuronal PKC activity. Diminished PKC activity reduces the phosphorylation of Na^+-K^+ATPase, leading to a decrease in nerve conduction and nerve regeneration. PKC inhibition should enhance perfusion and improved nerve function. The positive effect of PKC inhibition on nerve conduction may be due to improved nerve blood flow rather than improvement to nerve N^+-K^+ATPase defects.

N^+-K^+ATPase is an essential component of the sodium pump, and has an important role in maintaining cell functions such as regulation of cell volume, excitability, cytoplasmic enzyme activity and contractility.[81] N^+-K^+ATPase levels are reported to decrease in vascular and neuronal tissues during diabetes or high glucose exposure.[82–84] PKC can regulate N^+-K^+ATPase levels in some tissues by the phosphorylation/dephosphorylation of its α-subunit and act to either stimulate or inhibit its activity, depending on the system studied.

Four main hypotheses are postulated to explain the development of microvascular complications. They are:
1. Increased polyol pathway flux
2. Increased advanced glycation endproduct (AGE) formation
3. Activation of protein kinase C (PKC) isoforms
4. Increased hexosamine pathway flux.

Increased Polyol Pathway Flux

Aldose reductase {alditol: $NAD(P)^+$ 1-oxidoreductase, EC (1.1.1.21)} is the first enzyme in the polyol pathway. It is a cytosolic, monomeric oxidoreductase that catalyzes the NADPH-dependent reduction of a wide variety of carbonyl compounds, including glucose. Metabolism of glucose by this pathway is a very small percentage of total glucose use. But in a hyperglycemic environment, increased intracellular glucose results in its increased enzymatic conversion to the polyalcohol sorbitol, with concomitant decreases in NADPH. In the polyol pathway, sorbitol is oxidized to fructose by the enzyme sorbitol dehydrogenase, with NAD^+ reduced to NADH **(Figure 65.3)**.

Oxidation of sorbitol by NAD^+ increases the cytosolic NADH : NAD^+ ratio, thereby inhibiting activity of

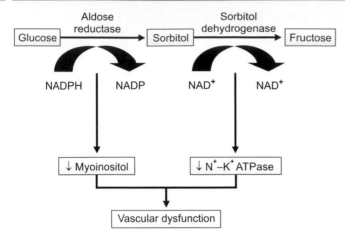

Figure 65.3 Possible mechanisms of the polyol effect on cellular function and redox potential

the enzyme glyceraldehyde-3-phosphate dehydrogenase (GAPDH), and increasing concentrations of triose phosphate.[85] Raised triose phosphate concentrations could increase formation of both methylglyosal, a precursor of advanced glycation endproducts (AGEs) and DAG, thus activating PKC. It has also been proposed that reduction of glucose to sorbitol by NADPH consumes NADPH. As NADPH is required for regenerating reduced glutathione (GSH), this could induce or exacerbate intracellular oxidative stress. Decreased levels of GSH have been found in the lenses of transgenic mice that overexpress aldose reductase, and this is the most likely mechanism by which increased flux through the polyol pathway has deleterious consequences.[86]

Studies of inhibition of the polyol pathway *in vivo* have yielded inconsistent results. In a five-year study in dogs, aldose reductase inhibition prevented diabetic neuropathy, but failed to prevent retinopathy or thickening of the capillary basement membrane in the retina, kidney and muscle.[87] Several negative clinical trials have questioned the relevance of this mechanism in humans.[88] The positive effect of aldose reductase inhibition on diabetic neuropathy has, however, been confirmed in humans in a rigorous multidose, placebo-controlled trial with the potent aldose reductase inhibitor zenarestat.[89]

Increased Intracellular Formation of Advanced Glycation Endproducts

Advanced glycation endproducts (AGEs) are found in increased amounts in diabetic retinal vessels[90] and renal glomeruli.[91] Intracellular hyperglycemia is the primary initiating event in the formation of both intracellular and extracellular AGEs.[92] The potential importance of AGEs in the pathogenesis of diabetic complications is apparent by the observation in animal models that two structurally unrelated AGE inhibitors partially prevented various functional and structural manifestations of diabetic microvascular disease in retina, kidney and nerve.[93-95]

Production of intracellular AGE precursors damages target cells by three general mechanisms. First, intracellular proteins modified by AGEs have altered function. Second, extracellular matrix components modified by AGE precursors interact abnormally with other matrix components and with the receptors for matrix proteins (integrins) on cells. Third, plasma proteins modified by AGE precursors bind to AGE receptors on endothelial cells, mesangial cells and macrophages, inducing receptor-mediated production of reactive oxygen species. This AGE receptor ligation activates the pleiotropic transcription factor NF-κβ, causing pathological changes in gene expression.

AGE formation alters the functional properties of several important matrix molecules. AGE formation on extracellular matrix not only interferes with matrix-matrix interactions, but also interferes with matrix-cell interactions.

Blockade of receptor of advanced glycation endproducts (RAGE), a member of the immunoglobulin superfamily with three immunoglobulin-like regions on a single polypeptide chain, suppressed macrovascular disease in an atherosclerosis—prone type 1 diabetic mouse model in a glucose- and lipid-independent fashion.[96]

Activation of Protein Kinase C

The protein kinase C (PKC) family comprises at least 11 isoforms, nine of which are activated by the lipid second messenger DAG. Intracellular hyperglycemia increases the amount of DAG in cultured microvascular cells and in the retina and renal glomeruli of diabetic animals **(Flow chart 65.4)**.

In early experimental diabetes, activation of PKC-β isoforms has been shown to mediate retinal and renal blood flow abnormalities[97] perhaps by depressing nitric oxide production and/or increasing endothelin-1 activity. Abnormal activation of PKC has been implicated in the decreased glomerular production of nitric oxide induced by experimental diabetes,[98] and in the decreased production of nitric oxide in smooth muscle

Flow chart 65.4 Schematic presentation on the effect of hyperglycemia on diacylglycerol (DAG) synthesis and protein kinase C (PKC) activation

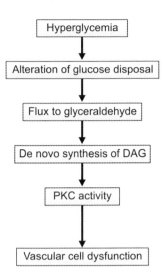

cells that is induced by hyperglycemia.[99] Activation of PKC also inhibits insulin-stimulated expression of the messenger RNA for endothelial nitric oxide synthase (ENOS) in cultured endothelial cells.[100] Hyperglycemia increases endothelin-1 stimulated MAP-kinase activity in glomerular mesangial cells by activating PKC isoforms.[101]

In addition to affecting hyperglycemia-induced abnormalities of blood flow and permeability, activation of PKC contributes to increased microvascular matrix protein accumulation by inducing expression of TGF-β_1, fibronectin and type IV collagen both in cultured mesangial cells[102] and in glomeruli of diabetic rats.[103] This effect seems to be mediated through inhibition of nitric oxide production by PKC **(Flow chart 65.3)**.[104]

Treatment with an inhibitor specific for PKC-β significantly reduced PKC activity in the retina and renal glomeruli of diabetic animals. Concomitantly, treatment significantly reduced diabetes-induced increases in retinal mean circulation time, normalized increases in glomerular filtration rate and partially corrected urinary albumin excretion. Treatment of a mouse model of type 2 diabetes (db/db) with a β-isoform-specific PKC-inhibitor ameliorated accelerated glomerular mesangial expansion.[105]

Increased Flux through the Hexosamine Pathway

Shunting of excess intracellular glucose into the hexosamine pathway might also cause several manifestations of diabetic complications.[106] In this pathway, fructose-6-phosphate is diverted from glycolysis to provide substrates for reactions that require uridine diphosphate (UDP)-N-acetylglucosamine, such as proteoglycan synthesis and the formation of O-linked glycoproteins. Inhibition of the rate-limiting enzyme in the conversion of glucose to glucosamine-glutamine: fructose-6-phosphate amidotransferase (GFAT)-blocks hyperglycemia-induced increases in the transcription of TGF-α, TGF-β_1[105] and PAI-1.[107] This pathway also plays an important role in hyperglycemia-induced and fat-induced insulin resistance.[108,109]

The prevalence of most microvascular complication is high even during the diagnosis of diabetes.[110] However, it is possible to make a very early diagnosis of these pathological process at work by measuring various early markers of microvascular complications. Once diagnosed, regular monitoring and proper management is the key to prevent complications.

SUMMARY

Microvascular complication of diabetes is a major health concern. Understanding regarding pathogenesis of microvascular complication is very essential. Four main hypotheses are postulated to explain the development of microvascular complications. They are increased polyol pathway flux, increased advanced glycation endproduct (AGE) formation, activation of protein kinase C (PKC) isoforms; and increased hexosamine pathway flux. Various pathophysiological processes take place in the retina, kidney and nerve such as retinal, renal and endoneural blood flow changes, basement membrane thickening, increased vascular permeability and neovascularization. It is possible to make a very early diagnosis of these pathological processes by measuring various early markers of microvascular complications. When early diagnosis is augmented with regular monitoring and proper management, prevention becomes possible.

ACKNOWLEDGMENT

I acknowledge the help of my research assistant, Ms Mamtha B Nair for preparing this chapter.

REFERENCES

1. Diabetes Control and Complications Trial (DCCT) Research Group. The effect of intensive treatment of diabetes on the development and progression of long-term complications in

insulin-dependent diabetes mellitus. The Diabetes Control and Complications Trial Research Group. N Engl J Med. 1993;329:977-86.

2. United Kingdom Prospective Diabetes Study (UKPDS) Group. Intensive blood-glucose control with sulphonylureas or insulin compared with conventional treatment and risk of complications in patients with type 2 diabetes (UKPDS 33). United Kingdom Prospective Diabetes Study (UKPDS) Group. Lancet. 1998;352:837-53.

3. Farouque HM, O'Brien RC, Meredith IT. Diabetes and coronary heart disease—from prevention to intervention: Part 1. Aust NZJ Med. 2000;30:351-9.

4. Anonymous tight blood pressure control and risk of macrovascular and microvascular complications in type 2 diabetes (UKPDS 38). BMJ. 1998;317:703-11.

5. Bergstrand A, Bucht H. The glomerular lesions of diabetes mellitus and their electron microscope appearances. J Pathol Bacteriol. 1959;77:231-42.

6. Mogensen CE, Osterby R, Gundersen HJG. Early functional and morphologic vascular renal consequences of the diabetic state. Diabetologia. 1979; 17:71-6.

7. Williamson JR, Kilo C. Extracellular matrix changes in diabetes mellitus. In Scarpelli DG, Migaki G (Eds): Comparative pathobiology of major age-related diseases. Modern Aging Research (Vol 4). New York: Alan R Liss. 1984, pp. 269-88.

8. Merriam JC Jr, Sommers SC. Mammary periductal hyalin in diabetic women: Report of 20 cases. Lab Invest. 1957; 6:412-20.

9. Schoffling K, Federlin K, Ditschunheit H, et al. Disorders of sexual function in male diabetic. Diabetes. 1963;12:519-27.

10. Durand M, Durand A. Les alterations vasculaires dermohypodermiques des diabetiques: etude aux microscopes optique et electronique. Pathol Biol. 1966;l4:1005-19.

11. Johnson PC. Non-vascular basement membrane thickening in diabetes mellitus [Letter]. Lancet. 1981;2:932-3.

12. Vracko R, Thorning D, Huang TW. Basal lamina of alveolar epithelium and capillaries: quantitative changes with aging and in diabetes mellitus. Am Rev Respir Dis. 1979;120:973-83.

13. Tisher CC. Anatomy of the kidney. In Brenner BM, Rector FC Jr (Eds): The kidney (Vol 2), 2nd edn. Philadelphia: WB Saunders, 1981:3-75.

14. Robison WG Jr, Kador PF, Kinoshita JH. Retinal capillaries: basement membrane thickening by galactosemia prevented with aldose reductase inhibitor. Science. 1983; 221:1177-9.

15. Kelley C, D'Amore P, Hechtman HB, Shepro D. Microvascular pericyte contractility *in vitro*: comparison with other cells of the vascular wall. J Cell Biol. 1987;104:483-90.

16. Herman IM, D'Amore PA. Microvascular pericytes contain muscle and nonmuscle actins. J Cell Biol. 1985;101:43-52.

17. Shimomura H, Spiro RG. Studies on macromolecular components of human glomerular basement membrane and alterations in diabetes: decreased levels of heparan sulfate proteoglycan and laminin. Diabetes. 1987;36:374-81.

18. Beisswenger PJ, Spiro RG. Studies on the human glomerular basement membrane: composition, nature of the carbohydrate units and chemical change in diabetes mellitus. Diabetes. 1973;22:180-93.

19. Grant ME, Heathcote JG, Orkin RW. Current concepts of basement-membrane structure and function. Biosci Rep. 1981;1:819-42.

20. Sage H. Collagens of basement membranes. J Invest Dermatol. 1982;79 (Suppl 1):51S-9S.

21. Kimmelstiel P, Wilson C. Intercapillary lesions in the glomeruli of the kidney. Am J Pathol. 1936;12:83-98.

22. Mauer SM, Steffes MW, Ellis EN, et al. Structural-functional relationships in diabetic nephropathy. J Clin Invest. 1984;74:1143-55.

23. Steffes MW, Mauer SM. Diabetic glomerulopathy: a morphological approach to monitoring development, progression and reversibility. Diabetic Nephropathy. 1985;4:114-7.

24. Wiseman MJ, Saunders AJ, Keen H, Viberti G. Effect of blood glucose control on increased glomerular filtration rate and kidney size in insulin-dependent diabetes. N Engl J Med. 1985;312:617-21.

25. Rasch R. Prevention of diabetic glomerulopathy in streptozotocin diabetic rats by insulin treatment: albumin excretion. Diabetologia. 1980;18: 4l3-6.

26. Steffes MW, Brown DM, Basgen JM, Mauer SM. Amelioration of mesangial volume and surface alterations following islet transplantation in diabetic rats. Diabetes. 1980;29:509-15.

27. Schnider S, Aronoff SL, Tchou P, et al. Urinary protein excretion in prediabetic (PD), normal (N), and diabetic (D) Pima Indians and normal Caucasians (NC) [Abstract no.37]. Diabetes. 1977;26 (Suppl 1):362.

28. Myers BD, Winetz JA, Chui F, Michaels AS. Mechanisms of proteinuria in diabetic nephropathy: a study of glomerular barrier function. Kidney Int. 1982;21: 633-4l.

29. Wahl P, Deppermann D, Hasslacher C. Biochemistry of glomerular basement membrane of the normal and diabetic human. Kidney Int. 1982;21:744-9.

30. Parthasarathy N, Spiro RG. Effect of diabetes on the glycosaminoglycan component of the human glomerular basement membrane. Diabetes. 1982;31:738-4l.

31. Nakamura Y, Myers BD. Charge selectivity of proteinuria in diabetic glomerulopathy. Diabetes. 1988;37:1202-11.

32. Wolf G, Sharma K, Chen Y, Ericksen M, Ziyadeh FN. High glucose-induced proliferation in mesangial cells is reversed by autocrine TGF-beta. Kidney Int. 1992;42: 647-56.

33. Nakamura T, Fukui M, Ebihara I, Osada S, Nagaoka I, Tomino Y, et al. mRNA expression of growth factors in glomeruli from diabetic rats. Diabetes. 1993;42:450-6.

34. Sharma K, Ziyadeh FN. Renal hypertrophy is associated with upregulation of TGF-beta 1 gene expression in diabetic BB rat and NOD mouse. Am J Physiol. 1994;267: F1094-2001.

35. Shankland SJ, Scholey JW, Ly H, Thai K. Expression of transforming growth factor- beta 1 during diabetic renal hypertrophy. Kidney Int. 1994;46:430-42.

36. Pankewycz OG, Guan JX, Bolton WK, Gomez A, Benedict JF. Renal TGF-beta regulation in spontaneously diabetic NOD mice with correlations in mesangial cells. Kidney Int. 1994;46:748-58.

37. Bollineni JS, Reddi AS. Transforming growth factor- beta 1 enhances glomerular collagen synthesis in diabetic rats. Diabetes. 1993;42:1673-7.

38. Yamamoto T, Nakamura T, Noble NA, Ruoslahti E, Border WA. Expression of transforming growth factor-beta is elevated in human and experimental diabetic nephropathy. Proc Natl Acad Sci USA 1993;90:1814-8.

39. Suzuki S, Ebihara I, Tomino Y, Koide H. Transcriptional activation of matrix genes by transforming growth factor-beta1 in mesangial cells. Exp Nephrol. 1993;1:229-37.

40. Ziyadeh FN, Sharma K, Ericksen M, Wolf G. Stimulation of collagen gene expression and protein synthesis in murine mesangial cells by high glucose is mediated by autocrine activation of transforming growth factor-beta. J Clin Invest. 1994;93: 536-42.

41. Nakamura T, Miller D, Ruoslahti E, Border WA. Production of extracellular matrix by glomerular epithelial cells is regulated by transforming growth factor-beta 1. Kidney Int. 1992;41:1213-21.

42. Mackay K, Danielpour D, Miller D, Border WA, Robbins AR. The 260-kDa transforming growth factor (TGF)-beta binding protein in rat glomeruli is a complex comprised of 170- and 85-kDa TGF-beta binding proteins. J Biol Chem. 1992;267: 11449-54.

43. Vijay Viswanathan, Snehalatha C, Mamtha B Nair, Kumutha R, Ramachandran A. Levels of transforming growth factor-beta 1 in south Indian type 2 diabetic subjects (Unpublished data).

44. Tilton RG, Miller EJ, Kilo C, Williamson JR. Pericyte form and distribution in rat retinal and uveal capillaries. Invest Ophthalmol Vis Sci. 1985;26:68-73.

45. Petty RG, Pearson JD. Endothelium—the axis of vascular health and disease. JR Coll Physicians Lond. 1989;23:92-102.

46. Cogan DG, Toussaint D, Kuwabara T. Retinal vascular patterns IV. Diabetic retinopathy. Arch Ophthalmol. 1961; 66:366- 78.

47. Kuwabara T, Cogan DG. Retinal vascular patterns VI. Mural cells of the retinal capillaries. Arch Ophthalmol. 1963;69: 492-502.

48. Ashton N. Injection of the retinal vascular system in enucleated eyes in diabetic retinopathy. Br J Ophthalmol. 1950;34:38-41.

49. Arnqvist HJ, Ballerman BJ, King GL. Receptors for and effects of insulin and IGF-1 in rat glomerular mesangial cells. Am J Physiol. 1988;254:C411-6.

50. Striker GE, Killen PD, Farin FM. Human glomerular cells *in vitro*: isolation and characterization. Transplant Proc. 1980;12 (Suppl 1):88-99.

51. Kreisberg JI, Karnovsky MJ. Glomerular cells in culture. Kidney Int. 1983;23:439-47.

52. Ostermann H, van de Loo J. Factors of the haemostatic system in diabetic patients: a survey of controlled studies. Haemostasis. 1986;16:386- 416.

53. Moroose R, Hoyer LW. Von Willebrand factor and platelet function. Annu Rev Med. 1986;37:157-63.

54. Banga JD, Sixma JJ. Diabetes mellitus, vascular disease and thrombosis. Clin Haematol. 1986;15:465-92.

55. Jaffe EA, Hoyer LW, Nachman RL. Synthesis of von Willebrand factor by cultured human endothelial cells. Proc Natl Acad Sci USA. 1974;71:1906-9.

56. Bloom AL. The biosynthesis of factor VIII. Clin Haematol. 1979;8:53-77.

57. Gonzalez J, Colwell JA, Sarji KE, et al. Effect of metabolic control with insulin on plasma von Willebrand factor activity (VIII R-WF) in diabetes mellitus. Thromb Res. 1980;17: 261-6.

58. Paton RC, Kernoff PBA, Wales JK, McNicol GP. Effects of diet and gliclazide on the haemostatic system of non-insulin-dependent diabetics. BMJ. 1981;283:1018-20.

59. Porta M, Maneschi F, White MC, Kohner EM. Twenty-four hour variations of von Willebrand factor and factor VIII-related antigen in diabetic retinopathy. Metabolism. 1981;30:695-9.

60. Muntean WE, Borkenstein MH, Haas J. Elevation of factor VIII coagulant activity over factor VIII coagulant antigen in diabetic children without vascular disease: a sign of activation of the factor VIII coagulant moiety during poor diabetes control. Diabetes. 1985;34:140-4.

61. Aanderud S, Krane H, Nordy A. Influence of glucose, insulin and sera from diabetic patients on the prostacyclin synthesis *in vitro* in cultured human endothelial cells. Diabetologia. 1985;28:641-4.

62. Umeda F, Inoguchi T, Nawata H. Reduced stimulatory activity on prostacyclin production by cultured endothelial cells in serum from aged and diabetic patients. Atherosclerosis. 1989; 75:61-6.

63. Williamson JR, Chang K, Tilton RG, Prater C, et al. Increased vascular permeability in spontaneously diabetic BB/W rats and in rats with mild versus severe streptozocin-induced diabetes. Prevention by aldose reductase inhibitors and castration. Diabetes. 1987;36: 813-21.

64. Stasek JE Jr, Patterson CE, Garcia JG. Protein kinase C phosphorylates caldesmon 77 and vimentin and enhances albumin permeability across cultured bovine pulmonary artery endothelial cell monlayers. J Cell Physiol. 1992; 153:62-75.

65. Turner CE, Pavalko FM, Burridge K. The role of phosphorylation and limited proteolytic cleavage of talin and vinculin in the disruption of focal adhesion integrity. J Biol Chem. 1989;264:11938-44.

66. Werth DK, Niedel JE, Pastan I. Vinculin: a cytoskeletal substrate of protein kinase C. J Biol Chem. 1983;258:11423-6.

67. Ortola FV, Ballermann BJ, Anderson S, et al. Elevated plasma atrial natriuretic peptide levels in diabetic rats: potential mediator of hyperfiltration. J Clin Invest. 1987;80:670-4.

68. Doi T, Striker LJ, Quaife C, et al. Progressive glomerulosclerosis develops in transgenic mice chronically expressing growth hormone and growth hormone releasing factor but not in those expressing insulin like growth factor-I. Am J Pathol. 1988;131:398-403.

69. Fagin JA, Melmed S. Relative increase in insulin-like growth factor I messenger ribonucleic acid levels in compensatory renal hypertrophy. Endocrinology. 1987;120: 718-24.

70. Williamson JR, Chang K, Rowold E, et al. Sorbinil prevents diabetes-induced increases in vascular permeability but does not alter collagen cross-linking. Diabetes. 1985;34:703-5.

71. Grunwald JE, Riva CE, Martin DB, et al. Effect of an insulin-induced decrease in blood glucose on the human diabetic retinal circulation. Ophthalmology. 1987;94:1614-20.

72. Kohner EM, Hamilton AM, Saunders SJ, et al. The retinal blood flow in diabetes. Diabetologia. 1975;11:27-33.

73. Aiello LP, Avery RL, Arrigg PG, Keyt BA, Jampel HD, Shah ST, et al. Vascular endothelial growth factor in ocular fluid of patients with diabetic retinopathy and other retinal disorders. N Engl J Med. 1994;331:1480-7.

74. Vijay Viswanathan, Snehalatha C, Mamtha B Nair, Ramachandran A. Markers of endothelial dysfunction in hyperglycaemic Asian Indian subjects. Journal of Diabetes and its Complications. 2004;18:47-52.

75. Mamtha B Nair, Viswanathan Vijay, Snehalatha C, Mohan R Suresh, Ramachandran A. Flow-mediated dilatation and carotid intimal media thickness in south Indian type 2 diabetic subjects. DRCP. 2004;25:13-9.

76. Schambelan M, Blake S, Sraer J, Bens M, Nivez MP, Wahbe F. Increased prostaglandin production by glomeruli isolated from

rats with streptozotocin-induced diabetes mellitus. J Clin Invest. 1985;75:404-12.

77. Craven PA, Caines MA, DeRubertis FR. Sequential alterations in glomerular prostaglandin and thromboxane synthesis in diabetic rats: relationship to the hyperfiltration of early diabetes. Metabolism. 1987;36:95-103.

78. Williams B, Schrier RW. Glucose-induced protein kinase C activity regulates arachidonic acid release and eicosanoid production by cultured glomerular mesangial cells. J Clin Invest. 1993;92:2889-96.

79. DeRubertis FR, Craven PA. Activation of protein kinase C in glomerular cells in diabetes. Mechanisms and potential links to the pathogenesis of diabetic glomerulopathy. Diabetes. 1994; 43:1-8.

80. Cameron NE, Cotter MA. Metabolic and vascular factors in the pathogenesis of diabetic neuropathy. Diabetes. 1997; 46:S31-7.

81. Vasilets LA, Schwarz W. Structure-function relationships of cation binding in the Na^+K^+-ATPase. Biochim Biophys Acta. 1993;1154:201-22.

82. Greene DA, Lattimer SA, Sima AA. Sorbitol, phospho-inositides, and sodium-potassium-ATPase in the pathogenesis of diabetic complications. N Engl J Med. 1987;316:599-606.

83. Macgregor LC, Matschinsky FM. Altered retinal metabolism in diabetes II. Measurement of sodium-potassium -ATPase and total sodium and potassium in individual retinal layers. J Biol Chem. 1986;261:4052-8.

84. Winegrad AI. Banting Lecture 1986. Does a common mechanism induce the diverse complications of diabetes? Diabetes. 1987;36:396-406.

85. Williamson JR, et al. Hyperglycemic pseudohypoxia and diabetic complications. Diabetes. 1993; 42:801-13.

86. Lee AY, Chung SS. Contributions of polyol pathway to oxidative stress in diabetic cataract. FASEB J. 1999; 13:23– 30.

87. Engerman RL, Kern TS, Larson ME. Nerve conduction and aldose reductase inhibition during 5 years of diabetes or galactosaemia in dogs. Diabetologia. 1994;37: 141-4.

88. Sorbinil Retinopathy Trial Research Group. A randomized trial of sorbinil: an aldose reductase inhibitor in diabetic retinopathy. Arch Ophthalmol. 1990;108:1234-44.

89. Greene DA, Arezzo JC, Brown MB. Effect of aldose reductase inhibition on nerve conduction and morphometry in diabetic neuropathy. Zenarestat Study Group, Neurology. 1999;53:580-91.

90. Stitt AW, et al. Advanced glycation endproducts (AGEs) colocalize with AGE receptors in the retinal vasculature of diabetic and of AGE-infused rats. Am J Pathol. 1997;150:523-8.

91. Horie K, et al. Immunohistochemical colocalization of glycoxidation products and lipid peroxidation products in diabetic renal glomerular lesions. Implication for glycoxidative stress in the pathogenesis of diabetic nephropathy. J Clin Invest. 1997;100: 2995-9.

92. Degenhardt TP, Thorpe SR, Baynes JW. Chemical modification of proteins by methylglyoxal. Cell Mol Biol. 1998;44:1139-45.

93. Soulis-Liparota T, Cooper M, Papazoglou D, Clarke B, Jerums G. Retardation by Aminoguanidine of development of albuminuria, mesangial expansion, and tissue fluorescence in streptozocin-induced diabetic rat. Diabetes. 1991;40:1328-34.

94. Nakamura S, et al. Progression of nephropathy in spontaneous diabetic rats is prevented by OPB-9195: a novel inhibitor of advanced glycation. Diabetes. 1997;46:895-99.

95. Hammes HP, et al. Aminoguanidine treatment inhibits the development of experimental diabetic retinopathy. Proc Natl Acad Sci USA. 1991;88:11555-9.

96. Park L, et al. Suppression of accelerated diabetic atherosclerosis by the soluble receptor for advanced glycation endproducts. Nature Med. 1998;4:1025-31.

97. Ishii H, et al. Amelioration of vascular dysfunctions in diabetic rats by an oral PKC beta inhibitor. Science. 1996;272:728-31.

98. Craven PA, Studer RK, DeRubertis FR. Impaired nitric oxide-dependent cyclic guanosine monophosphate generation in glomeruli from diabetic rats. Evidence for protein kinase C-mediated suppression of the cholinergic response. J Clin Invest. 1994; 93:311-20.

99. Ganz MB, Seftel A. Glucose-induced changes in protein kinase C and nitric oxide are prevented by vitamin E. Am J Physiol. 2000;278:E146-52.

100. Kuboki K, et al. Regulation of endothelial constitutive nitric oxide synthase gene expression in endothelial cells and *in vivo* a specific vascular action of insulin. Circulation. 2000;101:676-81.

101. Glogowski EA, Tsiani E, Zhou X, Fantus IG, Whiteside C. High glucose alters the response of mesangial cell protein kinase C isoforms to endothelin-1. Kidney Int. 1999;55:486-99.

102. Studer RK, Craven PA, DeRubertis FR. Role for protein kinase C in the mediation of increased fibronectin accumulation by mesangial cells grown in high-glucose medium. Diabetes. 1993;42:118-26.

103. Koya D, et al. Characterization of protein kinase C-beta isoform activation on the gene expression of transforming growth factor-beta, extracellular matrix components, and prostanoids in the glomeruli of diabetic rats. J Clin Invest. 1997;100:115-26.

104. Craven PA, Studer RK, Felder J, Phillips S, DeRubertis FR. Nitric oxide inhibition of transforming growth factor-beta and collagen synthesis in mesangial cells. Diabetes 1997;46:671-81.

105. Koya D, et al. Amelioration of accelerated diabetic mesangial expansion by treatment with a PKC-beta inhibitor in diabetic db/db mice, a rodent model for type 2 diabetes. FASEB J. 2000;14:439-47.

106. Kolm-Litty V, Sauer U, Nerlich A, Lehmann R, Schleicher ED. High glucose-induced transforming growth factor-beta 1 production is mediated by the hexosamine pathway in porcine glomerular mesangial cells. J Clin Invest. 1998; 101:160-9.

107. Du XL, et al. Hyperglycaemia-induced mitochondrial superoxide overproduction activates the hexosamine pathway and induces plasminogen activator inhibitor-1 expression by increasing Sp1 glycosylation. Proc Natl Acad Sci USA. 2000;97:12222-6.

108. Marshall S, Bacote V, Traxinger RR. Discovery of a metabolic pathway mediating glucose-induced desensitization of the glucose transport system. Role of hexosamine biosynthesis in the induction of insulin resistance. J Biol Chem. 1991;266:4706-12.

109. Hawkins M, et al. Role of the glucosamine pathway in fat-induced insulin resistance. J Clin Invest. 1997; 99:2173-82.

110. Viswanathan Vijay, Seena R, Lalitha S, Snehalatha C, Jayaraman Muthu, Ramachandran A. Significance of microalbuminuria at diagnosis of type 2 diabetes. Int J Diab Dev Countries. 1999;18:5-6.

Chapter 66

OCULAR COMPLICATIONS IN DIABETES

M Rema, R Pradeepa

CHAPTER OUTLINE

- Introduction
- Mediators and Mechanisms of Ocular Damage in Diabetes Mellitus
- Extraretinal Ocular Manifestations
- Retinal Manifestations
- Summary

INTRODUCTION

Diabetes poses a major health problem globally and is one of the top five leading causes of death in most developed countries and substantial evidences suggest that it will reach epidemic proportions in developing and newly industrialized countries.[1] Complications of diabetes are the major causes of morbidity and mortality in persons with type 1 and type 2 diabetes. Although the pathogenesis differs in the two forms of diabetes, the pathophysiology of microvascular complications appears to be similar. Diabetes particularly affects tissues in which glucose uptake increases during hyperglycemia, leading to raised intracellular glucose concentration causing cumulative and progressive tissue damage in the retina through the summation of microvascular occlusions.[2]

Of the many complications of diabetes, visual impairment is perhaps the most feared. Diabetic individuals are more prone to visual disability than those without diabetes. Eye disease represents an end-organ response to a generalized medical condition. All structures of the eye are susceptible to harmful effects of diabetes.[3]

In India with the epidemic increase in incidence of diabetes mellitus, diabetic retinopathy is fast becoming an important cause of visual disability. In an epidemiological study conducted in urban South India, the Chennai Urban Rural Epidemiology Study (CURES), the overall prevalence of diabetes was 17.6%.[4] Visual disability from diabetes represents a significant public health problem and foremost attention has to be paid to the retinal complications of diabetes mellitus, as one in four diabetic subjects develop diabetic retinopathy (DR) in the Indian scenario. This chapter will discuss namely about the extraretinal complications of diabetes mellitus **(Table 66.1)**.

MEDIATORS AND MECHANISMS OF OCULAR DAMAGE IN DIABETES MELLITUS

Diabetes has wide ranging effects on metabolism which indicates that there are many potential mediators of ocular tissue damage in long-standing disease, probably due to prolonged exposure to high glucose levels (hyperglycemia). Three hallmark international multicenter trials namely, the Diabetes Control and Complications Trial (DCCT)[5], the United Kingdom Prospective Diabetes Study (UKPDS)[6] and the Kumamoto trial[7] have demonstrated that intensive glycemic control helps to minimize/prevent diabetic eye complications. Currently,

TABLE 66.1	Ophthalmic abnormalities of diabetes mellitus
Structure	*Manifestations*
Extraretinal	
Orbit and lids	• Orbitorhinomucormycosis • Orbital cellulitis • Chalazion • Hordeolum externum (stye) • Hordeolum internum • Xanthelasma • Blepharoptosis • Blepharitis
Extraocular muscles	Cranial nerve palsies • Third nerve palsy (oculomotor) • Fourth nerve palsy (trochlear) • Sixth nerve palsy (abducens) • Seventh nerve/Bell's palsy (facial)
Conjunctiva	• Microcirculation changes • Microaneurysms
Cornea	• Generalized alterations • Corneal Sensitivity
Pupil and iris	• Pupillary abnormalities • Generalized alterations • Iris neovascularization
Angle structures	• Open-angle glaucoma • Angle closure glaucoma • Neovascular glaucoma (NVG)
Lens	• Cataract formation • Refractive changes
Vitreous	• Asteroid hyalosis • Vitreous contraction • Posterior vitreous detachment
Optic nerve	• Papillopathy • Anterior ischemic optic neuropathy (AION) • Optic neuritis • Optic atrophy
Retinal	
Retina	• Diabetic retinopathy • Lipemia retinalis • Retinal vein occlusion

four major biochemical pathways have been hypothesized to explain the mechanism of diabetic eye diseases all starting initially from hyperglycemia-induced vascular injury which has been reviewed in a recent article.[8] These mainly include: (1) Enhanced glucose flux through the polyol pathway, (2) Increased intracellular formation of advanced glycation endproducts (AGEs), (3) Activation of protein kinase C (PKC) isoforms, (4) Stimulation of the hexosamine pathway. Recent studies have suggested that these mechanisms seem to reflect a hyperglycemia-induced process initiated by superoxide overproduction by mitochondrial electron transport chain.[9]

Increased Polyol Pathway

In diabetic subjects with uncontrolled blood sugars, the activity of the polyol pathway noninsulin-dependent metabolic pathway of glucose is increased. This pathway consists of two steps: the reduction of glucose-to-sorbitol by aldose reductase and NADPH, followed by oxidation of sorbitol-to-fructose by sorbitol dehydrogenase and NAD^+.[10] Sorbitol, which cannot be transported through the lens membrane accumulates in the lens tissue creating a hypertonic condition, to maintain osmotic equilibrium. This alters the membrane permeability resulting in the loss of several important molecules including glutathione, magnesium, and potassium.

Sorbitol accumulation in the lens and in the nerves seems to be an important factor in the development of cataract and in the slowing down of nerve conduction in diabetic individuals. However, the mechanisms may be different, aldose reductase-induced osmotic stress appears to be the causative mechanism of diabetic cataract, whereas aldose reductase-induced oxidative stress the rationale of neuronal dysfunction.[11] Sorbitol accumulation has also been observed in corneal epithelium, which may result in corneal abnormalities. Recent studies also suggest that the polyol pathway may play a role in early structural abnormalities of retinal microangiopathy. Cellular damage may occur due to increased production of glycating sugars, resulting in AGE formation, and/or depletion of reduced glutathione, resulting in oxidative damage. The polyol pathway is a dream target in retinopathy treatment because excess aldose reductase activity has been proposed to be a mechanism for human diabetic retinopathy.[12] The long-term trial of Sorbinil—an inhibitor of aldose reductase, reported that it delayed the rate of progression of the number of microaneurysms but did not prevent the worsening of diabetic retinopathy.[13]

Increase Advanced Glycation Endproducts Formation

Glucose can react with epsilon amino-group of lysine in the protein resulting in formation of an adduct. This process is called nonenzymatic glycation and it can occur at an accelerated rate in diabetes due to chronic hyperglycemia. This nonenzymic glycated protein undergoes a series of chemical modification resulting in advanced glycation endproducts (AGEs).[14] AGEs can also arise from:

- Intracellular auto-oxidation of glucose-to-glyoxal
- Decomposition of the Amadori product (glucose-derived amino-1-deoxyfructose lysine adducts) to 3-deoxyglucosone and fragmentation of glyceraldehyde-3-phosphate and dihydroxyacetone phosphate to methylglyoxal.

The AGEs so formed can induce a variety of pathological changes which include damaging the structural proteins (collagen) and extracellular matrix components. These AGE-modified proteins bind to specific receptors—receptor for advanced glycation endproducts (RAGE) in the cell membrane of macrophages, endothelial cells and trigger a signaling cascade leading to the release of proinflammatory cytokines and adhesion proteins that favor thrombosis and eventually capillary occlusion. In addition, retinal endothelial AGE-receptor binding appears to mediate increased vascular permeability, probably through the induction of vascular endothelial growth factor (VEGF).

AGEs play a vital role in the complex pathogenesis of basement membrane thickening in diabetic retinopathy and might have a role in the degenerative changes of the lens in diabetic patients. Increased levels of AGEs have been observed in both senile and diabetic cataractous lenses.[15] It is reported that in diabetic subjects accumulation of AGEs in the basement membrane, particularly laminin, may play a causative role in the corneal epithelial disorders.[16] Administration of antioxidants[17] has shown to partially prevent various functional and structural manifestations of retina in animal models but has not been successful in reducing the clinical manifestations of diabetic retinopathy. Beneficial effects in the retinal vasculature of diabetic rats have also been observed with other inhibitors of AGE formation, including pyridoxamine and benfotiamine.[18] However, this could not be extrapolated to humans due to toxic effects and derivatives of it are being currently tried.

Increased Protein Kinase C Activation

The protein kinase C (PKC) family is a large group of structurally related enzymes that require for their activation, phosphatidyl serine/diacylglycerol (DAG)/ free fatty acids and/or Ca^{2+} ions in addition to Mg^{2+}. PKC isoforms (especially α and δ) are activated by the lipid second messenger DAG, synthesized *de novo* from increased intracellular glucose, leading to decreased tissue blood flow by reducing production of nitric oxide

(potent vasodilator). PKC also enhances vascular permeability and neovascularization in the eye through expression of VEGF. Strategies to block formation of VEGF by intravitreal injection has been tried because systemic anti-VEGF factors would have clinical disadvantages as the formation of new blood vessels is beneficial to other areas with diabetic vasculopathies as the coronary bed and the lower limbus.[19] Increase in PKC levels has been shown to alter many cellular functions including alterations in collagen synthesis, action of stimulating hormones and growth factor receptor recycling. Activation of PKC also alters the expression of endothelium-derived vasoactive factors such as the potent vasoconstrictor peptide endothelin-1 (ET-1), which has been identified in many retinal cells such as the capillary endothelial cells and pericytes[20] leading to vasoconstriction and retinal ischemia.

Helig et al[21] have demonstrated that the inhibition of hyperglycemia-induced superoxide in mice prevents diabetes-induced activation of the PKC pathway. The β-isoform of PKC has been identified to be specific to diabetic retinopathy and the inhibition of this isoform of PKC has been shown to block the VEGF-mediated processes.[22] PKC-β inhibitors have been tried in severe nonproliferative diabetic retinopathy[23] and macular edema[24] but have not been advocated yet for clinical practice. Recently, the safety and efficacy of the orally administered PKC-β isoform-selective inhibitor ruboxistaurin (RBX) has been evaluated by the PKC-DRS study group in subjects with moderately severe to very severe NPDR.[23] The study showed that RBX was well tolerated and reduced the risk of visual loss but DR progression may not be significantly reduced. The effect of another PKC inhibitor, PKC412 orally administered at doses of 100 mg/d or higher was studied and reported that it may significantly reduce diabetic macular edema (DME) and improve visual acuity.[24]

Hexosamine Pathway

Activation of the hexosamine pathway by hyperglycemia may result in various changes in both gene expression and in protein function that together contribute to the pathogenesis of diabetic vascular complications. This pathway is also one of the possible mechanisms involved in diabetic keratopathy. Recently studies have reported that hyperglycemia could cause diabetic vascular complications by shunting glucose into the hexosamine pathway leading to hyperglycemia-induced and lipidemia-induced insulin resistance and induction of synthesis of growth factors.[25] Nakamura et al[26] have demonstrated that the excessive glucose flux through the hexosamine pathway may direct retinal neurons to undergo apoptosis in a bimodal fashion and highlights that this pathway may be involved in retinal neurodegeneration in diabetes.

EXTRARETINAL OCULAR MANIFESTATIONS

Individuals with diabetes are generally prone to infections of any kind and at any site predisposing them to acute infections, which is normally of bacterial origin in the orbit and eyelids.

Orbit

Orbitorhinomucormycosis

Mucormycosis is a rare opportunistic infection caused by fungi of the family Mucoracae, which characteristically affects diabetic patients with ketoacidosis or immunosuppression.[27] This aggressive and fatal infection acquired by inhalation of spores, gives rise to upper respiratory infection, which then spreads to the contiguous sinuses and subsequently to the orbit and the brain. Mucormycosis presents with gradual-onset of facial and periorbital swelling, ptosis, diplopia and visual loss which may lead to complications such as retinal vascular occlusion, multiple cranial nerve palsies and cerebrovascular occlusions.

Figure 66.1 shows a 55-year-old woman with orbitorhinomucormycosis. The left eye presented with periorbital swelling, complete ptosis, proptosis and external ophthalmoplegia. Fundus examination showed multiple cotton-wool spots with disk pallor in the left eye **(Figure 66.2)**.

Treatment of Orbitorhinomucormycosis includes management of acidosis and aggressive surgical intervention under amphotericin B administered both systemically and locally. Wide excision of devitalized and necrosed tissue with correction of underlying

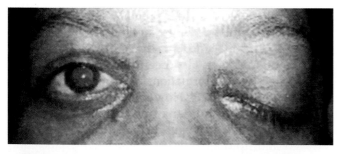

Figure 66.1 Orbitorhinomucormycosis of the left eye showing ptosis and periorbital swelling

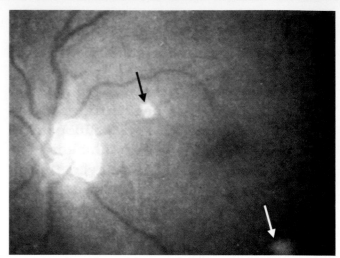

Figure 66.2 Left eye: Fundus picture shows cotton-wool spots with disk pallor

metabolic effects, is the only practicable mode of intervention.

Orbital Cellulitis

This condition is commonly seen in diabetes from any focus of infection in the body. Bacterial orbital cellulitis is a life-threatening infection of the soft tissue behind the orbital septum. It may be caused by the extension of preseptal cellulitis which may be sinus-related in some cases, local spread from adjacent dacryocystitis, midfacial or dental infection, hematogenous spread or following retinal, lacrimal or orbital surgery. Orbital cellulitis presents with severe malaise, fever, pain, visual impairment, unilateral, tender, warm and red periorbital and lid edema, proptosis, painful ophthalmoplegia and optic nerve dysfunction.[28]

To manage this condition: (1) Identify focus of infection and treat suitably; (2) Optic nerve function should be monitored every 4 hours, steroids should be used under cover of antibiotics; (3) Surgical intervention should be considered, if there is poor response to antibiotic therapy. Decreasing vision, orbital or sub-periosteal abscess and an atypical picture, may merit diagnostic biopsy.

Lids

Chalazion

Chalazion (Meibomian cyst) is a chronic, sterile, lipogranulomatous inflammatory lesion caused by blockage of meibomian gland orifices and stagnation of sebaceous secretions.[29] Chalazion is a painless, round,

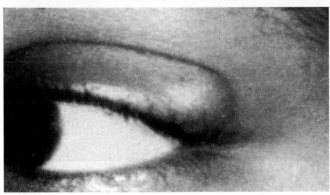

Figure 66.3 Chalazion in the upper lid of the left eye

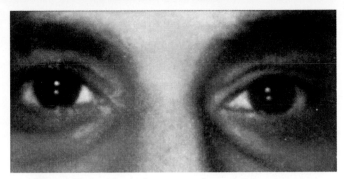

Figure 66.4 Xanthelasma on the medial upper and lower lids

smooth swelling within the tarsal plate of variable size which may be multiple or bilateral. Management of chalazion requires incision and curettage under cover of antibiotics and good glycemic control. In an acute stage, topical and systemic antibiotics may be required before incision. **Figure 66.3** shows a 40 years women presenting with chalazion on left lateral upper lid.

Hordeolum Externum (Stye)

Stye is a suppurative inflammation of one of the Zeis glands caused by *Staphylococcus*. Pain along the lid margin is followed by a swelling, which characterizes it from chalazion where swelling is painless, unless infected. The gland becomes hard, swollen and tender subsequently forming an abscess. Multiple lesions may also be present. Hordeola are found more frequently in persons who have uncontrolled diabetes, chronic blepharitis, seborrhea and increased serum lipids. Application of antibiotic ointment prevents recurrences. Hot compresses and epilation of the lash associated with the infected follicle may hasten resolution.

Hordeolum Internum

Hordeolum internum is an abscess caused by an acute staphylococcal infection of the meibomian gland. It is a tender, painful swelling within the tarsal plate, occurring less frequently but presents as a more violent inflammation than the stye. The lesion may enlarge and then discharge either posteriorly through the duct or through the conjunctiva. An incision and curettage may be required if a residual nodule remains after the acute infection has subsided after treatment with suitable antibiotics.[29]

Xanthelasma

This condition occurs more frequently in diabetic patients with elevated serum lipid levels, but does not

pose a threat to vision. Xanthelasma does not occur as a result of diabetes *per se*, but may reflect poor diabetic control.[27] It is a yellowish, subcutaneous plaque consisting of cholesterol and lipids which are usually located at the medial aspects of the eyelids. Destruction with carbon dioxide or argon laser is preferred to excision for cosmetic reasons. However, recurrences are possible if the disturbance in lipid metabolism persists. **Figure 66.4** illustrates xanthelasma on the medial part upper and lower lids of a 32-year-old male subject.

Blepharoptosis

Ptosis is an abnormally low position of the upper lid which may be unilateral or bilateral, partial or complete, congenital or acquired. The various causes for this condition include innervational defect such as third nerve palsy and oculosympathetic palsy (neurogenic), myopathy of the levator muscle itself or neuromyopathic (myogenic), defect of the levator aponeurosis (aponeurotic) or gravitational effect of a mass or scarring (mechanical). No alterations occur in the pupil, unlike in other third nerve palsies. The degree of lid closure is influenced by duration of diabetes and is considered to be more prevalent in type 1 diabetic individuals particularly in those with retinal involvement.[30]

The management of ptosis is variable, consequent to the causes. In neurogenic ptosis, patient should be treated on conservative lines for 6 to 9 months. Myogenic ptosis responds to corticosteroid, immunosuppressive therapy, plasmapheresis and thymectomy. In aponeurotic and mechanical ptosis, the deformity is usually corrected by surgery.

Blepharitis

Chronic blepharitis is common in diabetic patients due to uncontrolled hyperglycemia, reflecting general proneness to infections. This condition is a chronic

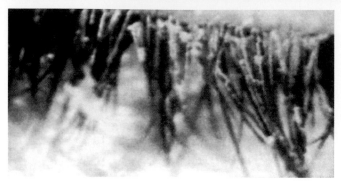

Figure 66.5 Scurf or debris found amid eyelashes in patient with blepharitis

inflammation of the lid margin. Clinically, it occurs in two forms, squamous and ulcerative blepharitis. Squamous blepharitis is characterized by the appearance of fine whitish scales around the roots of lashes, which can be easily removed without ulceration. While in ulcerative blepharitis, the lid margins are ulcerated and infection is more deeply seated and involves the hair follicles destroying some and distorting others in the process. If untreated the ulceration may extend to involve the whole lid margin and the inevitable sequelae of fibrosis leads to deformities of the lids. Scurf or debris, found amid eyelashes in a male patient with blepharitis **(Figure 66.5)**.

Management of blepharitis consists of appropriate removal of the crust, application of specific antibiotic ointment depending on the sensitivity of the organism and massage of the lid margin. Systemic tetracyclines and mechanical expression of the meibomian glands are the mainstay of treatment for squamous blepharitis.

Lacrimal Glands

Hyperglycemia can affect the nerves supplying the lacrimal gland. Diabetes has been reported to affect the lacrimal gland by decreasing tear secretion, forming a less uniform lipid layer and reducing tear break-up time.[31] Rubinstein et al reported that tear secretion is reduced only in type 2 subjects though the effect of age needs consideration.[32] Patient presents with complaints of dry eyes leading to irritation. As a sequel of lack of tears, the patient is at a higher risk of developing corneal ulcers, hence, proper lubrication using tear substitutes should be advised.

Conjunctiva

Microcirculatory changes occur in diabetic individuals, which are a reflection of general microvascular disturbance of diabetes.[33] Conjunctival microcirculation changes may manifest as microaneurysms, vasoconstriction, diurnal variation in venous dilation, vessel distension, increased tortuosity, fusiform dilatation, arteriole wall thickening, sludging of blood in vessels and capillary proliferation. Microaneurysms are often seen adjacent to the limbus and occasionally can be observed in nondiabetic individuals also. The diurnal variation in venous dilatation is independent of blood glucose level or time of insulin therapy.[34]

The conjunctival alterations are more common in adult diabetic individuals suggesting that the vasculature becomes more susceptible with age. In contrast, in a study conducted in pediatric diabetic patients conjunctival microabnormalities existed in all pediatric type 1 diabetic subjects in varying degrees despite their relatively young age.[35] Isenberg et al[36] have reported that conjunctival oxygen tension in diabetic patients had significant correlation with the level of conjunctival hypoxia and the degree of retinal involvement.

Cornea

Generalized Alterations

Diabetes has impact on every layer of the cornea and is often more susceptible to injury and heals more slowly in diabetic individuals than the normal individuals. The sorbitol pathway is believed to be an important factor in some corneal manifestations of diabetes. It has a significant effect on morphological, metabolic, physiological, and clinical aspects of the cornea. Morphological changes occur in the corneal epithelium, epithelial basement membrane and basement membrane complexes, stroma, and endothelium. Myriad primary and postoperative manifestations are caused due to the homeostasis of these structures in both the nonstressed and the stressed cornea. The corneal epithelium may exhibit changes including a decrease in the number of cells, thinning and basement membrane alterations affecting epithelial adherence and epithelialization. Clinically, this can lead to many diabetic patients having epithelial keratitis. Corneal epithelial lesions can be observed in approximately one-half of asymptomatic patients with diabetes mellitus. Recent studies suggest that the polyol pathway may play a role in the pathogenesis of these disorders.[37]

Corneal complications such as tear film dysfunction, elevated glucose in tears, neurotrophic ulcers, corneal edema, wrinkles in Descemet's membrane and decrease in corneal sensitivity have also been reported in diabetic individuals.[34] Type 2 diabetic individuals when compared with the healthy control group, showed decreased tear film break-up time, increased rate of staining with fluorescein sodium on the cornea and abnormal conjunctival epithelium.[38]

In the experimental scenario changes were observed in the morphologic features of the collagen within Descemet's membrane in diabetes induced rats.[39] Minute folds in Descemet's membrane probably represent an alteration in the tissue fluid level of the cornea. These folds increase with age in both normal and diabetic subjects, with female diabetic subjects being more prone. Little is known about the effects on corneal stroma. Some studies have reported stomal edema following vitrectomy to be associated with diabetes but others dispute this statement.

In addition to the morphological changes in the epithelium and endothelium, an increase in corneal thickness in diabetic individuals has also been reported.[40] This change may be observed early in the course of the disease and related to severity of the retinal involvement.

Corneal Sensitivity

Studies have demonstrated that diabetic individuals have decreased corneal sensitivity[41], making them more vulnerable to corneal trauma. The reduction in sensitivity is part of the diabetic peripheral neuropathy and due to inactivation of the trigeminal nerves and their branches in the cornea, which in effect increases the conduction time. It also decreases tear secretion, which in turn increases tear film osmolarity and reduces goblet cell density. The other factors involved in the pathogenesis are accumulation of sorbitol within the lamellae of the Schwann cell, causing mechanical compressive or toxic damage to the axon and partial demyelination of the nerve due to abnormal lipid metabolism.

Studies have clearly demonstrated the existence of neuropathy in diabetic cornea, both in an animal model and in the humans.[35] Diabetic keratopathy has been thought to represent a form of corneal neuropathy, which emerges subsequent to the undue stress like intraocular surgery or photocoagulation. These lesions are transient and clinically resemble the keratopathy seen in staphylococcal keratoconjunctivitis. The morphology of corneal nerves has been found to be altered in diabetic rats and humans.[42] These morphological alterations are probably implicated in the development of neurotrophic corneal ulcerations with diabetes.

Measurement of corneal sensitivity may be a useful tool in the early diagnosis of diabetic neuropathy. Ruben et al measured corneal sensitivity in diabetic patients undergoing photocoagulation for proliferative retinopathy and reported that both type 1 and type 2 diabetic individuals showed significantly decreased sensitivity and that there was no significant change following photocoagulation.[43] Decreased corneal sensitivity contribute to a host of complications observed in the epithelium of the diabetic individual including recurrent erosions, slowed wound repair, predisposition to abrasions, neurotrophic corneal ulceration, transient punctuate diabetic keratopathy, epithelial desquamation and defective re-epithelialisation. In established cases, re-epithelization should be promoted by use of lubricants and patching. Newer treatment modalities include use of topical nerve growth factor,[44] aldose reductase inhibitor CT-112[45] and amniotic membrane transplantation.[46]

Pupil and Iris

Pupillary Abnormalities

The pupillary abnormalities in diabetic individuals include decreased light reflexes both at the onset and during the course of diabetes mellitus, decreased hippus during continuous illumination and increased miosis or failure to dilate normally in the dark. Some diabetic pupils resemble the Argyll Robertson syndrome (non-syphilitic) and dilate poorly with anti-muscarinics but exhibit supersensitivity with sympathomimetic drugs.[47] These pupillary dysfunctions are closely associated with long duration and poor control of diabetes, and accounted for by either myopathy or neuropathy, or maybe both. The sequence of events in pupillary dysfunction in diabetes mellitus described by Alio et al[47] is summarized in **Flow chart 66.1**.

Other speculated causes for pupillary dysfunctions reported include rigidity of iris and distension of the pigment epithelium from the formation of vacuoles. Both these are inferred from the observation that the pupil motility depends on the glucose levels.

Generalized Alterations

Hyperglycemia can also cause proliferation of the iris pigments causing melanosis of the iris and overgrowth of the posterior pigment epithelium that extends over the edge of the pupil in the margin area forming an apron known as 'ectropion uveae'. These conditions are normally a sequel to iris neovascularization although it

Flow chart 66.1 The sequence of events in pupillary dysfunction in diabetes mellitus[47]

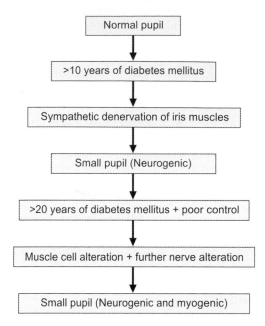

has been observed in cases without rubeosis also. Diabetic subjects are also predisposed to moderate-to-severe iritis, in which inflammation primarily affects the iris. It is characterized by a thick plastic exudative discharge with a tendency for bleeding from the iritis causing hyphema.[48]

Iris Neovascularization

Diabetic individuals are prone to both morphologic and vascular alterations. Iris neovascularization (rubeosis iridis) is known to occur due to frequent occlusion of small vessel elements. It develops as tiny dilated capillary tuffs or red spots around the pupillary margin and may be missed unless examined carefully under high magnification. The new vessels grow radially over the surface of the iris towards the angle, sometimes joining dilated blood vessels at the collarette. At this stage intraocular pressure (IOP) may be still normal in some cases and the new vessels may regress either spontaneously with good metabolic control and pan-retinal photocoagulation of the retina.[49]

Rubeosis is common in individuals with advanced diabetes with invariable proliferation of blood vessels in the retina and it has been estimated that less than 5% of individuals with retinal proliferation who are not laser treated may develop this condition.[50] Neovascular glaucoma may eventually develop which is a painful

and vision debilitating condition. Many studies have reported regression of neovascularization of iris following panretinal photocoagulation or by repair of a detached retina.

Angle Structures

Open-Angle Glaucoma

Open-angle glaucoma has reported to be two times more common in diabetic subjects than in the general population.[50] The pathologic mechanism leading to this condition is microscopic blockage of the trabecular meshwork. Open-angle glaucoma is an asymptomatic, progressive optic neuropathy characterized by enlarging optic disk cupping and visual field loss. The Blue Mountain Eye Study reported that the prevalence of open-angle glaucoma was increased in people with diabetes and ocular hypertension (elevated intraocular pressure in the presence of normal optic disks and visual fields) was also more common in diabetic individuals.[51]

Management of open-angle glaucoma in diabetic individuals includes a complete work-up and then treating by topical and systemic hypotensive agents taking into view their general medical condition. Early detection of optic nerve damage can be efficiently assessed by computerized visual fields charting and using newer imaging techniques like ocular coherence tomography (OCT). The OCT depicts cross-sectional image and can accurately assess the thickness of retinal nerve fiber layer (RFNL), optic cup disk ratio and peripapillary rim of the optic disk.

Angle Closure Glaucoma

Diabetes may be associated with angle closure glaucoma due to an increase in lens thickness in diabetic patients and autonomic dysfunction which may lead to a more dilated pupil.[52] This form is comparatively rare among persons with diabetes. It presents with severe pain, reduced visual acuity, congestion of the globe, increased IOP, corneal edema and aqueous flare due to leakage of proteins from the iris new vessels. Management is aimed mainly at relieving pain. Medical management is with systemic or topical hypotensive agents except miotics. Visual acuity recovers with medical treatment.

Neovascular Glaucoma

Neovascular glaucoma (NVG) from diabetes, although not nearly as common, inflicts devastating consequences on vision and is a serious condition occurring as a result of iris neovascularization. The leading cause of NVG is retinal vein occlusion, which accounts for 36% of all cases. Diabetes is the second in frequency accounting for 32% of all cases and 95% of bilateral cases.[53] Those with long-standing diabetes (>10 years), proliferative retinopathy and cataract have higher risk of developing NVG. Due to the increase in prompt application of panretinal photocoagulation, the prevalence of NVG is decreasing.[49]

Lens

The changes that may occur to the diabetic lens are: (i) The formation of cataracts and (ii) Alterations to its curvature and refractive index which result in refractive changes (dynamic changes).

Cataract Formation

Cataract is more prevalent and occurs at a younger age in diabetic individuals than in the general population. Peterson et al[54] have demonstrated that cataract is observed 15 to 25 times higher in diabetic patients under 40 years of age. It is a major cause of visual impairment and blindness, particularly in type 2 diabetes. The overall risk of cataract formation for all ages is 2 to 4 times greater in the diabetic subjects than in the nondiabetic subjects.[55] Posterior subcapsular cataract is particularly common in diabetic patients than other morphological types of cataract.[56]

Longer duration of diabetes, poor metabolic control, increased severity of retinopathy, older age at examination and diuretic usage in type 1 patients results in higher prevalence of cataract whatever age at examination. Increased severity of retinopathy, diuretic usage, lower intraocular pressure, smoking and lower diastolic blood pressure in type 2 patients were significantly associated with higher prevalence of cataract.[55]

Typically, these are snowflake opacities, polychromatic crystals and vacuoles in the lenticular cortex. The cataract can progress rapidly until the whole lens is cloudy, or reverse with appropriate treatment. The two types of cataract in diabetic individuals are (i) True diabetic and (ii) Senile type cortical cataracts. The general mechanism of both types of cataracts is related to sorbitol pathway. The 'snowflake' or 'juvenile diabetic' cataract characteristic of poorly controlled type 1 diabetes is very uncommon. These cataracts are bilateral, and rarely affect the vision. They often have a rapid onset, appear as white punctate or stellate opacities, and can resolve without treatment.

The senile type of cataract in the diabetic patient is identical and clinically alike in appearance as presented in the aged population. The rapidity of development is remarkable, especially with uncontrolled severe hyperglycemia. Dense cataracts often preclude a proper examination of retina which may result in undiagnosed vision threatening retinopathy.

Cataract surgery (phacoemulsification and intracapsular implantation of an intraocular plastic lens) is often effective in both cases, but may be compromised by coexistent retinopathy and postoperative complications including anterior-chamber inflammation and posterior capsule opacification.[57] Of patients undergoing surgery for senile type of cataract, 4.2% were found to be undiagnosed diabetic patients as reported by Caird et al,[58] Rema et al[59] have shown that 44% of type 2 diabetic subjects had progression of diabetic retinopathy after extracapsular cataract extraction and IOL implantation. In a few diabetic subjects, diabetic retinopathy was diagnosed for the first time after cataract surgery, i.e. 7 of 88 eyes that were not known to have retinopathy preoperatively.

Refractive Changes

The dynamic alterations including changes in lenticular status either hydration or dehydration, as a result of changes in the osmolality of the aqueous from either a rise or fall in blood glucose and the shape of lens and/or its refractive index, results in fluctuating refractive errors and variable vision. These sudden refractive shifts are frequently the presenting symptom for a newly diagnosed diabetic person. Acute, severe or even moderate hyperglycemia may cause this shift either towards hyperopia (transient nature) or myopia (more permanent nature). Many studies have reported that hyperopic shift is more common than the myopic one.[60] Transient refractive changes are commonly seen and may persist for a few weeks. Myopia may be due to an increase in thickness and curvature of the crystalline lens that occurs in diabetic patients, which is reversed after control of diabetes. Sometimes on an intensive control with insulin, there is a tendency towards hypermetropia following institution of therapy. The change in the refractive error is probably due to the alteration in the aldose reductase/sorbitol pathway.

Extraocular Muscles

Cranial Nerve Palsies

Cranial nerve palsies are some dramatic complications in uncontrolled diabetes. Presentation of such neuropathy, however, is of serious concern to the individual, because the presenting symptom is usually disturbing diplopia occasionally accompanied by pain in the eye. Cranial nerve palsies usually occur in isolation but can be seen as a multiple presentation and interestingly, diabetic cranial neuropathies are exclusively seen in adults. The cause of cranial neuropathies in diabetic patients is thought to be a combination of vascular and metabolic problems leading to a disruption of axonal transport and vascular permeability.[61]

Third Nerve Palsy (Oculomotor)

The third cranial nerve innervates the pupil, levator palpebrae, inferior and superior and medial rectus muscles. Diabetes affects the vasa nervosum which runs in the center of the nerves, occasionally leading to occlusion of vasa nervosum. This occlusion affects the central nerve fibers sparing the superficial pupillary fibers, thus resulting in "pupil sparing third nerve palsy". It is often associated with periorbital pain or ipsilateral headache which may occasionally be the presenting feature of diabetes.[62] Diabetes-associated third nerve palsy is manifested by unilateral ptosis and exotropia. The patient has bizarre defects in ocular mobility including elevation of upper eyelid on attempted adduction or depression in the affected eye. The pupil is spared in diabetes related occulomotor palsies, however, other causes have to be ruled out by a complete neurological examination and perhaps CT and MRI scans.

Fourth Nerve Palsy (Trochlear)

This condition is rare when compared to III nerve palsy. The IV cranial nerve supplies the superior oblique muscle. Although the most common cause of trochlear palsy is trauma, it can also be affected in diabetes, hypertension, tumors, vascular lesions, multiple sclerosis and meningitis. A patient with a trochlear nerve palsy typically has a vertical diplopia, worse on gaze away from the affected eye and at near. A torsional component may also be present (excyclotorsion). The patient usually adopts a contralateral head tilt to correct diplopia and bilateral involvement is common. Park's three step test and Double Maddox Rod test are useful in defining the extent of palsy. Diplopia charting and Hess charting can be done to determine the severity of diplopia.[62]

Sixth Nerve Palsy (Abducens)

In abducens nerve palsy, there is a horizontal diplopia, worse on gaze to the affected side and with distance vision. There is a limitation of abduction of the eye in question and the patient may exhibit a tilt of the head to the affected side to minimize diplopia.[62] Movement of the eye laterally past the midline is restricted or absent. The onset may be sudden and there is neither visual loss nor visual field loss. The sixth nerve has a long intracranial course and multiple causes of palsy necessitating careful neurological evaluation. A retrospective population-based case-control study of patients with new onset of neurologically isolated sixth nerve palsy concluded that there is a 6-fold increase in odds of having diabetes in cases of sixth nerve palsy over controls.[63]

Seventh Nerve/Bell's Palsy (Facial)

Bell's palsy, an idiopathic facial nerve palsy, is the most common cause for acute facial nerve paralysis and diabetic patients are four times more likely to develop this condition.[64] Patients with a facial nerve palsy present with a weakness on one side of the face.

Clinical features depend upon the level of lesion (Lower motor neuron or upper motor neuron) and whether one or both facial nerves are affected. The lower motor neuron lesion presents with weakness of all muscles of facial expression, deviation of angle of mouth, dribbling of saliva on the affected side, deepening of nasolabial fold, weakness of frowning (frontalis muscle) and eye closure (orbicularis oculi muscle) and signs of corneal exposure. There may be loss of taste on anterior 2/3rd of tongue in some lesions. Upper motor neuron lesion presents with weakness of lower half of face on opposite side of lesion with sparing of frontalis and orbicularis oculi muscles.

The prognosis for cranial nerve palsies is good, with function usually being restored over a period of 6 to 9 months. Nerve palsies that do not resolve after approximately six months are most probably not of diabetic origin. Physiotherapy is the mainstay of management of cranial nerve palsies. Nonsurgical management includes use of Fresnel prisms if the angle of deviation is small, uniocular occlusion to avoid diplopia. In case of abducens palsy, botulinum toxin injection may be injected into the uninvolved lateral rectus muscle to avoid contracture before the deviation improves/stabilizes. Surgical management is usually not earlier than six months from the date of onset.[62] Trochlear nerve palsy usually recovers completely within 6 to 8 months. A careful orthoptic evaluation should be made, followed either by superior oblique strengthening, inferior oblique weakening or classical Harada-Ito procedure. In case of facial palsy, the commonly employed, treatment modalities include eye patching and lubrication to protect the cornea.[65] In non-resolving type of facial palsy, tarsorrhaphy or medial canthoplasty may be done as a permanent procedure. Steroids are generally agreed to be beneficial in facial palsy.[66]

Diabetes can also affect autonomic nerve function. The most common clinical manifestation in the eye is an exaggerated miosis from a lack of sympathetic tone. Parasympathetic dysfunction can lead to a more dilated pupil. The diabetic patient may have light-near dissociation, where the pupil's near reflex is greater than the light reflex. Bilateral light-near dissociation is usually seen in type 1 diabetic subjects, although may also be seen in type 2 diabetic patients of long duration. This occurs due to pupillary autonomic denervation[67] and may represent a selective neuropathy involving pupillomotor parasympathetic nerve fibers. Amplitudes of accommodation may also be reduced.[61]

Vitreous

Asteroid Hyalosis

This condition is characterized by small but striking, highly refractile 'stars' (asteroids) in the vitreous. It appears as cream-white spherical bodies distributed throughout the vitreous either randomly or in chains or sheets. It rarely causes any visual symptoms and are usually found on routine examination. Opacity studies suggest that asteroid hyalosis are composed of calcium soaps together with various lipoids. They are usually unilateral (in 75% of cases) and occur mostly in elder persons and are said to be common in males than females. This condition is reported to be common in diabetic individuals, according to earlier reports.[68] It has been stated that 5.4% of the diabetic individuals have these bodies. Yazar et al have demonstrated that asteroid hyalosis can also cause artefactual lowering of axial length measurement, leading to significant error in calculations of intraocular lens power.[69]

Vitreous Contraction

Instability of the vitreous is caused due to loss of gel state without dehiscence at the vitreoretinal interface, which may induce traction of the vitreous in cases of proliferative diabetic retinopathy (PDR). Viterous body consists of hyaluronic acid, which can change its configuration as a result of ionic interactions causing swelling and shrinkage of the vitreous, which eventually results in structural and volumetric alterations in the vitreous. These alterations will produce traction upon the structures which are attached to the vitreous cortex

such as the new vessels present in PDR and contribute to progression of retinopathy either by traction on the new vessels or by inducing a rupture of the new vessels causing a vitreous hemorrhage.

Liquefaction/Posterior Vitreous Detachment

Posterior vitreous detachment (PVD) is a phenomenon, which occurs from degenerative changes in the vitreous and is significantly more common in diabetic subjects, even in eyes without retinopathy.[70] Pischel et al[71] reported that this condition is present in 60% of all patients over 50 years of age. Normally, there is no effect on visual acuity, but the patient experiences a brief episode of photopsia. Clinically, acute bilateral occurrence of PVD is generally rare.

Optic Nerve

Optic nerve dysfunction may present itself in various clinical characteristics including optic disk swelling (diabetic papillopathy), optic atrophy, optic neuritis and ischemic optic neuropathy [Anterior ischemic optic neuropathy (AION) and nonarteritic AION]. In a study conducted in diabetic patients, ischemic optic neuropathy was the predominant form of optic nerve lesions (59.20%) followed by secondary optic atrophy, postischemic optic neuropathy (33.40%) and retrobulbar optic neuritis (7.40%).[72]

Papillopathy

Diabetic papillopathy is an uncommon condition characterized by transient visual dysfunction coupled with optic disk swelling occurring in both type 1 and type 2 diabetic subjects. It generally affects the type 1 diabetic individuals in the second and third decade who have diabetes for over 10 years. The etiology is unknown but theories postulate that retinal vascular leakage into and surrounding the optic nerve and disruption of axoplasmic flow resulting from microvascular disease of the optic nerve head vasculature may be responsible for this condition.[73] In most cases, the papillopathy is bilateral (50% of cases) and is thought to be a manifestation of ischemia. When severe, it is very similar in appearance to papilledema caused by raised intracranial pressure. Any loss of vision, which is usually moderate at worst, tends to recover in about six months. Prognosis is relatively good despite lack of specific treatment. In most cases, spontaneous resolution occurs within several months, with stabilization or improvement of visual acuity, although mild optic atrophy may still develop.

Anterior Ischemic Optic Neuropathy

Anterior ischemic optic neuropathy (AION), one of the most common and visually crippling diseases in the middle-aged and elderly, is due to acute ischemia of the optic nerve head. AION is defined as segmental or generalized infarction within the prelaminar or laminar portions of the optic nerve caused by occlusion of short posterior ciliary arteries. Clinically, AION is of two types: (1) Arteritic AION caused due to giant cell arteritis and (2) Nonarteritic AION caused due to other risk factors.[74] AION affects diabetic patients of all ages. Diabetic subjects are more prone to develop bilateral AION.[75]

Arteritic AION: Arteritic AION associated with temporal arteritis is an ophthalmic emergency because this condition is likely to cause rapid, visual disability, which is almost always preventable if treated immediately.[74] In untreated patients, the incidence is 30 to 50%, of which one-third develop bilateral involvement. This disease has a predilection for medium sized and larger arteries, particularly the superficial temporal, ophthalmic, posterior ciliary and proximal part of the vertebral. Prognosis is very poor as visual loss is usually permanent although, very rarely, administration of large doses of systemic corticosteroids may be associated with partial visual recovery. Management involves taking a temporal artery biopsy and ESR and supporting with anti-inflammatory drugs.

Nonarteritic AION: Nonarteritic anterior ischemic optic neuropathy (NAION) refers to an idiopathic ischemic process of the anterior portion of the optic nerve. The typical presentation is sudden and painless visual loss, relative afferent pupil defect, a pale swollen optic disk and an inferior altitudinal hemianopsia.[76] Visual loss is frequently discovered on awakening, suggesting that nocturnal hypotension may play an important role.[77] The other associated risk factors include altered optic disk morphology, advanced age, hypertension, diabetes mellitus, hypercholesterolemia, collagen vascular disease and cataract surgery. It has been observed that 24% of subjects in the Ischemic Optic Neuropathy Decompression Trial Study had diabetes.[78] Currently, there is no effective long-term treatment for this condition, although any underlying systemic factors should be treated and reduction of risk factors such as smoking should be encouraged.[62,76] About 40% of the patients may have some improvement in central vision. There is approximately 30 to 50% chance of the fellow eye getting affected. However, recurrence in the same eye is very rare.[62] It is also important to differentiate it from the arteritic type to aid management.

Optic Neuritis

Optic neuritis is one of the most common causes of sudden vision loss in the young subjects and occurs with higher frequency in diabetic individuals. This condition is an inflammatory, infective or demyelinating process affecting the optic nerve. The hypothesized etiological classification is outlined as: (1) Demyelinating—the most common cause, (2) Parainfectious—following a viral infection or immunization, (3) Infectious—may be sinus related or cat-scratch fever, syphilis, Lyme disease, cryptococcal meningitis in AIDS patients and herpes zoster and (4) autoimmune-associated with systemic autoimmune diseases.[62] In diabetic subjects, along with autoimmune mechanism, ischemia and nutritional deficiencies are also implicated.[79] Usually, it affects only one eye, but may be extensive involving the chiasma and even the adjacent brain tissue.

Clinical features of demyelinating optic neuritis include subacute monocular visual impairment and may be discomfort in and around the eye, which often worsens due to movement of the eye. In some patients, frontal headache and tenderness of the globe are observed. Colors may appear "washed out". In para-infectious type, presentation is usually 1 to 3 weeks following a viral infection or immunization, frequently affecting more children than adults.

Management is probably not essential if visual loss is mild. The pain and discomfort due to this condition recedes after a few days. The vision usually improves in about 85% of patients after a period of weeks or even months.[79] However, when visual loss is severe and bilateral involvement is observed, intravenous steroids can be considered. It has been demonstrated in the optic neuritis treatment trial (ONTT) that there may be better and faster improvement in patients treated with intravenous steroids, especially in those who have extensive disease.[80] It has to be followed by oral steroids. Initiating therapy only with oral steroids can lead to deleterious effects.

Optic Atrophy

Optic atrophy often results from arterial blood flow insufficiency associated with some systemic vascular disease (cardiovascular disease, hypertension, or diabetes mellitus). The lack of adequate blood perfusion pressure can create conditions leading to anoxia and death of the nerve fiber layer with a resultant visual field defect.[81] It usually occurs as a sequel of AION, optic neuritis, severe ischemia, internal carotid disease, central retinal artery occlusion, and retinal artery branch occlusion. As all these conditions are more common in diabetic patients, they are at higher risk of developing optic atrophy.

The patient merely presents with loss of vision. The clinical picture varies according to the extent of damage of optic nerve, the signs include white or dirty grey, slightly raised disk with poorly delineated margins caused due to gliosis and decrease in number of small blood vessels.[79] The prognosis is very poor as there is no treatment to redeem vision. Hence, utmost care should be taken to prevent any damage to the other 'seeing eye'.

RETINAL MANIFESTATIONS

The most distressing effects of diabetes on the eye with regard to visual prognosis are on the retina. The retinal vascular system appears to be the prime target. Retinal complications due to diabetes include diabetic retinopathy, the most severe of the several ocular complications of diabetes, lipemia retinalis and retinal vein occlusion.

Diabetic Retinopathy

Diabetic retinopathy (DR) is a common complication of diabetes posing a serious threat to vision, and is seen in both type 1 and type 2 diabetes. The clinical hallmarks of DR include capillary dilatation, microaneurysms, increased vascular permeability leading to edema, and endothelial cell proliferation. This condition may occur with or without the other systemic complications of diabetes and its incidence increases with duration of diabetes.

Classification and Prevalence

Classically, retinopathy has been graded as nonproliferative diabetic retinopathy (NPDR) and proliferative diabetic retinopathy (PDR). Progression from mild-to-moderate, and then to severe, NPDR indicates progressive ischemia in the retina and an increased risk for the development of PDR[82] characterized by the growth of new blood vessels on the retina and posterior surface of the vitreous. Proliferative diabetic retinopathy (PDR) is an advanced and severe form of retinopathy. **Figures 66.6 and 66.7** show the color and fundus fluorescein angiography photographs of a male diabetic patient aged 57 years with extensive neovascularization at the optic disk.

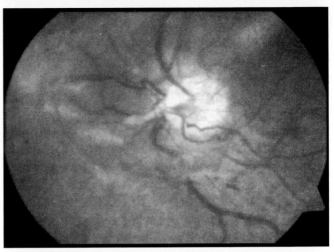

Figure 66.6 Optic disk with neovascularization

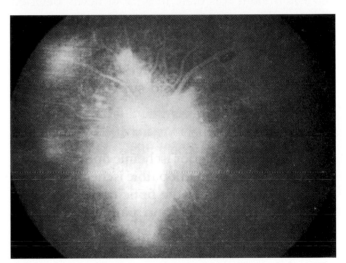

Figure 66.7 Late frame of fundus fluorescein angiography showing extensive dye leakage at the optic disk from new vessels

In the Indian scenario, the prevalence of DR is lower compared to most other populations. The prevalence of DR in a clinic cohort of 6792 type 2 diabetic patients was 34.1% which included 30.8% with NPDR, 3.4% with PDR and 6.4% had diabetic macular edema.[83] DR may be present even at the time of diagnosis due the insidious onset of type 2 diabetes. In a study of consecutive 500 newly diagnosed type 2 diabetic patients, it was observed that 7.3% already had diabetic retinopathy at the time of diagnosis of diabetes[84], whereas in the UKPDS,[85] the prevalence of diabetic retinopathy at the time of diagnosis of diabetes was 35%. In a recently conducted Chennai Urban Rural Epidemiology Study (CURES) eye study; the first population-based study, which used four-field stereoretinal photographs and

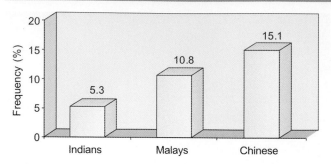

Figure 66.8 Prevalence of retinopathy in the Asian young diabetes study (ASDIAB)[87]

TABLE 66.2	Risk factors associated with the development of diabetic retinopathy
Systemic factors	*Ocular factors*
Age	Posterior vitreous
Sex	detachment
Duration of diabetes	Old chorioretinopathy
Poor glycemic control	Cataract surgery
Hypertension	
Pregnancy	
Renal disease	
Raised triglycerides	
and hematocrit	
Smoking	
Alcohol	
Obesity	

ETDRS grading to document DR in the Indian population, the overall prevalence of DR in urban population was 17.6%. Among the known diabetic subjects, 20.8% had DR while it was there in 5.1% of newly detected diabetic subjects.[4]

In another population-based study in Chennai (India), the Chennai Urban Population Study (CUPS), which included both known and newly detected diabetic individuals among the middle and lower socioeconomic groups, 17.5% had nonproliferative diabetic retinopathy while 1.5% had proliferative diabetic retinopathy.[86]

In a study done in young diabetics in Asia called as ASDIAB, the prevalence of DR was least among Indians (5.3%) as compared to other ethnic groups like Malays (10%) and Chinese (15.1%) **(Figure 66.8)**.[87] Higher levels of fasting C-peptide and glucagon stimulated C-peptide among the Indians in this study, may partly explain the lowest prevalence of DR in this group.

Risk Factors

The onset and progression of DR may be influenced by many systemic factors and ocular factors **(Table 66.2)**. In a large clinic-based study conducted in Chennai, it was shown that NPDR and PDR increased with increasing duration of diabetes. In this study, in type 2 diabetic subjects of 20 years or longer duration, 73% had NPDR and 11.9% had PDR.[83] In the CURES eye study severity of retinopathy proportionally increased with length of duration of diabetes and it has been observed that for every five year increase in duration of diabetes, the risk for DR increased by 1.89 times.[4] In Joslin clinic patients, there appears to be excess females over males in the older-onset group, however, among those with PDR, males equal females in number[88] while in the clinic cohort in Chennai, DR appeared to be more prevalent in the males compared to females at a ratio of 2 : 1.[83]

Recent data from epidemiological studies and clinical trials have shown that hyperglycemia is associated with increased incidence and progression of diabetic retinopathy in both type 1 and 2 diabetes.[5-7] Hyperglycemia, as measured by glycated hemoglobin levels, is a significant risk factor for the progression of diabetic retinopathy.[89] It has been shown in the CURES eye study[4] that there was a linear trend in the prevalence of retinopathy with increase in quartiles of HbA_{1c} [trend Chi square: 51.6, p<0.001] as shown in **Figure 66.9**.

Hypertension—an established risk factor for retinopathy has been hypothesized, to damage the retinal capillary endothelial cells by increase in sheer stress of the blood flow. In CURES eye study, conducted on 26,001 individuals in Chennai, among diabetic subjects with hypertension the prevalence of DR was higher (18.8%) but this did not reach statistical significance.[4] In the UKPDS, hypertensive patients with type 2 diabetes assigned to tight control had a 34% reduction in progression of retinopathy.[90]

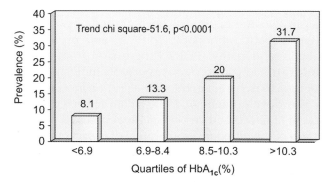

Figure 66.9 Prevalence of retinopathy in quartiles of HbA_{1c} levels—the Chennai Urban Rural Epidemiology Study (CURES)[4]

Dyslipidemia, independent of glycemia, has also been shown to be associated with an increased risk of developing retinopathy in the WESDR and Early Treatment Diabetic Retinopathy Study (ETDRS), although the results have not been consistent.[91] An association of diabetic macular edema in type 2 diabetic subjects with increased LDL levels has been shown in earlier study by Rema et al.[92] It has also been shown that in type 2 diabetic subjects, there is an increase in the lipid peroxidation in erythrocyte cell membrane and plasma and this is accentuated in patients with diabetic complications.[93] An association of DR has been observed with total cholesterol and serum triglycerides even after adjusting for age, as age by itself is a significant risk factor for hyperlipidemia in the CURES eye study. Diabetic macular edema also showed a strong correlation with high LDL levels in the study.[94] The role of oxidant stress in the causation of DR is being increasingly recognized.[95,96]

Microalbuminuria has been associated with the presence of retinopathy in persons with diabetes and may be a marker for the risk of developing proliferative retinopathy.[97] In the CURES eye study, proteinuria was present in 29.2% of the subjects with DR.[4] Other studies have shown a varying prevalence of DR from 75 to 86% in diabetic subjects with nephropathy.[98]

Local factors such as uveitis and cataract extraction may also accelerate the progression of DR.[99] In a retrospective analysis of type 2 diabetic subjects who underwent cataract surgery, Rema et al have reported that 44% had progression of DR after cataract surgery and this was mainly in patients who underwent extracapsular cataract extraction with IOL implantation.[59]

Recent studies have provided evidence that control of hyperglycemia is important to prevent diabetic retinopathy, however, some patients develop DR despite good control and others escape retinopathy despite poor control. This suggests the role of genetic factors in susceptibility to retinopathy.[100] Various studies have shown an association of genetic factors with retinopathy.[101-103] In a study conducted in 322 type 2 diabetic families, Rema et al reported that there was a familial clustering of diabetic retinopathy among siblings of diabetic probands with and without DR. The odds ratio was 3.5 suggesting that siblings of the probands with DR had 3.5 times higher risk of developing retinopathy.[104] Recently, a study done on 249 Mexican-American type 2 diabetic siblings of probands with DR showed that the severity of DR aggregates in families rather than the incidence of DR itself.[105]

Screening of Diabetic Retinopathy

As individuals with sight-threatening retinopathy may not have symptoms, lifelong evaluation for retinopathy by retinal screening of diabetic individuals is a valuable and necessary strategy.[106] To prevent diabetes related visual impairment, the treatment must be appropriately timed and rigorous.[107] **Table 66.3** outlines the recommended diabetic eye examination schedule. Sight-threatening diabetic retinal disease (STDRD) can be effectively identified using the direct ophthalmoscopy, indirect ophthalmoscopy coupled with biomicroscopy with 70 D lens and seven standard field stereoscopic 30° fundus photography (gold standard). However, digital color photography has now replaced this cumbersome mode of screening. Nonmydriatic cameras are effective for screening at physicians' office but not sensitive enough to pickup changes like microaneurysms and subtle neovascularization.

Recently several new, noninvasive techniques promise to improve diagnostic sensitivity, one such technique is the optical coherence tomography (OCT). This method correlates well with fundus fluorescein angiography (FFA). This noninvasive technique helps to study the cross-sectional anatomy of the retina, to obtain high resolution cross-sectional images of the macula and for evaluation and follow-up of patients with diabetic macular edema. OCT provides objective and quantitative measurements that are not possible with other techniques. **Figures 66.10A to H** depict an

TABLE 66.3	Diabetic eye examination schedule	
Type of diabetes	*Recommended initial eye examination*	*Routine minimum follow-up**
Type 1	5 years after onset or during puberty	Yearly
Type 2	At time of diagnosis of diabetes	Yearly
Pregnancy in pre-existing diabetes	Prior to conception or early in first trimester	Three months or more frequently as indicated by the physician six weeks postpartum

* Abnormal findings necessitate more frequent follow-up examinations

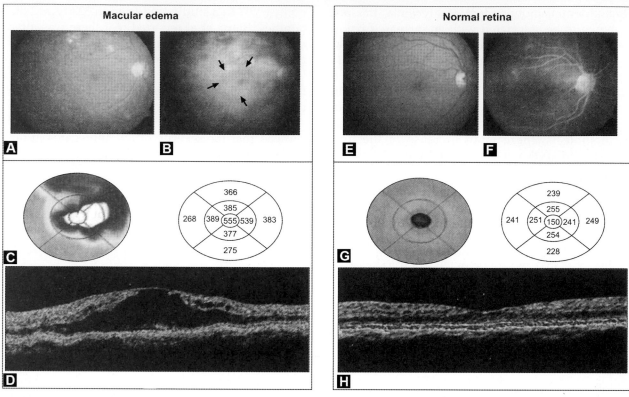

Figures 66.10A to H Comparison of OCT images in macular edema and normal retina. (A) Color photography of the right eye of a male diabetic subject shows exudates in the macular region. An area of retinal thickening can be seen within the exudative ring (B) Fundus fluorescein angiography (FFA) of the same eye shows diffuse dye leak all around the fovea as indicated by black arrows (C) The color thickness map shows evidence of fluid collection as indicated by the red color and the thickness of foveal region is 555 m (D) A single OCT image through the foveal region of the same patient shows disruption of foveal contour. Increased retinal thickness and extensive fluid accumulation is observed in the neurosensory retina (E) Right eye of a normal individual shown for comparison (F) FFA normal fovea and peri-foveal network (G) The color reflection map shows a normal foveal depression and color within normal range (H) A single OCT line scan of the macula region shows normal foveal contour. The foveal thickness is 150 m

OCT image in an individual with macular edema. Other newer diagnostic techniques include retinal thickness analyser, GDx VCC digiscope, etc. which need further refinement.

Surgical interventions include laser photocoagulation therapy and vitreoretinal surgery. Two large randomized and controlled clinical trials demonstrated that laser photocoagulation therapy decreases visual disability due to DR by 90%, if instituted at the correct stages.[108-110] In a clinic-based study conducted in 261 eyes of 168 type 2 diabetic subjects who underwent panretinal photocoagulation (PRP) at Chennai (India) 73% eyes maintained ≥6/9 at one-year follow-up. Visual acuity at baseline and duration of diabetes played a significant role in determining the post-PRP visual acuity.[111] Vitreous surgery may allow visual rehabilitation in many eyes that are otherwise untreatable.

Further details on diabetes retinopathy (DR) are dealt with in Chapter 67.

Lipemia Retinalis

One of the rare ophthalmological complications of hypertriglyceridemia is lipemia retinalis, which may be seen in unregulated diabetic individuals with diabetic coma. The retinal photograph shows retinal vessels with "milky" chylomicron-rich plasma. The retinal vessels may be distended affecting the blood flow. Davies in 1955[112] has reported that roughly 5/6 of cases of lipemia retinalis occur in diabetic subjects. This condition develops when serum triglyceride levels exceed 2.5 g/100 ml, more likely in levels between 3 and 3.5 g/100 ml. Even though lipemia retinalis does not cause significant visual loss, a recent study has demonstrated that it may be associated with vascular pathology, such as a branch retinal vein occlusion with marked exudative response and decreased visual acuity.[113] Reversal of this condition can be achieved by lowering triglycerides levels or by controlling ketosis without a sequel.

Retinal Vein Occlusion

Retinal vein occlusion (RVO) is one of the common retinal vascular diseases responsible for visual disability.[114] Visual loss can vary from mild or severe and the two complications related with a poor visual outcome include macular edema and severe retinal ischemia. Although RVO is not a complication of diabetes *per se*, this condition is said to occur more frequently in diabetic individuals compared to nondiabetic individuals. RVO is classified into branch-RVO, central-RVO and hemi-RVO. Arteriolosclerosis is an important contributing factor for branch-RVO and the other factors associated with increased risk for RVO include advancing age, systemic disorders (diabetes, hypertension, hyperlipidemia) and increased intra-ocular pressure. In a clinic-based study conducted in Chennai, the overall prevalence of RVO was 0.6% in type 2 diabetic subjects. This study also showed that diabetic retinopathy was found to be significantly higher in the subjects with RVO (73.5%) compared to those without RVO (27.4%)[115] in patients with type 2 diabetes.

SUMMARY

- As ocular complications in diabetes represents an end organ response to a generalized metabolic abnormality affecting all structures of the eye, routine, repetitive, lifelong, expert clinical examination after dilatation is essential for the fundamental ophthalmic care of the patient with diabetes.
- The most serious threat to vision is diabetic macular edema and proliferative retinopathy, which are treatable by laser, thus identification and timely treatment of these two conditions are mandatory to preserve vision.
- In diabetic individuals especially type 2 diabetes mellitus, open-angle glaucoma is two times more frequent than normal individuals, hence evaluation for glaucoma by optical coherence tomography (OCT) and field testing is essential.
- Optimal ophthalmic care for diabetic individuals must include diligent evaluation and treatment of concomitant systemic disorders like hypertension, nephropathy that influence the development,

progression and ultimate outcome of ocular manifestations.
- Optimization of these systemic considerations through an intensive, multidisciplinary, health care team-based approach will maximize the ophthalmic and general health of these individuals.

REFERENCES

1. King H, Aubert RE, Herman WH. Global burden of diabetes (1995-2025): prevalence, numerical estimates, and projections. Diabetes Care. 1998;21:1414-31.
2. Taguachi T, Brownlee M. The biochemical mechanisms of diabetic tissues damage (Chapter 47). In Pickup JC, Williams G (Eds). Textbook of Diabetes, 3rd edn. USA: Blackwell Publishing Company 2003, p 47.1.
3. Cavallerano J. Ocular manifestations of diabetes mellitus. Optom Clin. 1992; 2:93-116.
4. Rema M, Premkumar S, Anitha B, Deepa R, Pradeepa R, Mohan V. Prevalence of Diabetic Retinopathy in Urban India: The Chennai Urban Rural Epidemiology Study (CURES) Eye Study, I. Invest Ophthalmol Vis Sci. 2005;46:2328-33.
5. The Diabetes Control and Complications Trial (DCCT) Research Group. The effect of intensive treatment of diabetes on the development and progression of long-term complications in insulin-dependent diabetes mellitus. N Eng J Med. 1993;329:977-86.
6. United Kingdom Prospective Diabetes Study (UKPDS) Group. Intensive blood-glucose control with sulphonylureas or insulin compared with conventional treatment and risk of complications in patients with type 2 diabetes (UKPDS 33). Lancet. 1998;352:837 53.
7. Ohkubo Y, Kishikawa H, Araki E, et al. Intensive insulin therapy prevents the progression of diabetic microvascular complications in Japanese patients with non-insulin-dependent diabetes mellitus: a randomized prospective 6-year study. Diabetes Res Clin Pract. 1995;28:103-17.
8. Balasubramanyam M, Rema M, Premanand C. Biochemical and molecular mechanisms of diabetic retinopathy. Current Science. 2002; 83:1506-14.
9. Brownlee M. Biochemistry and molecular cell biology of diabetic complications. Nature.2001;414:813-20.
10. Bosquet F, Grimaldi A. Role of the polyol pathway in the occurrence of degenerative complications of diabetes. Presse Med. 1986;15:879-83.
11. Chung SS, Ho EC, Lam KS, Chung SK. Contribution of polyol pathway to diabetes-induced oxidative stress. J Am Soc Nephrol. 2003;14 (8 Suppl3):S233-6.
12. Dagher Z, Park YS, Asnaghi V, et al. Studies of rat and human retinas predict a role for the polyol pathway in human diabetic retinopathy. Diabetes. 2004;53:2404-11
13. Sorbinil Retinopathy Trial Research Group. A randomized trial of sorbinil— an aldose reductase inhibitor in diabetic retinopathy. Arch Ophthalmol. 1990;108: 1234-44.
14. Stitt AW. The role of advanced glycation in the pathogenesis of diabetic retinopathy. Exp Mol Pathol. 2003 ;75:95-108.
15. Zarina S, Zhao HR, Abraham EC. Advanced glycation end products in human senile and diabetic cataractous lenses. Mol Cell Biochem. 2000;210;29-34.

16. Kaji Y, Usui T, Oshika T, et al. Advanced glycation endproducts in diabetic corneas. Invest Ophthalmol Vis Sci. 2000 ;41:362-8.

17. Kowluru RA, Tang J, Kern TS. Abnormalities of retinal metabolism in diabetes and experimental galactosemia. VII. Effect of long-term administration of antioxidants on the development of retinopathy. Diabetes. 2001;50:1938-42.

18. Cameron NE, Gibson TM, Nangle MR, et al. Inhibitors of advanced glycation end product formation and neurovascular dysfunction in an experimental diabetes. Ann NY Acad Sci. 2005;1043:784-92

19. Duh E, Aiello LP. Vascular endothelial growth factor and diabetes: the agonist versus antagonist paradox. Diabetes. 1999;48:1899-906.

20. Way KJ, Katai N, King GL. Protein kinase C and the development of diabetic vascular complications. Diabet Med. 2001;18:945-59.

21. Helig CW, Concepcion LA, Riser BL, et al. Overexpresson of glucose transporters in rat mesangial cells cultured in a normal glucose milieu mimics the diabetic phenotype. J Clin Invest. 1995;96:1802-14.

22. Aiello LP, Rusell SE, Davis, et al. Amelioration of retinal haemodynamics by a PKC-â selective inhibitor (LY 333531) in patients with diabetes. Results of Phase 1 safety and pharmodynamic clinical trial. Invest Opthalmol Vi Sci. 1999;40(suppl):192

23. The PKC-DRS Study Group. The effect of ruboxistaurin on visual loss in patients with moderately severe to very severe nonproliferative diabetic retinopathy: initial results of the protein kinase C {beta} inhibitor diabetic retinopathy study (PKC-DRS) multicenter randomized clinical trial. Diabetes. 2005;54:2188-97.

24. Campochiaro PA; C99-PKC412-003 Study Group. Reduction of diabetic macular edema by oral administration of the kinase inhibitor PKC412. Invest Ophthalmol Vis Sci. 2004;45:922-31.

25. Nerlich AG, Sauer U, Kolm-Litty V, et al. Expression of glutamine: fructose-6-phosphate amidotransferase in human tissues: evidence for high variability and distinct regulation in diabetes. Diabetes. 1998;47:170-8.

26. Nakamura M, Barber AJ, Antonetti DA, et al. Excessive hexosamines block the europrotective effect of insulin and induce apoptosis in retinal neurons. J Biol Chem. 2001;23;437-48.

27. L'Esperance FA, James WA. The eye and diabetes mellitus. In Ellenberg M, Rifkin H (Eds). Diabetes Mellitus: Theory and Practice, 3rd edn. New York: Medical Examination Publishing, 1983, pp. 727-58.

28. Kanski JJ. Chapter 17 (Orbit). In Clinical Ophthalmology: a systemic approach, 5th edn. Butterworth- Heinmann 2003, pp. 568-9.

29. Nema HV, Nema N. Chapter 24 (Diseases of the lids). In Textbook of Ophthalmology , 3rd edn. New Delhi: Jaypee Brothers Medical Publishers, 2003; pp. 289-92.

30. Henkind P. The eye in diabetes mellitus: signs, symptoms and their pathogenesis. In Mausolf FA (Ed): The Eye and Systemic Disease. St Louis: CV Mosby, 1980, pp. 187-203.

31. Inoue K, Kato S, Othara C, et al. Ocular and systemic factors relevant to diabetic keratoepitheliopathy. Cornea. 2001;20:798-801.

32. Rubinstein MP. Diabetes: the anterior segment, and contact lens wear. Contact Lens J. 1987;15:4-11.

33. Cheung AT, Ramanujam S, Greer DA, et al. Microvascular abnormalities in the bulbar conjunctiva of patients with type 2 diabetes mellitus. Endocr Pract. 2001; 7:358-63.

34. Ditzel J, Beaven DW, Renold AE, et al. Early vascular changes in diabetes mellitus. Metabolism. 1960;9:400

35. Cheung AT, Price AR, Duong PL, et al. Microvascular abnormalities in pediatric diabetic patients. Microvasc Res. 2002;63(3):252-8.

36. Isenberg SJ, McRee WE, Jedrzynski MS. Conjunctival hypoxia in diabetes mellitus. Invest Ophthalmol Vis Sci. 1986;27:1512-5.

37. Sanchez-Thorin JC. The cornea in diabetes mellitus. Int Ophthalmol Clin. 1998;38:19-36.

38. Jin J, Chen LH, Liu XL, et al. Tear film function in non-insulin dependent diabetics. Zhonghua Yan Ke Za Zhi. 2003;39:10-3.

39. Rehany U, Ishii Y, Lahav M, Rumelt S. Collagen pleomorphism in Descemet's membrane of streptozotocin-induced diabetic rats: an electron microscopy study. Cornea. 2000;19(3):390-2.

40. Pierro L, Brancato R, Zaganelli E. Correlation of corneal thickness with blood glucose control in diabetes mellitus. Acta Ophthalmol. 1993;71:169-72.

41. McNamara NA, Brand RJ, Polse KA, Bourne WM. Corneal function during normal and high serum glucose levels in diabetes. Invest Ophthalmol Vis Sci. 1998;39:3-17.

42. Rosenberg ME, Tervo TM, Immonen IJ, Muller LJ, Gronhagen-Riska C, Vesaluoma MH. Corneal structure and sensitivity in type 1 diabetes mellitus. Invest Ophthalmol Vis Sci. 2000;41(10):2915-21.

43. Ruben ST. Corneal sensation in insulin dependent and non-insulin dependent diabetics with proliferative retinopathy. Acta Ophthalmol. 1994;72:576-80

44. Bonini S, Lambiase A, Rama P, et al. Topical treatment with nerve growth factor for neuropathic keratitis. Ophthalmology. 2000;107:1347-51.

45. Hosotani H, Ohashi Y, Yamada M, Tsubota K. Reversal of abnormal corneal epithelial cell morphologic characteristics and reduced corneal sensitivity in diabetic patients by aldose reductase inhibitor, CT-112. Am J Ophthalmol. 1995;119:288-94.

46. Kruse FE, Rohrschneider K, Volcker HE. Multilayer amniotic membrane transplantation for reconstruction of deep corneal ulcers. Ophthalmology 1999;106:1504-10.

47. Alio J, Hernandez I, Millan A, Sanchez J. Pupil responsiveness in diabetes mellitus. Ann Ophthalmol. 1989;21:132-7.

48. Shulman P. Diabetes: its effects on the body and the eye. Optom Wkly. 1972;63: 951-8.

49. Kanski JJ, Chapter 9 (Glaucoma). In Clinical Ophthalmology — A Systemic Approach, 5th edn. Butterworth-Heinmann 2003, pp. 233-6

50. Liang JC. Diabetic eye disease. In Wilensky JT, Read JE (Eds): Primary Ophthalmology. New York: Grune and Stratton.1984; pp. 193-210.

51. Mitchell P, Smith W, Chey T, et al. Open-angle glaucoma and diabetes: the Blue Mountains eye study. Australia: Ophthalmology. 1997;104:712-8.

52. Schertzer RM, Wang D, Bartholomew LR. Diabetes mellitus and glaucoma. Int Ophthalmol Clin. 1998;38:69-87.

53. Brown GC, Magargal LE, Schachat A, et al. Neovascular glaucoma. Etiologic considerations. Ophthalmology. 1984;91:315-20.

54. Bernth-Petersen P, Bach E. Epidemiologic aspects of cataract surgery III: frequencies of diabetes and glaucoma in a cataract population. Acta Ophthalmol (Copenh). 1983;61(3):406-16.

55. Klein BE, Klein R, Moss SE. Prevalence of cataracts in a population-based study of persons with diabetes mellitus. Ophthalmology. 1985;92:1191-6.

56. Rowe NG, Mitchell PG, Cumming RG, Wans JJ. Diabetes, fasting blood glucose and age-related cataract: the Blue Mountains eye study. Ophthalmic Epidemiol. 2000;7:103-14.

57. Towler HMA, Lightmen S. Chapter 49 (Clinical features and management of diabetic eye disease). In Pickup JC, Williams G (Eds). Textbook of Diabetes, 3rd edn. USA: Blackwell Publishing Company 2003, p 49.1.

58. Caird FI, Pirie A, Ramsell TG. Diabetes and the Eye. Oxford: Blackwell Scientific Publications, 1969.

59. Rema M, Geetha M. Outcomes of laser therapy for diabetic retinopathy in Type II diabetes mellitus patients after cataract surgery. Proceedings of Vitreo-Retinal Society of India, February 8-10, Goa, 2002.

60. Eva PR, Pascoe PT, Vaughan DG. Refractive change in hyperglycaemia: hyperopia, not myopia. Br J Ophthalmol. 1982;66:500-5.

61. Pardo G. Neuro-ophthalmological manifestations of diabetes mellitus. Int Ophthalmol Clin. 1998;38:213-26.

62. Kanski JJ, Chapter 18 (Neuro-opthalmology). In Clinical Ophthalmology –A Systemic Approach, 5th edn. Butterworth-Heinmann. 2003, pp. 596-636.

63. Patel SV, Holmes JM, Hodge DO, Burke JP. Diabetes and hypertension in isolated sixth nerve palsy: a population-based study. Ophthalmology. 2005;112:760-3.

64. Abraham IL, Ossting J, Hart AAM. Bell's palsy: factors affecting the prognosis in 200 patients with reference to hypertension and diabetes mellitus. Clin Otolaryngol. 1987;12:349-55.

65. Hughes GB. Practical management of Bell's palsy. Otolaryngol Head Neck Surg. 1990;102:658-63.

66. Jabor MA, Gianoli G. Management of Bell's palsy. J La State Med Soc. 1996;148(7):279-83.

67. Cahill M, Eustace P, de Jesus V. Pupillary autonomic denervation with increasing duration of diabetes mellitus. Br J Ophthalmol. 2001; 85:1225-30.

68. Bergren RL, Brown GC, Duker JS. Prevalence and association of asteroid hyalosis with systemic diseases. Am J Ophthalmol. 1991;111:289-93.

69. Yazar Z, Hanioglu S, Karakoc G, et al. Asteroid hyalosis. Eur J Ophthalmol. 2001;11:57-61.

70. Foos RY, Kreiger AE, Forsythe AB, Zakka KA. Posterior vitreous detachment in diabetic subjects. Ophthalmology. 1980;87:122-8.

71. Pischel DK. Detachment of the vitreous as seen by slit lamp examination, with notes on the technique of slit lamp microscopy of the vitreous cavity. Amer T Ophthalmol. 1953;36:1497-507.

72. Ignat F, Barascu D, Perovic I, Munteanu A. Optic nerve lesions in diabetes mellitus. Oftalmologia. 2002;(3):39-43.

73. Keely KA, Yip B. Diabetic papillopathy: two case reports in individuals with adult onset diabetes mellitus. J Am Optom Assoc. 1997;68(9):595-603.

74. Hayreh SS. Anterior ischemic optic neuropathy. Clin Neurosci. 1997;4:251-63.

75. Brogelli S, Valentini G. Anterior ischemic optic neuropathy in type I diabetes. Metab Pediatr Syst Ophthalmol. 1986;9:90-3.

76. Buono LM, Foroozan R, Sergott RC, et al. Nonarteritic anterior ischemic optic neuropathy. Curr Opin Ophthalmol. 2002;13:357-61.

77. Desai N, Patel MR, Prisant LM, et al. Nonarteritic anterior ischemic optic neuropathy. J Clin Hypertens. 2005,7.130-3.

78. Ischemic Optic Neuropathy Decompression Trial Study Group. Characteristics of patients with nonarteritic anterior ischemic optic neuropathy eligible for the ischemic optic neuropathy decompression trial. Arch Ophthalmol. 1996;114:1366-74.

79. Murthy GG. Non-retinal ocular complications of diabetes mellitus. In Ophthalmology Today (Vol IV).2003, pp. 108-9.

80. Beck RW. Optic Neuritis Study Group. The Optic Neuritis Treatment Trial: three year follow-up results. Arch Ophthalmol. 1995;113:136-7.

81. Wolf MA. Vascular implications of optic atrophy. J Am Optom Assoc. 1992;63:395-403.

82. Klein R, Klein BEK, Moss SE, et al. The Wisconsin epidemiological study of diabetic retinopathy X . The 4-year incidence and progression of diabetic retinopathy when age at diagnosis is less than 30 years. Arch Ophthalmol. 1989;107:244-9.

83. Rema M, Ponnaiya M, Mohan V. Prevalence of retinopathy in noninsulin-dependent diabetes mellitus at a diabetes centre in southern India. Diabetes Res Clin Pract. 1996;34:29-36.

84. Rema M, Deepa R, Mohan V. Prevalence of retinopathy at diagnosis among Type 2 diabetic patients attending a diabetic centre in South India. Br J Ophthal. 2000;84:1058-60.

85. Kohner EM, Aldington SJ, Stratton IM. United Kingdom Prospective Diabetes Study, 30: diabetic retinopathy at diagnosis of non-insulin-dependent diabetes mellitus and associated risk factors. Arch Ophthalmol. 1998 ;116:297-303.

86. Rema M, Shanthirani CS, Deepa R, Mohan V. Prevalence of diabetic retinopathy in a selected south Indian population: the Chennai Urban Population Study (CUPS). Diabetes Res Clin Pract. 2000;50:S252.

87. Rema M, Mohan V. Retinopathy at diagnosis among young Asian diabetic patients: ASDIAB Study Group. Diabetes. 2002; 51(suppl 2):A206-7.

88. Aiello LM, Rand LI, Briones JC, Wafai MZ, Sebestyen JG. Diabetic retinopathy in Joslin Clinic patients with adult-onset diabetes. Ophthalmology. 1981;88:619-23.

89. Klein R, Klein BE, Moss SE, Cruickshanks KJ. Relationship of hyperglycemia to the long-term incidence and progression of diabetic retinopathy. Arch Intern Med. 1994;154:2169-78.

90. United Kingdom Prospective Diabetes Study Group. Tight blood pressure control and risk of macrovascular and microvascular complications in type 2 diabetes (UKPDS 38). BMJ. 1998;317:708–13.

91. Ferris FL 3rd, Chew EY, Hoogwerf BJ. Serum lipids and diabetic retinopathy. Early Treatment Diabetic Retinopathy Study Research Group. Diabetes Care. 1996;19:1291-3.

92. Rema M, Mohan V, Susheela L, et al. Increased LDL cholesterol in non-insulin- dependent diabetes with maculopathy. Acta Diabetologica Latina. 1984;21:85--9.

93. Sundaram RK, Bhaskar A, Vijayalingam S, Viswanathan M, Rema M, Shanmugasundram KR. Antioxidant status and lipid peroxidation in type II diabetes mellitus with and without complications. Clinical Science. 1996;90: 255-60.

94. Rema M, Srivastava BK, Anitha B, Deepa R, Mohan V. Association of Serum Lipids with Diabetic Retinopathy in Urban South Indians: the Chennai Urban Rural Epidemiology

Study (CURES) Eye Study-2. Diabetic Medicine. 2006;23:1029-36.

95. Anusha P, Vijayalingam S, Shanmugasundaram KR, Rema M. Oxidative stress and the development of diabetic complications: antioxidants and lipid peroxidation in erythrocytes and cell membrane. Cell Biology International. 1995;19:987-93.

96. Rema M, Mohan V, Anusha B, Shanmugasundaram KR. Does oxidant stress play a role in diabetic retinopathy? Indian J Ophthalmol. 1995;43:17-21.

97. Cruickshanks KJ, Ritter LL, Klein R, Moss SE. The Ocular Complications in Association of Microalbuminuria with diabetic retinopathy. The Wisconsin Epidemiologic Study of Diabetic Retinopathy. Ophthalmology. 1993;100:862-7.

98. Vijay V, Snehalatha C, Ramachandran A, Viswanathan M. Prevalence of proteinuria in non-insulin-dependent diabetes. J Assoc Physicians India. 1994;42:792-4.

99. Knuimam MW, Welborn TA, McCann VJ, Stanton KG, Constable IJ. Prevalence of diabetic complications in relation to risk factors. Diabetes. 1986;35:1332-3.

100. Radha V, Rema M, Mohan V. Genes and diabetic retinopathy. Indian J Ophthalmol. 2002;50:5-11.

101. Hawrami K, Rema M, Mohan V, et al. A genetic study of retinopathy in south Indian type 2 (non-insulin-dependent) diabetic patients. Diabetologia. 1991;31:441-4.

102. Hawrami K, Hitman GA, Rema M, et al. An association in non-insulin-dependent diabetes mellitus subjects between susceptibility to retinopathy and tumor necrosis factor polymorphism. Hum Immunol. 1996;46:49-54.

103. Kumaramanickavel G, Sripriya S, Vellanki RN, et al. Tumor necrosis factor allelic polymorphism with diabetic retinopathy in India. Diabetes Res Clin Pract. 2001;54:89-94.

104. Rema M, Saravanan G, Deepa R. Familial clustering of diabetic retinopathy in South Indian Type 2 diabetic patients. Diabet Med. 2002;19:910-6.

105. Hallman DM, Huber JC Jr, Gonzalez VH, et al. Familial aggregation of severity of diabetic retinopathy in Mexican Americans from Starr County Texas. Diabetes Care. 2005;28:1163-8.

106. Namperumalswamy P, Nirmalan PK, Ramaswamy KM. Developing a screening program to detect sight threatening retinopathy in south India. Diabetes Care. 2003;26:1831-5.

107. Kohner EM, Barry PJ. Prevention of blindness in diabetic retinopathy. Diabetologia. 1984;26:173-9.

108. The Diabetic Retinopathy Study Research Group. Photocoagulation treatment of proliferative diabetic retinopathy: clinical application of DRS findings. Report No 8. Ophthalmology. 1981;88:583-600.

109. Early Treatment Diabetic Retinopathy Study (ETDRS) Research Group: Photocoagulation for macular edema: ERDRS Report 1. Arch Ophthalmol. 1985;103:1796-806.

110. Early Treatment Diabetic Retinopathy Study Research Group. Early photocoagulation for diabetic retinopathy: ETDRS Report 9. Ophthalmology. 1991;98 (Suppl):766-85.

111. Rema M, Sujatha P, Pradeepa R. Visual Outcomes of Pan-retinal Photocoagulation in Diabetic Retinopathy at one-year Follow-up and associated Risk Factors. Indian J Ophthalmol. 2005; 53:93-9.

112. Davies WS. Idiopathic lipemic retinalis. Arch Ophthalmol. 1955, 53:105-8.

113. Nagra PK, Ho AC, Dugan JD Jr. Lipemia retinalis associated with branch retinal vein occlusion. Am J Ophthalmol 2003;135:539-42.

114. Recchia FM, Brown GC. Systemic disorders associated with retinal vascular occlusion. Curr Opin Ophthalmol. 2000;11:462-7.

115. Rema M, Prathiba V, Pradeepa R. Retinal vein occlusion and associated risk factors in type 2 diabetes mellitus: a case control study. Proceedings of the 61st Annual Conference of All India Ophthalmological Society (AIOC), New Delhi 2003 (Abstract): p. 298.

Chapter 67

DIABETIC RETINOPATHY

P Namperumalsamy, Kim Ramasamy, Dhananjay Shukla, Vasumathy Vedantham, Chandramohan Kolluru

---

CHAPTER OUTLINE

- Introduction
- Clinical Features
- Classification
- Prevalence of Diabetic Retinopathy—Indian Scenario
- Pathogenesis
- Evaluation
- Management
- Summary

INTRODUCTION

Diabetic retinopathy is the most common cause of newly diagnosed legal blindness amongst the working population in industrialized world today. Type 1 diabetic patients have retinopathy of varying severity, approximately 25% of the diabetic patients have the sight-threatening levels of retinopathy.[1] The common causes of visual impairment in diabetic retinopathy include macular edema and complications due to proliferative diabetic retinopathy. Owing to the fact that the majority of diabetic subjects have type 2 disease, wherein macular edema is more common, it follows that macular edema accounts for more vision impairment than proliferative retinopathy in diabetic patients.[2]

According to the available epidemiological data from WHO (2004, **Table 67.1**), approximately 64 million persons are suffering from diabetes, of them, one-third were from India. It is estimated that this figure will go up to 300 millions of world population by the year 2030 **(Table 67.1)**, of them >79 million will be in India. In addition, there will be a large reservoir of undetected cases in India, bringing the true prevalence of disease among adults somewhere from 9 to 11%. According to

ICMR, the prevalence of diabetes ranges from 10% in urban and 4% in rural population. The factors attributed to these large numbers of diabetic population in India are urbanization, industrialization, unhealthy diet, and sedentary lifestyle.

According to WHO reports, 2% of diabetic patients become blind after 15 years and 10% develop severe visual disability.[1] Diabetic retinopathy is often asymptomatic in the early stages when it is amenable for treatment and visual loss is a late symptom.

TABLE 67.1	Prevalence of diabetes mellitus (WHO)	
Country	Year 2000 (in million)	Year 2030 (in million)
India	31.7	79.4
China	20.8	42.3
USA	17.7	30.3
Indonesia	8.4	21.3
Japan	6.8	8.9
Pakistan	5.2	13.9

Ref: Wild S, Roglic G, Green A, Sicree R, King H. Global prevalence of diabetes, estimates for the year 2000 and projections for 2030. Diabetes Care. 2004;27:1047-53.

Currently, the disease is detected too late to prevent blindness. Duration of diabetes mellitus seems to have a direct association with the prevalence of diabetic retinopathy than the severity of the disease. In IDDM, the prevalence of diabetic retinopathy is almost 97.5%. If the duration is 15 years or more, then in NIDDM, it is about 80%.[3]

This chapter aims at providing an overview of the various salient features, pathogenesis, current and future medical management options in diabetic retinopathy.

CLINICAL FEATURES

Symptoms

Subjects without retinopathy, nonproliferative diabetic retinopathy without significant macular lesions or proliferative diabetic retinopathy with neovascularization but without its sequelae are usually asymptomatic. Those with maculopathy may complain of metamorphopsia and varying degrees of visual impairment depending on the severity of maculopathy and foveal involvement. Black spots, floaters, blurred vision or sudden visual loss is usually seen in patients with vitreous hemorrhage, depending on the location and amount of bleeding. Distorted vision maybe experienced when fibrous tissue distorts the macula or when a traction retinal detachment partially involves the macula.

Signs[4,5]

Findings in the Retina

• *Hemorrhages and microaneurysms:* Microaneurysms are small saccular or fusiform capillary dilatations easily seen as small red dots with the direct ophthalmoscope. Microaneurysms alone (without hemorrhage) do not appear to contribute substantially to the risk of retinopathy progression. However, scattered, blotchy intraretinal hemorrhages do predict risk of progression to proliferative diabetic retinopathy **(Figure 67.1)**.

• *Venous beading:* Venous beading refers to irregular constriction and dilatation of venules in the retina. Venous beading is a good predictor of risk of retinopathy progression, if present in two of the four midperipheral retinal quadrants.

• *Soft exudates:* Soft exudates, also called *cotton wool spots* are areas of nerve fiber ischemia or infarction. They appear as opaque gray or white areas in the

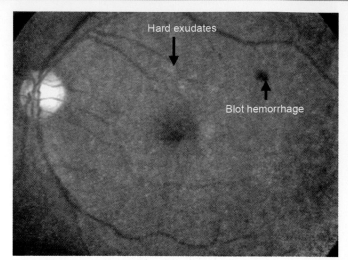

Figure 67.1 Mild nonproliferative diabetic retinopathy (NPDR): Few scattered retinal hemorrhages and hard exudates

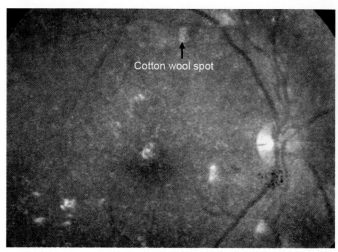

Figure 67.2 Moderate nonproliferative diabetic retinopathy (NPDR): More retinal hemorrhages, hard exudates and cotton wool spots

nerve fiber layer with soft or feathery edges. They have poor predictive value for retinopathy progressing to more severe levels **(Figure 67.2)**.

• *Hard exudates:* Hard exudates are lipid and lipoprotein deposits and result from leakage from abnormally permeable microaneurysms or capillaries in the retina **(Figure 67.1)**. Therefore, these lesions are often accompanied by retinal edema. Elevated blood cholesterol levels are associated with increased severity and extent of hard exudates.

• *Intraretinal microvascular abnormalities:* Some investigators believe that they are pre-existing

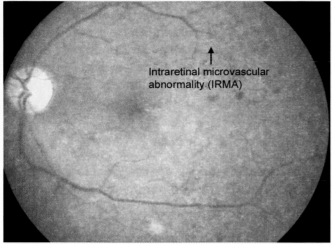

Figure 67.3 Severe NPDR: Multiple retinal hemorrhages, microaneurysms and intraretinal microvascular abnormalities (IRMA)

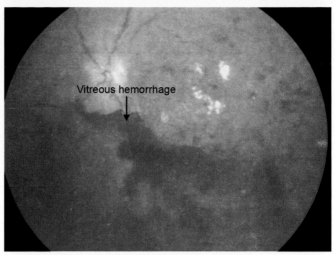

Figure 67.5 Advanced proliferative diabetic retinopathy: Vitreous hemorrhage

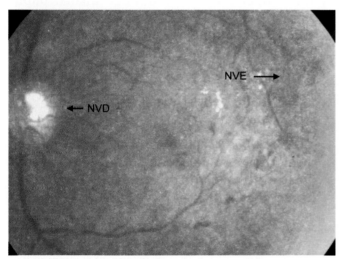

Figure 67.4 Proliferative diabetic retinopathy (PDR): Neovascularization of the disk (NVD) and neovascularization elsewhere (NVE)

dilated vessels (shunt vessels) while others believe that they may represent preproliferative stage. Clinically, they appear as dilated, telangiectatic capillaries within the retina **(Figure 67.3)**. They strongly indicate increasing hypoxia, the likelihood of retinopathy progression to proliferative retinopathy, even if present in only on mid peripheral field.

- *New vessels:* These vessels usually arise from retinal veins and often begin as a collection of multiple fine vessels. When they arise on or within one disk diameter of the optic nerve head, then they are referred to as neovascularization of the disk (NVD). When these arise further than one disk diameter away, then they are called neovascularization elsewhere (NVE). Unlike normal retinal vessels, NVD and NVE both leak fluorescein into the vitreous **(Figure 67.4)**.

The new vessels grow along the posterior hyaloid at the junction of ischemic and nonischemic retina. With increasing vitreous contraction, early posterior vitreous detachment occurs and new vessels are lifted up and result in vitreous hemorrhage **(Figure 67.5)** as well as traction on the underlying retina. If a total posterior vitreous detachment occurs at this stage, then the new vessels regress spontaneously into fibrous proliferations and hemorrhages settle down.

Otherwise, continued vitreous traction results in recurrent vitreous hemorrhage and progressive increase in tractional membranes and detachment.

- *Tractional retinal detachment:* Tractional retinal detachments **(Figure 67.6)** are usually confined to the posterior pole, most prominently along the vascular arcades. The contour of the detachment is concave and the clinical course is typically stationary (only about 15% progress to involve the macula). Vitrectomy is generally reserved for cases in which the macula is involved or is clearly threatened by progressive retinal detachment. Less commonly, tractional bands may cause secondary retinal breaks and rhegmatogenous retinal detachment.

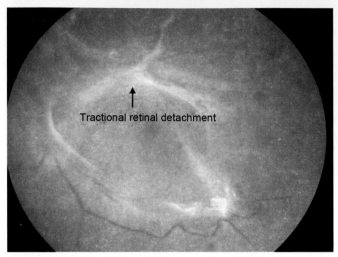

Tractional retinal detachment

Figure 67.6 Advanced proliferative diabetic retinopathy: Tractional retinal detachment

CLASSIFICATION

Diabetic retinopathy is broadly classified as:[6]
- Nonproliferative diabetic retinopathy (NPDR)
- Proliferative diabetic retinopathy (PDR).

Nonproliferative Diabetic Retinopathy (NPDR)

- *Mild NPDR:* At least one microaneurysm and few hemorrhages
- *Moderate NPDR:* Presence of microaneurysms and hemorrhages along with soft exudates, venous beading and intraretinal microvascular abnormalities (IRMA)
- *Severe NPDR:* Any one of the following:
  i. Hemorrhage and microaneurysms in four quadrants
  ii. Venous beading in two or more quadrants
  iii. IRMA in at least one quadrant.

Proliferative Diabetic Retinopathy (PDR)

- *Early PDR:* New vessels at disk (NVD) and new vessels elsewhere (NVE) without vitreous hemorrhage or pre-retinal hemorrhages.
- *High-risk PDR:*
  i. NVD greater than half disk area
  ii. NVD and vitreous hemorrhage
  iii. NVE greater than half disk area with vitreous hemorrhage.

To facilitate communication between retina specialists and health care professionals, a new grading system has been recently proposed; this is derived from the ETDRS[6] and the Wisconsin Epidemiologic Study of Diabetic Retinopathy[7] studies. This simplified grading system identifies five levels of DR which can be assessed by direct ophthalmoscopy through dilated pupils (Table 67.2).[8]

Diabetic Macular Edema

The most common cause of visual loss in diabetic retinopathy in type 2 diabetic subjects is macular edema. This can occur both in nonproliferative and proliferative diabetic retinopathy. The prevalence of macular edema in IDDM is 4%[9] and in NIDDM patients, it is about 5.1% in Indian diabetic subjects.[10]

Clinically significant macular edema (CSME) occurs if there is thickening of the retina involving the center of the macula or the area within 500 μ of it, if there are hard exudates at or within 500 μ of the center of the macula with thickening of the adjacent retina, or if there is a zone of retinal thickening one disk area or larger in size, any part of which is within one disk diameter of

TABLE 67.2	International clinical diabetic retinopathy disease severity scale[10]
Proposed disease severity level	*Dilated ophthalmoscopy findings*
No apparent retinopathy	No abnormalities
Mild nonproliferative DR	Microaneurysms only
Moderate nonproliferative DR	More than just microaneurysms, but less than severe NPDR
Severe nonproliferative DR	• No signs of PDR, with any of the following: • More than 20 intraretinal hemorrhages in each of four quadrants • Definite venous beading in two or more quadrants • Prominent intraretinal microvascular anomalies in one or more quadrants PDR, one or more of the following: • Neovascularization • Vitreous or preretinal hemorrhage

NPDR: Nonproliferative diabetic retinopathy; PDR: Proliferative diabetic retinopathy

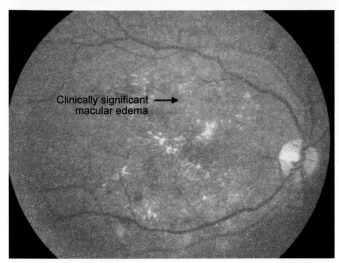

Figure 67.7 Clinically significant macular edema (CSME): Retinal thickening or adjacent hard exudates

the center of the macula.[6] This definition of CSME generally refers to the threshold level at which laser photocoagulation is carried out **(Figure 67.7)**.

In the simplified grading scale **(Table 67.3)**, macular edema has two major levels: Absent and present.[8] If diabetic macular edema is present, it is divided into mild (some retinal thickening or hard exudates in the posterior pole, but distant from the center of the macula), moderate (retinal thickening or hard exudates approaching the center of the macula but not the center)

and severe (retinal thickening or hard exudates involving the center of the macula.

PREVALENCE OF DIABETIC RETINOPATHY— INDIAN SCENARIO

Although there is an explosion of diabetes in India, the prevalence of DR in India is lower compared to the other populations.[11-13] The prevalence of DR in a cohort of 6792 type 2 diabetic patients attending a diabetes center at Chennai, Tamil Nadu, India (1996) screened using a combination of retinal photography and clinical examination by retinal specialists was 34.1%. This included 30.8% with NPDR, 3.4% with PDR and 6.4% had maculopathy.[14] As DR may be present even at the time of diagnosis of type 2 diabetes due to the insidious onset of this disease, a study of consecutive 448 newly diagnosed (South Indian) type 2 diabetic patients reported that 7.3% already had diabetic retinopathy.[15]

Recent population-based studies have reported the prevalence of the DR in urban India.[16-19] In a population-based study conducted at Hyderabad (Andhra Pradesh, India), the overall prevalence of DR in self-reported diabetic subjects was 22.4%[16] and a marginally higher prevalence of DR (26.8%) was reported among self-reported diabetic subjects aged 50 years and older from Palakkad (Kerala, India).[17] However, these studies have been restricted only to self-reported diabetic subjects. In the Chennai Urban Population Study (CUPS)

TABLE 67.3	International clinical diabetic macular edema disease severity scale[6]
Two major levels, with subcategories for diabetic macular edema are	
Proposed disease severity level	**Findings observable upon dilated ophthalmoscopy**
Diabetic macular edema absent	No retinal thickening or hard exudates in posterior pole
Diabetic macular edema present	Some retinal thickening or hard exudates in posterior pole
If diabetic macular edema is present, then it can be categorized as	
Proposed disease severity level	**Findings observable upon dilated ophthalmoscopy***
Diabetic macular edema present	• *Mild diabetic macular edema* Some retinal thickening or hard exudates in posterior pole but distant from the center of the macula • *Moderate diabetic macular edema* Retinal thickening or hard exudates approaching the center of the macula but not involving the center • *Severe diabetic macular edema* Retinal thickening or hard exudates involving the center of the macula

*Hard exudates are indicative of current or previous macular edema. Diabetic macular edema is defined as retinal thickening and this requires a three-dimensional assessment that is best performed by using slit-lamp biomicroscopy and/or stereo fundus photography with dilated pupils.

involving two residential areas representing the lower and middle income group, overall prevalence of DR was 19% (21.1% in middle income group compared to 14.3 % in the low income group).[18] In the Chennai Urban Rural Epidemiology Study (CURES) eye study, the first population-based study conducted both in self-reported and newly diagnosed diabetic subjects using four-field stereo retinal photograph reported the overall prevalence of DR as 17.6%.[10] Among the known diabetic subjects, 20.8% had DR while 5.1% of newly detected diabetic subjects had DR. Known diabetic subjects had higher frequency of all the grades of retinopathy compared to newly detected cases. Diabetic macular edema (DME) in the total diabetic population was 5.0% while among the known diabetic subjects it was 6.3% and 1.1% among the newly diagnosed diabetic subjects.[10]

The finding from the studies in India shows that the prevalence of DR in Indians is lower when compared to the Europeans. However, given the large number of diabetic subjects in India (31.7 million), even with the lower prevalence rates (17.6%), this would translate to over 5.6 million subjects with DR, causing an heavy economic burden.

PATHOGENESIS

The understanding of the pathogenesis of the disorder is essential and fundamental to the formulation of new treatment modalities that could effectively replace the current treatment option, namely photocoagulation.

The retina is unique in its tremendous metabolic capacity, which on an unit-weight basis exceeds any tissue in the body even the cerebral cortex in terms of glucose oxidation and oxygen uptake. It is therefore possible that the initial biochemical lesions that lead to diabetic retinopathy might occur in the neural or the glial cells of the retina, with secondary involvement of the vessels. Thus, these metabolic lesions occur much before the vascular lesions that is prior to the onset of clinically evident retinopathy.

High glucose levels are probably the most important pathogenetic factor in diabetic retinopathy. Two important multicentric clinical trials, the Diabetes Control and Complications Trial (DCCT) and the United Kingdom Prospective Diabetes Study (UKPDS) conclusively demonstrated that intensive glycemic control slows the onset and progression of diabetic retinopathy and other vascular complications in both type 1 and 2 diabetes.[19,20] However, the variation in the development of retinopathy among individuals with differing glycemic control might possibly relate to putative genetic and familial factors. Various Studies have identified that there is a strong familial and genetic predisposition for the etiology of DR.[21-24] In a study conducted in 322 Type 2 diabetic families, Rema et al[24] reported that there was a familial clustering of diabetic retinopathy among siblings of diabetic probands with and without DR. The odds ratio was 3.5 suggesting that siblings of the probands with DR had 3.5 times higher risk of developing retinopathy. The pathways involved in hyperglycemia are the sorbitol pathway and the nonenzymatic glycosylation of proteins leading to advanced glycation endproducts (AGE proteins) but conclusive evidence of these are lacking.

In addition, elevated BP is also an independent risk factor as proved by the UKPDS.[20] Recent studies have thrown light on the mechanisms by which hypertension increases the risk of development of diabetic retinopathy.[25] These include hypertension-induced vascular stretching that results in the increased expression of vascular endothelial growth factor (VEGF) and its receptors and the enhancement of retinal endothelial damage.

The other most important factor in pathogenesis of diabetic retinopathy is the alteration in the biochemistry. The role of growth factors has garnered the maximum attention, with numerous candidate molecules having been investigated as potential mediators of diabetic retinal vascular complications. These include basic fibroblastic growth factor (BFGF), growth hormone (GH), insulin like growth factor-I (IGF-I), connective tissue growth factor (CTGF), prostacyclin stimulating factor (PSF), hepatocyte growth factor (HGF) and vascular endothelial growth factor (VEGF).[26] The role of IGF-I is favored by the fact that diabetic retinopathy virtually never occurs before puberty and the occurrence of certain florid cases of proliferative diabetic retinopathy (PDR) that do not respond to photocoagulation but respond to hypophysectomy. These growth factors may be involved in retinal fibrosis, matrix deposition, biphasic changes in retinal blood flow and angiogenesis all of which happen in diabetic retinopathy. Neovascularization in all probability results from an alteration of the normal balance between the natural promoters of angiogenesis as mentioned above and the natural inhibitors in favor of the proangiogenic molecules.

Of all the molecules, the VEGF is the most extensively studied molecule and is the principal focus of novel treatments for PDR.[27] It has been proved that physiologic concentrations of VEGF increase retinal vascular permeability, which in turn is a hallmark of intraocular neovascularization. Furthermore, intraocular levels of VEGF decrease after adequate treatment of retinal neovascularization with panretinal photocoagulation. Experimental inhibition of VEGF production or binding to its receptor results in an antiproliferative effect that has been demonstrated in various animal models. The signal transduction pathways that are initiated by the binding of VEGF to its receptor endothelial cells result in the activation of protein kinase C (PKC). Experimental work has proved that inhibition of PKC *in vivo* reduces ischemic retinal neovascularization.[28] Both intravitreal and oral forms of PKC inhibitor have been shown to block VEGF induced increases in retinal vascular permeability in animals and to normalize the retinopathy induced changes in retinal blood flow in both animals and humans.

Laboratory and clinical research is now focussed on the prevention of retinal vascular leakage and retinal neovascularization by a modulation of the pathogenetic mechanisms of these growth factors.

The principal inhibitors of angiogenesis are the pericytes that release transforming growth factor-β (TGF-β) upon contact with the endothelial cells and failure of this naturally occurring inhibition of proliferation is also of importance in PDR. Hence, the loss of pericytes (that is pathologic hallmark of diabetic retinopathy) would lead to loss of inhibition of endothelial cell proliferation that in turn would lead to localized endothelial proliferation that are seen as microaneurysms clinically. The second most important inhibitor of retinal nevoascularization is the vascular basement membrane. Hence, the increased basement membrane thickness which is another hallmark of diabetic retinopathy could facilitate proliferation by removing the pericyte processes from their contact with the endothelial cells.[29]

Regardless of the above mentioned inciting mechanisms, the lesions of diabetic retinopathy seem to stem from both abnormalities of blood (sticky blood hypothesis) and blood vessel wall (sticky vessel hypothesis) leading to increased leukostasis (leukocytes attached to the endothelial wall) that occurs very early and universally in diabetes. This would lead in turn to physical blockage of the capillary tubes, endothelial dysfunction and apoptosis and the consequent fall in tissue perfusion leading to ischemic retinal damage.[30]

Sticky blood hypothesis: The leukocytes in diabetes are less deformable and demonstrate upregulation of

integrins (ligands for vascular adhesion molecules) on their surface and adhere more strongly to cultured endothelial cells under experimental conditions. All this could facilitate leukostasis.[30]

Sticky vessel hypothesis: The vessels (endothelium) could itself be more sticky and support to this comes from studies that have suggested that these cells in diabetes have increased expression of adhesion molecules, especially the intercellular adhesion molecule-I (ICAM-I) on their surface in response to hyperglycemia.[30]

The relative importance of all these factors is still to be elucidated with new factors being discovered regularly. Current advances and ongoing research is likely to throw up more candidates for the pathogenesis of diabetic retinopathy in the near future.

EVALUATION

Diabetic retinopathy changes can be evaluated clinically by several methods. A dilated pupil is essential to evaluate diabetic retinopathy adequately. A direct ophthalmoscope can be used as a screening tool to evaluate the fundus. The advantage of this method is that it provides a magnified view of the retina, allowing greater visualization of the structures. However, since the view is two-dimensional, macular edema and early neovascularization cannot be adequately evaluated. Also, the field of view is so narrow that neovascularization outside of the most posterior aspects of the fundus can be missed.

Indirect ophthalmoscopy is an excellent screening method for evaluating a large area of the fundus three dimensionally. However, the low magnification with this method makes it difficult to evaluate small areas of new vessels or to evaluate macular edema.

Slit-lamp biomicroscopy using a 78D or 90D lens is the examination technique of choice for evaluating diabetic retinopathy. This technique provides three-dimensional viewing of the fundus with excellent magnification that allows evaluation of macular edema and neovascularization over a wide field. It is helpful to use this technique for presence of diabetic macular edema. Disadvantages include the fact that the eyes must be dilated and performing the technique with accuracy requires much experience.

Fluorescein angiography with color fundus photography is another useful method for evaluating diabetic retinopathy. During the technique of fundus fluorescein angiography (FFA), the patient is given an

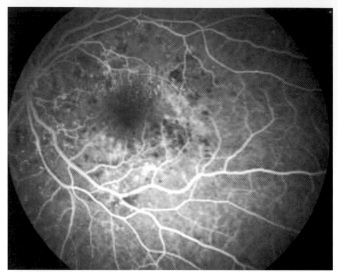

Figure 67.8 Fluorescein angiogram showing macular microaneurysms seen as hyperfluorescent dots

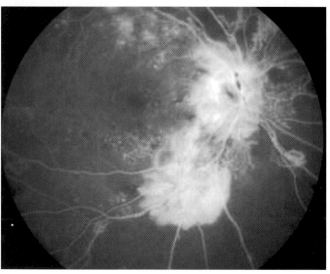

Figure 67.9 Fluorescein angiogram showing NVD and NVE right eye: Extensive capillary dropout in the nasal retina

injection of 5 to 10 ml of fluorescein dye intravenously. Rapid sequence photographs using filters matched to the spectral response of fluorescein *in vivo* are than taken immediately after injection of the dye and are continued periodically for 15 to 20 minutes. This technique can helps to determine the presence of capillary closure (which frequently cannot be determined by other clinical techniques), the presence of macular edema, the location of leaking microaneurysms and capillaries and the presence of neovascularization **(Figures 67.8 and 67.9)**. The disadvantages of this technique include risk of an allergic reaction and the additional cost.

Recently, digital retinal photography using digital image analyzing system has been used for screening purposes using nonmydriatic cameras, which are designed to allow photography of the fundus through an undilated pupil. This has the potential benefit of permitting retinal evaluation without the need for pupillary dilation, while providing a permanent record for later evaluation. However, these benefits are limited by the frequent difficulties of achieving adequate pictures through small pupils and through cataracts. Obtaining useful photographs can be difficult, even for the experienced ophthalmic photographer, though the results can be improved by dilating the pupils. It is difficult to evaluate microaneurysms, macular edema and early neovascularization. These photographs should be analyzed by an ophthalmologist who is experienced at evaluating diabetic retinopathy. This technique should be used only as a screening method to help identify patients who may need more extensive evaluation using one or more of the techniques described.

Role of optical coherence tomography (OCT): OCT is a technique that utilizes a noncontact, noninvasive device to project a near infrared light beam (820 nm) onto the retina which in turn gets reflected from the boundaries between the retinal microstructures. The interferometer in the instrument then compares the echo time delay of the light that is reflected from the various retinal layers with that of light of the same wavelength that is reflected from a reference mirror at a known distance. The interferometer then integrates several data points over 2 mm of depth to construct a real time tomogram of retinal structures using a false color scale. The hot colors (white, red, etc.) represent areas of high reflectivity while the cooler colors (blue, black, etc.) represent areas of low reflectivity. **Figure 67.10** represents the OCT of a normal eye.

Optical coherence tomography is a valuable tool in cases of diabetic retinopathy wherein a cross-sectional view of the retina is obtained.[31] It yields information that is complementary and sometimes even superior to conventional techniques such as fluorescein angiography.

Briefly, the applications of OCT in diabetic retinopathy are:

- *Defining the type of macular edema:* The types could be a sponge-like retinal thickness, cystoid macular edema **(Figure 67.11)** vitreomacular traction. Recognition of these types is crucial since the first and second types respond to focal or grid laser photocoagulation, while the third type necessitates surgical intervention.[31]

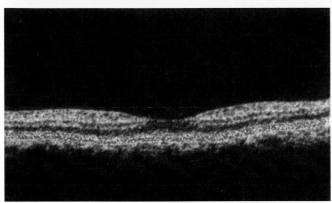

Figure 67.10 Normal optical coherence tomography (OCT)

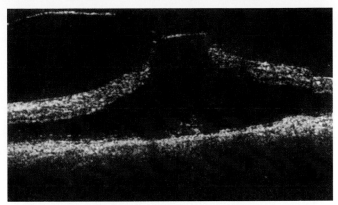

Figure 67.12 Diabetic macular edema with vitreous traction

Control of Systemic Risk Factors

Glycemic Control

Two major trials have demonstrated the effect of intensive blood glucose control in reducing the incidence and progression of DR. In Diabetes Control and Complications Trial (DCCT), risk for development of retinopathy was reduced by 76% in the intensive therapy (with the aim of maintaining blood glucose and glycosylated hemoglobin as close to normal range as possible), compared with the conventional group.[19] In United Kingdom Prospective Diabetic Study (UKPDS), patients who were assigned to intensive glucose control had a 25% risk reduction in microvascular endpoints, including the need for retinal laser photocoagulation. Epidemiological analysis of UKPDS data showed that for every percentage point decrease in glycosylated hemoglobin levels, there was a 35% reduction in the risk of microvascular complications.[20]

Both in type 1 and type 2 diabetes, strict glycemic control plays an important role, not only in prevention but also in the reversal of some of the changes of diabetic retinopathy.[20]

Blood Pressure (BP) Control

In the Wisconsin Epidemiologic Study of Diabetic Retinopathy (WESDR), progression of retinopathy was associated with higher diastolic BP at baseline and an increase in diastolic BP over a 4-year follow-up period. The recommended BP is systolic 135 mm Hg and diastolic 85 mm Hg.

UKPDS has shown that with right control of BP, patients had a 34% reduction in progression of retinopathy and a 47% reduced risk of deterioration in visual acuity of 3 lines.[32] Angiotensin converting enzyme (ACE) inhibitors when used to control blood pressure

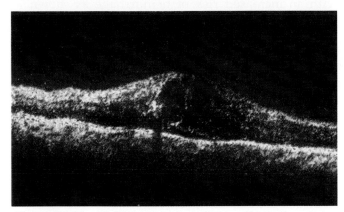

Figure 67.11 Diabetic macular edema with cystic spaces

- *Monitoring response to therapy:* Since it quantified retinal thickness, then it helps in the tracking of tissue alteration overtime following a therapy.
- *Detection of surgically treatable lesions:* These include lesions that are amenable to vitrectomy such as vitreomacular, traction causing recalcitrant macular edema **(Figure 67.12)** lamellar macular holes, taut posterior hyaloid membrane (wherein the vitreous stretches across the macula like a taut membrane that causes edema despite no demonstrable antero-posterior traction).

MANAGEMENT

Management of diabetic retinopathy include:
- Control of systemic risk factors
- Laser photocoagulation
- Vitreous surgery
- Potential pharmacological therapies
- Screening for diabetic retinopathy.

in type 1 diabetes was found to have a beneficial effect in progression of diabetic retinopathy. However in UKPDS, the beneficial effects of BP control were seen both with beta-blockers and ACE inhibitors with no statistically significant difference between them.

So a tight control of blood pressure in diabetes has a role in prevention and progression of diabetic retinopathy.

Lipid Control

Among insulin using patients in the WESDR, the presence of retinal hard exudates was significantly associated with increased serum cholesterol levels.[33] In Early Treatment of Diabetic Retinopathy Study (ETDRS), patients who have elevated serum cholesterol and low density lipoprotein levels at baseline were more likely to have retinal hard exudates than those with normal levels.[5] Lipid lowering recommendations are currently given to all patients with diabetes and elevated cholesterol irrespective of retinopathy status.

Renal Disease and DR

Lot of cross-sectional[34,35] and longitudinal studies[36,37] showed a relationship between proteinuria or micro-albuminuria and retinopathy. Patients with progressive renal dysfunction need to be monitored closely for rapidly worsening retinopathy. Conversely, rapidly progressive retinopathy, especially in a patient with long history of diabetes and where retinopathy has been previously stable, should suggest the need for renal evaluation.

Exercise and DR

Aerobic exercises in diabetic patients improve or maintain cardiovascular function, increase levels of HDL, help in weight reduction, increase insulin sensitivity, and help in controlling blood glucose levels. In general, people with proliferative diabetic retinopathy (PDR) should avoid anaerobic exercise and exercise that involves straining, jarring, near maximal isometric contractions or Valsalva-type maneuvers such as high impact aerobics, jogging or heavy weight training. Beneficial low-risk exercises are stationary cycling, low intensity machine rowing, swimming and walking.

Pregnancy and Diabetic Retinopathy

Progression of DR in pregnancy is a transient pheno-menon and the long-term progression of DR does not appear to be increased by pregnancy. Risk factors for retinopathy progression during pregnancy include baseline severity of retinopathy, glycemic control, duration of diabetes and concomitant hypertension. Panretinal laser photocoagulation (PRP) should be carefully considered for pregnant diabetic patients as they approach PDR. The treatment of high-risk PDR is same as in nonpregnant patients. Although vaginal delivery is associated with Valsalva maneuvers, it has not been associated with significant increased risk of vitreous hemorrhage in pregnancy patients with PDR.[38]

Anticoagulation and Thrombolysis

The use of aspirin in diabetic patients is not associated with an increased risk of hemorrhage as shown in the ETDRS and has no demonstrated impact on the progression of retinopathy or macular edema.[39]

Smoking and DR

The effects of smoking on DR are unclear.[38] In the Indian context, smoking has not been associated with diabetic retinopathy as only 17.5% patients smoked in the CURES eye study. Nevertheless, since smoking has deleterious influence on the cardiovascular system and the development of nephropathy, smoking in patients with diabetes should be discouraged.

Influence of Anemia

In patients with diabetic retinopathy, those with low hemoglobin levels have a five-fold increase in risk of developing severe retinopathy compared with those with high hemoglobin levels.[38] So all diabetic with retinopathy and anemia should receive appropriate treatment for correction for anemia.

Antioxidant Intake

Vitamins such as C, E and β-carotene have been shown to have protective effect from development of diabetic retinopathy.[40] Due to the potential for side effects with high dose vitamin supplementation, it is advised that patients do not ingest levels of vitamins in excessive of generally recommended doses until definite evidence is established by prospective clinical interventional studies.

Laser Photocoagulation

Laser photocoagulation is used to treat both diabetic retinopathy and diabetic macular edema. The goal of macular laser photocoagulation for diabetic macular

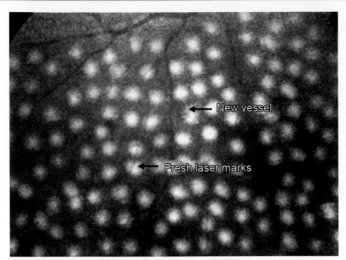

Figure 67.13 Proliferative diabetic retinopathy: Immediate post-PRP laser treatment

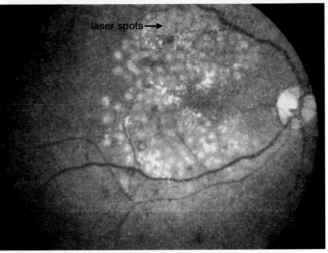

Figure 67.14 Clinically significant macular edema: Immediate post-focal laser treatment

edema is to limit vascular leakage through a series of focal laser burns at leaking microaneurysms or grid laser burns in regions of diffuse breakdown of the blood retinal barrier. The rationale of panretinal photoagulation for diabetic retinopathy is to ablate ischemic areas of the peripheral retina and thereby reduce the induction of angiogenic growth factors. Results of the diabetic retinopathy study demonstrated that panretinal photocoagulation **(Figure 67.13)** effectively reduces the risk of vision loss in a majority (60%) of patients with PDR.[41] The ETDRS results showed that macular laser photocoagulation reduced the risk of vision loss by 50% for patients with clinically significant diabetic macular edema **(Figure 67.14)**.[42,43] Macular focal and grid laser photocoagulation is indicated for clinically significant diabetic macular edema and panretinal photocoagulation is indicated for high-risk PDR.[44]

A study conducted retrospectively evaluating 96 eyes for the effect of various risk factors on the final visual outcome after laser photocoagulation for clinically significant macular edema (CSME) in diabetic retinopathy reported that advanced age of the patient, large size of CSME and poor baseline visual acuity were found to be significantly associated with poorer outcome.[45] To evaluate the visual outcome of PRP, a study conducted in 261 eyes of 160 type 2 Indian diabetic subjects with PDR showed that visual acuity at baseline, duration of diabetes and proteinuria played a significant role in determining the post-PRP visual acuity.[46]

Vitreous Surgery

Timely application of laser photocoagulation with reapplication needed is the mainstay of treatment to reduce visual loss. However, despite timely treatment and preventive regimens, a substantial number of patients will develop complications of progressive retinopathy and may need surgical intervention. The Diabetic Retinopathy Vitrectomy Study (DRVS)[47] established the indications for vitrectomy in diabetic patients by mid 1980s. Since then, because of newer instrumentation and improved surgical techniques these indications have been refined and expanded to a large extent. The main objectives of surgery in diabetic retinopathy are to neutralize and when possible eliminate the components that have led to the visual loss.

Objectives are:
• Removal of axial opacities such as nonclearing vitreous hemorrhages.
• Relieve anteroposterior traction and relieve tangential traction as in tractional retinal detachment and remove fibrinoid membranes from the vitreous and also to save the eye from harmful effects of glaucoma.

The indication and timing of pars plana vitrectomy for diabetic retinopathy continue to evolve, but have not changed conceptually, With the improvement in both instrumentation and surgical techniques, more difficult cases are now being considered and postoperative recovery of vision is more consistent.

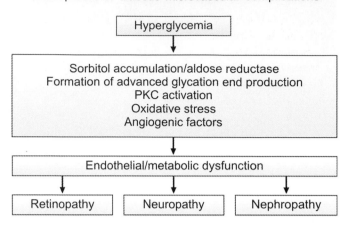

Although the postvitrectomy visual acuity outcomes are favorable compared to the natural history of diabetic retinopathy, they are still poor compared to the potential efficacy of preventive measures such as improved control of glucose and timely application of laser treatment.

Potential Pharmacological Therapies

Because of the limitations of current treatments, new pharmacological therapies are being developed, targeting the underlying biochemical mechanisms that cause diabetic retinopathy/diabetic macular edema **(Flow chart 67.1)**.

Role of Sorbitol Accumulation and Use of Aldose Reductase Inhibitors (ARIs)

The hyperglycemia of diabetes leads to an increased flux through the polyol pathway, resulting in elevated levels of sorbitol.[48] The ensuing disruption of the osmotic balance in the cell is believed to result in cellular damage which may be important in the loss of integrity of the blood retinal barrier, among other complications.

Clinical trials of ARI (sorbinil, ponalrestat and tolrestat) have been conducted for the treatment of DR.[49] Unfortunately, ARIs have shown little therapeutic promise for DR thus far.

Role of Advanced Glycation End Products (AGEs) and Use of Age Inhibitors

Carbohydrates interact with protein side chains in a nonenzymatic fashion to form Amadori products and these may subsequently form AGEs, especially in the presence of high glucose.[50] Excessive formation of AGEs has been proposed as another biochemical link between diabetes and the development of microvascular complications. AGEs may affect such functions as enzyme activity, binding of regulatory molecules, and susceptibility of proteins to proteolysis. The chronic interaction of these products with at least one specific cell surface receptor for AGEs (AGE-specific receptor) may perpetuate a proinflammatory signaling process and a proatherosclerotic state in vascular tissues. These processes may result in disruptions of retinal hemodynamics and/or damage to vascular endothelial cells. The inhibition of AGE formation using compounds such as aminoguanidine has been investigated to prevent some of the diabetic vascular abnormalities. The utility of these compounds for the prevention of DR remains to be proven in humans.

Role of the Protein Kinase C (PKC) Pathway and Use of PKC Inhibitors

PKC activity and levels of diacylglycerol (DAG), an activator of PKC are increased after exposure of vascular tissues to elevated glucose. PKC activity is also increased after exposure of vascular endothelial cells to oxidative stress, another mechanism implicated in the development and progression of diabetic microvascular complications. Ruboxistaurin (LY333531), a specific inhibitor of PKC-beta 1 and 2[51] has been shown to prevent and reverse microvascular complications in animal models of diabetes[52] to block neovascularization associated with retinal ischemia[53] and to inhibit the effect of VEGF on retinal permeability and endothelial cell growth.[28] In patients with minimal DR, ruboxistaurin reversed retinal blood flow abnormalities and was well tolerated.[54] PKC412 inhibits the alpha, beta and gamma isoforms, resulting in inhibition of ischemia-induced angiogenesis. Pharmacodynamic studies of PKC412 have reported some adverse outcomes, which may reflect PKC412's relative lack of specificity.

Role of Oxidative Stress and Use of Antioxidant Compounds

Production of reactive oxygen species (ROS) has been implicated in the development of diabetic complications. Diabetes may cause ROS production through glucose auto-oxidation, increased flux through the polyol pathway and increases in protein glycation.[55] ROS may activate aldose reductase and PKC and increase AGE production and DAG formation.

Inhibition of superoxide production can effectively block sorbitol accumulation, AGE formation and PKC activation, the predominant three mechanisms of diabetes induced vascular damage. Tocopherol also inhibits hyperglycemia-induced DAG production and PKC.[56] Tocopherol prevents retinal hemodynamic abnormalities in diabetic rats. In patients with type 1 diabetes and little or no baseline retinopathy, retinal blood flow was significantly increased after four months of tocopherol therapy.

Role of Angiogenic Factors and Use of Antiangiogenic Agents

VEGF is a key mediator of angiogenesis in the retina.[57] Clinical studies have shown that VEGF levels increase in patients as they progress from non-proliferative DR to active PDR. Successful panretinal photocoagulation has been found to reduce intraocular VEGF levels by 75% in patients treated for ocular neovascularization.[58] This suggests that specific inhibition of VEGF activity may prevent retinal neovascularization and associated blood flow abnormalities.

The role of VEGF in retinal neovascularization has also prompted the development of VEGF specific inhibitors such as antibodies to VEGF. These antibodies may be especially useful for the prevention of neovascularization during the very early stages of PDR. An endogenous inhibitor of angiogenesis is pigment endothelium derived factor (PEDF). PEDF inhibits angiogenesis induced by a wide variety of growth factors in addition to VEGF.[59] These findings suggest that PEDF may be useful as a primary intervention in the treatment of early DR.

Intravitreal Steroids

Diabetic macular edema is the major cause of partial blindness. Recently, triamcinolone acetonide has been used to treat the diabetic macular edema. Corticosteroids are known to attenuate effects of VEGF hence it is thought that intravitreal injection may be an efficient delivery route to treat diabetic macular edema. However, with the dose of 4 mg/0.1 ml triamcinolone acetonide repeated intravitreal injections are required once the triamcinolone crystals disappeared clinically. To overcome this problem, recently fluocinolone acetonide sustained release intravitreal implants were used. Preclinical studies demonstrated lack of any major ocular toxicity of intravitreal triamcinolone or fluocinolone sustained release implants. However, periodical ocular examination is needed to rule out steroid induced glaucoma or cataract formation.

Other Potential Therapies for Retinopathy Prevention

Somatostatin activity is linked with the progression of DR[60] and hypophysectomy has been proposed as an intervention for severe treatment resistant DR. Consequently, somatostatin has been evaluated for the treatment for DR.[61] In a recent trial of patients with severe nonproliferative DR or early PDR, therapy with octreotide (a somatostatin analog) decreased the need for retinal photocoagulation compared with conventional treatment.

Screening for Diabetic Retinopathy

Screening examination is performed to detect asymptomatic treatable condition. It is widely accepted that screening for diabetic retinopathy represents both good clinical practice and cost-effective health care. The natural history of the disease is known and early detection and treatment of retinopathy has been shown to be effective in preventing visual impairment.[62] With appropriate medical and ophthalmological interventions, including good glycemic and blood pressure control, it has been estimated that blindness may be prevented in at least one eye in 60 to 70% of cases with maculopathy and 90% of cases of proliferative retinopathy. The disability caused by blindness and partial sight, as well as the social costs in terms of loss of earning capacity and the required social support are considerable. It is important that all diabetic patients are screened for evidence of diabetic retinopathy. Lack of screening may also result in costly compensation claims.

Effectiveness of Different Screening Methods

There have been a number of studies assessing the effectiveness of different screening modalities. Examination techniques that have been used to detect diabetic retinopathy include direct and indirect ophthalmoscopy, stereoscopic mydriatic and non-mydriatic fundus photography and most recently telemedicine techniques. The gold standard for screening usually is seven field stereo fundus photographs read by trained graders as was done in the ETDRS.[42]

Ophthalmoscopy

Ophthalmoscopy is a useful screening procedure, easy to use and accessible to ophthalmologists and other

TABLE 67.4	Recommended eye examination schedule	
Type of diabetes mellitus	Recommendation time of first examination	Routine minimum follow-up
Type 1, IDDM	5 years after onset or during puberty	Yearly
Type 2, NIDDM	At time of diagnosis	Yearly
During pregnancy	Prior to pregnancy for counseling Early in first trimester	Each trimester If indicated more frequently up to 3–6 months postpartum

physicians and requires no specialized equipment. Compared with fundus photography, ophthalmoscopy by an experienced examiner was found to agree with grading by fundus photography (Gold Standard) 85% of the time. In the hands of primary care physicians, ophthalmoscopy was less sensitive than fundus photography in detecting both any DR and sight-threatening DR (sensitivity 63 vs 79% and 66 vs 87%, respectively).[63] With additional training, however, ophthalmologic screening by primary care physicians may be a clinically acceptable and cost-saving strategy to refer patients for evaluation by an ophthalmologist. Ophthalmoscopy compared favorably with fundus photography, with 100% sensitivity for referral or follow-up within one year.[64]

Fundus Photography and Telemedicine

Investigators have evaluated the potential for the use of digital cameras to obtain fundus images through nondilated pupils. The sensitivity and specificity of these nonstereoscopic digital screening methods have most often been compared with the ETDRS seven standard field images. Overall, these methods are in substantial agreement with the ETDRS classification for the grading of diabetic retinopathy and in fair to moderate agreement for the grading of diabetic macular edema.[65,66]

Recent studies showed that for 45° or 45 degree field nonstereoscopic color digital fundus photographs of each eye could be transmitted over the Internet and be used with great accuracy for the screening of DR.[67] These methods have also been shown to have good sensitivity and specificity when using a centrally based trained grader.

Current Guidelines

Recent data indicate that annual dilated eye examinations should be implemented from the initial diagnosis of both type 1 and type 2 diabetes. Referral to an experienced ophthalmologist is required if any

TABLE 67.5	Eye examination follow-up
Abnormality	Follow-up
None or few microaneurysms	Yearly
Mild and moderate NPDR	Every 6 months
Severe NPDR	4 months
Severe NPDR with CSME	2 months
PDR	2 months

level of diabetic macular edema, severe nonproliferative diabetic retinopathy, or PDR is detected in the examination. Regular follow-up is also essential to ensure early detection, even if no diabetic retinopathy was found initially; this is especially important for high-risk patients. Adherence to American Diabetes Association guidelines for annual ophthalmic examination is poor, ranging only from 34 to 65%. Even among patients at high-risk for vision loss (pre-existent diabetic retinopathy or long duration of diabetes), the rates of adherence were only 61 and 57%, respectively. These findings suggest a need for practitioner and patient education about diabetic retinopathy and its consequences. Screening is important not only for the detection of sight-threatening retinopathy, but also for the detection of any retinopathy so that particular effort can be made to improve blood pressure and glycemic control.

An appropriate follow-up schedule for all diabetic patients and for patients with various clinical staging of DR is given in the **Tables 67.4 and 67.5**.

SUMMARY

Diabetes and diabetes-related micro- and macrovascular complications are assuming increased importance in recent times. Diabetic retinopathy, the common cause of vision impairment in diabetes is often missed at the stages when it is amenable for treatment due to a asymptomatic phase before excellent treatment modalities such as lasers are available at present to retain the existing vision though not to restore the lost vision. Available data suggest that better control of hyperglycemia, blood pressure and hyperlipidemia will prevent development of complications of diabetes. With the available recent knowledge on pathogenic mechanisms, within the near future, pharmacologic treatment will likely be available to treat and prevent the progression of diabetic retinopathy.

Because new pharmacological approach to management is directed towards the early stage of diabetic retinopathy, it is extremely important to set stages for early detection by screening and creating awareness among patients and physicians. The interdisciplinary co-operation and team approach of ophthalmologist, diabetologist and primary care physicians will go a long way to identify these patients at risk of vision loss and prevent blindness. Blindness from diabetic retinopathy is largely preventable with timely detection and appropriate intervention therapy.

ACKNOWLEDGMENTS

The authors would like to acknowledge the support of the Technology Information, Forecasting and Assessment Council-Centre of Relevance and Excellence (TIFAC-CORE) in Diabetic Retinopathy Project, Aravind Eye Care System, Madurai, Tamil Nadu, India and also to Dr Dinesh K Sahu for his assistance.

REFERENCES

1. Klein R, Klein BE, Moss SE. Visual impairment in diabetes. Ophthalmol. 1984;91:1-9.
2. Klein R, Klein BE, Moss SE, Davis MD, DeMets DL. The Wisconsin epidemiologic study of diabetic retinopathy IV. Diabetic macular edema. Ophthalmol. 1984; 91:1464-74.
3. Klein R, Klein BE, Moss SE, Cruckshanks KJ. The Wisconsin Epidemiological Study of Diabetic Retinopathy XVII. The 14-year incidence and progression of diabetic retinopathy and associated risk factors in type 1 diabetes. Ophthalmol. 1998; 105:1801-15.
4. Davis MD, Fisher MR, Gangnon RE, et al. Risk factors for high-risk proliferative diabetic retinopathy and severe visual loss: early treatment diabetic retinopathy study (ETDRS) Report 18. Invest Ophthalmol Vis Sci. 1998;39:233-52.
5. Chew EY, Klein ML, Ferris FL, et al. Association of elevated serum lipid levels with retinal hard exudates in diabetic retinopathy. Early Treatment Diabetic Retinopathy Study (ETDRS) Report 22. Arch Ophthalmol. 1996;114:1079-84.
6. Early Treatment Diabetic Retinopathy Study Research group. Grading diabetic retinopathy from stereoscopic color fundus photographs: an extension of the modified Airlie House classification: early treatment diabetic retinopathy study (ETDRS) Report 10. Ophthalmol 1991;98 (Suppl):786-806.
7. Klein R, Klein BE, Moss SE. How many steps of progression of diabetic retinopathy are meaningful? The Wisconsin Epidemiologic Study of Diabetic Retinopathy. Arch Ophthalmol. 2001;119:547-53.
8. Wilkinson CP, Ferris FL 3rd, Klein RE, Lee PP, Agardh CD, Davis M, Dills D, Kampik A, Pararajasegaram R, Verdaguer JT. Global diabetic retinopathy Project Group. Proposed international clinical diabetic retinopathy and diabetic macular edema disease severity scales. Ophthalmol. 2003;110:1677-82.
9. Rema M, Mohan V, Ramachandran A, Viswanathan M. Retinopathy in Insulin Dependent Diabetes Mellitus (IDDM) in South India. Journal of Association of Physicians of India. 1988;36:703-5.
10. Rema M, Premkumar S, Anitha B, Deepa R, Pradeepa R, Mohan V. Prevalence of diabetic retinopathy in urban India: the Chennai Urban Rural Epidemiology Study (CURES) eye study I. Invest. Ophthalmol. Vis Sci. 2005;46:2328-33.
11. Varma R, Torres M, Pena F, Klein R, Azen SP. Los Angeles Latino Eye Study Group. Prevalence of diabetic retinopathy in adult Latinos: the Los Angeles Latino eye study. Ophthalmol. 2004;111:1298-306.
12. Broadbent DM, Scott JA, Vora JP, Harding SP. Prevalence of diabetic eye disease in an inner city population: the Liverpool Diabetic Eye Study Eye. 1999;13:160-5.
13. Nagi DK, Pettitt DJ, Bennett PH, Klein R, Knowler WC. Diabetic retinopathy assessed by fundus photography in Pima Indians with impaired glucose tolerance and NIDDM. Diabet Med. 1997;14:449-56.
14. Rema M, Ponnaiya M, Mohan V. Prevalence of retinopathy in noninsulin dependent diabetes mellitus at a diabetes centre in southern India. Diabetes Res Clin Pract. 1996;34:29-36.
15. Rema M, Deepa R, Mohan V. Prevalence of retinopathy at diagnosis among Type 2 diabetic patients attending a diabetic centre in South India. Br J Ophthalmol. 2000;84:1058-60.
16. Dandona L, Dandona R, Naduvilath TJ, McCarthy CA, Rao GN. Population based assessment of diabetic retinopathy in an urban population in southern India. Br J Ophthalmol. 1999; 83:937-40.
17. Narendran V, John RK, Raghuram A, Ravindran RD, Nirmalan PK, Thulasiraj RD. Diabetic retinopathy among self reported diabetics in southern India: a population based assessment. Br J Ophthalmol. 2002 ;86:1014-8.
18. Rema M, Shanthirani CS, Deepa R, Mohan V. Prevalence of diabetic retinopathy in a selected South Indian Population: the Chennai Urban Population Study (CUPS). Diabetes Res Clin Pract. 2000;50:S252.
19. The diabetes control and complications trial research group. The effect of intensive treatment of diabetes on the development and progression of long-term complications in insulin-dependent diabetes mellitus. N Engl J Med. 1993;329:977-86.
20. Intensive blood-glucose control with sulfonylureas or insulin compared with conventional treatment and risk of complications in patients with type 2 diabetes (UKPDS 33). United Kingdom Prospective Diabetes Study (UKPDS) Group. Lancet. 1998;352:837-53.
21. Hawrami K, Rema M, Mohan V, et al. A genetic study of retinopathy in south Indian type 2 (noninsulin dependent) diabetic patients. Diabetologia. 1991;31: 441-4.
22. Hawrami K, Hitman GA, Rema M, et al. An association in non-insulin-dependent diabetes mellitus subjects between

susceptibility to retinopathy and tumor necrosis factor polymorphism. Hum Immunol. 1996;46:49-54.

23. Kumaramanickavel G, Sripriya S, Vellanki RN, et al. Tumor necrosis factor allelic polymorphism with diabetic retinopathy in India. Diabetes Res Clin Pract. 2001;54:89-94.

24. Rema M, Saravanan G, Deepa R. Familial clustering of diabetic retinopathy in South Indian Type 2 diabetic patients. Diabet Med. 2002;19:910-16.

25. Efficacy of atenolol and captopril in reducing risk of macrovascular and microvascular complications in type 2 diabetes (UKPDS 39). United Kingdom Prospective Diabetes Study Group. BMJ. 1998;317:713-20.

26. Wunderlich K, Senn BC, Todesco L, Flammer J, Meyer P. Regulation of connective tissue growth factor gene expression in retinal vascular endothelial cells by angiogenic growth factors. Graefes Arch Clin Exp Ophthalmol. 2000;238:910-15.

27. Pe'er J, Folberg R, Itin A, Gnessin H, Hemo I, Keshet E. Upregulated expression of vascular endothelial growth factor in proliferative diabetic retinopathy. Br J Ophthalmol. 1996; 80:241-5.

28. Aiello LP, Bursell SE, Clermont A, Duh E, Ishii H, Takagi C, et al. Vascular endothelial growth factor-induced retinal permeability is mediated by protein kinase C in vivo and suppressed by an orally effective beta-isoform-selective inhibitor. Diabetes. 1997;46:1473-80.

29. Frank RN. On the pathogenesis of diabetic retinopathy: a 1990 update Ophthalmology. 1991;98:586-93.

30. Stanford MR. The pathogenesis of diabetic retinopathy. Br J Ophthalmol. 2004;88:444-5.

31. Panozzo G, Gusson E, Parolini B, Mercanti A. Role of OCT in the diagnosis and follow-up of diabetic macular edema. Semin Ophthalmol. 2003;18:74-81.

32. Tight blood pressure control and risk of macrovascular and microvascular complications in type 2 diabetes (UKPDS 38). United Kingdom Prospective Diabetes Study Group. BMJ. 1998;317:703-13.

33. Klein BE, Moss SE, Klein R, Surawicz TS. The Wisconsin Epidemiological Study of Diabetic Retinopathy XIII. Relationship of serum cholesterol to retinopathy and hard exudates. Ophthalmol. 1991;98:1261-5.

34. Savage S, Estacio RO, Jeffers B, Schrier RW. Urinary albumin excretion as a predictor of diabetic retinopathy, neuropathy, and cardiovascular disease in NIDDM. Diabetes Care. 1996;19:1243-8.

35. Klein R, Klein BE, Moss Se, et al. The Wisconsin Epidemiology Study of Diabetic Retinopathy V. Proteinuria and retinopathy in a population of diabetic persons diagnosed prior to 30 years of age. In Friedman Ea, L'Esperance Jr FA (Eds): Diabetic Renal-Retinal Syndrome 3. Orlando FL: Frune and Stratton, 1986.

36. Mathiesen ER, Rohn B, Storm B, et al. The natural course of microalbuminuria in insulin-dependent diabetes: a 10-year prospective study. Diabet Med. 1995;12:482-7.

37. Park JY, Kim HK, Chung YE, et al. Incidence and determinants of microalbuminuria in Koreans with type 2 diabetes. Diabetes Care. 1998;21:530-4.

38. Aiello LP. Systemic considerations in the management of diabetic retinopathy. Am J Ophthalmol. 2001;132:760-76.

39. Chew EY, Klien ML, Murphy RP, et al. Effects of aspirin on vitreous/preretinal hemorrhage in patients with diabetes mellitus. Early Treatment Diabetic Retinopathy Study (ETDRS) Report 20. Arch Ophthalmol. 1995;113:52-5.

40. Mayer-Davis EJ, Bell RA, Reboussin BA, et al. Antioxidant nutrient intake and diabetic retinopathy: the San Luis Valley Diabetes Study. Ophthalmol. 1998; 105:2264-70.

41. The Diabetic Retinopathy Study (DRS) Research Group. Preliminary report on the effects of photocoagulation therapy: DRS Report 1. Am J Ophthalmol. 1976; 81:383-96.

42. Early Treatment Diabetic Retinopathy Study Research Group. Photocoagulation for diabetic macular edema. Early Treatment Diabetic Retinopathy Study (ETDRS) Report 1. Arch Ophthalmol. 1985;103:1796-806.

43. Early Treatment Diabetic Retinopathy Study Research Group. Early photocoagulation for diabetic retinopathy (ETDRS) Report 9. Ophthalmol. 1991;98 (Suppl): 766-85.

44. Early Treatment Diabetic Retinopathy Study Research Group. Treatment techniques and clinical guidelines for photocoagulation of diabetic macular edema. Early Treatment Diabetic Retinopathy Study (ETDRS) Report 3. Ophthalmol. 1987;94: 761-74.

45. Gupta A, Gupta V, Dogra MR, Pandav SS. Risk factors influencing the treatment outcome in diabetic macular edema. Indian J Ophthalmol. 1996;44:145-8.

46. Rema M, Sujatha P, Pradeepa R. Visual outcomes of panretinal photocoagulation in diabetic retinopathy at one-year follow-up and associated risk factors. Indian J Ophthalmol. 2005; 53:93-9.

47. Diabetic Retinopathy Vitrectomy Study Research Group. Early vitrectomy for severe vitreous hemorrhage in diabetic retinopathy: four-year results of a randomized trial. Diabetic Retinopathy Vitrectomy Study (DRVS) Report 5. Arch Ophthalmol. 1990;108:958-64.

48. Gabbay KH. Hyperglycemia, polyol metabolism, and complications of diabetes mellitus. Annu Rev Med. 1975;26: 521-35.

49. Sorbinil Retinopathy Trail Research Group. A randomized trial of sorbinil: an aldose reductase inhibitor, in diabetic retinopathy. Arch Ophthalmol. 1990;108:1234-44.

50. Friedman EA. Advanced glycosylated end products and hyperglycemia in the pathogenesis of diabetic complications. Diabetes Care 1999;22 (Suppl 2):B65-71.

51. Jirousek MR, Gillig JR, Gonzalez CM, Heath WF, McDonalt JH III, Neel DA, Rito CJ, Singh U, Stramm LE, Melikian-Badalian A, Baevsky M, Ballas LM, Hall SE, Winneroski LL, Faul MM: (S)-13- [(dimethylamino) methyl}-10,11,14,15-tetrahydro-4,9:16,21-dimetheno-1H,13H-dibenzo [e,k] pyrrolo[3,4-h][1,4,13] oxadiazacyclohexadecene-1,3(2H)-dione(LY333531) and related analogues: isozyme selective inhibitors of protein kinase C beta. J Med Chem. 1996;39:2664-71.

52. Ishii H, Jirousek MR, Koya D, et al. Amelioration of vascular dysfunctions of diabetic rats by oral PKC-beta inhibitor. Science. 1996;272:728-31.

53. Danis RP, Bingaman DP, Jirousek MR, Yang Y. Inhibition of intraocular neovascularization caused by retinal ischemia in pigs by PKC-beta inhibition with LY333531. Invest Ophthalmol Vis Sci. 1998;39:171-9.

54. Aiello LP, Bursell S, Devries T, Alatorre C, King GL, Ways K. Protein kinase C selective inhibitor LY333531 ameliorates abnormal retinal hemodynamics in patients with diabetes (Abstract). Diabetes. 1999;48:A19.

55. Giugliano D, Ceriello A, Paolisso G. Oxidative stress and diabetic vascular complications. Diabetes Care. 1996;19:257-67.

56. Kunisaki M, Bursell SE, Clermont AC, Ishii H, Ballas LM, Jirousek MR, Umeda F, Nawata H, King GL. Vitamin E prevents diabetes-induced abnormal retinal blood flow via in the diacylglycerol-protein kinase C pathway. Am J Physiol. 1995;269: E239-46.

57. Miller JW, Adamis AP, Aiello LP. Vascular endothelial growth factor in ocular neovascularization and proliferative diabetic retinopathy. Diabetes Metab Rev. 1997;13:37-50.

58. Aiello LP, Avery RL, Arrigg PG, Keyt BA, Jampel HD, Shah ST, et al. Vascular endothelial growth factor in ocular fluid of patients with diabetic retinopathy and other retinal disorders. N Engl J Med. 1994;331:1480-7.

59. Dawson DW, Volpert OV, Gillis P, Crawford SE, Xu H, Benedict W, Bouck NP. Pigment epithelium-derived factor: a potent inhibitor of angiogenesis. Science. 1999;285:245-8.

60. Grant MB, Mames RN, Fitzgerald C, Hazariwala KM, Cooper-DeHoff R, Caballero S, Estes KS. The efficacy of octreotide in the therapy of severe nonproliferative and early proliferative diabetic retinopathy. Diabetes Care. 2000; 23:504-9.

61. McCombe M, Lightman S, Eckland DJ, et al. Effect of long-acting somatostatin analogue (BIM23014) on proliferative diabetic retinopathy: a pilot study. Eye. 1991;5:569-75.

62. Diabetic Retinopathy Study Research Group. Photocoagulation treatment of proliferative diabetic retinopathy. Clinical application of Diabetic Retinopathy Study Findings, DRS Report 1. Ophthalmol. 1981;88:585-600.

63. Moss, Scot E, et al. Comparison between ophthalmoscopy and fundus photography in determining severity of diabetic retinopathy ophthalmology 1985;92(1):62-7.

64. Griffith SP, Freeman WL, Shaw CJ, Mitchell WH, Olden CR, Figgs LD, Kinyoun JL, Underwood DL, Will JC. Screening for diabetic retinopathy in a clinical setting: a comparison of direct ophthalmoscopy by primary care physicians with fundus photography. J Fam Pract. 1993;37:49-56.

65. Newsom R, Moate B, Casswell T. Screening for diabetic retinopathy using digital colour photography and oral fluorescein angiography. Eye. 2000;14:579-82.

66. Bursell SE, Cavallerano JD, Cavallerano AA, Clermont AC, Birkmire-Peters D, Aiello LP, Aiello LM. Stereo nonmydriatic digital-video color retinal imaging compared with early treatment diabetic retinopathy study (ETDRS) seven standard field 35-mm stereo color photos for determining level of diabetic retinopathy. Ophthalmology. 2001;108:572-85.

67. Gomez-Ulla F, Fernandez MI, Gonzalez F, Rey P, Rodriguez M, Rodriguez-Cid MJ, Casanueva FF, Tome MA, Garcia-Tobio J, Gude F. Digital retinal images and tele-ophthalmology for detecting and grading diabetic retinopathy. Diabetes Care. 2002;25(8):1384-9.

Chapter 68

DIABETES AND KIDNEY

AL Kirpalani

CHAPTER OUTLINE

- Introduction
- Epidemiology
- Risk Factors for Diabetic Nephropathy
- Predicting the Development and Progression of Nephropathy
- Pathology
- Pathogenesis

- Pathogenesis of Histological Lesions
- Clinical Course and Natural History
- Management
- Post-transplant Diabetes Mellitus (PTDM)
- Other Renal Manifestations in Diabetics
- Summary

INTRODUCTION

Diabetic nephropathy (DN), a relatively common microvascular complication of both type 1 and type 2 DM contributes maximally to the pool of patients with chronic renal failure.

It is defined clinically as the presence of persistent proteinuria in a diabetic patient usually with retinopathy, elevated blood pressure and declining glomerular function, in the absence of UTI, other renal disease and/or heart failure.

Historically, the two most important milestones have been the recognition of albumin in the urine as a sign of severe renal disease by Richard Bright in 1836 and the identification of the classic lesion of diabetic nephropathy—the nodular glomerular intercapillary lesions described by Kimmelstiel and Wilson in 1936. Much research has gone into the understanding of the pathophysiology and the management of patients with diabetic nephropathy.

It is heartening that recent evidence indicates that diabetic nephropathy may be preventable and the deterioration of renal function can be controlled.

EPIDEMIOLOGY

Figures from the US Renal Data System over the last three decades has shown a continual increase in the incidence of renal failure among patients with diabetes, predominantly with type 2 DM. This trend has been observed both in developed and developing countries.[1]

It is commoner to see more patients of type 2 DM with nephropathy, than those with type 1 DM (9:1) even though the incidence of nephropathy is higher in patients with type 1 DM (30%), when compared to patients with type 2 DM (20%) and this is attributed to the fact that the prevalence of type 2 DM in the general population is very much higher.

Earlier, it was thought that risk of renal complications was considerably lower among patients with type 2 DM than among patients with type 1 DM, but recent data suggests that the incidence of ESRD in patients with type 2 DM has increased dramatically and the reason for this change is due to availability of better management options for hypertension and coronary artery disease in diabetic patients. As a result, more patients with type 2 DM live long enough for nephropathy and ESRD to develop. ESRD in patients with type 2 DM is therefore a disease of medical progress.

RISK FACTORS FOR DIABETIC NEPHROPATHY

Duration of Disease

The incidence of proteinuria and glomerulosclerosis increases as a function of the duration of diabetes, in both type 1 and type 2 DM up to 20 to 25 years of disease after which there is a decline in the number of patients developing renal disease.

Gender

There is a greater prevalence of nephropathy in men, when compared to women (between 1.1 to 1.7:1) and when this is coupled with the fact that women are diagnosed to have diabetes 1.5 times more frequently than men in these places indicates that men are at a greater risk of developing renal disease than women.

Racial and Other Factors

Certain racial and ethnic groups like Asians, West Indians, Pima Indians and Hispanic Americans have a higher incidence of diabetic nephropathy. This may relate to their predisposition to develop diabetes more frequently and at an earlier age than other populations as well as to the altered Na^+ excretion, lesser renal blood flow and increased vascular resistance observed in them.

Genetic Influence

A familial clustering of diabetic nephropathy has been demonstrated in all recent studies on the subject.[2] The cumulative incidence overt proteinuria in siblings of patients with advanced diabetic nephropathy is 71.5% after 25 years compared with 25.4% in siblings of patients without persistent proteinuria.

The possible genetic factors are[3]:
- *Expression of HLA*: The presence of A2 antigen increases the relative risk of development of micro-albuminuria by 2.25 times.
- *Polymorphism of an angiotensinogen converting enzyme (ACE)*: The most studied polymorphisms of the renin-angiotensin system are those in the precursor molecule, angiotensinogen, in the final enzymatic step, the ACE gene and in the receptor of the main agonist of the system, angiotensin II (AT2 receptor).[3] The angiotensinogen gene, which is located on chromosome 1, has been extensively studied in patients with hypertension and in those with atherosclerotic complications. The most studied gene in renal medicine is the ACE genotype. An important polymorphism in this gene, located in the intron 16 of chromosome 17, is that defined by the presence (insertion or I) or absence (deletion or D) of a 278-base pair sequence. The D allele is a risk allele because it is associated with increased ACE activity, hypertension and perhaps increased cardiovascular risk.
- The pharmacogenetics of the ACE gene (i.e. the possibility of predicting the renoprotective response to ACE inhibitors) is an equally important issue. The angiotensinogen gene has been studied as a predictor of poor response to ACE inhibition, as has the D allele, but further, larger studies are required before they can be gauged as predictors of response to therapy. The presence of DD genotype might identify type 1 diabetic patients in whom diabetic nephropathy progresses at a faster rate. The effect of therapeutic RAS blockade on the rate of deterioration of renal function in such patients is under debate, with some studies showing beneficial effect while others have not been able to duplicate these results.[4,5]
- *Polymorphism of nephrin gene*: Nephrin is a transmembrane protein located specifically at the slit diaphragm separating the podocyte foot processes and is currently under study to define its role in the pathogenesis of diabetic nephropathy. The absence of nephrin and the slit diaphragm causes massive proteinuria in both animal models and humans.[6] The expression of nephrin gene, nephrin mRNA and nephrin protein are downregulated in patients with both type 1 and type 2 DM and also altered in its distribution. Nephrin loss and redistribution precedes the development of glomerular lesions and is an early event in the onset of diabetic nephropathy.

In addition to the nephrin gene, possible genetic alterations may be seen in:
- Angiotensinogen gene
- AT II, type I receptor gene
- Aldolase reductase gene
- Apolipoprotein E gene

which may predispose to diabetic nephropathy.

Degree of Metabolic Control

Hyperglycemia is an important factor in the development and evolution of diabetic nephropathy. Patients who adequately controlled their blood glucose (as measured by glycosylated hemoglobin), developed less glomerulosclerosis than the patients whose diabetes was poorly controlled.

The concept of hyperglycemic memory, where gene expression is turned on or turned off *in vivo* during periods of poor glycemic control, explains the occurrence of persistent renal damage during subsequent periods of normal glucose control. This concept has been clinically documented in the DCCT, wherein the beneficial effect of intensive insulin therapy persisted for 4 to 5 years during follow-up, when compared to the conventional therapy group, inspite of identical glycosylated Hb levels during this period.[7]

Smoking is an independent risk factor for the development of microvascular complications of diabetes and is also independently related to increased urinary albumin excretion.

PREDICTING THE DEVELOPMENT AND PROGRESSION OF NEPHROPATHY

Identification of the factors predicting the onset of nephropathy in patients with diabetes and the factors predicting the progression of disease in the group of patients already having established nephropathy at an early age would not only provide incentive for more intensive follow-up of such patients, but also would provide clues for the design of therapeutic approaches based on particular factors.

Factors Predicting Risk of Nephropathy in Patients with Diabetes[8]

- *Family history of nephropathy*: In a family with two or more siblings with DM, the onset of nephropathy in one sibling, raises the risk of nephropathy in other siblings by fourfold. Thus, family history of nephropathy defined by dipstick positive proteinuria, predicts development of microalbuminuria.
- *Poor glycemic control*: Poor glycemic control is a strong determinant of progression to microalbuminuria[7] and normoalbuminuric patients who progress to microalbuminuria have significantly higher levels of HbA_{1c}.
- Increase in urinary albumin excretion even when values are in the normal albuminuric range is an independent risk factor for the development of microalbuminuria. Therefore, it is important to analyze albuminuria relative to earlier readings, rather than using the cut off for microalbuminuria as an absolute indicator to identify the population at risk.

- *Increased GFR*: A supranormal GFR (hyperfiltration) has been proposed as an early marker of progression to microalbuminuria in patients with diabetes[8]; controversy remains as to whether it is a predictor of microalbuminuria.[9] A positive correlation exists between initial hyperfiltration and subsequent increase in albuminuria and clinical nephropathy.[10] Glomerular hyperfiltration is attributed to:
  - Increased renal plasma flow especially in patients with poor blood glucose control and high protein intake.
  - An elevation in glomerular transcapillary hydraulic pressure difference.
  - Increased total glomerular surface area leading to an increased glomerular intrafiltration coefficient, in the early stages of diabetic nephropathy.
- The pattern of blood pressure, monitored by ambulatory blood pressure measurements (ABPM) is a predictor of nephropathy in type 1 diabetes. Patients with microalbuminuria have a higher nocturnal blood pressure than normoalbuminuric diabetic patients. Diabetic patients with a rise in systolic blood pressure during sleep have a greater risk to progress to microalbuminuria. The risk of progression to microalbuminuria is higher in those patients who have a 'non-dipper' status (i.e. a positive sleep/awake systolic blood pressure ratio) compared to those with a dipping pattern of systolic blood pressure.[11,14]

Factors Predicting Progression of Disease in Patients with Established Diabetic Nephropathy

- *Microalbuminuria*: Until recently, the risk of progression from microalbuminuria to proteinuria over a period of 6 to 14 years was thought to be as high as 80% and hence microalbuminuria was regarded as a strong and reliable predictor of nephropathy. With recent data, it has come to be recognized that there is no correlation between microalbuminuria and renal lesions on biopsy and microalbuminuria is seen in both advanced lesions and early mild lesions. Microalbuminuria is better regarded more as a marker than as a predictor of nephropathy.[12] Among the patients with microalbuminuria, 30-45% progress to proteinuria over a period of 10 years, 30% become normoalbuminuric and the rest continue to have microalbuminuria without progression.[13]

- *Hypertension*: Systemic hypertension strongly predicts both the progression from microalbuminuria to proteinuria and the subsequent decline of GFR. Hypertension and diabetes mellitus exhibit a complex and multifactorial interrelationship, and effective antihypertensive therapy delays the progression of renal disease in both type 1 and type 2 DM.
- A family history of nephropathy, hypertension and/or insulin resistance are considered to be predictors of progression.
- *Serum lipids*: Proteinuric diabetic patients have an unfavorable lipid profile, with elevated plasma total cholesterol (TVLDL and TLDL) and elevated plasma triglycerides. Also, Apo B-lipoprotein which is associated with VLDL and LDL and the highly atherogenic Lp (a) whereas the lipoprotein Apo A-l associated with HDL cholesterol is decreased, resulting in high total cholesterol / HDL cholesterol ratio. This markedly increases both cardiovascular risk and the risk of progression of nephropathy.[15]
- Smoking.

PATHOLOGY

Gross

The kidney of a diabetic patient may be increased, decreased or normal in size. In the early stages, it is invariably increased, particularly in patients with hyperfiltration (supranormal GFR). With progression of glomerulosclerosis and resultant scarring and loss of nephrons, reduction in kidney size occurs, but not grossly enough to result in bilateral contracted kidneys. This statement, however, most befits type 1 DM. In type 2 DM, it is not unusual to find shrunken kidneys at end stage.

Light Microscopy

Glomeruli

The glomeruli show a range of findings varying from the diffuse lesion with mesangial sclerosis to a nodular lesion sometimes combined with microaneurysms, exudative hyalinosis and the "capsular drop". In the early stages, the glomerular volume is enlarged by 70% and filtration surface area increases by 80%.

The diffuse lesion is characterized by a widespread increase in eosinophilic —PAS positive material within the mesangium (as seen in **Figure 68.1**). This is occasionally associated with hypercellularity. Uniform thickening of the capillary walls is common. These changes progress uniformly, paralleling the duration of disease, when the combination of mesangial expansion and thickened glomerular basement membrane (GBM) reduces filtration surface area by compromising patency of capillary lumina. Typical ischemic changes can be seen occasionally in glomeruli, mirroring the contribution of arteriosclerosis to the disease process. (For comparison, a section of the normal kidney with three normal glomeruli is shown in **Figure 68.2**).

Nodular glomerular intercapillary lesions described by Kimmelstiel and Wilson **(Figure 68.3),** are characterized by the accumulation of homogeneous eosinophilic material within the mesangium, appearing as a rounded accentuation of mesangial expansion which is usually

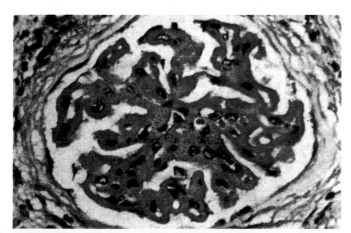

Figure 68.1 Single glomerulus showing diffused mesangial thickening patent capillaries and basement membranes of normal thickness and irregularly thick basement membranes in early diabetic (H & E x 80) nephropathy (H & E x 320)

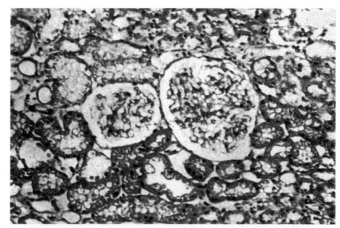

Figure 68.2 Normal kidney showing glomeruli with normal cellularity

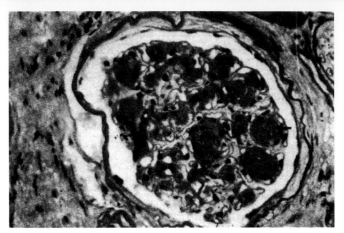

Figure 68.3 The classical Kimmelsteil-Wilson lesion (homogeneous nodular intercapillary eosinophilic material within the mesangial) seen in overt diabetic nephropathy (PAS x 200). *(Reprinted with permission from" Interpretation of Renal Biopsies" by Dr Arun Chitale)*

acellular. In most cases of advanced nephropathy, two populations of nodular lesions exist—smaller more numerous nodules arising secondary to continued mesangial expansion of the diffuse lesion and the larger, often solitary and laminated variants originating in relation to microaneurysms.

Exudative hyalinosis lesion or the "fibrin cap" is characterized initially by accumulation of hyaline eosinophilic homogeneous material between endothelial cells and the GBM of the capillary loops, progressing to occlude the capillary lumen. The overlying epithelial cells are often injured. These lesions are seen in 60% of cases of diabetic nephropathy and are not specific as they are also demonstrated in FSGS, reflux nephropathy and other forms of glomerulonephritis.

The "capsular drop" lesion is identified as a round eosinophilic accumulation of material between the basement membrane and parietal epithelial cell of the Bowman's capsule and is quite a characteristic of diabetic nephropathy.

Tubules

The tubules generally mirror the glomerular changes, with appearance of atrophic tubules in obsolescent glomeruli. The tubules are characterized by reduced size of epithelial cells and diminished luminal diameters, but the thickness of the tubular basement membrane is greater than expected for the degree of atrophy.

Blood Vessels

Both arteries and arterioles show typical changes of arteriosclerosis and arteriolosclerosis, respectively, which are manifested as varying degrees of intimal thickening and reduplication of the elastic lamina. Hyaline arteriolosclerosis occurs early and more frequently in diabetic renal disease and is characterized by striking hyaline deposition in arterioles (both afferent and efferent limbs). Using microangiography, the presence of microaneurysms in intrarenal vasculature, similar to that seen in retinopathy, have been documented.

Interstitium

Interstitial fibrosis is common and is accompanied by infiltration of chronic inflammatory cells (T cells and macrophages). Presence of interstitial fibrosis, particularly when associated with an inflammatory infiltrate correlates with renal survival. The degree of interstitial fibrosis correlates inversely with GFR.

All these changes described in the glomeruli, the tubules, the interstitium and the blood vessels are inter-related, although the progression in each compartment is not stereotypic for all patients.

Electron Microscopy Appearances

Glomerular Capillary Wall

Characteristically seen are the thickening of the GBM and the variable effacement of epithelial cell foot processes. Thickening of the GBM is considered as the earliest change in diabetic nephropathy and it has been demonstrated that this occurs as a result of excess material from epithelial cells rather than from endothelial cells. Changes seen in the foot processes are variable. Widening of the foot processes appears with the onset of microalbuminuria, but does not correlate with the degree of proteinuria. However, widening of filtration slits also occurs early and correlates with the GFR. There is an absolute loss in the number of visceral epithelial cells with concurrent mesangial expansion which makes the remaining cells spread out to cover the increased surface area.

Mesangium

Mesangial widening and mesangial nodules are due to increased mesangial matrix synthesis and decreased degradation secondary to cross-linking of glycosylated collagens. Increase occurs both in the amount of mesangial matrix and also the mesangial cells with increase in matrix being greater than the increase in cells. The major component of increased matrix is type IV collagen; also increased are type V and type VI collagen, laminin and fibronectin.

Immunofluorescence

The typical finding is the occurrence of linear staining along the glomerular capillary walls with IgG. The intensity of staining varies among individual patients and does not correspond to severity of the glomerular lesion. There are reports of capillary wall staining with IgM, C3, fibrinogen and albumin.

Hyalinosis or the exudative lesions stain brightly with IgM and C3. Linear staining with IgG and albumin is seen along the tubular basement membrane and Bowman's capsule, especially in advanced cases. This staining was thought to reflect structural changes in renal extracellular membranes, permitting entrapment of serum proteins as a result of changes in permeability.

PATHOGENESIS

Metabolic Pathways

Hyperglycemia and Non-enzymatic Glycosylation

There is a positive relationship between the abnormal glycemic milieu of diabetes and its microvascular complications. The evidence for a straightforward casual relationship between hyperglycemia and renal disease is not clear yet. The development of clinically overt renal disease is not linearly related to the duration of diabetes and affects between 35 and 50% of patients, depending on the type of diabetes. The majority of diabetic patients do not develop renal failure and although some histological damages occur in their kidneys, renal function essentially remains normal until death. Therefore, it appears that in humans, hyperglycemia is necessary but not sufficient to cause the renal damage that leads to kidney failure and that other factors are needed for the clinical manifestation of the syndrome.

Non-enzymatic reactions between glucose and the lysine-amino terminus of circulating and structural proteins give rise to two major classes of glycation products. Relatively short-lived proteins form a Schiff base which undergoes an Amadori rearrangement, with the formation of a stable, but still chemically reversible, sugar protein adduct. In addition structural proteins that turn over at a much slower rate, such as collagen,

imbibe different products derived from slow reactions of dehydration, degradation and undergoes rearrangement of the Amadori adducts to form chemically irreversible advanced glycation end products.

The three principal mechanisms by which non-enzymatic glycosylation seems to be involved in the pathogenesis of diabetic complications are as follows:

- Advanced glycation end products (AGEs) alter signal transduction pathways involving ligands on the extracellular matrix.
- Advanced glycation end products alter the level of soluble signals such as cytokines, hormones and free radicals via (AGE) specific cellular receptors.
- Intracellular protein glycation by glucose, fructose and other metabolic pathway intermediates can directly affect protein function in target tissues.

The Polyol Pathway

In the renal medullary cells, aldose reductase is involved in the generation of sorbitol, an organic osmolyte, from glucose in response to the high salinity in the medullary interstitium. Sorbitol would aid in preventing osmotic stress. It has been argued, that in diabetes, more glucose becomes available for reduction by aldose reductase in tissues where glucose uptake is insulin independent. Therefore an increased sorbitol and/or a reduced intracellular myoinositol concentration would contribute to diabetic complications, probably by upsetting osmoregulation in these cells. Effects of AGE on matrix function are summarized in **Table 68.1**.

Protein kinase C System

The protein kinase C system is distributed in cells ubiquitously and is involved in the transduction of extracellular signals such as growth factors, hormones and prostaglandins. Diacylglycerol (DAG) is the main regulatory activator of protein kinase C which in turn activates Na-K ATPase. In glomeruli and mesangial cells,

TABLE 68.1	Effects of AGE on matrix function	
	Function	*Effect*
Collagen	Type IV collagen assembly	Decrease
	Endothelial cell adhesion	Decrease
	Intermolecular spacing	Increase
Matrix	Arterial wall elasticity	Decrease
	Arterial wall fluid filtration	Increase
Laminin	Binding of type IV collagen	Decrease
	Stimulation of nerve growth	Decrease

DAG is produced in increased amounts via a *de novo* synthetic pathway, thus leading to protein kinase C activation.

Biochemical Abnormalities of Extracellular Matrix

Diabetic glomerulopathy is characterized by an excessive accumulation of glomerular basement membrane and mesangial matrix. This is due to both increased collagen synthesis and due to reduced activity of several renal cortical enzymes involved in collagen breakdown. An increase in hydroxylysine as well as an elevation of the glucose and galactose disaccharide units attached to hydroxylysine residues has been found.

Glucotoxicity

Direct pathogenetic effects of glucose itself have also been described.

Endothelial Function

The possible mediators by which diabetes may affect endothelial function include direct glucotoxicity, the polyol pathway, the protein kinase C system, prosta-glandins, advanced glycation end products and growth factors.

The mechanisms by which altered metabolic pathways may operate for the pathogenesis of DN are summarized in **Flow chart 68. 1**.

Hemodynamic and Related Pathways

Intraglomerular Hypertension (IGHTN)

Glomerular hypertension in diabetes occurs due to either decreased afferent arteriolar resistance or increased efferent arteriolar resistance or both. The onset of IGHTN causes endothelial, mesothelial and podocyte injury, resulting in glomerulosclerosis. The decrease in functioning of nephrons further elevates IGHTN resulting in a vicious cycle and thus greatly influences the rate of progression of glomerular damage.

The Role of Ca^{2+} and K^+ Channels

Afferent arteriolar dilatation in early stages of DNL is associated with its diminished responses to a variety of vasoconstrictor stimuli. Since, the vascular tone of afferent arterioles depends on Ca^{2+} influx into vascular smooth muscle cells through voltage-gated Ca^{2+}

Flow chart 68.1   The Metabolic Pathways: Algorithm showing the various metabolic pathways producing end organ damage [Hemodynamic and Related Pathways (Intraglomerular Hypertension IGHTN)]

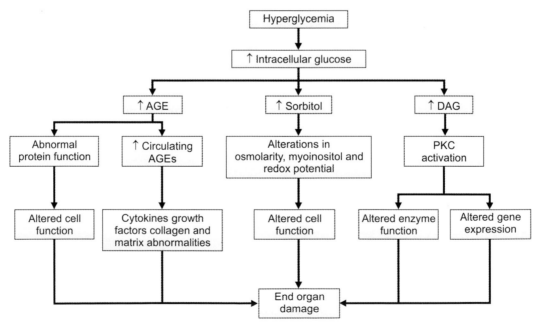

AGE: Advanced glycation end products
PKC : Protein kinase C
DAG: Diacylglycerol

channels, there is functional impairment of these channels secondary to hyperglycemia. This impairment is corrected by normalization of extracellular glucose level.[16]

Similarly, there is a functional overexpression of K^+ channels promoting hyperpolarization and at the same time decreasing Ca^{2+} influx through voltage—gated channels, resulting in afferent arteriolar vasodilatation.[17]

The Role of Tubuloglomerular Feedback

The juxtaglomerular apparatus helps in the maintenance of single nephron GFR (SNGFR), by adjusting afferent arteriolar resistance through the tubuloglomerular feedback, thus playing an important role in renal autoregulation and homeostasis of body fluid and electrolytes. The fractional reabsorption of fluid and electrolytes in the proximal tubule is increased in early diabetes relating probably to increased Na^+/glucose co-transport. Thereby, electrolyte concentration at the macula densa falls, resulting in increased SNGFR due to afferent arteriolar dilation mediated by tubuloglomerular feedback.[18,19]

The Role of Myogenic Autoregulation

In the normal kidney, increasing perfusion pressure causes myogenic constriction of preglomerular resistance vessels, especially the afferent arterioles, thereby preventing increase in glomerular pressure, when the systemic pressure is elevated. This response of the afferent arterioles is attenuated in diabetes and is normalized by inhibition of prostaglandin synthesis. This suggests that the impaired response is prostaglandin-mediated. The functionally impaired voltage-gated Ca^{2+} channels may also contribute to the attenuated arteriolar myogenic response.

The Role of Insulin

Insulinopenia results in impaired Ca^{2+} movement through voltage-gated Ca^{2+} channels. Insulin deficiency thus negates the effects of vasoconstrictor agents, on the afferent arteriole. Studies have revealed that insulin, at physiological concentration, causes afferent arteriolar constriction and efferent arteriolar dilation.[20]

The Role of Atrial Natriuretic Peptide (ANP)

ANP levels are consistently elevated in diabetic patients in parallel with the degree of metabolic control. ANP causes afferent arteriolar dilation and efferent arteriolar constriction, thereby causing glomerular hypertension and glomerular hyperfiltration. ANP also contributes to glomerular hypertension by antagonizing the vasoconstrictor action of angiotensin II and norepinephrine on the afferent arterioles.[21]

The Role of Renin Angiotensin System (RAS)

Although diabetic nephropathy is regarded as a low renin state, accumulating evidence shows that intrarenal RAS plays a very important role in its pathophysiology. Measuring plasma renin activity does not mirror the activity of RAS in the kidney. Hyperglycemia activates intrarenal RAS, causing local production of angiotensin II which increases renal vascular resistance, reduces renal blood flow and may exert negative feedback on systemic renin release. Angiotensin II, locally produced, contributes to intraglomerular hypertension by preferentially constricting the efferent arterioles as compared to afferent arterioles.[22]

Familial/Genetic Pathways

Insights into the predisposition to and mechanisms of diabetic renal disease, and possibly the attendant cardiovascular disease have come from studies of cell membrane cation transport systems. High rates of red cell sodium-lithium counter transport have been found to be an independent determinant of proteinuria as well as essential hypertension. Furthermore, an association between elevated sodium-lithium countertransport and reduced insulin sensitivity has been reported in type 1 DM.

With advances in molecular technology, a number of gene loci have been investigated to try to explain the genetic susceptibility to diabetic nephropathy. Associations have been shown between specific haplotypes of two candidate genes (insulin and angiotensin-converting enzyme) and diabetic nephropathy.

PATHOGENESIS OF HISTOLOGICAL LESIONS

The glomerular filtration barrier comprises of three layers of the capillary wall namely the innermost fenestrated vascular endothelium, the glomerular basement membrane and the podocyte layer facing the urinary space. The fenestrae of the vascular endothelial cells are between 70 to 100 nm in diameter allowing direct contact between blood plasma and the GBM.

The GBM is an acellular matrix made of large proteins such as type IV collagen and proteoglycans (mainly heparan sulfate) where the molecules exhibit a complex intermolecular and intramolecular interaction making the GBM a unique permeable scaffold that provides the capillary wall with tension, strength and flexibility. The GBM acts as a macromolecular filter with both, charge and size—selective feature. The anionic charge selectivity of GBM is mainly due to proteoglycans rich in heparan sulphate. Finally, podocytes with cell bodies in the urinary space, cover the outer aspect of the GBM, by the foot processes and the foot processes from two adjacent podocytes form an interdigitating sheath embedded within the GBM matrix. Between the foot processes there is narrow slit with a quite constant width of 400 nm. This slit contains an ultrathin membrane called the slit diaphragm which is the ultimate filter for plasma macromolecules.

Electron microscopic studies of mouse and rat kidney tissue and of humans have shown that the slit diaphragm has a three dimensional protein structure of highly ordered and periodic cross bridges, resulting in a zipper-like pattern with rod-like units extending foot processes to a linear central bar running parallel to the cell membranes.

Nephrin, originally described as a peculiar protein of the slit diaphragm, is a 1241-AA containing trans-membrane protein.[6] The extracellular portion contains 8 Ig motifs, characteristic of proteins participating in cell to cell interactions and one fibronectin type III-like molecule, while the intracellular portion has nine tyrosine residues typical of signaling molecules that could become phosphorylated during ligand binding to nephrin and could initiate a signaling cascade through phosphorylation of other proteins. The predicted structure and the biochemical properties of nephrin suggest that it could form dimers through homophilic interactions spanning the slit diaphragm forming its backbone.

Nephrin is anchored to the podocyte foot processes by two other proteins namely CD2AP and podocin which are important for the stability of the complex. Similarly, Neph I molecules span the slit diaphragm, associated with each other and also interact with nephrin through extracellular domains and are anchored to the zona occludens (ZO-1) of the podocyte foot processes and to podocin (schematically depicted in **Figure 68.4**).

The interaction between nephrin, Neph I, podocin, CD2AP and ZO-1 conform to the zipper-structure proposed by Rodewald and Karnovsky in 1974 and results in pores varying between 4 and 14 nm across the slit diaphragm which effectively hinder the traversal of proteins of the size of albumin into the urine.[4,23,24]

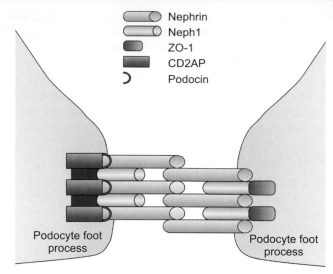

Figure 68.4 Schematic representation of the interaction of some molecular components of the glomerular slit diaphragm. Adapted from "Seminars in Nephrology", vol. 24, 2 March 2004 (© 2004 Elsevier Inc) (Permission awaited)

The actual structure of the slit diaphragm is very complex and is, as yet unresolved, but with cloning and identification of some of the proteins involved in it, the mystery of the slit diaphragm has begun to be unraveled.

Diabetic nephropathy, like other glomerulopathies is characterized by the early development of proteinuria followed later by a decline in GFR in association with glomerulosclerosis. Mechanisms underlying the loss of selectivity of the glomerular filtration barrier and the harmful effects of excessive filtered proteins on the proximal tubule are under study.

CLINICAL COURSE AND NATURAL HISTORY

The natural history of renal involvement has been better defined in type 1 DM than in type 2 DM, partly because the usual relatively acute onset of diabetes in the former allows for a more precise timing of observed clinical and physiologic events.

The diagnosis of diabetic nephropathy is usually based on clinical evidence. In the typical course, the development of proteinuria is slow; at first it is intermittent, and thereafter, becomes permanent and increasing. The onset of overt proteinuria is often associated with hypertension and declining glomerular filtration rate. If diabetic retinopathy is also present and other causes of clinical proteinuria can be excluded, there is no cause for a renal biopsy as approximately

95% of type 1 patients with these criteria have diabetic nephropathy. In fact, in proteinuric patients with type l DM for more than ten years, diabetic nephropathy is highly likely even in the absence of significant diabetic retinopathy. However, in type 2 DM, especially in patients without retinopathy, the incidence of other renal diseases may exceed 25% and renal biopsy may be a more important diagnostic tool.

Both, type 1 DM and type 2 DM patients are at risk of developing nephropathy. However, ESRD is less common in type 2 DM patients, in part because type 2 DM patients with signs of renal dysfunction have a very high cardiovascular mortality, and die before ESRD can manifest. Nonetheless, because the prevalence of type 2 DM is much greater than that of type 1 DM the total contribution of type 2 DM to ESRD far exceeds that of type 1 DM. The renal disease is often more dramatic and rapidly progressive in young type 1 DM patients compared to type 2 DM patients.

Definitions of Stages of Renal Involvement in Type 1 DM

Early Phase (Covert Nephropathy)

Stage I   Early hypertrophy-hyperfunction.

Stage II   Silent stage with normal albumin excretion, but histologically glomerular lesions are evident.

Stage III   Microalbuminuria (typically found >7 years of onset of DM).

Late Phase (Overt Nephropathy)

Stage IV   Overt diabetic nephropathy with clinical proteinuria (typically found after 15-18 years of DM).

Stage V   End-stage renal failure (typically found after approximately 25 years of diabetes).

Early Phase

After diagnosis of diabetes, a clinically silent phase of variable duration occurs. During this period, however, important abnormalities of renal functions and structure take place.

Glomerular filtration rate (GFR) is found to be elevated on an average by 20 to 40% above that of age matched normal subjects, both in adults and children with IDDM.[25,26] Data for NIDDM are controversial, with some groups reporting normal and others, supranormal GFR values.[27,28]

Hyperfiltration is related to the degree of control of blood glucose, at least within the range of normal levels to moderate hyperglycemia.

Higher blood glucose values tend to be associated with normal or low GFR. Intensified insulin treatment and good metabolic control bring the GFR toward normal levels after a period of weeks to months in both type 1 and type 2 DM. The increased GFR and renal plasma flow (RPF) are accompanied by an increase in kidney size of approximately 20% and a good correlation between GFR and kidney volume has been described in patients with IDDM. The prognostic significance of glomerular hyperfiltration remains uncertain. A positive correlation between initial hyperfiltration and subsequent increase in albuminuria and the development of clinical nephropathy was described in two retrospective studies[8,29] but no prospective study has yet been conducted.

Although in this silent phase, patients do not, by definition, demonstrate clinically detectable proteinuria. The use of a sensitive radioimmunoassay for urinary albumin has shown that in several circumstances, a proportion of patients with relatively early diabetes have elevated supranormal rates of albumin excretion.

Phase of Microalbuminuria

Microalbuminuria has now been documented and widely accepted as an important marker not only of early diabetic renal disease, but also of early vascular complications, including early mortality[30] **(Table 68.2)**.

Diabetic kidney disease is defined as the presence of clinical or dipstick positive proteinuria. Microalbuminuria not only predicts the later development of nephropathy in patients with diabetes,[31] but is also a

TABLE 68.2	Diagnostic definition of macro-, micro- and normoalbuminuria		
Condition	24 hr urinary albumin excretion	Overnight urinary albumin excretion rate	Albumin creatinine ratio
Macroalbuminuria	> 300 µg/day	> 200 µg/mt	>0.2
Microalbuminuria	30-300 µg/day	20-200 µg/mt	0.02–0.2
Normoalbuminuria	< 30 µg/day	< 20 µg/mt	<0.01

pointer to detect or predict other complications such as proliferative retinopathy.

In addition, microalbuminuria is strongly associated with cardiovascular risk and coronary heart disease in patients with diabetes.

Techniques of Measurement and Monitoring

Timed urinary collections (24 hours or overnight) remain the gold standard. However, they are cumbersome to the patient. For large scale screening, the use of early morning albumin creatinine ratio is a convenient and reliable method. Several factors such as strenuous exercise, urinary tract infection and menstruation can give a false positive result and should be kept in mind. As the prevalence of microalbuminuria in type 1 diabetes is low before five years duration, annual screening should be initiated at this point. In type 2 diabetes, screening should commence at the time of diagnosis. Detection of microalbuminuria facilitates the identification of high risk patients and should lead to a thorough evaluation of other diabetic complications such as retinopathy and silent cerebrovascular and cardiovascular ischemia, as well as a high level of attention regarding the general risk profile of the patient such as glycemic control serum lipids and smoking.

Steps and parameters for detection and confirmation of micro albuminuria are present in **Flow chart 68.2.**

Late Phase

Clinical Nephropathy

The onset of the clinical phase of diabetic nephropathy is signaled by the appearance of persistent proteinuria (total protein excretion of > 0.5 g/day), which corresponds to an albumin excretion rate greater than ~ 200 mg/ml (i.e. 300 mg/day). A phase of intermittent dipstick positivity of urine for protein precedes persistent proteinuria, but this most likely corresponds to the late phases of high microalbuminuria, with values intermittently breaking through the clinical threshold.[32]

The value of the term and concept of intermittent proteinuria is limited to it, being an indication for quantitative measurements of urinary albumin.

In those patients in whom persistent proteinuria develops, there is a progressive decline of the GFR to end stage renal failure. The fall in GFR appears to be linear with time in all patients but the rate of decline varies over an approximately four-fold range among individual patients.

Arterial pressure is very likely to be elevated in diabetic patients with established nephropathy. A small proportion (~ 25%) of patients may still have blood pressures within the so-called normal range at the onset of persistent proteinuria, although it may have risen within the normal range from previous lower levels

Flow chart 68.2 Screening for microalbuminuria: Algorithm on the approach to microalbuminuria

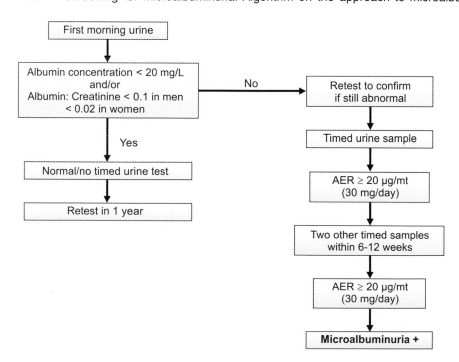

before the onset of proteinuria.[33,34] The degree of proteinuria in patients with diabetes is usually in the subnephrotic range, but heavy protein excretion and nephrotic syndrome may occur and this is related to a poorer renal outcome. These patients present with massive edema, hypoalbuminemia, hyperlipidemia with or without hypertension and a normal serum creatinine. The presence of concomitant retinopathy in these patients points to the presence of diabetic renal disease and obviates the need for a biopsy. In the absence of retinopathy, however, a kidney biopsy may be warranted; the common underlying lesion being membranous or membranoproliferative glomerulonephritis which may reverse with appropriate intervention.

Diabetic retinopathy is present in virtually all patients with type 1 DM and nephropathy. In advanced renal disease, retinopathy is usually severe with new vessel formation. Indeed, the absence of retinopathy should lead to careful consideration of other non-diabetic causes of proteinuria and renal disease. Whereas nearly all patients with nephropathy have retinal changes, the reverse is not true. Retinopathy, even of the proliferative type may occur in the absence of proteinuria and renal disease.

End-stage Renal Failure

The development of uremia in patients with diabetes is compounded by a number of other complications. Fluid retention and edema occur relatively early in the development of renal failure, in the absence of hypoalbuminemia. The variable contributions of cardiac insufficiency and of vasomotor defects secondary to neuropathy and peripheral vascular disease is well-recognized. Depressed renal function further compromises disposal of water and solutes and impairs osmotic diuresis, especially in the face of rapid compartmental shifts of fluid secondary to variations in blood glucose. Hyperkalemia may develop, partly as a result of the hyporeninemic hypoaldosteronism common in patients with advanced diabetic nephropathy, which may itself aggravate the metabolic acidosis of chronic renal failure. This is caused by sclerosis of the juxtaglomerular apparatus along with coincident autonomic dysfunction.

Peripheral neuropathy affects the majority of diabetic patients with renal failure. Uremia itself is a cause of neuropathy. It is likely to contribute to the severity of symptoms in a number of cases. Foot sepsis leading to amputation may occur, a development that is probably due to a combination of neural and arterial

disease. Autonomic neuropathy especially postural hypotension, make the treatment of hypertension troublesome. Diabetic diarrhea and gastroparesis causing nausea and vomiting are hard to distinguish from the gastrointestinal symptoms of uremia. Impotence and profuse sweating are also common manifestations of autonomic neuropathy. Arterial disease such as Monckeberg's sclerosis of medium-sized arteries are present in almost all diabetic patients with advanced renal disease. Disturbances of lipid metabolism characteristic of diabetes and uremia combined with arterial hypertension contribute to the development of severe sclerotic damage in the kidneys.

MANAGEMENT

The clinical syndrome termed diabetic nephropathy is characterized by persistent albuminuria, BP elevation, a relentless decline in GFR and a high risk of cardiovascular morbidity and mortality. Diabetic nephropathy has become the leading cause of ESRD in the world, thus imposing a great burden on the affected individual and society. So far, therapy in diabetic nephropathy has focused more on slowing the progression of renal disease once the stage of microalbuminuria has set in.

Renoprotection in a diabetic patient now envisages a multiple risk factor intervention strategy-based both on inhibiting disease progression mechanisms and on early detection and possibly, prevention from kidney damage in normoalbuminuric, normotensive diabetic patients. Studies have revealed various clinical, cellular and genetic markers that may help to identify those patients falling into this group.[35]

The strategy for the multiple risk factor intervention is based on the proven and the plausible mechanisms of progression of renal disease. (The recommended therapeutic interventions listed herewith according to their level of recommendations).

Level 1 [highest] recommendations are based on the primary analysis of one or more large clinical trials that are prospective randomized and controlled. Level 2 [intermediate] recommendations are based on a secondary analysis of one or more of the trials that provide level 1 recommendations, high-quality case controlled studies or randomized controlled trials involving relatively small number of patients. The level 3 [lowest] recommendations are based on observational studies or studies in experimental renal disease. Treatment has been dealt with according to the stage of diabetic renal disease.

Renoprotective Strategies According to Stage of Diabetic Nephropathy

Pre-CKD

- Adequate blood pressure control
- Adequate glycemic control
- ACEI / ARBs.

Stage 1

- Adequate blood pressure control
- Adequate glycemic control
- ACEI / ARBs.
- Avoid toxic agents
  - Pharmacological
  - Non-pharmacological
- Metabolic control: Control of hyperinsulinemia and hyperlipidemia.

Stage 2: Same as stage 1.

Stage 3

- Control blood pressure (level 1)
- ACE inhibitor therapy (level 1)
- ARB (level 2)
- Control blood glucose levels (level 1)
- Control blood lipids
  - Level 1 for cardiovascular benefit
  - Level 2 for renal benefit
- No cigarette smoking
  - Level 1 for cardiovascular benefit
  - Level 2 for renal benefit
- Control hyperinsulinemia
  - Level 2 for cardiovascular benefit
  - Level 3 for renal benefit
- Antiplatelet therapy.

Stage 4

All measures mentioned in stage 3 plus
- Dietary intervention
- Protein intake: level 1
- Salt intake: level 3
- Fluid intake: level 2
- Control plasma homocysteine
  - Level 2 for cardiovascular benefit
  - Level 3 for renal benefit
- Avoid use of NSAIDs
- Avoid hypokalemia
- Level 1 for general benefit
- Level 3 for renal benefit
- Correct anemia: Level 2 for renal benefit
- Control hyperphosphatemia: Level 3 for renal benefit
- Use antioxidants

  - Vit C 200 mg daily
  - Vit E
- Estrogen replacement therapy.

Stage 5

- Renal replacement therapy.

Control of Blood Glucose

In the past, there has been much discussion whether improved control of hyperglycemia translates into better cardiovascular and renal outcomes. Today, this has been proven both for type 1 diabetes in the DCCT trial as well as for type 2 diabetes in the Kumamoto trial and UKPDS (United Kingdom Prospective Diabetes Study), respectively. It has become clear that it is absolutely necessary to use an integrated approach controlling the entire spectrum of risk factors such as hypertension, smoking, dyslipidemia, etc. The risk of progression of nephropathy in the "at-risk-population", defined as an increment in urinary albumin excretion rate was decreased with intensified glycemic control. Furthermore, the DCCT[7] and UKPDS trials[36] have documented the progressive beneficial effect of intensive metabolic control on the development of microalbuminuria and overt proteinuira.

It has been suggested that, for type 1 diabetes, the HbA_{1c} goal should be within 2% of the upper limits of normal. In children, however, a tighter control of blood glucose is advocated as an HbA_{1c} of greater than 1.5 is seen to be associated with a greater risk of development and progression of retinopathy and nephropathy. However, no clear cut guidelines exist for type 2 diabetes though it may be prudent to maintain a tight blood glucose level in these patients.

Improved Glycemic Control

The role of intensified traditional insulin treatment: Intensified insulin treatment delays the onset and slows the progression of nephropathy in type 1 diabetic patients. The UK-PDS study showed that in type 2 diabetic patients, intensified insulin treatment significantly decreases the risk of microvascular, but not macrovascular disease. It is not sufficient to correct only fasting hyperglycemia or HbA_{1c} concentrations.

Rather, in addition, correction of postprandial hyperglycemia is necessary to reduce the incidence of cardiovascular disease in type 2 diabetic patients. This new recognition of the importance of postprandial hyperglycemia is not surprising in view of the observations[37] that despite of normal fasting blood glucose concentrations, a high blood glucose level after an oral glucose tolerance test was associated with excess cardiovascular mortality. This is particularly relevant in type 2 diabetes as it is characterized by lack of the first phase insulin response and an overshooting compensatory second phase response. The net result is that, the beta cell response to glucose is sluggish and delayed when a blood glucose concentration is either rising or falling.[38] This loss of early phase insulin secretion is an important and early event in the natural history of type 2 diabetes. Because a normal pattern of insulin secretion is essential for the effective control of postprandial metabolism, a rational basis for the development of agents that target early-phase insulin release exists.

Conventional oral hypoglycemic agents may not target, or adequately control, postprandial glycemia. Moreover, the use of long-acting sulfonylureas is to be avoided because of the high risk of hypoglycemia due to the altered insulin metabolism in renal failure. The short-acting sulfonylureas may still have utility. The emergence of new classes of oral agents (with a more specific mode of action) such as the meglitinide analogs (repaglinide, nateglinide and mitiglinide) specifically addresses postprandial hyperglycemia. They could also prove effective in combination with a thiozolidinedione, a drug class that targets insulin resistance. By increasing both the supply and physiological effectiveness of circulating insulin in patients with type 2 diabetes, such a secretagogue/ sensitizer combination therapy regimen may be an improvement on the efficacy of either agent in monotherapy. Both meglitinides and thiozolidinedione can be safely used in mild-to-moderate renal insufficiency and thus may help to postpone the use of insulin in susceptible population.[39] These abnormalities, i.e. impaired early insulin response and late hyperinsulinemia precede the onset of overt type 2 diabetes and are independent predictors of type 2 diabetes.

The development of insulin resistance is a defense mechanism against the development of late postprandial hyperinsulinemia, so to speak to prevent deleterious hypoglycemia. Recently, the fast-acting insulin analog Lispro has permitted the prevention of postprandial hyperglycemia and late hyperinsulinemia.[40] With glinides, i.e. insulin secretagogues, one can restore the early phase of insulin secretion after an oral glucose load and the glycemic response can be almost normalized.[41] In addition, pioglitazone and rosiglitazone, by their property to improve insulin resistance, may help to decrease the progression of nephropathy.[43]

When oral glycemic agents fail, the results are poorer if one adds long-acting insulin at night time compared with a mixture of lispro and intermediate acting insulin.[42] Lispro is thus far better than regular insulin, in either type 1 and type 2 diabetes, in the control of postprandial hyperglycemia. The new direct-acting insulin as part has similar effects.

It has to be realized that hypoglycemia or normalization of a previously high blood glucose value may be the first indicator of underlying diabetic nephropathy and patients with overt nephropathy may not require hypoglycemic agents. Therefore, there appear to be two subsets of patients—those who no longer need hypoglycemic agents and are euglycemic as azotemia advances, and those who continue to require hypoglycemic agents well into advanced uremia. The second group of patients need repeated readjustment of doses because of frequent swing between hypo and hyperglycemia and in general have a shorter survival with less chances of reaching renal transplantation than the euglycemic group.

Control of Blood Pressure

The belief that blood pressure control is important in slowing the progression of renal disease has been strongly held for decades. This belief was not confirmed till 1994 when the MDRD study published its results.[44] In those with proteinuria over 1 gm/day, a blood pressure of 125/75 mm Hg slowed progression of renal disease better than the usual blood pressure goal (135/ 85 mm Hg). Those with minor proteinuria (< 1 gm/day) generally had slow rates of GFR decline (~ 3 to 4 ml/ mt/year) and this rate of GFR decline was affected little by the low blood pressure goal. Nevertheless, anti hypertensive therapy significantly slowed the increase in proteinuria over time that typically occurs in diabetic nephropahty.[45]

Methods for Blood Pressure Control

Blood pressure is taken in the sitting position and after the patient has taken the morning's antihypertensive medication.[46]

Recommended antihypertensive regimens:
- Nonpharmacological
  - Restrict salt intake
  - Lose excess weight
  - Avoid alcohol
- Pharmacological.

Stated below is a stepwise sequence that may be used until the patient reaches his or her blood pressure goal:

- Low dose ACEI therapy plus dietary salt restriction.
- Moderate dose ACEI therapy plus dietary salt restriction.
- Moderate dose ACEI therapy plus dietary salt restriction plus diuretic.
- ACEI, diuretic and non-dihydropyridine calcium channel blocker (ND-CCB): The combination of an ACEI and a ND-CCB is more antiproteinuric at the same blood pressure level than either drug taken alone.[47] The dihydropyridine CCBs (D-CCB) are not recommended in patients with renal disease, unless the D-CCBs are required for direct BP control.[48]
- ACEI, diuretic, clonidine: This combination is recommended for individuals receiving insulin (clonidine does not affect glucoregulation) and for those having difficulty with β blockers.
- ACEI, diuretic, β blocker: This combination is appropriate for patients with coronary artery disease.
- ACEI, diuretic, α-1 blocker: If triple therapy does not achieve the blood pressure goal, the patient should be re-evaluated for drug and dietary compliance. If that evaluation is negative and sustained, hypertension is present on ambulatory blood pressure monitoring and secondary causes of hypertension especially renal artery stenosis should be sought.[49]

If the evaluation for secondary causes of hypertension is negative, a more intensive triple therapy is recommended. The initial step is to step-up the diuretic dose. A further increase is ACEI therapy is not recommended to achieve the blood pressure goal. Rather, high-dose ACEI therapy should be reserved for those who have achieved their proteinuria goal.[50] If more intensive triple therapy does not achieve blood pressure goal, quadruple antihypertensive therapy is recommended.

RAS Blockade and Renoprotection

There is now compelling evidence that renin angiotensin system (RAS) blockade is renoprotective, independent of its antihypertensive effects, in both diabetic and nondiabetic nephropathies.[51] Three options are available: ACEI alone, ARBs alone or ACEI combined with ARBs.

ACEI Therapy

In diabetic nephropathy, ACEI is renoprotective in both the early nephropathy (microalbuminuria) of both type 1 and 2 diabetes and in the overt nephropathy of the type 1 diabetes.[50] Evidence for ACEI renoprotection in overt nephropathy of type 2 diabetes is less clear. Given the broad health benefits of chronic ACEI therapy observed in the Heart Outcomes Prevention Evaluation (HOPE) trial, ACEI therapy in pre-CKD stage 1 nephropathy might be worthwhile.[52]

Renoprotection in humans has been documented using four different ACEI (enalapril, captopril, benazepril and ramipril) and renoprotection is regarded as a class specific effect of ACEI.[53] However, there are pharmacological differences among ACEI that could be biologically significant.[54] Trials show that the amount of ACEI therapy needed to achieve renoprotection is modest (e.g. 3.0 mg ramipril, 5 mg enalapril daily, 10 mg benazepril or 25 mg captopril twice daily). Whether larger doses of ACEI confer, additional renoprotection is unknown.[55]

Goal of ACEI therapy: ACEI induced nephroprotection is shown by improved blood pressure control and particularly by decreased proteinuria.[56] However, ACEI drugs are not particularly potent antihypertensive agents in patients with chronic renal insufficiency. Thus, their renoprotection may probably relate to their antiproteinuric effects and the ability to attenuate other actions of angiotensin II.[57] Presently, it is not clear whether increasing the ACEI dose to high levels (e.g. 4 to 8 times the recommend starting dose) increases its antiproteinuric effects. The trials of ACEI therapy in congestive heart failure suggest that high-dose ACEI therapy is better than low dose therapy in prolonging patient survival.[58]

Determinants of the antiproteinuric response to ACEI: The ACE genotype may influence progression of renal disease and the effect of ACE inhibition to decrease proteinuria and slow progression of renal disease.[59] Re-evaluation of the REIN study has shown that ACEI therapy in those homozygous for the deletion (D) polymorphism showed greater reduction in proteinuria and greater slowing of GFR decline than those homozygous or heterozygous for the insertion (I) polymorphism.

ACEI therapy should be withheld if the patient has >33% increase in serum, creatinine from base line value and/or hyperkalemia, on initiation of the drug. It would be prudent, however, to rule out K^+ compliance in diet (by a 24 hour urine $K^+ < 40$ meq/ day) or acidosis as a cause of increase in the serum K^+ concentration before discontinuing ACEI.

ARB Therapy

Randomized parallel crossover studies carried out in types 1 and 2 diabetic patients with covert or overt nephropathy have demonstrated that ARBs and ACEI have similar beneficial effect on proteinuria, blood pressure and renal hemodynamics.[60,61]

ARBs have a favorable side effect profile compared to ACEI as they are less likely to cause cough, angioedema or hyperkalemia.[62] The renoprotective dose for ARBs is being evaluated, however, additional dose titration studies are needed to obtain the maximum benefit of this valuable new class of compounds.

Dual Renin-Angiotensin Therapy System Blockade

The rationale for a combination therapy with ARBs and ACEI is based on the assumption that nonclassic pathways of renin angiotensin aldosterone system (RAAS) produce a substantial amount of angiotensin II.[63] During long-term ACEI treatment, the phenomenon of 'ACE-escape' evolves, i.e. plasma levels of angiotensin II and aldosterone returning to pre-treatment levels.[64] Various clinical trials have demonstrated that dual blockade of the RAAS is superior to the maximal recommended dose of ACEI with regard to lowering of proteinuria and blood pressure in diabetic patients with nephropathy.[65-67]

Dietary Measures

The concept of using one fixed prescription suitable for all patients of diabetic nephropathy is obsolete. The diet of every patient needs to be individualized depending on the tendency to retain or lose salt, serum potassium, serum protein and cholesterol levels, overall nutritional status and urine volume. If the patient is to be prevented from going into a state of negative nitrogen balance due to protein restriction, it is important to ensure an intake of at least 30 to 35 kcal/kg/day to fulfill his energy requirements, an intake of at least 20 gm 'first class' proteins and adequate vitamins in the diet. This may result in increasing hyperglycemia necessitating increased insulin or OHA doses. The serum protein and cholesterol need to be regularly monitored and appropriate dietary modification offered. The avoidance of malnutrition is especially important in CKD stage 4 and 5 due to their susceptibility to infection. Patients with a better nutritional status during dialysis have better outcomes and reduced tendency to infections after transplant. A low serum albumin and cholesterol may not directly be a consequence of inadequate dietary intake alone but may also reflect an underlying pro-inflammatory state. This is evidenced by an increase in C-reactive peptide, transferrin, pre-albumin and other pro-inflammatory markers in stage 4 and 5 CKD. This 'malnutrition-inflammation axis' significantly contributes to atherosclerosis and cardiovascular morbidity and mortality.

Protein Intake (Level 1)

Based on the meta analyses and secondary analyses of the randomized trials, it can be concluded that protein restriction slows progression of renal disease by about 0.5 ml/mt/year.[70] When patients are initiated on a dietary protein intake of 0.6 g/kg ideal body wt/day, the average achieved dietary protein intake is 0.7-0.8 kg/lBW/day. This and lower levels of dietary protein intake are associated with slowed renal disease progression.[68] In patients with heavy proteinuria, however, for each gram of proteinuria exceeding 3 g/day, protein intake should be increased by 1 gm daily.[69] A high protein diet can raise blood pressure, increase pathogenic blood lipids, promote proteinuria and progressive renal damage.[71] Periodic monitoring of dietary protein intake should be undertaken by measuring 24 hours urine urea and creatinine. The benefit of low protein diet in the MDRD study occurred in those with GFRs between 12.5 and 55 ml/mt/1.73 m^2. Whether it is beneficial to introduce low protein diet at higher levels of GFR is unknown. However, given the diet's safety and probable efficacy, the low protein diet can be recommended even in early progressive renal disease, especially in type 1 diabetes.[71]

Salt Intake (Level 2)

In the MDRD study, baseline urinary sodium excretion was not detected to be an independent risk factor for the progression of renal disease.

Nevertheless, high salt intake can override the antiproteinuric effects of ACEI and calcium channel blocker therapy, and this could promote renal disease progression. The JNC VII recommends an upper limit of salt intake of 100 mEq/day (i.e. 6 gm of salt) for adequate blood pressure control.

Fluid Intake

An analysis of the MDRD study revealed a significant association between high fluid intake and a more rapid progression of renal disease. The magnitude of the association is relatively large. The difference in GFR decline, adjusted for covariate of renal disease progression is 1-1.5 ml/mt/yr greater in those in the highest quartile of 24 hours urine volume (> 2.85 L) compared with those in the lowest quartile of 24 hours urine volume (< 2.0 L).

Potassium Intake

Patients with overt diabetic nephropathy may have a low or high serum potassium. Hyperkalemia is due to (a) decreased renal K^+ clearance, (b) hyporeninemic-hypoaldosteronism which may be associated with type IV renal tubular acidosis, (c) concurrent acidosis, (d) catabolic stress or (e) uncontrolled hyperglycemia. In addition, therapy with potassium- sparing diuretics, beta-blockers, NSAIDS and ACEI-ARB's may precipitate hyperkalemia. Hypokalemia is usually secondary to diuretics or excessive extra-renal K^+ losses. It is best to avoid sustained potassium depletion which can be the cause of progressive interstitial fibrosis[72] and renal hypertrophy, apparently through the induction of growth factors.[73]

Dietary K^+ intake should be tailored according to the body's needs. Patients should generally receive not more than 40 to 60 mEql of potassium per day. K^+ containing foods such as citrus fruits, chocolates, nuts and dairy products should be avoided. Leaching of vegetables by cutting into small pieces, boiling and discarding the eluted water prior to cooking is a useful maneuver to reduce their K^+ content. Correction of acidosis by oral sodium bicarbonate alone is enough to normalize K^+. K^+ binding resins such as calcium resonium can be used in the short term but tend to cause GI upset over a long period of time. Uncontrolled severe hyperkalemia will, however, necessitate dialysis.

Control of Blood Lipids

The third report of the National Cholesterol Education Program (NCEP); Adult Treatment Panel III; states that diabetes is a coronary heart disease equivalent.[74]

These recommendations along with those of the American Diabetes Association (ADA), suggest that patients with diabetes and renal disease should be treated with
- An adequate life style modification.
- Diet with total fat intake 25 to 35% of total calories, saturated fats <7% of total calories, cholesterol < 200 mg/day, daily fiber intake 20 to 30 g/day and
- Hypolipidemic drugs, if LDL cholesterol is ≥ 130 mg% in the absence of vascular complications or ≥ 100 mg% in their presence or if triglycerides are > 200 according to individual clinical presentations. The hypolipidemic drugs should be statins if the

main lipid abnormality is LDL cholesterol elevation; fibrates are contraindicated if renal disease is moderate or severe. The combination of statins and fibrates should not be considered because the risk of myositis is inappropriately high in these patients.[75] An encouraging role of statins in the early stages of diabetic nephropathy, independent of their cholesterol lowering strategies is being purported. By inhibiting the HMG CoA reductase activity, statins reduce the synthesis not only of cholesterol, but also of a number of nonsterol metabolites derived from the same pathway in particular, mavalonic acid. These nonsterol metabolites are clinically involved in the transduction of signals derived from membrane receptors and modulate renal function by regulating the organization of the actin cytoskeleton, smooth muscle contraction, stress fiber formation, cell-migration and cytokinesis, cell proliferation and protection against apoptosis.[76,77] Thus, statins could play an important role in reducing kidney damage, including proliferation of mesangial cell in early nephropathy.[78]

Antiplatelet Therapy

A position statement of the ADA on aspirin therapy in diabetes[79] gives the following recommendations:
- Use aspirin therapy as a secondary prevention strategy in men and women who have diabetes and evidence of large vessel disease.
- Consider aspirin therapy as a primary prevention strategy in high risk men and women with type 1 and 2 diabetes; this includes diabetic subjects with the following:
  - A family history of coronary artery disease
  - Cigarette smoking
  - Obesity
  - Albuminuria (either micro or macro)
  - Dyslipidemia (cholesterol > 200 mg / dl, LDL > 100 mg/dl, HDL cholesterol < 45 mg/dl in men and < 55 mg/dl in women, triglycerides > 200 mg/dl)
  - Age > 30 yrs.
- Clopidogrel may be used in place of aspirin.
- GP lib / IIIa receptor antagonists are under study: While the ADA advises aspirin therapy to all diabetic patients with micro or macroalbuminuria, controversy still remains regarding the safety of aspirin in uremia,[80] the need for adequate gastroprotection and the probable increased risk of renal impairment.[81] Whether clopidogrel would provide a perfect answer to these problems remains to be seen.

Control of Hyperphosphatemia

Dietary phosphorus restriction (~800 mg of elemental phosphorus daily) and phosphate binders are recommended to maintain serum phosphate level within the normal range.

Correction of Anemia

In a randomized trial that demonstrated slower progression of renal disease with correction of anemia by erythropoeitin therapy, the achieved hematocrit was 32% in the erythropoeitin group and 25% in the control group.[82] The goal hemoglobin of 11 to 12 gm/dl seems appropriate. This is also the hemoglobin goal for renal patients in the National Kidney Foundation Dialysis Outcomes Quality Index (DOQI) guidelines. The renoprotective effect of anemia correction is greater in non-diabetics than diabetic patients and may require initiation of erythropoietin therapy before the serum creatinine exceeds 4.0 mg/dl.[82] There is some evidence, though not too convincing, that those in ESRD receiving erythropoietin should avoid normalization of hemoglobin levels, i.e. Hb above 12 gm% or PVC > 40% as there appears to be a greater incidence of cardiovascular morbidity and mortality in such patients.

Control of Hyperinsulinemia

Weight reduction and exercise in obese patients decrease insulin resistance in patients with elevated C-peptide levels. Therefore, these therapies can be recommended as general health measures. In addition, hyperinsulinemia may promote progression of glomerular sclerosis.[83] Whether more aggressive measures to reduce insulin resistance, such as therapy with PPARg agonists or biguanides should be recommended in patients with high C-peptide levels and evidence of progressive glomerulopathy is not yet clear.

Control of Plasma Homocysteine Levels

Hyperhomocystinemia develops as GFR falls, apparently as a result of changes in renal metabolism rather than decreased urinary excretion.[84] Hyperhomocysteinemia is a risk factor for microalbuminuria in diabetic patients.[85] Normalization of plasma homocysteine is difficult in advanced renal insufficiency despite high dose folic acid therapy and supplementation with vitamin B_6 and B_{12}.[86]

Renal Replacement Therapy in Patients with Diabetes and End-stage Renal Disease

More than 35% of all new patients starting dialysis are for diabetic nephropathy, making it the single largest cause of end-stage renal disease.

The modality used may be hemodialysis (HD), peritoneal dialysis (PD) or kidney transplant. In the past, the nephrologist looked upon these three modalities to be used separately for each patient depending on which one appeared to be best suited for the individual patient. This, however, has changed and the present approach is to use all three modalities appropriately, interchanging them depending on the suitability at a particular time. This has made it possible to prolong the patient's life and improve the quality of life one offers to the patient. Practically, however, most patients will be initiated on one or the other forms of dialysis. The concept of pre-emptive kidney transplantation is emerging but the paucity of organs makes it a remotely possible option to begin with. Later on, however, with planning, matching and availability, the probability of switching over to kidney transplantation definitely holds promise.

When to Initiate RRT

Current guidelines emphasize initiation of dialysis prior to the appearance of frank uremic manifestations (at creatinine clearance equal to 9-14 ml/mt for a 70 kg patient). To prevent insidious malnutrition. In diabetic patients, dialysis should be initiated at a higher creatinine clearance, usually about 15 ml/mt unlike the ESRD due to other renal diseases which may well tolerate creatinine clearances of 10 ml/mt or less before being forced to initiate dialysis. There are several reasons for early initiation of dialysis in diabetic patients. Renal function deteriorates rapidly in this group. Hypertension, which is associated with rapid acceleration of diabetic retinopathy, is often difficult to control when the creatinine clearance falls below 15 ml per minute. Uremic symptoms may manifest at a less advanced degree of renal insufficiency in diabetic than in nondiabetic patients.

The Choice of Hemodialysis (HD) Versus Peritoneal Dialysis (PD)

Long-term peritoneal dialysis in diabetic patients may complicate control of blood glucose because deranged glucose homeostasis is stressed further by the large amount of glucose administered via the dialysis solution. In addition, glucose adsorption from the abdominal cavity decreases appetite. Many patients on PD have great difficulty in ingesting the recommended amount of protein (1.2 g per kg daily). On the other hand, the incidence and severity of hypoglycemic episodes is reduced in continuous ambulatory peritoneal dialysis (CAPD) compared to that in hemodialysis patients due to the constant presence of glucose in the abdomen. Rates of infection (peritonitis, exit site and tunnel infections) and rates of catheter replacement are similar between diabetic and nondiabetic patients. Coexisting blood vessel disease often hinders the creation of an adequate, long lasting vascular access for hemodialysis. In diabetic patients, the survival rates of both AV fistulas and grafts are substantially reduced. Because of autonomic nervous system dysfunction or cardiac diastolic dysfunction, diabetic patients may be at an increased risk for hypotension during dialysis. The poor vascular access and risk of hypotension combine to cause diabetic patients to receive an inadequate quantum of dialysis in terms of fractional urea clearance (kt/v), than their nondiabetic counterparts. There is no difference in the rate of progression of retinopathy between patients treated with HD and those treated with PD. Although visual impairment impedes training to perform the exchange procedure properly, blind diabetic patients can be trained to perform CAPD without a helper. When properly instructed, the risk of developing peritonitis is only slightly greater than in the visually competent ones.

For either modality of dialysis, improvement in nutrition and the clearance of small solutes by increasing dialysis time and efficiency, together with meticulous management and prevention of cardiovascular and infection related morbidity, may lead to a substantial improvement in patient survival **(Table 68.3)**.

Hemodialysis: The Problem of Vascular Access

The necessity for vascular access in patients with renal failure may be temporary or permanent.[87] A temporary access is established into a large vein (internal jugular, femoral or less desirably subclavian). The construction of a permanent vascular access permits repeated angioaccess for months-to-years. An ideal permanent access delivers a flow adequate for the dialysis prescription (~300 ml/min), lasts a long time and has a low complication rate. The autologous AV fistula comes closest to satisfying these criteria because it has the best five year patency rate and during this period requires fewer interventions than other access methods. Prosthetic AV grafts are constructed by the insertion of a subcutaneous tube in a straight, curved or loop configuration between an extremity artery and vein. The placement of a cuffed double-lumen silicone elastomer catheter (e.g. perm-cath device) or a pair of cuffed single-lumen catheters (e.g. Tesio catheter) into an internal jugular vein for permanent access is also done in selected circumstances.

Widespread microvascular disease, advanced and relatively early atherosclerosis, higher rates of infection and lower blood pressures make the incidence of complications of vascular access placement higher in diabetic patients compared to their nondiabetic counterparts. Access failure is infact, the commonest cause of hospitalization in HD patients.

Stenosis: More than 85% of AV graft thromboses are associated with a hemodynamically significant stenosis. The most common cause of stenosis in AV grafts is myointimal hyperplasia, which usually occurs at or distal to the graft-vein anastomosis. In the AV fistula, the cause of stenosis tends to be more varied and may be due to turbulence, pseudoaneurysm formation and needle-stick injury. Early detection permits correction

TABLE 68.3	Dialysis modalities for diabetic ESRD (End-stage Renal Disease)	
Modality	*Advantages*	*Disadvantages*
Hemodialysis	Very efficient Frequent medical follow-up No protein loss in dialysate	Access problems Greater incidence of hypotension Prone to hypoglycemia Predialysis hyperkalemia
CAPD	Good cardiovascular tolerance No need for A-V access Less hypoglycemia, good control of serum potassium	Peritonitis, exit site infection Protein loss in dialysate Increased intra-abdominal pressure effects

*CAPD: Continuous ambulatory peritoneal dialysis

of stenosis (by angioplasty or surgical revision) prior to thrombosis and extends the useful life of the access.

Thrombosis: Thrombosis of the fistula occurs either soon after constriction or as a late event. Early thrombosis results from technical factors. Poor flow precedes late thrombosis in most cases, but hypotension or hypercoagulability may also precipitate thrombosis.

Ischemia or edema of the graft extremity: Ischemia distal to an AV access can occur at any time (hours-to-months) following access construction. This is particularly common in diabetic patients especially in the elderly subjects and those with vascular anomalies. Pain of the hand on exercise, a steal effect or the appearance of non-healing ulcers usually requires surgical intervention. With the usual radiocephalic side-to-side fistula, the radial artery anastomosis regularly steals blood flow from the ulnar artery system. Converting the side-of-artery to an end-of-artery anastomosis may be used to treat ischemia due to steal.

Edema of the hand results from increased pressure in the veins draining the hand. Treatment consists of converting the anastomosis from the side-of-vein to an end-of-vein opening or by selectively tying off the affected veins.

Pseudoaneurysm: The incidence of pseudoaneurysms appear similar in the diabetic and nondiabetic dialytic population. Infection of a pseudoaneurysm may, however, be more common in the former.

Infections: Infections of the AV fistula are usually staphylococcal and should be treated in the same manner as subacute endocarditis. Prompt therapy with anti-staphylococcal antimicrobials after local and blood cultures have been obtained is often curative. Patients who develop septic embolus during dialysis may need surgical closure.

Graft infection occurs in 5 to 20% of cases. Most infections are staphylococcal, but rarely gram-negative organisms such as *E. coli* may be cultured. Local infection of a graft can be treated with antibiotics and by resection of the infected portion. A graft placed within 30 days that becomes infected should always be removed.

Congestive heart failure: The AV fistula or the AV graft occasionally can cause a high output congestive heart failure. The concomitant ischemic heart disease and diastolic dysfunction places the diabetic patient at a greater risk of cardiac dysfunction. Surgical narrowing, banding or closure of the fistula or graft, however, should be done only after cardiac studies have shown marked changes in cardiac output following transient occlusion of the fistula.

Problem of cardiovascular instability: Intradialytic hypotension is far more common in the diabetic dialysis dependent population than in the normoglycemic ESRD patients. The causes of this include:

- Autonomic neuropathy rendering the mechanisms counteracting the hypotension toothless. The patient is therefore, unable to recruit sympathetic activity to offset these effects.
- Concomitant diastolic dysfunction due to left ventricular hypertrophy and ischemic heart disease.
- Poor myocardial contractility.

Malnutrition: Whatever the mode of dialysis therapy, diabetic patients generally show evidence of wasting and malnutrition. It has recently been documented that there exists a 'malnutrition - inflammation axis' linking malnutrition and atherosclerosis. Paradoxically obese patients have a longer survival and those with very low serum cholesterol (below 100 mg%) have poorer survival in ESRD patients on dialysis. Uremia itself makes for a proinflammatory and proatherogenic mileu. Among the various proinflammatory markers are low albumin, low pre-albumin, high transferrin and high C reactive protein. In addition, cytokine activation brought about by bioincompatible hemodialysis membranes may worsen malnutrition and hasten the process of atherosclerosis.

Many factors contribute, namely poor food intake, diabetic gastroparesis and enteropathy and the catabolic stress associated with frequent intercurrent illness. Diabetic gastroparesis can be associated with poor food intake and unpredictable nutrient absorption, the result can be hypoglycemia alternating with hyperglycemia. In such patients, small, frequent feeding may improve symptoms.

Peritoneal Dialysis

Chronic peritoneal dialysis is of two types; CAPD and automated peritoneal dialysis (APD). CAPD typically involves four 2.0 to 2.5 L dwells daily, with each lasting 4 to 8 hours. In APD, 3 to 10 dwells are delivered nightly using an automated cycler and each dwell is 1 to 2 liters. In the daytime, the patient usually carries a dwell which is drained each night before cycling recommences; this is called continuous cycling peritoneal dialysis (CCPD). Alternatively, the patient is left dry during the day and this is termed nocturnal intermittent peritoneal dialysis (NIPD).

During the course of a peritoneal dialysis dwell, three transport processes occur simultaneously:

- *Diffusion:* Uremic solutes and potassium diffuse from the peritoneal capillary blood down the concentration gradient into the dialysate, whereas glucose, lactate and to a lesser extent calcium diffuse in the opposite direction.
- *Ultrafiltration:* Simultaneously, the relative hyperosmolarity of the dialysate leads to ultrafiltration of water and associated solutes across the membrane.
- *Absorption:* Also simultaneously, there is constant absorption of water and solutes from the peritoneal cavity both directly and indirectly through the lymphatic system.

Complications of PD

Peritonitis: At least two of the following three conditions should be present:

- Symptoms and signs of peritoneal inflammation.
- Cloudy peritoneal fluid with an elevated peritoneal fluid cell count (more than 100 cells per ml) with predominantly (i.e. more than 50%) neutrophils.
- Demonstration of bacteria in the peritoneal effluent by Gram's stain or culture.
- The most common symptom of peritonitis is abdominal pain. However, peritonitis should be suspected whenever a chronic peritoneal dialysis patient suffers from generalized malaise, particularly if nausea, vomiting or diarrhea is also present.

The most common organisms isolated include *Staphylococcus epidermis, S. aureus, coliforms, Pseudomonas;* whereas mycobacteria and fungi may be found in severe cases.

Other infective complications such as catheter exit site infection and catheter tunnel infection seen in all patients in CAPD, are more common in diabetes.

Lipid abnormalities: Typically these patients have high total and LDL cholesterol, high triglycerides and lipoprotein (a) levels. Compared with HD, the most striking differences are the high apoB protein and LDL cholesterol levels, which are usually normal in hemodialysis patients. Thus, the lipoprotein profile of peritoneal dialysis is markedly atherogenic.

Protein loss: PD is associated with significant loss of protein across the peritoneum. This is about 0.5 to 1 g/L of dialysate drained. Hence, with 10 liters exchanged per day, up to 5 to 10 gm of protein are lost. The major component of the protein losses is albumin, but IgG accounts for up to 15%. This is especially disadvantageous in the already malnourished and immuno-compromised diabetic ESRD population. Therefore, measurements of both peritoneal and urinary protein losses need to be evaluated and appropriate dietary corrections made by increasing the oral protein intake.

Electrolyte disturbances: It is common to see hypo or hypernatremia, hypokalemia, hypo/hypercalcemia or elevated lactate levels in these patients.

Special Problems in Diabetic Patients on Dialysis

Control of Blood Glucose

In uremic patients, insulin secretion by the β cells of the pancreas is reduced and the responsiveness of the peripheral tissues to insulin is depressed. On the other hand, the rate of insulin catabolism (both renal and extrarenal) is decreased and therefore the half life of any insulin present in the circulation is prolonged. All these abnormalities are only partially corrected by dialysis. Furthermore, the clinical presentation of hyperglycemia is modified due to the absence of the safety valve effect of glucosuria. Hyperglycemia is especially a problem in patients on PD due to significant but variable glucose absorption across the peritoneum. This along with the resultant hyperinsulinemia are important risk factors for the development of atherosclerosis. The deposition of advanced glycated end products (AGE) in the peritoneal membrane is associated with an increase in peritoneal permeability and excessive protein loss in the dialysate.

Hypertension and Peripheral Vascular Disease

The incidence of hypertension is high in diabetic dialysis patients. Control of high blood pressure is very important for the prevention of cardiovascular sequelae and deterioration of vision. Most diabetic patients have volume sensitive hypertension that can be controlled by appropriate sodium and fluid restriction and by removal of excess extracellular fluid by dialysis.

The incidence of stroke is also higher in diabetic dialysis patients than in their nondiabetic counterparts. Although the use of aspirin has been shown to reduce the risk of stroke in nonuremic patients, the benefit of such therapy in diabetic dialysis patients is unknown and the use of aspirin theoretically increases the risk of intraocular and gastrointestinal hemorrhage.

Eye Diseases in Diabetic Subjects on Dialysis

Retinopathy is present almost universally in every diabetic patient starting dialysis. The early stage of background retinopathy, with leakage and occlusion of small retinal blood vessels can cause visual loss if the macular area is involved. Slowing the progression of this stage requires careful control of blood pressure and blood glucose. Despite the use of heparin in HD, there is no evidence that the progression of retinopathy in diabetic patients on HD differs from that of diabetics on peritoneal dialysis.

Other less common causes of blindness in diabetic patients on dialysis include macular edema, glaucoma, cataracts and corneal disease. In addition, conjunctivitis, keratitis, band keratopathy and glaucoma are other ophthalmologic problems seen in this population on dialysis.

Bone Disease

Among diabetics with ESRD, a dynamic bone disease is common. The bone disease is characterized by a low bone formation rate, which is presumably due to the high circulating levels of somatostatin inhibitors in affected patients. This low bone formation rate is believed to predispose diabetic patients to aluminium toxicity; diabetic patients on dialysis have been shown to accumulate bone aluminium at a faster rate than their nondiabetic counterparts.

Kidney Transplantation in Diabetic Patients

There is little question that kidney transplantation alone or combined with pancreas transplantation is the treatment of choice for end-stage renal disease secondary to diabetic nephropathy. Live donor kidney transplantation in diabetic recipients is associated with a survival advantage compared with cadaveric transplantation; however, both forms of transplantation offer a pronounced survival advantage over chronic dialysis.

Pre-operative Assessment

The propensity for the premature development of atherosclerosis in diabetic patients mandates careful screening for overt and covert vascular disease.

Coronary Artery Disease

The possibility of covert CAD should be considered in every diabetic transplant candidate. In most transplantation programs, all diabetic patients undergo screening with an exercise stress test to help in determining that which patients should undergo further evaluation with catheterization. The stress test is usually supplemented with thallium or sestamibi scintigraphy or echocardiography to increase its specificity. In some centers, these patients undergo an oral or intravenous dipyridamole-thallium stress test or a dobutamine stress echocardiography, designed to simulate the lesions amenable to bypass or angioplasty, which should be treated before transplantation. In a few centers, each diabetic patients needing transplant is evaluated by coronary angiography.

Cerebrovascular and Peripheral Vascular Disease

The increased susceptibility of diabetic transplant recipients to cerebrovascular and peripheral vascular disease mandates particular attention to these issues in the pre-transplantation evaluation. A history of cerebrovascular events or intermittent claudication or presence of carotid bruit may need further evaluation by MR angiography before transplant. Additionally, a radiological search for calcification and/or occlusion of the internal or external iliac circulation to which the donor kidney would have to be anastomosed may be justified, specially since this can now be established without an invasive procedure using MR angiography.

Infections

Patients should be free of significant infections such as peritonitis, osteomyelitis or unhealed foot ulcerations at the time of transplantation. An actively infected/pyelonephrotic kidney contraindicates transplant and may require pretransplant nephrectomy. All such complications need to be treated prior to transplantation.

Pre-emptive Transplantation

For patients with diabetic nephropathy, transplantation should be strongly considered before the initiation of dialysis (GFR 20 ml/mt or a serum creatinine of 4-5 mg/dl). Early transplantation can obviate the need for dialysis access, can prevent episodes of congestive heart failure and volume overload and can correct hypertension. Early transplantation may slow retinopathy and correct neuropathy secondary to uremia, which can exacerbate with worsening diabetic nephropathy.

Insulin Requirements

After successful transplantation, the hyperglycemic stage re-emerges due to normalization of insulin degradation by the normal donor kidney and the carbohydrate intolerance induced by corticosteroids, cyclosporine and tacrolimus may lead to increased insulin requirements and cause noninsulin-dependent diabetic patients to require large doses of insulin. Patients should be forewarned about this possibility.

Postoperative Complications

Several studies have shown no significant difference in major postoperative complications in diabetic as compared to non-diabetic patients, especially with regard to wound complications. Postoperative ileus, nausea and vomiting are more common due to coexisting diabetic enteropathy.

Graft Dysfunction

Rejection: The incidence of rejection and cyclosporine toxicity in diabetic patients is not different from that in nondiabetic patients. Therapy with high dose corticosteroids used for the reversal of ongoing rejection is frequently accompanied by poor blood sugar control and requires close monitoring.

Pseudorejection: In patients with poor blood sugar control, hypovolemia can cause elevations in BUN and creatinine and mimic a rejection episode. Functional outlet dysfunction due to neurogenic bladder also occurs more frequently in diabetes.

Urinary tract infection (UTI): UTI is more common in diabetic recipients because of the higher incidence of neurogenic bladder and poor glycemic control. Prophylaxis with daily double strength trimethoprim-sulfamethoxazole is recommended in some centers.

Long-term complications:
• *Peripheral vascular disease:* Many other complications of diabetes such as peripheral vascular disease and neuropathy may continue to progress after transplant. Although many ischemic foot ulcers are secondary to microvascular disease, macrovascular occlusion secondary to atherosclerotic plaques is not uncommon.
• *Retinopathy:* Stabilization of retinopathy is common after transplantation with most patients experiencing no change in visual acuity or showing some improvement.
• *Neuropathy:*
  – Diabetic gastropathy is common and gastroparesis is best treated with metaclopramide or cisapride/mosapride. Diabetic diarrhea can be treated with oral or transdermal clonidine.
  – Neurogenic bladder is a frequent complicating factor after transplantation. Intermittent self catheterization may be necessary in some patients.
  – Orthostatic hypotension with supine hypertension is common secondary to autonomic neuropathy and may be transiently exacerbated after successful transplantation, particularly if the patient had been in a fluid positive state before transplantation. Orthostatic hypotension typically resolves as the hematocrit rises. This process can be expedited with erythropoietin injections if necessary.

Hypertension: Hypertension is common after transplantation and may be due to the effects of cyclosporine or tacrolimus, retained native kidneys or rarely renal artery stenosis at the site of anastomosis of the transplanted kidney.

Bone disease: Diabetic transplant recipients are particularly susceptible to osteoporosis and its consequences and a fracture rate of up to 40% has been described on a long-term follow-up. Ideally, lumbar spine and hip bone mineral density should be measured by dual X-ray absorptiometry at the time of transplantation and at yearly intervals thereafter. The biphosphonates represent the most effective means of prevention and treatment.

Pregnancy: Pregnant diabetic transplant recipients (usually patients of nephropathy following type 1 diabetes) represent a particularly high risk group. Prematurity is universal and deterioration of graft function is common.

Kidney-Pancreas Transplantation

To provide the pancreatic islets needed to produce insulin and cure diabetes, it is necessary to transplant both the exocrine and endocrine pancreas. Three patient groups can be considered for whole organ pancreas transplantation :
• Pancreas alone (PA) for patients who have not yet developed advanced kidney disease.
• Simultaneous pancreas–kidney transplantation (SPK) for patients with renal failure.
• Pancreas transplant after kidney transplantation for patients who have previously undergone successful kidney transplantation.

POST-TRANSPLANT DIABETES MELLITUS (PTDM)

New onset diabetes mellitus after transplantation is characterized by decreased insulin secretion and increased insulin resistance secondary to the effects of immunosuppression. Several factors that are closely associated with the development of type 2 diabetes in the general population are also frequently noted in the kidney transplant population as well. These include obesity, increased age, increased BMI, family history of DM, abnormal glucose tolerance and African-American descent.[88]

Effect of Immunosuppressives on Blood Glucose

It has been well-recognized that steroids can cause glucose intolerance, insulin resistance and frank hyperglycemia. The effect of steroids on the development of new-onset DM is dose-dependent, with lower steroid maintenance doses being associated with lower rates of DM. The calcineurin inhibitors like cyclosporine and tacrolimus (tacrolimus > cyclosporine) have also been shown to be diabetogenic. The exact mechanism of DM induced by tacrolimus and cyclosporine is not known. They affect the synthesis and secretion of insulin through reversible toxicity to the β cells.[89] In addition, insulin release may be independently affected by cyclosporin A (CsA), because CsA also inhibits the release of insulin in response to a glucose challenge.[90] CsA also affects peripheral glucose tolerance, presumably through a mechanism of insulin resistance. There is also evidence that both the calcineurin inhibitors may act directly on the transcriptional regulation of insulin gene expression in β cells.[91]

ADA Diagnostic Criteria for New Onset DM After Transplant and Goals for Glycemic Control[92]

Diagnostic Criteria

Symptoms of diabetes plus RBS > 200 mg/dL
    Or
Fasting plasma glucose >126 mg/ dL
    Or
2 hr post glucose > 200 mg/dL in an oral GT test

Goals for Glycemic Control

Preprandial   PG 90-130 mg/dL
Postprandial   PG < 180 mg/dL
HbA$_{1C}$ <7%

The American Society of Nephrology recommends that blood glucose should be monitored at least every week from month 1 to month 3 posttransplant, at least every 2 weeks from month 4 to month 6 and after the first 6 months, at least monthly.[93]

Management and Treatment

The ADA recommends that tight glycemic control should be attempted if the patient is not at risk for complications caused by hypoglycemia. For transplant recipients in whom nonpharmacological therapy has failed, monotherapy with an oral agent may be initiated[88] although insulin may be considered as the first option.

Options include glucoside inhibitors, biguanides, meglitinides, sulfonylureas and thiazolidinediones. Meglitinides may be the safest option other than insulin for transplant recipients with renal impairment. For patients failing monotherapy with an oral agent, combination therapy may be considered as the next step,[88] failing which insulin should be initiated. All patients with new onset DM, should be routinely monitored for complications, including retinopathy and neuropathy. Tight control of blood pressure and blood lipids are recommended.

OTHER RENAL MANIFESTATIONS IN DIABETICS

Renal Papillary Necrosis

Diabetes has long been associated with renal papillary necrosis; its prevalence in autopsy cases averages 4.4 % (Mujais 1984), but this figure may be an underestimate since diabetes has been found in up to 50% patients with renal papillary necrosis. It tends to occur in long-standing disease and affects both kidneys in up to 65% of patients. When it is unilateral, the contralateral kidney becomes involved in the ensuing years. It is more frequent in women, particularly those with recurrent urinary tract infection. It may manifest as acute renal failure or be nearly asymptomatic and follow a more indolent course with bouts of urinary infection and/or renal colic. Microscopic hematuria and sterile pyuria are also more common when this condition is present. Proteinuria is often present but is usually modest (< 2 g/24h). The urographic appearances of moth-eaten calyces and 'ring-shadow' image of the necrotic papilla are highly suggestive of this condition.

The management of acute papillary necrosis is compounded by the need to maintain adequate metabolic control. If obstruction is present, its relief is urgent and mandatory and this will often determine the success of associated antibiotic therapy. In the chronic indolent form, the use of NSAIDs may further compromise medullary circulation and should be avoided. Radiological contrast is also best avoided.

Sonography and MRI (using gadolinium if necessary) are the mainstay of diagnostic procedures.

Autonomic Neuropathy of the Bladder

It is difficult to ascertain the true prevalence of autonomic neuropathy of the bladder in diabetes because of its insidious onset. The first abnormality is impairment of sensation, with decreased awareness of bladder distention. As a result, micturition occurs at progressively larger bladder volumes and this together with progressive damage of the parasympathetic innervation of the detrusor, leads to weaker bladder contraction, incomplete emptying, and increasing residual volume. Involvement of the efferent sympathetic innervation to the trigone may lead to functional incompetence of the vesicoureteral junction and incomplete relaxation of the internal sphincter during micturition.

On detection of autonomic bladder dysfunction, the patient should be trained to perform voluntary regular voiding even in the absence of subjective urge. Intermittent or temporary catheterization and associated parasympathomimetic drug treatment with bethenechol may help to reduce bladder distention and recovery of detrusor function.

Urinary Tract Infections in Diabetic Patients

A large proportion of UTI are asymptomatic in the diabetic patients and their pathogenic role is not clear. However, in patients with diabetic nephropathy even asymptomatic infection may be associated with worsening of renal function and efforts should be directed to its eradication. Upper urinary tract infections can lead to severe complications in the diabetic patient. Perinephric abscesses, which can be bilateral, are more frequent in diabetic patients and may have an insidious onset followed by persistent fevers and rigors. Infections of the kidney with anaerobic gas-forming organisms are more common in diabetic patients. Emphysematous pyelonephritis **(Figure 68.5)** is more frequent in women and is usually caused by *Escherichia coli*, although *Candida* species and *Cryptococcus* have also been reported. The infection is bilateral in approximately 10% of cases. Severe ascending infection can lead to the formation of multiple intrarenal abscesses **(Figure 68.6)**, usually cortical, which may be difficult to treat and require prolonged hospitalization and parenteral antibiotics.

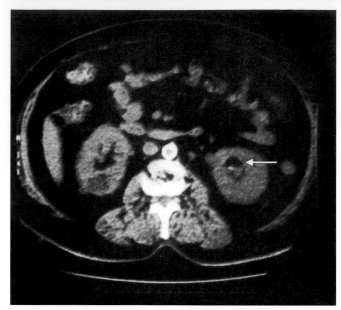

Figure 68.5 Emphysematous pyelonephritis: The figure shows a plain CT image of a diabetic patient with severe pyelonephritis and multiple gas shadows within the renal cortex (depicted by an arrow)

Acute Renal Failure in Diabetic Patients

- *Toxicity induced by radiologic contrast agents :* Diabetic nephropathy patients are at high risk of acute exacerbation of their renal dysfunction (defined as a ≥1.0 mg/dl rise in serum creatinine) after the administration of both ionic and nonionic radiographic contrast media. The incidence is as high 76% after intravenous pyelography and 23% after angiography[94] in patients with serum creatinine of ≥2.0 mg/dl. In diabetic patients with normal renal function, the risk is minimal. Measures such as adequate hydration both before and after contrast administration, minimal contrast dose, use of newer isosmotic nonionic contrast, use of N-acetyl cysteine both before and after contrast, sodium bicarbonate infusions and hemofiltration after contrast administration may substantially reduce the incidence of contrast nephropathy.[95]
- *Rhabdomyolysis:* Diabetic patients who have prolonged coma due to hyperosmolar encephalopathy, severe hypoglycemia, fascitis and myonecrosis may develop acute renal failure due to rhabdomyolysis. This may be a cause of unexplained acute renal failure in the appropriate clinical setting.

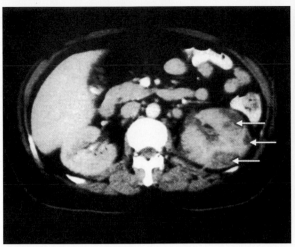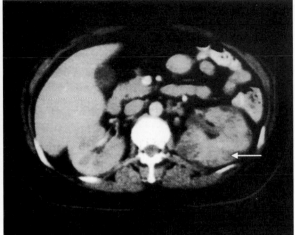

Figure 68.6 Multiple renal abscesses: The figure shows a plain CT image of a diabetic patient with severe pyelonephritis, multiple abscesses within the renal cortex and fraying of the renal outline (depicted by an arrow)

Other Glomerular Diseases in Diabetic Patients

The overall prevalence of nondiabetic glomerular disease in proteinuric diabetic patients is reported to range between 8 to 37%. Membranous nephropathy is the glomerular disease which has been most often described with diabetes.

Nondiabetic renal disorders, warranting a kidney biopsy:

- Severe microscopic hematuria and/or red cell casts.
- Duration of type 1 DM less than 10 years at onset of proteinuria.
- Biochemical or clinical evidence of a multisystem disorder (such as positive ANA, ANCA, HIV, Hep B, Hep C, ASO).
- Absence of retinopathy: Retinopathy is almost invariably present in proteinuria of diabetic origin, with concordance rates of 90 to 95% in type 1 patients. Retinopathy seems to be more severe in those with overt nephropathy. In type 2 DM, the concordance rate with diabetic glomerulopathy is about 85% in proteinuric patients with retinopathy, but is 40 to 60% in those without retinopathy.

SUMMARY

The kidneys of diabetic patients are vulnerable to recurrent episodes of infection, glomerulonephritis, higher incidence of acute renal failure and above all the chronic kidney disease known as diabetic nephropathy. These diseases shorten the lifespan of the diabetic patient and are the cause of recurrent hospitalization with compromised quality of life. The incidence of chronic kidney disease due to diabetic nephropathy is significantly rising even as the average life span of the diabetic increases due to better glycemic control and lower incidence of coronary artery and cerebrovascular disease. Therefore, more and more diabetic patients are likely to spend the later part of their lives in a chronic dialysis program and become candidates for kidney or kidney-pancreatic transplantation. The nephrologist is confronted not only with the care of end-stage renal disease due to diabetes but also with the more important role of preventing the development of diabetic nephropathy as well as preventing the progression of established nephropathy from the relatively innocuous stage 1 to the fatal stage 5 of this disease. In this chapter, we endeavor to outline the current clinical approach of the nephrologist in dealing with the diabetic patient.

REFERENCES

1. United States Renal Data System. Excerpts from US Renal Data System Annual Data Report: Atlas of end stage renal disease in the United States. Am J Kidney Dis. 2000; 36: S1-279.
2. Seaquist ER, Goetz FC, Fich S, et al. Familial clustering of diabetic kidney disease. N Engl J Med. 1989; 320: 1161-5.
3. Parving HH. Nephrology forum: diabetic nephropathy—prevention and treatment. Kidney Int. 2001; 60: 2041-55.
4. Staessen JA, Ginnochio G, Wang JG, et al. Genetic variability in the renin-angiotensin system: prevalence of alleles and genotypes. J Cardiovasc Risk. 1997;4:401-22.
5. Kunz R, Bork JP, Fritsche L, et al. Association between the angiotensin converting enzyme —insertion (deletion

polymorphism and diabetic nephropathy: a methodologic appraisal and systematic review). J . M Sec Nephrol. 1998; 9:1653-63.

6. Hotzman LB, St. John PL, Kovari IA, et al . Nephrin localises at the slit pode of the glomerular epithelial cell. Kidney Int. 1999; 56: 1481-99.

7. The diabetes control and complications trial research group : effect of intensive therapy on the development and progression of diabetic nephropathy in the DCCT. KI 1995; 47: 1703-20.

8. Mogensen CE, Christansen CK . Predicting diabetes in insulin dependent patients. N Engl J Med. 1984; 311: 89-93.

9. Rundberg S, Persson B, Dahlquist G. Increased glomerular filtration rate as a predictor of diabetic nephropathy: an eight year prospective study. Kidney Int. 1992; 41: 822-8.

10. Poulsen PL, Hansen KW, Mogensen CE. Ambulatory blood pressure in the transition from normo to microalbuminuria. A longitudinal study. Diabetes 1994; 43:1248-53.

11. Lurbe E, Redon J, Kesania A, et al. Increase in nocturnal blood pressure and progression to microalbuminuria in type I diabetes. N Engl J Med. 2002; 347: 797-805.

12. Viberti GC, Hill RD, Jarret RJ, et al. Early detection of patients at risk of developing diabetic nephropathy. Acta Endocrinol (Copenh) .1982; 100: 550-5.

13. Caramori ML, Fioretto P, Mauer M : the need for early predictors of diabetic nephropathy risk. Is albumin excretion rate sufficient? Diabetes. 2000; 49: 1399-408.

14. Hebert L, Kusek J, Greene T, et al. Effects of blood pressure control on progressive renal disease in blacks and whites. Hypertension. 1997; 30: 428-35.

15. Jandeleit - Dahm K, Cao Z, Cox AJ, et al. Role of hyperlipidemia in progressive renal disease: focus on diabetic nephropathy. Kidney Int. 1999; 56 (suppl 71): 531-6.

16. Brenner BM, Lawler EV, Mackenzie HS . The hyperfiltration theory a paradigm shift in nephrology. Kidney Int. 1996; 49: 1774-7.

17. Ikenaga H, Bast JP, Fallet RW, Carmines PK. Exaggerated impact of ATP-sensitive K^+ channels on afferent arteriolar diameter in diabetes mellitus. J Am Soc Nephrol. 2000; 11: 1199-207.

18. Barajas L, Powers K, The structure of the juxtaglomerular apparatus (JGA) and the control of renin secretion: an update. J Hypertension. 1984; 2 (suppl 1): 3-12.

19. Briggs JP, Schnermann J. The tubuloglomerular feedback mechanism: functional and biochemical aspects. Ann Rev Physiol. 1987; 49: 251-73.

20. Johnson PC. The myogenic response. In Bohr DF, Somlyo AP, Sparks HV Jr, (Eds): Handbook of Physiology ; The cardiovascular system: vascular smooth muscle. Am Physiol Soc, Bethesda MD 1980;2(2):409-42.

21. Scholey JS, Meyer TW. Control of glomerular hypertension by insulin administration in diabetic rats. J Clin Invest. 1989; 83:1384-9.

22. Laragh JH, Atlas SA. Atrial natriuretic hormone : a regulator of blood pressure and volume homeostasis. Kidney Int. 1988; 34: S64-71.

23. Rodewald R, Karnovsky MJ. Porous substructure of the glomerular slit diaphragm in the rat and mouse. J Cell Biol. 1674; 60:423-33.

24. Velming L, Vande Pijl J, Lemkes H, et al. The DD genotype of the ACE gene polymorphism is associated with progression of diabetic nephropathy to endstage renal failure in IDDM. Clin Nephrol. 1999; 51:133-40.

25. Ditzel J, Swhraztz M. Abnormal glomerular filtration in short-term insulin treated diabetic subjects. Diabetes. 1967;16:264-7.

26. Mogersen CE. Glomerular filtration rate and renal plasma flow in short-term juvenile diabetes mellitus. Scand J Clin Lab Invest. 1971;28:91-100.

27. Vora J, Thomas DM, Dean J, et al. Renal function and albumin excretion rate in 62 newly presenting noninsulin-dependent diabetics. Kidney Int. 1990; 37: 245.

28. Loon N, Nelson R, Myers BD. Glomerular barrier abnormality in new onset NIDDM in Pima Indians. Kidney Int. 1990; 37: 513.

29. Mogensen CE. Early glomerular hyperfiltration in insulin - dependent diabetics and late nephrapathy. Scand J Clin Lb Invest. 1986; 46: 201-6.

30. Dineen S, Gerstein H.C. The association of microalbuminuria and mortality in non-insulin -dependent diabetes mellitus. A systematic overview of the literature. Arch Intern Med. 1997; 157:1413-8.

31. Adler AL, Stratton IM, Neil HA ,et al. Association of systolic blood pressure with macrovascular and microvascular complication of type 2 diabetes (UKPDS 36) prospective observational study. BMJ 2000; 321: 412-9.

32. Jerume J, Cooper ME. Spectrum of proteinuria in type I and II diabetes. Diabetes Care. 1987; 10: 419-27.

33. Wiseman MJ, Viberta GC. Glycemia, arterial pressure and microalbuminuria in type 1 diabetes. Diabetologia. 1984; 26: 401-5.

34. Jensen T, Borch-Johnsen K, Deckert T . Changes in blood pressure and renal function in patients with type 1 insulin-dependent diabetes mellitus prior to clinical diabetic nephropathy. Diabetes Res. 1987; 4: 159-62.

35. Parving HH : Renoprotection in diabetes : genetic and non-genetic risk factors and treatment. Diabetologia. 1998; 41: 745-9.

36. UK prospective diabetes study group. Efficacy of atenolol and captopril in reducing risk of macrovascular and microvascular complications in type 2 DM : UKPDS 39. Br. Med J 1998; 713-720.

37. Pfeifer M, Halter J, Porte D Jr. Insulin secretion in diabetes mellitus. Am J Med. 1981; 70: 579-8.

38. Ehrman D, Breda E, Cavaghan M, et al. Insulin secretory responses to rising and falling glucose concentration are delayed in subjects with impaired glucose tolerance. Diabetologia. 2002; 45: 509-17.

39. Dornhorst A . Insulinotropic meglitinide analogues. Lancet. 2001; 358: 1709-16.

40. Bruttomesso D, Pianta A, Mari A ,et al. Restoration of early rise in plasma insulin levels improves the glucose tolerance of type 2 diabetic patients. Diabetes. 1999; 48: 99-105.

41. Uchino H, Niwa M, Shimizu T. Impairment of early insulin response after glucose load, rather than insulin resistance is responsible for post prandial hyperglycemia seen in obese type 2 diabetes : assessment using nateglinide, a new insulin secretagogue. Endocr J. 2000; 47: 639-41.

42. Ruggenenti P, Dodesini A, Flores C ,et al. Insulin lispro is better than regular insulin in limiting post prandial hyperglycemia and fully prevents meal induced hyperfiltration in type 2 diabetics with overt nephropathy. Diabetes. 2002; 51 (suppl 2): A191,775-p.

43. Isshiki K, Haneda M, Koya D ,et al. Thiazolidinedine compounds ameliorate glomerular dysfunction independent

of their insulin sensitizing action in diabetic rats. Diabetes. 2000; 49: 1022-32.

44. Klahr S, Levey A, Bek J, et al. The effects of dietary protein restriction and blood pressure control on the progression of chronic renal disease. N Engl J Med. 1994; 330: 877-84.

45. Hebert L. Target blood pressure for antihypertensive therapy in patients with proteinuric renal disease. Curr Hypertens Rep. 1999; 1: 454-60.

46. Yarrows S, Julins S, Pickering T. Home blood pressure monitoring. Arch Intern Med. 2000; 160: 1257-61.

47. Bakns G, Williams B. Effects of angiotensin converting enzyme inhibitors and calcium antagonists combination on proteinuria in diabetic nephropathy. Kidney Int. 1998; 54: 1283-9.

48. Tarif N, Bakris G. Preservation of renal function: the spectrum of effects by calcium channel blockers. Nephrol Dial Transplant 1997; 12: 2244-50.

49. The sixth report of the joint national committee on prevention, detection evaluation and treatment of high blood pressure. Arch Intern Med 1993; 118: 129--38.
The seventh report of the joint national committee on prevention, detection evaluation and treatment of high blood pressure. JAMA 2003; 289: 2560-72.

50. Ruggenenti P, Pema A, Benimi R ,et al. In chronic nephropathies, prolonged ACE inhibitors can induce remission. Dynamics of time-dependent changes on GFR. J Am Soc Nephrol. 1999; 10: 997-1006.

51. Brenner B, Taal M . Renoprotective benefits of RAAS inhibition: from ACE to angiotensin II antagonists. Kidney Int 2000; 57: 1803-17.

52. Yusuf S, Sleight P, Pogue J. Effects of an angiotensin converting enzyme inhibitor, ramipril on cardiovascular events in high risk patients. N Engl J Med 2000; 342:145-53.

53. Ots M, Mackenzie H, Troy J ,et al. Effects of combination therapy with enalapril and losartan on the rate of progression of renal injury in rats with 5/ 6 renal mass ablation. J Am Soc Nephrol. 1998; 9: 224--30.

54. Furberg C, Herrigton D, Psaty BM . Are drugs within a class interchangeable? Lancet. 1999; 354:1202-4.

55. Hebert L . Renoprotective therapy : how good can it get? Kidney Int. 2000; 57: 343-4.

56. Maschio G, Alberti D, Jannis G ,et al. Effect of angiotensin converting enzyme inhibitor benazepril on the progression of chronic renal insufficiency. N Engl J Med. 1996; 334: 939-45.

57. Ruggmenti P, Reena A, Mosconi L, et al. Randomised placebo controlled trial of effect of ramipril on decline in glomerular filtration rate and risk of terminal renal failure in proteinuric, non-diabetic nephropathy. Lancet. 1997; 249:1857-63.

58. Hobbs R. High or low doses of ACE inhibitors for heart failure? Results of the atlas study. Cleve Chin J Med. 1998; 65: 539-42.

59. Pema A, Ruggmenti P, Testa A ,et al. ACE genotype and ACE inhibitors - induced renoprotection in chronic proteinuric nephropathies. Kidney Int 2000; 57: 274-81.

60. Anderson S, Tarnow L, Roosing P, Parving HH. Renoprotective effects of angiotensin type II receptor blockade in type 1 diabetic patients with diabetic nephropathy. Kidney Int. 2000; 57: 601-6.

61. Anderson S, Jacobsen P, Tarnow L, Rossing P, Parving HH. Time course of the antiproteinuric and antihypertensive effect of losartan in diabetic nephropathy. Nephrol Dial Transplant. 2003; 18: 293--7.

62. Tarrif N, Bakris G. Angiotensin II receptor blockade and progression of nondiabetic renal disease. Kidney Int. 1997; 52 (Suppl): 567-70.

63. Hilgers KF, Mann JF. ACE inhibitors versus AT receptor antagonist in patients with chronic renal disease. J Am Soc Nephrol. 2002; 13: 1100-8.

64. Cao Z, Bornet F, Cardido R, et al. Angiotensin type 2 receptor antagonism confers renal protection in a rat model of progressive renal injury. J Am Soc Nephrol. 2002; 13:1773-87.

65. Agarwal R. Add on angiotensin receptors blockade with maximized ACE inhibitors. Kidney Int. 2001; 59: 2282-9.

66. Jacobsen P, Anderson S, Rossing K, et al. HH : dual blockade of the renin-angiotensin system in type I patients with diabetic nephropath. Nephrol Dial Transplant 2002; 17:1019-24.

67. Jacobsen P, Anderson S, Rossing K, Jansen BR, Parving HH : Dual blockade of the renin-angiotensin system versus maximal recommended dose of ACE inhibitors in diabetic nephropathy. Kidney Int. 2003; 63: 1874--80.

68. Levey A, Greene T, Beck G et al. Dietary protein restriction and the progression of chronic renal disease : what have all the results of the MDRD study shown ? J Am Soc Nephrol. 1999; 10: 2426-39.

69. Maroni B, Staffeld C, Young V, et al. Mechanisms permitting nephritic patients to achieve nitrogen equilibrium with a protein restricted diet. J Clin Invest 1997; 99:1479-87.

70. Walser M, Mitch W, Maroni B, et al. Should protein intake be restricted in predialysis patients ? Kidney Int 1999; 55: 771-7.

71. Dullaart R, Van Dormaal J, Beusekamp B, et al. Long-term effects of protein restricted diet on albuminuria and renal function in IDDM patients without clinical nephropathy and hypertension. Diabetes Care. 1993; 16: 483-92.

72. Cremen W, Bock K. Symptoms and causes of chronic hypokalemic nephropathy in man. Clin Nephrol. 1997;7:112.

73. Ray P, McCune B, Gomez R, et al. Renal vascular induction of TGF - â2 and rennin by potassium depletion. Kidney Int 1993; 44: 1006-13.

74. Executive summary of the third report of the National Cholesterol Education Program (NCEP) Expert Panel on detection, evaluation and treatment of high blood cholesterol in adults. JAMA. 2001; 285: 2486-97.

75. American Diabetes Association : Management of dyslipidemia in adults with diabetes. Diabetes Care 2003; 26 (1): 583-6.

76. Cavarape A, Endlich N, Assaloni R, Bartoli E, Parekh N, Endlilich K. Rho kinase inhibition blunts renal vasoconstriction induced by distinct signaling pathways *in vivo*. J Am Soc Nephrol. 2003; 14: 37-45.

77. Sharpe CC, Hendry BM. Signaling focus on Rho in renal disease. J Am Soc Nephrol. 2003; 14: 261-4.

78. Danesh FR, Sadeghi MM, Amro N, et al. 3 hydroxy 3 methyl glutatyl CoA reductase inhibitors prevent high glucose induced proliferation of mesangial cells via modulation of Rho GTPase/ p21 signaling pathway: implications for diabetic nephropathy. Proc Natl Acad Sci .USA. 2002; 99: 8301-5.

79. American diabetes association : Aspirin therapy in diabetes. Diabetes Care. 2003; 26 (Suppl 1): 587-8.

80. Noris M, Remuzzi G : Uremic bleeding : Closing the circle after 30 years of controversies? Blood. 1999; 94: 2569-74.

81. Forced CM, Ejerbald E, Lindblad P, Blot WJ, et al. Acetaminophen, aspirin and chronic renal failure. N Engl J Med 2001; 345:1801-8.

82. Kuriyama S, Tomonari H, Yoshida H et al : Reversal of anemia by erythropoietin therapy retards the progression of chronic renal failure, especially in nondiabetic patients. Nephron 1997; 77: 176-185.

83. Kubo M, Kiyohara Y, Kato, et al. Effect of hyperinsulinemia on renal function in a general Japanese population : the Hisayama study. Kidney Int. 1999; 55: 2450-2.

84. Refsum H, Veland P, Nygard O, et al. Homocysteine and cardiovascular disease. Annu Rev Med. 1998; 49: 31-62.

85. Hoogeveen E, Kostense P, Jager A, et al. Serum homocysteine level and protein intake are related to risk of micro-albuminuria. The HOVIN study. Kidney Int. 1998; 54: 203-9.

86. Touam M, Zingraft J, Jingers P, et al. Effective correction of hyperhomocysteinemia in hemodialysis patients by intravenous folic acid and pyridoxine therapy. Kidney Int. 1999; 56: 2292-2296.

87. Konner K, Hulbert - Sheraon TE, Rory EC. Tailoring the initial vascular access for dialysis patients. Kidney Int. 2002; 62: 329-38.

88. Davidson J, Wilkinson A, et al. New-onset diabetes after transplantation: 2003 International consensus guidelines. Transplantation 2003; 75: 5513-5524.

89. Werr MR, Fink JC. Risk for post transplant diabetes mellitus with current immunosuppressive medications. Am J Kidney Dis. 1999; 34: 1-13.

90. Neilsen JH, Nerup J. Direct effects of cyclosporin A on human pancreatic beta-cells. Diabetes 1986; 35: 1049--1052.

91. Redman JB, Olson LK, Robertson RP. Effects of FK 506 on human insulin gene expression, insulin mRNA levels and insulin secretion in HIT-T15 cells. J Clin Invest. 1996; 98: 2786-93.

92. Mariana Markel. New onset diabetes mellitus in transplant patients : pathogenesis, complications and management. Am J Kid Dis .2004; 43 (6): 953-65.

93. Kasiske BL, Harmon WE, et al. Recommendations for the outpatient surveillance of renal transplant recipients. J Am Soc Nephrol. 2000; 11; S1-86

94. Allaqaband S, Timuluri R, Gupta A, Malik AM. Prospective study of N-acetylcysteine, fenoldopam and saline for prevention of radiocontrast induced nephropathy. Catheter Cardiovasc Intern. 2002; 57:279-83.

95. Fishbane S, Durham JH, Marzo K. Prevention of radiocontrast induced nephropathy. J Am Soc Nephrol. 2004; 15: 251-60.

Chapter 69

NEUROLOGICAL COMPLICATIONS OF DIABETES

Ashok Kumar Das, Prasanth G, Thomas Mathew

CHAPTER OUTLINE

- Neurological Complications in Diabetes—An Overview
- Diabetic Peripheral Neuropathy
- Conclusion
- Summary

NEUROLOGICAL COMPLICATIONS IN DIABETES—AN OVERVIEW

Diabetes is a metabolic disease that affects multiple systems. Even within the nervous system the manifestations of this disease can be wide and varied. The special metabolic and exacting nutritional requirements of neurons make them vulnerable to even minor alterations in the milieu. Diabetes affects the nervous system both directly as well as indirectly. Insulin deficiency and hyperglycemia can be directly pathogenic while the microvascular and macrovascular damage in diabetic individuals contributes to indirect damage. Diabetic neuropathy is the commonest and best-characterized neurological complication of diabetes.[1] The prevalence of neurological problems in a diabetic population may be as high as 50%.[2] The possible neurological manifestations attributed to diabetes are summarized in **Table 69.1**. The main emphasis of this chapter is on diabetic peripheral neuropathy.

DIABETIC PERIPHERAL NEUROPATHY

Neuropathy is the most frequent symptomatic complication of diabetes and potentially one of the most disturbing. The consequences of diabetic neuropathy can extend to several other systems. The early recognition and appropriate management of neuropathy in the patient with diabetes is important because:

- Half of the cases may be asymptomatic and can be recognized only by focused testing, which includes quantitative sensory and autonomic function testing and also nerve conduction studies when appropriate.
- Effective treatment options are available which not only provide symptomatic relief but also retard the progression of the disease to a great extent.
- Autonomic neuropathy is a common presentation, which can lead to life-threatening complications.

Definition

The presence of symptoms and or signs of peripheral nerve dysfunction in people with diabetes after the exclusion of other causes.[1]

This definition implies that all patients with peripheral nerve dysfunction and diabetes do not have diabetic peripheral neuropathy. Studies such as the famous Rochester diabetic study showed that upto 10% of neuropathy in diabetics had a nondiabetic causation.[3] Confirmation of the etiology may require quantitative electrophysiology, sensory, and autonomic function testing.

TABLE 69.1	Neurological complications of diabetes
Complications	*Comment*
• Cerebrovascular diseases	• Macrovascular complications

• Immune peripheral neuropathy
  – CIDP
  – Perineuritis
	• Risk of stroke 2–3 times that of general population
	• Predisposition

• Diabetic peripheral neuropathies (sensorimotor, autonomic)	• Discussed in detail below
• Diabetic muscle infarction	• Type I (80%) > type 2 (20%). Most common site is the thigh—presents with severe pain; resolves by 6–8 weeks
• Cranial nerve palsies	• Cranial nerves 3 and 6 are most commonly involved secondary to microangiopathy • Increased incidence of 7th nerve palsy seen in diabetics
• Cognitive dysfunction in diabetics	• Increased incidence of Alzheimer's disease in diabetics • Vascular dementia is also more common in diabetics • Mixed type dementias occur in diabetics

• Acute complications
  – Hypoglycemia
  – Hyperglycemia
  – Diabetic ketoacidosis
  – Hyperosmolar nonketotic coma (HONK)
	• Hypoglycemia causes various neuroglycopenic and autonomic symptoms
	• Hyperglycemia per se is associated with versive seizures
	• Ketosis may develop altered consciousness, cerebral edema
	• HONK cerebral infarctions, seizures and global cerebral dysfunction features

Prevalence

The prevalence approaches 50% among those who have had the disease for more than 25 years.[1] Large proportions of diabetic patients seen for routine diabetic care have neuropathy but that the diagnosis is often overlooked. One of the largest published series reported a prevalence of 7.5% at the time of diagnosis of diabetes, with the prevalence increasing steadily thereafter with no plateau.[3] Most patients with diabetic neuropathy are asymptomatic. Many patients do not manifest a single type of diabetic neuropathy but rather a mixture of neuropathic features often dominated by one or another subtype. The prevalence of asymptomatic diabetic neuropathy with subtle changes detected by quantitative testing may approach 60 to even 100% depending on the definition and the techniques used.[4]

Neurologic complications occur equally in type 1, type 2 and also in secondary causes of diabetes. The most important risk factors for the development of neuropathy are the long duration and increased severity of hyperglycemia. Other implicated factors are shown in **Table 69.2.**

TABLE 69.2	Risk factors for the development of diabetic neuropathy
	• Male sex • Increased height • Smoking • Retinopathy • Microalbuminuria • Alcoholism

Classification

There are numerous schemes for the classification of diabetic neuropathy. But none of them are complete. This is because most patients do not fit neatly into any single category but instead have several overlapping clinical features. For instance, many diabetics with distal, primarily sensory polyneuropathy can also be shown to have autonomic dysfunction, usually in the form of vasomotor disturbance in the limbs and abnormalities of sweating. The most popular classification is the one proposed by Thomas, which divides the neuropathies into generalized and focal types **(see Table 69.3).**[5]

TABLE 69.3	Classification of diabetic neuropathies
Generalized symmetric polyneuropathies	Focal and multifocal neuropathies
• Acute sensory • Chronic sensorimotor • Autonomic	• Cranial • Truncal • Focal Limb • Proximal motor (amyotrophy) • Coexisting CIDP

TABLE 69.4	Reversible and irreversible diabetic neuropathies

Reversible
- Mononeuropathies
  - Femoral
  - Cranial nerve palsies (III, IV and VI)
  - Truncal Radiculopathies
- Pressure palsies
  - Median
  - Ulnar
  - Lateral popliteal nerve

Irreversible neuropathies
- Chronic sensorimotor neuropathy
- Autonomic neuropathy

The neuropathies may also be classified as symmetric versus asymmetric[6] and progressive versus nonprogressive[7] neuropathies (Natural History) and reversible and irreversible neuropathies **(Table 69.4)**.

Hyperglycemic neuropathy: Seen in patients with poor diabetic control wherein they suffer from uncomfortable sensations from the lower limbs which resolves rapidly when glycemic control is achieved. The mechanism is not known, but the recovery is too rapid to ascribe to nerve fiber regeneration or remyelination.

Natural History

There are two categories of diabetic neuropathy:
1. Progressive neuropathies
2. Nonprogressive neuropathies

Diabetic symmetric peripheral neuropathy and autonomic neuropathy exhibit a progressively worsening course while most of the mononeuropathies, radiculopathies and acute painful neuropathies including the cranial neuropathies have a self-limiting course. Progression is influenced by the glycemic control.

Electrophysiology may be used to monitor the progression of diabetic neuropathy. As diabetic neuropathy is predominantly an axonopathy, serial measurement of the CMAP amplitude would be a better indicator of the progression than the nerve conduction velocity.

Pathogenesis

The pathogenesis of diabetic neuropathy is multifactorial. The various pathogenic factors are interrelated and together contribute to the development and progression of the syndrome.[8] The actual process of neuropathic progression is dynamic, with nerve degeneration and regeneration occurring spontaneously and simultaneously. The net balance between these processes determines whether the neuropathy progresses, regresses or stabilizes **(Flow chart 69.1)**.

The chief mechanisms involved in the pathogenesis of diabetic neuropathy are:
- Hyperglycemia (metabolic)
- Local nerve ischemia (vascular)
- Neurotrophic factor deficiency
- Immune mechanisms.

Hyperglycemia

The results from the Diabetes Control and Complications Trial (DCCT) convincingly demonstrated that hyperglycemia and insulin deficiency contribute to the development of diabetic neuropathy.[9] Hyperglycemia is believed to contribute to nerve damage chiefly through the polyol pathway.

Increased availability of glucose increases its metabolism by the enzyme aldose reductase (a part of the polyol pathway) leading to intracellular accumulation of sorbitol **(Flow chart 69.2)**. This accumulation of sorbitol produces a reciprocal decrease in levels of myoinositol and taurine to the point that they become insufficient for normal intracellular metabolism.[10] Myoinositol and taurine depletion causes reduced Na^+/K^+ adenosine triphosphatase activity and slows nerve conduction velocity.[11] Moreover, sorbitol accumulation also results in a reduction of nicotinamide-adenine dinucleotide phosphate (NADPH) and glutathione stores in the cell.[12] This may impair the cell's ability to detoxify reactive oxygen species and other agents causing oxidative cell injury.

Hyperglycemia *per se* promotes the formation of reactive oxygen species by auto-oxidation of glucose and formation of advanced glycation end products.[13] Glycation of proteins secondarily leads to complications by the uptake of these modified substances by certain receptors. These receptors for advanced glycation end products (RAGE) is an immunoglobulin that inter-

Flow chart 69.1 Current view of pathogenesis of neuropathy

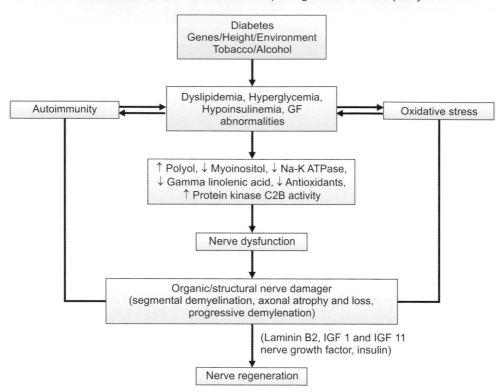

Flow chart 69.2 The sorbitol pathway

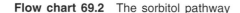

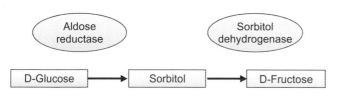

nalizes these abnormal proteins and causes cellular toxicity.

Local Nerve Ischemia

The role of local nerve ischemia in the development of diabetic neuropathy is unclear.[14] Sural nerve biopsies from diabetic patients reveal many changes suggestive of local vascular disease including basement membrane thickening, endothelial cell proliferation and vessel occlusions.[15] Nerve blood flow is reduced in diabetic rats.[16] Some studies show a reduction in nerve blood flow in diabetic patients, but others do not.[17,18]

A recent study done in rats has shown that therapeutic neovascularization using human umbilical cord blood-derived endothelial precursor cells (EPCs)

reversed diabetic neuropathy.[19] VEGF gene transfer was reported to increase nerve conduction velocity and nerve blood flow in diabetic animals.[20] Ischemia may also induce oxidative stress in the nerve, increasing the production of reactive oxygen species.

Neuropathic Factor Deficiency

Neuropathic factors are involved in the development, maintenance, and regeneration of responsive elements of the nervous system. The best studied of these is nerve growth factor (NGF), a protein that promotes the survival of sympathetic and small fiber neural crest-derived sensory neurons in the peripheral nervous system. In diabetic animal models both NGF production and retrograde transport appear to be impaired.[21-23] In a human study, abnormal expression of NGF in skin keratinocytes correlates with early manifestations of small fiber sensory oral tissues and that damage may be selective force may provide a link between the immune and vascular theories of causation of neuropathy. Further evidence of the inflammatory response is increased nuclear factor-kB in Schwann cells and in neural microvessels. Among type 1 diabetes, antibodies

TABLE 69.5	Treatment of diabetic neuropathy based on the pathogenetic mechanisms		
Abnormality	Compound/Drug	Aim of treatment	Status
• Polyol pathway ↑	Aldose reductase inhibitors (sorbinil, tolrestat, epalrestat, zopolrestat, zenarestat, fidarestat)	Nerve sorbitol ↓	Most of the trials are disappointing. Epalrestat marketed in Japan
• Myoinositol ↓	Myoinositol	Nerve myoinositol ↑	Equivocal
• Oxidative stress ↑	Alpha lipoic acid	Oxygen free radicals ↓	Effective in RCTs; trials ongoing
• Nonenzymatic glycation ↑	Aminoguanidine	AGE accumulation ↓	Withdrawn due to side effects
• Protein kinase C ↑	Ruboxistaurin (PKC inhibitor)	Increases NBF (Nerve blood flow)	Promising; Phase 3 trials ongoing
• GLA synthesis ↓	Gamma linolenic acid	EFA metabolism ↑	Withdrawn

to autonomic structures {autoantibodies to sympathetic ganglia (CF-SG), vagus nerve (CF-VN) and adrenal medulla (CF-ADM)} are often found.[24-26] There is evidence to believe that autoimmune mechanisms are more involved in pathogenesis of neuropathy in type 1 than in type 2 diabetes.

Other Mechanisms

Other abnormalities noted in nerves of diabetic patients include—increased activity of protein kinase C, decreased synthesis of gamma linolenic acid, etc.[27] understanding these mechanisms has enabled us to develop treatment options specifically targeting these abnormalities **(Table 69.5)**.

Poly (ADP-ribose) polymerase (PARP) activation, a downstream effector of free radical and oxidant-induced DNA single-strand breakage, is an important mechanism in the pathogenesis of diabetes complications. PARP activation leads to: (1) NAD^+ depletion and energy failure, (2) Changes in transcriptional regulation and gene expression, and (3) Poly ADP-ribosylation and resulting inhibition of the glycolytic enzyme glyceraldehyde 3-phosphate dehydrogenase, with concomitant activation of several major pathogenetic mechanisms, i.e. nonenzymatic glycation, protein kinase C, and hexosamine pathway. PARP inhibitors have been tried in animal studies and they have demonstrated improvement in rat models of early diabetic neuropathy.[28]

It has been noted in many studies that the small unmyelinated nerve fibers are more affected than the larger peripheral nerves. As to why small fibers more vulnerable, it has been postulated that the high density of ion channels at the nodes of Ranvier may protect myelinated fibers in the early stages of the disease.[29]

Clinical Features

Clinical features depend on the type of neuropathy. It has to be kept in mind that most patients have overlapping features of multiple types.

Acute Sensory Neuropathy

Acute sensory neuropathy is rare, tends to follow periods of poor metabolic control (e.g. ketoacidosis) or sudden change in glycemic control (e.g. insulin neuritis). It is characterized by acute onset of severe sensory symptoms with marked nocturnal exacerbation but few neurologic signs on examination of the legs. Affected patients typically complain of severe and often unrelenting leg pain, which may be worse at night. Cutaneous hyperesthesia is a common and disturbing complication. Patients may report that they cannot tolerate the sensation of sheets or clothing touching their feet. Positive symptoms dominate the clinical picture. This type of neuropathy is at times associated with weight loss for which the term diabetic cachexia is often used. It is a self-limiting entity and usually remits by six months to two years.

Distal Symmetric Polyneuropathy (Chronic Sensorimotor Neuropathy)

It is the most common type of diabetic neuropathy. It is a predominant sensory neuropathy with subclinical autonomic neuropathy. Motor dysfunction is less common but does occur. The condition has an insidious onset and typically affects the most distal lower extremities first, resulting in a stocking pattern of sensory loss.[30] The process starts in the toes, and extends up the legs; upper extremities are involved in the later stages, beginning with the fingertips.

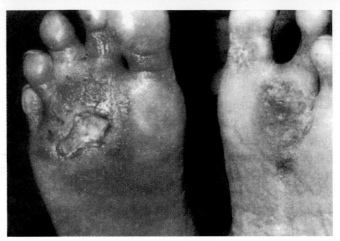

Figure 69.1 Neuropathic ulcers

Earliest manifestations are loss of pain and temperature sensations due to small fiber affliction.[31] This may predispose the patient to injury and possible foot ulceration **(Figure 69.1)**. Large fibers are involved later and result in loss of vibration and proprioception and even sensory ataxia in more severe cases. Sensory fiber degeneration may cause paresthesias, dysesthesias and at times neuropathic pain. The latter may be described as a burning sensation, sharp stabbing pain (type C fiber involvement) or a severe, deep, aching feeling (A delta fiber type involvement).

Motor involvement is usually minor and restricted to distal segments of extremities, but the resulting foot deformity abnormally redistributes weight bearing, contributing to callosities and ulcers. Examination may show sensory loss especially to pain and temperature, rarely wasting and weakness and diminished ankle and knee reflexes.

It is important to note that most patients with distal symmetric polyneuropathy are asymptomatic or only mildly symptomatic and the syndrome may be detected only by careful physical examination. The most serious consequence of distal symmetric neuropathy is the development of diabetic foot problems like neuropathic ulceration, neuropathic edema and Charcot's arthropathy. These may ultimately lead to refractory infections, gangrene, and sepsis with loss of foot the whole limb or in many cases, even life. Hence, the need to recognize this entity and treat it aggressively. The common differential diagnoses in this setting are leprosy, amyloidosis, Charcot Marie Tooth disease, vitamin B_{12} deficiency, alcoholism, and peripheral vascular disease **(Figure 69.1)**.

When pain is the predominant symptom, other differentials must be considered **(Table 69.6)**.

Proximal Motor Neuropathies—Diabetic Amyotrophy

This syndrome usually develops in people more than 50 years of age and is associated with poor glycemic control. Men are affected more than women. The cardinal feature is wasting of the thigh with or without pain. On examination, there is readily demonstrable weakness of the iliopsoas, obturator, and adductor magnus with relative preservation of power in the gluteus maximus and the hamstrings. The patient cannot rise up from a sitting position but toe or heel standing may be surprisingly well preserved. The onset may be gradual or acute. This syndrome may present symmetrically or asymmetrically and there is some disagreement as to whether the two types of presentation are distinct syndromes.[31] Recovery is the rule; pain begins to subside after three months and weakness usually resolves by 12 months. In some cases, an immune-mediated epineural microvasculitis has been demonstrated in nerve biopsies. Electrophysiology reveals a lumbosacral plexopathy. The important differential diagnoses are diseases of the nerve root, spinal cord and the cauda equina.

When an unusually severe, predominantly motor neuropathy and progressive polyneuropathy develops in diabetic patients, one must consider CIDP. The diagnosis of CIDP is often overlooked and the patient

TABLE 69.6	Pain syndromes other than neuropathy—common in diabetics
Differential diagnosis	*Comment*
• Claudication	Common in diabetics; differentiate with Doppler study
• Morton's neuroma	Usually unilateral, more in females, pain increases on pressure
• Fasciitis	Plantar fasciitis common, calcaneal spur on X-ray, usually unilateral, tenderness over the sole
• Osteoarthritis	Secondary to diabetes. Improves with rest, X-ray shows sclerotic changes
• Radiculopathy	Root pains, malignancies must be considered in elderly

simply labeled as having diabetic neuropathy: progressive symmetric or asymmetric motor deficits, progressive sensory neuropathy in spite of optimal glycemic control together with typical electrophysiological findings, and an unusually high cerebrospinal fluid protein level all suggest the possibility of an underlying treatable demyelinating neuropathy. As immunomodulatory therapy with combinations of corticosteroids, plasmapheresis, and intravenous immune globulin can produce a relatively rapid and substantial improvement in neurological deficits and electrophysiology in some cases of CIDP; referral to a neurologist is indicated if this diagnosis is suspected. The other possibilities to be considered are monoclonal gammopathies, circulating antiantibodies and inflammatory vasculitides.

Thoracolumbar Neuropathy/Radiculopathy

This complication is also commoner in older diabetic patients. It presents with intermittent chest or abdominal pain in a nerve root distribution and may be associated with a dermatomal pattern of sensory loss. During acute presentation, there may be misdiagnosis of acute abdomen or as malingering. There may be local bulging due to the weakness of abdominal muscles. Recovery is expected in less than 6 months and symptoms rarely persist more than one to two years. The muscle bulging almost always resolves.

Cranial Nerve Palsies

The cranial nerves most commonly involved are the third nerve followed in frequency by the fourth and sixth cranial nerves.[31] They are thought to occur due to a microvascular infarct, which, in the majority, resolves spontaneously over several months. They may present with eye pain, diplopia, and in the case of third nerve involvement, ptosis. Pupil is usually spared. Recovery takes place within three to six months and relapse is very rare. The most important differential diagnosis is aneurysm of the posterior communicating artery where ptosis and pupillary dilatation are common. There is weak association between diabetes and lesions of 7th and 8th nerves.[7]

Compression Neuropathies

Mononeuropathies may have a sudden onset and can occur as a result of involvement of the median (5.8% of all diabetic neuropathies), ulnar (2.1%), radial (0.6%), and common peroneal nerves.[32] Among the compression neuropathies, the most common is the Carpal-Tunnel syndrome. They are more common in diabetes when compared with those without diabetes. Carpal-Tunnel syndrome results in paresthesias, and numbness of the lateral 3½ fingers. There may be associated weakness of thenar muscles. The ulnar nerve compression can cause numbness of fourth and fifth fingers and wasting of interossei. Medial and lateral plantar entrapments decrease sensation in the inside and outside and of the feet respectively. The increased prevalence of Carpal-Tunnel syndrome in diabetes may be related to repeated undetected trauma, metabolic changes or accumulation of fluid or edema. The physician should be aware that the symptoms may spread to the whole hand or arm and the signs may extend beyond those subserved by the entrapped nerve. Entrapments may require decompression, but initial management should be expectant with strong reassurance to the patient for recovery entrapment neuropathies should be differentiated from mononeuropathies due to vasculitis and subsequent ischemia or infarction of individual nerves. These isolated peripheral nerve lesions involve particularly ulnar, median, radial, femoral and lateral cutaneous nerves of the thigh. The important differentiating points are summarized in **Table 69.7**.

Diabetic Autonomic Neuropathy (DAN)

Prevalence data for DAN range from 1.6 to 90% depending on the tests used, populations examined, and type and stage of disease.

An autonomic neuropathy is common in patients with longstanding diabetes. The symptoms of autonomic neuropathy can be extremely disagreeable and disabling if several occur together. Gustatory sweating is the commonest autonomic disturbance, followed by postural hypotension, impotence, diarrhea, bladder hypotonia and gastroparesis. The development of autonomic neuropathy is less clearly related to poor metabolic control than somatic neuropathy and

TABLE 69.7	Differentiation between entrapment neuropathies and mononeuropathies	
Feature	Entrapment	Mononeuritis
Onset	Gradual	Sudden
Pain	Chronic	Acute
Multiple nerves involved	Rare	Common
Course	Persists without intervention	Resolves
Treatment	Rest/Splint/Surgery	Physical

improved control rarely results in amelioration of symptoms. More than a fourth of patients with insulin-dependent diabetes may have evidence of autonomic dysfunction at the time of diagnosis.[33] Patients with symptomatic autonomic neuropathy and reduced heart rate variability have a significantly reduced 10-year survival rate.[34]

Within 10 years of developing overt symptoms of autonomic neuropathy, 30 to 50% of patients are dead—many from sudden cardiorespiratory arrest, the cause of which is unknown. Patients with postural hypotension have the highest subsequent mortality. The symptoms and signs arising from autonomic neuropathy affecting various systems are summarized below:

- *Cardiovascular neuropathy (CAN)*, the presence of autonomic neuropathy may limit an individual's exercise capacity and increase the risk of an adverse cardiovascular event during exercise. Sudden death and silent myocardial ischemia have been attributed to CAN in diabetes. Resting and stress thallium myocardial scintigraphy is an appropriate non-invasive test for the presence and extent of macrovascular coronary artery disease in these individuals. Reduced cardiovascular autonomic function, as measured by heart rate variability (HRV), was strongly (relative risk is doubled) associated with increased risk of silent myocardial ischemia and mortality.[35] Other features include:
- Symptoms such as cough, nausea, dyspnea, fatigue and giddiness[32]
- Postural hypotension
- Resting tachycardia
- Fixed heart rate
- Sudden cardiorespiratory arrest.

Diabetic autonomic neuropathy is associated with abnormalities in the distribution of cardiac sympathetic innervation, so that even in the absence of ischemia the risk of arrhythmia is very high. A simple marker of CAN is prolongation of QT interval with a value more than 430 ms being a marker for increased risk of arrhythmias.[32]

As clinical examination alone is inadequate to rule out CAN, additional tests are required—the recommended ones are R-R variation, valsalva maneuver, and postural blood pressure testing. This battery of three recommended tests for assessing CAN can be readily performed in the average clinic, hospital, or diagnostic center with the use of available technology.[1]

At time of diagnosis of type 2 diabetes and within 5 years after diagnosis of type 1 diabetes (unless an individual has symptoms suggestive of autonomic dysfunction earlier), patients should be screened for CAN. Knowledge of early autonomic dysfunction can encourage patient and physician to improve metabolic control and to use therapies, such as ACE inhibitors and β-blockers that are proven to be effective for patients with CAN.

Quantitative autonomic function testing (QAFT) should be performed when planning an exercise program for individuals with diabetes about to embark on a moderate to high-intensity exercise program, especially those at high-risk for underlying cardiovascular disease and also as a part of the preanesthetic work-up in appropriate setting.

Gastrointestinal: The manifestations include:
- Dysphagia due to esophageal atony
- Gastroparesis which presents as abdominal fullness, nausea, vomiting, and unstable diabetes
- Constipation due to colonic atony
- Diarrhea, which is relatively uncommon, rarely severe, painless, and not associated with bleeding, may have nocturnal exacerbations
- Fecal incontinence may be a rare feature.

There are no true population-based studies using radioisotopic techniques that quantify gastric emptying in diabetic patients, but cross-sectional studies have indicated that—50% of outpatients with long-standing diabetes have delayed gastric emptying and up to 76% of diabetic outpatients indicate that they have one or more gastrointestinal symptom, the most common of which is constipation.

Genitourinary: The abnormalities in this system are:
- Difficulty in micturition, urinary incontinence
- Recurrent infections due to an atonic bladder
- *Impotence:* A complete work-up for impotence in men should include history (medical and sexual); psychological evaluation; hormone levels; measurement of nocturnal penile tumescence; tests to assess penile, pelvic, and spinal nerve function; cardiovascular autonomic function tests; and measurement of penile and brachial blood pressure
- Retrograde ejaculation.

Genitourinary bladder dysfunction has been shown in 43 to 87% of individuals with type 1 diabetes. Diabetic women have a five-fold higher risk of unrecognized voiding difficulty compared with nondiabetic women. The history and physical are generally noncontributory, and the patient should be referred to a urologist for urodynamic studies.

The prevalence of erectile dysfunction in diabetic men ranges from 27 to 75%.

Sudomotor: Manifestations in this system are:
- Gustatory sweating
- Nocturnal sweating without hypoglycemia
- Anhidrosis which leads to fissures/cracks in the feet

Vasomotor abnormalities present with:
- Dependent edema
- Cold feet—due to loss of skin vasomotor response
- Bullous formations.

Pupillary abnormalities are:
- Decreased pupil size
- Resistance to mydriatics
- Delayed or absent response to light.

Diagnosis

The diagnostic methods for the detection of diabetic neuropathy can be divided into traditional and newer ones.

Traditional Methods

Clinical examination of neuropathy is subjective and has limitations in assessing diabetic neuropathy. The intra- and inter-rater variability limits the reproducibility and the reliability of test results.[36] Moreover, routine clinical examination detects abnormalities at a relatively advanced age. Nevertheless, a meticulous clinical examination should never be neglected in the work-up of any diabetic patient. A number of devices have been devised to detect sensory abnormalities and allow quantitation of the deficit **(Table 69.8)**.

All patients with diabetes should be screened annually for DPN by examining pinprick, temperature, and vibration perception (using a 128 -Hz tuning fork), 10 g monofilament pressure sensation at the distal halluces, and ankle reflexes. Combinations of more than one test have >87% sensitivity in detecting DPN. Loss of 10 g monofilament perception and reduced vibration perception predict foot ulcers.

TABLE 69.8	Devices to detect sensory abnormalities
Device	*Sensory modality assessed*
• Biothesiometer/ Vibrameter	Vibration perception threshold
• Semmes-Weinstein monofilaments	Light touch sensation
• Thermotest	Thermal threshold
• Pinchometer or series of weighted needles	Pain

TABLE 69.9	Tests for detection of autonomic neuropathy		
		Normal	*Abnormal*
• Heart rate variation during deep breathing		>15	<10
• Heart rate variation on standing			
– 15 seconds after standing		>15	<12
– 30:15 ratio		1.04	<1.00
• Heart rate change during Valsalva		>1.21	<1.2
• Postural fall in systolic BP		<10	>30

The earliest and the most sensitive abnormality in patients with autonomic neuropathy is a decrease in the heart rate variability during deep breathing. This is followed by alterations in the heart rate on standing and then the valsalva maneuver. Postural hypotension is a late event. There are more sophisticated equipment for autonomic tests that are used as research tools, e.g. high-resolution infrared cameras to measure papillary diameter in dark, etc. The tests employed for the detection of autonomic neuropathy are given in **Table 69.9**.

Standard Electrophysiological Methods

Standard electrophysiological methods have also been used extensively to diagnose and follow the progression of diabetic polyneuropathy. However, because there is little demyelination in the early stages, changes in the maximal conduction velocity are gradual.[37] Furthermore, whole nerve electrophysiology exclusively measures function in large-diameter neurons, and the spectrum of nerve fibers involved in diabetic neuropathy includes both large and small diameter fibers.[38] Thus electrophysiology, particularly conduction velocity alone, may provide a poor measure of early dysfunction in some patients.[39]

Newer Methods

Several highly sensitive methods are being developed for the early detection of diabetes, so that early intervention can be done.

Skin punch biopsy and immunohistochemical staining for peripheral axons: Skin punch biopsy offers a relatively easy, sensitive and less invasive alternative to whole nerve biopsy.[40] Typically, skin punch biopsy specimens (3 to 4 mm in diameter) are obtained with the patient under local lidocaine anesthesia, with a sterile technique.[41] The tissue is cut into 52 µm frozen sections and processed for immunohistochemistry using antibodies to human protein gene product 9.5 (PGP 9.5). This approach provides reliable and intensive staining of small diameter axons innervating the skin. Fiber density can be readily quantified with reported inter-observer agreement as high as 96%.[42] Holland et al reported a strong correlation between reductions in intradermal nerve fiber density and estimate of severity of clinical symptoms in patients with peripheral neuropathy associated with a wide range of conditions, including diabetes.[39]

Quantitative sensory testing (QST): Quantitative sensory procedures facilitate early diagnosis and accurate assessment of diabetic neuropathy.[43] In QST, standardized sensory testing instruments are used to control and deliver specific stimuli at designated intensities to test sensory thresholds, defined as the minimum stimulus energy detectable 50% of the time. QST is noninvasive, requires about 10 minutes per session, and can be conducted with nonprofessional personnel after a brief training period. A variety of instruments have been developed for QST; The biothesiometer **(Figure 69.2)** and the Semmes-Weinstein monofilament **(Figure 69.3)** are commonly used. The computer-assisted sensory evaluation (CASE) IV device is one of the most effective.

Electrophysiologic testing: When properly trained and monitored, electrophysiology has proved an effective

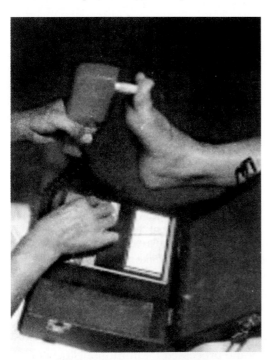

Figure 69.2 Biothesiometer

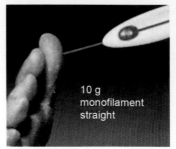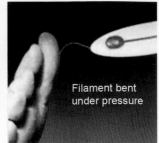

Figure 69.3 Semmes-Weinstein monofilament

end point in several multicenter studies of diabetic neuropathy.[44] The assessment of response area, rather than amplitude, the calculation of the distribution of velocities and the use of multistimulus collision techniques may enhance the sensitivity of electrophysiology to activity in small-diameter myelinated fibers. However, reliable implementation of these techniques has proven difficult.

Peripheral nerve imaging: Eaton et al suggested that the endoneural edema reflected magnetic resonance imaging of peripheral nerves may initiate the deterioration, that is later detected in electrophysiologic testing and neurologic examination.[45] The strength of MRI imaging of peripheral nerves include the ability to target specific areas, the lack of invasiveness, and the feasibility of repeat procedures. Limitations are the costs and as yet unproven diagnostic sensitivity.

Composite Measures for Diagnosis and Assessment of Diabetic Neuropathy

Assessment of the onset and progress of diabetic neuropathy may be enhanced by the use of composite measures that combine information from QST, electrophysiology, and signs and symptoms into a single score. This composite provides a single score based on results from multiple tests and expresses the degree of abnormality as a percentile task. This scoring system is highly effective for diagnosis and continuing assessment of diabetes, but it is also very time consuming. Many scoring systems have been developed, but the best known the NIS (LL)+7, developed by Dyck et al[46] **(Table 69.10)**.

Management

The most important step in the management of any diabetic neuropathy is strict glycemic control. The DCCT and UKPDS trials have shown that meticulous control of blood sugar not only decreases the risk of

TABLE 69.10	Neuropathy disability score (NDS)

Parameter	Scoring

• Vibration perception threshold
  128-Hz tuning fork; apex of big toe: normal = can distinguish
  vibrating/not vibrating
• Temperature perception on dorsum of the foot: using a beaker of warm or ice water
• Pin-Prick
  Apply pin proximal to big toe nail just enough to deform the skin; trial pair = sharp,
  blunt; normal, can distinguish sharp/not sharp
	Normal = 0
	Abnormal = 1

• Achilles reflex	Present = 0 Present with reinforcement = 1 Absent = 2
(modified from Dyck et al[46])	NDS Total out of 10

developing neuropathy but also slows the progression in established neuropathy. Measures aimed at improvement of lipid and blood pressure indices, and the avoidance of cigarette smoking and excess alcohol consumption, are recommended for the prevention of other complications of diabetes though there are no clear prevention studies involving these.

Treatment Options

In view of the multifactorial nature of the pathogenesis, multiple treatment options may be needed to provide optimum relief to a patient of diabetic neuropathy **(See Table 69.2)**. Needless to say the very fact that so many options are available points to the fact that none of them are ideal. Some degree of trial and error may be required before striking the ideal combination for the management of a particular patient. A list of various therapeutic strategies tried in diabetic neuropathies is given below with a brief description of some of them.

Aldose reductase inhibitors: Aldose reductase inhibitors reduce the flux of glucose through the polyol pathway, inhibiting tissue accumulation of sorbitol and fructose and preventing reduction of redox potentials. Alrestatin, the first aldose reductase inhibitor studied, was shown to improve sensory impairment scores in one study.[47] But in other studies no objective benefits were noted.[48] Patient selection may have complicated interpretation of these trials because more severe neuropathy may be irreversible. Sorbinil, another widely studied ARI, generated more promising clinical effects. In a double blind cross over trial, treatment with sorbinil resulted in a small but significant improvement in both motor and sensory conduction velocities compared with placebo.[49] Additional studies have demonstrated minor improvements in test results but failed to demonstrate progressive benefit with long-term therapy.[50] In a placebo-controlled, double blind study of another ARI, tolrestat,[51] diabetic patients with asymptomatic neuropathy, as defined by at least one pathologic cardiovascular reflex were treated for one year.[52] Patients who received tolrestat had significant improvement in autonomic function tests as well as in vibration perception, whereas placebo-treated patients showed deterioration in most of the parameters studied.

Human IVIG: Some studies[52] have shown improvement of distal sensorimotor neuropathy with IVIG treatment and works as an immunomodulator.

Gamma linolenic acid: It preserves prostaglandin E2 and is believed to increase the nerve blood flow.

Aminoguandine: It is an inhibitor of AGE formation. Trials in animals have shown improved nerve conduction in diabetic neuropathy.

Alpha lipoic acid: It is a derivative of octanoic acid, which is normally present in the food, and is also synthesized by the liver. It acts as a thiol replenishing and redox-modulating agent and has to be used parenterally.

Capsaicin: An alkaloid found in red pepper depletes the tissue of substance P a mediator of pain. Best used for localized pain syndromes.

Protein kinase C inhibition: Protein kinase C has been implicated in the pathogenesis of microvascular complications. An inhibitor (LY333531), now named ruboxistaurin, has shown promise in preliminary studies and more extensive studies are going on.

TABLE 69.11	Management of autonomic dysfunction syndromes

Dysfunction	Treatment
• Diabetic gastroparesis	Frequent small meals; prokinetic drugs, e.g. Cisapride, domperidone, metoclopromide, erythromycin, rarely surgery
• Diabetic constipation	Stimulant laxatives, e.g. Senna, dulcolax
• Diabetic diarrhea	Loperamide, codeine, tetracyclines, erythromycin
• Neuropathic bladder	Manual pressure, Crede's method, intermittent self catheterization, antibiotics for infection
• Erectile dysfunction	Sex therapy, psychotherapy, counseling; Drugs—yohimbine, sildenafil, vardenafil, tadalafil; Intracavernosal injection of vasoactive agents, e.g. alprostadil, phentolamine, papaverine, vacuum tumescence devices
• Vaginal dryness	Vaginal lubricants
• Sudomotor dysfunction	Emollients and skin lubricants, scopolamine, glycopyrrolate, botulinum toxin, vasodilators
• Postural hypotension	Head end elevation, gradual rising from the bed, pressure stockings; fludrocortisone (up to 1 mg/day), midodrine (2.5-10 mg /day)

Others:
- N-acetyl L-carnitine
- Myoinositol
- ACE inhibitors
- Calcium channel blockers
- Nerve growth factors
- Gangliosides
- Continuous insulin infusions.

Management of Autonomic Neuropathy

Attention to strict glycemic control can alleviate autonomic neuropathy to some extent.[53] Other studies have found benefits with ACE inhibitors, spirono-lactone, aldose reductase inhibitors, beta- blockers and anticholinergics in various forms of autonomic neuropathy. Multifactorial intervention also helps in controlling DAN.[54]

The management of autonomic dysfunction syndromes is summarized below in **Table 69.11**.

Management of Entrapment Neuropathies/ Mononeuropathies

The main stay of nonsurgical treatment for entrapment neuropathies is rest, placement of a splint and anti-inflammatory medication. Surgical treatment is indicated when conservative methods fail, e.g. sectioning of the volar carpal ligament of Carpal-Tunnel syndrome. The management of mononeuropathies involves reassurance and physical therapy. Most of them resolve spontaneously. Carbamazepine is particularly useful for the pain of entrapment neuropathies.

Managing the pain of diabetic neuropathies: Control of pain is one of the most difficult management issues in

diabetic neuropathy. Many different pain syndromes have been described reflecting pathology at different levels of the neuraxis. There is no single correct approach to the management of any given patient, with painful neuropathy. Often it requires patience on the part of the patients and physicians who must try a variety of different medications on a trial and error basis until a satisfactory regimen is established. The general principles in the management of painful neuropathy include:
- Carefully listening to the patient's complaints
- Explanation and reassurance
- Treatment targeted at the dominant symptoms
- Timing of medications to suit the maximal intensity of pain and to decrease the side effects.

The various oral drugs used in the management of diabetic painful neuropathy are shown in **Table 69.12**.

Other drugs tried for the treatment of painful neuropathies include ibuprofen (600 mg qid), sulindac (200 mg bid), and mexiletene (150–400 per day).

Newer Agents for the Management of Diabetic Neuropathy

Pregabalin: This structural analog of gabapentin has recently been confirmed to be useful in painful diabetic neuropathy in a randomized controlled trial. In contrast to gabapentin, which is usually given in three daily doses, pregabalin is effective when given twice daily. Topiramate, another anticonvulsant used in complex partial seizures, was recently shown to be efficacious in the management of neuropathic pain.

Duloxetine: The Food and Drug Administration have recently approved the 5-hydroxy tryptamine and

TABLE 69.12	Response of specific pain syndromes to oral drugs		
Drug class	Drugs	Dose (mg per day)	Side effects
• Tricyclic antidepressants	Amitryptiline	25–150	++++
	Imipramine	25–150	++++
• SSRIs	Paroxetine	40	+++
	Citalopram	40	+++
• Anticonvulsants	Gabapentin	900–1800	++
	Pregabalin	150–600	++
	Carbamazepine	200–400	+++
	Topiramate	Upto 400	++
• Opioids	Tramadol	50–400	+++
	Oxycodone CR	10–60	++++

norepinephrine reuptake inhibitor duloxetine for the treatment of neuropathic pain.[55]

NMDA antagonists: This is a relatively new class of drugs and includes dextromethorphan and memantine. Preliminary studies of both agents suggest some efficacy in painful diabetic neuropathy, although further studies are required.

There are a lot of nonpharmacological therapies that have been tried with limited success, including sympathectomy, spinal cord blockade and electrical spinal cord stimulation. Another procedure is transcutaneous electric nerve stimulation (TENS).

Many physicians initiate treatment with either a tricyclic or an anticonvulsant. The choice of which particular drug to use within these general classes of agents may depend on the individual side effect profiles. A guide to the use of a particular agent might be based on the type of pain syndrome-the C fiber pain versus the A-delta fiber pain as shown in **Table 69.13**.

Once initiated, the drugs should be increased until the maximum dose or until side effects become prohibitive before trying other therapies. Sometimes, a

TABLE 69.13	Comparison of C-Fiber and A delta fiber mediated pain syndromes	
C Fiber Pain	A-Delta Fiber Pain
---	---
Seen in the initial stages; characterized by burning, lancinating types of pain; associated with dysesthesias, allodynia, and hyperalgesia	Deep-seated type of pain seen in later stages of the disease. Described as a dull aching pain
Treatment options: Clonidine (sympathetic blockade), and Capsaicin	Treatment options: Continuous insulin infusion, opioids, tricyclics, antiepileptics, TENS, calcitonin

combination of tricyclic antidepressants plus an anticonvulsant is effective. If this regimen is ineffective and the pain is burning and restricted to particular anatomic site or reflects allodynia (a marked hypersensitivity of the skin), it is reasonable to add capsaicin to the regimen. If the pain is still refractory to therapy, then other drugs discussed above may be tried as well as nonpharmacologic treatments.[24] In cases of severe pain, certain agents may be used in combination (e.g. an antidepressant and an anticonvulsant) or combined with a topical or nonpharmacological treatment. All patients with DPN, whether symptomatic or not, are at increased risk of foot ulceration and should be considered for pediatric referral and foot care education (**Flow chart 69.3** for management algorithm of DPN).

CONCLUSION

Despite advances, it is found that diabetic neuropathy still does not get the attention it deserves. A recent community-based study in the US found that physicians underestimate neuropathy in many patients with type 2 diabetes who are under their care and thus may be missing potential opportunities for early intervention. Physicians prospectively identified only 31 and 66% of patients with mild/moderate and severe neuropathy, respectively. The same study also showed a prevalence of neuropathy as high as 37% in a population of type 2 diabetics.[56] It is very important for all doctors, especially primary care physicians to look for and recognize diabetic neuropathy. Early diagnosis with clinical tests or simple inexpensive methods such as monofilament tests can go a long way in preventing the limb-threatening and life-threatening consequences of neuropathy.

Future management of diabetic neuropathy will be more specific with developments in the field of immunotherapy and nerve growth factors. A large

Flow chart 69.3 Management of symptomatic DPN (from Diabetic Neuropathies) (A statement by the American Diabetes Association. Diabetes Care. 2005;28:956-62)

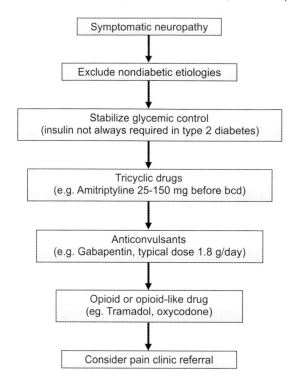

number of neurotrophic factors that exert specific effects on the specific populations in the peripheral nervous system have been discovered. Among the most promising agents are nerve growth factor, brain-derived neurotrophic factor, neurotrophin (NT)-3 and (NT)-4/5), insulin like growth factor (IGF)-II, and glial cell-derived neuroptrophic factor. Of these NGF and the IGF's have been tested most extensively in animal models of diabetic neuropathy, with encouraging results. Recombinant human nerve growth factor (rh-NGF) has been tested in phase II clinical trials for treatment of patients with diabetes and the results have been encouraging. Phase in trials of rh-NGF have been completed and clinical trials of other neurotrophic factors are likely to be conducted in the next few years.[57] It was once said that all we could do for patients with diabetic neuropathy was commiserate with them. But things are changing and we can now offer more hope. Proximal neuropathies are likely to be inflammatory or vasculitis and generally respond to immunotherapy. A large, definitive clinical trial of the various forms of immunotherapy versus placebo therapy is needed. Distal symmetric polyneuropathy remains a therapeutic challenge, but ongoing trials, particularly those targeted

at specific nerve fiber deficits, hold great promise for arrest and even reversal of the disorder.

SUMMARY

Diabetic neuropathy is a common but underdiagnosed complication of both type 1 and type 2 diabetes. Popularly classified as symmetric and asymmetric neuropathies, the common types include acute sensory neuropathy, chronic sensorimotor neuropathy, diabetic amyotrophy, autonomic neuropathy and various focal neuropathies including cranial mononeuropathies. Multiple biochemical abnormalities have been described in the nerves of diabetic subjects, which may be the direct tissue toxic consequence of hyperglycemia or secondary to the microvascular damage, which accompanies the disease process. In addition recent studies have implicated immunological abnormalities contributing to the development of diabetes peripheral neuropathy (DPN). Diabetic autonomic neuropathy can have multisystem involvement and may be the cause for significant morbidity and mortality in diabetic patients. Patients with peripheral neuropathy must be considered at risk for insensitive foot ulceration and must receive preventive education and podiatric care. Diagnosis of DPN involves clinical tests plus the use of certain simple tools, which help to objectively quantify the ongoing process. Electrophysiology may have a supportive role especially to rule out other etiologies. Current management of DPN is mostly symptomatic with the use of tricyclic antidepressants or antiepileptics for pain and general measures to take care of the foot. Autonomic neuropathy requires appropriate organ specific interventions for symptom control. Newer drugs are coming up which target the various pathophysiologic processes involved in diabetic neuropathy but most of these are in the experimental stages as of now.

REFERENCES

1. Andrew JM Boulton, Arthur I Vinik, et al. Diabetic Neuropathies: a statement by the American Diabetes Association. Diabetes Care. 2005; 28:956-62.
2. Zahar AH, Sofi FA, Laway BA, Masoodi SR, Shah NA, Dar FA. Profile of neurological complications in Diabetes: retrospective analysis of 1294 cases. Ann Saudi Med. 1997;17(1);20-5.
3. Dyck PJ, Katz KM, Kames JL, Litchy WJ, Klein R, Pach JM. The prevalence by staged severity of various types of diabetic neuropathy, retinopathy and nephropathy in a population based cohort: the Rochester Diabetic Neuropathy study. Neurology. 1993;43:817-24.

4. Thomas PK, Tomlinson DR. Diabetic and hypoglycemic neuropathy. In Dyck PJ, Thomas PK, Griffin JW, Low PA, Podulso (Eds): Peripheral neuropathy. Philadelphia :WB Saunders. 1993; pp.1219--50.

5. Thomas PK. Classification, differential diagnosis, and staging of diabetic peripheral neuropathy. Diabetes. 1997;46(Suppl 2):S54-7.

6. Asbury AK. Disease of the peripheral nervous system. In Fauci, Braunwald, Isselbacher. et al (Eds): Harrison's Principles of Internal Medicine, 14th edn. USA: McGraw-Hill. 1998;Chapter 381: 2457-68.

7. Watkins PJ, Edmonds ME. Clinical features of diabetic neuropathy. In Pickup JC, Williams G (Eds): Textbook of Diabetes, 2nd edn. London: Blackwell Science Ltd. 1997;Chapter 50:2-3.

8. Stevens MJ, Feldmen EL, Greene DA. The etiology of diabetic neuropathy: the combined roles of metabolic and vascular defects. Diabet Med. 1995;12:566-79.

9. Diabetes Control and Complications Trial (DCCT) Research Group. The effect of intensive treatment of diabetes on the development and progression of long term complications in insulin-dependent diabetes mellitus. N Engl J Med. 1993;329:977-86.

10. Greene DA, Lattimer SA. Impaired rat sciatic nerve sodium potassium adenosine triphosphatase in acute streptozotocin diabetes and its correction by dietary myoinositol supplementation. J Clin Invest. 1983;72:1058-63.

11. Greene DA, Sima AA, Stevens MJ, Feldman EL, Lattimer SA. Complications: neuropathy, pathogenetic considerations. Diabetic Care. 1992;15(12):1902-25.

12. Nagamatsu M, Nickander KK, Schmelzer JD, et al. Lipoic acid improves nerve blood flow, reduces oxidative stress and improves distal nerve conduction in experimental diabetic neuropathy. Diabetes Care. 1995;18:1160-7.

13. Hunt JV, Dean RT, Wolff SP. Hydroxyl radical production and auto-oxidative glycosylation: glucose anti oxidation as the cause of protein damage in the experimental glycation model of diabetes mellitus and ageing. Biochem J. 1988;256:205-12.

14. Feldman EL, Stevens MJ, Greene DA. Pathogenesis of diabetic neuropathy. Clin Neurosci. 1997;4:365-70.

15. Dyck PJ, Lais A, Karnes JL, et al. Fiber loss is primary and multifocal in sural nerves in diabetic polyneuropathy. Ann Neurol. 1986;19:425-39.

16. Low PA, Tuck RR, Takeuchi M. Nerve microenvironment in diabetic neuropathy. In Dyck PJ, Thomas PK, Winegard AL, Porte D (Eds): Diabetic Neuropathy. Philadelphia: WB Saunders. 1987; 16:266-78.

17. Theriault M, Dort J, Sutherland G, Zochodne DW. Local human sural nerve blood flow in diabetic and other polyneuropathies. Brain. 1997;120:1131-8.

18. Testaye S, Harris N, Jakubowski JJ, et al. Impaired blood flow and arteriovenous shunting in human diabetic neuropathy: a novel technique of nerve photography and fluorescein angiography. Diabetologica. 1993;36:1266-74.

19. Naruse K, Hamada Y, et al. Therapeutic neovascularization using cord blood-derived endothelial progenitor cells for diabetic neuropathy. Diabetes, 2005;54:1823-8.

20. Schratzberger P, Walter DH, Rittig K, Bahlmann FH, Pola R, Curry C, Silver M, Krainin JG, Weinberg DH, Ropper AH, Isner JM. Reversal of experimental diabetic neuropathy by VEGF gene transfer. J Clin Invest. 2001;107:1083-92.

21. Hellweg R, Hartung HD. Endogenous levels of nerve growth factor (NGF) are altered in experimental diabetes mellitus: a possible role for NGF in the pathogenesis of diabetic neuropathy. J Neuroscience Res. 1990;26:258-67.

22. Anand P, Terenghi G, Warner G, et al. The role of endogenous nerve growth factor in human diabetic neuropathy. Nat Med. 1996;2:703-7.

23. Said G, Goulon-Goeau C, Lacroix C, Moulonquet A. Nerve biopsy findings in different patterns of proximal diabetic neuropathy. Ann Neurol. 1994;35:559-69.

24. Vinik AL, Milicevic Z. Preventive measures and treatment options for diabetic neuropathy. Contemp Intern Med. 1994;16:41-2.

25. Vinik AL, Leichter SB, Pittenger GL, et al. Phospholipid and glutamic acid decarboxylase antibodies in diabetic neuropathy. Diabetes Care. 1995;18:1225-32.

26. Ejskjaer N, Arift S, Dodds W, et al. Prevalence of autoantibodies to autonomic nervous tissue structures in Type 1 diabetes mellitus. Diabetic Med. 1999;16: 544-9.

27. Aron IV. Diabetic neuropathy : pathogenesis and therapy. The Am J Med. 1999;107(2B):19-24s.

28. Li F, Drel VR, et al. Low-dose poly (ADP-Ribose) polymerase inhibitor-containing combination therapies reverse early peripheral diabetic neuropathy. Diabetes. 2005;54:1514-22.

29. Waxman SG. Determinants of conduction velocity in myelinated nerve fibers. Muscle Nerve. 1980;3:141-50.

30. Greene DA, Sima AAF, Pfeifer MA, Albers JW. Diabetic neuropathy. Ann Rev Med. 1990;4:303-7.

31. Pourmand R. Diabetic Neuropathy. Neurol Clin. 1997;15:569-76.

32. Bloomgarden ZT. Diabetic Retinopathy and Neuropathy. Diabetes Care. 2005;28:963-70.

33. Dryberg T, Benn J, Christiansen JS, et al. Prevalence of diabetic autonomic neuropathy measured by simple bedside tests. Diabetologica. 1981;20:190-4.

34. Sampson MJ, Wilson S, Karginni S, et al. Progression of diabetic autonomic neuropathy over a decade in insulin dependent diabetes. QJ Med. 1990;75: 635-46.

35. Vinik AL, Maser RE, Mitchell BD, Freeman R. Diabetic autonomic neuropathy (Technical Review). Diabetes Care. 2003;26:1553-79.

36. Suwanwalaikorns VA, Stansberry KB, et al. Quantitative measurement of cutaneous perception in diabetic neuropathy. Muscle Nerve. 1995;18: 574-84.

37. Arezzo JC. The use of electrophysiology for assessment of diabetic neuropathy. Neurosci Res Communications. 1997;21:13-23.

38. Yong RJ, Zhou YQ, Radriguez, et al. Variable relationship between peripheral somatic and autonomic neuropathy in patients with different syndromes of diabetic neuropathy. Diabetes. 1986; 35:192-7.

39. Holland NR, Stocks A, Hauer P, et al. Intraepidermal nerve fibre density in patients with painful neuropathy. Neurology. 1996;48:708-11.

40. Kennedy WR, Weldelschafer-Crabb G, Johnson T. Quantification of epidermal nerves in diabetic neuropathy. Neuropathy. 1996;47:1042-8.

41. McCarthy BG, Hsieh ST, Stocks A, et al. Cutaneous innervation in sensory neuropathies: evaluation by skin biopsy. Neurology. 1995;45: 1848-55.

42. Holland NR, Carwford TO, Hauer P, et al. Small-fiber sensory neuropathies clinical course and neuropathology of idiopathic cases. Ann Neurol. 1998;44:47-59.

43. Arezzo JC. Quantitative sensory testing for diabetic peripheral neuropathy, Wilmington, DE: Center for advanced study of diabetes. 1988;2:3.

44. Nicolucci A, Carinici F, Cavaliere D, et al. A meta--analysis of trials on aldose reductase inhibitors in diabetic peripheral neuropathy. Diabetic Med. 1996; B:1017-26.

45. Eaton RP, Quails C, Bicknell J, et al. Structure-function relationship with peripheral nerves in diabetic neuropathy: the hydration hypothesis. Diabetologica. 1996;39:439-46.

46. Dyck PJ, Melton LJ, O'Brien PC, Service FJ. Approaches to improve epidemiological studies of diabetic neuropathy: insights from the Ractstel Diabetic Neuropathy Study. Diabetes. 1997; 46 (Suppl 2):S5-8.

47. Faglius J, Jamson S. Effects of aldose reductase inhibitor treatment in diabetic polyneuropathy: a clinical and neurophysiological study. J Neurol Neurosurg Psychiatry. 1981;44:991-1001.

48. Handelsman TJ. Clinical trial of an aldose reductase inhibitor in diabetic neuropathy. Diabetes. 1981;30:459-64.

49. Young RJ, Ewing DJ, Clarke BF. A controlled trial of sorbinil, an aldose redutase inhibitor, in chronic painful diabetic neuropathy. Diabetes. 1983;32:938--42.

50. Judgewitsch R, Japsan J, Polonsky J. Aldose reductase inhibitors improves nerve conduction velocity in diabetic patients. N Engl J Med. 1983;308:119-25.

51. Bovlton AJM. Effects of Tolrestat: a new aldose reductase inhibitor, on nerve conduction and paraesthetic symptoms in diabetic neuropathy (Abstract). Diabetologica. 1986;29:521.

52. Krendel DA, Costigan DA, Hopkins LC. Successful treatment of neuropathies in patients with diabetes mellitus. Arch Neurol. 1995;52:1053-61.

53. Diabetes Control and Complications Trial Research Group. The effect of intensive diabetes therapy on measures of autonomic nervous system function in the Diabetes Control and Complications Trial (DCCT). Diabetologia. 1998; 41:416-23.

54. Gaede P, Vedel P, Larsen N, Jensen GV, Parving HH, Pedersen O. Multifactorial intervention and cardiovascular disease in patients with type 2 diabetes. N Engl J Med. 2003;348:383-93.

55. Wernicke J, Rosen AS, Lu Y, Iyengar S, Lee TC. Superiority of duloxetine over placebo in the treatment of diabetic neuropathic pain demonstrated in two studies (Abstract). Diabetes. 2004;53 (Suppl 2):A24.

56. Hermann W, Kennedy L. Underdiagnosis of peripheral neuropathy in type 2 diabetes. Diabetes Care. 2005;28:1480-1.

57. Apfel SC. Neurotrophic factor in the therapy of diabetic neuropathy. Am J Med. 1999;107(2B): 345-413.

Chapter 70

DIABETES MELLITUS AND GASTROINTESTINAL SYSTEM

Subrat Kumar Acharya

CHAPTER OUTLINE

- Introduction
- Diabetes and the Gut
- Epidemiology of Gastrointestinal (GI) Symptoms in Diabetes
- Diabetic Gastroparesis
- Diabetic Diarrhea
- Anorectal Dysfunction
- Other Gastrointestinal (GI) Symptoms
- Health-related Quality of Life Issues

- Liver Disease and Diabetes
- Nonalcoholic Fatty Liver Disease
- Hepatocellular Carcinoma
- Gallbladder Diseases
- Diabetes and Pancreas
- Therapeutic Modulation of Gastric Emptying
- Gut Peptides
- Conclusion

INTRODUCTION

The relationship between gastrointestinal tract and diabetes is fascinating. Postprandial blood glucose concentrations are both a determinant of, as well as determined by, the delivery of nutrients from the stomach into the small intestine. Furthermore, the prevalence of upper gastrointestinal (GI) symptoms, which occur frequently in diabetic patients are related to glycemic control. The whole GI tract including hepatobiliary system manifest effects of diabetes-induced damage **(Table 70.1)**, yet by modulating the rate of gastric emptying, interventions have the potential to become mainstream therapies in the treatment of diabetes. This complementary relationship has implications for both physiological regulation of gut function and the management of patients with diabetes. Gastrointestinal symptoms such as nausea and vomiting, heartburn, abdominal pain, diarrhea, constipation and fecal incontinence are common in patients with diabetes. Diabetes gastroenteropathy is a clinically relevant problem. In addition to the increased morbidity it causes, it results in severely impaired metabolic control, which in turn increases the risk of hyper or hypoglycemia. Moreover, the poorly controlled blood glucose level increases the risk of secondary diabetes complications, namely, retinopathy, nephropathy, neuropathy and cardiovascular disease. Gastrointestinal symptoms may also cause malnutrition in patients with diabetes, which together with the disturbed immune defense in diabetes, may cause intercurrent infections. Gastrointestinal symptoms in patients with diabetes are attributed to disturbed gastrointestinal motility. Gastrointestinal dysmotility in diabetes is believed to be caused by autonomic neuropathy and/or hyperglycemia. The neuroendocrine

TABLE 70.1	Effect of diabetes on gastrointestinal tract
Esophagus	Esophageal motility disorder
	Esophageal reflux disease
Stomach	Impaired gastric emptying
	Gastroparesis
	Diabetic dyspepsia
Small bowel	Diarrhea
	Intestinal pseudo-obstruction
Large bowel	Constipation
Anorectal	Fecal incontinence
Liver	Nonalcoholic fatty liver disease
	Hepatocellular carcinoma
Gallbladder	Gallstone disease
	Cholecystoparesis
	Emphysematous gallbladder
Pancreas	? Pancreatic cancer
Miscellaneous	Unexplained abdominal pain

system of the gut secretes peptides/amines that play an important role in regulating gastrointestinal motility. It is conceivable, therefore, that a disturbance in this regulatory system may contribute to the pathogenesis of gastrointestinal complications in diabetes. There is also increasing support for the concept that the modulation of gastric emptying could be used to optimize glycemic control in diabetes This review addresses all these issues.

DIABETES AND THE GUT

It is known that glycemic control alters several gastrointestinal functions such as gastric emptying, gastric myoelectric activity, antroduodenal motor activity, gastric visceral sensation and the colonic response to feeding. *Diabetic enteropathy* refers to all the gastrointestinal complications of diabetes and may include dysphagia, heartburn, nausea and vomiting, abdominal pain, constipation, diarrhea and fecal incontinence.[1]

EPIDEMIOLOGY OF GASTROINTESTINAL (GI) SYMPTOMS IN DIABETES

The first community based epidemiological studies on GI dysfunction in diabetics were performed in Germany and Finland.[2,3] These studies had surprising results. The only gastrointestinal problem with higher prevalence in diabetics than in controls was constipation, use of laxatives and history of gallbladder surgery. A recent questionnaire-based community study reported more diarrhea, fecal incontinence, dysphagia and postprandial fullness among diabetics than among controls.[4] In this study, 95% of the patients had type 2 diabetes. Epidemiological studies attempted to identify risk factors for developing gastrointestinal symptoms among diabetic subjects and an association of poor glycemic control and gastrointestinal symptom complexes was seen.

DIABETIC GASTROPARESIS

As early as 1937, Ferroir reported that, in diabetic patients, stomach contractions were slow, lack vigor, and die out quickly, and that treatment with insulin alleviates secretory and motor abnormalities without resulting in hypoglycemia. Kassender recognized asymptomatic gastric retention in diabetes in 1958 and coined the term *gastroparesis diabeticorum*. More recently, the term *diabetic dyspepsia* has been used to reflect the spectrum of postprandial symptoms in diabetes attributable to upper gastrointestinal dysfunctions including those associated with delayed gastric emptying. Hence, nausea, vomiting and early satiety are classical symptoms of gastroparesis, the term dyspepsia in addition reflects bloating, fullness, and pain in the upper abdomen. There is no clear association between length of disease and the onset of delayed gastric emptying. Gastroparesis affects both type 1 (insulin-dependent) and type 2 (noninsulin-dependent) forms of diabetes.

Symptoms and Signs

Nausea and vomiting, often accompanied by weight loss and early satiety, are common gastrointestinal symptoms among patients with diabetes. Episodes of nausea and vomiting may last for days to months or may be cyclical in nature. Diabetic gastroparesis is frequently associated with retinopathy, nephropathy, peripheral neuropathy and other forms of autonomic dysfunction including abnormal pupillary responses, anhidrosis, gustatory sweating, orthostatic hypotension, impotence, retrograde ejaculation and dysfunction of the urinary bladder. The diagnosis of gastroparesis may be confirmed by demonstrating gastric emptying delay during a 4-hour scintigraphic study.

Pathophysiology

Abnormal gastrointestinal motility in diabetes is multifactorial. The factors involved in pathophysiology of diabetic gastroparesis are shown in **Table 70.2**.

TABLE 70.2	Causes of diabetic gastroparesis

- Autonomic neuropathy
- Intrinsic neuropathy
- Excitatory and inhibitory nerves
- Interstitial cells of Cajal
- Acute elevations in blood glucose
- Psychosomatic factors

All these factors are associated with abnormal motor and sensory function.

Autonomic Neuropathy

Abnormal gastric motility results in impaired gastric contractility or abnormal myoelectrical control. This syndrome is more often seen in type 1 (or insulin-dependent) diabetes mellitus. The majority of patients have associated peripheral neuropathy or autonomic neuropathy. Earlier these changes were attributed to vagal dysfunction. Vagal neuropathy was considered a likely cofactor preventing the gastric accommodation response. However, now it has been seen using single photon emission computed tomography imaging that patients with diabetes and vagal neuropathy show normal postprandial changes in gastric volume.

Enteric Neuropathy

The enteric nerves have been studied in experimental animal models of diabetes. These nerves appear morphologically normal in diabetic models. However, it has been seen that there may be reduced substance P, increased VIPergic (inhibitory neurotransmitter) and increased calcitonin gene-related peptide (sensory transmitter) intrinsic neurons. These may contribute to abnormal fluid and electrolyte handling in the gut.

Abnormal Interstitial Cells of Cajal

It has been seen that the pacemaker cells in the walls of the upper digestive tract are abnormal in experimental diabetic models and this was also confirmed in a single patient with diabetes. These electrophysiological disturbances are associated with long-standing diabetes. This results in reduced volume of interstitial cells of Cajal in the antrum and fundus.

Effect of Changes in Blood Glucose

Alterations in glycemic control also alter glucose counter regulatory hormones which may directly affect gastrointestinal motility. These include growth hormone, cortisol, glucagon, glucagon-like peptide 1, epinephrine and somatostatin. These also contribute to motor dysfunction. Glycemia influences the rate of emptying. Acute changes in blood glucose concentrations affect gastric motility in diabetes; hyperglycemia slows gastric emptying whereas hypoglycemia may accelerate it; blood glucose concentrations may also influence symptoms.

Pylorospasm

Human studies at Mayo Clinic had shown earlier that diabetic gastroparesis is associated with pylorospasm.[5] This data had suggested that inhibition of pyloric tone may be a novel approach to therapy of gastroparesis. This might be achieved by restoring nitrergic innervation, replacing the cellular effects of nitric oxide by enhancing cGMP in pylori muscle with a phosphodiesterase-5 inhibitor-like Sildenafil or blocking the excitation of pyloric tone with injection of botulinum toxin.

Psychological Factors

Lutsman et al[6] have provided evidence that symptoms in diabetes are significantly influenced by psychological factors.

Treatment of Diabetic Gastroparesis

Treatment options are limited and rely on dietary modifications, judicious use of available pharmacological agents, and occasionally surgical or endoscopic placement of gastrostomies or jejunostomies **(Table 70.3)**. The general points include control of blood sugar and restoration of hydration.[7-15]

Current pharmacological agents for treating gastroparesis include metoclopramide, erythromycin,

TABLE 70.3	Management strategies for diabetic gastroparesis

- Improvement in glycemic control
- Dietary changes: Small low fat meals, devoid of indigestible fiber
- Dopamine antagonists: Metoclopramide, domperidone
- Substituted benzamides: Mosapride, itopride
- Motilin agonist: Erythromycin
- If severe dehydration: Parenteral nutrition, enteral nutrition
- In refractory chronic cases:
  - Endoscopic/Surgical gastrostomy
  - Endoscopic/Surgical jejunostomy
  - Gastric electrical stimulation (GES) with a high-frequency/low-energy stimulus
  - Near total gastrectomy and Roux-en-Y anastomosis

cisapride, mosapride, itopride and domperidone. Antidopaminergic gastrointestinal prokinetics (bromopride, clebopride, domperidone, levosulpiride and metoclopramide) have been exploited clinically for the management of motor disorders of the upper gastrointestinal tract, including functional dyspepsia, gastric stasis of various origins and emesis. The prokinetic effect of these drugs is mediated through the blockade of enteric (neuronal and muscular) inhibitory D2 receptors. It has been suggested that the serotonergic (5-HT4) component of some antidopaminergic prokinetics may enhance their therapeutic efficacy in gastrointestinal disorders, such as diabetic dyspepsia and diabetic gastroparesis.

To normalize gastric and intestinal propulsion, erythromycin at a dose of 3 mg/kg body weight given intravenously appears to be effective in acute cases. Subsequently the patient can be switched on to oral erythromycin. Erythromycin stimulates gastric motility and enhances its emptying. It has no effect on sensory function. During the acute phase, liquids and blenderized solids should be given as their gastric emptying is faster than the solids. Frequent monitoring of blood sugar is essential. Other prokinetic agents can be used as adjunctive therapy. These include metoclopramide which has a central antiemetic activity. During acute administration, it increases gastric emptying of liquids in diabetic gastroparesis but its long-term efficacy is restricted by a decline in its efficacy and its predisposition to development of extrapyramidal syndrome. Erythromycin also loses much of its stimulatory effect after the first few weeks of treatment possibly due to down-regulation of motilin receptor expression. If there is no response to prokinetic therapy and the motor dysfunction is limited to the stomach, then gastric bypass with a jejunal feeding tube can be done. Such tubes allow restoration of normal nutritional status.

Surgical therapies: The surgical therapies which have been tried are gastrostomy, jejunostomy, gastric pacing/stimulation, and gastrectomy or surgical drainage procedures.

Gastric pacing: Diabetic gastroparesis has been attributed to impaired myoelectrical activity in antrum. Hence, it has been postulated that gastric pacing will correct and entrain gastric slow wave activity and therefore improve gastric emptying. Two approaches have been proposed: Stimulation with an attempt to capture pacesetter potentials and use of only stimulation rather than pacing (high frequency gastric electrical stimulation). Gastric pacing offers promise for patients with medically refractory gastroparesis but awaits further investigation.

DIABETIC DIARRHEA

Diabetic diarrhea affects around 3.7% of diabetes predominantly patients with IDDM.[16] It is more common in men than in women. Diabetic diarrhea is often nocturnal and may have steatorrhea associated with it. The diarrhea may be cyclical with normal intervening periods as is the case with upper gastrointestinal symptoms. The natural history of lower GI symptoms and factors influencing symptom turnover in diabetes mellitus are unknown. A study has determined the natural history of GI symptoms in diabetes mellitus over a 3-year period in 892 subjects with diabetes.[17] It was seen that symptoms more often fluctuated than persisted, but the prevalence at recruitment and 3 years later was similar. In this study, multivariate analysis showed that abnormal sweating and diabetic foot problems predicted symptom turnover for abdominal pain (OR=2.01), and paresthesia (pins and needles) and foot problems predicted fecal incontinence (OR=2.24), but not constipation or diarrhea. Symptom turnover in constipation was associated with depression and neuroticism, and depression was associated with abdominal pain. The odds for symptoms persisting were not generally related to type or duration of diabetes, or self-rated glycemic control. The natural history of GI symptoms in diabetes suggests that symptoms may either persist or fluctuate, but the prevalence is constant because symptom onset is balanced by disappearance. Glycemic control does not seem to predict symptom change.

The mechanisms of chronic diarrhea, a frequent symptom in diabetes mellitus, are multifactorial and complex **(Table 70.4)**, although small intestinal bacterial overgrowth and autonomic neuropathy seem to play a major role.[18,19] Diabetic diarrhea is frequently due to celiac sprue, bacterial overgrowth in the small bowel, or fecal incontinence in conjunction with anorectal dysfunction; however, in almost 50% of the patients, these causes can be excluded, and abnormal intestinal

TABLE 70.4	Causes of diabetic diarrhea

- Drug-induced metformin
- Celiac sprue
- Bacterial overgrowth
- Fecal incontinence
- Diabetic autonomic neuropathy

motility or secretion is postulated to be one of the likely causes of the diarrhea. Small intestinal bacterial overgrowth should be actively searched for because of its high frequency in diabetic diarrhea, facility of diagnosis, and often successful treatment with antibiotics. In diabetic diarrhea, marked abnormalities are found in the motor patterns of the small intestine. There may be abnormalities of Phase 2 and 3 contractions in the motor pattern. However, whole gut transit times and mouth-to-cecum times are often similar to healthy controls. The pathogenesis of diarrhea is because of decreased intestinal resorption rather than intestinal dysmotility as adrenergic function is impaired because of autonomic neuropathy.

A practical algorithm based on three sequential assessments would be: first, tests of blood and stool specimens and flexible sigmoidoscopy to detect evidence of malabsorption or disease in the distal colon; second, small bowel aspirate and biopsy if the results of initial blood or stool tests are abnormal or anorectal function tests if those test results are normal; and, finally, measurement of gastrointestinal transit or therapeutic trials with opioids, clonidine hydrochloride, and rarely, cholestyramine resin or octreotide acetate.

The management involves use of adrenergic agonists to stimulate intestinal absorption of fluids or electrolytes (Table 70.5). The α 2 adrenergic agonist clonidine (0.1-0.6 mg twice daily) reverses peripheral adrenergic resorptive abnormalities. Octreotide (50 to 75 μg subcutaneously daily) has also been used to treat refractory cases.[20] However, by decreasing intestinal transit time, it may in a few cases predispose to small bacterial overgrowth and paradoxical resurgence of diarrhea.

TABLE 70.5	Management strategies for diabetic diarrhea

- Strict glycemic control
- Avoid medications like—biguanides, α-glucosidase inhibitors, tetrahydrolipostatins
- Symptomatic measures—codeine sulfate, diphenoxylate with atropine, loperamide, psyllium hydrophilic mucilloid
- Adrenergic agonists—clonidine
- Octreotide, somatostatin
- Oral quinolones to treat superimposed bacterial overgrowth syndrome

ANORECTAL DYSFUNCTION

Fecal incontinence is defined as the involuntary loss of stool at any time of life after toilet training. It is a socially and psychologically devastating condition for patients and their families, and a topic which both patients and physicians are reluctant to approach. Patients with long-standing diabetes mellitus have increased incidence of fecal incontinence and severely impaired function of both the anal sphincters and the rectum. These findings could be attributed to the increased incidence of microangiopathy and autonomic and peripheral neuropathy observed in this subset of diabetic patients. In contrast to earlier concepts which promoted the concept that high stool volumes overwhelm normal continence mechanisms, recent studies indicate that the vast majority of diabetic patients with fecal incontinence have normal or only moderately increased daily stool volumes, but exhibit multiple abnormalities of anorectal sensory and motor functions.[21,22] These changes are not observed in continent diabetic patients. In diabetic subjects, hyperglycemia is associated with reduction in maximal and plateau anal squeeze pressures and the rectal pressure/volume relationship (compliance) during barostat distension. Hyperglycemia has no effect on the perception of rectal distension. In patients with diabetes, acute hyperglycemia inhibits external anal sphincter function and decreases rectal compliance, potentially increasing the risk of fecal incontinence.[23,24] Treatment consists of pharmacologic and dietary interventions to modulate diarrhea, and biofeedback techniques to improve rectal sensory thresholds and striated muscle responsiveness of continence mechanisms. This dual approach is often successful and is free of risks. Surgery may be the best option for cases refractory to medical treatment.

OTHER GASTROINTESTINAL (GI) SYMPTOMS

Colon Related

The colon is frequently involved in diabetes. The most common gastrointestinal complaint is constipation, rarely chronic intestinal pseudo-obstruction may also occur. Severe constipation may lead on to sequelae like stercoral ulcer, perforation, volvulus and over flow diarrhea.

Unexplained Abdominal Pain

Diabetic radiculopathy may cause unexplained upper abdominal pain in patients with diabetic neuropathy. The diagnosis may be supported by an abnormal electromyography (EMG) of the anterior abdominal wall muscles when compared with an EMG of thoracic paraspinal muscles.

Esophageal Dysfunction

Delayed esophageal transit and abnormal esophageal motility occur frequently in patients with long-standing diabetes, and the prevalence of gastroesophageal reflux disease also appears to be increased. In healthy volunteers, marked hyperglycemia decreases lower esophageal sphincter pressure but increases the duration of peristaltic waves. Abnormal esophageal motor activity is so common in patients with diabetic autonomic neuropathy that the absence of this sign in persons with gastrointestinal symptoms leads to a doubt on the diagnosis of diabetic gastroenteropathy. Diabetic autonomic neuropathy leads to absence of coordinated peristaltic activity and the presence of many low-amplitude, double-peaked, and tertiary contractions. Such esophageal disturbances are frequently asymptomatic, although dysphagia can be seen in as many as one-third of patients. Frequently, they are asymptomatic because of concomitant sensory diabetic neuropathy.

HEALTH RELATED QUALITY OF LIFE ISSUES

Morbidity from GI symptoms in diabetes is considered to be high, but there is a scarcity of studies which have quantified the impact of GI symptoms in diabetes on health-related quality of life. Available data suggest that there is a clinically significant decrease in quality-of-life scores in diabetes compared with population norms across all subscales.[25] The impact on quality of life in diabetes is predominantly observed in type 2 diabetes. Individually all GI symptom groups are significantly associated with poorer quality of life in diabetes, independent of age, gender, smoking, alcohol use, and type of diabetes.

LIVER DISEASE AND DIABETES

There is compelling evidence to suggest a link between liver disease and diabetes. The link suggests that: (1) Liver disease causes diabetes; (2) Diabetes contributes to or causes liver disease. The liver diseases which bear testimony to it are hepatitis C, nonalcoholic fatty liver disease, hepatocellular carcinoma.

Hepatitis C

There is strong evidence of an association between chronic hepatitis C and diabetes. Third National Health and Nutrition Examination Survey (NHANES III) done in USA showed that the rate of diabetes among those 40 years of age and older was three times higher among those with hepatitis C virus infection compared with those who did not have hepatitis C virus infection.[26] Another study in cirrhotics being evaluated for transplantation showed that, diabetes mellitus was present in 50% of 34 patients with hepatitis C compared with only 9% of 66 patients with cirrhosis caused by other conditions.[27]

Epidemiological studies in the form of case control studies and cohort studies have shown that hepatitis C virus (HCV) infection is independently associated with type 2 diabetes mellitus.[28-30] The association of HCV with diabetes is seen even before the onset of cirrhosis.[31] This association is in marked contrast to patients with **hepatitis B** virus (HBV) infection who do not have an increased prevalence of diabetes.[32]

There is growing evidence in medical literature to call hepatitis C as a metabolic disease.[33] Alterations in hepatic lipid and carbohydrate metabolism are commonly observed in chronic hepatitis C. The hypothesis explaining the connection between HCV and the onset of type 2 diabetes is being gradually formed. One of the suggested possibilities is: insulin resistance may just be a consequence of steatosis. Hepatic steatosis is recognized as a component of the metabolic syndrome, a condition that arises from insulin resistance and that precedes the onset of type 2 diabetes.[34] Chronic hepatitis C is associated with hepatic steatosis to a greater extent than other etiology of chronic liver disease. Transgenic mouse and cellular models of hepatitis C have demonstrated a highly reproducible occurrence of lipid accumulation in liver which further suggests that metabolic alterations resulting in fat accumulation in hepatocytes can be a direct effect of HCV.[35] Intracellular fat accumulation by itself causes insulin resistance. Interventions reducing intracellular triglyceride content improve insulin sensitivity. Hence, the connection between hepatitis C and diabetes could be secondary to the ability of HCV to induce hepatic steatosis. The second hypothesis is that direct effect of HCV proteins has a direct effect on insulin-signaling pathways. Insulin action is mediated by binding to the cell-surface insulin receptor, a ligand-activated tyrosine kinase. After insulin binding, the receptor undergoes autophosphorylation with activation of kinase activity. The signal is transmitted by subsequent tyrosine phosphorylation of a family of insulin-receptor substrates (IRS) (IRS-1, IRS-2, IRS-3 and IRS--4). After tyrosine phosphorylation, the IRS proteins serve as docking sites for src homology (SH) domain proteins, which transmit the signal to the downstream molecules that control glucose metabolism, lipid metabolism, and cell growth and differentiation.

There is also evidence to suggest that rapid fibrosis progression occurs in the presence of diabetes and hepatic steatosis in chronic hepatitis C.[36-38] Studies evaluating the temporal relationship of steatosis with the onset of diabetes in hepatitis C would greatly facilitate interventions that prevent the development of steatosis and would have the potential to prevent HCV-associated type 2 diabetes and to slow the progression of the disease itself.

NONALCOHOLIC FATTY LIVER DISEASE

Nonalcoholic fatty liver disease (NAFLD) is being increasingly recognized as a common liver disorder that represents the hepatic manifestation of the metabolic syndrome, an aggregate of disorders related to obesity, insulin resistance, type II diabetes, hypertension and hyperlipidemia. Nonalcoholic steatohepatitis (NASH) is the progressive form of liver injury that carries a risk for progressive fibrosis, cirrhosis, and end-stage liver disease. Hepatocellular carcinoma (HCC) is a documented complication in an as yet unknown percentage of cases of NASH. The clinical diagnosis is based on the presence of the insulin resistance syndrome and exclusion of alcohol abuse as well as viral, autoimmune, genetic, and drug-induced liver diseases.

NAFLD is associated with insulin resistance, which may be evident clinically with obesity, type 2 diabetes mellitus, and hypertriglyceridemia. NASH has been associated with type 2 diabetes mellitus and glucose intolerance, with or without superimposed obesity. Type 2 diabetes, hyperglycemia, and glucose intolerance have been described in 20 to 75% of adult patients with NASH. Wanless and Lentz reported that a history of type 2 diabetes was associated with a 2.6-fold increase in the prevalence of NASH.[39] The association between type 2 diabetes and NASH is greatest in morbidly obese patients. Although NAFLD is known to occur in overtly lean individuals, which indicates that excessive adiposity is not required for the development of NAFLD, the severities of insulin resistance and NAFLD tend to parallel each other, and the greatest prevalence of type 2 diabetes occurs in patients with NAFLD and cirrhosis. This observation suggests that insulin resistance and NAFLD may be related pathogenically. Experiments in mice demonstrate that insulin resistance and NAFLD result from a chronic inflammatory state that is characterized by increased levels of TNF-α. Although diabetes and obesity were initially held culpable, insulin resistance (IR) is now considered the fundamental operative mechanism. IR is probably the "first step" in nonalcoholic steatohepatitis. Essentially, it is hypothesized that high circulating insulin levels are associated with defective fatty acid oxidation in mitochondria, resulting in intracytoplasmic accumulation of triglycerides. This accumulated fat then incites an inflammatory and fibrotic response. Oxidative stress may be the elusive "second" of possibly multiple steps in the progression of steatosis to fibrosing steatohepatitis. Factors that modulate the life expectancy of patients with NASH are not known, but older age, obesity, diabetes mellitus, and AST/ALT>1 have been shown to be significant predictors of severe liver fibrosis.[40]

HEPATOCELLULAR CARCINOMA

There is also a well-documented association between diabetes and hepatocellular carcinoma (HCC). Earlier epidemiologic studies showed no association between DM and HCC,[41] whereas subsequent studies indicate a significant association between HCC and DM.[42] As early as 1986, Lawson et al noted a 4-fold greater incidence of diabetes among patients with HCC in Scotland compared with controls.[43] The observation was confirmed in both Italy and Sweden.[44,45] However, the temporal association between DM and HCC in these studies is unclear. Because the development of chronic liver disease may lead to glucose intolerance and occasionally diabetes, the study of the risk of chronic liver disease and HCC from DM requires longitudinal cohort studies that exclude most cases of chronic liver disease at the time the identification of diabetes is made. In a longitudinal cohort study, El-Serag et al[46] provided the evidence that long-standing diabetes is followed by the development of liver disease and HCC, suggesting a causative role for diabetes mellitus. It appears that it is type 2 rather than type 1 diabetes that leads to liver disease. The pathophysiology underlying the increased risk of chronic nonalcoholic liver disease and HCC with diabetes is not certain. Whether HCC occurs because of insulin resistance, which leads to NASH progressing to cirrhosis, or whether the stimulatory effects of insulin on hepatocyte growth lead more directly to neoplasia, remains unclear till date.

GALLBLADDER DISEASES

There is convincing evidence of an increased prevalence of gallstones in patients with diabetes mellitus, from both autopsy and epidemiological studies.[47] The chemical composition of these stones has not been investigated, but it is generally accepted that they are rich in cholesterol. Diabetics tend to be obese and to have hypertriglyceridemia, and both of these conditions are associated with an increased risk of gallstones.

Gallstones

Diabetic patients do have a higher prevalence of gallstones than the normal population, and diabetic women have a higher prevalence of gallstones than non-diabetic women. In a recent case-control study, Santis et al[48] have shown that the prevalence of diabetes in the subjects affected by gallstone disease was significantly higher than that in controls (11.6% vs 4.8%), and that diabetes was frequent, even according to sex (18.3% vs 9.9% for men and 9.3% vs 2.6% for women). Several observations suggest an association between diabetes and gallstone disease. Gallbladder motor function abnormalities and supersaturated bile have been described in patients with diabetes. The fasting gallbladder volume of diabetic subjects is greater than the control subjects. The postprandial gallbladder ejection fraction is reduced in diabetic subjects, and may predispose such patients to gallstone formation. It is generally believed that patients with diabetes, at least those with maturity-onset diabetes, secrete a supersaturated bile. However, in the few studies that have compared diabetes with age- and weight-matched controls, neither the type 1 nor the type 2 diabetes have been shown to secrete a more lithogenic bile than controls. Therefore, the secretion of lithogenic bile by diabetes does not explain satisfactorily the higher frequency of gallstones in this population.

Biliary sepsis tends to be more severe in diabetic patients. In addition to severe bouts of cholecystitis and ascending cholangitis, unusual infections with gas-producing organisms and rare abscesses due to *Yersinia enterocolitica* have been reported. Presence of type 2 diabetes also predisposes to emphysematous gall-bladder. An increased incidence of *sclerosing cholangitis* has also been reported in diabetic patients.[49] Despite the increased severity of cholecystitis and cholangitis in diabetic patients, however, it is not recommended that diabetic patients with asymptomatic gallstones undergo prophylactic cholecystectomy.

Diabetic Cholecystoparesis

Type 2 diabetic patients have an impaired absolute gallbladder emptying (as assessed by cholescintigraphy) and only a minor reduction in net volume changes (as assessed by ultrasonography). The reduced gallbladder postprandial turnover in diabetes reflects stasis of the gallbladder contents and contributes to the effect of cholesterol nucleation promoting factors in enhancing cholesterol crystal precipitation and gallstone formation, as well as a reduced efficiency of the gallbladder in eliminating its contents, including cholesterol crystals.

The exact mechanisms for the impairment in postprandial gallbladder emptying in diabetics are not known. It is reported that type 2 diabetic patients with gallstones, fasting serum insulin and daily average insulin levels are higher than in type 2 diabetic patients without gallstones. Several studies have recently pointed to the effect of blood glucose concentrations in the regulation of gastrointestinal motility both in healthy subjects and in diabetics. In healthy volunteers acute hyperglycemia dose-dependently inhibits both cholecystokinin (CCK) and meal-stimulated gallbladder emptying, as well as CCK-stimulated pancreatic polypeptide secretion, suggesting impaired cholinergic activity during hyperglycemia. In healthy subjects, acute hyperglycemia and also euglycemic hyperinsulinemia have been shown to reduce basal duodenal bilirubin output and inhibit gallbladder emptying stimulated by infusion of low-dose CCK, producing plasma CCK levels similar to those seen after a low-fat meal. This inhibitory effect was more pronounced during hyper-glycemia than during euglycemic hyperinsulinemia. Higher levels of plasma CCK seem to overcome the inhibitory effect of glucose and insulin. In type 1 diabetes, euglycemia, the gallbladder contraction in response to CCK is not different from controls, whereas during hyperglycemia it is significantly reduced.

Erythromycin, and some of its analogs, are potent motilin receptor agonists and will stimulate gastro-intestinal motor activity in many species, including humans. It has been reported that erythromycin stimulates gallbladder emptying in humans, in both normal subjects and those with gallstone disease. Cisapride is a gastrointestinal prokinetic agent that increases gastrointestinal motility by stimulating the release of acetylcholine from cholinergic nerve endings. Cisapride has also been shown to decrease the fasting and postprandial gallbladder volumes.[50]

DIABETES AND PANCREAS

Tropical chronic pancreatitis (TCP) is generally a disease of youth and early adulthood.[51] Over 90% of patients develop the illness prior to the age of 40 years. The disease typically presents with abdominal pain, severe malnutrition, and exocrine or endocrine insufficiency.

Steatorrhea is rare owing to a generally very low fat intake. Endocrine insufficiency is an inevitable consequence of TCP and is often classified as a specific cause of diabetes called fibrocalculous pancreatic diabetes.[52-54] Pancreatic calculi develop in over 90% of these patients. The pathology is characterized by large, intraductal calculi, marked dilation of the main pancreatic duct, and gland atrophy. FCPD is considered in detail in another chapter. In the western world, alcoholic chronic pancreatitis (ACP) is the common type of chronic pancreatitis.

Endocrine insufficiency with secondary diabetes is a consequence of long-standing chronic pancreatitis. Islet cells appear to be relatively resistant to destruction in chronic pancreatitis. When diabetes occurs in chronic pancreatitis, both insulin-producing β-cells and glucagon-producing α-cells are destroyed, unlike type 1 diabetes mellitus, in which β-cells are selectively destroyed. Deficiency of insulin and glucagon in chronic pancreatitis leads to a brittle type of diabetes. In patients with diabetes due to chronic pancreatitis, compensatory endogenous release of glucagon in response to hypoglycemia is absent. Exogenous administration of insulin in these patients may therefore lead to prolonged and severe hypoglycemia.

Diabetes mellitus appears to be nearly as common as steatorrhea in patients with far-advanced chronic pancreatitis. In one study, the median time to develop diabetes was 19.8 years, 11.9 years, and 26.3 years in patients with alcoholic, late-onset idiopathic, and early-onset idiopathic chronic pancreatitis, respectively.[55] A recent study reported development of diabetes in 9.6 years in TCP patients.[56] Shorter median times of 6 to 10 years have been observed in others. Ultimately, 40 to 70% of patients will develop diabetes after prolonged follow-up in ACP and upto 90% in TCP. Microangiopathic complications are as common in patients with diabetes associated with chronic pancreatitis (FCPD) as in patients with type 1 diabetes, if corrected for disease duration.[57-63]

According to the published data, about 70% of patients with pancreatic cancer have impaired glucose tolerance (IGT) or frank diabetes, whereas 30% do not. Adenocarcinoma of the pancreas is two to four times more common in diabetic alcoholics than in the general population. In some cases, it is difficult to determine whether the diabetes antedates or is caused by the malignancy, and recent data suggest that the relationship between pancreatic cancer and diabetes may be an epiphenomenon and that diabetes is not a risk factor for pancreatic malignancy.[64,65]

Oral Hypoglycemic Drugs and Gastrointestinal Symptoms

Gastrointestinal symptoms are commonly reported as side effects of drugs, including oral hypoglycemics, particularly metformin and α-glucosidase inhibitors. However, due to the high background incidence of gastrointestinal symptoms it may be very difficult to distinguish between spontaneous and truly drug-related gastrointestinal symptoms. In a study evaluating 956 subjects with type 2 diabetes, logistic regression analysis showed that metformin use was independently associated with chronic diarrhea and fecal incontinence.[66] Use of sulfonylureas is associated with mild abdominal pain, but not with any other gastrointestinal symptom. The mechanism causing diarrhea in diabetes patients taking metformin is not clear. Increased intestinal motility can be a possible mechanism.

THERAPEUTIC MODULATION OF GASTRIC EMPTYING

The potential for modulation of the rate of gastric emptying to be therapeutically useful in the control of postprandial hyperglycemia in diabetic patients is now being explored. In type 1 diabetes, interventions that improve the coordination between nutrient absorption and the action of exogenous insulin would be expected to be beneficial; in patients with type 1 diabetes and delayed gastric emptying, both the rate of emptying and the HbA$_{1c}$ improved after 6 months of treatment with the prokinetic drug levosulpiride, a D$_2$-dopamine receptor antagonist. Conversely, when gastric emptying was increased with cisapride, postprandial blood glucose levels increased; HbA$_{1c}$ concentration was unchanged after 8 weeks of treatment, possibly because the acceleration of gastric emptying was modest. In type 2 diabetes, slowing the absorption of nutrients should prove to be effective, in line with the delayed release of insulin characteristic of this disorder; for example, an increase in meal viscosity using guar gum, and parenteral administration of the human amylin analog, pramlintide (AC137), reduce postprandial blood glucose concentrations in type 2 diabetes, predominantly by slowing gastric emptying.[67]

GUT PEPTIDES

Extensive research during the past three decades has identified two gut hormones, glucagon-like peptide-1 (GLP-1) and glucose-dependent insulinotropic peptide

(GIP, also known as gastric inhibitory polypeptide) that are important in postprandial glucose metabolism.[68,69] Both peptides are incretins; they are secreted during carbohydrate absorption and increase insulin secretion. Since they are potent insulin secretagogues, GIP and GLP-1 have received considerable attention as potential diabetes therapeutics. However, only GLP-1 exerts insulinotropic properties when administered to patients with type 2 diabetes. However, the effect of GLP-1 on postprandial blood glucose concentrations is mediated predominantly by slowing gastric emptying. The usefulness of GLP-1 in clinical practice awaits the development of an analog of sufficiently long half-life to be effective by subcutaneous injection or by an alternative route.

CONCLUSION

Disordered gastrointestinal function in diabetes has been attributed to irreversible autonomic neuropathy, and changes in upper-gut motor and sensory function. Prolonged as well as acute hyperglycemia appears to affect every region of the gastrointestinal tract. Gastrointestinal symptoms affecting esophagus to anorectum are common in patients with diabetes. Of these, the most trouble some are diabetic gastroparesis, diarrhea and fecal incontinence. Clinical symptoms of enteric diabetic autonomic neuropathy are more common in older patients with long-standing insulin-dependent diabetes, poor glucose control, and symptoms of cardiovascular or peripheral neuropathy. At present, the treatment of these conditions is ungratifying for the physician. However, better understanding of enteric nervous system will greatly facilitate progress in treatment of diabetic enteropathy. Besides, association of diabetes mellitus with NAFLD and hepatitis C infection has been established. Diabetics also have been shown to have higher frequency of gallstones. On the other hand, primary GI tract diseases like chronic pancreatitis leads to diabetes mellitus.

REFERENCES

1. Feldman M, Schiller ER. Disorders of gastrointestinal motility associated with diabetes mellitus. Ann Intern Med. 1983;98:378-84.
2. Enck P, Rathmann W, Spiekermann M, et al. Prevalence of gastrointestinal symptoms in diabetic patients and non-diabetic subjects. Z Gastroenterol. 1994;32:637-41.
3. Janatuinen E, Pikkarainen P, Laakso M, Pyorala K. Gastrointestinal symptoms in middle-aged diabetic patients. Scand Gastroenterol.1993;28:427-32.
4. Bytzer P, Talley NJ, Leemon M, et al. Prevalence of gastrointestinal symptoms associated with diabetes mellitus: a population-based survey of 15,000 adults. Arch Intern Med. 2001;161:1989-96.
5. Mearin F, Camilleri M, Malagelada JR. Pyloric dysfunction in diabetics with recurrent nausea and vomiting. Gastroenterology. 1986;90:1919-25.
6. Lustman PJ, Anderson RJ, Freedland KE, et al. Depression and poor glycemic control: a meta- analytic review of the literature. Diabetes Care. 2000;23:934-42.
7. Tonini M, Cipollina L, Poluzzi E, Crema F, Corazza GR, DePonti F. Clinical implications of enteric and central D2 receptor blockade by antidopaminergic gastrointestinal prokinetics. Aliment Pharmacol Ther. 2004;15:379-90.
8. Gentilcore D, O'Donovan D, Jones KL, Horowitz M. Nutrition therapy for diabetic gastroparesis. Curr Diab Rep. 2003;3:418-26.
9. Smith DS, Ferris CD. Current concepts in diabetic gastroparesis. Drugs. 2003;63:1339-58.
10. Talley NJ. Diabetic gastropathy and prokinetics. Am J Gastroenterol. 2003;98:264-71.
11. Maganti K, Onyemere K, Jones MP. Oral erythromycin and symptomatic relief of gastroparesis: a systematic review. Am J Gastroenterol. 2003 ;98:259-63.
12. Lata PF, Pigarelli DL. Chronic metoclopramide therapy for diabetic gastroparesis. Ann Pharmacother. 2003;37:122-6.
13. Jones MP, Maganti K. A systematic review of surgical therapy for gastroparesis. Am J Gastroenterol. 2003;98:2122-9.
14. Lin Z, Forster J, Sarosiek I, McCallum RW. Treatment of diabetic gastroparesis by high-frequency gastric electrical stimulation. Diabetes Care. 2004;27:1071-6.
15. Watkins PJ, Buxton-Thomas MS, Howard ER. Long-term outcome after gastrectomy for intractable diabetic gastroparesis. Diabet Med. 2003;20:58-63.
16. Lysy J, Israeli E, Goldin E. The prevalence of chronic diarrhea among diabetic patients. Am J Gastroenterol. 1999;94:2165-70.
17. Talley NJ, Howell S, Jones MP, Horowitz M. Predictors of turnover of lower gastrointestinal symptoms in diabetes mellitus. Am J Gastroenterol. 2002;97:3087--94.
18. Valdovinos MA, Camilleri M, Zimmerman BR. Chronic diarrhea in diabetes mellitus: mechanisms and an approach to diagnosis and treatment. Mayo Clin Proc. 1993;68:691-702.
19. Virally-Monod M, Tielmans D, Kevorkian JP, Bouhnik Y, Flourie B, Porokhov B, Ajzenberg C, Warnet A, Guillausseau PJ. Chronic diarrhoea and diabetes mellitus: prevalence of small intestinal bacterial overgrowth. Diabetes Metab. 1998;24:530-6.
20. Meyer C, O'Neal DN, Connell W, Alford F, Ward G, Jenkins AJ. Octreotide treatment of severe diabetic diarrhoea. Intern Med J. 2003;33:617-8.
21. Wald A. Incontinence and anorectal dysfunction in patients with diabetes mellitus. Eur J Gastroenterol Hepatol. 1995;7:737-9.
22. Russo A, Botten R, Kong MF, Chapman IM, Fraser RJ, Horowitz M, Sun WM. Effects of acute hyperglycaemia on anorectal motor and sensory function in diabetes mellitus. Diabet Med. 2004;21:176-82.
23. Cooper ZR, Rose S. Fecal incontinence: a clinical approach. Mt Sinai J Med. 2000;67:96-105.
24. Epanomeritakis E, Koutsoumbi P, Tsiaoussis I, Ganotakis E, Vlata M, Vassilakis JS, Xynos E. Impairment of anorectal

function in diabetes mellitus parallels duration of disease. Dis Colon Rectum. 1999;42:1394-400.

25. Talley NJ, Young L, Bytzer P, Hammer J, Leemon M, Jones M, Horowitz M. Impact of chronic gastrointestinal symptoms in diabetes mellitus on health-related quality of life. Am J Gastroenterol. 2001;96:71-6.

26. Mehta SH, Brancati FL, Sulkowski MS, Strathdee SA, Szklo M, Thomas DL. Prevalence of type 2 diabetes mellitus among persons with hepatitis C virus infection in the United States. Ann Intern Med 2001;133:592-599.

27. Allison ME, Wreghitt T, Palmer CR, Alexander GJ. Evidence for a link between hepatitis C virus infection and diabetes mellitus in a cirrhotic population. J Hepatol 1994;21:1135-1139.

28. Mason AL, Lau JY, Hoang N, Qian K, Alexander GJ, Xu L, Guo L, Jacob S, Regenstein FG, Zimmerman R, Everhart JE, Wasserfall C, Maclaren NK, Perrillo RP. Association of diabetes mellitus and chronic hepatitis C virus infection. Hepatology. 1999;29:328-33.

29. Caronia S, Taylor K, Pagliaro L, Carr C, Palazzo U, Petrik J, O'Rahilly S, Shore S, Tom BD, Alexander GJ. Further evidence for an association between non-insulin-dependent diabetes mellitus and chronic hepatitis C virus infection. Hepatology. 1999;30:1059-63.

30. Grimbert S, Valensi P, Levy-Marchal C, Perret G, Richardet JP, Raffoux C, Trinchet JC, Beaugrand M. High prevalence of diabetes mellitus in patients with chronic hepatitis C. A case-control study. Gastroenterol Clin Biol. 1996;20:544-8.

31. Knobler H, Schihmanter R, Zifroni A, Fenakel G, Schattner A. Increased risk of type 2 diabetes in noncirrhotic patients with chronic hepatitis C virus infection. Mayo Clin Proc. 2000;75:355-9.

32. Fraser GM, Harman I, Meller N, Niv Y, Porath A. Diabetes mellitus is associated with chronic hepatitis C but not chronic hepatitis B infection. Isr J Med Sci. 1996;32:526-30.

33. Weinman SA, Belalcazar LM. Hepatitis C: a metabolic liver disease. Gastroenterology. 2004;126:917-9.

34. Marchesini G, Brizi M, Bianchi G, Tomassetti S, Bugianesi E, Lenzi M, McCullough AJ, Natale S, Forlani G, Melchionda N. Nonalcoholic fatty liver disease: a feature of the metabolic syndrome. Diabetes. 2001;50:1844-50.

35. Lerat H, Honda M, Beard MR, Loesch K, Sun J, Yang Y, Okuda M, Gosert R, Xiao SY, Weinman SA, Lemon SM. Steatosis and liver cancer in transgenic mice expressing the structural and nonstructural proteins of hepatitis C virus. Gastroenterology 2002;122:352--65.

36. Ratziu V, Munteanu M, Charlotte F, Bonyhay L, Poynard T. Fibrogenic impact of high serum glucose in chronic hepatitis C. J Hepatol. 2003;39:1049-55.

37. Hu KQ, Kyulo NL, Esrailian E, Thompson K, Chase R, Hillebrand DJ, Runyon BA. Overweight and obesity, hepatic steatosis, and progression of chronic hepatitis C: a retrospective study on a large cohort of patients in the United States. J Hepatol. 2004;40:147-54.

38. Hickman IJ, Powell EE, Prins JB, Clouston AD, Ash S, Purdie DM, Jonsson JR. In overweight patients with chronic hepatitis C, circulating insulin is associated with hepatic fibrosis: implications for therapy. J Hepatol. 2003;39:1042-8.

39. Wanless I, Lentz J. Fatty liver hepatitis (steatohepatitis) and obesity: an autopsy study with analysis of risk factors. Hepatology. 1990;12:1106-10.

40. Angulo P, Keach J, Batts K, Lindor K. Independent predictors of liver fibrosis in patients with nonalcoholic steatohepatitis. Hepatology. 1999;30:1356-62.

41. Ragozzino M, Melton LJ III, Chu CP, Palumbo PJ. Subsequent cancer risk in the incidence cohort of Rochester, Minnesota, residents with diabetes mellitus. J Chronic Dis. 1982;35:13-9.

42. Kingston ME, Ali MA, Atiyeh M, Donnelly RJ. Diabetes mellitus in chronic active hepatitis and cirrhosis. Gastroenterology 1984;87:688-94.

43. Lawson DH, Gray JMB, McKillop C, Clarke J, Lee FD, Patrick RS. Diabetes mellitus and primary hepatocellular carcinoma. Q J Med. 1986;234:945-55.

44. LaVecchia C, Negri E, DeCarli A, Franceschi S. Diabetes mellitus and the risk of primary liver cancer. Int J Cancer. 1997;73:204-7.

45. Adami HO, Chow WH, Nyren O, Berne C, Linet MS, Ekbom A, Wolk A, McLaughlin JK, Fraumeni JF. Excess risk of primary liver cancer in patients with diabetes mellitus. J Natl Cancer Inst. 1996;88:1472-7.

46. El-Serag HB, Tran T, Everhart JE. Diabetes increases the risk of chronic liver disease and hepatocellular carcinoma. Gastroenterology. 2004;126:460-8.

47. Chapman BA, Wilson IR, Frampton CM, et al. Prevalence of gallbladder disease in diabetes mellitus. Dig Dis Sci. 1996;41:2222-8.

48. De Santis, A, Attili, AF, Ginanni Corradini S, et al. Gallstones and diabetes: a case-control study in a free-living population sample. Hepatology. 1997;25:787-90.

49. Lillemoe KD, Pitt HA, Cameron JL. Sclerosing cholangitis. Adv Surg. 1988,21.65-92.

50. Dhiman RK, Arke L, Bhansali A, Gupta S, Chawla YK. Cisapride improves gallbladder emptying in patients with type 2 diabetes mellitus. J Gastroenterol Hepatol. 2001;16:1044-50.

51. Mohan V, Pitchumoni CS. Tropical Chronic Pancreatitis. In The Pancreas (Vol 1). Beger HG, Warshaw AL, Buchler MW, Carr-Locke DL, Neoptolemos JP, Russell C, Sarr MG (Eds). London: Blackwell Science. 1998. pp. 688-97.

52. Mohan V, Nagalotimath SJ, Yajnik CS, Tripathy BB. Fibrocalculous Pancreatic Diabetes. Diabetes Metabolism Reviews. 1998;14:153-70.

53. Mohan V, Premalatha G. Fibrocalculous Pancreatic Diabetes. International Journal of Diabetes. 1995;3:71-82.

54. Mohan V, Rema M, Susheela L, et al. Tropical pancreatic diabetes in south India: heterogeneity in clinical and biochemial profile. Diabetologia. 1985;28:229-32.

55. Layer P, Yamamoto H, Kalthoff L, et al. The different courses of early- and late-onset idiopathic and alcoholic chronic pancreatitis. Gastroenterology. 1994; 107:1481.

56. Mohan V, Barman KK, Rajan VS, Chari ST, Deepa R. Natural history of endocrine failure in tropical chronic pancreatitis: a longitudinal follow-up study. Journal of Gastroenterology and Hepatalogy. 2005;20:1927--34.

57. Rema M, Rajendran B, Mohan V, Ramachandran A, Viswanathan M, Kohner EM. Retinopathy in Tropical Pancreatic Diabetes. Archives of Ophthalmology. 1985;103:1487-9.

58. Ramachandran A, Mohan V, Kumaravel TS, et al. Peripheral neuropathy in tropical pancreatic diabetes. Acta Diabetologica Latina. 1985;23:135-40.

59. Mohan V, Ramachandran A, Viswanathan M. Two case reports of macrovascular complications in fibrocalculous pancreatic diabetes. Acta Diabetol. 1989;26:345-9.

60. Mohan V, Premalatha G, Padma A, et al. Fibrocalculous pancreatic diabetes—long-term survival analysis. Diabetes Care. 1996;19:1274-8.

61. Shelgikar KM, Yajnik CS, Mohan V. Complications in fibrocalculous pancreatic diabetes—the Pune and Madras experience. International Journal of Diabetes in Developing Countries. 1995;15:70-5.

62. Mohan V, Premalatha G, Sastry NG. Peripheral vascular disease in noninsulin dependent diabetic mellitus in south India. Diabetes Res Clin Pract. 1995;27:235-40.

63. Barman KK, Padmnabhan M, Premalatha G, Deepa R, Rema M, Mohan V. Prevalence of diabetic complications in fibrocalculous pancreatic diabetic patients and type 2 diabetic patients: a cross- sectional comparative study. Journal of Diabetes and its Complications. 2004;18:264-70.

64. Saruc M, Pour PM. Diabetes and its relationship to pancreatic carcinoma. Pancreas. 2003;26:381-7.

65. Frye JN, et al. Pancreatic cancer and diabetes: is there a relationship? A case-controlled study. Aust NZJ Surg. 2000;70:722-4.

66. Bytzer P, Talley NJ, Jones MP, Horowitz M. Oral hypoglycaemic drugs and gastrointestinal symptoms in diabetes mellitus. Aliment Pharmacol Ther. 2001;15:137-42.

67. Christopher K, Rayner, Melvin Samsom, Karen L, Jones Michael Horowitz. Relationships of upper gastrointestinal motor and sensory function with glycemic control. Diabetes Care. 2001;24:371-81.

68. Vahl TP, D'Alessio DA. Gut peptides in the treatment of diabetes mellitus. Expert Opin Investig Drugs. 2004;13:177-88.

69. El-Salhy M. The possible role of the gut neuroendocrine system in diabetes gastroenteropathy. Histology and Histopathology. 2002;17:1153--61.

Chapter 71

SKIN DISEASES AND DIABETES

Sarita Bajaj, Ashok Kumar Bajaj

CHAPTER OUTLINE

- Introduction
- Skin Markers of Diabetes Mellitus
- Cutaneous Infections

- Foot Infections
- Miscellaneous Manifestations
- Cutaneous Complications of Therapy
- Summary

INTRODUCTION

Cutaneous disorders associated with diabetes mellitus (DM) are thought to occur in about 30% of patients during the course of their disease,[1-4] but a recent study[5] has documented prevalence rate of skin diseases to be 60% in (unselected) diabetic subjects consecutively attending an outpatient clinic.

The cutaneous signs of diabetes are the manifestations of multiple factors. Abnormal carbohydrate metabolism, other altered metabolic pathways, atherosclerosis, microangiopathy, neuron degeneration, and impaired host mechanisms all play a role. Cutaneous manifestations generally appear subsequent to the development of diabetes, but may be the first presenting sign or even precede the diagnosis by many years.

The cutaneous findings can be classified into four major groups: (1) Skin diseases associated with diabetes, such as necrobiosis lipoidica, diabetic dermopathy, and diabetic bullae; (2) Cutaneous infections; (3) Cutaneous manifestations of diabetic complications, such as neuropathic foot ulcers; and (4) Skin reactions to diabetic treatment.[6] Diabetic bullae, limited joint mobility and waxy skin and diabetic dermopathy are virtually diagnostic of diabetes. For all these, recognition is the key to treatment and prevention.

SKIN MARKERS OF DIABETES MELLITUS (TABLES 71.1 AND 71.2)

Necrobiosis Lipoidica Diabeticorum

- Rare
- Best known skin lesion associated with diabetes
- Unknown etiology
- Not related to diabetic status or duration
- Usually pretibial site
- A therapeutic challenge.

Necrobiosis lipoidica diabeticorum (NLD) is relatively rare, even in diabetic patients, in whom it has been reported to occur in 0.3 to 1.6%.[7] Only 11 to 65% of patients with NLD have diabetes at the time of cutaneous diagnosis.[8,9] Of those without diabetes, approximately 90% eventually develop diabetes, have abnormal glucose tolerance, or report one or both parents with diabetes.[7] Consequently, nondiabetic patients with NLD should be evaluated and followed for development of diabetes.

TABLE 71.1	Diabetes mellitus and skin manifestations	

Necrobiotic disorders

    Necrobiosis lipoidica diabeticorum

    Disseminated granuloma annulare

Vascular changes

    Diabetic dermopathy

    Diabetic foot

Changes in collagen and skin constituents

    Scleredema

    Dupuytren's contracture

    Limited joint mobility and waxy skin

    Infections

    Bacterial

    Candidiasis

    Erythrasma

    Dermatophytosis

Neuropathy

    Trophic ulcer

    Pathological gustatory sweating

    Peripheral neuropathy

Miscellaneous

Diabetic bullae

Genital pruritus

Acanthosis nigricans

Skin tags

Vitiligo

Perforating dermatoses

Lichen planus

Nail disorders

Hair disorders

Metabolic disorders

Eruptive and other xanthomata

Carotinemia

Porphyria cutanea tarda

Hemochromatosis

Rare syndromes

Werner's syndrome

Partial lipodystrophy

Glucagonoma

Reactions to antidiabetic drugs

Sulfonylureas

Biguanides

Insulin

TABLE 71.2	Virtually diagnostic markers of diabetes mellitus

- Diabetic bullae
- Syndrome of limited joint mobility and waxy skin
- Diabetic dermopathy

NLD occurs three times more commonly in female than in male patients and is associated with both type 1 diabetes mellitus (T1DM) and type 2 diabetes mellitus (T2DM). The lesion is uncommonly observed in blacks or orientals. The average age of onset is 34 years.[7]

The fully developed clinical appearance is diagnostic: Non-scaling plaques with yellow atrophic centers, surface telangiectasia, and a violaceous or erythematous border that may be raised **(Figure 71.1)**. The lesion may vary in size from a papule less than a centimeter to larger plaques several centimeters in dimension. Multiple or bilateral lesions are found in

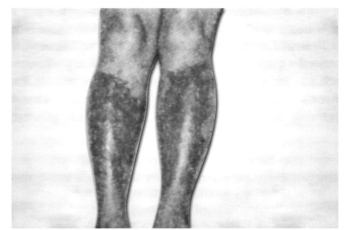

Figure 71.1 Large plaques of necrobiosis lipoidica diabeticorum over both shins

the majority of cases. Whereas most lesions of NLD present on the pretibial and medial malleoli, about 15% of lesions are found elsewhere including the hands, forearms, abdomen, face or scalp. When NLD occurs in areas other than lower extremities the patient is less likely to have diabetes. Ulceration is reported in about one-third of leg lesions: Mostly in large ones following minor trauma.[7]

NLD can usually be diagnosed by a dermatologist on clinical appearance alone. If the diagnosis is not certain, a biopsy will reveal the characteristic changes of granulomatous inflammation and degeneration in collagen and elastic fibers associated with altered extracellular matrix deposition.[10]

The pathogenesis of NLD is still not clearly understood. However, diabetic microangiopathy associated with neuropathy may contribute to the necrobiosis of collagen.

NLD has not as yet been demonstrated to have any consistent relationship to diabetic control. About 20% of patients show spontaneous regression of the lesions. Intralesional triamcinolone injection and occlusive dressing with potent topical steroids over the active margins prevent progression, but the role of oral corticosteroids is not ascertained as yet. Efficacy of aspirin and dipyridamole has been questioned by double blind trials, but pentoxifylline has shown encouraging results.[11]

The successful management of ulcers rests on control of diabetes and prevention and treatment of secondary infection by suitable antibiotics. When conservative treatment fails, split thickness grafting is a therapeutic option.

Granuloma Annulare

- Association with diabetes not clear
- Benign
- Asymptomatic
- Self-limiting dermatosis.

Granuloma annulare (GA) was first described by Fox[12] in 1895. It is an inflammatory disease of unknown etiology characterized clinically by dermal papules and plaques and histologically by collagen degeneration and granulomatous inflammation.

Clinically, the well-recognized subtypes of GA are localized, generalized, subcutaneous and perforating GA. The localized form consists typically of skin-colored or pink papules in an annular configuration on the distal upper and lower extremities particularly overlying bony prominences. They are asymptomatic and nearly three quarters of all cases will resolve spontaneously. Generalized GA typically involves the arms, chest, abdomen and thighs with sparing of the face. Spontaneous resolution is much less common than in localized GA.

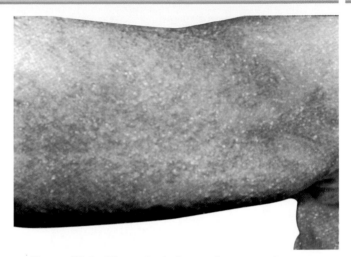

Figure 71.2 Disseminated granuloma annulare over upper arm

The disseminated form can appear and disappear rapidly **(Figure 71.2)**. There is also a perforating form which can be associated with diabetes.[13]

All forms of GA share common histological features and the histopathological similarity to necrobiosis lipoidica would imply a shared etiology and both conditions may coexist in the same patient. Pathogenesis of GA may involve a cell-mediated immune mechanism. An analysis of 100 cases of generalized GA showed an association with diabetes in 21% of cases (as compared with 9% of localized GA). In another series of some 1100 patients approximately 120 were reported to have coexistent diabetes and GA.[13]

Although localized GA frequently resolves spontaneously without scarring, the generalized variant has a more protracted course with rare spontaneous resolution. Sporadic therapeutic success has been reported with topical, systemic, and intralesional steroids; isotretinoin; chlorambucil; freezing; chloroquine; potassium iodide; niacinamide; chlorpropamide; dapsone; antimalarials; as well as psoralen +UVA exposure.[14,15]

Diabetic Dermopathy (Shin Spots, Pigmented Pretibial Patches)

- Most common cutaneous finding
- Asymptomatic
- Pretibial location
- Cutaneous sign of microvascular disease.

In 1964, Melin[16] and later Bindley[17] described the existence of atrophic hyperpigmented 5 to 12 mm lesions occurring on the pretibial area of the lower legs.

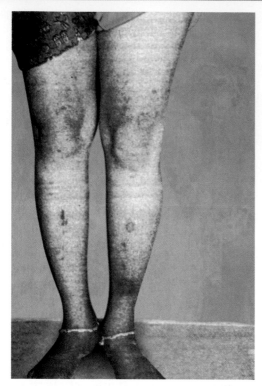

Figure 71.3 Multiple lesions of diabetic dermopathy on the legs

Affecting 7 to 70% of diabetic subjects predominantly men over the age of 50, diabetic dermopathy, also known as shin spots and pigmented pretibial papules, is considered the most common cutaneous manifestation of DM.[6,18] Diabetic dermopathy, however is not pathognomonic of diabetes because 20% of nondiabetic persons may develop similar lesions.

The lesions start as small red papules that subsequently undergo atrophic changes 1 to 2 weeks later. These irregularly round or oval, circumscribed, hyperpigmented, shallow lesions vary in number from few to many. They are usually bilateral, but are not symmetrically distributed **(Figure 71.3)**. They are asymptomatic and often are overlooked by patient and physician alike.[19,20]

These lesions appear to be consistent with posttraumatic atrophy and postinflammatory hyperpigmentation in poorly vascularized skin. When several are present, they may be a cutaneous sign of microvascular disease in other tissues. Their presence in patients seen for other conditions should prompt an evaluation for diabetes mellitus. The frequency of these lesions increases with the duration of diabetes and severity of diabetes. The genesis of shin spots is unclear. The frequency of changes over bony prominences suggests that trauma may be a modifying factor, especially in diabetic patients with neuropathy. Evidences also exist for and against the role of microangiopathy.

The lesions of diabetic dermopathy may resolve spontaneously, even as new lesions arise. Treatment should focus on the patient's diabetes. No treatment for these nonulcerated lesions is required except for protection from trauma.[6]

Diabetic Bullae

- Clinically distinct diabetic marker
- Occur suddenly
- Acral distribution
- Resolve spontaneously
- Unknown etiology
- In long-standing diabetes
- Retinopathy in 75%.

The sudden spontaneous appearance of one or more tense blisters, generally on the acral portions of the body is a rare, but specific event in diabetes. Since its first description in 1930[21] only about 100 cases of this condition have appeared in the published literature. In a recent study,[22] 12 patients have been described over a period of 8 years emphasizing the fact that it is not as uncommon as believed to be.

Approximately 0.5% of diabetic patients develop diabetic bullae or bullosis diabeticorum. The characteristic history is the appearance of multiple, painless, bullae varying in size from half to several centimeters and occurring spontaneously without antecedent trauma, often overnight. Location is variable with reports of involvement of the fingers, toes, hands, feet, arms and rarely the trunk.

However, they are more commonly seen on the distal extremities, particularly on the feet and lower legs **(Figure 71.3)**. They contain clear sterile fluid with eosinophilic material and a few polymorphs, and occur on a noninflammed base. The lesions dry up to form a dark or black crust.[23]

Most patients are with long-standing diabetes with peripheral neuropathy and nephropathy. Coexistent retinopathy occurs in 75% of patients. The age group of affected patients has varied from 17 to 79 years. Males are more commonly affected than females with a ratio of approximately 2:1.[24] The abnormalities of carbohydrate metabolism are not proportionate to the clinical presentation. There have been a few reports of diabetic bullae leading to the diagnosis of DM[25] **(Figure 71.4).**

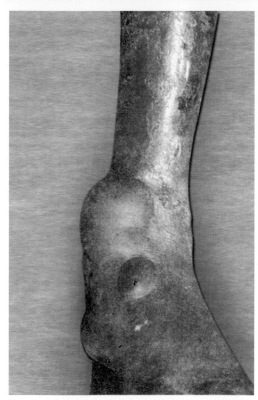

Figure 71.4 Large diabetic bullae around the ankle

Histological reports are varied. Several authors have reported an intraepidermal level of split varying from suprabasilar to subcorneal. Others have reported the split subepidermally varying from the lamina lucida to immediately beneath the lamina densa. The etiology of diabetic bullae is unknown, but does not seem to be an immunologically mediated.

The differential diagnosis includes bullous pemphigoid, epidermolysis bullosa acquisita, porphyria cutanea tarda, bullous impetigo, erythema multiforme, and coma blisters. Bullosis diabeticorum remains a diagnosis of exclusion with negative immunofluorescent studies, porphyrin levels and cultures.

The bullae heal spontaneously in 2 to 5 weeks but may recur in the same or new anatomic locations.[6] If large and symptomatic, then the bullae can be aspirated with an intact blister roof providing a physiologic wound covering.

Diabetic Thick Skin

Three forms of diabetic thick skin have been identified. First, diabetics in general have an asymptomatic, often unnoticed, but measurable increase in skin thickness. Second, the diabetic hand syndrome (syndrome of limited joint mobility, cheiroarthropathy, waxy skin and stiff joints, scleroderma-like syndrome, and diabetic sclerodactyly) consists of scleroderma-like skin changes in the fingers with limited joint mobility. Third, diabetic scleredema is distinct from the self-resolving scleredema adultorum of Buschke seen in children after a streptococcal infection.

Quantitative estimations of skin thickness have been determined by microscopic measurement, caliper measurement, ultrasonography, and radiologic investigation.[25] Normally, skin thickness varies based on body site, age and sex. Typically, the skin thickens until adulthood then decreases in thickness after age 20. Several groups have found an increase in skin thickness of the forearm in T1DM in comparison with age and sex-matched nondiabetic controls.[6]

Limited Joint Mobility (Diabetic Hand Syndrome)

- Collagen disease seen only in diabetes
- Limitation of joint mobility
- Thickness and waxiness of skin
- Asymptomatic
- Harbinger of microvascular disease.

Rosenbloom and Frias[26] first described in 1974 a clinical syndrome consisting of two major components: Limitation of mobility, primarily of the joints of the hands and thickening and stiffness of the skin most marked on the dorsa of the fingers. Limited joint mobility (LJM) is the earliest clinically apparent long-term complication of diabetes in children and adolescents. It occurs in all forms of diabetes, classical type 1, nonautoimmune type 1 and type 2 diabetes mellitus.[27] LJM may be the harbinger of a subset of young people who are at 400 to 600% greater risk for developing retinopathy, nephropathy, neuropathy and hypertension.[28]

The abnormal waxiness and thickness of the skin appears in about one-third of patients with LJM. More predictable in the severe cases, although at times evident without joint involvement. Clinical clues that the skin on the dorsum of the fingers is thickened include pebbled or rough skin (Huntley's papules: **Figure 71.5**), which are multiple grouped minute papules on the extensor surfaces of the fingers, on or near the knuckles or periungual areas.[6]

Joint stiffness begins in the metacarpophalangeal and proximal interphalangeal joints of the fifth finger and extends medially. The distal interphalangeal joints and larger joints may also be involved, most commonly the wrist and the elbow, but also the ankles, cervical and

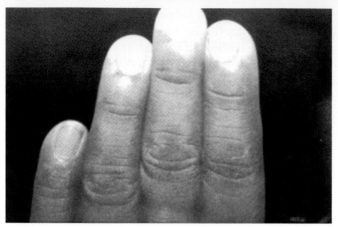

Figure 71.5 Huntley's papules (pebbled appearance) on the dorsa of distal phalanges

thoracolumbar spine. The limitation of movement initially involves active and later passive extension. Flexion limitations may occur in the end stage. The limitation is painless, unresponsive to physical therapy and nondisabling. Apart from periarticular thickening radiographs of the joints reveal no intrinsic abnormality.[11]

Limited joint mobility can be demonstrated by inability to flatten the hand on a tabletop and by failure of palmar approximation (the prayer sign: **Figure 71.6**). The patient places the hands together in prayer position with the forearm parallel to the floor. Normal placement allows for juxtaposition of all the fingers as well as the palm. Staging of LJM is useful for patient follow-up and in reporting relationships to other complications and control criteria.

The Brink Starkman[28] classification is as follows:

Stage 0   No abnormality

Stage I   Skin thickening without contractures

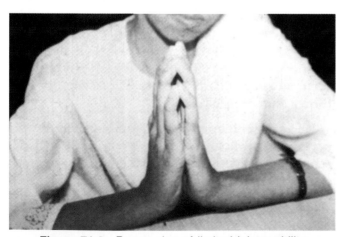

Figure 71.6 Prayer sign of limited joint mobility

Stage II   Bilateral fifth finger contracture
Stage III   Other fingers involved bilaterally
Stage IV   Fingers plus wrist involvement
Stage V   Fingers, wrist and other joint involvement.

Clinically, LJM can be differentiated from scleroderma by the absence of Raynaud's phenomenon, ulceration, tapering, calcinosis of the fingers, and the lack of visceral involvement.[4]

Although contractures of the joints seem related to duration of hyperglycemia particularly in those with insulin dependence, it is probable that if a patient is to develop this complication, he does so by the end of the first decade of disease. There is less agreement as to the relationship of the syndrome to diabetes control.

Scleredema Diabeticorum

- Poorly controlled obese T2DM
- Associated with retinopathy
- Extensive skin involvement
- Resistant to treatment.

Scleredema diabeticorum (SD) is a diffuse non pitting induration of the skin with loss of skin markings occurring in 2.5 to 14% of obese diabetics,[18] most of them who are poorly controlled and in need of insulin. Conversely, 94% of adult patients with scleredema have diabetes. The thickened skin in scleredema pits, if pressure is applied forcefully for 30 seconds, and it may display a Peau d'orange appearance usually with a modest erythematous tinge. Although usually asymptomatic, neck discomfort and back pain may accompany severe cases of this chronic disorder. If the deltoid area is involved, patients may experience a decreased range of motion of the upper extermity.[26]

SD shares certain characteristics with sclerederma adultorum of Buschke but also has distinct differences. Like the classic type, the condition often involves the nape of the neck, upper chest, back, and arms, with occasional extension to the face and abdomen.[18] The cutaneous problem is not only generally more widespread than in the classic type, but also has little tendency to resolution. There is usually no prodromal infection. For SD, there seems to be a moderate correlation with microangiopathy (retinopathy).[20]

The histology is identical in both types and characterized by marked thickening of the dermis with swollen collagen bundles separated by wide clear spaces previously occupied by mucin and by an increased number of mast cells.

Scleredema does not respond to increased diabetic control. The use of potent topical and intralesional

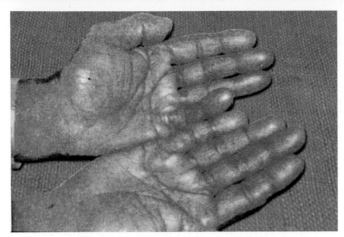

Figure 71.7 Dupuytren's contracture

steroids have been reported, however, the lesion is essentially permanent, causes little morbidity apart from limitation of movement. There is no specific treatment.[29]

Dupuytren's Contracture

- Long-standing diabetes
- Male predominance
- Older patients
- Greater occurrence of retinopathy.

Dupuytren's contracture (DC) typically affects the third and fourth fingers and is characterized by palmar fascial thickening or nodules. It is recognized in 1 to 13% of middle-aged or elderly normal individuals.[30] The prevalence of DC in diabetes varies from 1.6 to 63% in different series, but patients with diabetes and DC tend to be older with long-standing disease. There is a genetic predisposition and an increased frequency in diabetic, epileptic and alcoholic persons. Although diabetic subjects are more prone to DC, the clinical picture **(Figure 71.7)** and course of the disease is indistinguishable from other patients with this disorder. There is a male predominance with the onset delayed in women.

Retinopathy occurs significantly more frequently in those patients who have DC than in those without.[30] Presence of either LJM or DC may be associated with the presence of microangiopathy.

Presistent pain may be relieved by ultrasound treatment or heat, along with stretching exercises. Local steroid injections may provide symptomatic relief but do not alter the clinical course. Conservative surgical fasciotomy is required to restore function, if limitation of the fingers develops.

CUTANEOUS INFECTIONS

- Recurrent genital candidiasis
- Carbuncle
- Extensive erythrasma
- Rhinocerebral mucormycosis.

Skin infections occur in 20 to 50% of those with diabetes.[5,7] Poor diabetes control might be the cause or the consequence of the concurrent infection. The infectious disorders can be of fungal or less commonly bacterial origin.[5] Factors that would render a diabetic patient more susceptible to increased morbidity from skin infections include uncontrolled hyperglycemia, ketoacidosis, abnormal microcirculation, peripheral vessel disease, diabetic neuropathy, decreased phagocytosis and killing activity, impaired leukocyte adherence, delayed chemotaxis, an impaired T-cell mediated immune response, a dry skin, hypohidrosis and trauma.[14,18]

Diabetic subjects have an increased incidence of infections due to *Candida albicans*, *Corynebacterium minutissimum* and soft tissue infections of the lower extremities. They are also more susceptible to some rare infections including rhinocerebral mucormycosis, malignant pseudomonas external otitis and the deep mycosis.

Therapy for infections in diabetic patients in poor control is often not successful until hyperglycemia is corrected which in turn is aggravated by infection requiring an increase in the dose of insulin to establish control.

Candida Infections

Little controversy exists about the association of *Candida albicans* infection especially of the female genitalia, which occurs with greater severity and frequency in poorly controlled diabetes. The presence of pruritus vulvae and the coexistence of culture proven candida in a nonpregnant woman can alert clinicians to the onset of diabetes. It is marked by leukorrhea, intertriginous erythema with scaling, satellite papules, pustules and superficial erosions **(Figure 71.8)**.

Lesions may also occur in places such as the corners of the mouth (perleche), axilla, inframammary region, groin, abdominal or other skin fold. Angular stomatitis may be caused by increased concentration of salivary glucose.[25] Balanitis, balanoposthitis, and phimosis **(Figure 71.9)** may be less common than candida infections in women, but are presenting manifestations of diabetes in uncircumcised men.[31]

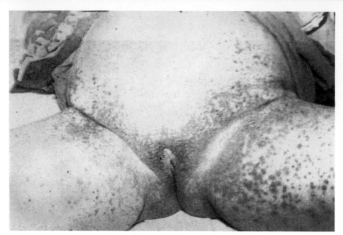

Figure 71.8 Intertriginous candidal infection of groins showing satellite lesions

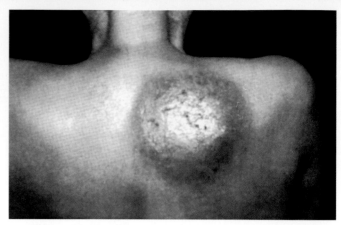

Figure 71.10 A large carbuncle on the upper back

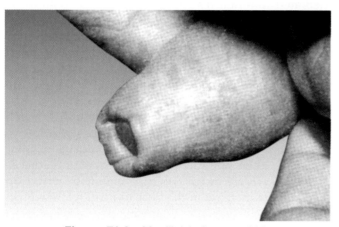

Figure 71.9 Monilial balanoposthitis

Frequently recurrent, candidal paronychia presents as painful nail-fold erythema, swelling, and separation from the nail margin with subsequent nail dystrophy. Pseudohyphae and spores on potassium hydroxide preparation support a candidal diagnosis. Purulent drainage may indicate a secondary bacterial involvement. Less common than paronychia, another site of candidal infection of the hands is of the web space between the middle and fourth fingers (erosio interdigitalis blastomycetica) or between the fourth and fifth toes due to occlusion and retention of moisture.

A classic cutaneous complication in childhood diabetes and occasionally in diabetic adults, candidiasis presents as white, curd like patches (thrush) on the buccal mucosa and tongue.

Successful treatment of these candida infections includes normalization of the blood glucose and the use of topical antifungal medication. Oral fluconazole and ketoconazole therapy is sometimes required. Because maceration and skin breaks can serve as portals of entry for bacteria leading to cellulitis and potentially serious limb-threatening infections, tinea pedis should be aggressively managed in cases with diabetes.[6]

Bacterial Infections

Common bacterial infections of the diabetic skin usually caused by *Staphylococcus aureus* and hemolytic streptococci, include impetigo, folliculitis, furunculosis, carbuncle, ecthyma, cellulitis and erysipelas; can be more severe and widespread.

Carbuncle characteristically occurs as an extremely painful lesion at the nape of the neck, the back or thighs **(Figure 71.10)**. Fever and malaise are often present and the patient may appear quite ill. The involved area is red, swollen and multiple pustules soon appear on the surface draining externally around multiple hair follicles **(Figure 71.11)**. The lesion heals leaving a permanent scar. It is imperative to assess all patients for diabetes.

In diabetes, erysipelas of the legs is often complicated by bullous lesions leading to diabetic gangrene and necrotizing fasciitis. Although infection due to *Staphylococcus* is apparently no more frequent in well-controlled diabetics, it remains good practice to exclude this disease in any patient with recurring or resistant furunculosis or folliculitis.[31]

Extensive erythrasma, caused by gram-positive *Corynebacterium minutissimum*, occurs with increased frequency in elderly, obese patients with diabetes. Clinically, it is manifested by tan-red, fine, scaly patches in intertriginous areas **(Figure 71.12)**.

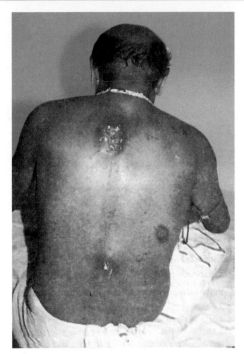

Figure 71.11 Multiple carbuncles on the back

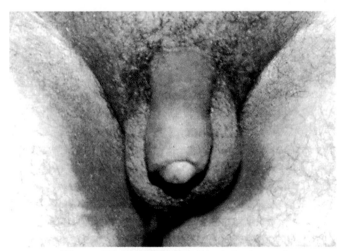

Figure 71.12 Brownish black lesions of erythrasma in the groins

Fatal in over 50% of patients, 25% malignant otitis externa caused by *Pseudomonas aeruginosa*, especially in elderly diabetic men can progress to chondritis, osteomyelitis and bacterial meningitis.

Phycomycetes Infections

Hyperglycemia can allow usually nonpathogenic organisms to establish an infection in traumatized skin occasionally resulting in gangrene and loss of limb. Patients with diabetes who have leg ulcers or non healing surgical wounds may have a complicating phycomycete infection. This infection should be suspected when leg ulcers or post-traumatic lesions do not respond to therapy.

Patients with uncontrolled diabetes and ketosis may be predisposed to deep fungal infections or rhino-cerebral mucormycosis of the turbinates, septum, palate, maxillary and ethmoid sinuses. Treatment consists of correction of acid-base imbalance, aggressive debridement of necrotic tissues, and intravenous amphotericin.[4]

FOOT INFECTIONS

Problems of the feet in diabetic subjects are discussed elsewhere in this book. The sum total of angiopathy, neuropathy and cutaneous infection results in the process known as *diabetic foot*. In addition, trauma is of great importance. Foot infections are usually of mixed aerobic, facultative and anaerobic organisms usually requiring broad-spectrum antibiotics against all these forms of organisms. Leg ulcer infection can rapidly progress to gangrene and amputation. Prophylactic care of the diabetic foot is essential.

MISCELLANEOUS MANIFESTATIONS (FIGURES 71.13 TO 71.18)

Acanthosis Nigricans

• Cutaneous marker of insulin resistance
• Velvety hyperpigmentation in flexural areas.

In acanthosis nigricans (AN) velvety, hyperpigmented (brown, yellow or gray) thickened plaques are seen in body folds such as the axilla **(Figure 71.13)** under the breasts, neck **(Figure 71.14)** and the groin. Other locations include the umbilicus, areolae, submammary regions, and hands (tripe hands).[7] Although, it may be familial and benign, it has long been recognized as a cutaneous marker for a heterogeneous group of endocrine disorders that are characterized by insulin resistance, viz. obesity, diabetes and polycystic ovarian disease.

In a study of 223 patients with AN, nearly 50% of patients in their fifth decade had type 2 DM, whereas only 4 of the 99 patients under age 29 had developed diabetes. Impaired glucose tolerance without a diagnosis of DM, however, was present in a larger proportion of the younger patients.[8] Because AN can also be seen as a complication of carcinoma (particularly

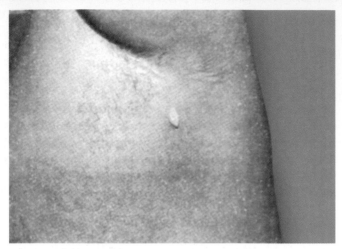

Figure 71.13 Acanthosis nigricans and skin tags in the axilla

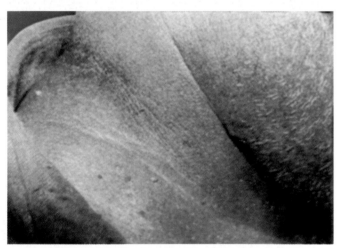

Figure 71.14 Acanthosis nigricans neck

of the stomach), secondary to medications, such as nicotinic acid or corticosteroids, and in various other endocrinopathies, work-up becomes necessary to rule out other underlying disorders.[6]

Insulin resistance contributes significantly to the pathogenesis of type 2 DM and has been implicated as the common denominator of most causes of AN whether by way of genetic defects of the insulin receptor or defects of postreceptor functions, antibodies or by obesity.[32] Insulin resistant diabetes has been associated with AN in various syndromes including total lipodystrophy. There is no correlation between the severity of insulin resistance and AN.

All patients with unexplained AN should be screened for insulin resistance.

Topical 5 to 10% salicylic acid ointment or tretinoin 0.05%, or systemic isotretinoin may be tried for cosmetic improvement.[18] Weight reduction is clearly of benefit. Clinical improvement with dietary fish oil supplementation has been reported.[6]

Skin Tags (Acrochordon, Soft Fibromas)

• Common in obese and elderly women
• Not a reliable diabetic marker.

Skin tags (ST) are small, soft, pedunculated, often pigmented lesions, usually occurring on the eyelids, neck and axillae **(Figure 71.13)**. The condition is very common; particularly in middle aged and elderly women. In obesity, ST are both commoner and more numerous.

Though some reports[33,34] suggest association of diabetes with skin tags, at present there is insufficient evidence to regard skin tags as a reliable diabetic marker.

Perforating Dermatoses

Patients with renal failure and/or type 1 DM or type 2 DM often have an acquired perforating dermatoses of the skin characterized by hyperkeratotic papules (2–10 mm diameter) with transepidermal eliminate on of degenerated material, such as collagen and elastin. Lesions occur primarily on the legs, but may also be found on the trunk and face. They are often very itchy with little tenderness and spontaneous resolution. Improvement has been achieved with topical retinoic acid, protection from scratching combined with good diabetic control and ultraviolet therapy.[35]

Xanthomas

Eruptive xanthomas **(Figures 71.15)** are firm, nontender, itchy, skin-colored or yellow papules (1–4 mm) often surrounded by an erythematous rim. Knees, elbows, back and buttocks are commonly involved. They appear suddenly in crops in less than 0.1% diabetic patients with poor control and raised triglyceride levels.[36] Often presenting as a Koebner phenomenon, the lesions may be tender.[14] Polyphagia in uncontrolled diabetes accelerates formation of very low density lipoprotein and increases chylomicrons.[6]

Other chronic diseases such as chronic biliary cirrhosis, nephrotic syndrome, chronic renal failure, myxedema, chronic pancreatitis and glycogen storage disease may show secondary eruptive xanthomata. Xanthomas and diabetes are also associated with

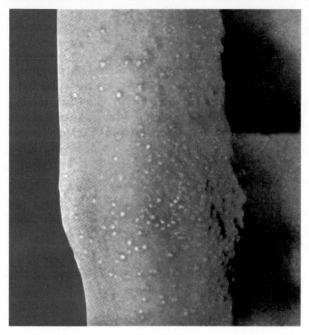

Figure 71.15 Eruptive xanthomas

hemochromatosis and total lipodystrophy. When carbohydrate and lipid metabolism is controlled, the lesions tend to resolve.

Multiple xanthomas may coalesce and form tuberous xanthomas.[6] Tendon xanthomata are more persistent, tender on pressure and often seen over the pressure areas such as knees, elbows and Achilles' tendon. They occur more frequently with hypercholesterolemia. Xanthelasma **(Figures 71.16A and B)** may be associated with hypercholesterolemia.

Vitiligo

Many theories exist to explain the cause of vitiligo. Genetic, autoimmune melanocytic self destruction, as well as abnormal neurogenic stimuli play an important etiological role.

There is an increased association of vitiligo with other endocrinopathies, specifically those associated with a proven or presumed autoimmune etiology. Vitiligo has been reported in T2DM as well T1DM making it difficult to advance autoimmune and genetic factors as the only explanation for their coexistence.[36] Vitiligo may precede the onset of clinically evident diabetes and also occurs more frequently in families of diabetic patients.

There appears to be no difference in the clinical course of vitiligo even if associated diabetes is well controlled **(Figure 71.17)**.

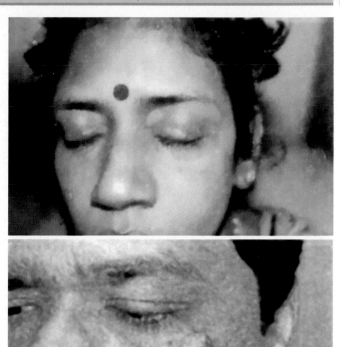

Figures 71.16A and B Xanthelasma palpebrarum

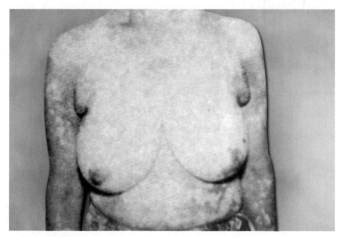

Figure 71.17 Extensive bilateral symmetrical lesions of vitiligo in a diabetic

Rubeosis faciei

Although difficult to quantify, flushed face of rubeosis faciei has been reported in 3 to 59% of diabetic subjects.

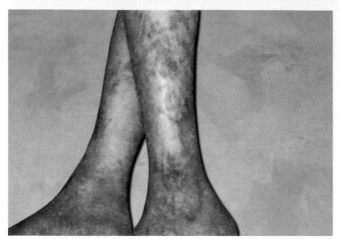

Figure 71.18 Papules and plaques of lichen planus over the legs

Blond and red-haired persons appear more erythematous because of reduced cutaneous melanin to obscure the erythema. The red color may be caused by microangiopathy, increased solar sensitivity, or dehydration. Tighter glucose control might improve the appearance.[7]

Lichen Planus

Numerous reports have studied the association of diabetes and lichen planus **(Figure 71.18)**, especially oral lichen planus. The prevalence of decreased glucose tolerance in patients with oral lichen planus varies widely between 1.6% and 85%.[6] *Fewer studies have examined the frequency of lichen planus is known to have diabetes.* Although most reports do not differentiate the types of diabetes, the reported rate vary from 0.55 to 5.76% of patients having clinical and less often histologic evidence of oral lichen planus.

Some authors argue that what seems clinically to be oral lichen planus may actually be lichenoid reactions to drugs, such as nonsteroidal anti-inflammatory drugs, antihypertensives and oral hypoglycemic agents.[37]

An increased incidence of diabetes and abnormal glucose tolerance has been claimed in patients with lichen planus but as yet there is no unequivocal evidence in favor of this association.[38]

Pruritus

Generalized pruritus is not associated specifically with diabetes, but if it occurs dry skin is commonly the cause and suitable emollients should be prescribed. When pruritus is present, it is usually localized. Localized anogenital pruritus (pruritus vulvae and balanitis) may be the presenting symptom of diabetes.[11]

Nail Changes

- Subtle yet valuable indicator of systemic disease
- Paronychia
- Periungual telangiectasia
- Yellow nails.

No nail changes are truly pathognomonic for diabetes, many do suggest that it be ruled out.

Paronychia may result in partial or total matrix destruction followed by permanent abnormality of the nail plate. A greenish-black discoloration may appear as a result of *Pseudomonas* colonization.

Hypertrophic thickening, darkening and surface irregularity (onychauxis) may be due to vascular insufficiency. Venous dilatation in the cutaneous microcirculation is an excellent indicator of functional microangiopathy and of long-term control of the diabetic.

Yellow discoloration of the nails may develop from many causes. In diabetes, yellow nails probably represent glycosylation end products.[39]

Hair Disorders

Diffuse thinning of the scalp hair is not unusual in uncontrolled diabetes and fine lanugo hairs on the back and arm may be seen in undernourished diabetic patients.

Achard-Thiers syndrome consists of obesity, hirsutism principally of the face, hypertension and diabetes.

Generalized hypertrichosis can be seen in the Lawrence-Seip syndrome.[40]

Hemochromatosis

Hemochromatosis is a clinical disorder referred to as "bronze diabetes" with chief components being diabetes, hepatic cirrhosis, hyperpigmentation of the skin, cardiomyopathy, arthritis and hypogonadism. Abnormal glucose tolerance is found in 60 to 80%.[41]

Kaposi's Sarcoma

Kaposi's sarcoma seen in AIDS patients bears no relation to diabetes. Diabetes mellitus has been reported with greater than expected frequency in Kaposi's sarcoma.[42]

Yellow Skin

Up to 10% of diabetic patients may show some yellow discoloration of the skin.[36] The cause of yellow skin remains in dispute. Possibilities include elevated serum carotene and one or more glycosylation end products which are noted to be yellow.[20]

Porphyria Cutanea Tarda

Diabetes mellitus has been found associated with porphyria in 8 to 22% of cases.[43] There is a higher association with men.

The cutaneous manifestations include bullae on light-exposed areas, excessive skin fragility, hypertrichosis, melanosis, scarring, alopecia and scleroderma-like plaques.

Werner's Syndrome

In this hereditary disorder of connective tissue, insulin resistant diabetes is found in at least one-third of the cases.

Premature aging affects many tissues and the disease is heralded in the first or second decades by premature graying of the hair and alopecia.[44]

Glucagonoma

At the time of presentation, patients with the glucagonoma syndrome have a triad of symptoms including glucose intolerance, normocytic normochromic anemia and a distinctive eruption termed necrolytic migratory erythema.[19] The dermatological component may precede other evidence of its existence, sometimes by several years.[36]

Clinically, there is a polymorphous, erythematous eruption with a peripheral scale. It waxes and wanes in a 7 to 14 day generalized cycle. Superficial vesiculation leads to erosions and necrosis, characteristically in the perioral area, around the genitals and in the anal orifice.

Systemic accompaniments include weight loss, weakness, diarrhea, anemia and mild nonketotic diabetes. A beefy red tongue, angular cheilitis, and nail hypertrophy also may be present.[19]

If surgical excision of the glucagonoma is possible, the eruption can be expected to clear within 48 hours after surgery.[40]

Pathological Gustatory Sweating

Marked facial sweating produced by eating food, especially cheese, can spread to the neck, shoulders, and upper chest in long-standing diabetics with neuropathy and nephropathy. Degeneration in the autonomic nervous system occurs in diabetes and it is suggested that aberrant regeneration accounts for gustatory sweating. *Gustatory sweating may resolve postrenal transplant suggesting an etiological role of nephropathy.* This condition often responds to treatment with atropine, clonidine, anticholinergic agents or topical glycopyrrolate.[6]

CUTANEOUS COMPLICATIONS OF THERAPY

- Sulfonylureas—a wide variety of skin eruptions
- Insulin
  - Allergy: immediate, delayed, biphasic with interrupted therapy
  - Faulty injection technique
  - Lipodystrophy.

Oral Hypoglycemic Agents

An allergic reaction occurs in 15% of patients taking sulfonylureas. Maculopapular rashes, lichenoid eruptions, morbilliform eruptions, generalized erythema, urticarial eruptions, exfoliative dermatitis, generalized erythema multiforme, Stevens-Johnson syndrome, toxic epidermal necrolysis and even photoallergic reactions have been attributed to sulfonylureas. Maculopapular rashes are usually seen during the first two months of therapy which often disappear while the patient is maintained on the drug.[28,36] The chlorpropamide alcohol flush may be seen in up to 1 to 30% of patients.[44]

Similar reactions have also been reported with metformin. Reports of cutaneous reactions are more limited in case of newer classes of antidiabetic drugs including acarbose and rosiglitazone.[6] One case of erythema multiforme caused by acarbose has been reported.

Insulin

Infection

Infection at sites of insulin injection is remarkably rare **(Figure 71.19)**. To minimize fingertip infection in patients monitoring their blood glucose, it is recommended that samples be obtained from the side of the fingers.[45]

Idiosyncratic Reactions

These are uncommon, but may lead to painful induration and pigmentation, keloids,[46] tattoos,[47] verrucous plaques resembling acanthosis nigricans,[48] purpura, and localized pigmentation[6] at the sites of injections of insulin.

Insulin Allergy

The incidence of insulin reaction varies from 10 to 56%.[49] There is an increase in insulin reaction with interrupted therapy. The purified or recombinant insulins are much less likely (0.1–0.2%) to induce generalized allergic

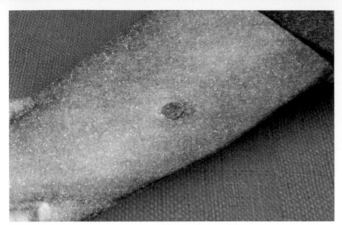

Figure 71.19 Infection at site of insulin injection

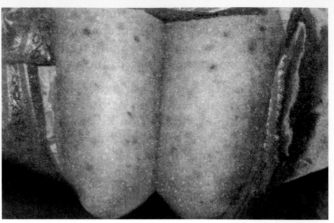

Figure 71.20 Pigmented atrophic and indurated papules on the thighs due to intradermal insulin injections

reaction. Insulin allergy could be due to the insulin molecule, proinsulin, preservatives (parabens) and additives (zinc).[36]

Insulin reactions may be immediate, e.g. urticaria, angioedema and rarely anaphylaxis. They may occur shortly after starting treatment or many years later. IgG antibody mediates this allergic reaction. Change of insulin to a more purified product is the treatment of choice. In some patients, serum sickness type reaction follows the immediate reaction.[28,36]

Delayed reactions occur in about 1% of patients within one month of therapy and most cases resolve in several weeks. An itchy nodule followed by hyper-pigmentation and even scarring may be seen. It is caused by cell-mediated immunity.[36]

Many cutaneous problems at the site of injection are not allergic but due to faulty technique. This is usually secondary to the insulin being administered intradermally rather than subcutaneously and result is local inflammation induration and occasionally in ulceration and scars **(Figure 71.20)**. A local reaction has also been reported in a patient allergic to latex caused by small amounts of latex rubber antigens in the insulin injection materials (insulin vial and syringe).[50]

Insulin Lipodystrophy

It may be atrophic or hypertrophic or even both may occur in the same patient. Insulin lipoatrophy is loss of fat at the sites of injection occurring in about 10% patients receiving conventional insulin. It is more common in females in areas of substantial fat deposition and occurs 6 to 24 months after starting injections. Although, it is usually present at the site of injection, it can occur at remote areas.[40]

These lesions seldom show complete, spontaneous resolution. Rotating the injection sites for prevention, and injections of highly purified or recombinant insulin into the periphery of the atrophic area may improve the lesion.[28] Because duration of injected insulin deposition may also be a complicating factor, Murao et al[51] suggest substituting rapidly acting insulin to avoid lipoatrophy.

Insulin Fat Hypertrophy

Clinically and histologically resembles a lipoma and occurs at the site of injection. It is more common in men with months or years of repeated injections into relatively avascular or anesthetic areas. Spontaneous resolution may occur if the injection site is rested or if purified insulin is injected. Intralesional steriods will cause local improvement but may eventually cause atrophy.[36] Since patients often prefer to inject into the hypertrophied sites because the skin overlying these areas is relatively hypoesthetic, it is necessary to inform the patient of the need to rotate sites of insulin administration to avoid areas of hypertrophy. It is important to recognize that the absorption of insulin may be slower when injected into a hypertrophied area, and this can affect diabetic control.[52]

SUMMARY

The cutaneous manifestations in diabetes mellitus are due to multiple factors like metabolic disturbances, chronic degenerative changes and complications due to therapy. Diabetic patients are more prone to develop bacterial, fungal and viral infections, Patients with recurrent furuncles or carbuncle should always be investigated for diabetes. Monilial balanoposthitis and vulvovaginitis as well as extensive ringworm infections are common amongst diabetic subject. Pruritus vulvae are quite frequent in diabetic females.

Eruptive exanthomas are a characteristic, but uncommon complication of diabetes with associated hypertriglyceridemia. The lesions come in crops and regress when hyperlipidemia is controlled.

Necrobiosis lipoidica is the most specific, but very rare manifestation of diabetes. Majority of the patients either have diabetes or develop diabetes later or have first degree relatives with diabetes. Diabetic dermopathy is the most common dermatosis associated with diabetes. Diabetic bullae are pathognomonic of diabetes. They are painless, noninflammatory bullae, and commonly appear spontaneously on the feet and hands. Granuloma annulare is another uncommon disorder and disseminated and diffuse granuloma annulare has strong association with diabetes.

Patients with various dermatoses-like acanthosis nigricans, generalized vitiligo, perforating dermatoses, skin tags, generalized pruritus and knuckle pebbles also need to be screened for diabetes.

REFERENCES

1. Braverman I. Cutaneous manifestations of diabetes mellitus. Med Clin North Am. 1971; 55:1019-29.
2. Jelinek JE. Skin disorders associated with diabetes mellitus. In Rifkin H, Porte D (Eds). Ellenberg and Rifkin's Diabetes Mellitus, Theory and Practice. NewYork: Elsevier 1990; pp. 838-49.
3. Hall SE, Sibbald RG. The skin in diabetes mellitus. In Pickup JC, Williams G (Eds): Chronic Complications of Diabetes. Oxford : Blackwell 1994;pp. 250-9.
4. Perez MI, Kohn SR. Cutaneous manifestations of diabetes mellitus. J Am Acad Dermatol. 1994; 30: 519-31.
5. Romano G, Moretti G, DiBenedetto A, et al. Skin lesions in diabetes mellitus: prevalence and clinical correlations. Diab Res Clin Prac. 1998; 39:101-6.
6. Ferringer T, Miller OF. Cutaneous manifestations of diabetes mellitus. Dermatol Clin 2002; 20: 483-92.
7. Paron NG, Lambert PW. Cutaneous manifestations of diabetes mellitus. Prim Care. 2000; 27: 371-83.
8. Stuart CA, Gilkison CR, Smith MM, et al. Acanthosis Nigricans as a risk factor for non-insulin dependent diabetes mellitus. Clin Pediatr. 1998; 37: 73-80.
9. O'Toole EA, Kennedy U, Nolan JJ, et al. Necrobiosis Lipoidica: only a minority of patients have diabetes mellitus. Br J Dermatol. 1999;140: 283-6.
10. Thiboutot DM. Dermatological manifestations of endocrine disorders. J Clin Endo Met. 1995; 80: 3082-7.
11. Jelinek JE. The skin in diabetes. Diabet Med. 1993;10 :201-13.
12. Fox TC. Ringed eruption of the finger. Br J Dermatol. 1895; 7:91-5.
13. Shapiro B, Albert M, Harrist TJ. Generalized granuloma annulare. Med Surg Dermatol. 1997; 4:217-8.
14. Jelinek JE. Cutaneous manifestations of diabetes mellitus. Int J Dermatol. 1994;33:605-17.
15. Dabski K, Winkelman RK. Generalized granuloma annulare: clinical and laboratory findings in 100 patients. J Am Acad Dermatol. 1989; 20:39-47.
16. Melin H. An atrophic circumscribed skin lesion in the lower extremities of diabetics. Acta Med Scand. 1964;176 (Suppl 423):1-75.
17. Bindley GW. Dermopathy in the diabetic syndrome. Arch Dematol. 1965;92 :625.
18. Sibbald RG, Landolt SJ, Toth D. Skin and diabetes. Endocrinol Metab Clin North Am. 1996;25:463-72.
19. Feingold KR, Elias PM. Endocrine-skin interactions. J Am Acad Dermatol. 1987;17:921-40.
20. Huntley AC. Cutaneous manifestations of diabetes mellitus. Dermatol Clinics. 1989;7:531-46.
21. Kramer DW. Early or warning signs of impending gangrene in diabetes. Med J Rec. 1930;132:338-42.
22. Lipsky BA, Baker PD, Ahroni JH. Diabetic bullae: 12 cases of a purportedly rare cutaneous disorder. Int J Dermatol. 2000; 39:196-200.
23. Rocca F, Pereyra E. Phlyctenar lesions in the feet of diabetic patients. Diabetes. 1963;12:220-2.
24. Basarab T, Munn SE, Mcgrath J, Russel Jone R. Bullosis diabeticorum: a case report and literature review. Clin Exp Dermatol. 1995;20:218-20.
25. Huntley AC. Cutaneous manifestations of diabetes mellitus. Diabetes Metab Rev. 1993;9:161-76.
26. Rosenbloom AI, Frias JL. Diabetes mellitus, short stature and joint stiffness: a new syndrome. Clin Res. 1974; 22 :92A.
27. Rosenbloom AL. Limited joint mobility in insulin dependent childhood diabetes. Eur J Pediatr. 1990;149:380-8.
28. Brink JS. The diagnosis and management of Type I diabetes mellitus. In Norman Lavin (Ed): Manual of Endocrinology and Metabolism. Boston: Little, Brown and Company. 1988; pp. 573-88.
29. Cole GW, Headley J, Skowsky R. Scleredema diabeticorum: a common and distinct cutaneous manifestation of diabetes mellitus. Diabetes Care. 1983;6:189-92.
30. Pal B, Griffiths ID, Anderson J, Dick WC. Association of limited joint mobility with Dupuytren's contracture in diabetes mellitus. J Rheumatol. 1987;14:582-5.
31. Meurer M, Szeimies RM. Diabetes mellitus and skin diseases. Curr Probl. 1991;20:11-23.
32. Rendon MI, Cruz PD, Sontheimer RD. Acanthosis nigricans: cutaneous marker of tissue resistance to insulin. J Am Acad Dermatol. 1989;21:461-9.
33. Kahana M, Grossman E, Feinstein A, Ronner M, Cohen M, Millet MS. Skin tags: a cutaneous marker for diabetes mellitus. Acta Dermatol Venereol. 1987;67:175-7.
34. Thappa DM. Skin tags as markers of diabetes mellitus: an epidemiological study in India. Tokyo: J Dermatology. 1995;22:729-31.
35. Rapini RP, Hebert AA, Drucker CR. Acquired perforating dermatoses : evidence for combined transepidermal elimination of both collagen and elastic fibers. Arch Dermatol. 1989;125:1074-8.
36. Sibbald RG, Schachter RK. The skin and diabetes mellitus. Int J Dermatol. 1984;23: 567-84.

37. Lozada-Nur F, Miranda C. Oral lichen planus: epidemiology, clinical characteristics, and associated diseases. Semin Cutan Med Surg. 1997;16:273-7.

38. Nigam PK, Singh G, Agarwal JK. Plasma insulin response to oral glycemic stimulus in lichen planus. Br J Dermatol. 1988;19:128-9.

39. Greene RA, Scher RK. Nail changes associated with diabetes mellitus. J Am Acad Dermatol. 1987;16:1015-21.

40. Mendelsohn S, Verbov J. Diabetes and the skin-a review. Br J Clin Prac. 1983;37:85-94.

41. Powell LW. Hemochromatosis and related iron storage diseases. In Wright R, Millward-Sadler GH, Alberti KGMM, Karran S (Eds): Liver and Biliary disease. London: Balliere-Tindall. 1985; pp. 936-82.

42. Digiovanna JJ, Sarai B. Kaposi's Sarcoma: retrospective study of 90 cases with particular emphasis on the familial occurrence, ethnic background and prevalence of other diseases. Am J Med. 1981;71:779-83.

43. Grossman ME, Bickers DR, Poh-Fitzpatrick MB, Deleo VA, Harber LC. Porphyria cutanea tarda: clinical features and laboratory findings in 40 patients. Am J Med. 1979;67:277-86.

44. Fitzgerald MG, Gaddie R, Malins JM, O'Sullivan DJ. Alcohol sensitivity in diabetics receiving chlorpropamide. Diabetes. 1962;11:40-3.

45. Ryar EA, Miller J, Skyler JS. Finger sepsis: possible complication of self monitoring of blood glucose concentration. Br Med J. 1983;286:1614-5.

46. Rutenberg J, Bookman JJ. Multiple keloids formed at the sites of insulin injections: a case report. Diabetes. 196;10:320-1.

47. Shelley WB, Shelley D, Burmeister V. Tattoos from insulin needles. Ann Intern Med. 1986;105:549-50.

48. Fleming MG, Simon SI. Cutaneous insulin reaction resembling acanthosis nigricans. Arch Dermatol. 1986;122:1054-6.

49. Paley RG, Tunbridge RE. Dermal reactions to insulin therapy. Diabetes. 1952;1:22.

50. Towse A, O'Brien M, Twarog F, et al. Local reaction secondary to insulin injection: a potential role for latex antigens in insulin vials and syringes. Diabetes Care. 1995;18:1195-7.

51. Murao S, Hirata K, Ishida T, et al. Lipoatrophy induced by recombinant human insulin injection. Intern Med. 1998;11:310-4.

52. Young RJ, Hannan WJ, Frier BM, Steel JM, Duncar LJ. Diabetic lipohypertrophy delays insulin absorption. Diabetes Care. 1984;7:479-80.

Chapter 72

BONE DISEASE IN DIABETES MELLITUS

D Sudhaker Rao

CHAPTER OUTLINE

- Introduction
- Pathogenesis of Bone Disease in Diabetes Mellitus
- Bone Mineral Density in Diabetes Mellitus
- Fractures in Diabetes Mellitus
- Approach to a Patient with Diabetes for Bone Disease
- Management of Low Bone Density and/or Osteoporosis in the Diabetic Population
- Monitoring of Therapy
- Special Circumstances
- Summary

INTRODUCTION

Diabetes mellitus is a common chronic condition that affects millions of aging population worldwide. It is associated with a variety of complications that are well known to practicing clinicians. However, the status of skeleton and its disorders in patients with diabetes mellitus has received very little attention. This is surprising because bone disease in diabetes mellitus is probably as old as the disease itself since descriptions of bone disease in diabetes can be traced as far back as the 1920s[1] and is as old as insulin itself.

There are several reasons for this situation. First, the traditional complications of diabetes dominate the clinical manifestations and require more immediate management whereas bone disease and fractures do not receive the required attention. Second, fractures are relatively uncommon random clinical events, and when they do occur, receive only orthopedic interventions with no concerted effort either to assess the background for fractures or to prevent them. Third, many vertebral fractures are asymptomatic and therefore, may not come to clinical attention; this in fact might underestimate the true prevalence of osteoporosis in diabetic patients. Fourth, most of the information related to bone in diabetes is centered on metatarsal fractures and Charcot joints, the pathogenesis of which is poorly understood. Finally, only recently has there been any systematic assessment of bone status in diabetes, largely facilitated by the availability of techniques to measure bone mass and thus assess fracture risk. Consequently, in the last five years several large population-based studies have demonstrated an increased risk of fractures in patients with diabetes mellitus both in type 1 and type 2 with or without low bone mass.[2-12]

PATHOGENESIS OF BONE DISEASE IN DIABETES MELLITUS

For the purposes of this review, the terms *bone disease* and *bone mass* are used rather loosely and interchangeably to encompass a variety of bone problems encountered in patients with diabetes mellitus—both type 1 and type 2. There are many reasons why diabetics are likely to develop bone disease and sustain fractures **(Table 72.1)**.[5,10,13] In type 1 diabetes for instance, patients

TABLE 72.1	Contrasting contributing factors to low bone mass and increased fractures, risk in patients with diabetes mellitus	
Type 1 diabetes	**Type 2 diabetes**	
Thin body size/frame	Large body size/frame (?protective)	
Low peak adult bone mass	Normal peak adult bone mass	
Advanced glycation of collagen	Advanced glycation of collagen	
Lower IGF-I	Higher IGF-1*	
Accelerated bone loss due to hypercalciuria	Attenuated age-related bone loss due to and increased bone resorption low bone turnover	
Hypercalciuria	?Hypercalciuria	

*IGF-1: Insulin-like growth factor 1

may not attain the full potential of peak adult bone mass because of lower IGF-1 levels and due to the catabolic effects of frequent uncontrolled hyperglycemia during critical growth period.[10,14] Since almost 40% of the skeletal calcium is accumulated between the ages of 10 to 15 years, precisely the time when diabetes control may not be optimal, developing diabetes at this critical juncture may adversely affect the potential to achieve peak adult bone mass. Poor nutrition, especially calcium and vitamin D, low body mass, overt or subclinical malabsorption such as cystic fibrosis or celiac sprue,[15-17] and hypercalciuria-induced negative calcium balance during periods of hyperglycemia[10,13] may all contribute to low bone mass and increased risk of fractures.

In contrast, the occurrence of bone disease in type 2 diabetes mellitus presents an apparent paradox[5] **(Table 72.1)**. Patients with type 2 diabetes are frequently obese, which is associated with higher bone density and lower fracture rates in a multitude of studies. Unlike patients with type 1 diabetes mellitus, type 2 diabetic patients have higher levels of IGF-I, which is known to stimulate bone formation. Indeed, there is suggestive evidence that age-related bone loss is attenuated and bone turnover is either normal or reduced in patients with type 2 diabetes mellitus.[18,19] Thus many patients with type 2 diabetes mellitus would be expected to have low risk of fractures. Yet, many epidemiologic studies have demonstrated otherwise.[2-12] It is possible that skeletal aging (not to be confused with the chronologic age of the patient) is accelerated in the presence of diabetes mellitus[18] somewhat analogs to the well-known phenomenon of accelerated atherosclerosis. Diabetes mellitus is known to cause advanced glycation of a variety of proteins (or AGE products) that may also include glycation of type-I collagen in bone and thus compromise its integrity.[14] Therefore, bone density at

relevant measurement sites may not reflect the true quality of the skeleton in patients with type 2 diabetes mellitus; in other words the quantity of bone may be normal but the quality is not.

There are a few abnormalities that are common to both types of diabetes that contribute to fractures. These include hypogonadism, neurovascular complications leading to poor bone quality and increased fragility, repetitive trauma, advanced glycation of proteins, especially type-I collagen in bone, osteoblast dysfunction and osteocyte apoptosis.

Other well-established risk factors associated with increased risk of fractures in nondiabetic patients[20,21] are also operative in patients with diabetes mellitus. With the increasing life expectancy of many diabetic patients, the age related decline in osteoblast function contributes to the pathogenesis of bone loss and fractures.[22] Since vitamin D depletion is common in the general population, it may not be surprising that a significant number of patients with diabetes may very well have associated vitamin D depletion and calcium malabsorption or both.[15,16,23] This is specifically relevant in the Indian context.[24] Both diabetes and vitamin D depletion are known to increase the risk of falls, fractures, and mortality.[25-27] Furthermore, peripheral vascular disease, neuropathy, loss of proprioception, balance and coordination that are common in this disease may also contribute to the bone disease and fractures. Reduced interstitial bone fluid flow as a result of diabetic microvascular disease may result in osteocyte apoptosis and reduced osteocyte density leading increased fragility of bone.[28] Interestingly, while increased levels of fructosamine are indicative of undiagnosed diabetes mellitus, a low level, which reflects frailty or poor nutrition, is associated with increased risk of hip fractures.[29]

TABLE 72.2	Bone mineral density in diabetes mellitus
Type of measurement	*Magnitude of difference*
Radiogrammetry (metacarpals) (7 studies in patients with type 1 DM)	2.5–10% lower
Single photon absorptiometry (forearm) (10 studies in patients with type 1 DM)	4–10% lower than control prevalence of low BMD* 13–70%
Dual energy X-ray absorptiometry (Type 2 diabetes)	BMD of calcaneum, distal forearm and femoral neck was 6–10% higher in type 2 diabetics than controls
Dual energy X-ray absorptiometry (Type 1 diabetes)	BMD of the spine and hip 4–6% higher than matched controls

*BMD: Bone mineral density

BONE MINERAL DENSITY IN DIABETES MELLITUS

Several different types of techniques and measurement sites were used to assess bone density in patients with diabetes mellitus and as could be expected the results have been contradictory **(Table 72.2)**. In general, bone density tends to be lower in patients with type 1 compared to type 2 diabetes mellitus most likely due to higher BMI and IGF-I of the latter. Bone density is also related to the duration of diabetes, insulin therapy and the presence of diabetic complications. Despite a higher bone density, fracture risk is greater in type 2 diabetes than in nondiabetics, implying a compromised bone quality.

FRACTURES IN DIABETES MELLITUS

Several prospective population-based cohort studies suggest that the risk of fractures in general and hip fractures in particular are increased in patients with diabetes. As the patients are living longer with improved treatment modalities, it is possible that the hip fracture risk will continue to increase in this population.[2-12] A systematic study of the prevalence of wrist, vertebral, and hip fractures, the three most common osteoporotic fractures, indicates that they are significantly higher in diabetic than in the nondiabetic population **(Table 72.3)**. The increased risk is most evident in patients with longer duration of diabetes (>10 years), those with retinopathy, and patients on insulin

TABLE 72.3	Epidemiology of fractures in diabetes mellitus (selected studies to illustrate the scope of the problem)		
Study	*Sample size number*	*Years of observation*	*Relative risk (Comments)*
Blue Mountain Eye Study (Australia)[2]	3654	2 years	5.9 (If on insulin) 5.4 (If retinopathy) 3.3 (If >10 y DM) 2.5 (If cataracts)
Iowa Postmenopausal Women Study[3]	32,089	11 years	12.3 (Type 1 DM) 1.7 (Type 2 DM) 1.6 (New DM)
Study of Osteoporotic Fractures (USA)[4]	9654	>10 years	2.7 (Foot) 1.94 (Humerus) 1.82 (Hip)
The Finnish Study[7]	124	Case-controlled cohort study	BMD is low both in type 1 and 2 DM fracture risk increased
The Norwegian Hip Fracture Study[9]	52,313	Observational study	5.81 (Women) 7.67 (Men)
Nord-Trondelag Health Survey[6]	35,444 (>50 y)	Observational Study	6.9 (Type 1 DM) 1.8 (Type 2 DM)

TABLE 72.4	Relative risk of different types of fractures in patients with diabetes mellitus	
Fracture site	*Women not on insulin RR (CI)*	*Women on insulin RR (CI)*
Hip	1.82 (1.24–2.69)	1.14 (0.42–3.08)
Proximal humerus	1.94 (1.24–3.02)	2.38 (0.97–5.81)
Distal forearm	0.93 (0.62–1.39)	1.52 (0.72–3.20)
Ankle	1.06 (0.65–1.72)	1.92 (0.85–4.34)
Foot	1.09 (0.64–1.84)	2.68 (1.18–6.06)
All nonvertebral	1.30 (1.10–1.53)	1.39 (0.97–1.98)
Vertebral	1.12 (0.69–1.83)	0.98 (0.30–3.20)

Statistically significant values are shown in bold face type

(Table 72.3). An interesting feature is that patients with diabetes appear to have higher incidence of fractures of the humerus and calcaneum;[2,11,30,31] the reasons for this are not readily apparent. Also, patients with diabetes sustain fractures at higher bone density than the nondiabetic population, implying that bone quality is compromised. The relevant data on fractures is summarized in **Table 72.4**.

The metatarsal fractures that frequently occur in diabetic subjects may not be related to the systemic effects of diabetes on the skeleton, but rather due to vascular and neuropathic complications of the disease.[32] Similarly, Charcot's joints are also in consequence of neurovascular compromise; the pathogenesis of both is poorly understood.

Nevertheless, awareness of these complications in an individual patient is important in clinical practice. Morbidity and mortality following hip fracture is increased in general population and may even be worse in patients with diabetes. Proper recognition and appropriate interventions are essential in avoiding osteoporosis and its consequences in patients with both type 1 and type 2 diabetes.

APPROACH TO A PATIENT WITH DIABETES FOR BONE DISEASE

Every diabetic patient should be assessed for risk factors for osteoporosis and fractures according to the guidelines established by several organizations for nondiabetic patients. These guidelines can be easily accessed through worldwide web almost instantaneously. The author prefers the guidelines developed by the National Osteoporosis Foundation (NOF; *www.nof.org*) or the International Society for Clinical Densitometry (ISCD; *www.iscd.org*). Diabetic patients who are particularly at risk for osteoporosis include postmenopausal women, elderly patients of either gender, patients with cystic fibrosis who may have additional contribution from malabsorption,[17] patients with clinical signs and symptoms of peripheral neuropathy and vascular disease, retinopathy, and propensity to falls.[25] Although the measurement of bone density at relevant sites remains the best available tool to assess fracture risk, interpretation of bone density results in diabetics is a challenging task. Bone density may not always be low especially in patients with type 2 diabetes but is frequently low in those with type 1. Unfortunately, the quality of bone, which may be abnormal despite normal bone density, cannot be estimated noninvasively at the present time. Therefore, patients may need treatment even at a higher bone density than the general population, if they have already sustained fractures.

Measurement of serum calcium, alkaline phosphatase, 25-hydroxyvitamin D and parathyroid hormone (PTH) is important to exclude both vitamin D depletion and secondary hyperparathyroidism.[33] In type 1 diabetes, it is important to measure 24-hour urine calcium to be sure that uncontrolled diabetes is not associated with significant hypercalciuria. Renal dysfunction is an independent risk factor for fractures in patients with diabetes. Fasting urine N-terminal telopetide (NTX) is a sensitive marker of bone resorption, but lacks specificity. Nevertheless, baseline measurement of fasting urine NTX and again after several weeks of antifracture therapy to assess response is reasonable. Spine X-rays should be performed only in those patients with a history of back pain or significant height loss (greater than 1–2 inches). However, routine X-rays of the spine may not be cost effective except if one has access to vertebral morphometry on bone density instruments.

MANAGEMENT OF LOW BONE DENSITY AND/OR OSTEOPOROSIS IN THE DIABETIC POPULATION

Adequate calcium and vitamin D nutrition should be assured by recommending a least 1,000 mg of elemental calcium for men, 1,200 mg for women on hormone therapy and 1,500 mg for women not on hormone therapy. Adequate vitamin D supplementation in the form of multivitamins or other supplements amounting to at least 600 to 800 IU of vitamin D should be recommended to all patients.[15] It should be kept in mind that every randomized clinical trial in osteoporosis was conducted with supplemental calcium and vitamin D.

Therefore, it is imperative to assure adequate calcium and vitamin D nutrition for optimal bone health and response to specific therapy.

In patients with vitamin D depletion (serum 25-hydroxyvitamin D levels <20 ng/dl) pharmacologic vitamin D therapy may be required before beginning specific therapy for osteoporosis. This author recommends 50,000 IU of vitamin D once a week for 8 to 12 weeks to replenish vitamin D stores followed by 600 to 800 IU of vitamin D/day for life. This strategy entails no harm and has the potential of reducing fractures in general and hip fractures in particular.[15]

For those who have evidence of decreased bone density and/or history of fractures, any of the currently approved drugs for osteoporosis in nondiabetic patients can be prescribed.[34,35] Although there is not a priori reason to believe that diabetic patients respond differently, rigorous therapeutic beneficial results with antifracture therapy in this population is not available. Special attention should be paid to renal dysfunction when using alendronate or risedronate, the two currently approved drugs, since bisphosphonates are cleared by the kidneys. Any decrease in renal function would compromise the elimination of the bisphosphonate. In general, patients with serum creatinine <2.0 mg/dl can be treated with bisphosphonates without too much problem, but follow-up should be more diligent and more frequent. Special attention should also be paid to the patients with overt or subclinical autonomic neuropathy or diabetic gastroparesis. In such cases, intravenous bisphosphonates can be considered provided renal function is not impaired and the dose is appropriately timed.[36]

Raloxifene, a selective estrogen receptor modulator, is also an effective therapy for postmenopausal women with decreased bone density.[37,38] In addition to preventing vertebral fractures, it offers other extraskeletal benefits that may be particularly relevant to the diabetic population. However, because of the potential increase in the incidence of venous thromboembolic events, it may not be an appropriate choice for a diabetic patient with increased risk of micro- and macrovascular events. Similarly, estrogen replacement therapy should be considered after evaluating the potential risk benefit ratio. However, with the recent women's health initiative study results, estrogen therapy may not be as attractive as it had been in the past.[39] Obviously, both estrogen and raloxifene can only be used in postmenopausal women.

Calcitonin, both parental and nasal, has been used with success in osteoporosis and is probably the safest therapy available.[40,41] However, it is also the weakest antifracture medicine. The parental form is also used in metatarsal and ankle fractures and in the management of Charcot joints. The analgesic effect of higher doses of subcutaneous calcitonin (200 units every 8 or 6 hours) is particularly attractive in patients with painful neuropathy and metatarsal fractures.

MONITORING OF THERAPY

Patients should be monitored with periodic measurements of urine NTX to assess the response to specific therapy and also to assure that bone turnover is not excessively suppressed, since diabetes mellitus itself is associated with decreased bone turnover, especially in the elderly. Treatment with bisphosphonates might further reduce bone turnover and increase the bone aging (not to be confused with chronologic age of the patient) and bone fragility. Periodic assessment of calcium and vitamin D by measuring PTH and 25-hydroxyvitamin D on a yearly basis is reasonable. Bone density should be performed at least two years after initiation of therapy and periodically thereafter. Fall prevention and regular exercise program are just as important as pharmacologic therapy and nutritional supplements. In patients with propensity to falls, hip protectors might offer the best nonpharmacologic therapy to prevent hip fracture. Corrective glasses for declining vision, prompt intervention for retinopathy and attention to foot care to prevent falls are essential to prevent fractures.

SPECIAL CIRCUMSTANCES

Apart from low bone density and increased risk of fractures, diabetic patients present with special bone problems. Metatarsal and ankle fractures occur with increased frequency in patients with diabetes and may not necessarily be associated with decreased bone density. Similarly, Charcot joint, the most devastating skeletal complication of diabetic mellitus, requires prompt treatment. The pathogenesis of these fractures is not well understood. Vascular insufficiency, neuropathy, local inflammatory cytokine production leading increased bone turnover, similar to that seen in regional accelerated phenomenon, unrecognized infection, and repetitive trauma may all contribute to the development of these complications. The often used descriptive term *diabetic osteopathy* probably should be restricted to these conditions rather than to the generalized decrease in bone density and other well-known osteoporotic fractures. Both the metatarsal fractures and Charcot joints can be treated with intravenous bisphosphonates pamidronate 60 mg every 3 to 6 months or zolidronic acid 4 mg once a year or at less frequent intervals depending upon the response of biochemical markers of bone turnover. Although no convincing long-term results are available, several reports have shown significant therapeutic benefit. Hopefully with the more frequent use of oral bisphosphonate to prevent bone loss, we may even be able to prevent these complications.

An emerging bone disease, commonly referred to as adynamic bone disease, characterized by a markedly reduced bone turnover is seen with increasing frequency in patients on maintenance hemodialysis.[42] Aluminum accumulation, advancing age, and diabetes are the three most risk factors for the development of this bone lesion in renal failure. However, the clinical relevance of this bone disease in the context of diabetic patients is yet to be determined. Since little is known about its pathogenesis a logical treatment strategy cannot be recommended, but cautious and judicious use of daily injection of PTH in those with PTH levels <100 pg/ml might be considered.[43] The author has treated one such patient with some success.

Delayed fracture healing is common in diabetic patients for a variety of reasons including poor bone quality, impaired osteoblast function, osteocyte apoptosis, and local cytokine-mediated bone resorption.[44,45] Compression fractures of dorsal vertebrae can occur in patients who develop hypoglycemic convulsions.[46]

SUMMARY

Diabetes is a chronic condition associated with a variety of systemic effects including vascular and tissue damage, advanced glycation of collagen, and bone cell dysfunction. With the availability of newer technology to detect osteoporosis much earlier than clinical fractures, it is possible to detect patients who are at the greatest risk for fractures and initiate therapy with bisphosphonates, which have been proven effective in several randomized controlled clinical trials. Assessment of vitamin D and calcium nutrition by appropriate biochemical measurements and insuring adequate calcium vitamin D nutrition is essential in the management of osteoporosis and fracture prevention in diabetics. Regular exercise program, fall prevention education, and wearing hip protectors are other nonpharmacologic modalities to prevent osteoporotic fractures in the diabetic population. For patients with metatarsal fractures and Charcot joints, intravenous bisphosphonates are an effective form of therapy. Monitoring patients from time-to-time to assess the effectiveness of treatment is recommended.

ACKNOWLEDGMENTS

The author sincerely thanks the following: Dr Fred Whitehouse, my mentor and a consummate teacher, for helpful discussions and constructive criticism, Drs Bhan, Gonzalez-Feldman and Levy, for critical reviewing of the earlier drafts of the manuscript, and Ms Charlene Jones for reference retrieval and manuscript preparation. This work was partly supported by the Indian Society for Bone and Mineral Research.

REFERENCES

1. Albright F, Reifenstein EC. The parathyroid glands and metabolic bone diseases: selected studies. Baltimore: The Williams and Wilkins Company, 1948.
2. Ivers RQ, Cumming RG, Mitchell P, Peduto AJ. Diabetes and risk of fracture: the Blue Mountains Eye Study. Diabetes Care. 2001;24:1198-203.
3. Nicodemus KK, Folsom AR, Iowa Women's HS. Type 1 and type 2 diabetes and incident hip fractures in postmenopausal women. Diabetes Care. 2001;24:1192-7.
4. Schwartz AV, Sellmeyer DE, Ensrud KE, et al. Older women with diabetes have an increased risk of fracture: a prospective study. J Clin Endocrinol Metab. 2001; 86:32-8.
5. Nelson DA, Jacober SJ. Why do older women with diabetes have an increased fracture risk? J Clin Endocrinol Metab. 2001;86:29-31.
6. Forsen L, Meyer HE, Midthjell K, Edna TH. Diabetes mellitus and the incidence of hip fracture: results from the Nord-Trondelag Health Survey. Diabetologia. 1999;42:920-5.
7. Tuominen JT, Impivaara O, Puukka P, Ronnemaa T. Bone mineral density in patients with type 1 and type 2 diabetes. Diabetes Care. 1999;22:1196-200.
8. Melchior TM, Sorensen H, Torp-Pedersen C. Hip and distal arm fracture rates in peri- and postmenopausal insulin-treated diabetic females. J Intern Med. 1994; 236:203-8.
9. Meyer HE, Tverdal A, Falch JA. Risk factors for hip fracture in middle-aged Norwegian women and men. Am J Epidemiol. 1993;137:1203-11.
10. Ziegler R. Diabetes mellitus and bone metabolism. Horm Metabol Res. 1992; 26:90-4.
11. Kelsey JL, Browner WS, Seeley DG, Nevitt MC, Cummings SR. Risk factors for fractures of the distal forearm and proximal humerus. The Study of Osteoporotic Fractures Research Group. Am J Epidemiol. 1992;135:477-89.
12. Van Daele PL, Stolk RP, Burger H, et al. Bone density in non-insulin-dependent diabetes mellitus. The Rotterdam Study. Ann Intern Med. 1995;122:409-14.
13. Bouillon R. Diabetic bone disease. Calcif Tis Internat. 1991;49:155-60.

14. Garay-Sevilla ME, Nava LE, Malacara JM, Wrobel K, Perez U. Advanced glycosylation end products (AGEs), insulin-like growth factor-1 (IGF-1) and IGF-binding protein-3 (IGFBP-3) in patients with type 2 diabetes mellitus. Diabetes Metab Res Rev. 2000;16:106-13.

15. Rao DS. Perspective on assessment of vitamin D nutrition. J Clin Densitometry. 1999;2:457-64.

16. Basha B, Rao DS, Han ZH, Parfitt AM. Osteomalacia due to vitamin D depletion in the US. Ame J Med. 2000;108:296-300.

17. Elkin SL, Fairney A, Burnett S, et al. Vertebral deformities and low bone mineral density in adults with cystic fibrosis: a cross-sectional study. Osteoporosis Int. 2001; 12:366-72.

18. Krakauer JC, McKenna MJ, Buderer NF, et al. Bone loss and bone turnover in diabetes. Diabetes. 1995; 44:775-82.

19. Hampson G, Evans C, Petitt RJ, et al. Bone mineral density, collagen type 1 alpha 1 genotypes and bone turnover in premenopausal women with diabetes mellitus. Diabetologia. 1998;41:1314-20.

20. Grisso JA, Kelsey JL, Strom BL, et al. Risk factors for hip fracture in black women. N Engl J Med. 1994;330:1555-9.

21. Cummings SR, Nevitt MC, Browner WS, et al. Risk factors for hip fracture in white women. N Engl J Med. 1995;332:767-73.

22. Parfitt AM, Han ZH, Palnitkar S, Rao DS, Shih MS, Nelson D. Effects of ethnicity and age or menopause on osteoblast function, bone mineralization, and osteoid accumulation in iliac bone. J Bone Miner Res. 1997;12:1864-73.

23. Parikh N, Durr J, Honasoge M, Phillips ER, Kimura J, Rao DS. Prevalence of vitamin D depletion among patients referred for evaluation of osteoporosis. J Bone Miner Res. 1999;14:S539.

24. Rao DS. Role of vitamin D and calcium nutrition in bone health in India. In Mithal A, Rao DS, Zaidi M (Eds): metabolic bone disorders. Lucknow, India: Indian Society of Bone and Mineral Research. 1998; pp. 71-6.

25. Wallace C, Reiber GE, LeMaster J, et al. Incidence of falls, risk factors for falls, and fall-related fractures in individuals with diabetes and a prior foot ulcer. Diabetes Care. 2002;25:1983-6.

26. Trivedi DP, Doll R, Khaw KT. Effect of four monthly oral vitamin D$_3$ (cholecalciferol) supplementation on fractures and mortality in men and women living in the community: randomised double blind controlled trial. Br Med J. 2003;326:469-71.

27. Gloth FM, Smith CE, Hollis BW, Tobin JD. Functional improvement with vitamin D replenishment in a cohort of frail, vitamin D deficient older people. J Am Geriatr Soc. 1995;43:1269-71.

28. Qiu SJ, Palnitkar S, Rao DS. Age-related changes in osteocyte density and distribution in human cancellous bone. J Bone Miner Res. 1999;14:S308.

29. Jamal SA, Stone K, Browner WS, Ensrud KE, Cummings SR. Serum fructosamine level and the risk of hip fracture in elderly women: a case-cohort study within the study of osteoporotic fractures. Ame J Med. 1998;105:488-93.

30. Kathol MH, el-Khoury GY, Moore TE, Marsh JL. Calcaneal insufficiency avulsion fractures in patients with diabetes mellitus. Radiology. 1991;180:725-9.

31. Hedlund LJ, Maki DD, Griffiths HJ. Calcaneal fractures in diabetic patients. J Diabetes and its Complications. 1998;12:81-7.

32. Cundy TF, Edmonds ME, Watkins PJ. Osteopenia and metatarsal fractures in diabetic neuropathy. Diabetic Med. 1985;2:461-4.

33. Tannenbaum C, Clark J, Schwartzman K, et al. Yield of laboratory testing to identify secondary contributors to osteoporosis in otherwise healthy women. J Clin Endocrinol Metab. 2002;87:4431-7.

34. Black DM, Cummings SR, Karpf DB, et al. Randomised trial of effect of alendronate on risk of fracture in women with existing vertebral fractures. Lancet. 1996; 348:1535-41.

35. McClung MR, Geusens P, Miller PD, et al. Effect of risedronate on the risk of hip fracture in elderly women. N Engl J Med. 2001;344:333-40.

36. Reid IR, Brown JP, Burckhardt P, et al. Intravenous zoledronic acid in postmenopausal women with low bone mineral density. N Engl J Med 2002; 346:653-661.

37. Barrett-Connor E, Grady D, Sashegyi A, et al. Raloxifene and cardiovascular events in soteoporotic postmenopausal women: Four-year results from the multiple outcomes of raloxifene evaluation (MORE) randomized trial [Article]. JAMA. 2002; 287:847-57.

38. Barrett-Connor E, Holbrook TL. Sex differences in osteoporosis in older adults with non-insulin dependent diabetes mellitus. JAMA. 1992; 268:3333-7.

39. Manson JE, Hsia J, Johnson KC, et al. Estrogen plus progestin and the risk of coronary heart disease. The New England Journal of Medicine. 2003; 349:523-34.

40. Adami H, Baroni MC, Broggini M, et al. Treatment of postmenopausal osteoporosis with continuous daily oral alendronate in comparison with either placebo or intranasal salmon calcitonin. Osteoporosis Int. 1993;3:21-7.

41. Adami H, Passeri M, Ortolani S, et al. Effects of oral alendronate and intranasal salmon calcitonin on bone mass and biochemical markers of bone turnover in postmenopausal women with osteoporosis. Bone. 1995;17:383-90.

42. Malluche HH, Faugere MC. Risk of adynamic bone disease in dialyzed patients. Kidney Internat. 1992;38:S62-7.

43. Neer RM, Arnaud CD, Zanchetta JR, et al. Effect of parathyroid hormone (1-34) on fractures and bone mineral density in postmenopausal women with osteoporosis. N Engl J Med. 2001;344:1434-41.

44. Loder RT. The influence of diabetes mellitus on the healing of closed fractures. Clin Orthop Rel Res. 1988;232:210-6.

45. Dixit PK, Ekstrom RA. Retardation of bone fracture healing in experimental diabetes. Indian J Med Res. 1987;85:426-35.

46. Nabarro JD. Compression fractures of the dorsal spine in hypoglycaemic fits in diabetes. Bri Med J Clin Res Ed. 1985;291:1320.

Chapter 73

RHEUMATOLOGICAL MANIFESTATIONS OF DIABETES MELLITUS

Ramnath Misra, Parshant Aggarwal

CHAPTER OUTLINE

- Introduction
- Hyperostosis
- Diabetic Cheiroarthropathy (Limited joint mobility syndrome)
- Diabetic Muscular Infarction
- Adhesive Capsulitis of the Shoulder (Periarthritis)
- Neuropathic Arthropathy

- Dupuytren's Contracture
- Palmar Flexor Tenosynovitis (Trigger finger)
- Osteopenia
- Carpal-Tunnel Syndrome
- Gout
- Osteoarthritis
- Conclusion

INTRODUCTION

Diabetes mellitus leads to complex metabolic disturbances leading onto a variety of alterations in connective tissue. Although cardiovascular, renal, ocular and neurological complications represent most severe long-term complications of diabetes mellitus (DM), many rheumatic syndromes occur more frequently in diabetic patients than in general population.[1,2] These syndromes may appear as independent disease processes or as modification in the course or frequency of common rheumatic conditions.[3] A classification of these varied manifestations based upon the underlying mechanisms and strength of the association[1] is given below **(Table 73.1)**.

HYPEROSTOSIS

Hyperostosis or metaplastic calcification is much more common in diabetes than in the general population. In

TABLE 73.1	Joint and bone conditions associated with DM

Characteristically associated with diabetes
   Diffuse idiopathic skeletal hyperostosis (DISH)
   Limited joint mobility syndrome
   Diabetic muscular infarction

Increased incidence in diabetes
   Adhesive capsulitis of the shoulder
   Neuropathic arthropathy
   Dupuytren's disease
   Palmar flexor tenosynovitis (trigger finger)
   Osteopenia

Probable association with diabetes
   Carpal-Tunnel syndrome
   Gout
   Osteoarthritis

diabetic subjects, the prevalence varies between 13 to 49% as compared to 1.6 to 13% in general population.[1,4,5] The entheseal regions (sites of ligament and tendon attachments with bone) are predominantly affected. It

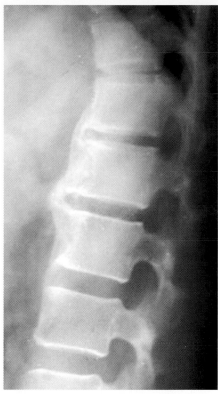

Figure 73.1 Diffuse idiopathic skeletal hyperostosis (DISH). The X-ray in the lateral view of lumbar spine shows calcification of anterospinal ligament resulting in joining or 'bridging' of four contiguous vertebrae

is a systemic condition and not just a reaction to local mechanical factors.[6] Hyperostosis may present as hyperostotic spondylosis (calcification of spinal ligaments), hyperostosis frontalis interna (abnormal deposition of bone on inner aspect of frontal bone) or anywhere else in the body.[1] Calcification of the spinal ligaments is the commonest and is known as diffuse idiopathic skeletal hyperostosis (DISH). Clinically, deposition of new bone is usually asymptomatic apart from increasing stiffness in the neck, back or peripheral joints. Symptomatology are milder than that would be expected from the extent of radiological involvement. The radiological diagnostic criteria includes bridging of four contiguous vertebral bodies by new bone formation in the absence of degenerative disk disease and the absence of inflammatory sacroiliac or facet changes **(Figure 73.1)**.[7] Rarely fractures through the bony bridges may occur which are difficult to diagnose and treat.[8] This condition is more likely associated with other metabolic derangements such as hyperuricemia, obesity, dyslipidemia and elevated growth hormone levels.[5,6] Hyperinsulinemia for prolonged periods is

believed to promote new bone growth, particularly at the entheseal sites in DISH.[6] There is no specific medical therapy hence emphasis is on controlling the metabolic imbalance. Physical therapy can be of help.[9]

DIABETIC CHEIROARTHROPATHY (LIMITED JOINT MOBILITY SYNDROME)

It is also known as the diabetic hand syndrome and has a strong association with diabetes. It is particularly seen in patients with long-standing type 1 diabetes but also occurs in patients with type 2 diabetes. In type 1 diabetics, the frequency varies widely from 9 to 50% of the patients.[3,10] There is an inability to extend metacarpophalangeal joints fully associated with thickening and tightening of skin of the dorsum of hands resembling the skin changes seen in systemic sclerosis.[1,3] The flexor tendon sheath may be thickened. Therefore, the patients has stiffness of fingers and reduction of manual dexterity leading onto difficulty in forming fist, weakness of grip and difficulty in fine movements.[11] There is limitation of both active and passive movements. It is evaluated by two simple tests—the inability to approximate the palmar surfaces of fingers and palms resulting in *the prayer sign* **(Figure 73.2)** and inability to flatten the palm against the surface of table—*the table top test*.[12] The condition generally begins on ulnar side and then spreads radially, rarely it may be a generalized phenomenon, affecting all the extremities. It may

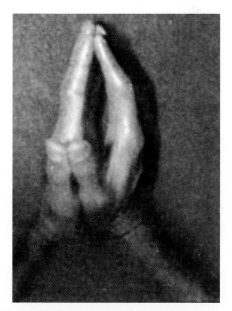

Figure 73.2 Diabetic cheiroarthropathy—*Prayer sign* showing inability to appose palmar surfaces of hands due to limitation of PIP and MCP extension

precede the onset of diabetes in some patients.[11] It can be distinguished from systemic sclerosis by the absence of Raynaud's phenomenon and serological markers.

The cause of cheiroarthropathy is not clear. The etiology is believed to be multifactorial, including genetic factors. Microangiopathy and direct metabolic changes including increased nonenzymatic glycosylation may be important in pathogenesis.[3,11]

The management mainly consists of reassurance and explanation with emphasis on strict diabetic control. The role of aldose reductase inhibitors is controversial.

DIABETIC MUSCULAR INFARCTION

Muscle infarction is a rare complication of diabetes seen more often in women. It usually occurs in patients with long-standing type 1 DM who have multiple end organ microvascular complications. The group of muscles of thigh and calves are commonly involved. It can cause bilateral involvement.[13,14] Typically, patient presents with acute onset of localized pain and tenderness. On examination, there is a palpable mass with swelling and induration of surrounding tissue and limited range of movement. Systemic evidence of infection is lacking, as is skin discoloration. Lesion generally persists for weeks followed by resolution over several weeks to months. Recurrence is reported in about 50%.[13]

Muscle enzymes like creatinine kinase levels have been reported to be normal in three-fourth of the patients, however, elevated levels may be found in first few days after acute muscle infarction. T2 weighted MR sequences are highly sensitive to pick-up acute changes, which show high intensity signal in involved muscle. Histological features consist of large areas of muscle necrosis and edema, there may be presence of regenerating muscle fibers and lymphocytic interstitial infiltration. However, changes are nonspecific. The condition has to be distinguished from several others listed in **Table 73.2**.

The underlying etiology is most likely diabetic microvascular disease although vasculitis has been suggested in some instances. Management consists of bed rest, analgesics and aggressive metabolic control.[13] Prognosis is good but there is increased risk of cardiovascular mortality.[1]

ADHESIVE CAPSULITIS OF THE SHOULDER (PERIARTHRITIS)

The association between diabetes and periarthritis of shoulder is well established with reported incidence

TABLE 73.2	Differential diagnosis of diabetic muscular infarction[14]

Vascular
    Hemorrhage
    Arterial occlusion
    Thrombophlebitis
    Hemangioma
    Lymph edema

Infections
    Pyomyositis
    Osteomyelitis
    Parasitic infestation
    Sarcoma

Miscellaneous
    Ruptured synovial cyst

between 11 to 19% in diabetic subjects as compared to 2 to 3% in age-matched controls; also bilateral involvement is more common in diabetic subjects than in nondiabetic subjects (33 to 44% vs 5 to 20%).[1] A recent series from India has reported an incidence of 17.9% in diabetic patients. Moreover of nondiabetic patients with adhesive capsulitis 23.3% had impaired glucose tolerance.[15] It presents with pain and restriction of shoulder joint movement. The glenohumeral joint is normal. Treatment includes physiotherapy, nonsteroidal anti-inflammatory drugs, local steroid injections and surgery.

NEUROPATHIC ARTHROPATHY

This results from impairment of joint sensation due to damage of sensory nerve supply of the joints. Repetitive trauma leads to cartilage and capsular damage leads onto a disorganized but painless joint.[16] First described in 1868, as a consequence of tabes dorsalis, it can be a consequence of many conditions but diabetes is the commonest cause in developed countries.[1] It affects 0.1 to 0.4% of diabetic patients, most frequently in the age group 50 to 69 years. There is no gender association but it tends to affect those with a longer duration of diabetes with majority of cases reported in literature having disease duration more than 10 years.[1,3,16] The most commonly affected joints are metatarsophalangeal (31.5%) followed by tarsometatarsal (27.4%), tarsal (21.8%), ankle (10.2%) and interphalangeal (9.1%).[3] Knee, wrist, elbow, shoulders and intervertebral joints are rarely involved. About 20% of cases have bilateral involvement.[16]

Clinical symptoms are much milder than expected on basis of radiological changes. The affected joints are subluxed with loose articular capsule and abnormal joint mobility with marked painless swelling. In advanced cases, marked deformities are seen. The clue to diagnosis is based on neurological finding of loss of joint and vibration sensation. Signs of peripheral neuropathy are present in all the cases. The overlying skin shows erythema, pigmentations and atrophic changes with skin ulceration.[17] The radiological findings include circumscribed osteoporosis, subluxation, osteolysis, fractures, periosteal reaction, arthrosis deformans and ankylosis.[3] Though the diagnosis is not difficult in a typical case, there may be considerable difficulty in distinguishing this condition from coexisting osteomyelitis. MRI plays an important role in diagnosing infectious process but can fail to distinguish between the two conditions.[1,18]

The pathogenesis is contributed by several factors with a dominating role played by peripheral neuropathy.[1,3,19] Other factors including microangiopathy, impaired autonomic nerve function[11,20] may be responsible.

Conservative management is indicated in most cases with emphasis on strict diabetic control. Bed rest and protection from weight bearing are helpful. Importance of foot hygiene cannot be overemphasized. Surgery is indicated for nonhealing ulcers, broad-spectrum antibiotics are essential when indicated. Amputation is indicated in only a few cases with severe microangiopathy or gangrene.[3,11]

DUPUYTREN'S CONTRACTURE

It is fairly common in diabetic patients with prevalence between 21 to 63% in diabetic patients as compared to 5 to 22% in general population.[21] The condition is associated with both type 1 and type 2 diabetes. It occurs more frequently in patients with long-standing disease. Dupuytren's contracture is milder in diabetic patients compared to nondiabetic persons. Surgery is rarely required. Middle and the ring finger are affected more frequently.[22]

PALMAR FLEXOR TENOSYNOVITIS (TRIGGER FINGER)

It results from stenosing tenosynovitis of digital flexors and is seen more commonly in type 1 DM patients with long-standing disease.[23] Intermittent locking of finger flexion movement is called as trigger finger. It may occur any time in the day but is more frequent in the morning while bending the fingers.[11] This phenomenon is related to cheiroarthropathy and Dupuytren's contracture. Within the flexor tendon sheath, a nodular swelling can often be palpated. Treatment consists of local corticosteroid injection that gives excellent response in most of the cases.

OSTEOPENIA

The association between diabetes and osteoporosis is controversial. Although most studies have shown lower bone mineral density in type 1 diabetic patients, bone mass in type 2 diabetic patients may be greater than in controls.[3,24] The mechanisms leading to decreased bone mineral density in type 1 diabetes are not clear. It has been found that low bone mass in patients with type 1 diabetes begins after the onset of disease. It has been postulated that decreased levels of insulin and insulin-related growth factors might be responsible.[1,24]

CARPAL-TUNNEL SYNDROME

The reported frequency of this syndrome in diabetic patients is as high as 25% and nondiabetic subjects with this syndrome may have an increased propensity to develop diabetes[1,11] but no controlled study has found a higher incidence in diabetic patients than in age and weight-matched controls.

GOUT

Definite association has not been proven and it might be possible that primary abnormality is obesity, which can lead onto gouty arthritis. Recent reports have failed to show association between the two.[15]

OSTEOARTHRITIS (OA)

Higher prevalence is reported in diabetic patients than in general population and the former have an earlier onset of OA.[15] Impaired glucose utilization in diabetic patients may alter glycosaminoglycan and proteoglycan production.[1] However, osteoarthritis in DM may be related to obesity than with diabetes itself.[11] None of the reports showing association between the two disorders have used weight-matched controls; thereby the association between the two is not conclusive.

CONCLUSION

Musculoskeletal manifestations are quite common in both forms of diabetes which may adversely affect the functional quality of life. These vary from milder tenosynovitis to severe destruction of the joints. The pathogenesis of these conditions have not been precisely elucidated. Till we are clearer about the exact mechanisms, it is advisable to prescribe a tighter metabolic control of the disease as hyperglycemia *per se* may be the basis of structural alternation of the cartilage and periarticular tissues leading to joint dysfunction.

REFERENCES

1. Crispin JC, Alcocer-Varela J. Rheumatological manifestations of diabetes mellitus. Am J Med. 2003;114:753-7.
2. Peterson KR, Edelman SV, Kim DD. Musculoskeletal complications of diabetes mellitus. Clin Diabetes. 2001;19:132-5.
3. Forgacs SS. Diabetes mellitus. In Hochberg MC, Silman AJ, Smolen JS, Weinblatt ME, Weisman MH (Eds): Rheumatology, 3rd edn. London: Mosby; 2003.pp.1977-82.
4. Forgacs S. Diabetes mellitus and rheumatic disease. Clin Rheum Dis. 1986;12:729-53.
5. Kiss C, Szilagyi M, Paksky A, Poor G. Risk factors for diffuse idiopathic skeletal hyperostosis: a case controlled study. Rheumatology. 2002;41:27-30.
6. Littlejohn GO. Insulin and new bone formation in diffuse idiopathic skeletal hyperostosis. Clin Rheumatol. 1985;4:294-300.
7. Littlejohn GO. More emphasis on the enthuses. J Rheumatol. 1989;16:1020-1.
8. Mata S, Fortin PR, Fitzcharles MA, et al. A controlled study of diffuse idiopathic skeletal hyperostosis. Clinical features and functional status. Medicine (Baltimore). 1997;76:104-17.
9. Littlejohn G. Diffuse idiopathic skeletal hyperostosis. In Hochberg MC, Silman AJ, Smolen JS, Weinblatt ME, Weisman MH (Eds). Rheumatology, 3rd edn. London: Mosby; 2003. pp. 1863-7.
10. Garza-Elizondo MA, Diaz-Jouanen E, Franco-Casique J, Alarcon-Segovia D. Joint contractures and scleroderma-like skin changes in the hands of insulin dependent juvenile diabetics. J Rheumatol. 1983;10:797-800.
11. Pal B. Rheumatic disorders and bone problems in diabetes mellitus. In Pickup JC, Williams G (Eds): textbook of diabetes, 3rd edn. Oxford: Blackwell Science; 2003. pp. 61.1-13.
12. Clarke C, Pisowicz A, Spathis G. Limited joint mobility in children and adolescents with insulin-dependent diabetes mellitus. Ann Rheum Dis. 1990;42:297-300.
13. Umpierrez GE, Stiles RG, Kleinblatt J, Krendel DA, Watts NB. Diabetic muscular infarction. Am J Med. 1996;101:245-50.
14. Rocca PV, Alloway JA, Nashel DJ. Diabetic muscular infarction. Semin Arth Rheum. 1993;22:280-6.
15. Sarkar RN, Banerjee S, Basu AK, Bandhopadhyay D. Rheumatological manifestations of diabetes mellitus. J Ind Rheumatol Assoc. 2003;11:25-9.
16. Sinha S, Munichoodappa CS, Kozak GP. Neuroarthropathy in diabetes mellitus. Medicine. 1972;51:191-210.
17. Forgacs S. Clinical picture of diabetic osteoarthropathy. Acta Diabetol Lat. 1976;13:111-9.
18. Wang A, Weinstein D, Greenfield L, et al. MRI and diabetic foot infections. Magn Reson Imaging. 1990;8:805-9.
19. Bruckner FE, Howell A. Neuropatic joint. Semin Arth Rheum. 1972;2:47-69.
20. Brower AC, Allman RM. Pathogenesis of the Neuropathic joint: neurotraumatic vs neurovascular. Radiology. 1981;139:349-54.
21. Holt PJL. Rheumatological manifestations of diabetes mellitus. Clin Rheum Dis. 1981;7:723-46.
22. Arkkila PE, Kantola IM, Viikari JS. Dupuytren's disease: association with chronic diabetic complications. J Rheumatol. 1997;24:153-9.
23. Benedetti A, Noacco C, Simonatti M. Diabetic trigger finger. N Engl J Med. 1982;306:1552.
24. Tuominen JT, Impivaara O, Puukka P, Ronnemaa T. Bone mineral density in patients with type 1 and type 2 diabetes. Diabetes Care. 1999;22:1196-200.

Chapter 74

SEXUAL DYSFUNCTION IN DIABETES

V Balaji, V Seshiah

CHAPTER OUTLINE

- Introduction
- Physiology of Penile Erection
- Etiology
- Clinical Features
- Clinical Evaluation
- Psychogenic or Organic
- Clinical Assessment

- Vascular Assessment
- Neurological Assessment
- Hormonal Assessment
- Treatment of Diabetic Erectile Failure
- Sexual Problems in Diabetic Women
- Conclusion
- Summary

INTRODUCTION

Sexual function is a complex blend of anatomic, neurologic, metabolic, endocrine and psychic factors more than any other human activity. Alterations in any one of the factors can result in sexual dysfunction. Though the exact prevalence of sexual dysfunction in general population is not known, the consensus is that this problem is not uncommon in male diabetic subjects. Amongst the systemic diseases, diabetes is unique in this regard. The prevalence of erectile dysfunction in male diabetic subjects varies between 30 to 70%, the average being 50% and increases as age advances.[1] Sexual dysfunction in a male diabetic subject may occur at an early age and could be the presenting symptom of diabetes.

PHYSIOLOGY OF PENILE ERECTION

The normal male sexual response consists of four phases of excitement, plateau (erection, ejaculation), orgasm and resolution. Factors required for the production and maintenance of an erection and for normal ejaculation to occur are given in **Table 74.1**. Failure of any one of these responses results in sexual dysfunction. The commonest sexual dysfunction that occurs in a male diabetic subject is erectile failure and in contrast to other complications of diabetes, erectile failure in a male diabetic subject can occur before and as well as years after diagnosis of diabetes. Rarely retrograde ejaculation (dry orgasm) may occur in a male diabetic subject with long duration of poorly controlled diabetes due to

TABLE 74.1	Factors required for the production and maintenance of an erection

- Adequate desire and arousal
- Adequate testosterone levels and endocrine status
- Anatomically normal penis
- Adequate arterial inflow
- Effective venous occlusive mechanism
- Integrity of autonomic and sensory neural pathways

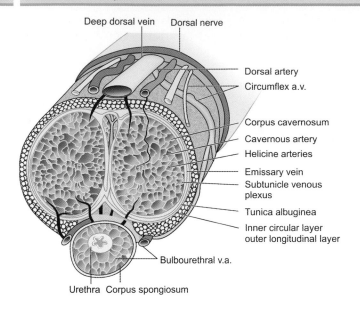

Figure 74.1 Structure of the erectile components of the penis with blood supply and innervation

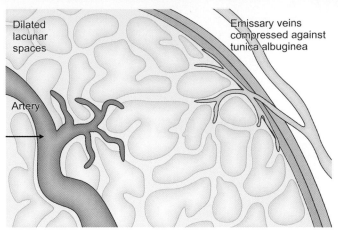

Figure 74.2 The erect state, following activation of efferent autonomic nerves, the elevated pressure in the lacunar space expands the trabecular structures against the tunica albuginea

dysfunction of the autonomic and somatic nervous systems. Though erectile failure occurs with increased frequency in a male diabetic subject due to diabetes *per se*, it is important to remember that any cause of erectile failure in nondiabetic men may also operate in diabetic males.

The structure of the penis includes two corpora cavernosa **(Figure 74.1)**. They are spongy channels capable of expanding to contain more blood at times of sexual arousal. Penile arteries occupy the central position in each unit. The veins are located near the surface of the organ. Erection depends upon the adequate filling of the paired corpora cavernosa with blood at systolic pressure by the cavernosal arteries. A number of corkscrew-shaped helicine arteries branch off from each cavernosal artery and empty into the interconnected sinusoidal (lacunar) spaces. At the time of arousal, these tonically contracted helicine arteries relax allowing the augmented blood flow to the lacunar spaces resulting in tumescence. Penile erection is initiated by a complex set of psychogenic, visual, olfactory, auditory and other stimuli. The cerebral cortex, processes the stimuli and the efferent impulses pass through spinal cord, sacral parasympathetic *(Nervi erigentes)* to the trabecular (sinusoidal spaces) smooth muscles. Release of neurotransmitter acetyl choline by the parasympathetic nerves mediates the relaxation of the trabecular smooth muscle. Acetyl choline acts on endothelial cells to release a second noradrenergic,

noncholinergic (NANC) neurotransmitter. The vasoactive intestinal polypeptide (VIP) was thought to be the final neurotransmitter earlier but the recent concept is that nitric oxide is the carrier of the NANC relaxation signal. Nitric oxide causes relaxation of the trabecular smooth muscles by stimulating guanylate cyclase to produce cyclic guanosine monophosphate (cGMP) which functions as the final messenger. The relaxed trabecular smooth muscles allow increased blood flow into the sinusoidal spaces. The increased blood flow expands the relaxed trabecular walls against the tunica albuginea, compressing the plexus of subtunical veins and restricting the venous drainage from the sinusoidal spaces. Erection is therefore a balance between adequate arterial inflow from the cavernosal arteries and the resistance to outflow of blood from the sinusoidal spaces by the effective veno-occlusive mechanism **(Figure 74.2)**. Detumescence is accomplished by the reversal of these processes, which depend upon sympathetic tone **(Figure 74.3)**.

ETIOLOGY

Causes of erectile failure may be enumerated as metabolic, psychogenic, endocrine, neurological, vascular, drug-induced or mixed **(Table 74.2)**. The organic causes are the commonest, comprising about 85% of the cases, psychological problems account for about 10% and in the remaining 5%, the cause remains unknown.[2] Failure to attain penile erection due to organic causes puts a man into strain and repeated unsuccessful attempts leads to psychological stress and the vicious cycle

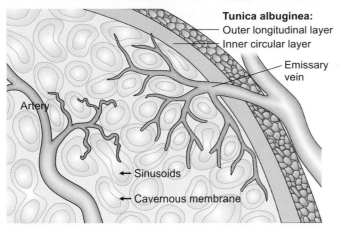

Figure 74.3 When the penis is in the flaccid state (left insert), the contracted corporal smooth muscle allows blood to drain from the erectile tissue to the subtunical venules under conditions of low outflow resistance

perpetuates. In any sexual dysfunction, psychogenic cause always exists and male diabetic subjects are no exception to this.

Metabolic Causes

Among the organic causes of erectile failure diabetes is the most important. The impact of diabetes and associated factors on sexual function is given in **Flow chart 74.1**.

Pathogenesis

In diabetes pathogenesis of erectile dysfunction is multifactorial. Neuropathy, accelerated atherosclerosis and alterations in the corporal tissues with smooth muscle degeneration, abnormal collagen deposition and endothelial dysfunction have all been implicated.[3] Increased oxidative stress, glycation, protein kinase C

TABLE 74.2	Causes of impotence

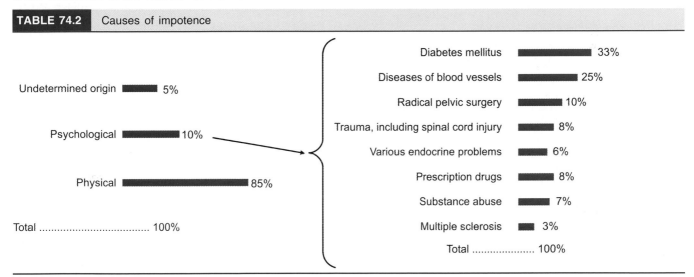

Flow chart 74.1 The impact of diabetes and associated factors on sexual function in men
(*Adapted from Textbook of Diabetes, 2nd edition*)

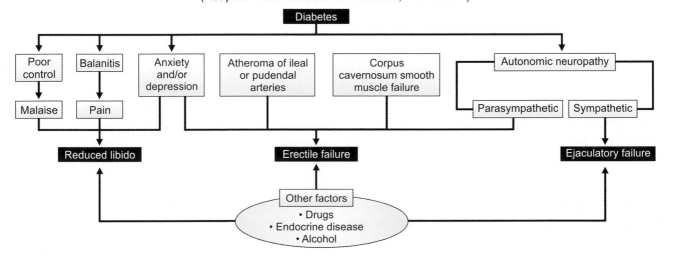

activity and aldose reductase may also act as causative factors.

Hormonal Causes

The role of hormonal disturbances leading to diabetic erectile failure is yet to be settled. There are differing opinions on this factor causing sexual dysfunction as testosterone levels and its response to hCG stimulation are found to be normal in many instances. Testicular biopsy studies showed more abnormalities when compared with nondiabetic controls and hence comes the concept of *diabetic testes.* In a study conducted at Govt General Hospital, Chennai, Tamil Nadu, India, on male diabetic subjects with erectile failure there were reduction in urinary testosterone levels and concomitant reduction in Leydig cell distribution in testicular biopsies.[4]

Spermatogenesis

Alterations in spermatogenesis appear closely associated with metabolic disturbances and to the presence of autonomic neuropathy. Damage to seminal vesicles is seen. Alterations in the sexual behavior and reduction in the weight of secondary sex glands is observed in diabetic animals. In these animals production of androgens and disturbance in spermatogenesis occurs as a result of altered gonadotropin pulsatility.

Neurogenic Causes

Increased incidence of erectile failure in a male diabetic subject seems to be primarily a result of diabetic autonomic neuropathy. This observation has been substantiated by bladder function studies. The pelvic parasympathetic nerves (Nervi erigentes) that lead to erection also innervate the bladder and involvement of those nerves is demonstrated by the abnormal cystometrogram.

Autonomic neuropathy assessment in male diabetic subjects with erectile failure revealed greater involvement of parasympathetic nerves and hence it is not surprising that erectile failure is the common sexual dysfunction in a male diabetic subject. Peptidergic nervous system also could be involved in diabetic erectile failure as it has been recently demonstrated in them a deficiency of vasoactive intestinal polypeptide (VIP) and nitric oxide in the penile tissue.

Vascular Causes

Both macro- and microvascular complications of diabetes may generate the clinical picture of diabetic erectile failure. Severe vascular lesions involving the distal aorta and iliac arteries as in Leriche's syndrome may also result in erectile failure. Small blood vessel disease (microangiopathy) may further interfere with normal penile function. Whether neuropathy in a male diabetic subject can influence vascular lesions with subsequent production of erectile failure is still subjudice. Invariably male diabetic patients with arterial occlusive disease secondary to arterioscleroses do also have corporal veno-occlusive disorder.

Drug-induced Erectile Failure

Since diabetic subjects receive a number of drugs for control of diabetes and its complications, they may suffer from the side effects of these drugs. Some of these drugs (methyl dopa, reserpine, atenolol, clonidine, pindolol, prazocin, verapamil and guanathidine) may cause erectile failure in a male diabetic subject. Withdrawal of these drugs may restore potency.

CLINICAL FEATURES

Diabetic sexual dysfunction can be differentiated into two distinct clinical entities namely: (i) Transient or temporary dysfunction, (ii) Progressive dysfunction. The transient type of dysfunction is characterized by a reduction in libido and a mild degree of erectile failure, both attributable to lethargy, tiredness and malaise due to disturbed metabolism at the onset of diabetes or during episodes of acute metabolic derangement termed as *phasic sexual indifference* which can also be found in other debilitating illnesses. The other type of sexual dysfunction which is organically determined by the vascular, neurogenic or hormonal derangement is characteristically progressive, irreversible and is distinctly termed as *diabetic erectile failure (impotence).* Some of the chronic diseases like hypertension, heart disease, lipid disorders, renal failure, liver disease besides diabetes also cause and precipitate erectile failure. Chronic smoking and alcohol also play contributing role.

CLINICAL EVALUATION

History and physical examination may indicate the probable cause of erectile failure. Hypertension, addiction to alcohol, smoking and concomitant endocrine diseases must be enquired and looked for. The protocol for diagnosis of erectile dysfunction proposed by Italian Diabetology Society's *Diabetic Neuropathy* Study Group (1996) is easy to follow **(Table 74.3).**

TABLE 74.3	Protocol for diagnosis of erectile dysfunction proposed by Italian Diabetology Society's *Diabetic Neuropathy* Study Group (1996)

Targeted questionnaire

Penile biothesiometry

Cardiovascular tests

PGE_1 drug stimulation

Patients → <40 years old: 5 µg

Patients → 40 years old: 10 µg

If the erectile response is absent

Repeat after 1 week with 10 or 20 µg PGE_1

Persistently absent

Refer to andrology unit for further investigation (Rigiscan, ultrasound, Doppler ultrasonography, invasive vascular tests)

If the erectile response is present

Oral and/or intracavernosal drug and/or psychological treatment

PSYCHOGENIC OR ORGANIC

The foremost is to distinguish between psychogenic and organic causes of erectile failure. In psychogenic erectile failure, the onset is abrupt, libido is diminished and nocturnal and special situation erection is present. A few factors that may help to differentiate is given in **Table 74.4**.

CLINICAL ASSESSMENT

- Examination of the genitalia is essential to detect primary penile abnormalities such as balanitis, phimosis, penile curvature and fibrosis from Peyronie's disease or congenital or traumatic conditions.

TABLE 74.4	Some factors that help to differentiate psychological from organic causes of erectile failure

	More likely to be	
	Psychological	*Organic*
Onset	Sudden	Gradual
Permanence	Intermittent or partial	Permanent and total
Spontaneous erections (Nocturnal or on waking, etc.)	Sometimes	Never
Psychological problems	May be overt	May be secondary
Organic causes	None apparent	May be apparent

- *Testicular sensation:* The simple and the easiest test is palpation (no pressure) of the testes for pain sensitivity. The sacral nerves that carry pain sensation are similar to the nerves involved in the process of erection. The loss of testicular pain sensitivity suggests neurogenic etiology.
- *Interruption of urination:* Ability to stop the urination for a few seconds and to resume again is yet another simple test to rule out organic erectile failure. This maneuver is possible only if the autonomic nervous system is intact.
- i. *Nocturnal penile tumescence (NPT) testing:* Normal individuals have penile erections 3 to 5 times in a night lasting for 15 to 30 minutes associated with rapid eye movement (REM) which occurs during sleep. Psychogenic impotent person will not show any alteration in this pattern but organic impotent person will have diminished frequency and duration of erections. The NPT can be monitored by special equipment.
- ii. *Stamp test:* Stamp test is a simple procedure for assessing nocturnal erections.[5] The patient is asked to stick a strip of postage stamps around the base of the penis overnight and asked to observe for the snapping of the stamp strip the next day morning. Snap indicates that he has had penile tumescence in the night and rules out organic cause. Both NPT and the stamp test may indicate engorgement but not the extent of firmness of the penis. The presence of nocturnal erection can also be assessed by monitoring maximal penile diameter using a snap gauge fastener.[6] These tests are generally regarded as proof of organic normality. They measure the tumescence and not rigidity.
- Papaverin injection into the cavernosa will elicit erection in psychogenic as well as in neurogenic causes of erectile failure. Erection will not occur in vasculogenic erectile failure.

VASCULAR ASSESSMENT

Recent noninvasive methods to assess vascular integrity have revolutionized the methods to diagnose the cause of erectile failure. Incidence of vascular lesions in the causation of erectile failure in a male diabetic subject is now found to be greater than that of a nondiabetic subject. Noninvasive methods like Doppler, penile plethysmography and pulse volume recorder have helped to diagnose a number of cases of vascular lesions. Invasive methods like contrast cavernosography and phallarteriography also have helped to pinpoint the lesions.

To assess vascular causes:
- Clinical assessment
- Penile pulses
- Peripheral pulses
- Penile systolic BP (Doppler)
- Penile/brachial pressure index (PPBI)

$$PPBI \quad \frac{Penile\ systolic\ BP}{Brachial\ systolic\ BP} \quad \begin{array}{l} Normal > 0.75\ Vascular \\ lesion\ is\ suspected\ if \\ < 0.6\ and\ > 1.2 \end{array}$$

- Penile plethysmography
- Penile pulse volume recording
- Contrast study

NEUROLOGICAL ASSESSMENT

A number of techniques and equipment are available for neurological assessment. Autonomic innervation of the corpora can be studied by recording electrical activity by intracavernosal electromyography. Investigations like perineal electromyography, sacral latency testing, dorsal nerve somatosensory evoked potential, vibration perception sensitivity are also helpful in assessing the neurological involvement. Recently introduced rigiscan technique has been found to be very useful in assessing tumescence and found to be related to autonomic neuropathy **(Figure 74.4)**.

To assess neurological causes:
- Clinical assessment for peripheral neuropathy
- Penile biothesiometry
- Cardiac autonomic reflex testing for autonomic neuropathy
- Nerve conduction velocities (pudendal nerve reflex latency)
- Sacral-evoked potential
- Genitocerebral-evoked potential.

Biothesiometer is a useful equipment to assess peripheral and penile neuropathies. One useful way to evaluate the nerves that carry sensation away from the penis is by the use of a technique called penile biotheisometry. This is a quantitative measure of the vibratory sense of the penis.

The device is placed on the tip of the finger, and slowly the frequency is increased until the vibration is felt. This is then used as a baseline to compare the vibration sense of the penis as well. It is a useful way to

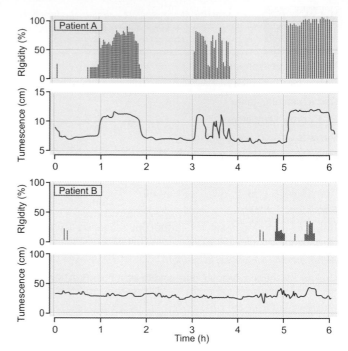

Figure 74.4 Nocturnal penile tumescence studies, using the Rigiscan device. Nocturnal penile tumescence studies, using the Rigiscan device, which allows simultaneous measurements of penis rigidity (expressed as a percentage of maximum) and tumescence (expressed as penile circumference). Patient A shows normal nocturnal erectile responses, while these are essentially absent in patient B. Erectile failure in patient A is therefore predominantly psychogenic in origin (*Adapted from Textbook of Diabetes, 2nd edition*)

detect early neuropathic disease in younger men, particularly in men with diabetes. It is also used in men who have had circumcisions and complain that the head of the penis has lost sensation.

HORMONAL ASSESSMENT

Androgens initiate and maintain growth and development of the male reproductive system and sexual behavior. Certain amount of testosterone is essential for adequate sexual response. Some impotent males have high prolactin levels, which possesses inhibitory effects on actions of testosterone. Other endocrine diseases of thyroid, pituitary and adrenal also affect the sexual functions. Correcting of any of the hormonal abnormality is likely to restore potency and cells for detailed endocrine work-up.

To assess hormonal causes:

Hormone Assay
- Testosterone
- FSH, LH
- Prolactin
- T3, T4
- Cortisol.

TREATMENT OF DIABETIC ERECTILE FAILURE (TABLE 74.5)

Step Care Approach Recommended for the Management of Diabetic Erectile Failure

Step I is correction of reversible factors like metabolic, drugs, malnutrition and further advice regarding avoidance of smoking and alcohol excess.

Step II is to tackle psychological problems contributing to sexual dysfunction. Advocate sensate focus therapy, noncoital sexual exercises as suggested by Master's and Johnson. Further, reduction of performance anxiety by reassurance will also help the patient to overcome this problem.

Step III (Medical Treatment) CNS stimulants such as yohimbine, strychnine and certain Ayurvedic preparation such as Mucuna pruriens have beneficial effect, which, however, is not long-lasting. Certain other medications like vasodilators, to correct vascular

TABLE 74.5	Treatment of erectile dysfunction

Metabolic control of diabetes

Psycho- or behavioral therapy

Drug treatment
- Yohimbine
- α_1-antagonists
- Local nitro derivatives
- Sildenafil
- Endourethral alprostadil

Intracavernosal injection
- Papaverine
- Alprostadil
- Phentolamine
- Moxisylte

External mechanical support
   Vacuum device

Revascularization surgery
   Venous
   Arterial

Penile prosthesis

insufficiency and testosterone for hormone deficiency and Sorbinil, gangliosides for neuropathy may be helpful.

There is a statistical decline of testosterone levels, particularly free testosterone, in aging men. While this fall is only moderate, aging men show clinical signs of hypogonadism (loss of muscle mass/strength, reduction in bone mass and an increase in visceral fat). Testosterone replacement or supplement therapy may improve bone mass, muscle mass, strength and frequently nocturnal erections as well in this age group. However, the effects on sexual function, mood and cognition are less clear, but may be meaningful in certain men. The identification of that segment of the aging male population that might possibly benefit from androgen supplementation remains unclear. Questions still remain regarding the magnitude and longevity of these potential beneficial effects. One has to bear in mind the long-term adverse effect of androgen on cardiovascular and prostrate diseases.

Sildenafil Citrate

This drug has virtually, sidelined all the other modalities of treatment for erectile failure. Sildenafil is a phosphodiesterase-5 inhibitor. With sexual arousal, nerve impulses are transmitted along noradrenergic, noncholinergic nerves (NANC) and nitric oxide synthase is activated releasing nitric oxide (NO). This produces smooth muscle relaxation around the blood vessels in the corpora cavernosa and trabecular network and erection is produced by marked increase in blood flow. This relaxation mechanism activated by NO involves guanylate cyclase and cyclic guanosine monophosphate (cGMP). This cGMP is hydrolyzed by the enzyme PDE-5. In erectile dysfunction, there is reduced cGMP in the tissues. Its normal hydrolysis by PDE-5 limits its availability further. The effect of sildenafil is therefore to increase availability of cGMP by inhibiting PDE-5, thereby reducing cGMP clearance **(Figure 74.5)**. Sildenafil action depends upon the activation of NO pathway, which is dependent on sexual arousal. It does not trigger erection as such but improves its quality by promoting the smooth muscle relaxation initiated by NO release.

Sildenafil has an onset of action of 30 to 60 minutes after taking orally and lasts for 4 hours. The initial dose could be 25 mg and increased gradually depending upon the response and not to exceed 100 mg per day. This drug is generally well tolerated but a few may develop headache, dyspepsia, flushing and transient color visual disturbance.[7] There is no evidence of

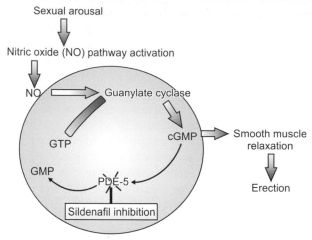

Sexual arousal

Nitric oxide (NO) pathway activation

Smooth muscle cell of corpus cavernosum

Figure 74.5 Schematic representation of action of sildenafil on phosphodiesterase-5 (PDE-5) and cyclic guanosine monophosphate (cGMP) in smooth muscle cell of corpora cavernosum. GTP, guanosine 5'-triphosphate; GMP, guanosine 5'–phosphate. (*Adapted from William D Alexander, Diabetes Annual 2002*)

adverse cardiovascular consequence among men treated with this agent.[8] Sildenafil is contraindicated in men taking nitrates because of potential serious hypotension, which may be fatal.[9]

Tadalafil

Tadalafil seems a good molecule for treatment in erectile dysfunction in both diabetic and nondiabetic male subjects. It has advantages over the available sildenafil in dosing schedule because of its long half-life, it can be used at any time of the day. The other main advantage is its specificity to the PDE-5. The dose recommended to start with is 10 mg and can be increased to 20 mg.

Vardenafil

Similar to tadalafil in action and dosage recommended.

Vasoactive Agents

Three drugs are commonly used: Papaverine (20–80 mg), Phentolamine (2–4 mg) and Prostaglandin E1 (20–40 µg).[10,11] A variety of combination of these drugs is practiced, papaverine alone, papaverine and phentolamine, prostaglandin alone, papaverine and prostaglandin or a mixture of papaverine, phentolamine and prostaglandin. These drugs bypass the impaired endothelial and neural mechanisms and are successful

TABLE 74.6	Recommended doses of drugs for intra-cavernosal injection	
Alprostadil	Starting dose	5–10 µg
	Incremental increases by	5 µg upto 20 µg
		10 µg upto 40 µg
Papaverine	Starting dose	10 mg
	Incremental increases by	5 mg upto 20 mg
		10 mg upto 60 mg

Combinations should start with combinations of minimum doses and increase by similar increments to those above. Combinations may also include phentolamine or VIP

in psychogenic and neurogenic erectile failure. The success rate for the papaverin alone is 36%, the combination of papaverin and phentolamine 68% and prostaglandin E1 alone 76%. The recommended doses of drugs for intracavernosal injection are given in **Table 74.6**.

Local papaverin injection has been found to be successful in producing short-term erection. A 25 to 30 mg of papaverin is injected with strict aseptic precautions, at the root of the penis about 2 inches away from the glands. The injection is given at 2, 5, 7 or 11 o' clock positions using an insulin syringe and needle. Of these, 5 and 7 o'clock positions are preferred. The injection is given on one or both the sides. Erection occurs within 10 to 30 minutes, when given on one side and within 5 to 10 minutes when given on both sides. While the erection subsides after ejaculation in most of the subjects, it persists for two hours or more in some. Side effects are minimal. Pain during intercourse can occur. Priapism is uncommon but can occur due to over zealous administration of higher doses of papaverin. The injection should not be repeated within two weeks. To relieve priapism, a butterfly needle is inserted into one of the corpora and 20 to 40 ml of blood is aspirated and 5 to 10 ml diluted α-agonist phenylephrine or noradrenalin is introduced. The α-agonists are contraindicated in persons taking monoamine oxidase inhibitors. The other method is to infuse 5 to 10 ml of 2000 units of heparin diluted in 200 ml of saline through a butterfly needle inserted into the corpora cavernosa. Rarely surgical decompression may be required.

Medicated Urethral System for Erection (MUSE)[12,13]

The intraurethral application of alprostadil is an alternative treatment for many men, and provides a less invasive alternative to intrapenile injection. Alprostadil is a prostaglandin-E preparation in a pellet form that is inserted with a plunger-like mechanism into the urethral opening. The plunger device is a thin plastic tube with a button at the top. Intraurethral therapy is associated with significantly less efficacy than direct injection of alprostadil. The efficacy may be increased by using an elastic band placed at the base of the penis. The associated side-effects include pain as well as systemic hypotension.

Erecaid System [Vacuum Constriction Devices (VCDs)][14]

The erecaid system consists of a cylindrical tube in which the penis is inserted and suction is applied from the other end by a hand-operated pump. This will result in expansion of the sinusoidal spaces and blood gushes in producing tumescence. A suction band is slipped at the root after penis has expanded. The band should not be kept for more than 30 minutes. The side effects associated with VCD therapy include penile pain, penile numbness, bruising and retarded ejaculation. The advantages of VCD therapy include its nonpharmacological nature, on-demand use, lack of contraindications and cost. The disadvantages of VCD therapy include their cumbersome utilization and minor local side effects.

Surgical Treatment

Microvascular Arterial Bypass and Venous Ligation

Surgical methods that are available for the treatment of erectile failure are by-pass surgery for vascular lesion, iliac-pudendal, pudendal-cavernous, pudendal-penile grafts. Surgery may achieve the goal of increasing arterial inflow and decreasing venous outflow.

Prosthesis (Penile Implants)

The final treatment option for erectile dysfunction is the surgical implantation of a malleable or inflatable penile prosthesis. This option is highly invasive and irreversible and should therefore be reserved for select cases failing other treatment modalities. However, under unique and uncommon circumstances, a penile implant could be selected as a primary option. When properly selected, penile prosthesis may be associated with high rates of patient satisfaction. Penile implant surgery is uncommonly associated with prosthesis infection, but such cases usually require explantation and may result in severe scarring and penile deformity.

The advantages of penile prosthesis implantation include relative efficacy and a long-term solution. The disadvantages of penile prosthesis include irreversibility, invasiveness, surgical complications and mechanical failure.

Various prosthesis like Carrion's (semirigid) and Balloon (inflatable) prosthesis are available for the management of erectile failure.

SEXUAL PROBLEMS IN DIABETIC WOMEN

The equivalent of impotence in a woman is absence of vaginal lubrication during intercourse.[15] They may also suffer from fatigue, depression, changes in perimenstrual blood glucose control, vaginitis, decreased sexual desire and an increased time to reach orgasm.

A distinct clinical entity *clitoral neuropathy* has been reported. This is usually mistaken for candidial vaginitis since it produces paresthesias over the genitalia.

It is quite easy to manage most of the sexual problems in female diabetic subjects. Systematic clinical approach in diagnosis is all that is required. A lubricant like KY Jelly additionally during intercourse helps overcome dry coitus.

Adequate control of diabetes and prompt treatment of candidial vaginitis relieves dyspareunia and orgasmic dysfunction.[16] Strict metabolic control and neurovitamins help overcome clitoral neuropathy in diabetic women.

CONCLUSION

Both women and men with diabetes are at increased risk for sexual dysfunction. In men, sexual dysfunction is related to somatic and psychological factors, whereas in women with diabetes, psychological factors are more predominant.[17] A diabetic subject presenting with sexual dysfunction requires utmost sympathy and deft handling. The patient and the spouse should be educated on the effects of the chronic disease on the sexual function and further counseled to adapt well to the new situation. The future for these unfortunate men is not all that gloomy as the treatment choice ranges from oral medications to injections, from psychological therapy to surgery and from external devices to internal ones.

SUMMARY

Sexual function is a complex blend of anatomic, neurologic, metabolic, endocrine and psychic factors more than any other human activity. The prevalence of erectile dysfunction in male diabetic subjects varies between 30 to 70%, the average being 50% and increases as age advances. Erection is a balance between adequate arterial inflow from the cavernosal arteries and the resistance to blood outflow from the sinusoidal spaces by the effective veno-occlusive mechanism.

Causes of erectile failure may be enumerated as metabolic, psychogenic, endocrine, neurological, vascular and drug induced or mixed. The organic causes are the commonest. Pathogenesis of erectile dysfunction is multifactorial. Neuropathy, accelerated athero-sclerosis and alterations in the corporal tissues, smooth muscle degeneration, abnormal collagen deposition and endothelial dysfunction have all been implicated.

Increased incidence of erectile failure in a male diabetic subject seems to be primarily a result of diabetic autonomic neuropathy. Both macro- and microvascular complications of diabetes may confound the clinical picture of diabetic erectile failure. Since diabetic subjects receive a number of drugs for control of diabetes and its complications, they may suffer from the side effects of these drugs. History and physical examination may indicate the probable cause of erectile failure.

The foremost is to distinguish between psychogenic and organic causes of erectile failure. In psychogenic erectile failure the onset is abrupt, libido is diminished and nocturnal and special situation erection is present.

Nocturnal penile tumescence studies, using the Rigiscan device, which allows simultaneous measure-ments of penis rigidity.

The first step in the approach is correction of rever-sible factors like metabolic, drugs, malnutrition and further advice regarding avoidance of smoking and alcohol excess. Tackle psychological problems contribut-ing to sexual dysfunction.

Sildenafil citrate has virtually, side-lined all the other modalities of treatment for erectile failure. Treatment choice ranges from oral medications to injections, from psychological therapy to surgery and from external devices to internal ones.

REFERENCES

1. Feldman HD, Goldstein I, Hatzichristou DG, et al. Impotence and its medical and psychosocial correlates: results of the Massachusetts Male Ageing Study. J Urol. 1994;51:54-61.

2. Lustman PJ, Clouse RE. Relationship of psychiatric illness to impotence in men with diabetes. Diabetes Care. 1990;13:893-5.

3. Saenz de Tejada I, Goldstein I. Diabetic penile neuropathy. Urol Clin North Am. 1988;15:17-22.

4. Seshiah V, Sam GP Moses, Prithikachary, Ashok Cherian, Rajendran N. Sexual Dysfunction in Diabetic Men. The Antiseptic. 1979;76:42-5.

5. Kumar TV, Seshiah V. Diabetes and sexual dysfunction: simple objective asessment and clinical correlation with peripheral and autonomic neuropathy. Diabetic Neuropathy. John Ward and Yoshio Goto (Eds): John Wiley and Sons Ltd.; 1990. pp. 429-37.

6. Bradley WE, Lin JT. Assessment of diabetic sexual dysfunction and cystopathy. Diabetic Neuropathy. 1987;15:146-54.

7. Boulton AJM, Selam JL, Sweeney M, Zeigler D. Sildenafil citrate for the treatment of erectile dysfunction in men with type II diabetes mellitus. Diabetologia. 2001;44:1296-301.

8. Shakir SA, Wilton LV, Boshier A, Layton D, Heeley E. Cardiovascular events in users of sildenafil: results from first phase of prescription event monitoring in England. BMJ. 2001;322:651-2.

9. Cheitlin MD, Hutter AM, Brindis RG, et al. Use of sildenafil (viagra) in patients with cardiovascular disease. Circulation. 1999;99:168-77.

10. Virag R. Intravenous injection of papaverine for erectile failure. Lancet. 1982;2:938.

11. Brindley GS. Cavernosal alpha blockade: a new treatment for investigating and treating erectile impotence. Br Psychol. 1983;143:332-7.

12. Padma-Nathan H, Hellstrom WJ, Kaiser FE, et al. Treatment of men with erectile dysfunction with transurethral alprostadil: medicated urethral system for erection (MUSE) Study Group. N Engl J Med. 1997;336:1-7.

13. Porst H. Transurethrale Alprostadil applikation mit MUSE™ (medicated urethral system for erection). Urologe (A). 1998;37:410-16.

14. Dutta TC, Eid JF. Vacuum constriction devices for erectile dysfunction: a long term, prospective study of patients with mild, moderate, and severe dysfunction. Urology. 1999;54: 891-3.

15. Paul Enzlin, et al. Sexual dysfunction in women with type 1 diabetes: a controlled study. Diabetes Care. 2002;25(4):672.

16. Jovanovic L. Sex and the woman with diabetes: desire versus dysfunction. IDF bulletin. 1998;43:23-8.

17. Paul Enzlin, et al. Prevalence and predictors of sexual dysfunction in patients with type 1 diabetes. Diabetes Care. 2003;26(2):409-14.

Chapter 75

IMPACT OF GLYCEMIC CONTROL ON COMPLICATIONS OF DIABETES MELLITUS

Ashok Kumar Das

CHAPTER OUTLINE

- Introduction
- Pathophysiological Effects of Hyperglycemia
- Historical Background— Early Trials
- Type 1 Diabetes Mellitus—Glycemic Control and Complications
- Type 2 Diabetes Mellitus—Glycemic Control and Complications
- Impact of Intensive Glycemic Control in the Critical Care Setting
- Recent Trials
- Recommendations for Glycemic Control
- Hazards of Intensive Glycemic Control
- Conclusion

INTRODUCTION

Diabetes Mellitus is a chronic disease affecting millions of people worldwide and is a leading cause of death, illness and disability. In the last decade considerable progress has been made in understanding the pathophysiology of type 1 and type 2 diabetes. At present, we cannot speak about a cure for diabetes. Cure is an appropriate future goal, especially for type 1 diabetes, for which progress in immunology, molecular biology and immunotherapy has been dramatic.[1]

As the longevity of the human population is increasing, the microvascular and macrovascular complications of DM is causing a major health burden Over the years, debate has continued concerning the role of hyperglycemia in the pathogenesis of the chronic complications of diabetes.

The *glucose hypothesis* assumed that glucose itself was the major mediator of these complications and that specific treatment of diabetes to reduce chronic hyperglycemia could significantly slow or prevent these complications. In experimental animals, studies have demonstrated a relationship between high blood glucose concentrations and conditions that resemble complications that occur in humans with long-standing diabetes.[2-4]

PATHOPHYSIOLOGICAL EFFECTS OF HYPERGLYCEMIA

The various mechanisms of glucose toxicity include:
- Increased production of advanced glycosylation end products
- Alterations in the sorbitol pathway
- Increased production of protein kinase C.

Nonenzymatically-mediated glycosylation of proteins occurs at a rate proportional to glucose concentration and the accumulation of these advanced glycosylation end products causes thickened basement membranes and an inactivation of endothelium-derived relaxing factor, which results in microvascular constriction and leakage and oxidation of low-density lipoproteins.

Peripheral hyperglycemia leads to intracellular hyperglycemia which increases flux through the polyol pathway. The increased production of sorbitol via this pathway results in a decrease in the uptake of myoinositol, which decreases Na^+-K^+-ATPase activity, leading to microvascular leakage and oxidation of low-density lipoproteins.

Hyperglycemia also induces the production of protein kinase C, which liberates vascular endothelial growth factor that promotes the formation of fragile new blood vessels and causes endothelial damage.

Many randomized controlled trials have demonstrated the effects of improved glycemic control on chronic complications of diabetes. These include two studies in patients with type 1 diabetes—the Diabetes Control and Complications Trial (DCCT) and the smaller Stockholm Diabetes Intervention Study (SDIS) and two studies in patients with type 2 diabetes, the United Kingdom Prospective Diabetes Study (UKPDS) and the smaller Kumamoto Study. Before the completion of these studies, a number of older, smaller randomized controlled trials were included in a meta-analysis, which also suggested a significant relationship between glycemia and complications.

HISTORICAL BACKGROUND—EARLY TRIALS

Retrospective and unrandomized prospective studies conducted in the early years have documented associations between both the duration and degree of hyperglycemia and the severity of microvascular complications.

Pirart in his follow-up of 4400 patients (both type 1 and type 2 diabetics) for up to 25 years showed that poor glycemic control was clearly related to a higher prevalence of retinopathy, neuropathy and nephropathy than in those with 'fair' and 'good' control.[5]

Prospective clinical trials conducted by: (1) Kroc collaborative study group[6] and (2) Steno study group[7] compared one or more forms of intensive insulin therapy with conventional therapy. None of these studies could show an amelioration of retinopathy with intensive therapy. Indeed, on the contrary, with intensive therapy a transient worsening of retinopathy was seen in the first 6 to 12 months.

Some of the studies demonstrated that intensive therapy did ameliorate the increase in urinary albumin excretion[8,9] but this was without any clear effect on the development of overt clinical nephropathy.

TABLE 75.1	The Stockholm Diabetes Intervention Study—major results	
	Standard Group (n = 54)	*Intensified Group (n = 48)*
Retinopathy	52%	27%
Nephropathy	18%	2%
Neuropathy	32%	14%

(Adapted from Reichard P, et al. The Stockholm Diabetes Intervention Study. J Int Med. 1991;230:304-9)

TYPE 1 DIABETES MELLITUS—GLYCEMIC CONTROL AND COMPLICATIONS

To prove the relationship between hyperglycemia and diabetic complications, it is essential to demonstrate that a randomized prospective intervention that lowered average blood glucose to levels near the normal range, could slow the onset or progression of the chronic complications of diabetes. Key advances in knowledge and technology that occurred in the late 1970s made such studies feasible.

The Stockholm Diabetes Intervention Study (SDIS) (Table 75.1)

This small scale but long-term trial initiated in 1982, compared the effects of intensified insulin treatment and standard treatment on the progression of microvascular complications of T1DM.[10] Patients enrolled had T1DM with unsatisfactory glycemic control, nonproliferative retinopathy and normal serum creatinine concentrations. Forty-eight patients were assigned to receive intensive insulin treatment and 54 patients were assigned to receive standard insulin treatment. Results of the 7.5 year follow-up were published in 1993[11] and showed significant reduction in the development of nephropathy, retinopathy and neuropathy in the intensified treatment group. Statistically significant difference was also found in pinprick sensitivity.

The Diabetes Control and Complications Trial (DCCT)

DCCT was designed to conclusively test the glucose hypothesis and resolve controversies raised by the earlier studies.

DCCT included 1,441 subjects with type 1 diabetes. Of these, 726 were in the primary prevention cohort and had a duration of diabetes <5 years, no retinopathy,

TABLE 75.2	Relative reduction in risk of clinical complications in diabetes patients given intensive therapy

Clinical complication	Relative risk reduction (%)
Albuminuria	
Microalbuminuria	35%
Macroalbuminuria	56%
Clinical Neuropathy	60%
Retinopathy	
Initial appearance	27%
Clinically significant	34-76%
Severe	45%

(Adapted from DCCT. The effect of intensive treatment of diabetes on the development and progression of long-term complications in noninsulin-dependent diabetes mellitus. N Eng J Med. 1993;327:977-86)

and normal albumin excretion at baseline. The remaining 715 were in the secondary intervention cohort and had a duration of diabetes <15 years, mild-to-moderate background retinopathy, and either normal albumin excretion or microalbuminuria at baseline.[12]

Subjects were randomly assigned either to intensive therapy or conventional therapy. Intensive therapy consisted of insulin administered either by continuous subcutaneous insulin infusion with an external insulin pump or multiple daily insulin injections (three or more injections per day). Insulin therapy was guided by self-monitoring of blood glucose (SMBG). Conventional therapy consisted of no more than two daily insulin injections; urine glucose monitoring or SMBG no more than twice daily.

The intensive group achieved a median HbA_{1c} of 7.2% versus an HbA_{1c} of 9.1% in the conventional group. On analyzing the results, risk reductions for microvascular and neurological end points were found to be dramatically significant **(Table 75.2)**.

DCCT and Retinopathy[13]

- Retinopathy was the primary outcome evaluated in the DCCT.
- Intensive therapy reduced the risk of total three step changes in retinopathy by 60% and the risk of developing at least one microaneurysm by 27%.
- Intensive therapy was associated with a 54% decrease in the incidence of retinopathy progression.
- Intensive therapy also had a beneficial effect in ameliorating the more severe retinopathy events.

- The risk of developing severe nonproliferative retinopathy was decreased by 46%.

DCCT and Nephropathy[14]

- Incidence of microalbuminuria showed a relative reduction of 34% over 6.5 years with intensive therapy.
- No significant difference was seen in the incidence of sustained microalbuminuria, macroalbuminuria and abnormal creatinine clearance.
- A relative reduction of 43% was seen in the incidence of microalbuminuria in the secondary prevention group.

DCCT and Neuropathy[14]

- Incidence of new confirmed clinical neuropathy reduced by 69%
- Progression of neuropathy reduced by 57%
- A 43% reduction of abnormal autonomic function was also seen.

DCCT and Macrovascular Disease[14]

Although the DCCT was not designed to evaluate the effects of glycemic control on macrovascular disease, some of its indicators were evaluated. Intensive insulin therapy was associated with a significant relative reduction (34%) in the development of hypercholesterolemia.

Intensive insulin therapy also reduced the relative risk of macrovascular disease (peripheral and cardiovascular disease) by 41%, but the difference was not significant, probably because of the small number of patients who developed macrovascular disease as the DCCT population consisted of relatively young patients.

Implications of DCCT

- DCCT conclusively showed that the improvement of glycemic control reduced nonproliferative and proliferative retinopathy, nephropathy and neuropathy.
- A key finding was that for every 1% reduction in HbA_{1c} there was a 30% reduction in microvascular complications.
- Improved glycemic control also slowed the progression of early diabetic complications.
- It is possible that intensive therapy can reduce macrovascular disease as well.
- The results also showed that the benefits of intensive therapy clearly outweigh the risk for most of the patients with type 1 diabetes.

Follow-up After DCCT

After the close of the DCCT, subjects in the conventional therapy group were offered intensive therapy and instructed in its use. Most were enrolled in the epidemiology of diabetes interventions and complications (EDIC) long-term observational study. EDIC compared the long-term effects of the intensive or conventional therapy provided during the DCCT on the development of retinal and renal complications of diabetes. Although the difference in median HbA_{1c} results between the groups narrowed and merged during follow-up, during the next eight years the impact of previous intensive therapy was sustained, with dramatically less progression of both retinopathy and nephropathy.

TYPE 2 DIABETES MELLITUS—GLYCEMIC CONTROL AND COMPLICATIONS

The natural history of microvascular complications in type 2 diabetes has been difficult to define because the disease may be present for many years before it is diagnosed, and the incidence and progression of complications may be influenced by multiple confounding factors including age and hypertension. Nevertheless, hyperglycemia is clearly associated with the presence and progression of microvascular complications in type 2 diabetes.[15]

The Wisconsin Epidemiological Study of Diabetic Retinopathy (WESDR)

The WESDR was a large epidemiologic study designed to identify the relationship between hyperglycemia and chronic complications. The initial trial focused on diabetic retinopathy, but a follow-up trial examined the frequency and progression of microvascular and macrovascular complications over a 10-year period. A strong correlation was reported between higher HbA_{1c} values and loss of vision, retinopathy, renal failure, lower-extremity amputation, myocardial infarction and overall mortality. The results showed that:
* Those with HbA_{1c} more than 87% were four times more likely to develop retinopathy than those with HbA_{1c} between 5.4 to 7.6%.
* Those with high HbA_{1c} were 4 to 6 times more likely to show progression of nonproliferative retinopathy.
* Risk of having developed proliferative retinopathy after 10 years was 14 times more in those with high base line HbA_{1c}.[16]

The United Kingdom Prospective Diabetes Study (UKPDS)[17]

The UKPDS was a 20 year prospective randomized intervention trial to determine whether patients with type 2 diabetes can attain clinical benefit with intensive glycemic control. More than 5000 patients with type 2 diabetes were recruited from about 23 hospital based clinics in England, Scotland and Northern Ireland and were randomized into intensive and conventional treatment groups. Of the 5102 patients in the trial, 4209 were randomly assigned; 342 to a metformin therapy group intended for obese patients and 3867 to therapy with insulin or sulfonylureas. Patients in both groups were further randomly assigned to intensive or conventional therapy. The goals for the patients in the conventional therapy group were a fasting plasma glucose concentration of <270 mg/dl and no symptoms of hyperglycemia. The goals for the patients in the intensive therapy group were a fasting plasma glucose concentration of <108 mg/dl and no symptoms of hyperglycemia.

The objectives were:
* To determine whether a policy of reducing hyperglycemia to near normal levels will reduce the risk of glycemic complication.
* To study the advantages and disadvantages of any specific therapy (insulin, sulfonylurea, or metformin).
* To ascertain whether a specific glycemic threshold is apparent.

Results of UKPDS

* A strong association was found between the major complications of diabetes and hyperglycemia.
* Each percent point reduction in HbA_{1c} was associated with a 35% reduction in microvascular complications **(Table 75.3)**.
* Ten year incidence of microvascular complication was 25% lower in patients receiving intensive treatment.
* Improved glycemic control did not conclusively reduce cardiovascular mortality but was associated with improvement with lipoprotein risk profile.

Effect on Individual Complications (Table 75.4)

UKPDS retinopathy result:
* In the intensively treated group, need for photocoagulation showed a reduction of 29% within six years of follow-up.

TABLE 75.3	The relative risk reduction per 1% reduction in HbA_{1c} levels[18,20]	
End point studied	Relative risk reduction %	P
Microvascular end points	52%	<0.0001
Fatal and nonfatal myocardial infarction	14	<0.0001
Fatal and nonfatal stroke	12	0.035
Cataract extraction	19	<0.0001
Amputation or death from PVD	43	<0.0001
Heart failure	16	0.016
Diabetes related deaths	21	<0.0001
Any diabetes related endpoint	21	<0.0001
All cause mortality	14	<0.0001

- The incidence of two-step progression on ETDRS scale lowered from 17.8 to 23%.
- There was a 24% lower cataract extraction rate in the intensive treatment group.
- No significant difference was seen in the incidence of decreased visual acuity, blindness and vitreous haemorrhage.[19]

UKPDS nephropathy results:
- Significant difference was seen in the incidence of microalbuminuria between the two groups within three years.
- There was a relative risk reduction of 33% over 9 years in the incidence of gross proteinuria.
- Relative risk reduction of 60% was seen in the incidence of two-fold rise in serum creatinine.
- Rates of renal failure and death from renal disease, however, did not differ.[20,21]

UKPDS neuropathy results:
- Incidence of VPT>25 volts from both toes was higher in the conventionally treated group after 9 years.

- No significant difference was seen in the incidence of absent knee and ankle reflexes.
- Incidence of impotence, abnormal cardiac autonomic function tests also did not differ significantly between the groups.

UKPDS and Macrovascular Complications

- 16% reduction was seen in the incidence of myocardial infarction in the intensive group
- There was a relative risk reduction of 46% in the incidence of sudden death.
- The incidence of fatal myocardial infarction, heart failure, angina, stroke, amputation and death from PVD was not lowered significantly.

Kumamoto Study

This study was a prospective randomized six-year trial in 110 nonobese Japanese patients who were randomized to receive either intensive or conventional insulin regimens. The goal of the intensive therapy was to maintain blood glucose levels close to normal, with HbA_{1c} concentrations of <7%.

After 6 years, 7.7% of patients in the intensive therapy group had developed retinopathy, compared with 32% of the patients who received conventional therapy. Intensive therapy patients had a 70% relative reduction in the risk of development or progression of nephropathy. The incidence of albuminuria was 9.6% among patients in the intensive therapy group whereas it was 30% in the conventional therapy group. Significant differences in nerve conduction velocities and vibratory sensation thresholds were also observed between the two groups.

These results demonstrate the effectiveness of improved glycemic control in individuals of different ethnicity.

TABLE 75.4	Microvascular complications[20]			
Endpoint	Primary prevention group	Secondary prevention group	RR reduction
Retinopathy			
Incidence	1.2/100 patient years	4-7/100 patient years	76%
Role of progression	3-7/100 patient years	7-8/100 patient years	54%
Early worsening	13.1%	7.6%	
Nephropathy (Microalbuminuria)	Reduction from 3.4 to 2.2/100,000 patient years	5.7 to 3.6/100,000 patient years	
Neuropathy			
Incidence	3.1/100 patient years	9.8/100 patient years	69%
Progression	7.0/100 patient years	16.1/100 patient years	57%

(Adapted from UKPDS (33). Lancet. 1998;45:1289-98)

TABLE 75.5	Mortality in infusion vs control group[22]		
	Infusion (n=306)	Control (n=314)	P
In hospital mortality	9.1%	11.1%	ns
Three-months mortality	12.4%	15.6%	ns
One-year mortality	18.6%	26.1%	0.0273

Macrovascular Disease in Type 2 Diabetes

Strong association of hyperglycemia with coronary artery disease has been shown in various cross-sectional longitudinal studies. Selected evidence for association between hyperglycemia and peripheral vascular disease was seen in WESDR, but limited association was seen in UKPDS.

Diabetes Mellitus, Insulin-Glucose Infusion in Acute Myocardial Infarction (DIGAMI) Study

The DIGAMI study compared intensive glycemic control in diabetic patients with AMI with conventional treatment.[22] Three hundred six patients were included in the insulin infusion group who received insulin infusion for at least 24 hours (Blood sugar maintained between 126–180 mg/dl) followed later by subcutaneous insulin four times a day. Three hundred fourteen patients were included in the control group. The results are shown in **Table 75.5**.

Greatest mortality benefit was seen in those not on insulin before and those at low cardiac risk. Significant benefit was seen by three months itself (relative mortality reduction of 52%). Thus intensive insulin therapy provides mortality benefit.

IMPACT OF INTENSIVE GLYCEMIC CONTROL IN THE CRITICAL CARE SETTING

Hyperglycemia is common in critically ill patients, and occurs even in those who have not previously had diabetes. Pronounced hyperglycemia or relative insulin deficiency in these patients can lead to various complications like sepsis, critical illness polyneuropathy, etc.

In nondiabetic patients with protracted critical illnesses, high serum levels of insulin-like growth factor-binding protein-1, which reflect an impaired response of hepatocytes to insulin are seen, and is associated with increased mortality.

Van Den Berghe et al performed a prospective, randomized, controlled trial to determine whether maintenance of blood glucose levels below 110 mg/dl with intensive insulin therapy could reduce morbidity and mortality in critically ill-patients.[23]

Analysis of the results from this study showed that:

- Intensive insulin therapy reduced the duration of intensive care but not the overall length of stay in the hospital.
- The greatest reduction in mortality involved deaths due to multiple-organ failure with a proven septic focus.
- Intensive insulin therapy also reduced overall in-hospital mortality by 34%, bloodstream infections by 46%, acute renal failure requiring dialysis or hemofiltration by 41%, the median number of red-cell transfusions by 50%, and critical-illness polyneuropathy by 44%.
- Significantly fewer patients in the intensive-treatment group required prolonged ventilatory support and renal replacement therapy.
- The various markers of inflammation was elevated to a lesser extent when strict blood sugar levels were maintained.

RECENT TRIALS

The various issues regarding glycemic control like the impact of more intensive glycemic control, the impact of earlier intervention, and the potential added benefit of specific classes drugs in reducing cardiovascular complications or sustaining pancreatic β-cell function are being addressed in many of the recent trials. They include:

- The Veterans Affairs Diabetes Trial (VADT), which is addressing the question of whether intensive glycemic control will improve cardiovascular morbidity and mortality in older men with type 2 diabetes.[24] In this trial, 1,792 subjects are being followed for 5 to 7 years, with a goal HbA$_{1c}$ in the intensive group of 6% and is slated to conclude in 2008.
- The Action to Control Cardiovascular Risk in Diabetes (ACCORD) trial, which is also addressing the impact of strict glycemic control on cardiovascular morbidity and mortality.

RECOMMENDATIONS FOR GLYCEMIC CONTROL

Based on these studies, the American Diabetes Association (ADA) recommends[25] that goal preprandial

TABLE 75.6	Recommendations for glycemic control by American Diabetes Association (ADA) and American College of Endocrinology (ACE)			
Biochemical index	Normal value	Goal value		Additional intervention suggested by ADA
		ADA	ACE	
Preprandial blood glucose control (mg/dl)	<100	90-130	<110	<80 or >140 (whole blood)
Postprandial blood glucose control (mg/dl)	<140	180	<140	b
Bedtime glucose	<110	100-140 (whole blood)	a	<100 or >160
HbA$_{1c}$ (%) ≤	<6	<7	<6.5	>8

a: Plasma values unless otherwise indicated

b: ADA was unable to reach consensus on a recommendation

(Adapted from ASHP. Therapeutic position statement on strict glycemic control in patients with diabetes. Am J Health Syst Pharm. 2003;60:2357-62)

plasma glucose is 90 to 130 mg/dl and postprandial glucose goal is <180 mg/dl. Normal HbA$_{1c}$ is less than six. Goal is less than seven. The ADA target for blood pressure is <130/80. The American Association of Clinical Endocrinology recommends preprandial glucose targets of <110, postprandial, <140 and HbA$_{1c}$ < to 6.5.[26] They also recommend blood pressure goal of <130/85. HbA$_{1c}$ measurements are suggested every three months. Blood sugar testing in type 1 diabetics or pregnant women with diabetes are suggested at least three times a day. The frequency of glucose monitoring for type 2 diabetics is not known but should be sufficient to facilitate achievement of the glucose goals **(Table 75.6)**.

HAZARDS OF INTENSIVE GLYCEMIC CONTROL

Although strict glycemic control will benefit a majority of patients, it may be difficult to achieve in all patients because of the risks associated with severe hypoglycemia. Intensive therapy may not be appropriate for patients with a history of repeated severe hypoglycemic episodes or for those who display a lack of hypoglycemic awareness. Diabetes care for patients younger than 18 years requires consideration of complicated physical and emotional growth needs. Intensive therapy is also inappropriate for patients without the cognitive ability or the motivation required to adhere to the regimen.

Adverse effects often seen with intensive blood glucose control include:
- Hypoglycemia
- Weight gain
- Restrictions on lifestyle

- Increased short-term costs
- Inconvenience, discomfort, etc.
- Hypertension.

CONCLUSION

Chronic hyperglycemia plays a causative role in the pathogenesis of diabetic microvascular complications. The risk of developing specific complications of diabetes such as retinopathy, nephropathy and neuropathy is clearly associated with the degree and duration of hyperglycemia. The DCCT in type 1 diabetes and the UKPDS in type 2 diabetic patients have conclusively proven that intensive glycemic control can delay the onset as well as the progression of the dreaded complications of diabetes. Treatment to restore glycemia to near normal levels should be a reasonable goal for both patients and the treating physicians.

REFERENCES

1. Prevention of Type 1 diabetes mellitus. American Diabetes Association position statement. Diabetes Care. 1990;13(9):1026-7.
2. Engerman RL, Kern TS. Progression of incipient diabetic retinopathy during good glycemic control. Diabetes. 1987;36:802-12.
3. Kern TS, Engerman RL. Arrest of glomerulopathy in diabetic dogs by improved glycemic control. Diabetologia. 1990;33:522-5.
4. Cohen AJ, McGill PD, Rossetti RG. Glomerulopathy in spontaneously diabetic rat: impact of glycemic control. Diabetes. 1987;36:944-51.
5. Pirart J. Diabetes mellitus and its degenerative complications: a prospective study of 4,400 patients observed between 1947 and 1973. Diabetes Care. 1978;1:168-88, 268-81.

6. Kroc Collaborative study Group. Blood glucose control and the evolution of diabetic retinopathy and albuminuria. N Engl J Med. 1984;311:365-72.

7. Lauritzen T, Frost-Larsen K, Larsen HW, et al. The Steno study group. Two year experience with continuous subcutaneous insulin infusion in relation to retinopathy and neuropathy. Diabetes. 1985;34 (suppl 3):74-9.

8. Feldt-Rasmussen B, Mathiesen ER, Deckert T. Effect of two years of strict metabolic control on progression of incipient nephropathy in insulin-dependent diabetes. Lancet. 1986;2:1300-4.

9. Reichard P, Rosenqvist V. Nephropathy is delayed by intensified insulin treatment in patients with insulin-dependent diabetes mellitus and retinopathy. J Int Med. 1989;226:71-87.

10. Reichard P, Berglund B, Britz A. Intensified conventional insulin treatment retards the microvascular complications of IDDM. The Stockholm' Diabetes Intervention Study (SDIS) after 5 years. J Intern Med. 1991;230:101-8.

11. Reichard P, Nilsson BY, Rosenqvist V. The effect of long-term intensified insulin treatment on the development of microvascular complications of diabetes mellitus. N Engl J Med. 1993;329:304-9.

12. The Diabetes Control and Complications Trial (DCCT) Research Group. The diabetes control and complications trial. Design and methodological considerations for the feasibility phase. Diabetes. 1986;35:530-45.

13. The Diabetes Control and Complications Trial (DCCT) Research Group. Diabetes control and complications trial: results of feasibility study. Diabetes Care. 1987;10:1-19.

14. The Diabetes Control and Complications Trial (DCCT) Research Group. DCCT Update Symposium. Presented at the 53rd Annual Meeting of the American Diabetes Association. Las Vegas, Nevada, 13th June, 1993.

15. Liu QZ, Knowler We, Nelson RG, et al. Insulin treatment, endogenous insulin concentration and ECG abnormities in diabetic Pima Indians cross-sectional and prospective analysis. Diabetes. 1992;41:1141-50.

16. Klein R. Hyperglycemia and microvascular and macrovascular disease in diabetes. Diabetes care. 1995;18:258-71.

17. Leslie RD, et al. United Kingdom Prospective Diabetes Study (UKDPS). What now or so what? Diabetes metabolisom research previews. 1999;15(1):65-71.

18. The United Kingdom Prospective Diabetes Study (UKPDS 35). BMJ. 2000;321: 405-12.

19. Stratton IM, Kohner EM, Aldington SJ, et al. The United Kingdom Prospective Diabetes Study (UKPDS 50). Risk factors for incidence and progression of retinopathy in type 2 diabetes over 6 years from diagnosis. Diabetologia. 2001;44(2):156-63.

20. The United Kingdom Prospective Diabetes Study (UKPDS) group. Intensive blood glucose control with sulphonyl ureas or insulin compared with conventional treatment and risk of complication in patients with type 2 diabetes (UKPDS 33). Lancet. 1998;45:1289-98.

21. The United Kingdom Prospective Diabetes Study (UKPDS) group. Tight blood pressure control and risk of microvascular and macrovascular complications in type 2 diabetes (UKPDS 38). BMJ. 1998;317:703-13.

22. Malurberg K, Ryden L, et al. Randomised trial of insulin glucose infusion followed by subcutaneous insulin treatment in diabetic patients with acute myocardial infarction (DIGAMI study). Effect of mortality at 1 year. J Am Coll Cardiol.1995;26: 57-65.

23. Van Den Berghe G, et al. Intensive insulin therapy in the surgical intensive care unit. N Engl J Med. 2001;345:1359

24. Abraira C, Duckworth W, McCarren M, Emanuele N, Arca D, Reda D, Henderson W, for the participants of the VA Cooperative Study of Glycemic Control and Complications in Diabetes Mellitus Type 2: design of the cooperative study on glycemic control and complications in diabetes mellitus type 2. J Diabetes Compl. 2003 17:314-22.

25. Standards of Medical Care for Patients with Diabetes Mellitus: classification, diagnosis and screening. American Diabetes Association. Diabetes Care. 2004;27:515-35.

26. Feld S, et al. American Association of Clinical Endocrinologists and the American College of Endocrinology. Medical Guidelines for the Management of Diabetes Mellitus: the AACE System of Intensive Diabetes Self-Management. Endo Pract. 2002; 8:40-83.

Section 11

DIABETES THROUGH LIFE AND EVENTS

Chapter 76

DIABETES MELLITUS IN NEONATES AND INFANTS

PSN Menon

CHAPTER OUTLINE

- Introduction
- Transient Neonatal Diabetes Mellitus
- Permanent Neonatal Diabetes Mellitus
- Conclusion
- Summary

INTRODUCTION

Diabetes mellitus (DM) is not uncommon in children, but its onset in infancy is rare and diagnosis is frequently missed. The lack of awareness about the occurrence of this disease in infancy by most primary care physicians contributes to the low reported prevalence. A transient hyperglycemic state (defined as blood sugar more than 125 mg/dl) can be observed in neonates with sepsis or respiratory distress syndrome, and those receiving parenteral glucose solutions and occasionally in premature infants. This often returns to normal following appropriate therapy with withdrawal of fluids or reducing the strength of the glucose infusion.

In this chapter, hyperglycemia in the first year of life is presented, focusing on transient and permanent forms of diabetes mellitus in newborn period and infancy. The clinical presentation, pathophysiology, diagnostic evaluation, and management of these entities are discussed.

TRANSIENT NEONATAL DIABETES MELLITUS

Neonatal diabetes mellitus (NDM) is a very rare condition. It is defined as hyperglycemia occurring in the first few months of life that lasts for more than two weeks and requires insulin therapy.[1,2] It is distinct from autoimmune type 1 diabetes mellitus, which manifests after the first 3 to 6 months of life.[3] Little is known about NDM, especially its long-term course. This syndrome is also known as congenital neonatal diabetes mellitus, pseudodiabetes, congenital temporary diabetes and infantile glycosuria. Most cases resolve spontaneously by a few months, and hence, this entity is called as transient neonatal diabetes mellitus (TNDM).[4]

Epidemiology

Very little is known about the prevalence or incidence of TNDM. A German study reported an incidence of neonatal diabetes of about 1 in 450,000 to 600,000 births.[1] There are no published studies from India and developing countries except for a few case reports.[5-8] Approximately, one-third of patients with NDM has TNDM followed by recurrence. It does not share any of the markers of autoimmunity such as ICA, GAD_{65} or IA_2 antibodies.[2]

Etiopathogenesis

The etiology of TNDM is obscure. It is being increasingly recognized as a genetic disease with disturbances in the genes regulating islet organogenesis and function including insulin secretion.[3,9] This is suggested by the occurrence of NDM in twins and several pairs of triplets and half-siblings.[1,10,11] There is family history of type 1 diabetes mellitus in about one-third of the cases.[12] A long-term survivor has become a parent of a boy with TNDM.[1] There is case report of two first cousins, one with transient and the other with permanent forms of diabetes of newborn from Saudi Arabia.[13] Although this condition has been reported in an infant of a mother with impaired glucose tolerance, it is clear that these infants are generally not predisposed to neonatal diabetes. Flat glucose tolerance curves have been observed in some mothers.

The majority of TNDM maps to a locus on chromosome 6q24, a region in which the ZAC (zinc finger protein associated with apoptosis and cell cycle arrest) gene is located.[9] Some of them ameliorate only to recur in later life with characteristics of type 2 DM. The transmission is always from the father, himself being affected.[14] Paternal uniparental disomy for chromosome 6 has been described in some cases.[15] Other abnormalities include paternally inherited duplication of 6q24 and a methylation defect at CpG island overlapping exon of ZAC.[16,17] These variable patterns of TNDM suggest a disorder of imprinting with overexpression.

Pancreatic islet cells in autopsy studies have been described as normal, reduced or even excess.[18] Data from studies on pancreas in fetuses and neonates suggest that the most likely etiology of this disorder is a maturational delay of the adenyl cyclase-cyclic adenosine monophosphate (cAMP) system in islets mediating insulin secretion or its rapid destruction by an overactive cAMP-phosphodiesterase system.[18] Pagliara et al showed that in infants with TNDM, administration of glucose and tolbutamide failed to elicit any significant insulin release during the diabetic phase, whereas intramuscular injection of caffeine benzoate, a phosphodiesterase inhibitor, evoked considerable secretion.[18] Thus, it is possible that some cases of TNDM are the result of a quantitative rather than qualitative difference in the regulation of perinatal insulin secretion. Infants with TNDM have a delayed maturation of the β-cell similar to the precocious maturation seen in infants of diabetic mothers.

Insulin, C-peptide and insulin-like growth factor-1 (IGF-1) levels are low in these infants during the diabetic phase and become normal with clinical recovery.[12,19,20] IGF-2 levels are normal. Insulin is an anabolic hormone and growth factor *in utero*, and an important determinant of fetal growth.[21] Most of the entities associated with TNDM are characterized by being small for gestational age (SGA) at birth.[10,20,22,23] Mutation in insulin receptor is responsible for fetal growth retardation seen in insulin resistance syndromes, such as leprechaunism and Rabson-Mendenhall syndrome.[24]

- Neonatal diabetes mellitus is defined as hyperglycemia occurring in the first few months of life that lasts for more than 2 weeks and requires insulin therapy
- Incidence is about 1:450,000 to 600,000 births
- Etiologic mechanism is incompletely understood
- Majority of TNDM maps to a locus on chromosome 6q24
- Maturational delay of cAMP mediated insulin release is the likely pathophysiology.

Clinical Features

The average age of onset is two weeks, but the range of onset may be within hours of birth to 6 weeks. Onset in most cases is in the first month of life, but in approximately 15 to 20 percent of cases, the onset was between 1 and 3 months of life.[1] Boys and girls are equally affected. Infants are typically term and small for gestational age (SGA) and rarely large. These babies are prone for birth asphyxia. Rarely, hypoglycemia may precede the onset of diabetes in these neonates.[4,5] They have characteristic "open-eyed alert facies" and are emaciated with marked subcutaneous fat wasting.[25] Onset is usually sudden with severe dehydration without any history of vomiting and diarrhea. Urine output may increase because of osmotic loss. They may also present with "honeyed nappies", polydipsia and polyuria. In these infants, urinary tract infection and septicemia should be promptly looked for.[25] **Table 76.1** summarizes the clinical features of TNDM.

TABLE 76.1	Clinical features of transient neonatal diabetes mellitus (TNDM)

- Small for gestational age (SGA)
- Proneness for birth asphyxia
- Emaciation with marked loss of subcutaneous fat
- Open-eyed alert facies
- Severe dehydration (without vomiting/diarrhea) of acute onset
- Polyuria, polydipsia
- Honeyed nappies
- Proneness for infections, such as urinary tract infection, septicemia
- Need for insulin to correct hyperglycemia for a short period

TABLE 76.2	Laboratory investigation in transient neonatal diabetes mellitus (TNDM)

- Hyperglycemia: Blood sugar levels, random more than 200 mg/dl
- Glycosuria
- Absent or mild ketonemia or ketonuria
- Low baseline insulin, C-peptide, IGF-1 levels
- Glucagon stimulation test with estimation of insulin and C-peptide levels

TNDM is also associated with Wolcott-Rallison syndrome (multiple epiphyseal or spondyloepiphyseal dysplasias and renal anomalies), hyperuricemia and celiac disease.[1] Evidence of renal impairment not corrected by rehydration suggests the possibility of WR syndrome, which can be confirmed by radiological demonstration of epiphyseal dysplasia. Macroglossia is frequently seen with TNDM and paternal uniparental disomy for chromosome 6.[11,20,22,23,26,27] NDM has been reported with other dysmorphic features including large fontanels, hypospadias, umbilical hernia and inguinal hernia.[26]

Diagnosis

The diagnosis of TNDM is based on a clinical presentation with high index of suspicion or detection of hyperglycemia and glycosuria on routine laboratory testing **(Table 76.2)**. The blood glucose levels can range from 200 to 2000 mg/dl, and the rate of rise of glucose may be very rapid. Ketonuria is usually absent and mild ketonuria does not rule out the diagnosis. Insulin, C-peptide and IGF-1 levels are low during the diabetic phase.

Clinical course can be predicted by sequential glucagon stimulation tests.[20] It also helps assess β-cell function. After obtaining baseline sample for insulin and C-peptide levels, glucagon 30 μg/kg is administered intravenously. Samples are drawn at 5 and 15 minutes for insulin and C-peptide estimations. While the glucagon-mediated insulin and C-peptide response is minimal during diabetic phase, it increases with clinical recovery indicating improving β-cell function and remission. Parents of infants with appreciable insulin response can be reassured that chances of spontaneous recovery are very high. On the other hand, an absent insulin response in an infant with prolonged insulin requirement should prompt the clinician to make a diagnosis of permanent neonatal diabetes and look for causes, such as pancreatic dysgenesis. A chromosome 6

anomaly, if present, is strongly in favor of transient form of disease.[17]

Differential Diagnosis

The identity of reducing substances in the urine of a young infant failing to thrive must be established in order to rule out the possibility of galactosuria or lactosuria. Glucose intolerance may be seen in infants with severe prematurity, sepsis and respiratory distress syndrome. Glycosuria may occur in renal tubular dysfunction associated with Fanconi's syndrome, tyrosinosis and galactosemia. The presence of hyperglycemia as well as glycosuria will establish the diagnosis of DM. Diseases of the central nervous system and overwhelming stress must be suspected in infants with hyperglycemia. Confirmation of septicemia by screening tests is essential in newborns with lethargy and failure to thrive.

Complications

These infants are prone to severe dehydration, hypothermia, urinary tract infections and septicemia. During insulin therapy, they may develop repeated hypoglycemic attacks.

- Most affected neonates are small for gestational age (SGA) with osmotic polyuria, dehydration and hyperglycemia with characteristic open-eyed alert facies.
- Ketoacidosis when present is mild.
- Transient hyperglycemic states should be excluded by careful evaluation.
- Insulin, C-peptide and IGF-1 levels are low in TNDM.
- Antibodies to insulin, islet cells and other markers of type 1 DM are absent.
- Clinical course can be predicted by sequential glucagon stimulation tests.

Management

Management consists of adequate hydration, insulin therapy, and monitoring. Dehydration should be promptly corrected with isotonic saline, and the excessive osmotic loss associated with severe hyperglycemia should be managed with appropriate fluids.

Insulin is the mainstay of the therapy. The response to exogenous insulin is quick and dramatic. These infants are quite insulin sensitive and administration of small frequent doses of insulin and close monitoring are essential to prevent rapid drop in blood sugar levels. The daily requirement of insulin may fluctuate considerably. The initial doses of short acting insulin should be conservative, about 0.25 to 0.5 units per kg/per dose administered subcutaneously. The doses may be repeated every 4 hours, if the blood sugar levels do not fall. Alternatively, if indicated (as in severe hyperglycemia), insulin can be administered as continuous intravenous infusion. Doses can range from 0.025 to 0.2 units/kg/hr for more insulin resistant infants. Blood sugar levels should be gradually reduced to 80 to 100 mg/dl/hr and insulin doses adjusted accordingly. Blood glucose should be monitored every hour, if insulin is given intravenously; and 2 hourly, if given subcutaneously until hyperglycemia is controlled. Once the condition of the infant and hyperglycemia are settled, insulin should be changed to longer acting insulin preparations (NPH or lente insulin) and preferably given twice daily. Administration of ultra-lente insulin has been tried to prevent hypoglycemia.[28] Insulin pump may provide a valuable tool to administer insulin.[29] Experience with newer insulin analogs are limited in these children. Insulin adjustments and blood sugar monitoring should be done as in cases of type 1 DM.

The newborn can be discharged home on insulin therapy and closely followed up to avoid hypoglycemia. Many parents are unprepared and reluctant to manage these children at home. Hence, parents and caregivers of these infants should receive counseling and diabetes education, in addition to the normal care of the newborn. As pancreatic function improves, insulin requirement decreases. While such an infant is on insulin, results of withdrawal of injections from time to time may be observed. The most useful indication of the continuing need for insulin is the failure to maintain expected weight gain on an adequate calorie intake. In some infants, insulin can be withdrawn after several weeks to months when it is observed that the exogenous insulin induces hypoglycemia, and its omission is not associated with hyperglycemia. However, hyperglycemia and insulin dependency have been reported to persist up to 5 years with subsequent resolution.[1] Thus, the course of TNDM is highly variable.

There have been case reports of treatment of TNDM with oral antidiabetic drugs, such as chlorpropamide (sulfonylurea that stimulates insulin secretion by the pancreatic cells).[30] After the initial hyperglycemia was controlled, insulin was tapered, and chlorpropamide was added. Gradually, the dose was increased from 2 to 12 mg/per day. Subsequently, when pancreatic function improved, chlorpropamide was stopped.

Breastfeeding should be ensured and baby should be nursed as frequently as possible. While on insulin, artificial milk should be given when breastfeeding cannot be established. Regular weaning can be started by 4 months of age.

Monitoring

Although strict blood monitoring is essential to avoid hypoglycemia during insulin therapy, very strict control of blood sugar is not desirable. The goals of management are to keep urine free of sugar and ketones, and maintain adequate growth of infant. During home insulin therapy, blood sugar and/or urine sugar should be monitored as in type 1 DM. In young infants with diabetes, glycosylated hemoglobin levels must be interpreted with caution because hemoglobin F can interfere with some assays. Sequential glucagon stimulation testing should be performed to assess insulin and/or C-peptide response in these infants with hyperglycemia in order to predict their clinical course and chances of spontaneous remission. On follow-up visits, their anthropometric measurements and developmental assessment should be carried out.

Long-term Outcome

Course of TNDM is highly variable, since diabetes may recur after a prolonged period.[31] Thus, one should be careful to consider a remission permanent, and neonatal diabetes should probably be considered as a prediabetic state. A study reported that among newborn infants with DM, diabetes was transient in about 50% of cases. Approximately 20% of them had TNDM with later recurrence at 7 to 20 years. The remaining 30% had permanent neonatal diabetes mellitus.[1] Most children with TNDM in remission have no evidence of β-cell dysfunction or insulin resistance in the fasting state. Measures of insulin response to intravenous glucose loading are often normal, but suggest future recurrence if profoundly abnormal.[32] The presence of HLA-DR3 and DR4 antigens increases the likelihood of permanent diabetes mellitus. The overall prognosis for general health and normal intellectual development is usually good.

- Management consists of adequate hydration, insulin therapy, and monitoring.
- Parents should receive counseling and diabetic education in addition to normal care of newborn.
- Ensure breastfeeding and good nutrition for good catch-up growth.
- The course of TNDM is highly variable. About 20% has recurrence at 7 to 20 years.

PERMANENT NEONATAL DIABETES MELLITUS

Epidemiology

Permanent neonatal diabetes mellitus (PNDM) is very rare. The exact incidence or prevalence is not known. A study from Sultanate of Oman reported an incidence of 1.788 per 100,000 live births/year compared to 1 in 500,000 reported from Germany.[1,33] This high incidence is probably due to the high degree of consanguinity in Oman. Autosomal recessive form of inheritance is reported from Oman.[33,34] A clinic based study done in south India reported PNDM to be prevalent among 1 in 8,661 of all diabetic patients or 1 in 125 type 1 diabetic patients.[35]

Etiology

The possible causes are pancreatic dysgenesis and type 1 DM. Pancreatic agenesis is more common, and includes a spectrum of developmental functional anomalies ranging from mild hypoplasia to complete agenesis. These functional anomalies of pancreas include both exocrine and endocrine insufficiencies. Pancreatic dysgenesis can be classified as mild, moderate, and severe types.

Type 1 autoimmune DM is uncommon in neonatal period. There are no clinical or autoimmune evidence of congenital infection at birth. Islet cell antibodies are unusual, and HLA DR3/DR4 associations are rare.[36] Histopathological features of the pancreas are different from those seen in classical type 1 DM. Slowly deteriorating insulin secretion and C-peptide production leading to diabetes is known with infantile cystinosis.[37]

Genetic Regulation of Pancreatic Islet Development

A number of differentiation, transcriptional and growth factors, and hormones influence embryonic development of pancreas.[2,38-40] Among the transcriptional factors, the homeodomain protein PDX-1 (Pancreas and Duodenum homeoboX-1, also known as IDX-1, STF-1 or insulin promoter factor IPF-1) is a regulator of insulin gene transcription expressed in developing pancreatic bud. Null mutation of PDX-1 in mice results in failure of growth and differentiation of pancreatic bud leading to pancreatic agenesis. A homozygous point mutation in this gene has been described in a patient with pancreatic agenesis indicating that this gene is critical for human pancreas development.[41] There was evidence of both exocrine and endocrine pancreatic dysfunction with absence of pancreatic tissue on imaging studies.[41] Interestingly, heterozygosity for PDX-1 mutation is associated with later onset of DM, as occurs in maturity-onset diabetes of youth (MODY).[42,43]

PNDM can also be caused by mutations in key components of insulin secretion, such as glucokinase (GCK) and KCNJ11 gene. Homozygous mutations of glucokinase result in PNDM.[44] Permanent neonatal diabetes can result from complete deficiency of glucokinase activity. They are characterized by intrauterine growth retardation (IUGR), permanent insulin requiring diabetes from first day of life and hyperglycemia in both parents.[45] Autosomal recessive inheritance and enzyme deficiency are typical.

Activating mutations in KCNJ11 gene encoding for the Kir6.2 subunit of the β-cell ATP-sensitive (K^+) channel have recently been shown to be a common cause of PNDM. Germline mutations of Kir6.2 were the most frequent cause of PNDM in cohort studies.[46,47] Family history of diabetes is present in a few patients, and some affected children had neurological features, including muscle weakness, motor delay, and epilepsy. Insulin secretory response to tolbutamide was present in a few patients tested, but not to glucose or glucagon. Ketoacidosis is common with marked hyperglycemia, and patients require insulin therapy.[48]

PNDM can also be caused by mutations in eukaryotic translation initiation factor-2 alpha kinase3 (EIF2AK3) and forkhead box P-3.[46] PNDM caused by a mutation of the HNF-1β (hepatocyte nuclear factor 1-β) gene associated with neonatal polycystic dysplastic kidneys has been reported recently.[49] A novel gene for neonatal diabetes has been mapped to chromosome 10p12.1-p13 in a recent study.[50] These neonates have low levels of circulating C-peptide and low or undetectable insulin in the presence of severe hyperglycemia unresponsive to insulin infusion.

- PNDM is rare; incidence 1.8 per 100,000 to 500,000 in various studies
- Most likely causes are pancreatic agenesis and type 1 DM
- A homozygous mutation in transcription factor PDX-1 (IPF-1) is associated with pancreatic agenesis indicating its role in pancreatic islet cell development
- PNDM can be caused by mutations in key components of insulin secretion, such as glucokinase (GCK) gene and Kir6.2 subunit of KCNJ11 gene, which regulates b-cell ATP-sensitive (K^+) channel
- This subgroup of patients may respond to tolbutamide on follow-up.

Clinical Features

Patients with PNDM usually present within the first three months of life and require insulin therapy. In most cases, the cause is unknown. The clinical presentation varies according to the etiology. Milder cases of pancreatic dysgenesis usually present as incidental hyperglycemia and glycosuria of infancy and childhood in which mild hyperglycemia is detected in infants and children during intercurrent illnesses, such as pneumonia, otitis media, and gastroenteritis. They lack the usual symptoms of polyuria, polydipsia, and polyphagia. Hyperglycemia resolves with resolution of the acute process.[51] The absence of typical features of TNDM, such as SGA and lack of need for insulin should make one suspect mild pancreatic dysgenesis rather than TNDM.

Patients with moderate pancreatic dysgenesis initially present similar to infants with TNDM, with features of IUGR, failure to thrive, acute onset of severe dehydration along with osmotic polyuria and polydipsia (early onset type PNDM). The cases reported by Bappal et al[34] were of IUGR, diabetic ketoacidosis and parental consanguinity, whereas diarrhea, fever, lethargy, poor feeding, poor weight gain, dehydration and tachypnea were common in the group reported by Soliman et al.[33] Ketoacidosis when it occurs is generally mild. Dysmorphic features are usually not present. Severe forms of pancreatic dysgenesis are extremely rare. Most of these children are SGA, do not survive neonatal period and have multiple associated anomalies, and evidence of fat malabsorption.

In type 1 autoimmune DM, infants are of normal weight. They may manifest at any time during infancy, but most often later in infancy, usually after 180 days after birth (late onset type PNDM). Onset is insidious characterized by polyuria, polydipsia, polyphagia and failure to thrive. They may also present acutely with ketoacidosis. Most children with early onset type of PNDM have "protective" HLA genotype of type 1 DM and are less likely to have autoimmune markers.[36]

Diagnosis

Diagnosis of pancreatic dysgenesis is usually clinical, based on demonstration of both endocrine and exocrine dysfunction of pancreas. These infants are SGA, and develop hyperglycemia, glycosuria, and acute onset dehydration within few weeks of life. Diabetes keto-acidosis is a common feature in Asian infants even though less common in West.[8] C-peptide secretion is absent or minimal at the time of presentation and

metabolic control of the disease. Diagnosis is usually established by demonstrating hyperglycemia; insulin (and IGF-1) levels when measured are low and respond poorly to oral or intravenous glucose.

The pointers toward diagnosis in these infants are persistent need for insulin beyond several months of age, subnormal insulin response to oral or intravenous glucose and glucagon stimulation test, low IGF-1, abnormal stools, and failure to gain weight despite high caloric intake and reasonably good control of blood sugar with insulin. A reasonable approach to the diagnosis of exocrine insufficiency in infants includes stool smear for fat droplets, 72 hr stool fat balance studies, serum immunoreactive trypsinogen, and fecal chymotrypsin or elastase. Alternatively, a clinical response to pancreatic enzyme replacement can also be tried. Abdominal ultrasonography and other modes of imaging can confirm the diagnosis of pancreatic agenesis. Hypertriglyceridemia is a common association in type 1 DM. Anti-insulin antibodies, anti-islet cell antibodies, and/or anti-GAD antibodies may be present.

Differential Diagnosis

Persistent hyperglycemia (blood sugar in excess of 200 mg/dl) should lead to a diagnosis of DM and initiation of appropriate therapy. However, it should be remembered that all hyperglycemias in infancy are not due to abnormal β-cell function. A common cause in the pediatric age group is administration of high dose of steroids as seen in patients of nephrotic syndrome, leukemia, asthma or arthritis. Endogenous excessive production of cortisol as in adrenal hyperplasia is a rare cause of hyperglycemia in infants. Pheochromocytoma and some primary CNS tumors can be associated with hyperglycemia. Polyuria and polydipsia are associated with diabetes insipidus. Features of malabsorption seen in pancreatic dysgenesis may also be associated with cystic fibrosis and celiac disease.[4] Patients with PNDM are less likely to have IUGR and are older at diagnosis, and have higher initial insulin requirements compared to TNDM, but no clinical feature is reliable in distinguishing PNDM from TNDM on an individual case basis. No chromosome 6 abnormalities are known in PNDM so far.[17]

Complications

Patients with pancreatic dysgenesis, in addition to the complications of diabetes, are prone to complications secondary to deficiency of nutrients and fat-soluble vitamins, severe protein-energy deficiency and growth

TABLE 76.3	Complications of permanent neonatal diabetes mellitus (PNDM)
Acute	• Ketoacidosis • Hypoglycemia • Insulin allergy • Susceptibility to infection
Intermediate	• Growth failure • Osteopenia • Delayed puberty • Lipodystrophy
Chronic	• Retinopathy • Nephropathy • Neuropathy • Cataract

failure. Long-term follow-up of PNDM over 20 years showed very few complications.[52] The growth and development are generally unaffected. Complications of type 1 DM in infants can be acute and long-term as in case of older children. They are listed in **Table 76.3**.

• Mild, moderate and severe forms of pancreatic agenesis have been described
• Markers of type 1 autoimmune DM may be present in those who initially manifest with DM after 3 to 6 months of life
• Both exocrine and endocrine pancreatic deficiencies can be established by investigations.

Management

Principle of management of type 1 DM in infants are same as that of older children. Initial management of hyperglycemia is similar to TNDM. Insulin pump may be a useful tool in the initial phase. After stabilization of blood sugar in infants, long acting insulin is given subcutaneously twice or more daily. Blood sugars are monitored regularly and dosage of insulin changed accordingly. Hypoglycemia should be carefully watched for. Periodic estimation of glycosylated hemoglobin is essential to monitor glycemic control.

The possible role of sulfonylurea in the management of PNDM is under investigation. Patients with mutations in the KCNJ11 gene encoding Kir 6.2 had insulin secretory response to tolbutamide but not to glucose or glucagon. Glibenclamide was introduced in increasing doses to investigate whether sulfonylurea could replace insulin. Insulin was discontinued at a glybenclamide dose of 0.3-0.4 mg/kg without any deterioration in blood glucose and stabilization of HbA_{1c} Apparently insulin-dependent patients with mutation in Kir6.2 may be managed on oral sulfonylurea with sustained metabolic control instead of insulin injections.[46]

Feeding of the infant should be ensured. No special diets are required. Infants can be given home made food. Calories should be adequate to maintain growth and development of the infant. Treatment of pancreatic dysgenesis with exocrine deficiency consists of management of diabetes by maintaining a diet with adequate fat intake along with optimal pancreatic enzyme replacement. Stool consistency and frequency, weight gain, and linear growth should be used to titrate the appropriate amount of enzyme replacement. Diet should be supplemented with fat-soluble vitamins, especially A and E. Other vitamins and micronutrients are also essential. Prothrombin time, partial thromboplastin time and fat-soluble vitamin levels should be monitored periodically to ensure compliance and adequacy of supplementation. Management of type 1 DM essentially follows the same guidelines in older children. The stress should be on diabetic education and psychosocial support to the families.

CONCLUSION

Most newborns and infants with hyperglycemia have transient diabetes of the newborn and spontaneous remission is likely. The insulin and C-peptide responses to glucagon improve with remission and recovery. Recurrence of hyperglycemia later in childhood should alert the clinician to the possible diagnosis of pancreatic dysgenesis rather than TDNB. Long-term follow-up is necessary for arriving at a final diagnosis.

SUMMARY

Diabetes mellitus is uncommon in newborn period and infancy. The two common forms described are the transient and permanent types of neonatal diabetes mellitus. Transient neonatal diabetes mellitus (TNDM) is defined as hyperglycemia occurring in the first few months of life that last more than two weeks and require insulin therapy. Most affected neonates are small for gestational age (SGA) with osmotic polyuria, dehydration, and hyperglycemia with characteristic open-eyed alert facies. Ketoacidosis when present is mild. The most likely etiology is a maturational delay of the cAMP-mediated insulin release. A genetic basis has been ascribed to a locus on chromosome 6q24 in which the ZAC gene is located. Insulin, C-peptide and IGF-1 levels are low in these infants, and antibodies to insulin or islet cells or other markers of autoimmune type 1 DM are absent. Clinical course can be predicted by sequential glucagon stimulation tests. The response to exogenous insulin is rapid and rewarding with good catch-up growth.

Permanent neonatal diabetes mellitus (PNDM) is relatively rare. The most likely etiology includes pancreatic agenesis and type 1 DM. Pancreatic agenesis has an early onset, and is usually characterized by signs and symptoms of malabsorption. Ketoacidosis is common. Homozygous deletion in the PDX-1 gene is a known association indicating its role in islet cell development. Mutations in key components of insulin secretion, such as glucokinase and KCNJ11 gene are shown to be common causes of PNDM. Markers of type 1 DM may be present in those initially present with DM after 3 to 6 months of life. IUGR is less common, and insulin requirements are high in PNDM. Even though insulin is the mainstay of therapy, sulfonylurea may have a role in the follow-up management in a selected few. The course of neonatal DM is highly variable. Diabetes is transient in about half of the patients with spontaneous resolution. Another 20% have recurrence at around 7 to 20 years whereas 30% have PNDM from onset. The variable course requires appropriate caution in providing counseling of parents with a diabetic newborn.

REFERENCES

1. von Muhlendahl KE, Herkenhoff H. Long-term course of neonatal diabetes. N Eng J Med 1995;333: 704-8.
2. Sperling MA. Neonatal diabetes. In Menon RK, Sperling MA (Eds): Pediatric Diabetes. Boston: Kluwer Academic Publishers; 2003. pp 215-25.
3. Hathout EH, Sharkey J, Racine M, et al. Diabetic autoimmunity in infants and preschoolers with type 1 diabetes. Pediatr Diabetes 2000;1:131-4.
4. Menon PSN, Khatwa UA. Diabetes mellitus in newborns and infants. Indian J Pediatr 2000;67: 443-8.
5. Rais N, Joshi M. Transient neonatal diabetes mellitus. Indian J Pediatr 1988;55:979-82.
6. Merchant R, Irani A, Nagar P. Transient diabetes mellitus in early infancy. Indian Pediatr 1985;22: 529-32.
7. Popat YO, Jethwani MG, Vaidya HD, et al. Diabetes mellitus in infancy. Indian Pediatr 1994;31: 1005-6.
8. Seth A, Sharda S, Narula MK, Aneja S, Taluja V. Diabetes mellitus in an infant. Indian J Pediatr 2004;71:947.
9. Shield JPH, Temple IK. Neonatal diabetes mellitus. Pediatr Diabetes 2002;3:109-12.
10. Ferguson AW, Milner RDG. Transient neonatal diabetes mellitus in sibs. Arch Dis Child 1970;45: 80-3..
11. Coffey JD Jr, Killelea DE. Transient neonatal diabetes mellitus in half sisters: a sequel. Am J Dis Child 1982;136:626-7.
12. Gentz JC, Cornblath M. Transient diabetes of the newborn. Adv Pediatr 1969;16:345-63.
13. Mathew PM, Hann RW, Hamdan JA. Neonatal diabetes in first cousins. Clin Pediatr (Phila) 1988; 27:247-51.
14. Temple IK, Gardner RJ, MacKay DJG, Barber JC, Robinson DO, Shield JP. Transient neonatal diabetes: widening the understanding of the aetiopathogenesis of diabetes. Diabetes 2000;49:1359-66.
15. Whiteford ML, Narendra A, White MP, et al. Paternal uniparental disomy for chromosome 6 causes transient neonatal diabetes. J Med Genet 1997;34:176-8.
16. Temple IK, Shield JP. Transient neonatal diabetes: a disorder of imprinting. J Med Genet 2002;39: 872-5.
17. Metz C, Cave H, Bertrand AM, et al. Neonatal diabetes mellitus: chromosomal analysis in transient and permanent cases. J Pediatr 2002;141:483-9.
18. Pagliara AS, Karl IE, Kipnis DB. Transient neonatal diabetes: delayed maturation of the pancreatic beta-cell. J Pediatr 1973;82:97-101.
19. Halliday HL, Reid MM, Hadden DR. C-peptide levels in transient neonatal diabetes. Diabet Med 1986;3:80-1.
20. Blethen SL, White NH, Santiago JV, Daughaday WH. Plasma somatomedins, endogenous insulin secretion, and growth in transient neonatal diabetes mellitus. J Clin Endocrinol Metab 1981;52:144-7.
21. Menon RK, Sperling MA. Insulin as a growth factor. Endocrinol Metab Clin North Am 1997;25: 633-47.
22. Schiff D, Colle E, Stern L. Metabolic and growth patterns in transient neonatal diabetes mellitus. New Eng J Med 1972;287:119-22.
23. Salerno MC, Gasparini N, Sandomerico ML, et al. Two interesting cases of transient neonatal diabetes mellitus. J Pediatr Endocrinol 1994;7:47-52.
24. Longo N, Wang Y, Smith SA, et al. Genotype-phenotype correlation in inherited severe insulin resistance. Human Mol Genet 2002;11:1465-75.
25. Romano AA. The infant of a diabetic mother and diabetes in the first year of life. In Lifshitz F (Ed): Pediatric Endocrinology (3rd edn). New York: Marcel Dekker Inc; 1996. pp 567-81.
26. Battin M, Yong C, Phang M, Daaboul T. Transient neonatal diabetes mellitus and macroglossia. J Perinatol 1996;16:288-91..
27. Christian SL, Rich BH, Loebl C, et al. Significance of genetic testing for paternal uniparental disomy of chromosome 6 in neonatal diabetes. J Pediatr 1999;134:42-6.
28. Mitamura R, Kimura H, Murakami Y, et al. Ultralente insulin treatment of transient neonatal diabetes mellitus. J Pediatr 1996;128:268-70.
29. Polak M, Shield J. Neonatal and very-early-onset diabetes mellitus. Semin Neonatol 2004;9:59-65.
30. Kuna P, Addy DP. Transient neonatal diabetes mellitus: treatment with chlorpropamide. Am J Dis Child 1979;133:65-6.
31. Weimerskirch D, Klein DJ. Recurrence of insulin-dependent diabetes mellitus after transient neonatal diabetes: a report of two cases. J Pediatr 1993;122:598-600.
32. Shield JP, Temple IK, Sabin M, et al. An assessment of pancreatic endocrine function and insulin sensitivity in patients with transient neonatal diabetes in remission. Arch Dis Child Fetal Neonatal Ed 2004; 89(4):F341-3.
33. Soliman AT, elZalabany MM, Bappal B, et al. Permanent neonatal diabetes mellitus: epidemiology, mode of presentation, pathogenesis and growth. Indian J Pediatr 1999;66:363-73.

34. Bappal B, Raghupathy P, De Silva V, *et al*. Permanent neonatal diabetes mellitus: clinical presentation and epidemiology in Oman. Arch Dis Child Fetal Neonatal Ed. 1999;80:209-12.

35. Sen SK. Premalatha G, Mohan V. Infantile type 1 diabetes mellitus (onset less than one year of age): a report of eight patients. Intern J Diabet Develop Countr. 2003;22:103-6.

36. Iafusco D, Stazi MA, Cotichini R, et al. Permanent diabetes mellitus in the first year of life. Diabetologia 2002;45:798-804 erratum Diabetologia 2003;46:140.

37. Filler G, Amendt P, von Bredow MA, et al. Slowly deteriorating insulin secretion and C-peptide production characterizes diabetes mellitus in infantile cystinosis. Eur J Pediatr 1998;157:738-42.

38. Humphrey RK, Smith MS, Tuch BE, et al. Regulation of the pancreatic cell differentiation and morphogenesis. Pediatr Diabetes 2002;3:46-63.

39. Sander M, German MS. The beta cell transcription factors and development of the pancreas. J Mol Med 1997;75:327-40.

40. Yamaoka T, Itakura M. Development of pancreatic islets. In J Mol Med 1999;3:247-61.

41. Stoffers DA, Zenkin NT, Stanojevic V, et al. Pancreatic agenesis attributable to a single nucleotide deletion in the human IPF1 gene coding sequence. Nat Genet 1997;1997:15-106.

42. Habener JF, Stoffers DA. A newly discovered role of transcription factors involved in pancreas development and the pathogenesis of diabetes mellitus. Proc Assoc Am Physicians 1998;110:12-21.

43. Fajans SS, Bell GI, Polonsky KS. Molecular mechanisms and clinical pathophysiology of maturity-onset diabetes of the young. New Eng J Med 2001;345:971-80.

44. Njolstad PR, Sovik O, Cuesta-Munoz A, et al. Neonatal diabetes mellitus due to complete glucokinase deficiency. NEJM 2001;344:1588-92.

45. Njolstad PR, Sagen JV, Bjorkhaug L, et al. Permanent neonatal diabetes caused by glucokinase deficiency: inborn error of the glucose-insulin signaling pathway. Diabetes 2003;52:2854-60.

46. Sagen JV, Raeder H, Hathout E, et al. Permanent neonatal diabetes due to mutations in KCNJ11 encoding Kir6.2: patient characteristics and initial response to sufonylurea therapy. Diabetes 2004; 53:2713-8.

47. Gloyn AL, Cummings EA, Edghill EL, et al. Permanent neonatal diabetes due to paternal germline mosaicism for an activating mutation of the KCNJ11 gene encoding the Kir6.2 subunit of the beta-cell potassium adenosine triphosphate channel. J Clin Endocrinol Metab 2004;89:3932-5.

48. Gloyn AL, Pearson ER, Antcliff JF, et al. Activating mutations in the gene encoding the ATP-sensitive potassium-channel subunit Kir6.2 and permanent neonatal diabetes. New Eng J Med 2004;350:1838-49.

49. Yorifuji T, Kurokawa K, Mamada M, et al. Neonatal diabetes mellitus and neonatal polycystic, dysplastic kidneys: phenotypically discordant recurrence of a mutation in the hepatocyte nuclear factor-1beta gene due to germline mosaicism. J Clin Endocrinol Metab 2004;89:2905-8.

50. Sellick GS, Garrett C, Houlston RS. A novel gene for neonatal diabetes maps to chromosome 10p12.1-p13. Diabetes 2003;52:2636-8.

51. Schatz DA, Kowa H, Winter WE, et al. Natural history of incidental hyperglycemia and glycosuria of childhood. J Pediatr 1989;115:676-80.

52. Dorchy H. Permanent neonatal diabetes mellitus: lack of diabetic complications after a 20-year follow-up. Eur J Pediatr 1992;151(2):151.

Chapter 77

DIABETES IN CHILDREN

Aspi J Irani

CHAPTER OUTLINE

- Introduction
- Etiology
- Clinical Presentation
- Diagnosis
- Stages of Diabetes in Childhood
- Day-to-day Management
- Growth and Pubertal Development
- Diabetes Related Emergencies in Children
- Patient Education
- Psychosocial Aspects

INTRODUCTION

Diabetes is the commonest endocrine-metabolic disease of childhood. Childhood diabetes includes a variety of clinical conditions related to hyperglycemia and glycosuria of which type 1 diabetes is by far the commonest. For the child, this diagnosis implies a lifetime on insulin injections with frequent pricks for blood glucose testing, restrictions in diet and physical activity, regular visits to the doctor and living in constant fear of hypoglycemia and ketoacidosis. The child with diabetes is deprived of the normal pleasures and carefree existence that one associates with this phase of life, hence emotional and psychological problems are common.

Prior to the discovery of insulin, childhood diabetes was a fatal disease. Insulin injections keep the child alive but cannot match the intricate physiological profile of endogenous insulin production; this inability to completely normalize the metabolic milieu is the chief factor responsible for the considerable long-term morbidity associated with this disease.

ETIOLOGY

Type 1 Diabetes is still by far the commonest variety of diabetes seen in children. In recent years, there has been an increase in the incidence of type 2 diabetes in this age group.

Type 1 diabetes can present at any age, the earliest reported case being less than a week old[1], but it is rare below the age of 9 months. There are two peaks of age at onset, the first being at 5 years and the other during puberty. There does not appear to be a sex predilection, but in areas of high prevalence, males are affected slightly more than females.[2] The onset of the disease shows a seasonal variation with maximum number of cases presenting during the winter months. The incidence varies considerably between countries. It is highest in Finland (30-40/100,000) followed by Sardinia, Canada and Sweden and it is lowest in China and Japan (1/100,000).[3,4] There is a considerable variation in different races living in the same environment and in the same race in different environments.[5] This only serves to underscore the importance of both genetic and environmental factors acting together in the genesis of this disease. Epidemics of type 1 diabetes are also known to occur.[4] Maternal ingestion of smoked mutton or of foods containing high amounts of protein and nitrosamines[6,7] or of coffee and sugar during pregnancy[8]; and failure to breast-feed or early introduction of cow's milk in infant diet[9,10] have all been blamed from time-to-time but there is no consistent or conclusive evidence to implicate any of these factors. Older maternal age, maternal pre-eclampsia, neonatal respiratory disease and jaundice due to blood group incompatibility were found to be perinatal risk factors for subsequent type 1 diabetes in the EURODIAB study.[11]

The incidence of childhood onset type 1 diabetes is rapidly increasing in many parts of the world, especially in children below the age of five years.[12] Type 1 diabetes is caused by autoimmune destruction of the β-cells in the pancreas.[13,14] It is more likely to develop in children with certain HLA genes (B8, B15, DR3, DR4, and particularly DQB1*0302, DQB1*0201, DQA1*0301 and DQA1*0501) which control related immune responses. Other, as yet unidentified, genetic factors[15] outside the HLA system are also certain to be involved since the risk of developing diabetes in a HLA identical sibling of an index case is only 1:7. Autoantibodies directed against various β-cell antigens and against insulin viz. islet cell antibodies or (ICAs), antibodies to glutamic acid decarboxylase or GAD65, tyrosine phosphatases IA-2, IA-2B and insulin autoantibodies or IAAs can be detected in serum several years before onset of clinical disease and serve as markers for the autoimmune process. The exact nature of the environmental factors that initiate autoimmunity in genetically susceptible children is not known but certain viruses[16], particularly rubella, coxsackie B4, CMV, mumps and adenovirus and dietary toxins (cow's milk protein exposure in early infancy) have been implicated. Children with type 1 diabetes are also prone to other autoimmune disorders such as Hashimoto's thyroiditis, Graves' disease, Addison's disease, vitiligo, pernicious anemia and celiac disease. A few cases of type 1 diabetes (about 5%) are not associated with any evidence of autoimmunity and are classified as type 1B (nonimmune-mediated). Higher proportion of type 1B cases have been reported from Lucknow, Uttar Pradesh, India by Bhatia et al (Chapter 33).

Other Varieties of Diabetes in Childhood

Classical Type 2 Diabetes[17-19]

There has been an increasing incidence of type 2 diabetes in childhood and adolescence in the past decade. In one study, as many as 33% of diabetics presenting between 10 to 19 years were found to be of the type 2 variety. Ramchandran from South India reported on a series of 18 children below 15 years of age with type 2 diabetes, the youngest being 9 years old.[17] Important clinical features that differentiate type 2 from type 1 diabetes include a strong family history of type 2 diabetes in a first or second degree relative (present in 80%), overweight or obesity, presence of acanthosis nigricans (seen in over 70%), and the absence of ketoacidosis. Ketoacidosis, however, does not exclude type 2 diabetes. It may be the presenting feature in 5 to 25% of adolescents with type 2 diabetes. Features of polycystic ovarian syndrome and/or presence of hypertension or lipid disorders in a given case should make one suspect type 2 diabetes. Many cases are asymptomatic and may be picked-up on screening. It is recommended that all Indian children above the age of 10 years who are overweight and have any one of the following risk factors should be screened: family history of type 2 diabetes in first or second degree relative, presence of *acanthosis*, dyslipidemia, hypertension or polycystic ovaries. For screening in Indian children, both fasting as well as two hour post glucose values are recommended.

HLA antigens and autoimmune markers of β-cell destruction are typically associated with type 1 diabetes but it must be kept in mind that these may be present in 3 to 27% of type 2 diabetics while 20% of type 1 diabetics may not have any such antibodies. Fasting insulin or C-peptide levels are usually normal or elevated but not to the extent expected for the degree of hyperglycemia in type 2 diabetes whereas the levels would be low in type 1. Presence of other autoimmune diseases in the patient or family members[20] would make the diagnosis of type 1 diabetes more likely. C-peptide levels measured after two years duration of disease, if found to be below 0.6 ng/mL in fasting state and below 1.5 ng/mL at 90 min after a standardized nutritional meal challenge would favor a diagnosis of type 1 diabetes.

Diet and exercise therapy may control hyperglycemia in some cases. In other cases, oral hypoglycemic agents may be added and the drug of choice in children is metformin. When it is difficult to distinguish type 1 from type 2 diabetes, insulin should be started as it would be effective in both varieties. After one year of onset of diabetes if the insulin dose requirement is below 0.3 units/kg body weight, type 2 diabetes is very likely and a trial of metformin should be considered.

Maturity Onset Diabetes of the Young (MODY)

This refers to noninsulin dependent diabetes developing below the age of 25 years and characterized by β-cell dysfunction with defective insulin release but minimal or no defects in insulin action.[21] There is a strong family history with autosomal dominant inheritance in all the subtypes described so far. Each subtype has a distinct chromosomal association. Molecular diagnostic testing which is currently available only in research laboratories is necessary for specific classification. These children unlike those with early onset type 2 diabetes are not obese. The disease is often, but not always mild. Some patients may eventually require insulin and may also develop microvascular complications in later life.

Miscellaneous

A number of pancreatic and endocrine diseases, metabolic disorders, malformation syndromes, chromosomal and genetic disorders and drugs may be associated with glucose intolerance or frank diabetes in children.[22] Most of these entities are very rare and moreover only a small percentage of children under these conditions would develop diabetes. The commoner ones are described briefly here.

Fibrocalculous pancreatic diabetes (FCPD): This is a tropical disease of uncertain etiology. It is characterized by pancreatic fibrosis and formation of calculi in the lumen of the pancreatic ducts. There is extensive damage of the acini and islets so that diabetes is invariably associated with dysfunction of exocrine pancreas. Patients may have a history of recurrent abdominal pain since early childhood. The patients as a rule have radiopaque pancreatic calculi before the onset of diabetes. Malnutrition is often associated.

Cystic fibrosis: This is an autosomal recessive disorder characterized by chronic obstruction and infection in the airways, maldigestion due to pancreatic insufficiency, biliary cirrhosis, and excessive salt loss in sweat. It is common in Caucasians, occurring in 1 in 2500 live births but is extremely rare in our country. Patients with this debilitating disease develop diabetes after the age of 10 years due to fibrosis and disruption of the islets in the pancreas. Onset of diabetes below the age of five years has also been reported. These patients are insulin requiring but generally ketosis resistant.

Surgery for hyperinsulinemia: Hyperinsulinemia is the commonest cause of persistent hypoglycemia in the newborn. Whereas a few cases can be managed medically with diazoxide, the majority require 95% pancreatectomy. Postoperatively, transient hyperglycemia and rarely permanent diabetes can occur especially during periods of stress or if the patient has to be continued on diazoxide.[23] In some cases, hyperinsulinemia does not respond to subtotal pancreatectomy and a total pancreatectomy may be required at a later date with resultant permanent diabetes.

Congenital rubella syndrome: Children with this syndrome have mental retardation, microcephaly, sensorineural deafness, congenital cataracts and congenital heart disease. About 10% develop type 1 diabetes in the early second decade of life. An interesting feature in these patients is the presence of various anti-islet antibodies since infancy and the slow progression of β-cell destruction.

Diabetes following transient neonatal diabetes: It is now well documented[24,25] that children who had transient diabetes in the neonatal period may develop an insulin-dependent variety of diabetes in the late first decade or early second decade of life. Hence, close follow-up and appropriate counseling is essential in these patients. These type 1 diabetic patients have low insulin requirements and absence of islet cell antibodies and HLA markers.

Obesity syndromes (Prader Willi, Laurence Moon Biedl): These syndromes have associated diabetes, usually type 2 in 10% of cases. Obesity, mental retardation and hypogonadism are common to both syndromes. Children with Prader-Willi also display hypotonia, short stature, and abnormally small hands and feet. About 60 to 70% of them have an interstitial microdeletion involving chromosome 15q11-13. Laurence Moon Biedl syndrome is associated with retinitis pigmentosa, polydactylism and a spectrum of renal anomalies. *Alstrom syndrome*[26] is another syndrome characterized by infantile obesity, with blindness due to infantile cone and rod retinal dystrophy, infantile cardiomyopathy, sensorineural deafness and slowly progressive chronic nephropathy. Type 2 diabetes develops in the second decade of life. The inheritance is autosomal recessive.

Wolfram syndrome: This is an autosomal recessive disorder characterized by diabetes insipidus, type 1 diabetes mellitus without autoimmune markers, optic atrophy and sensorineural deafness, (DIDMOAD syndrome).[27,28] The initial presentation is usually with diabetes mellitus. These children often also have marked dilatation of the urinary tract and in some cases there may be progressive neurodegeneration after adolescence.

Mongolism: Type 1 diabetes as well as hypothyroidism occurs with greater frequency in these children than in the general population. The prevalence of diabetes is estimated to be 2.1% and that of hypothyroidism is 16 to 28%. Though most of these children require insulin, a few of them may behave like type 2 diabetes.

Turner's syndrome: Like Mongolism, it is also associated with autoimmune thyroid disease and with carbohydrate intolerance which occurs in 15% during childhood and may progress to frank diabetes in over 60% during early adult life.

Thalassemia major: About 6% of children develop diabetes during the second decade or later.[29] The etiopathogenetic factor is hemosiderosis, which causes both insulin resistance at the level of the liver and insulin deficiency from destruction of the β-cells in the pancreas. The increased incidence of viral injury to the liver on account of multiple transfusions may be a contributory factor.

Drug induced: L-Asparginase used in treatment of childhood acute lymphoblastic leukemia causes a dose-related pancreatitis that can lead to transient or permanent diabetes.

Corticosteroid drugs in high doses over prolonged periods as used in nephrotic syndrome, leukemia or severe asthma can cause a reversible hyperglycemia.

Diazoxide given in hypertension or hyperinsulinemia can lead to transient diabetes.

Patients receiving alpha-interferon have been reported to develop diabetes with islet cell antibodies and in certain instances severe insulin deficiency.

Siep-Berardinelli syndrome: This is an autosomal recessive disorder with congenital generalized lipodystrophy, acromegaloid facies, thickened skin, large hands and feet, muscular hypertrophy, tall stature, hepatomegaly due to fatty infiltration, acanthosis nigricans, hirsutism, and in many cases mental retardation. There is marked hyperlipidemia. Diabetes secondary to insulin resistance develops in adolescence. Syndromes with partial lipodystrophy involving distinct areas of the body (Köbberling-Dunnigan syndrome, Mandibuloacral dysplasia) are also associated with insulin resistance.

CLINICAL PRESENTATION

The clinical onset of diabetes in a child is often rapid with symptoms being present for only a few days or weeks preceeding diagnosis. The early symptoms include polyuria, nocturia, polydipsia, polyphagia,

TABLE 77.1	When to suspect diabetes in a child

- Typical early symptoms: Polyuria, polydipsia, polyphagia, weight loss, weakness
- Secondary enuresis
- Weight loss and weakness despite eating well
- History of ants collecting around urine
- Vaginal candidiasis
- Polyuria in a child with clinical dehydration
- Respiratory distress without positive findings on examination of respiratory or cardiovascular systems
- Typical acetone odor in the breath
- In the differential diagnoses of coma and acute abdomen

weight loss and fatigue. A few patients may complain of muscle cramps and pruritus. Although these symptoms are very typical, the possibility of diabetes is often not considered because of a lack of awareness **(Table 77.1)**. Some patients may be suspected to have diabetes when ants are seen collecting around the urine. A recent onset of enuresis in a previously toilet-trained child and vaginal candidiasis in prepubertal girls are important additional clues to the diagnosis. Recurrent pyogenic skin infections are rarely a presenting feature in childhood. A proportion of cases may present with features of diabetic ketoacidosis particularly when diagnosis is delayed (infra).

Sooner or later in the course of the illness when ketosis develops, there is anorexia, abdominal pain and vomiting. Abdominal rigidity and distention may also be present which has at times led to the mistaken diagnosis of surgical acute abdomen. At this stage, the child is dehydrated while respiration becomes rapid and deep (Kussmaul's respiration) due to acidosis. There is a peculiar "acetone" fruity odor to the breath. Polyuria in a dehydrated child and respiratory distress in the absence of any clinical signs in the respiratory or cardiovascular systems must suggest the diagnosis of diabetes. Once ketosis sets in, progression to drowsiness, disorientation and finally coma may be rapid.

In some children, the onset may be catastrophic with ketoacidosis developing within a few days whereas in a few others there may be mild symptoms for over six months prior to diagnosis.

DIAGNOSIS

In a child with typical symptoms of polyuria, polydipsia, polyphagia, unexplained weight loss or ketosis a single random venous plasma glucose level at or above

11.1 mmol/L should clinch the diagnosis. In these cases, a glucose tolerance test is not only unnecessary but is also contraindicated as excessive hyperglycemia can result.

To confirm the diagnosis in the rare mildly symptomatic patient with nondiagnostic elevation of random plasma glucose, an oral glucose tolerance test (OGTT) is essential. It should be performed after the child has been on a high carbohydrate diet (200 gm/m2/day) for the preceding three days. The child should not have suffered from a febrile illness in the past two weeks and must be off all drugs that can affect blood glucose. The test is performed in the morning after an eight hour overnight fast. The recommended glucose load is 1.75 gm/kg to a maximum of 75 gm, administered in 250 to 300 ml of water over a period of 5 minutes. The test is said to be positive if (1) fasting venous plasma glucose is >7 mmol/L, (2) two hour post glucose value is >11.1 mmol/L. These abnormal results are to be confirmed by repeat testing on a different day. If the fasting value is <7 mmol/L but the two hour value is >7.7 mmol/L and <11.1 mmol/L, the patient is said to have impaired glucose tolerance (IGT). Only 0 to 10% of children with IGT may develop diabetes in future, hence no intervention other than weight control is recommended for these patients.

Susceptibility to type 1 diabetes in a child with normal OGTT can be ascertained with a fair degree of certainty by (1) studying the HLA type, (2) looking for presence and titer of islet cell autoantibodies, insulin autoantibodies, autoantibodies to GAD65 and to tyrosine phosphatases, (3) estimation of the first phase insulin release on intravenous glucose tolerance testing. This work-up is recommended only for research purposes for there is as yet no accepted therapy that can be offered to arrest the progression of the disease.

Entities that are Sometimes Confused with Diabetes in a Child

Conditions associated with polyuria: Diabetes insipidus, renal tubular acidosis, psychogenic polydipsia.

Conditions with reducing substances/glucose in urine (Renal glycosuria, Fanconi syndrome): None of the above conditions will have hyperglycemia as a feature, thus making it easy to distinguish them from diabetes mellitus.

Stress hyperglycemia: During acute severe illnesses, some children may develop hyperglycemia. At times, there may also be ketoacidosis on account of vomiting and starvation. These parameters return to normal on recovery from the primary illness and a normal OGTT done after 4 to 6 weeks would settle the issue.

Transient neonatal diabetes: This is a rare disorder seen in full-term, but small for gestational age babies in the first six weeks of life and is due to delayed maturation of normal insulin release. These babies require insulin for variable periods ranging from 14 days to 18 months after which there is complete recovery. The differentiation from permanent diabetes is initially difficult but becomes evident on follow-up. Family history of type 1 diabetes, HLA typing of the infant, detection of pancreatic auto-antibodies if present and serial C-peptide estimations may enable an earlier differentiation.

STAGES OF DIABETES IN CHILDHOOD

There are typically four stages in the evolution of childhood diabetes from clinical presentation when 10 to 20% of the β-cells are still producing insulin, to the stage of total diabetes characterized by complete absence of insulin production in the body.

Stage of Metabolic Recovery

On account of the accumulated metabolic deficit, there are high levels of stress hormones and compensatory hyperphagia. As the child emerges from the "starvation amidst plenty" situation, insulin requirement is fairly high at the time of diagnosis ranging from 1 to 1.5 units/kg/day. With treatment, the symptoms improve dramatically. There is a rapid weight gain. At this stage, the liver may enlarge due to deposition of glycogen, peripheral edema may occur, transient cataracts are described, variations in visual acuity are common and some patients may complain of temporary hair loss.

Partial Remission or "Honeymoon" Phase

After the first few days or weeks, insulin requirement drops to less than 0.5 units/kg/day in 60 to 70% of children. If this stage is not anticipated, it may be heralded by recurrent episodes of hypoglycemia. This is invariably a temporary phase due to regression of the inflammatory changes in the islets allowing the remaining β-cells to function better. Insulin sensitivity also increases once hyperglycemia is controlled and levels of stress hormones decline. A few children may actually be able to maintain reasonably good blood glucose values without any insulin though it is not advisable to omit insulin altogether. This phase lasts longer in adolescents than in children. Attempts to arrest the disease process at this stage with the use of immuno-suppressants and immunomodulators have not been successful.[30] However, the remission phase can be prolonged with institution of intensified management at the very outset.[31,32]

Intensification Phase

Insulin requirement begins to rise again, 3 to 12 months later, as β-cell destruction progresses relentlessly. This may happen gradually over weeks or months or it may be abrupt, precipitated by infection or other forms of stress. Parents should be informed in advance about this, so that they do not blame other factors for the apparently deteriorating glycemic control.

Total Diabetes

This is the stage when endogenous insulin production is negligible and no longer plays a significant role in glucose homeostasis. It is usually reached in two years after clinical onset of the disease.

DAY-TO-DAY MANAGEMENT

In the day-to-day management of childhood diabetes, there are four therapeutic measures each needing equal emphasis namely insulin therapy, meal planning, planned physical activity and monitoring. The proper application and integration of these measures are essential for good diabetes control. Since the responsibility for day-to-day management at home rests on the patient's family, education in self-care skills together with psychosocial support are very crucial.

Goals

- Freedom from symptoms of hyperglycemia and clinically significant hypoglycemia
- No episodes of DKA
- No school absenteeism on account of diabetes-related problems
- Adoption of a healthy lifestyle with regard to diet and exercise
- Educated in self-management
- Emotional well-being (child and family members)
- Normal growth and physical development. No obesity
- Majority of pre-meal blood glucose levels between 70 to 140 mgs% (higher targets, up to 160 in children below five years of age and those who tend to have a seizure with hypoglycemia)
- $HbA_{1c} < 8\%$; average blood glucose < 150 mg%
- Normal serum lipids
- Absence of microvascular complications on screening tests.

The blood glucose and glycosylated hemoglobin targets would have to vary from case-to-case depending on the age of the child, the proneness to severe hypo-glycemia[33] and the ability and willingness of the parents and the child to comprehend and to implement various levels of self-management.

The initial management at diagnosis must be under observation in a hospital setting, if the patient is dehydrated or below the age of six years or if the parents are very anxious, disturbed, illiterate or of low intelligence or in case telephone facility is not available in the home. All other cases can be managed on an outpatient basis.

Effective management of childhood diabetes requires a team approach. The team must comprise of a pediatric diabetologist, dietitian, psychiatrist or clinical psychologist, patient educator and social worker. The team must provide comprehensive care not merely for "the diabetic child" but for "the child who also has diabetes", and for the family members.

Insulin Therapy

Which Insulin?

Source: Insulin from animal sources are still available in our country and are a boon for the poor patient. Synthetic insulin made by recombinant DNA technology (including synthetic human insulin and its analogs) are now being widely used. The child with diabetes is started on the insulin preparation that the family can afford. Thus, a poor patient can be prescribed animal insulins and a well-off patient, human insulin or insulin analogs. Patients who are already on porcine insulin and doing well, need not be switched to human insulin. The indications for changing to a less antigenic source of insulin are insulin allergy, extensive lipoatrophy and suspected immunoresistance.

Time action profile: Short-acting insulins are used alone in the management of DKA, for insulin supplements on sick days and in the insulin pump therapy. For conventional day-to-day management, a combination of short-acting insulin and intermediate-acting insulin (preferably NPH when the two are to be mixed in the same syringe) is used. In the multi-dose basal-bolus insulin regimens, regular insulin or a short-acting analog is used for the bolus component whereas an intermediate-acting insulin or the long-acting insulin analog, insulin glargine or detemir to provide basal insulin requirement.

Role of insulin analogs: The short-acting insulin analogs lispro and aspart have certain advantages over regular insulin[34,35] like (1) more flexible life style from immediate pre-prandial dosing schedule, (2) improved glycemic control by synchronizing insulin and food absorption, (3) reduced risk of post-prandial, nocturnal, or severe hypoglycemia, (4) low risk of exercise-induced hyperglycemia with exercise more than three hours post-prandial and (5) above all, in a fussy child who often refuses food after taking the insulin shot, these insulins can be injected immediately after a meal. On the negative side, there is the higher cost and the theoretical risk of unknown teratogenicity.

The long-acting insulin analogs, glargine and detemir,[36] are now commercially available in India. These provide better basal insulinemia than the intermediate-acting preparations as they are virtually peakless, may work for 24 hours in most patients and have minimum day-to-day variability in absorption and action. They are associated with less risk of overnight hypoglycemia because they do not have a peak of activity as do NPH and ultralente and this has been confirmed in studies in the pediatric age group.

However, these insulins are much more expensive. Insulin glargine being acidic cannot be mixed with any other insulin, hence the patient should be willing to take four injections a day, three of short-acting and one of glargine.

In the future, oral insulin, inhaled insulin and nasal insulin are likely to enter the market and may provide a less painful route for taking premeal insulin boluses.

Pre-mixed insulins: They are not of much use in children as the proportion of the two components would have to be varied from time-to-time.

Which Regimen?

The *one injection a day regimen* in which a mixture of short-acting and intermediate-acting insulins is given before breakfast has several disadvantages. It gives a single large peak of insulin with risk of hypoglycemia in the late afternoon and early evening hours. It does not permit flexibility for any of the meals. The action wears off after 16 to 18 hours so that the patient remains underinsulinized in the pre-dawn period when insulin requirement is high. This regimen, however, does work in a few children who are in the honeymoon phase. An occasional patient during this phase may require only intermediate-acting insulin or insulin glargine once a day.

The most popular regimen in little children is the *two injections a day or split-mixed regimen.* The injections are given 20 to 30 minutes before breakfast and dinner, each being a mixture of short- and intermediate-acting insulins in the ratio 1:2 or 1:3 for the morning dose and 1:1 or 1:2 for the evening dose. The starting dose may be 0.5 to 1.0 units/kg/day if the patient is not ketotic and 1.0 to 1.5 units/kg/day in case there is ketosis. Subsequently, the dose is fine-tuned as discussed in the section on home monitoring. The advantage of this regimen is that the patient is more or less evenly insulinized throughout the 24 hours. The patient also enjoys some flexibility for the evening meal. In children who have an early dinner (at about 6 pm), the evening intermediate-acting insulin may peak at or shortly after midnight when insulin requirement is lowest while its action wanes after 2 to 3 am when the physiological need is high. To counter this, either the evening NPH can be replaced with long-acting insulin or the evening dose may be split to provide short-acting before dinner and NPH at bedtime (*the three injections a day regimen*).

Basal bolus regimens or multidose insulin (MDI) regimens were devised to mimic endogenous insulin production and provide flexibility in timing and contents of meals. The patient injects regular insulin or a short-acting insulin analog before each of the three major meals to provide premeal bolus insulin and one or two injections of intermediate acting insulin (pre-breakfast and bedtime) or a long-acting analog are taken to cover basal needs. Alternately, a single night-time injection of insulin glargine can be used for the basal component. Some youngsters do very well on doses of insulin lispro or aspart before each major meal and NPH insulin at bedtime. 40 to 50% of the days dose is needed for the basal component and the remaining is divided between the three boluses depending on the carbohydrate content of each meal. This regimen, even without intensification of other aspects of management is worth trying in children who are not well-controlled with the split-mixed insulin regimen. The child's refusal to accept three or more injections should be the only deterrent.

The *open loop insulin pump or continuous subcutaneous insulin infusion* (CSII) serves the same purpose as the basal bolus regimens but has the added advantages of using regular insulin or short-acting insulin analogs (the insulins with the least variability in day-to-day absorption) for both bolus and basal requirement. Further, the pump can be programed to supply variable basal rates which is particularly important for the early night (lower rate), the pre-dawn period (higher rate) and during exercise (lower rate). Transient elevations of blood glucose can be managed with small bolus injections without fear of superimposing it on a peak of long-acting insulin activity. In carefully selected children including toddlers, CSII has now been shown to give improved metabolic control with significantly lower insulin doses while reducing the risk of DKA and profound hypoglycemia.[37-39] Two types of the insulin pumps are available in India. This mode of therapy should be considered selectively in patients who are motivated, intelligent, willing to perform at least 5 blood glucose tests each day, can learn carbohydrate counting and have 24 hours physician back-up on telephone.

Who Injects?

All children above the age of eight years must be encouraged to inject themselves but only under the supervision of their parents. Self injection is less painful and psychologically less traumatic for the child. Children usually accept self injection when they see their peers doing it either at the childhood diabetes center or at camps for diabetic children. In younger children, the responsibility for injecting the child must be shared by both parents.

Injection devices: Disposable syringes have very fine needles, the injection is virtually painless in view of the silicone coating of the needles and there is very little dead space, hence less wastage of insulin. These syringes also work out very economical as most patients reuse them a number of times till the needle tip becomes blunt. Handling with clean hands, capping the needle by non-touch technique and storing in the butter compartment of the refrigerator are some of the precautions taken to keep these syringes sterile for repeated use. There should be no role for glass syringes with steel needles in the management of childhood diabetes. The pen injector is a boon for older children on the multidose regimens especially when the afternoon dose is to be administered in school or college. This device cannot be recommended as a routine since it is not possible to alter the ratio of short- and inter-mediate-acting insulins when the two are to be given simultaneously and also because insulin cartridges are significantly more expensive than insulin vials. Children with fear of needles may find the automatic injectors helpful as the needle is hidden from view and is inserted through the skin quickly by a spring loaded trigger.

Insulin dose depends on age, body weight, duration of diabetes and stage of pubertal development. Most patients need 0.6 to 1.5 units/kg/day with the higher dose range in the initial days after diagnosis and during the pubertal years. The dose would have to be periodically modified based on blood glucose results, food intake, exercise, state of physical and mental health.

Injection sites: The thighs and the anterior abdominal wall are the preferred sites in children, as self injection is convenient in these regions and the areas are relatively large allowing for proper site rotation. The abdominal site is preferred when the interval between injection and meal has to be short as insulin injected at this site is absorbed significantly faster than from the thigh. The abdomen is also preferred when physical activity involving the lower limbs is planned soon after the insulin dose. When parents administer the injection they can use the buttocks or arms. Insulin absorption from the abdomen and the buttocks is more predictable than from the extremities.

Meal Planning

Children with diabetes need careful meal planning (1) to ensure normal growth, (2) to match the time action curve of exogenously administered insulin, (3) to limit swings between hyperglycemia and hypoglycemia, (4) to prevent or delay the long-term macrovascular and microvascular complications of diabetes and (5) to inculcate good eating habits for the future.

To ensure normal growth, the caloric requirement is calculated using the same formula as for nondiabetic children: 100 cal/kg for the first 10 kg plus 50 cal/kg for the next 10 kg plus 20 cal/kg for the rest. Additional calories for catch-up growth would be required for the first 4 to 6 weeks after diagnosis. Any formula gives only a rough estimate, hence initially the child's usual eating habits and appetite can be used as an additional guide and during follow-up evaluation, the growth curve is the best indicator of caloric need. The meal prescription needs to be reviewed every six months on account of the rapid growth and frequent changes in activity and daily schedule during childhood. Caloric restriction is indicated mostly for obese children.

To match the time action curve of injected insulin, in patients on the conventional split-mixed insulin regimen, timings as well as carbohydrate and calorie content for each meal must be fairly constant from day-to-day. It is traditionally recommended that 20% of the total calories should be consumed at breakfast, 25% at lunch and at dinner and 10% at each of the three mid meal snacks. School going young children may consume 25% at breakfast and 20% for lunch in recess time. A separate meal plan would be required for weekly holidays and also for the vacation months. In patients on the multidose, basal-bolus insulin regimens, frequent snacks and rigid meals are not essential as the insulin regimen can be designed to match food intake. Thus, it is possible to suit individual needs and preferences. The insulin regimen and dose is decided after finalizing a meal plan acceptable to the child and family rather than trying to impose a meal plan to match a standard insulin prescription.

To minimize swings *in blood glucose levels,* meals should be frequent and small rather than few and large. Complex carbohydrates and foods with a low glycemic index must be preferred while highly refined carbohydrates must be restricted as much as possible except in treatment of hypoglycemia and to cover short activity bursts. Diets high in fiber of the soluble variety, have been shown to lead to a flatter blood glucose curve, to reduce insulin requirement and also to help in lowering total and LDL-cholesterol. A dietary fiber intake of up to 2 gm /100 kcal of food intake appears to be beneficial in children. In our society, this is not difficult with our routine preference for whole fruits, vegetables, legumes, oats, beans and whole-grain cereals. Brown rice and pasta can also be tried. Growing children on a high fiber diet require supplements of calcium, iron and zinc. High fiber diets can cause flatulence, abdominal cramps and discomfort. Bulky high fiber foods may not be suitable for children below the age of five years for they have a smaller capacity for food and so require a more energy dense diet.

To prevent or delay development of macrovascular and to a certain extent microvascular complications, the fat, protein and salt content of the diet needs to be regulated.

The diet should not include excess fat (>30% of total calories). Saturated fats must account for not more than 10% of the total calories, 10 to 15% should come from monounsaturated fats and the rest from polyunsaturated fats. To achieve this, patients should avoid high fat snacks such as potato chips, french fries, burgers, cakes and pastries and full fat dairy products such as butter, cream, full fat cheese. Baking, boiling and grilling should be used in food preparation instead of frying. Importance must be given to the quantity of cooking oil used which should not be more than 0.5 kg/person/month. Cholesterol intake needs to be restricted to 250 to 300 mg/day. This can be achieved by using skim milk (except in children below age of 5 years as skim milk is very low in vitamin A and in calories), restricting eggs to 4 to 5 per week, using

vegetable oils in cooking, cutting down on red and brown meats and preferring fish and poultry. Of the essential fatty acids, omega 3 and omega 6, the former is present in small quantities and in limited number of foods namely fish and fish oils, linseed and mustard oil, rajma and urad dals, fenugreek or methi seeds, walnuts and green leafy vegetables, while the latter is present in a larger variety of foods of daily use. An ideal ratio of omega 6:omega 3 is 4.0, hence care must be taken to incorporate omega 3 containing foods in the diet.

Protein intake should be aimed at 15 to 20% of the total calories. Protein rich foods of animal origin tend to be high in saturated fat while those of vegetable origin such as beans and legumes are associated with fiber and complex carbohydrate and hence are to be preferred. There is evidence that progression of diabetic renal disease can be delayed by timely protein restriction. In overt nephropathy, proteins are restricted to 8 to 10% of total calories.

Children with type 1 diabetes are at higher risk for developing hypertension than their nondiabetic counterparts, hence it would be prudent to use salt in moderation. Diabetic children are likely to consume more sodium as emphasis is on salty rather than sweet food. Regular blood pressure monitoring is essential and at the first sign of hypertension, a sodium-restricted diet must be instituted.

Other diet issues: Routine vitamin or mineral supplements are unnecessary for children who observe the prescribed meal plan. Supplementation becomes necessary only in patients with food faddism, in obese children on a restrictive diet, and if there is coexistent celiac disease, IgA deficiency, pernicious anemia or achlorhydria, conditions which are known to occur more commonly in patients with type 1 diabetes.

Most children can do without sweeteners, hence the use of artificial sweeteners must not be advised as a routine especially as their safety has been a subject of controversy.[40] Sugar has traditionally been forbidden in a diabetic child's diet, but a small amount of sucrose mixed with other foods does not significantly affect blood glucose rise after a meal.

The glycemic index of sucrose is 69 which compares favorably with that of bread or potatoes which is 71. A maximum of 15 grams of sucrose can be permitted, provided that the patient is not overweight and the intake is spread throughout the day rather than consumed all at once and it is fitted into the dietary allowance and not in addition to the normal diet. Based on the concept of glycemic index, it is also reasonable to occasionally allow ice-creams and chocolates in prevention of exercise-induced and nocturnal hypoglycemia.

In view of the above observations, the use of special "diabetic" chocolates and sweets appears unnecessary. Not only do they contain the same amount of calories as sucrose but also the fructose and sorbitol which are used in them as sweeteners can cause osmotic diarrhea and abdominal discomfort. Further, in poorly-controlled diabetics these sugars can lead to a considerable rise in blood glucose as they would be rapidly released into the blood stream rather than being stored as glycogen.

In order that the meals should not be monotonous, patients on conventional insulin regimens must be provided with an extensive dietary exchange list and taught how to use the list for variety in the diet. Patients on intensified management are taught carbohydrate counting and algorithms are established for their individual insulin, carbohydrate ratio bringing even greater flexibility in their meals. The meals advised for diabetic children are to be very nutritious and tasty and represent the ideal diet for any normal healthy person. Hence, the entire family must be encouraged to eat the same meals not only to ensure the child's compliance with the meal plan but also in the interest of their own long-term health.

At the outset, patients should be encouraged to weigh foods for a clearer understanding of portion sizes. This practice ought to be repeated for a few days in every six months to refresh the memory.

Adolescents must be instructed to study the influence of various foods on their blood glucose levels with the help of home blood glucose monitoring. This will encourage them to take a more active and informed role in self-management.

The role of meal planning in prevention of hypoglycemia must be explained to the patient. A meal plan for sick days when the child is anorexic and/or vomiting must be provided. These issues are discussed in the section on "emergencies".

The toddler and pre-school child presents a peculiar problem. After nine months of age, the growth rate slows down so that food requirement also decreases and the toddler begins to get fussy and disinterested in meals. Mothers get worried at this change in the child's appetite and try to force or coax him to eat. As negativism is a feature at this age, the toddler responds with food refusal and vomiting. This intensifies the problem for the parent who will in turn aggravate it by even greater pressure. This situation can be averted with proper counseling. There should be no forcing, no coaxing, no anxiety displayed over the child's appetite and no attempts to feed the child by diverting his attention as each of these measures is certain to prove counterproductive. There should be no bribes or bargaining at mealtimes as this can encourage manipulative behavior. Parents must avoid offering food items which they know the child dislikes rather than backtracking after a protracted battle with the child. Food should be decorated and presented in an attractive manner. Meal times must always be pleasant. All household members must eat the same meals and at the same time because children eat best by imitation. No junk foods or other items that are undesirable for the diabetic child should be brought into the house for it is easier to avoid temptation than to fight it.

Planned Physical Activity

Regular exercise is important for a diabetic child because of the long-term benefits that it confers. It gives the child a sense of well-being and improves self esteem. It increases insulin sensitivity leading to a gradual reduction in insulin requirement. It helps in weight control and has beneficial effects on blood lipids and on cardiopulmonary function.

During exercise, there is rapid absorption of insulin from the injection site due to increased blood flow in the exercising limb. This dampens hepatic glycogenolysis and gluconeogenesis and promotes over utilization of glucose. Thus, in an adequately controlled patient, sporadic or unaccustomed exercise can precipitate hypoglycemia. Hypoglycemia may occur during or shortly after exercise. It can also develop up to several hours after the activity as muscle and liver continue to take up glucose from the blood stream to replenish their depleted glycogen store. To prevent this, various measures have been recommended which are discussed in the section on hypoglycemia.

In a poorly controlled diabetic, exercise can lead to a paradoxical rise in blood glucose and worsening of ketosis. This happens because insulin levels continue to remain inadequate while levels of stress hormones rise leading to unrestrained glycogenolysis and neoglucogenesis. At the same time, the increased glucose pouring in the blood stream cannot be utilized by the muscles for lack of insulin. Hence, exercise cannot substitute insulin in diabetes management.

Aerobic, low resistance high movement type of exercises (running, cycling) are beneficial while high resistance low movement exercises (weight lifting) can cause a rise in blood pressure and are better avoided. Activities during which a sudden attack of hypoglycemia can prove fatal (e.g. swimming, rock climbing) should be undertaken only under supervision. Children should develop an interest in some activity that does not need a partner or partners so that these can be pursued regularly without dependence on others.

Monitoring

This includes routine home monitoring by the patient and periodic, long-term monitoring of the diabetic state during clinic visits.

Home Monitoring

There are three steps namely testing, recording and taking corrective action. Most parents, even those who are uneducated, can be taught the first two steps.

Testing: Patients must test their blood glucose and urine acetone at home. The availability of spring loaded trigger devices for painless blood letting has made blood testing more acceptable to children. Many children above 10 years of age can actively participate in testing. Blood glucose test strips can be read visually or with a reflectance meter. The tests must be performed before each major meal, at bedtime and at 2 to 3 am. At the outset, all these tests are done daily. After stabilization they can be done on two days each week. Patients on intensified management must check post meal blood glucose also. Urine acetone must be checked once daily as a routine but on sick days or whenever blood glucose is over 300 mg%, it must be looked for with each blood test. Majority of parents are very keen to do their best for their children and hence blood glucose monitoring is not difficult to implement in childhood diabetes. Urine glucose testing may still have a role in patients who cannot afford strips or refuse to test blood glucose often enough; who can be advised to routinely test urine and resort to blood test whenever the urine glucose is ++ on sick days and to confirm clinically suspected hypoglycemia.

Alternate site testing meters are now available which have the advantages that a very small volume of blood is required and a variety of surfaces other than the finger tips can be used for blood letting which are less painful as they have fewer nerve endings. However, these alternate sites are not appropriate for confirming hypoglycemia as there is a lag of about 30 minutes between the readings at the finger tip and the forearm.

A blood ketone monitoring strip and meter (the precision Xtra meter) is also now available and this should make the home management of sick days more precise. This meter measures primarily β-hydroxy-butyric acid while urine ketone measures acetoacetic acid. A blood value of 0.6 mmol/L is normal, 0.6 to 1.5 mmol/L indicates moderate ketosis and 1.6 to 3 mmol/L is considered high.

Two devices for continuous glucose monitoring are available: the Glucowatch - Cygnus and the MiniMed Continuous Glucose Monitoring System (CGMS). The former is worn on the wrist and works on the principle of reverse iontophoresis. It measures glucose in the subcutaneous interstitial fluid and gives a display in every 20 minutes with an alarm for hypoglycemia and for high glucose levels. A hypoglycemia alarm makes intensive management less risky in children. The CGMS is the size of a pager and is connected to a subcutaneous electrode which measures and records interstitial glucose levels in every five minutes over a period of 72 hours. It does not display any glucose values during the time it is worn but after disconnecting, the data can be downloaded on to a computer and analyzed for glucose trends in relation to various events of the day, such as food and exercise. Both these devices can be very helpful in managing children with brittle diabetes with frequent hypoglycemia and hypoglycemia unawareness and for children on intensive management.

Recording: The home blood glucose monitoring results must be recorded in a diary along with the timing and severity of hypoglycemic episodes, if any, during the course of the day. The most important but often neglected part of the record is the "comments column". Here, the patient writes down at the end of each day if any aberration in meals, activity or stress could have accounted for abnormally high or low glucose values during the day. The "comments column"is very important because it teaches the patient to think logically about his treatment plan.

Blood glucose meters can also store several readings and can provide averages over a period of time. The readings from some meters can be downloaded on a computer and analyzed for overall mean, mean for a particular time period of the day and standard deviation.

Taking corrective action: When three consecutive readings at a given time are outside the target range for the patient without any obvious errors in diet, activity or stress, the dose of the insulin covering that period should be revised. For this, the patient must be taught which insulin controls which test result (see **Table 77.2**). Adjustment is made at the rate of 10% of the current dose at a time. This is termed "pattern adjustment algorithm".

Patients on intensified management also need to learn algorithms for pre-meal insulin supplements.

TABLE 77.2	Correlation between insulin and glucose
Insulin	Test result under its control
Patient on 2 Injection Regimen	
Morning short-acting	Pre-lunch blood glucose
Morning intermediate-acting	Pre-dinner blood glucose
Evening short-acting	Bedtime blood glucose
Evening intermediate-acting	3 am and pre-breakfast blood glucose
Patient on Multidose Insulin Regimen	
Morning short-acting	Post-breakfast and pre-lunch blood glucose
Noon short-acting	Post-lunch and pre-dinner blood glucose
Evening short-acting	Bedtime blood glucose
Evening intermediate/long-acting	2-3 am and pre-breakfast blood glucose
Morning intermediate/long-acting	Pre-dinner blood glucose after post-lunch is normalized

Whenever pre-meal blood glucose is outside the target range the interval between the insulin dose and the meal may be reduced or even eliminated if blood glucose is below the target or extended up to 60 minutes if the value is above the target. Further, the insulin dose can be stepped-up by 1 unit for every 'X' mg % that blood glucose is above the target (where 'X' = 1500 divided by the patient's usual total daily dose). In addition, the pre-meal insulin dose can be adjusted according to the anticipated carbohydrate content of the meal that is to follow for which a knowledge of the patients insulin, carbohydrate ratio must be known.

Clinic Monitoring

This is required for assessment of the degree of control over a long-term, to evaluate patients' self-management skills and emotional well-being, for early detection of complications and for reinforcement of patient education. The old view that children with diabetes are protected from microvascular complications in the prepubertal years[41] may no longer be valid.[42]

- On reporting to the clinic, the child should take his insulin shot and test his blood glucose under supervision of the clinic staff, so that the errors in his techniques can be detected and corrected. The same blood sample can be simultaneously checked with the clinic equipment to confirm that the patient's equipments are functioning reliably.
- A careful history is obtained to elicit symptoms attributable to hyperglycemia (especially nocturia and weakness) or clinically significant hypoglycemia. Any school absenteeism on account of diabetes should be noted.

- The home monitoring records are scrutinized noting the frequency of testing and whether any corrective action is being taken. Dose adjustments or a change in regimen may be advised based on these records.
- *Growth charting:* The child's height and weight must be carefully charted and compared with previous readings. It is also advisable to chart the mid parental height on the graph. This value is obtained by halving the sum of the parents heights in centimeters plus 13 in the case of a male child and the sum of the heights minus 13 in females. If the child's current height when extrapolated to 18 years falls within +/– 8 cm of the corrected mid parental height, it indicates that the child is probably growing according to the family growth potential. A reasonably well-controlled child would have normal height and weight velocity. A sudden increase in weight with slow down in height velocity may be a clue to presence of hypothyroidism. Mere increase in weight may indicate that the patient is overeating and also over-insulinizing himself or it may signal recent onset of hypothyroidism. Weight loss could be due to poor control of diabetes, onset of hyperthyroidism, associated chronic disease like tuberculosis, celiac disease or an eating disorder.
- Injection sites should be inspected for lipodystrophic changes. If lipohypertrophy is found, education in systematic site rotation needs to be reinforced and injecting in the affected site should be strictly avoided till it has returned to normal. Extensive lipoatrophy calls for a switch to a less antigenic insulin, either porcine or human as the case may be.
- *Evaluation for limited joint mobility[43] (LJM):* This is done by feeling the skin over the fingers for

waxiness, thickening and toughness and then asking the patient to approximate his palms as if doing a "namaste" to see if the metacarpophalangeal and proximal interphalangeal joints of the opposing fifth fingers touch. Presence of LJM may be a marker, albeit inconsistent, of developing microvascular complications at other sites. LJM may later spread to the more medial fingers followed by the wrist, the elbow and then other large joints and the spine. A recent study[44] has shown a significant reduction in frequency of LJM in children in 1998 as compared to children screened in 1976.

- Blood pressure must be recorded. If the reading is above the 95th percentile for age and sex in a child or above 130/85 mm of mercury in an adolescent, the patient should be started on treatment with ACE inhibitors. Ambulatory blood pressure monitoring may show alterations before clinic blood pressure readings become abnormal. These include a loss of nocturnal fall in blood pressure, and an increased frequency of blood pressure readings above the 95th percentile for age and sex.[45]

- An enlarged and firm thyroid gland in a diabetic child would indicate presence of autoimmune thyroiditis. Less than half of such children will become hypothyroid and an even smaller number will develop Graves' disease. Mere presence of a goiter in the absence of disturbed thyroid function tests does not call for any treatment. Slowing of height velocity, weight gain, frequent unexplained hypoglycemia and significant decline in insulin requirement should suggest the possibility of clinical hypothyroidism.

- Evidences of other endocrine/autoimmune diseases must be sought. Addison's disease should be suspected if there is unexplained hypoglycemia, declining insulin requirements, skin pigmentation, lethargy and weight loss. Celiac disease must be suspected in a child who has abdominal pain, distension, loose stools, evidences of malabsorption, resistant iron deficiency anemia or failure to thrive. Alopecia areata, vitiligo, hypoparathyroidism and autoimmune hepatitis are occasionally associated with type 1 diabetes.

- In all older children and adolescents, an inquiry into symptoms of peripheral neuropathy (numbness, pain, cramps and paresthesia) and symptoms suggestive of genitourinary or gastrointestinal autonomic neuropathy must be made. Ankle jerks should be tested and sensations in the lower limbs must be evaluated. If any abnormalities are detected

in the screening tests, a more detailed evaluation should follow.

- Foot examination.

- Dilated eye fundus examination performed by highly-trained personnel is important at diagnosis of diabetes to exclude cataracts and other disorders and subsequently, it should be repeated annually (to look for early signs of diabetic retinopathy) after two years duration of disease in children with pubertal onset of diabetes while in those with prepubertal onset screening should commence after five years duration of diabetes, at age of 11 years or at onset of puberty (whichever is earlier).[46] Diminishing vision and optic atrophy should suggest the diagnosis of Wolfram syndrome.

- The child and the parents should be separately interviewed and encouraged to speak out their feelings and difficulties. This helps to detect any underlying conflicts or emotional disorders which may be contributing to poor control.

- The patient should meet the dietitian so that the diet prescription can be reviewed in the light of the child's recent weight gain and growth pattern and also to accommodate any changes in daily schedule.

- Finally, the educator spends time with the patients reinforcing education and assessing the patient's knowledge and ability to apply the same in day-to-day living. Teenagers are counseled about the harmful effects of smoking and the beneficial effects of regular physical activity. Advice regarding vaccinations must be provided as a preventive measure against infectious diseases. Vaccines for chickenpox, hepatitis A, typhoid and influenza[47] which are optional in India must be offered to those diabetic patients who can afford them.

- *Laboratory evaluation:*
  - Fasting/random blood glucose should be checked at each clinic visit with the same sample being tested by the patient with his home monitoring equipment.
  - Glycosylated hemoglobin should be estimated once in 3 to 6 months. Its importance lies in the fact that it is the only objective long-term indicator of diabetes control and that it is not patient dependent. Any discrepancy between the glycosylated hemoglobin and the patient's home monitoring records would mean that there is lack of accuracy or cheating in home blood tests. This test also gives the patient an objective goal to aim at.

- Serum lipids can be checked once within six months of initial diagnosis and if normal, the measurement should be repeated at mid-puberty and whenever the patient reports in poor metabolic control. Lipid abnormalities could be due to poorly-controlled diabetes, familial hyperlipidemia or associated hypothyroidism. If abnormal results are obtained, family screening for hyperlipidemia should be undertaken.
- Urine should be tested for microalbuminuria once in a year. In children with prepubertal onset of diabetes, this screening should begin after five years of the disease or at the age of 11 years or at puberty (whichever is earlier) while in those with pubertal onset, screening should be undertaken after two years of onset.[48] The test can be performed either on a 24-hour urine sample or a timed overnight sample or a spot first morning sample. An abnormal screening test must be repeated on two more occasions as studies have shown that as many as 33% of adolescents with microalbuminuria may revert to normoalbuminuria over a period of time. Patients with microalbuminuria should be initiated into intensified management. If it persists after 6 to 12 months of improved glycemic control, the patient should be started on ACE inhibitors or angiotensin II receptor antagonists and advised dietary protein restriction to not more than 1.0 to 1.2 g/kg/day.[49]
- Serum TSH and anti-thyroid auto antibodies should be checked once a year. The presence of antibody is not an indication for treatment[50] unless the TSH, T4 and T3 levels confirm malfunctioning of the thyroid gland. About 25 to 50% of children with type 1 diabetes will test positive for anti-thyroid antibodies: antithyroperoxidase and antithyroglobulin (prevalence of which increases with age), but the majority of these patients are euthyroid. The patient who is antibody positive should be explained the early symptoms of hypothyroidism or hyperthyroidism and told to report back if these appear. Overt hypothyroidism occurs in 1 to 5% of patients. Hyperthyroidism is less common, may be transient, occasionally precedes hypothyroidism or vice versa.
- In centers where facilities are available, screening for other autoimmune disorders may be undertaken. Adrenocortical antibodies and anti-21-hydroxylase antibodies are found in 1.6 to 2.3% of type 1 diabetics, but symptomatic Addison's disease is rare.[51,52] Gastric parietal cell antibodies are found in up to 18% of type 1 diabetes patients and 7% of these are likely to develop pernicious anemia.[53,54] Anemia unresponsive to iron therapy must lead to investigation for pernicious anemia or celiac disease (CD). The incidence of CD in type 1 diabetes is 1.0 to 6.4% which is 2 to 10 times higher than in the general population.[55] Antiendomysium antibodies (EMA) and tissue transglutaminase antibodies (tTGA) are highly specific and sensitive screening tests. Typical findings on jejunal biopsy and improvement on a gluten free diet on clinical, antibody and histopathological parameters would confirm the diagnosis. Sixty percent of cases are detectable at the onset of diabetes but a further 40% will be picked-up on follow-up screening. Seroconversion can occur upto eight years after diabetes onset, hence annual or once in two years screening seems reasonable. The risk of long-term complications of CD (iron deficiency, short-stature, osteoporosis, neuropsychiatric disorders, fertility problems, GIT malignancies) is the same in symptomatic and in asymptomatic cases and is proportionate to the time of exposure to gluten, hence the importance of early screening and intervention.[56]

GROWTH AND PUBERTAL DEVELOPMENT

The Mauriac syndrome is an extreme example of diabetic dwarfism. This syndrome which is rarely encountered these days[57] is the result of poorly-controlled diabetes of long-duration. It is characterized by stunted-growth, hepatomegaly, obesity, pallor, a thickened skin and delayed puberty. Skeletal maturation is severely retarded in all cases. These children have exaggerated growth hormone response to stimuli but their IGF-1 levels are markedly reduced. With treatment, the hepatomegaly resolves promptly and growth improves but in some cases poor growth may continue despite improved control. Sudden onset or rapid progression of retinopathy may occur in some patients with initiation of therapy.

The effect of less severe degrees of hyperglycemia on linear growth has been difficult to define. Children who are well-controlled on conventional therapy have a final adult height that appears to be normal and not significantly different from the calculated target[58,59] except when the onset of diabetes has been in the first five years of life.[60,61] On switching over to intensified therapy, some children who were thought to be growing normally on conventional therapy were found to register an acceleration in linear growth. Studies on identical twins who were discordant for IDDM have shown that adult height is reduced by an average of two inches if onset of diabetes was before puberty but not when onset was during or after puberty.[62] From these observations, it may be concluded that the metabolic derangements of diabetes have a negative impact on growth, the extent of which depends on the level of control and the age of onset, but well-controlled children can expect to attain a normal adult height.

There are multiple factors that could potentially affect growth in children with diabetes. These include:

- Lack of adequate insulin replacement.
- Inadequate insulin delivery to the liver despite peripheral hyperinsulinemia which happens even in the intensively treated patients. This results in reduced production and bioactivity of IGF-1. However, IGF-1 concentration in prepubertal and pubertal diabetic children has not been shown to correlate consistently with growth velocity.[63]
- Elevated levels of the catabolic stress hormones.
- Dietary inadequacy coupled with loss of calories in urine due to glycosuria.
- Psychosocial deprivation.
- Associated diseases: Hypothyroidism, celiac disease, eating disorders or chronic infections particularly tuberculosis. These must be considered and excluded in any child with poor growth or growth arrest.

Growth Hormone (GH), IGF-1 and Insulin Resistance during Puberty

With the onset of puberty, there is normally a spurt in GH secretion. This leads to a selective insulin resistance, restricted to insulin action on peripheral glucose utilization. In non-diabetic subjects, this acts as a stimulus for increased insulin release which in turn stimulates IGF-1 production by its action on the GH receptor in the liver and increases IGF-1 bioactivity by virtue of its inhibitory action on the IGF-1 binding protein, IGFBP-1.[64] IGF-1 which is partly responsible for the enhanced growth during pubertal years also regulates GH secretion by a negative feedback. In a diabetic on subcutaneous insulin, delivery of insulin to the liver is always deficient as insulin is absorbed from the subcutaneous space into the systemic circulation in contrast to direct portal delivery of endogenously produced insulin.[65] Thus, both the level as well as bioactivity of IGF-1 remains low. This could affect growth and it also results in markedly elevated levels of GH[66] in the absence of appropriate negative feedback, leading to insulin resistance. Some studies have shown that recombinant IGF-1 given at night may be effective in suppressing GH levels and may be a more physiological method of overcoming the dawn phenomenon.[67]

Even intensified insulin therapy with multidose insulin or with the external insulin pump does not normalize growth hormone level or IGFBP-1 level whereas direct infusion of insulin into the portal circulation has been shown to give the desired result.[65]

However, the bulk of data seems to indicate that IGF-1 concentrations in prepubertal and pubertal diabetic children do not predict growth velocity.[63]

Pubertal Changes in Diabetic Children

Poorly-controlled diabetic children have delayed bone age and hence delayed onset of puberty. Once menarche occurs poor control may be associated with irregular cycles or secondary amenorrhea.[68] Delayed puberty and irregular cycles are, however, not seen in well-controlled diabetes where the timing and sequence of appearance of secondary sex characteristics is normal.

Testosterone levels are normal in diabetic children at puberty but DHEAS levels are low suggesting a dissociation of pubarche and adrenarche[69] and levels of sex hormone binding globulin are also lower than in normal subjects resulting in higher levels of free testosterone. Girls with irregular cycles or prolonged periods of amenorrhoea have lower levels of sex hormone binding globulin, higher androstenedione and an elevated LH / FSH ratio.[68,70] They also have low levels of IGF-1 and higher levels of IGFBP-1. There is evidence that ovarian cells have IGF-1 receptors highlighting its importance in ovarian maturation and normal ovarian cycling. Girls with IDDM may have a higher incidence of polycystic ovarian change on pelvic ultrasound.[68]

DIABETES RELATED EMERGENCIES IN CHILDREN

Hypoglycemia

Hypoglycemia is the commonest and most feared acute complication of diabetes in children. Hypoglycemia may be classified as mild, moderate and severe.[71] *Mild hypoglycemia* refers to presence of neuroendocrine symptoms and signs[72,73] such as tremors, tachycardia, palpitations, sweating, pallor, abdominal pain and excessive hunger. The child is not confused or disoriented at this stage and if old enough, can take remedial steps on his own. These early symptoms may be absent (patients in tight glycemic control or patients with long standing diabetes and autonomic neuropathy), they may go unrecognized (in infants or during sleep) or treatment may be delayed (child engrossed in play, unavailability of sugar) in which case the child may progress to the next stage of *moderate hypoglycemia* when symptoms due to neuroglucopenia develop. These include headache, mood changes, irritability, altered behavior, decreased attentiveness and drowsiness. The patient is confused and disoriented, will frequently be uncooperative or belligerent and is in no position to help himself. If coma and/or convulsions follow, it is referred to as *severe hypoglycemia.*

Even without intervention, not all patients progress to the third stage. The counter-regulatory hormones particularly epinephrine lead to a rebound rise that may persist for several hours. This may be mistakenly interpreted as an indication for stepping-up insulin dose leading to the so called Somogyi phenomenon.

Causes and Prevention

Hypoglycemia can result from alterations in diet, exercise or insulin.

Eating late or eating less is common in children. Little children often refuse to eat meals on time using this ploy to bully their parents. The short-acting insulin analogs, lispro and aspart, are a boon for mothers with this predicament as they can be injected immediately after the child has eaten. The child may be detained at school or stranded in traffic and so miss his meal. To safeguard against this, school teachers must be suitably instructed and the child should always carry a snack (fruit or biscuits) in a hand bag when he is traveling. Manipulative behavior, food fads and eating disorders may be the causes of hypoglycemia especially in adolescents. During gastroenteritis or other illnesses with poor oral intake, if there is impending or mild hypoglycaemia, mini-dose glucagon (10 μg per year of age subcutaneously followed half an hour later by double the dose only if there is no response) has been shown to be effective and safe.[74]

Over exercising or exercising at unaccustomed times can lead to hypoglycemia not only during or shortly after exercise but in the case of prolonged aerobic activity, hypoglycemia may develop several hours later.[75] A common cause of hypoglycemic seizures in sleep is unplanned excessive physical activity during the evening. The following simple preventive measures must be enforced: (1) insulin should not be injected in the exercising limb if the exercise is to commence soon after injection, (2) an additional snack comprising 10 to 15 gm of complex carbohydrate must be consumed for every half hour of vigorous exercise or (3) if the exercise is planned well in advance, the insulin dose covering the exercise and post exercise period can be reduced by an arbitrary amount. This can be standardized for a given child by studying the pre-and post-exercise blood glucose levels on a few occasions, (4) following vigorous evening exercise, the patient should have 50% extra carbohydrate for the bedtime snack and monitor the bedtime as well as 3 am blood glucose and (5) if possible, exercise should be avoided at the time of peak insulin action.

Excess insulin administration on the part of the patient may be accidental due to reversal of doses of short-acting and intermediate-acting insulins; reversal of morning and evening doses; incorrect technique of measuring insulin or syringe-insulin mismatch. It may result from injection in lipohypertrophic areas or from attempts at achieving consistent euglycemia. It may be intentional[76] with suicidal intent or as an attention seeking measure. A hot water bath or sitting in a tub of hot water for 1 to 2 hours after injecting insulin can hasten the absorption and lead to hypoglycemia. In view of the small insulin requirement in children even one extra unit would amount to a very large percentage change in insulin dose.

Studies have shown a lower incidence of hypoglycemia with the short-acting insulin analogs because of better matching of insulin action and food absorption.[77] Similarly, use of insulin glargine as basal insulin has also been shown to result in reduced hypoglycemic episodes especially at night while giving improved glycemic control.[78,79]

Excess insulin administration on the part of the doctor could be due to switching to less antigenic insulins without dose reduction, attempting to fix the insulin dose during hospitalization, failure to anticipate the honeymoon phase, failure to detect hypothyroidism or Addison's disease or failure to identify the Somogyi phenomenon. Insulin doses fixed in hospital tend to be on the higher side in view of the higher level of stress and absence of physical activity.

Rigidly controlled children are more prone to hypoglycemia. Minor variations in rate of insulin absorption due to exercise, local heat, massage or random site rotation from one region to another, or a small variation in the percentage of bound and free insulin may trigger hypoglycemia.

Rigidly controlled patients are also more likely to experience severe hypoglycemia.[80] As the brain increases fractional extraction of glucose from plasma in adaptation to low normal blood glucose levels, the responses of sympathetic centers in the ventromedial hypothalamus to falling blood glucose are delayed and reduced (loss of hypoglycemia awareness). Another reason is the unavailability of ketones since hyperinsulinemia suppresses ketogenesis.

Recent studies have shown a significant and sustained reduction in rate of severe hypoglycemia with CSII without any deterioration in the level of glycemic control even in pre-school children and toddlers.[81,38]

Night-time hypoglycemia[82-84] often goes undetected. Autonomic symptoms may not be sufficient to awaken the child and hence severe hypoglycemia is commonest at night. Night-time hypoglycemia must be suspected in a child with a history of restless sleep, night sweats, nightmares, confusional states, seizure or enuresis or if the child wakes up experiencing lethargy, impaired thinking, altered mood or headaches. Family members must be instructed to be alert to unusual sounds or activity during patient's sleep. Night-time hypoglycemia must be suspected if the early morning blood glucose level is <60 mg /dl with ketonuria and if the 2 to 4 am glucose is <50 to 60 mg/dl. The incidence of night-time hypoglycemia can be reduced by avoiding aggressive pre-meal insulin supplement at bedtime, performing periodic 3 am blood glucose estimations to adjust overnight basal insulin dose and taking necessary precautions to prevent the delayed effect of prolonged exercise. Children with a bedtime blood glucose below 100 mg% are more likely to have nocturnal hypoglycemia[85] hence, they should take an extra snack at bedtime and recheck blood glucose at 3 am. Uncooked corn starch mixed with liquids or with solid foods or in the form of snack bars at bedtime has been shown to reduce risk of nocturnal hypoglycemia. Similarly, sugar containing high fat ice-creams too are effective as the protein and fat in the ice-cream ensures a slow release and absorption of sugar through the night. Alanine which stimulates glucagon release and terbutaline which raises epinephrine levels may have a role in hypoglycemia prevention.[86]

Treatment

Prompt action is a must when hypoglycemia is suspected. It is always better to confirm the clinical suspicion with a blood glucose test but this should not be an excuse to delay treatment. Mild symptoms responds to ingestion of 10 to 15 gms of carbohydrate given in the form of 2 to 3 teaspoons of sugar, 4 to 6 ounces of unsweetened fruit juice or carbonated drinks, or 1 tablespoon of honey. The response takes 10 to 15 minutes. If there is no response, then a second dose should be given. Chocolates and ice-creams should not be used as their fat content could retard absorption of available sugar and their regular use would contribute to obesity and to the temptation to feign hypoglycemia.

Children with moderate hypoglycemia would have to be coaxed to have any of the the oral agents listed above. Putting the child's hands around the cup and to guide the cup to the mouth reduces the chances of the drink being rejected. Alternatively glucagon can be used. Glucagon is given intramuscularly or deep subcutaneously in the deltoid region or the anterolateral thigh. The dose is 0.25 to 0.5 mg. in children below 5 years, 0.5 to 1.0 mg in children between 5 to 10 years and 1.0 mg in those above 10 years. The precise dose can be calculated as 10 to 20 µg/kg. The lower dose is nearly as effective and carries much less risk of inducing vomiting. Vomiting is common after glucagon but since it raises blood glucose for half an hour, the child need not eat immediately after coming around.

The comatose or convulsing patient must be given either glucagon or preferably intravenous dextrose. A bolus dose of 25% dextrose, 1 to 2 ml/kg body weight is given slowly over a few minutes followed by an infusion of 10% dextrose at 5 ml/kg/hour till the child can accept orally. Clinical improvement takes 10 to 15 minutes with the former and 1 to 5 minutes with the latter. Repeated doses will not hasten recovery unless blood glucose measurements show persistent hypoglycemia. If for some reason parenteral therapy is not possible in an unconscious or uncooperative child, glucose or sugar can be dissolved in a small amount of water to make a paste which can then be applied between the patient's cheek and gum.

Since the rise in blood glucose with oral or parenteral glucose is short-lived, the patient should eat a snack of complex carbohydrates (bread, cereal, milk) comprising approximately 10% of his daily calorie quota after initial treatment.

Certain points need to be stressed: (1) The child's diabetic state must not be kept a secret from school teachers, close friends and other significant persons with whom the child comes in contact, (2) these persons must be trained in recognition and first aid management of hypoglycemia, (3) the child must carry a diabetes identification card and 3 teaspoons of sugar on his person all the time.

Adverse Effects

Short-term effects: Mild hypoglycemia is chiefly of nuisance value. Moderate hypoglycemia interferes with normal thinking and can lead to accidents and injuries. It can make swimming or riding a bicycle hazardous. It can cause embarrassment because of uncontrolled behavior in public. After recovering from the physical symptoms, impaired cognitive function may persist for many more hours thus affecting school performance. Transient hemiparesis has been described but is rare and has a benign course.[87, 88] Severe hypoglycemia can culminate in a seizure but deaths due to hypoglycemia are exceptional. There is strong circumstantial evidence that the phenomenon of "dead in bed" referring to unexpected deaths occurring during sleep in patients with diabetes could be due to altered ventricular repolarization during hypoglycemia resulting in serious cardiac arrhythmia. Data from prepubertal subjects has shown that QTc prolongation can occur with fall in potassium and elevation of adrenaline during night-time hypoglycemia.[89-91]

Long-term effects: Severe hypoglycemia must be avoided at any cost in children particularly those below the age of five years as repeated or prolonged episodes can cause irreparable damage to the developing brain.[92] The brain of a young child has a very high glucose requirement for its metabolism and as a source of membrane lipids and protein synthesis. When glucose is unavailable, the brain normally uses ketone bodies as an alternative fuel. In a diabetic child, since hypoglycemia is due to hyperinsulinemia ketone production is suppressed. Deprived of both fuels, the cerebral structural substrates may be broken down to support brain metabolism at the expense of brain growth. The resultant brain damage may be overt or subtle. In one study, 80% of children with more than five episodes of severe hypoglycemia had EEG abnormalities.[93,94] Lower IQs have been correlated with recurrent severe hypoglycemia. Adolescents with diabetes have poorer performance on cognitive function testing, poorer verbal skills and reading ability especially if the onset of diabetes was before the age of five years.[95,96] Hypoglycemia associated with seizure activity is more likely to cause neurological dysfunction than if there is coma without seizure.[97] It is not known why some children develop a seizure while others with the same level of blood glucose do not. If a patient has had a hypoglycemic seizure his target levels of blood glucose need to be raised.

Recurrent hypoglycemia may cause hunger with overeating and resultant obesity. Frequent hypoglycemia have a deleterious effect on the morale of child and family members. Fear of hypoglycemia can lead to chronic overeating and deliberate underinsulinization.

Complications of Treatment

Glucagon often causes dose-related abdominal pain, nausea and vomiting. There is danger of aspiration with forced feeding of glucose solution in a comatose child. Giving an excess of intravenous glucose can rarely lead to hyperosmolar coma or may even cause sudden death due to abrupt rise in osmolarity.[98]

Diabetic Ketoacidosis

Diabetic ketoacidosis (DKA) is defined as severe uncontrolled diabetes requiring emergency treatment with intravenous fluids and insulin. It is characterized biochemically by blood glucose >250 mg%, serum ketones >3 mmol/L, serum bicarbonate <15 mEq/L and venous pH <7.3. Rarely, partially-treated patients may present with near-normal glucose values and this is referred to as "euglycemic ketoacidosis". The term "diabetic coma" is misleading as most patients with DKA are not unconscious. DKA is the commonest reason for hospitalization and the commonest diabetes-related cause of death in children with diabetes.[99]

Causes

DKA may be the initial presenting manifestation of diabetes in a new case. This occurs in 25 to 40% of cases because of a delay in diagnosis.

In a known diabetic, DKA may be due to:

- *Failure to administer insulin:* Insulin omission may be due to various reasons, e.g. it could be due to poverty, the patient being unable to afford insulin or the patient may have switched over to homeopathy, ayurveda or naturopathy. It could be an attention seeking measure, a manifestation of denial of diabetes or rebellion against it, an attempt at suicide or an occasional oversight as diabetes is pushed into the background of adolescent life. Insulin omission may be an attempt to lose weight and hence eating disorders or weight manipulation should be important considerations in an adolescent girl with DKA.
- *Stress in the form of infection, vomiting, nervous stress or trauma:* Failure to educate patients in management of "sick days" can be a serious lapse on the part of the medical team as this is a very important cause of DKA. A common sequence is infection, fever or anorexia, skipping of meals and unwise withholding of insulin.

Overeating *per se* never causes DKA. It can only lead to hyperglycemia.

High dose glucocorticoids, certain antipsychotics (olanzepine),[100] interferon alfa, diazoxide and salbutamol overdose (usually as infusion, rarely oral)[101] have all been reported to induce DKA in patients without previous diagnosis of type 1 diabetes. Certain inborn errors of metabolism (in particular, methylmalonicaciduria) may present with a metabolic emergency resembling DKA.[102]

Diagnosis

DKA must be suspected clinically in any child with the typical symptoms of hyperglycemia (polyuria, polydipsia, polyphagia, weakness and weight loss) who shows evidences of (1) dehydration, (2) rapid, deep breathing due to acidosis, (3) abdominal pain with distention and vomiting, (4) a peculiar fruity odor to the breath and (5) drowsiness or in some cases, coma. The diagnosis can be easily confirmed with bedside tests for blood glucose and urine acetone using strips and meters. This should not take more than a few minutes. Treatment must be started immediately on the basis of these results as the single most important factor that correlates with mortality in DKA is the duration of the process. While initiating treatment, blood and urine samples must be sent to the laboratory and an ECG should be obtained (see **Table 77.3**).

Treatment

When the patient presents in coma with obtunded airway reflexes, or has an ileus, certain emergency measures (endotracheal intubation, gastric decompression) may have to be instituted. Thereafter, the first priority is to replenish circulating blood volume with isotonic fluids.

Fluid replacement must be slow and cautious to avoid precipitating cerebral edema.[103-108]

The maintenance requirement is calculated as 1500 ml/m² irrespective of age or 100 ml/kg for the first 10 kg plus 50 ml/kg for next 10 kg, plus 20 ml/kg above 20 kg. This amount is given uniformly over 24 hours.

TABLE 77.3	Baseline investigations in a child with DKA

- Blood tests—CBC, glucose, ketones, electrolytes, pH, bicarbonate, gases, phosphate, BUN, creatinine, osmolarity, hemoglobin, culture
- Urine tests—Glucose, ketones, albumin, culture
- ECG for potassium status

The deficit in a typical case of DKA is 6 to 10% of body weight. The higher value of 10% applies only for children below the age of 2 years. A bolus of not more than 10 ml/kg must be given in the first hour and this amount may be repeated only if hypovolemic shock persists. The remaining deficit should be corrected slowly over 36 to 48 hours. An objective rule is that if the plasma osmolarity is >320 mOsmol/L, the deficit should be corrected over 36 hours and if it is >340 mOsm/L, the correction should be even slower, over 48 hours. If corrected serum sodium (calculated by adding 1.6 mEq/L to the observed value for every 100 mg/dl elevation of blood glucose above the level of 100 mg/dl) is in the hypernatremic range, rehydration should be further prolonged to 72 hours.

The ongoing losses which includes the urine output in the first five hours after starting treatment or till such time as glycosuria ceases, plus the volume of vomitus or gastric aspirate if any, can be ignored altogether.

For initial hydration, normal saline is used because an isotonic solution is necessary for replenishing the extra-cellular space and to ensure a gradual decline in plasma osmolarity thereby guarding against cerebral edema. After the initial 1 to 2 infusions, a switch to half-strength saline would serve to replenish free water but some consider it safer to continue normal saline for a longer period till blood glucose is below 250 mg/dl so as to allow osmotic equilibrium to be established more gradually. It is important to ensure that the corrected serum sodium rises as blood glucose level falls. The use of large amounts of 0.9% saline has also been associated with the development of hyperchloremic metabolic acidosis.[109] There is no data to support the use of colloids or of solutions more dilute than 0.45% saline in the management of childhood DKA. Because the severity of dehydration may be difficult to determine and can be overestimated, it is recommended that the amount of fluid infused per day should not exceed 1.5 to 2 times the usual daily requirement.

When blood glucose approaches 250 mg/dl, 5% dextrose should be added to the infusion and at 150 mg/dl, 10% dextrose is added so that the insulin infusion can be continued without risk of hypoglycemia till such time as the acidosis is corrected. Addition of carbohydrate is also necessary as a substrate for insulin action so that fatty acid breakdown can be halted. In those rare children who have severe vomiting and blood glucose below 250 mg/dl at presentation, the initial drip itself would have to incorporate 5% dextrose.

Potassium replacement: Total body potassium is considerably depleted in all cases of DKA even though initial serum level may be normal or at times high. Further, serum potassium always declines markedly with initiation of therapy as renal function improves leading to potassium loss in urine while correction of acidosis and action of insulin moves the ion intracellularly. For these reasons, potassium replacement must be started early, after the initial 20 ml/kg of intravenous fluids. When the initial serum potassium is below 3 mEq /L potassium must be given immediately irrespective of renal function, as insulin therapy may induce arrhythmias and respiratory muscle weakness. If the patient is hyperkalemic at presentation, giving potassium before starting insulin may increase extracellular potassium further and precipitate life threatening arrhythmias. The rate of administration of potassium should be 20 to 30 mEq/L of intravenous fluids. It should not exceed 40 to 60 meq /L or 0.5 mEq/kg body weight/hour. If a higher rate or concentration is necessary, a central venous line and continuous ECG monitoring are required. Alternatively, multiple intravenous lines can be employed to prevent local venous irritation. Additional potassium may also be given by nasogastric tube. Potassium should ideally be replaced partly (2/3rd) as potassium chloride and partly (1/3rd) as potassium phosphate to prevent hyperchloremic acidosis and at the same time supplement phosphate. Potassium replacement should continue throughout IV fluid therapy.

Potassium phosphate is not available in our country. Fortunately, in a child with adequate renal function hyperchloremic acidosis does not occur. Phosphate depletion in DKA leads to deficiency of 2,3-DPG in the red blood cells with shift of the oxygen dissociation curve to the left but this effect is offset by the effect of acidosis which shifts the curve to the right. Thus, phosphate replacement too is not mandatory, provided injudicious use of bicarbonate is avoided.

Bicarbonate replacement is given only in a few selected cases. Once treatment is started with insulin and intravenous fluids, the ketoacid and lactic acid molecules are metabolized in the liver to bicarbonate. Thus, routine provision of bicarbonate may over correct acidosis precipitating true alkalosis. There is also the danger of causing acute hypokalemia and hypernatremia if bicarbonate is routinely supplied. Rapid correction of acidosis with bicarbonate may unmask the effects of 2,3-DPG depletion. The most important danger of routine bicarbonate administration is that of precipitating paradoxical CNS acidosis. This happens because bicarbonate does not cross the blood-brain barrier whereas the carbon dioxide formed by its interaction with H^+ ions can cross over especially after correction of acidosis and hyperventilation so that carbon dioxide can no longer be washed-out. Use of bicarbonate should thus be restricted to only those emergency situations with symptomatic hyperkalemia or cardiovascular instability or if pH <7.0. If indicated, 40 to 80 mEq/m^2 of bicarbonate may be given as a slow infusion over two hours. If bicarbonate is given, care must be taken to monitor serum potassium and ECG, provide additional potassium (13 mEq for 100 mEq bicarbonate) and replace normal saline with 1/2 strength saline in view of the additional sodium load.

Insulin therapy: It can be withheld until initial fluid expansion (first 1 hour), to allow for potassium addition to the drip and to give a more realistic starting glucose level. Only short-acting insulin is used so that adjustments made produce relatively quick results. Low (physiological) dose insulin regimens are employed as it acts by inhibition of lipolysis and gluconeogenesis without stimulating peripheral uptake of glucose. The latter effect seen with high doses used in the past is both dangerous (because it can lead to hypoglycemia and hypokalemia) and unnecessary (since blood glucose would fall in any case because of renal excretion and also because body tissues can use nonglucose substrates such as ketones for their energy needs).

Continuous insulin infusion is the method of choice in an intensive care set-up. A loading dose of 0.1 µ/kg body weight may be given and a continuous infusion is set up to provide 0.1 µ/kg/hour by adding 50 units of plain insulin to 500 ml of normal saline (run off 50-60 ml in order to saturate insulin binding sites in the infusion tubing). If blood glucose does not show the expected fall of 50 to 100 mg%/hour, the infusion rate is doubled. When blood glucose falls to 150 mg% the infusion rate must be halved but it should not be discontinued till acidosis has been corrected (pH > 7.3, bicarbonate >15 mEq/L) which usually takes more time than correction of hyperglycemia. With correction of acidosis, the infusion of insulin is continued till the next major meal is due, when the patient is given subcutaneous regular insulin 0.5 units/kg at least 30 minutes before the meal and before stopping the insulin infusion.

Where facilities for intensive care are not available, hourly intramuscular insulin injections can be employed. An initial dose of 0.25 units/kg is followed by 0.1 unit/kg/hour till acidosis is corrected. In a severely dehydrated patient, it may be advisable to give half of the first dose intravenously. This method is simpler and it shares most of the advantages of the low dose infusion method. Steady blood levels are reached in 2 to 4 hours.

Oral feeding can be started as soon as the patient is conscious, has no vomiting or abdominal distension, has normal bowel sounds, and is willing if not eager to eat. Thus, most patients will start feeding within 4 to 12 hours of initiation of therapy. Start with clear liquids followed by soft solids and finally full diet with patient's appetite and tolerance being the best guides. Potassium supplementation by the oral route must be continued till the patient returns to the pre-illness weight, since replenishment of tissue glycogen and protein stores, which occurs as the patient enters the anabolic state, would draw a considerable amount of potassium from the blood stream.

Insulin in the post acidosis phase: It is advisable to start with a mixture of regular and intermediate-acting insulin in two daily doses as soon as possible. In the first few days, the insulin requirement may be as high as 1.5 to 2 units/kg/day but this soon declines. A newly diagnosed patient should be sent home after basic self care education without attempting to achieve perfect control because blood glucose levels will show considerable improvement over the next few days away from the stresses of the hospital environment and also with the setting in of the honeymoon phase. In a known diabetic who has developed ketoacidosis the cause should be ascertained (omission of insulin /incorrect sick day management) and addressed before discharge from hospital.

Complications

Careful clinical and laboratory monitoring is important till the ketoacidosis has been corrected (see **Table 77.4**). The complications that may occur in a child with DKA are largely due to therapeutic errors (see **Table 77.5**). *Cerebral edema* is the most serious and frequently fatal complication of DKA. The incidence of clinically significant cerebral edema is 2-3%.[110, 111] The therapeutic errors that can lead to it are summarized in **Table 77.5**.

TABLE 77.4	Monitoring in DKA	
Parameter	*Frequency of checking*
Heart rate, respiratory rate and blood pressure	Hourly
Fluid intake and output chart	Hourly
Capillary blood glucose, preferably lab venous glucose	Hourly
Serum electrolytes and (in severe cases) ECG	Every 1-2 hours initially then every 2-4 hours
Blood urea, hematocrit, blood gases	Every 2-4 hours
CNS evaluation for warning signs/symptoms of cerebral edema (headache, slowing of heart rate, restlessness, irritability, increasing drowsiness, recurrence of vomiting, cranial nerve palsies, papillary changes, rising blood pressure, decreased oxygen saturation)	Hourly or more frequent

TABLE 77.5	Iatrogenic complications during management of DKA (The numbers in brackets refer to the therapeutic errors causing the complications)	
Therapeutic Errors	*Complications*
1. Delay in providing potassium	Hypokalemia (1, 2, 3)
2. Injudicious use of bicarbonate	Tissue hypoxia, alkalosis, hypernatremia, hypokalemia, CNS acidosis (2)
3. High dose insulin	Hypoglycemia (3)
4. Use of hypotonic solutions/too rapid hydration	Cerebral edema (2, 3, 4, 5)
5. Delay in starting IV infusion	Shock, intravascular thrombosis (5)
6. Nonprovision of phosphate ?	RBC 2,3-DPG deficiency (6)
7. Provision of excess phosphate	Hypocalcemic tetany (7)
8. Provision of excess chloride	Hyperchloremic acidosis (8)
9. Over treatment with potassium	Hyperkalemia (9)

There is evidence to support an association between severity of acidosis, greater hypocapnia and elevated serum urea nitrogen at diagnosis and the occurrence of cerebral edema. Further, a failure of serum sodium to rise as glucose concentration falls during therapy of DKA is more likely to be associated with the development of cerebral edema. This complication must be suspected in any child with sudden neurological deterioration after initial favorable response to treatment. It usually develops 4 to 12 hours after starting treatment. A close watch should be kept for the early signs of impending cerebral edema.[112] These are decreasing sensorium, severe headache, vomiting, disoriented or agitational behavior, deterioration in any of the vital signs (temperature, slowing pulse rate, respiration or increasing blood pressure), incontinence, pupillary changes, papilledema or a seizure. At the earliest sign, the rate of fluid administration should be reduced and supportive treatment, mannitol (0.25-1.0 gm/kg over 20 minutes to be repeated after 2 hours if necessary) and possibly dexamethasone should be given. Hypertonic (3%) saline, 5 to 10 ml/kg over 30 minutes may be an alternative to mannitol.[113] Symptomatic cerebral edema carries a high mortality. Early detection and prompt treatment has been shown to prevent death or neurological damage in 50% of cases. Mild, asymptomatic cerebral edema is perhaps present in all children with DKA.

Rhinocerebral mucormycosis : It must be suspected in any child who during or after treatment for DKA develops hemorrhagic lesions in the buccal mucosa with black, necrotic eschar on the palate or turbinate, a black necrotic discharge from the sinuses, proptosis, signs of cerebritis and cranial nerve palsies with fever. Early diagnosis is essential for successful treatment. A KOH preparation of the necrotic material will show nonseptate hyphae consistent with a diagnosis of mucor. Aggressive surgical debridement, amphotericin-B, good diabetes control and in some cases hyperbaric oxygen are the keys to successful treatment. Blindness, cranial nerve palsies and hemiparesis are common residues in survivors.

Other complications reported include intracranial thrombosis, aspiration pneumonia, adult respiratory distress syndrome, pneumomediastinum, and rhabdomyolysis. Hypothalamopituitary insufficiency (with growth hormone and/or TSH deficiency) have been reported as late sequelae.[114]

Prevention of DKA at presentation is possible only if a greater awareness of the symptoms of childhood diabetes is created amongst pediatricians, family physicians and the lay public so that the diagnosis is made at an early stage. A school and physician awareness campaign was shown to reduce the rates of DKA from 78% to nil over a six year period.[115]

In a known diabetic, the medical team must ensure that the patient does not omit insulin (intentionally or for lack of finance) and that all patients are given appropriate instructions on managing diabetes on sick days (see **Table 77.6**). Patient counseling and intensive education in self-management alongwith financial assistance in selected cases should be part of the management program. A 24-hour diabetes telephone help line[116] and adult supervision of insulin administration[117] have been shown to reduce the occurrence of DKA. The value of home measurement of beta-hydroxybutyrate for earlier diagnosis of DKA needs to be assessed. In patients on CSII, the occurrence of DKA can be reduced by instructing patients on keeping vials/pens of short-acting insulin for prompt administration in case of mechanical pump failure.

Recurrent DKA

Psychosocial rather than biomedical/physiological factors account for most cases of recurrent ketoacidosis. About 20% of pediatric patients account for 80% of all admissions for DKA.[118] Recurrent DKA is commoner in girls in the early teenage years. It is rare in the first two years after diagnosis and in adulthood. A younger age at onset of diabetes and pre-existing psychopathology before diabetes onset increase the risk. Families low in warmth and support, high levels of unresolved family conflict and lack of parental involvement in the diabetes care of the adolescent are all contributory factors.[119] The following steps would go a long way in preventing this tragic complication: (1) provide patients an opportunity to talk about their feelings and mental conflicts with a psychologist who should be a part of the diabetes management team, (2) hand over autonomy to the adolescent very gradually, only at their request and under ongoing parental supervision, (3) encourage constant regular touch between patient and the medical team, (4) help arrange for financial support in the case of needy patients and (5) most importantly, provide continuing ongoing diabetes education.[120]

Hyperglycemic nonketotic hypertonicity (HNKH) in children: This term is preferred to "hyperglycemic, hyperosmolar nonketotic coma" as coma occurs in less than 10% of cases. It is rare in children and only a handful of cases have been reported. It is distinguished from DKA

TABLE 77.6	Sick day guidelines

- Usual insulin doses must be continued even though appetite may be poor, unless blood glucose is <80 mg/dl, in which case omit regular insulin and reduce intermediate-acting by 20%
- Blood glucose and urine acetone must be checked in every 2-4 hours

  If blood glucose is >250 mg%, a supplemental dose of regular insulin must be taken immediately

Blood glucose	Urine acetone	Extra regular insulin (percentage of total dose taken on routine days)
>250 mg/dl	Absent or trace	10%
>250 mg/dl	Moderate or large	20%
>400 mg/dl	Absent or present	20%
<250 mg/dl	Absent or present	nil

- If it is not possible to eat the usual meals, plenty of liquids must be consumed in small and frequent sips : salty liquids when blood glucose is >250 mg% (e.g. milk without sugar, veg and non-veg soups, kanji and buttermilk) and sweet liquids when blood glucose is <100 mg% (milk with sugar, fruit juices, ice-cream, etc.).
- Hospitalization necessary if >2 supplemental doses of insulin are required, there are >2 vomits or in case of breathlessness or drowsiness

primarily by the lack of ketoacidosis. One proposed mechanism to explain this entity is the differential sensitivity of lipid and carbohydrate metabolism to the effects of insulin. Patients who develop HNKH have enough insulin to suppress lipolysis but not to promote glucose utilization. Therapy is similar to that for DKA with certain exceptions like boluses of insulin are not indicated, a switch to half-strength saline is made early, immediately after the first bolus of normal saline has established adequate tissue perfusion so as to correct the hypernatremia and the possibility of precipitating infections in particular pneumonia and urinary infections need to be considered more strongly.

PATIENT EDUCATION

Diabetes is the only chronic childhood disease in which the patient and the family members have to play the key role in day-to-day management. Patient education is thus a crucial aspect of the management plan. All patients must be taught:

- Procedures: Insulin injection technique including site rotation, home blood glucose testing, urine testing for glucose and acetone and glucagon administration.
- Prevention: Early recognition and first-aid management of the diabetes-related emergencies like hypoglycemia and ketoacidosis.
- Principles of meal planning and exercise planning and how these can be integrated into the child's lifestyle.
- Interpretation of home monitoring records for adjustments in the therapeutic regimen.
- For those opting for intensified management, the use of pre-meal insulin supplements, details of carbohydrate counting and (when indicated) details of operating the insulin pump and trouble shooting.

Education reduces the patient's dependence on doctors and brings down the cost of treatment besides the convenience it provides to the patient. It also gives the patient a sense of control over his disease. The level of education and consequently the therapeutic goals would have to vary from patient-to-patient depending on their capabilities and their desire to learn.

In the pre-adolescent, the management responsibility rests chiefly with the parents. Both parents must receive thorough and ongoing education. Little children should be made to help the parents initially by collecting the insulin syringe and vials in preparation for the injection, later they can learn how to mix insulin and they can help to keep a tab on site rotation. By 8 to 10 years, self injection under supervision should be encouraged. Children can also be taught to identify and report the early symptoms of hypoglycemia and they should know what they must do at such times. They should be aware that missing a meal can be dangerous and that extra snacks have to be taken before and after excessive physical activity. They can be taught which foods are best avoided, which can be taken freely and which can be had in measured amounts (i.e. the concept of forbidden, restricted and free foods).

The adolescent on the other hand, must learn all aspects of management but the parents too must be given equal attention as they would have to guide and supervise the adolescent at home. Adolescents can be actively involved in teaching of the parents as this approach gives a boost to their morale.

Skills acquired by the patient will invariably reduce with time and after initial interest patients tend to drift. Hence, periodic reinforcement of education is a must.

The medical team must interact with and train the patient's local pediatrician or physician to whom the patient may have to turn for guidance from time-to-time.

PSYCHOSOCIAL ASPECTS

The topic has been dealt with in detail in chapter 82 and problems in adolescent in Chapter 78.

Informing the School Authorities

Many schools are reluctant to accept a child with diabetes. This is due to misconceptions about childhood diabetes and a fear of the unknown. The usual concerns are that diabetes may be contagious, it would hamper the child's academic ability, the child would be very irregular in school, the child would not be able to participate in sports and the child would need special attention and care which the teachers would not be capable of rendering.

The school authorities must be sent a formal note incorporating relevant informations about childhood diabetes. It must be emphasized that besides taking daily injections, testing blood glucose, observing strict meal timings and certain precautions before and after physical activity the child with diabetes is no different from any other child in the school. It must be stressed that diabetes is not contagious and that it will not affect the academic performance or school attendance in a well controlled child. Teachers must be urged to make the child feel *normal* by treating him as they would treat any other child.

At the same time, it must be stated that teachers would have certain responsibilities to fulfill towards the child. They must be urged to ensure that meals are not missed or delayed and that the child takes his pre-exercise snack. They must encourage the child to participate in all sports activities but maintain strict supervision during swimming. They must allow time off for performing diabetic chores in an inconspicuous manner so as not to embarrass the child. They should be able to recognize the early symptoms of hypogly-cemia and provide first aid management for the same. Teachers must also be advised to look for and report to the parents any signs of poor diabetes control they may observe in the child such as excessive thirst or excessive urination or any emotional disturbance in the child. The contact numbers of members of the diabetes management team must be provided so that the school authorities can get in touch with them in case they have any unanswered queries or in an emergency.

Camps for Diabetic Children

Diabetic children with their families must be encouraged to attend holiday-cum-educational camps. The aim of these residential camps in our country has been to bring together the children, their family members and the entire medical team in a holiday atmosphere for reinforcement of education and counseling.[121] Some of the grown up childhood diabetics with their families must also attend and serve as role models for the newer cases. The camps are best conducted over a period of 3 to 4 days during the winter vacations at a holiday resort. Winter is the season when the weather is pleasant and water supply is less of a problem at holiday destinations in our country.

Camp activities should include:

Formal patient education: By means of lectures and demonstrations. Special sessions in small groups must be conducted for those whose learning abilities are known to be suboptimal.

Informal education: Educational games and competitions that not only reinforce education but also give the medical team a chance to assess how much of the formal education has been imbibed.

Learn as you perform under supervision sessions: Children take their insulin shots and test their blood glucose and urine acetone under supervision of the medical staff. This helps in perfecting techniques.

Opening out sessions: Separate sessions must be conducted for the parents, for children of different age groups and for adolescents in which they are encouraged to speak out their difficulties, their fears and views. Their misconceptions, if any, must be set to rest.

Sex education classes for adolescent: Must be arranged during the camp.

Games and entertainment programs to be presented by children: They can display their talents and help the parents to realize that there is more to their child than just his diabetes.

Camp exhibition in which all diabetes related paraphernalia are displayed and their role and method of use has been explained.

Research can be conducted at the camp as a large number of children are present at one time in one place. A fundus examination, blood pressure check and urinary microalbuminuria microbial testing must be done at the camp.

Awards can be presented to children in various age groups for best techniques, best blood glucose results, best performance in the camp quiz contest and so on to introduce an element of competitiveness.

Parents can sit together during the camp and discuss how they would like to work together to help their children, e.g. in obtaining employment.

Planned strenuous physical activities have not been a feature of camps in India as it is in the West. This is because of constraint of time and space. To partly compensate for this, adventure hikes and other sporting activities can be organized periodically for the older children to give them the confidence that no physical activity is beyond them and also to teach them how to manage their diabetes in such situations. Day camps are gaining popularity in Western countries because they are more economical and convenient, less time consuming and easier to plan and conduct. These should become a routine practice in small centers in our country which may not be able to organize full-fledged residential camps.

REFERENCES

1. Ivarsson A, Marner B, Lernmark A, et al. Nonislet pancreatic autoantibodies in sibship with permanent neonatal insulin-dependent diabetes mellitus. Diabetes. 1988;37:347-50.
2. Green A, Gale EAM, Patterson CC. Incidence of childhood-onset insulin dependent diabetes mellitus : the EURODIABACE study. Lancet. 1992;339:905-9.
3. Laporte RE, Tuomilehto J. The DiaMond project. Practical Diabetes Int. 1995;12:93.
4. WHO Diamond Project Group on Epidemics. Child diabetes, epidemics and epidemiology: an approach for controlling diabetes. Am J Epidemiol. 1992;135:803-16.
5. Bodansky HJ, Staines A, Stephenson C, et al. Evidence for an environmental effect in the etiology of insulin-dependent diabetes in a transmigratory population. Br Med J. 1992;304: 1020-2.
6. Symon DN, Hennessy ER, Small PJ. Smoked food in the diets of mothers of diabetic children. Lancet. 1984;2:514.
7. Dahlquist GG, Blom LG, Persson L, et al. Dietary factors and the risk of developing insulin-dependent diabetes in childhood. Br Med J. 1990;300:1302-6.
8. Pozilli P, Bottazzo GF. Coffee or sugar: which is to blame in IDDM ? Diabetes Care.1991;14:144-5.
9. Ellis TM, Atkinson MA. Early infant diets and insulin-dependent diabetes. Lancet. 1996;347:1464-5.
10. Gimeno SGA, Desouza JMP. IDDM and milk consumption. Diabetes Care. 1997;20:1256-60.
11. Dahlquist GG, Patterson C, Soltesz G. Perinatal risk factors for childhood Type 1 diabetes in Europe: The EURODIAB substudy 2 study group. Diabetes Care. 1999;22:1698-702.
12. The EURODIAB TIGER study group: recent trends in the incidence of Type 1 diabetes in European children. Diabetologia 1998;41(1):A21.
13. Atkinson MA, Maclaren NK. The pathogenesis of insulin-dependent diabetes mellitus. N Engl J Med. 1994;331:1428-36.
14. Speiling MA. Aspects of etiology, prediction and prevention of insulin-dependent diabetes mellitus in childhood. Pediatr Clin North Am. 1997;44:269-84.
15. Faas S, Trucco M. The genes influencing the susceptibility to IDDM in humans. J Endocrinol Invest. 1994;17:477-95.
16. Hyoty H, Hiltunen M, Knip M, et al. A prospective study of the role of coxsackie B and other enterovirus infections in the pathogenesis of IDDM. Diabetes; 1995. pp. 652-7.
17. Ramchandran A, Snehalata C, Satyavani K, et al. Type 2 diabetes in Asian-Indian urban children. Diabetes Care. 2003;26(4):1022-5.
18. Bhatia V. Recommendations: IAP task force for childhood prevention of adult diseases; Insulin resistance and type 2 diabetes mellitus in childhood. Ind Pediatr. 2004;41:443-57.
19. American Diabetes Association. Type 2 diabetes in children and adolescents. Diabetes care. 2000;23:381-9.
20. Tait KF, Marshall T, Carr-Smith J, et al. Clustering of autoimmune disease in parents of siblings from the Type 1 diabetes. Warren repository. Diab Med. 2004;21:358.
21. Velho G, Froguel P. Genetic, metabolic and clinical characteristics of maturity onset diabetes of the young. Eur J Endocrinol. 1998;138:233-9.
22. Batch JA, Werther GA. Unusual diabetes and diabetes in the context of other disorders. In Christopher J.H. Kelnar (Ed): Childhood and Adolescent Diabetes, Chapman and Hall Medical, London; 1994. pp. 397-417.
23. Spitz L, Bhargava R, Grant D, et al. Surgical treat of hyper-insulinemic hypoglycaemia in infancy and childhood. Arch Dis Child. 1992;67:201-5.
24. Weimerskirch D, Klein DJ. Recurrence of insulin-dependent diabetes mellitus after transient neonatal diabetes : a report of two cases. J Pediatr. 1993;122:598-600.
25. Shield JP, Baum JD. Is transient neonatal diabetes a risk factor for diabetes in later life? Lancet. 1993;341:693.
26. Russell-Eggitt IM, Clayton PT, Coffey R, et al. Alstrom syndrome. Report of 22 cases and literature review. Ophthalmology. 1998;105:1274-80.
27. Najjar SS, Saikaly MG, Zaytoun GM, et al. Association of diabetes insipidus, diabetes mellitus, optic atrophy and deafness: the Wolfram or DIDMOAD syndrome. Arch Dis Child. 1985;60:823-8.
28. Barrett TG, Bundey SE, MacLeod AF. Neurodegeneration and diabetes : UK nationwide study of Wolfram (DIDMOAD) syndrome. Lancet. 1995;346:1458-63.
29. DeSanctis V, Zurlo M, Senesi E, et al. Insulin- dependent diabetes in thalassemia. Arch Dis Child. 1988;63:58-62.
30. Bougnereo PF, Landais P, Boisson C, et al. Limited duration of remission of insulin-dependencies in children with recent onset type 1 diabetes treated with low dose cyclosporin. Diabetes. 1990;30:1264-72.

31. Steffes M, Tamborlane W, Becker D, et al. The effect of intensive diabetes treatment on residual B-cell function in the diabetes control and complications trial. Diabetes. 1996;45(2):18A.

32. Shah SC, Malone JI, Simpson NE. A randomized trial of intensive insulin therapy in newly diagnosed insulin-dependent diabetes mellitus. N Eng J Med. 1989;320: 550-4.

33. American Diabetes Association. Implications of the diabetes control and complications trial. Diabetes Care. 1993;16:1517-20.

34. Danne T, Deiss D, Hopfenmuller W, et al. Experience with insulin analogues in children. Hoerm Res. 2002;57(1):46-53.

35. Mohn A, Dunger DB, Chiarelli F. The potential role of insulin analogues in the treatment of children and adolescents with Type 1 diabetes mellitus. Diab Nutr Metab. 2001;14:349-57.

36. Danne T, Lyypke K, Walte K, et al. Insulin detemir is characterized by a consistent pharmacokinetic profile across age-groups in children, adolescents, and adults with type 1 diabetes. Diabetes Care. 2003;26:3087-92.

37. Boland EA, Grey M, Oesterle A, Fredrickson L, Tamborlane WV. Continuous subcutaneous insulin infusion: a new way to lower risk of severe hypoglycaemia, improve metabolic control, and enhance coping in adolescents with type 1 diabetes. Diabetes care. 1999;22:1179-84.

38. Litton J, Rice A, Friedman N, et al. Insulin pump therapy in toddlers and preschool children with type 1 diabetes mellitus. J Pediatr. 2002;141:490-5.

39. Willi SM, Planton J, Egede L, Schwarz S. Benefits of continuous subcutaneous insulin infusion in children with Type 1 diabetes. J Pediatr. 2003;143:796-801.

40. Saravis S, Schachar R, Zlotkin S, et al. Aspartame: effects on learning, behavior, and mood. Pediatrics. 1990;86:75-83.

41. Kostraba JN, Dorman JS, Orchard TJ, et al. Contribution of diabetes duration before puberty to the development of microvascular complications in IDDM subjects. Diabetes Care. 1989;12:686-93.

42. Donaghue KC, Fung ATW, Hing S, et al. The effect of prepubertal diabetes duration in diabetes microvascular complications in early and late adolescence. Diabetes Care. 1997;20:77.

43. Yosipovitch G, Loh KC, Hock OB. Medical pearl: scleroderma-like skin changes in patients with diabetes mellitus. J Am Acad. Dermatol. 2003;48:109-11.

44. Infante JR, Rosenbloom AL, Silverstein JH, et al. Changes in frequency and severity of limited joint mobility in children with type 1 diabetes mellitus between 1976-78 and 1998. J Pediatr. 2001:138:33-7.

45. Sochett E, Daneman D. Early diabetes-related complications in children and adolescents with type 1 diabetes: implications for screening and intervention. Endocrinol Metab Clin North Am. 1999;28:865-82.

46. ISPAD consensus guidelines 2000. Vascular complications; 2000. pp. 95-101.

47. Colquhoun AJ, Nicholson KG, Botha JL. Effectiveness of influenza vaccine in reducing hospital admissions in people with diabetes. Epidemiol and Infection; 1997. pp. 335-4.

48. Chiarelli F, Mohn A, Tumini S, et al. Screening for vascular complications in children and adolescents with type 1 diabetes mellitus. Horm Res. 2002;57(1):113-6.

49. DeFronzo RA. Diabetic nephropathy: etiologic and therapeutic considerations. Diabetes reviews. 1995;3:510-50.

50. Connors MH, Dunger DB, Chapel H, et al. Diminished thyroxine-binding globulin in pubertal diabetic children. Diabetes Care.1996;19:246-8.

51. Betterle C, Volpato M, Rees Smith B, Furmaniak J, Chen S, Zanchetta R, et al.II. Adrenal cortex and steroid 21-hydroxylase autoantibodies in children with organ-specific autoimmune diseases: markers of high progression to clinical Addison's disease. J Clin Endocrinol Metab.1997;82:939-42.

52. Peterson P, Salmi H, Hyoty H, Miettinen A, Ilonen J, Reijonen H, et al. Steroid 21-hydroxylase autoantibodies in insulin-dependent diabetes mellitus. Childhood diabetes in Finland (DiMe) study group. Clin Immunol Immunopathol. 1997;82:37-42.

53. Perros P, Singh RK, Ludlam CA, Frier BM. Prevalence of pernicious anemia in patients with type 1 diabetes mellitus and autoimmune thyroid disease. Diabet Med. 2000;17:749-51.

54. De Block CE, De Leeuw IH, Decochez K, Winnock F, Van Autreve J, Van Campenhout CM, et al. The presence of thyrogastric antibodies in first degree relatives of type 1 diabetic patients is associated with age and proband antibody status. J Clin Endocrinol Metab. 2001;86:4358-63.

55. Roldan MB, Barrio R, Roy G, Parra C, Alonso M, Yturriaga R, et al. Diagnostic value of serological markers for celiac disease in diabetic children and adolescents. J Pediatr Endocrinol Metab. 1998;11:751-6.

56. Toscano V, Conti FG, Anastasi E, Mariani P, Tiberti C, Poggi M, et al. Importance of gluten in the induction of endocrine autoantibodies and organ dysfunction in adolescent celiac patients. Am JGastroenterol. 1999;117:297-303.

57. Massarano AA, Smith CP. Mauriac syndrome in childhood diabetes. Practical Diabetes International. 1995;12:88-9.

58. Jackson KL. Growth and maturation of children with insulin-dependent diabetes mellitus. Pediatr Clin North Am. 1984;31:545-67.

59. Salardi S, Tonioli S, Tassoni P, et al. Growth and growth factors in diabetes mellitus. Arch Dis Child. 1987;62:57-62.

60. Brown M, Ahmed ML, Clayton KL, et al. Growth during childhood and final height in type 1 diabetes. Diabetic Med. 1994;11:182-7.

61. Wise JE, Kolb EL, Sauder SE. Effect of glycemic control on growth velocity in children with IDDM. Diabetes Care.1992;15:826-30.

62. Tattersall RB, Pyke DA. Growth in diabetic children: studies in identical twins. Lancet. 1973;2:1105.

63. Matthew H. Connors. Growth in the diabetic child, Pediatr Clin North Am. 1997;44:301-6.

64. Hilding A, Brismar K, Degerblad M, et al. Altered relation between circulating levels of insulin-like growth factor-binding protein-1 and insulin in growth hormone deficient patients and insulin-dependent diabetic patients compared to that in healthy subjects. J Clin Endocrinol Metab. 1995;80:2646-52.

65. Shisko PI, Kovaler PA, Goncharov VG, et al. Comparison of peripheral and portal (via the umbilical vein) route of insulin infusion in IDDM patients. Diabetes.1992;41:1042-9.

66. Pal BR, Matthews DR, Edge JA, et al. The frequency and amplitude of growth hormone secretory episodes as determined by deconvolution analysis are increased in adolescents with insulin-dependent diabetes mellitus and are unaffected by short-term euglycemia. Clin Endocrin. 1992;38:93-100.

67. Dunger DB, Cheetham TD, Crowne EC. Insulin-like growth factors (IGFs) and IGF-1 treatment in the adolescent with insulin-dependent diabetes mellitus. Metabol Clin Exper. 1995;44(4):119-23.

68. Adcock C, Perry LA, Lindsell DRM, et al. Menstrual irregularities are more common in adolescents with type 1 diabetes:association with poor glycemic control and weight gain. Diabetic Med. 1994;11:465-70.

69. Cohen HN, Paterson KR, Wallace AM, et al. Dissociation of adrenarche and gonadarche in diabetes mellitus. Clin Endocrin. 1984;20:717-24.

70. Holly JMP, Dunger DB, Edge JA, et al. Sex hormone binding globulin levels in adolescents with insulin- dependent diabetes mellitus. Diab Med. 1992b;7:371-4.

71. Bergada I, Suissa S, Dufresne J, et al. Severe hypoglycaemia in IDDM children. Diabetes Care. 1989;12:239-44.

72. Macfarlane PI, Walters M, Stutchfield P, et al. A prospective study of symptomatic hypoglycaemia in childhood diabetes. Diabetic Med. 1989;6:627-30.

73. McCrimmon RJ, Gold AE, Deary IJ, et al. Symptoms of hypoglycaemia in children with insulin-dependent diabetes mellitus (IDDM). Diabetologia. 1994;37(1):A165.

74. Haymond MW, Schreiner B. Mini-dose glucagons rescue for hypoglycaemia in children with type 1 diabetes. Diabetes Care. 2001;24:643-5.

75. MacDonald MJ. Post exercise late-onset hypoglycaemia in insulin-dependent diabetic patients. Diabetes Care. 1987;10:584-8.

76. Grunberger G, Weiner JL, Silverman R, et al. Factitious hypoglycaemia due to surreptitious administration of insulin. Ann Int Med. 1988;108:252-7.

77. Holleman F, Schmitt H, Rottiers R, et al. Reduced frequency of severe hypoglycaemia coma in well controlled IDDM patients treated with insulin lispro. Diabetes Care. 1997;20:1827-32.

78. Chase PH, Dixon B, Pearson J, et al. Reduced hypoglycemic episodes and improved glycemic control in children with type 1 diabetes using insulin glargine and neutral protamine hagedorn insulin. J Pediatr. 2003;143:737-40.

79. Schober E, Schoenle E, van Dyk J, et al. The pediatric study group of insulin glargine. Comparitive trial between insulin glargine and NPH insulin in children and adolescents with type 1 diabetes mellitus. J Pediatr Endocrinol Metab. 2002; 15:369-76.

80. Pramming S, Thorsteinsson B, Bendtson I, et al. Symptomatic hypoglycaemia in 411 type 1 diabetic patients. Diabetic Med. 1991;8:217-22.

81. Bode BW, Steed RD, Davidson PC. Reduction in severe hypoglycaemia with long-term continuous subcutaneous insulin infusion in type 1 diabetes. Diabetes Care. 1996;19:324-7.

82. Shalwitz RA, Farkus-Hirsch R, White NH, et al. Prevalence and consequences of nocturnal hypoglycaemia among conventionally-treated children with diabetes mellitus. J Pediatr. 1990;116:685-9.

83. Kaufman FR, Austin J, Neinstein A, et al. Nocturnal hypoglycaemia detected with the continuous glucose monitoring system in pediatric patients with Type 1 diabetes. J Pediatr. 2002;141:625-30.

84. Beregszaszi M, Tubiana-Rufi N, Benali K, et al. Nocturnal hypoglycaemia in children and adolescents with insulin-dependent diabetes mellitus: prevalence and risk factors. J Pediatr. 1997;131:27-33.

85. Whincup G, Milner RDG. Prediction and management of nocturnal hypoglycaemia in diabetics. Arch Dis Child. 1987;62:333-7.

86. Saleh TY, Cryer PE. Alanine and terbutaline in the prevention of nocturnal hypoglycaemia in IDDM. Diabetes Care. 1997; 20:1231-36.

87. Wayne EA, Dean HJ, Booth F, et al. Focal neurological deficits associated with hypoglycaemia in children with diabetes. J Pediatr. 1990;117:575-7.

88. Pocecco M, Ronfani L. Transient focal neurologic deficits associated with hypoglycaemia in children with insulin-dependent diabetes mellitus. Italian Collaborative Pediatric Diabetologic Group. Acta Pediatr. 1998;87:524-44.

89. Sovik O, Thordarson H. Dead-in-bed syndrome in young diabetic patients. Diabetes Care. 1999;22 (suppl 2):B40-2.

90. Marques JLB, George E, Peacey SR, Harris ND, Macdonald IA, Cochrane T, Heller SR. Altered ventricular repolarisation during hypoglycaemia in patients with diabetes. Diab Med. 1997;14:648-54.

91. Suys BE, Huybrechts S, De Wolf D, et al. QTc interval prolongation and QTc dispersion in children and adolescents with type 1 diabetes. J Pediatr. 2002;141:59-63.

92. Puczynski SS, Puczynski MS, Reich S, et al. Mental efficiency and hypoglycaemia. Develop and Behav Pediatr. 1990;11:170-4.

93. Eeg-Olofsson O. Hypoglycaemia and neurological disturbances in children with diabetes mellitus. Acta Paed. Scand. 1977;270(1):91-6.

94. Soltesz G, Acsadi G. Association between diabetes, severe hypoglycaemia and electroencephalographic abnormalities. Arch Dis Child. 1989;64:992-6.

95. Ryan C, Vega A, Drash A. Cognitive deficits in adolescents who developed diabetes early in life. Pediatrics. 1985;75:921-7.

96. Ryan CM, Atchinson J, Puczynski SS, et al. Mild hypoglycaemia associated with deterioration of mental efficiency in children with insulin-dependent diabetes mellitus. J Pediatr. 1990;117:32-8.

97. Kaufman FR, Epport K, Halvorson M. Neurocognitive functioning in children diagnosed with diabetes before age 10 years. Diabetes. 1997;46:67A.

98. Shah A, Stanhope R, Matthew D. Hazards of pharmacological tests of growth hormone secretion in childhood. Brit Med J 1992;304:173-4.

99. White NH, Henry DN. Special issues in diabetes management In Haire-Joshu D (Ed): management of diabetes mellitus; perspectives of care across the life span. Mosby Year Book; 1996. pp. 342-404.

100. Selva KA, Scott SM. Diabetic ketoacidosis associatedwith olanzepine in an adolescent patient. J Pediatr. 2001;138: 936-8.

101. Habib GS, Saliba WR, Cohen L. DKA associated with oral salbutamol overdose. Am J Med. 2002;113:701-2.

102. Ciani F, Donati MA, Tulli G. Lethal late onset cblB methylmalonic aciduria. Crit Care Med. 2002;28:2119-21.

103. Rosenbloom AL, Hanas R. Diabetic ketoacidosis (DKA): treatment guidelines. Clin Pediatr. 1996;35:261-6.

104. Harris GD, Fiordalisi I. Physiologic management of diabetic ketoacidemia. A 5-year prospective pediatric experience in 232 episodes. Arch Pediatr Adolesc Med. 1994;148:1046-52.

105. Harris GD, Fiordalisi I, Harris WL, et al. Minimizing the risk of brain herniation during treatment of diabetic ketoacidemia: a retrospective and prospective study. J Pediatr. 1990;117:22-31.

106. Roberts KB. Fluid mangement of children who have diabetic ketoacidosis. Pediatr Rev. 1995;16:304-5.

107. Edge JA, Dunger DB. Variations in the management of diabetic ketoacidosis in children. Diabet Med. 1994;11:984-6.

108. Dunger DB, Sperling MA, Acerini CL, et al. European Society for Pediatric Endocrinology/Lawson Wilkins Pediatric Endocrine Society Consensus Statement on Diabetic Keto-acidosis in Children and Adolescents. Pediatrics. 2004;113:133-40.

109. Oh MS, Carroll HJ, Uribarri J. Mechanism of normochloremic and hyperchloremic acidosis in diabetic ketoacidosis. Nephron. 1990;54:1-6.

110. Plotnick L. Insulin-dependent diabetes mellitus. Pediatr Rev. 1994;15:137-50.

111. Rosenbloom AL, Schatz DA. Diabetic ketoacidosis in childhood. Pediatr Ann. 1994;23:284-8.

112. Rosenbloom AL. Intracerebral crises during treatment of diabetic ketoacidosis. Diabetes Care. 1990;13:22-33.

113. Kamat P, Vats A, Gross M, et al. Use of hypertonic saline for the treatment of altered mental status associated with diabetic ketoacidosis. Pediatr Crit Care Med. 2003;4:239-42.

114. Dunlop KA, Woodman D, Carson DJ. Hypopituitarism following cerebral oedema with diabetic ketoacidosis. Arch Dis Child. 2002;87:337-8.

115. Vanelli M, Chiari G, Ghizzoni L, et al. Effectiveness of a prevention program for diabetic ketoacidosis in children. An 8-year study in schools and private practices. Diabetes Care. 1999;22:7-9.

116. Hoffman WH, O'Neill P, Khoury C, et al. Service and education for the insulin-dependent child. Diabetes Care. 1978;1:285-8.

117. Golden MP, Herrold AJ, Orr DP. An approach to prevention of recurrent diabetic ketoacidosis in the pediatric population. J. Pediatr. 1985;107:195-200.

118. Chas Skinner T. Recurrent diabetic ketoacidosis: causes, prevention and management. Hormone Research. 2002;57(1): 78-80.

119. Tattersall RB. Brittle diabetes revisited: the third Arnold Bloom Memorial Lecture. Diab Med. 1997;14:99-110.

120. Weissberg-Benchel J, Wirtz P, Glasgow AM, Turek J, Tynan WD, Ward J. Adolescent diabetes management and mismanagement. Diabetes Care. 1995;18:77-82.

121. Irani AJ, Dalal DG, Ajgaonkar VS. Camps for diabetic children. JAPI. 1995;1:54-7.

Chapter 78

DIABETES IN ADOLESCENTS AND YOUNG ADULTS

PG Raman, N Sudha, V Mohan

CHAPTER OUTLINE

- Introduction
- Types of Diabetes Seen in the Young
- Type 1 Diabetes
- Type 2 Diabetes in Young
- Maturity Onset Diabetes of Young

- Fibrocalculous Pancreatic Diabetes
- Malnutrition Modulated Diabetes Mellitus
- Diabetes Secondary to Endocrine Disorders
- Genetic Syndromes and Diabetes
- Polycystic Ovarian Syndrome
- Summary

INTRODUCTION

Diabetes in the young in India and other developing countries presents a diagnostic challenge to the physician, as several types of diabetes may be seen at younger age groups as shown in **Figure 78.1**. In a study of young diabetic patients (age at onset below 30 years) seen at a diabetes center in south India, some years ago it was seen that 57.7% had type 2 diabetes, 22% type 1 diabetes mellitus, 5% gestational diabetes mellitus (GDM), 4% fibrocalculous pancreatic diabetes (FCPD), and 1% malnutrition modulated diabetes mellitus (MMDM) or protein deficient diabetes mellitus (PDDM).[1] The corresponding figures from a clinic in north India were as follows: type 1 diabetes 36%, MMDM 32%, type 2 in young 13%, FCPD 11%, and autoimmune polyglandular syndrome (APS) 8%[2] **(Figure 78.2)**. In this chapter, different clinicopathological types of diabetes in the young will be discussed along with certain issues like psychosocial aspects, effect of puberty on glycemic control, physical activity, and dietary pattern. As the child with diabetes is often

deprived of the normal pleasures and carefree existence that is associated with this phase of life, emotional and psychological problems are inevitable. These have to be dealt with in addition to the clinical profile and management of diabetes.

TYPES OF DIABETES SEEN IN THE YOUNG

In western countries, till recently, the majority of diabetes in the young was type 1 diabetes while more recently increasing incidence of patients with type 2 diabetes is being reported. In India and other developing countries, diabetes in the young presents a fascinating spectrum, as there are so many forms of diabetes presenting at younger age groups as listed in below:

- Type 1 diabetes
  - Immune mediated
  - Nonimmune mediated (Idiopathic)
- Type 2 diabetes in the young
- Maturity onset diabetes of young (MODY)
- Fibrocalculous pancreatic diabetes (FCPD)

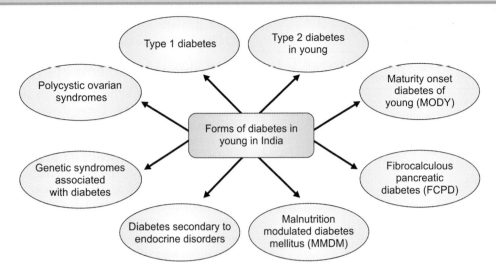

Figure 78.1   Forms of diabetes in young in India

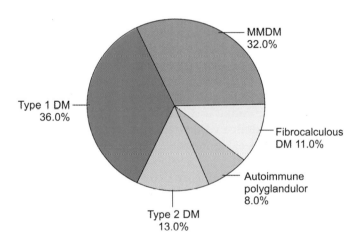

Figure 78.2   Distribution of clinical types among young onset diabetes in Northern India

- Malnutrition modulated diabetes mellitus (MMDM)
- Diabetes secondary to endocrine disorders
- Genetic syndromes associated with diabetes
- Polycystic ovarian syndrome (PCOS).

TYPE 1 DIABETES

This type of diabetes, formerly called insulin dependent diabetes mellitus (IDDM) results from total destruction of beta cells of the pancreas.[3] It is of two types: immune mediated and nonimmune or idiopathic. It is the most common form of diabetes in children and young adults in western countries. Its incidence is highest in Scandinavian countries, such as Finland (49/100,000 patient years) and lowest common in Japan (1/100,000 patient years). In India, the frequency is reported to be 10.5/100,000 patient years.[4]

Etiopathogenesis

The pathogenesis of immune mediated type 1 diabetes can be considered under different stages of the disease, such as genetic predisposition, environmental triggers, initiation of autoimmunity, prediabetic period, and finally, overt diabetes. This is considered in greater detail in Chapters 16 and 24, and hence, only a brief overview is given below. The genetics of type 1 diabetes is complex and almost 20 loci are believed to be involved. The most important of these is the histocompatibility (HLA) region, especially the DQ alleles.[5-8] The association of HLA-DR and HLA-DQ with type 1 is shown in **Table 78.1**.[7,9] Environmental triggers include viral infections (mumps, rubella, coxsackie-B and

TABLE 78.1	HLA-DR and HLA-DQ and the risk for type 1 diabetes mellitus[7,9]	
Risk	*Genotypes*	
Susceptible	DR3	DQA1 0301
	DR4	DQA 0501
	DR1	DQB1 0210
		DQB1 0302
Resistant	DR2	
	DR5	
	DQB1 0602	
	DQB1 0301	

TABLE 78.2	Prevalence of GAD antibodies in immune type 1 diabetes mellitus	
S.No.	Subject Group	Frequency of autoantibodies (%)
1.	Healthy controls	0.3–0.6
2.	First degree relatives of type 1 diabetes mellitus	3–4
3.	Patient with autoimmune endocrine disorders	1–2
4.	Patients with type 1 diabetes mellitus	55–85

cytomegalovirus), diet (milk proteins), drugs and toxins. Autoimmunity plays an important role and is related to specific T-cell cytotoxic responses against islet antigens. The prediabetic period is characterized by the presence of T-cell abnormalities and autoantibodies against islet cell antigens, which include cytoplasmic islet cell antibodies, insulin autoantibodies, antibodies against glutamic acid decarboxylase (GAD), and tyrosine phosphatase. Prevalence of GAD autoantibodies in immune type 1 diabetes is shown in **Table 78.2.** Finally, in the stage of overt diabetes, beta cell function rapidly declines and insulin dependent diabetes sets in.

Clinical Features

The peak age of onset of type 1 diabetes is around 11 years in females and 18 years in males. The clinical features of type 1 diabetes include polyuria, polydipsia, polyphagia, weight loss, fatigue, blurred vision, pyogenic skin infections and genital candidial infections. Between 10 and 30% of diabetic children may present with diabetic ketoacidosis at diagnosis.[10]

Puberty and Type 1 Diabetes Mellitus

The enhanced growth hormone secretion accounts for the decreased insulin sensitivity observed during normal puberty, as well as the deterioration in glycemic control occurring at this time. Dysregulation of growth hormone-IGF axis is well documented in type 1 diabetes mellitus. The main disturbance includes increased growth hormone secretion, paradoxically associated with decreased serum IGF-1 levels, which leads to impaired growth at puberty. Children who are well controlled have a final adult height that appears to be normal and not significantly different from the calculated target [11,12] except when the onset of diabetes has been is the first 5 years of life.[13,14] However, normal linear growth in type 1 prepubertal diabetes can be achieved with good control of diabetes.[15]

Psychological Problems in Type 1 Diabetes

Adolescents with type 1 diabetes are at high risk of psychiatric disorders. These disorders can occur at the time of diagnosis and include denial, anger, guilt, depression, and finally, acceptance. Fear of hypoglycemia, apprehension of complications and anxiety induced sexual dysfunction usually appear later. The emotional turmoil associated with the physical and psychosocial changes during adolescence plays a major role in deteriorating diabetes control at this stage. With psychological and social support and good diabetes education, fear of diabetes and its complications can be removed.[16] Impairment of cognitive function and hence learning problems are sometimes seen in children with diabetes.[17] Poor control of diabetes in early years is often associated with pre-existing behavior disorders.

The attitude of the parents towards the child has an important bearing on the child's psychosocial development. Some parents become over protective and, at the other extreme, there are a few parents who look upon the child as a burden and neglect the child. Over pampering can make it difficult for the child to attain social independence while negligence can lead to poor control of diabetes. Hence, the child not only needs good care from their parents but also concern and affection. Education and counseling on diabetes plays a major role in shaping the patient.

Social Problems

For adolescents, peer influences together with family support and supervision, play an important role in ensuring adherence to treatment and achieving good glycemic control. In adults, diabetes often complicates their marriages, their ability to cope with family and career pressures and often add to the financial burden due to costs of treatment. Parents must be cautioned against concealing their disease when marriage is being finalized as the consequences can be quite grave. All the pros and cons must be explained to the family of the proposed life partner, for which the medical team would also have to play an important role. Such a marriage is more likely to be successful. In case, a diabetic gets married to another diabetic, the chances of the offspring developing diabetes should be explained to both.

During pregnancy, the diabetes control tends to worsen due to release of counter-regulatory hormones and this could lead to aggravation of microvascular and macrovascular complications. Strict monitoring and good glycemic control is a must during pregnancy to prevent fetal and maternal complications.

The employment prospects of type 1 diabetic patients are better today than ever before. They can function well in managerial jobs as well as those requiring manual labor. However, a diabetic individual on insulin should not be assigned a job considered hazardous to himself or others, such as driving a vehicle or working at heights. Good education and vocational training can help in securing suitable jobs for patients with type 1 diabetes.

Management

The management of type 1 diabetes mellitus comprises of life long insulin, diet, exercise, and diabetes education.

Popular insulin regimens include:
1. Premixed insulin (30/70) BD doses and
2. Regular + NPH insulin BD doses
3. Multiple injection regimens (e.g. regular –regular – regular + NPH at night) are used in cases where good control cannot be achieved with BD regimes.

The diet therapy involves adherence to recommended total caloric intake based on body weight. The caloric distribution could be 55 to 60% carbohydrate, 25 to 30% fat and 15% protein. Daily caloric requirements is divided to provide 20% at breakfast, 30% at lunch, 25% at dinner (or vice versa), and the rest divided to midmorning early, evening (tea time) and bedtime snacks. Occasional allowances are permissible for special occasions.

The prevention of diabetic ketoacidosis is a must by educating type 1 diabetic patients to adhere to sick day rules to follow correct insulin dosage and taking adequate care of infections. During illness, insulin should not be skipped but short-acting insulin in small frequent doses should be taken. Urine should be checked for ketones. All type 1 diabetic patients should receive comprehensive self-management education, including self-monitoring of blood glucose (SMBG), recognition and management of hypoglycemia and lifestyle changes.

Prognosis

Compared to earlier times, survival of type 1 diabetic patients for 50 years or more is now feasible with good control of diabetes. When compared to nondiabetic subjects, the life span of type 1 diabetic individual is, however, reduced on an average by 10 to 15 years. Aggressive treatment with tight diabetes control can help in preventing the long-term complications of diabetes.

Prevention of Type 1 Diabetes Mellitus

Several trials have been done in prevention of type 1 diabetes mellitus, including the European Nicotinamide Diabetes Intervention Trial (ENDIT) and the Diabetes Prevention Trial (DPT) of North America. Vaccine strategies have also been tried for prevention of type 1 diabetes mellitus including BCG/Q fever vaccine. However, none of these have given conclusive evidence to justify their routine use in prevention of type 1 diabetes.

TYPE 2 DIABETES IN YOUNG

Prevalence

Until recently, type 1 diabetes was the only type of diabetes considered to be prevalent among children and adolescents, as very few have type 2 while other forms of diabetes are even more rare.

Recent data, however, indicate that the incidence and prevalence of type 2 diabetes in young is increasing world wide.[18] Type 2 is increasingly being reported in children from USA, Canada, Japan, Hong Kong, Australia, New Zealand, Libya, and Bangladesh.[19] In Pima Indians, a population known to have highest prevalence of diabetes, the prevalence rates of type 2 diabetes was 22.3 per 1000 in the 10 to 14 years age group and 50.9 per 1000 in 15 to 19 years of age group.[18,20-22] Clinic based studies from Chennai have been reported on type 2 diabetes in the young in India,[2,23] although its prevalence is still relatively low.

Etiopathogenesis

The emerging epidemic of type 2 diabetes mellitus among youth parallels the increasing prevalence of obesity in children and youth.[18,24-29] However, the prevalence of obesity in young Indian type 2 diabetic subjects has been found to be lower than that in Europeans.[2,24,30] Family history of diabetes has been found to be strongly associated with type 2 diabetes in young. Some studies estimate that 45 to 80% patients with type 2 diabetes in young have at least one parent with diabetes and 74 to 100% have first or second degree relative with type 2 diabetes.[25] Up to 62% of offspring of two diabetic parents in south India have been shown to have abnormal glucose tolerance.[31] Pima Indians

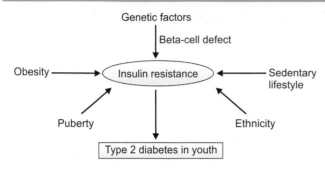

Figure 78.3 Factors associated with insulin resistance in type 2 diabetes mellitus in children. *(Adapted from* Reference 2)

show a "U" shaped relationship between birth-weight and the subsequent development of diabetes, with the lowest birth weight group (<2.5 kg) demonstrating a risk similar to that of the group with the highest birth weight.[32] Indeed, *in utero* fetal undernutrition has been found to be the strongest single risk factor for development of type 2 diabetes in Pima Indians. Fetal undernutrition leads to poor beta cell development, reduced insulin sensitivity, reduced insulin secretion, and increased insulin resistance.

Although the precise mechanisms responsible for the development of type 2 diabetes in children and adolescent are poorly understood, the initial abnormality is impaired insulin secretion, compounded with insulin resistance and more severe beta cell failure in course of time. Other risk factors like race, obesity, puberty and gender are associated with type 2 diabetes in young and predispose to the condition because of the augmentation of insulin resistance[33] **(Figure 78.3)**.

Among Asian Indians, there is evidence for increased insulin resistance and significantly higher insulin levels have also been reported in Asian Indians in UK.[34] During puberty, there is increased resistance to the action of insulin, resulting in hyperinsulinemia[35] and this can predispose to diabetes.

Lifestyle factors related in particular to excessive caloric intake and fat rich foods and sedentary behavior are often ingrained in the lifestyle of the child and family with type 2 diabetes, predisposing to earlier onset of diabetes in these families.

Screening Criteria

The screening criteria includes those who have BMI >85% for age and sex, weight or >120% of ideal body weight plus any two of the following risk factors:
  i. Family history of type 2 diabetes mellitus in first or second degree relatives.

  ii. Race and ethnicity (Asian Indian, American Indian, African Americans, Hispanic Americans).
 iii. Signs of insulin resistance or conditions associated with insulin resistance (acanthosis nigricans, hypertension, dyslipidemia and polycystic ovarian syndrome).

Clinical Features

The mean age of diagnosis is usually between 12 and 16 years, i.e. around puberty[35] with a higher frequency among females.[18,22,36] The clinical features distinguishing type 2 diabetes and type 1 diabetes are shown in **Table 78.3**. Type 2 diabetes is to be suspected, if the patient belongs to a race with high prevalence of type 2 diabetes, and is tuberal, obese; has acanthosis nigricans; has almost invariably a positive family history of type 2 diabetes. Elevated blood glucose is detected by routine screening procedures. The spectrum of disease at presentation may range from asymptomatic hyperglycemia to very rarely diabetic ketoacidosis (DKA) or hyperglycemic hyperosmolar state (HHS). Obesity is the hallmark of type 2 diabetes and a large majority of affected children are either obese or overweight at diagnosis.[18] Acanthosis nigricans, a cutaneous finding characterized by velvety hyperpigmented patches, typically seen at the base of neck, in the axilla and anogenital area is present in as many as 80 to 90% of children with type 2 diabetes. Other features include hirsutism, sleep apnea syndrome, polycystic ovarian syndrome, hypertension and dyslipidemia. **Figure 78.4** shows differential diagnosis of diabetes in youth in India.

Management

Diet and exercise plays a major role in the management of type 2 diabetes. Numerous cultural and socioeconomic barriers interfere with the implementation of dietary changes in youth with diabetes. Hence, dietary recommendations should be culturally appropriate and sensitive to family resources.

Increasing physical activity is an important component of the treatment plan, as it decreases the insulin resistance and helps in weight reduction. Ideally, the exercise should be done daily for about 30 to 40 minutes and the type of exercise should be customized for each patient. Metformin is currently recommended as the first oral agent to be used in obese young type 2 diabetic patients.[18,37] Other drugs are not yet approved, although several are undergoing clinical trials. A treatment algorithm is shown in **Figure 78.5**. The ultimate goal is to reduce risk of acute and chronic

TABLE 78.3	Differences between type 1 and type 2 diabetes
Type 1 diabetes	*Type 2 diabetes*
Majority are not overweight	Up to 85% may be overweight
Recurrent history of weight loss, polyuria, polydypsia	Mild—no weight loss
Acute onset	Insidious onset
30-40% have diabetic ketoacidosis	5-25% have mild ketosis at onset
Honeymoon (remission) seen frequently	Remission less common
Needs insulin for survival after remission hypoglycemic agents	Insulin is not needed for survival; Respond to oral
5% have first degree or second degree relatives with diabetes	45-80% have family history of diabetes mellitus
No acanthosis nigricans	80-90% show acanthosis nigricans
Immune markers, such as GAD, IA2, IA2B	85-98% no immune markers seen
Strong HLA association, endogenous C-peptide/ insulin levels low and no increase after oral or IV glucose administration	No HLA association C-peptide/insulin level normal or high and glucose stimulation increase the response
Associated with other autoimmune disorders of thyroid, adrenal vitiligo, pernicious anemia, prone to celiac disease	Not associated with autoimmune disorders

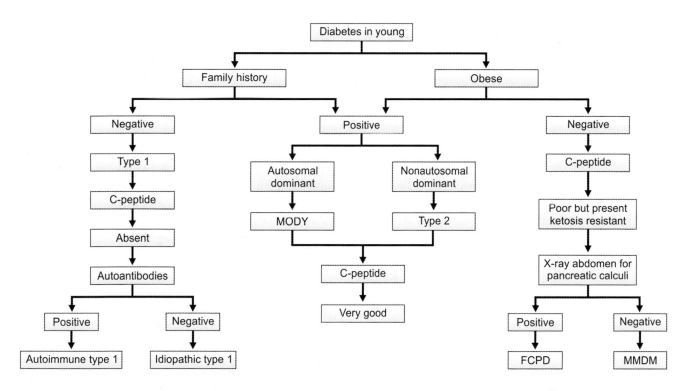

Figure 78.4 Differential diagnosis of diabetes in youth in India (Mohan et al[38])

complications associated with diabetes. Besides normalization of blood glucose, successful control of associated comorbidities, such as hypertension and hyperlipidemia is also important.

Prevention

The frequent association of type 2 diabetes with sedentary lifestyle and excessive caloric intake suggests that the condition may be prevented or delayed, if

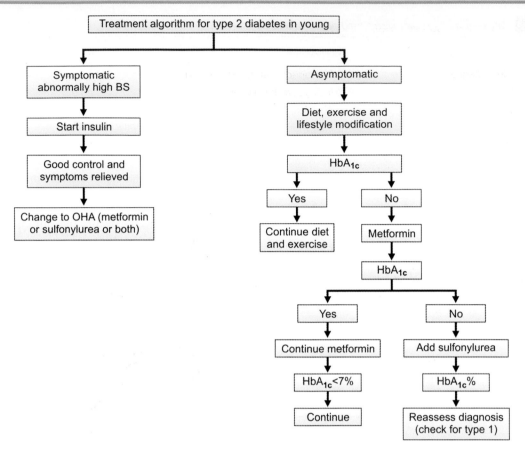

Figure 78.5 Treatment algorithm in type 2 diabetes mellitus in young

lifestyle changes, such as increasing physical activity and modifying diet are implemented in individuals at risk[38,39] particularly in those with a strong family history of diabetes.

MATURITY ONSET DIABETES OF YOUNG (MODY)

The term "MODY" was first introduced by Tattersal and Fajans[40] in their classic report, published in 1975 to denote a unique noninsulin dependent from of juvenile onset diabetes.

Autosomal dominant inheritance, including vertical transmission of diabetes through at least three generations is an important diagnostic criteria for MODY. This topic is discussed in greater detail in chapter 25 and hence only a brief review is given here.

Pathogenesis

The pathogenesis of MODY differs from type 2 diabetes in that it is monogenetic in origin and insulin secretory defects are more important than insulin resistance in

several forms of MODY. Patients with MODY show reduced secretion of insulin in response to a glucose load. Mohan et al[41] performed simultaneous studies of insulin and C-peptide responses to glucose load in subjects with MODY and matched groups of control (nondiabetic subjects). It was found that C-peptide responses to glucose load were lower in MODY, thereby providing evidence for decreased beta cell function. Individuals with this disorder have severely impaired insulin secretion but no evidence of pancreatic islet cell autoimmunity. Fajans et al[42] also reported that the insulin response declines with increasing duration of diabetes.

MODY has to be distinguished from another subgroup of type 2 diabetes called 'Early Onset NIDDM' (type 2 diabetes) described by Tripathy and Kar from India[72] and O'Rahilly et al.[43] **Table 78.4** shows the distinguishing features between the two types.

Clinical Features of Subtypes of MODY
Glucokinase (MODY 2)

Patients with glucokinase mutations have a unique phenotype with modest fasting hyperglycemia, which

TABLE 78.4	Differences between MODY and type 2 diabetes mellitus		
S.No.	Features	MODY	Type 2 DM
1.	Mode of inheritance	Monogenic; autosomal dominant	Polygenic
2.	Age at onset	<25 years by definition	Variable
3.	Penetrance	80-95%	Variable 10-40%
4.	Body habitus	Nonobese	Obese
5.	Metabolic syndrome	Usually absent	Usually present

is often present from very young age, but there is very little increase in glycemia with age.

Transcription Factor MODY (MODY 1, MODY 3 and MODY 5)

In contrast to glucokinase deficient MODY, patients with transcription factor mutations (HNF-1α, HNF-4α, HNF-1β and IPF1) have a normal fasting glucose level in childhood but develop progressive hyperglycemia in adolescence and early adulthood.

Since MODY is an important classical genetic model for study of etiology of type 2 form of diabetes, identification of many more MODY genes can be anticipated. The management of MODY is similar to that of type 2 diabetes.

FIBROCALCULOUS PANCREATIC DIABETES

Fibrocalculous pancreatic diabetes (FCPD) is a form of diabetes secondary to nonalcoholic chronic pancreatopathy of uncertain etiology, predominantly seen in tropical developing countries. Chapter 32 discusses FCPD in greater detail and, hence, only a brief outline is provided here. In the recent classification of diabetes of American Diabetes Association, FCPD has been reclassified as a secondary form of diabetes under "Diseases of exocrine pancreas."[44] This has also been ratified by the World Health Organization Consultation Group.[45] Various terms had been used for this condition but currently the term "Tropical calcific pancreatitis" (TCP) is used in gastroenterology to denote the prediabetic stage of FCPD or Pre-FCPD[46,47] and fibrocalculous pancreatic diabetes (FCPD) to denote the diabetes secondary to TCP more appropriately fibrocalculous pancreatopathy.

Several reports have confirmed the widespread occurrence of this syndrome in developing countries of the world, mostly located in the tropical zone. In India, FCPD has been described by several workers in Kerala,[48-50] Orissa,[51-53] Karnataka,[54] Tamil Nadu,[55-57] Nagpur,[58] Pune,[59] Tripura,[60] and other places in India.[61] In the clinical presentation of FCPD, majority of patients are lean, but cases with gross malnutrition are becoming uncommon. Most of the patients are aged between 10 and 30 years, when diagnosis is made, but FCPD may occur in infancy,[62] childhood[63] and the elderly.[64] The four cardinal features include abdominal pain, pancreatic calculi, steatorrhea and diabetes. One of the characteristic clinical features is that, despite requiring insulin for control, patients rarely become ketotic on withdrawal of insulin.[65] This is attributed to the partial preservation of beta cell function as shown by C-peptide studies.[66-68]

The etiopathogenetic mechanisms of FCPD still remain unclear. The hypotheses that have been proposed include cassava hypothesis, familial and genetic factors, oxidative stress and micronutrient deficiency, and these are discussed in detail in Chapter 32.

Regarding the management of FCPD, the principles of diet and exercise are the same as for the other types of diabetes except that a more liberal caloric and protein intake is advised because of the associated undernutrition. Although patients may initially respond to oral drugs, majority of patients sooner, rather later, need insulin for control of diabetes.

MALNUTRITION MODULATED DIABETES MELLITUS

At the International Workshop on Diabetes in the Tropics, held at Cuttack in October 1995, the term "malnutrition modulated diabetes mellitus (MMDM)" was coined to replace the earlier term protein-deficient diabetes mellitus (PDDM) to described a unique form of diabetes associated with undernutrition but absence of pancreatic pathology.[69,70]

The clinical association of diabetes associated with malnutrition was first described at Cuttack by Tripathy and colleagues[71,72] who can truly be considered to be the pioneers in this field. Large number of cases have subsequently been reported from Calcutta, Delhi, Chennai, Agra, Jhansi, Lucknow, Hyderabad and Nagpur and several other developing countries.[73] This condition is most fully described in Chapter 31 and, hence, only a brief review is given here.

Patients present with emaciation, asthenia, extreme weakness, paresthesias, superficial skin infection and dehydration. Most patients present between 12 and 20 years of age and are usually distinguished by extreme leanness. Body mass index is often less than 16 kg/m^2. Marks of malnutrition, such as skin and hair change, parotid enlargement, xerosis and angular stomatitis are seen in about 25% of the patients. The excellent scoring system for diagnosis of this condition by Tripathy and colleagues has nearly helped to diagnose this condition without any ambiguity. Family history of diabetes is present in only 5% of Cuttack cases, whereas it is 20% at Dhaka[74] [Bangladesh]. Pancreatic islet cell antibodies tested positive is 37.5% of these patients compared to 66% in type 1 and 25% in type 2 diabetic patients.[75,76] Basal insulin and C-peptide levels in MMDM were distinctly below normal but substantially above those seen in type 1 patients. Minute doses of intravenous insulin raised human growth hormone to a very high level compared to normals and any other class of diabetes with low BMI.[75] Absence of pancreatic calcification is essential for the diagnosis of MMDM, which is characterized by both insulinopenia and insulin resistance. The management of this type of diabetes includes high caloric diet (50-60 Kcal/kg) and the diet should liberal in carbohydrates and problem for restoration of energy and gain in weight. Insulin often in high doses is the mainstay of treatment.

DIABETES SECONDARY TO ENDOCRINE DISORDERS

The term "secondary diabetes" is defined as "any situation with diabetes, impaired glucose tolerance or hyperglycemia where a distinct pathology for the insulin secretory defect or resistance can be demonstrated unlike is case of classical type 1 or type 2 diabetes".

These include diabetes secondary to chronic pancreatitis, fibrocalculous pancreatopathy diabetes, surgical pancreatectomy, drug-induced diabetes,[77-79] various endocrine disorders associated with obesity and insulin resistance. However, in this section, we will

discuss only about the secondary diabetes due to endocrine disorders.

Various endocrine disorders like acromegaly (excess growth hormone),[80] gigantism, Cushing's syndrome (excess cortisol),[81] pheochromocytoma (adrenal medullary tumors),[82] glucagonoma syndrome (a cell tumor)[83] are associated with peripheral insulin resistance and glucose intolerance leading to secondary diabetes.

The clinical and laboratory evidence of autoimmunity or presence of other endocrine diseases will help us diagnose diabetes secondary to these disorders. Both basal and dynamic hormone testing are indicated whenever an endocrine syndrome is considered. In the management of secondary diabetes, curable conditions deserve appropriate treatment, whereas incurable genetic syndromes can only await the future prospects of gene therapy.

GENETIC SYNDROMES AND DIABETES

Diabetes mellitus is associated with over 100 well defined rare genetic syndromes but in total probably account for <1% of all cases of diabetes. Some of these are associated with abnormal insulin.[84,85] This can be classified as follows:

1. Genetic disorders affecting the pancreas: Hereditary, hemochromatosis, cystic fibrosis.
2. Inborn errors of metabolism: Roger's syndrome, alpha-1-antitrypsin deficiency.
3. Genetic syndromes associated with obesity and diabetes: Prader-Willi syndrome, Bardet-Biedl syndrome, Alstrom's syndrome.
4. Genetic syndromes associated with lipodystrophy: Leprechaunism,[86,87] Seip-Berardinelli syndrome.[88]
5. Cytogenetic disorders: Down's syndrome, Turner's syndrome and Klinefelter's syndrome.
6. Mitochondrial syndromes: MELAS syndrome, Ballviger-Wallace syndrome.

POLYCYSTIC OVARIAN SYNDROME

Polycystic ovary syndrome affects 5 to 10% of all premenopausal women and young girls. It is associated with obesity, hyperinsulinemia, hirsutism, acanthosis nigricans chronic anovulation and hyperandrogenism. Anovulatory women with PCOS have higher leutinizing hormone levels, compared to normal. If the patient is overweight, screening with oral glucose tolerance test should be performed, since more than 25% of obese women with PCOS will develop impaired glucose tolerance or overt diabetes by the age of 30 years.

SUMMARY

As already mentioned, the presence of various types of childhood diabetes, such as type 1 (immune and nonimmune), type 2 diabetes, MODY, FCPD, MMDM, secondary diabetes, genetic syndrome and PCOS presents a great diagnostic challenge to physicians in India. Epidemiologic evidence suggests that there is an emerging epidemic of type 2 diabetes in young, which presents a serious public health problem. The full effect of this epidemic will be felt, as these young diabetic individuals become adults and develop the long-term complications of diabetes. Health care providers must understand the implications of this and rise to the occasion to ensure the future health of young population. Preventive measures, such as lifestyle modification and routine screening for diabetes, particularly in those at high risk, are to be instituted early to stress the epidemic of type 2 diabetes in the young.

REFERENCES

1. Ramachandran A, Mohan V, Snehalatha C, et al. Clinical features of diabetes in the young as seen at a diabetes centre in South India. Diabetes Research and Clinical Practice. 1988;4:117-25.
2. Kochupillai N, Goswami R. Youth onset diabetes in India. Nature of diabetes and use of bovine insulin in their treatment. In Ahuja MM, Tripathy BB, Moses SGP, Chandalia HB (Eds): RSSDI Textbook of Diabetes Mellitus; 2002. pp. 255-8.
3. Atkinson MA, Maclaren NK. The pathogenesis of insulin dependent diabetes. N Engl J Med. 1994;331:1428-36.
4. Ramachandran A, Snehalatha C, Krishnaswamy CV, Madras IDDM Registry Group. Incidence of IDDM in children in urban population in Southern India. Diab Res Clin Pact. 1996;34:79-82.
5. Srikanta S, Ahuja MMS, Malaviya AN, Mehra NK, Vaidya MC. Type 1 diabetes mellitus in North India: HLA and autoimmunity. N Engl J Med. 1981;304:1175-6.
6. Srikanta S, Malaviya AN, Mehra NK, Vaidya MC, Geevargese PJ, Ahuja MMS. Autoimmunity in Type 1 diabetes. J Clin Immunol. 1981;1:169-73.
7. Bhatia E, Mehra NK, Taneja V, Vaidya MC, Ahuja MMS. HLA DR antigen frequencies in a north Indian type 1 diabetic population. Diabetes. 1985;8:565-7.
8. Bhatia E, Mehra NK, Malaviya AN, Ahuja MMS. HLA and autoimmunity in north Indian type 1 diabetic multiplex families. Horm Metabol Res. 1986;18:331-4.
9. The Diabetes Control and Complications Trial Research Group. The effect of intensive treatment of diabetes on the development and progression of long-term complications in insulin-dependent diabetes mellitus. N Engl J Med. 1993;329:977-86.
10. Harinarayanan CV, Srikanta S, Ahuja MMS. Childhood diabetes mellitus in developing countries-survey. Int J Diab Dev Countries; 1990. p. 10.
11. Chandalia HB, Sahasrabudhe T. Evaluation of linear growth in pre-pubertal insulin dependent diabetes. Int J Diab Dev Countries; 1990. p. 10.
12. Jackson KL. Growth and maturation of children with insulin dependent diabetes mellitus. Pediatr Clin North Am. 1984;31:545-67.
13. Salardi S, Tonioli S, Tassori P, et al. Growth and growth factors in diabetes mellitus. Arch Dis Child. 1987;62:57-62.
14. Brown M, Ahmed ML, Clayton KL, et al. Growth during childhood and final height in type 1 diabetes. Diabet Med. 1994;11:182-7.
15. Wise JE, Kolb EL, Sauder SE. Effect of glycaemic control on growth velocity in children with IDDM. Diabetes Care. 1992;15:826-30.
16. Rao PV. Diabetes education—international perspective. Int J Diab Dev Countries. 1997;17:99-103.
17. Holmes CS, Dunlap WP, Chen RS, Cornwell J. Gender differences in the learning status of diabetic children. J Consult Clin Psychol. 1992;60:698-704.
18. American Diabetes Association. Type 2 diabetes in children and adolescents. Pediatrics. 2000;105:671-80.
19. Barman KK, Mohan V. Type 2 diabetes in the young. In Dash RJ (Ed): New Vistas in Type 2 Diabetes. Chandigarh: Diabetes Education Society; 2001. pp. 52-72.
20. Fagot-Campagna A, Pettitt DJ, Engelgau MM, et al. Type 2 diabetes mellitus among North American children and adolescents: as epidemiological review and public health prospective. J Pediatr. 2000;136:664-72.
21. The Report of the Expert Committee on the diagnosis of classi-fication of diabetes mellitus. Diabetes Care. 1999;22:5-19.
22. National Diabetes Data Group. Classification and diagnosis of diabetes mellitus and other categories of glucose intolerance. Diabetes. 1979;28:1039-57.
23. Ramachandran A, Snehalatha C, Satyavani K, Sivasankari S, Vijay V. Type 2 diabetes in Asian-Indian urban children. Diabetes Care. 2000;26:1022-5.
24. Asmal AC, Dayal B, Jialal I, et al. NIDDM with young age at onset in blacks and Indians. S Afr Med J. 1981;60:93-6.
25. Glasner NC. Noninsulin dependent diabetes in childhood and adolescence. Pediatr Clinics North Am. 1997;44:307-37.
26. Young TK, Dean HS, Flett B, Wood-Steiman P. Childhood obesity in a population at high risk for type 2 diabetes. J Pediatr. 2000;136:365-9.
27. Rosenbloom AL, House DV, Winter WE. NIDDM in minority youth: research priorities and needs. Clin Pediatr. 1998;37:143-52.
28. Caprio S, Tamborlane WV. Metabolic impact of obesity in childhood. Endocrine Metab Clin North Am. 1999;28:731-47.
29. Gower BA, Nagy TR, Trowbridge CA, et al. Fat distribution and insulin response in prepubertal African and American and white children. Am J Clin Nutr. 1998;67:821-7.
30. Ramachandran A, Gallaghar TF, Mohan V, et al. Comparative study of clinical pattern of diabetes from two referral centres for diabetes in the USA and India. J Diabet Assoc Ind. 1986;26:83-8.
31. Viswanathan M, Mohan V, Snehalatha C, Ramachandran A. High prevalence of type 2 (noninsulin dependent) diabetes among offspring of conjugal diabetic parents in India. Diabetologia. 1985;28:907-10.

32. Petitt DJ, Nerson RC, Saad MF, et al. Diabetes and obesity in the offspring of Pima Indian women with diabetes during pregnancy. Diabetes Care. 1993;16:310-4.

33. Rosenbloom AL, Joe JR, Young RS, Winter WE. Emerging epidemic of type 2 diabetes in youth. Diabetes Care. 1999;22:345-54.

34. Mohan V, Sharp PS, Cloke HR, Burrin JM, Schemer B, Kohner EM. Serum immunoreactive insulin responses to a glucose load in Asian Indian and European type 2 (noninsulin dependent) diabetic patients and control subjects. Diabetologia. 1986;29:235-7.

35. Arslanian SA, Kalhan SC. Correlation between fatty acid and glucose metabolism: potential explanation of insulin resistance of puberty. Diabetes. 1994;43:908-14.

36. Dean JH, Young TK, Flett B, Wood-Steiman P. Screening for type 2 diabetes mellitus in aboriginal children in Northern Canada. Lancet. 1998;352:1523.

37. Hansen JR, Michael J, Fulop, Hunter MK. Type 2 diabetes mellitus in youth: a growing challenge. Clinical Diab. 2000;18:52-6.

38. Pinhas-Hamiel O, Standiford D, Hamiel D, et al. The type 2 family: a setting for development and treatment of type 2 diabetes mellitus. Arch Pediatr Adolesc Med. 1999;153:1063-7.

39. Trissler RJ. Type 2 diabetes on the rise in children: is the American lifestyle coming home to roost? Am Diet Association. 1999;99:1354.

40. Tattersall RB, Fajans SS. A difference between the inheritance of classical juvenile onset and maturity onset type diabetes of young people. Diabetes. 1975;24:44-53.

41. Mohan V, Snehalatha C, Ramachandran A, Jayashree R, Viswanathan M. C-peptide responses to glucose load in maturity onset diabetes of the young (MODY). Diabetes Care. 1985;8:69-72.

42. Fajans J. Maturity onset diabetes of young (MODY). Diab Metab Rev. 1989;5:579-606.

43. O'Rahilly S, Turner RC. Early onset type 2 diabetes vs maturity onset diabetes of youth: evidence for the existence of two discrete diabetic syndromes. Diabetic Med. 1988;5:224-9.

44. Report of the Expert Committee on the diagnosis of classification of diabetes mellitus. Diabetes Care. 1997;20:1183-97.

45. Alberti KGMM, Zimmet PZ. Definition, diagnosis and classification of diabetes mellitus and its complications. Part 1: diagnosis and classification of diabetes mellitus: provisional report of a WHO consultation. Diabet Med. 1998;78:539-53.

46. Mohan V, Alberti KGMM. Diabetes in the tropics. In Alberti KGMM, Defronzo RA, Keen H, Zimmet P (Eds): International Textbook of Diabetes Mellitus (2nd edn). Chichester: John Wiley and Sons Ltd.; 1997. pp. 171-81.

47. Mohan V, Premalatha G. Fibrocalculous pancreatic diabetes. Int J Diabetes. 1995;3:71-82.

48. Gee Varghese PJ. Pancreatic diabetes. Bombay: Popular Prakashan; 1968. pp. 110-5.

49. Gee Varghese PJ. Calcific pancreatitis. Bombay; Varghese Publishing House. 1985.

50. Balakrishnan V. Tropical pancreatitis (pancreatic tropicale). In Bernades P, Hugier M (Eds): Maladies du Pancreas Exocrine, Doin, Pairs; 1987. pp. 207-27.

51. Tripathy BB, Samal KC. Chronic calcific pancreatitis in the young in Orissa. In Balakrishnan V (Ed): Chronic Pancreatitis in India. Trivandrum: Indian Society of Pancreatology; 1987. pp. 87-96.

52. Tripathy BB. Epidemiology of tropical calcific pancreatitis. In Kumar N, Acharya SK (Eds): Tropical Calcific Pancreatitis. Trivandrum: Roussel Scientific Institute; 1994. pp. 12-28.

53. Tripathy BB, Samal KC. Overview and consensus statement on diabetes in tropical areas. Diabetes/Metab Rev. 1997;13:63-76.

54. Nagalotimath SJ. Pancreatic in Karnataka: a note on pathology. In Balakrishnan V (Ed): Chronic Pancreatitis in India. Trivandrum: Indian Society of Pancreatology; 1986. pp.105-11.

55. Viswanathan M. Pancreatic diabetes in India: an overview. In Podolsky S, Viswanathan M (Eds): Secondary Diabetes: The Spectrum of Diabetic Syndromes. New York: Raven Press; 1980. pp. 105-16.

56. Moses SGP, Kannan V. The clinical profile of undernourished diabetics aged 30 or less with associated complication in Madras. In Baba S, Goto Y, Fukui I (Eds): Diabetes Mellitus in Asia. Amsterdam: Excerpta Medica; 1976. pp. 259-62.

57. Mohan V, Mohan R, Susheela L, et al. Tropical pancreatic diabetes in South India: heterogeneity in clinical and biochemical profile. Diabetologia. 1985;28:229-32.

58. Pendsey SP, Doongaji SK, Vaidya MG. Clinical profile of fibrocalculous pancreatic diabetes (FPCD) from Vidarbha region. J Diab Assoc India. 1990;30:7.

59. Shelgikar KM, Yajnik CS, Mohan. Complications in fibrocalculous pancreatic diabetes—the Pune and Madras experience. Int J Diab Dev Countries. 1995;15:70- 5.

60. Bhattacharya PK, Mohan V. Fibrocalculous pancreatic diabetes in Tripura. The Antiseptic. 1990;87:161-5.

61. Anand BS. Clinical profile of chronic pancreatitis in Delhi. In Balakrishnan V (Ed): Chronic Pancreatitis in India. Trivandrum: Indian Society of Pancreatology; 1987. pp. 15-22.

62. Premalatha G, Mohan V. Fibrocalculous pancreatic diabetes in infancy—two case reports. Diabetes Res Clin Pract. 1990;25:137-40.

63. Mohan V, Ramachandran A, Vishwanathan M. Childhood onset fibrocalculous pancreatic disease. J Assoc Physicians India. 1989;37:342-5.

64. Mohan V, Suresh S, Suresh I, et al. Fibrocalculous pancreatic diabetes in the elderly. J Assoc Physicians India. 1989;37:342-5.

65. Yajnik CS, Shelgikar KM, Naik SS, et al. The ketosis resistance in fibrocalculous pancreatic diabetes: clinical observations and endocrine metabolic measurements during oral glucose tolerance test. Diabetes Res Clin Pract. 1992;15:149-56.

66. Sood R, Ahuja MMS, Karmarkar MG. Serum C-peptide levels in young ketosis resistant diabetics. Indian J Med Res. 1983;78:661-4.

67. Vannasaeng S, Nitiyanant TW, Vachayanrat A, et al. C-peptide secretion in clacific tropical pancreatic diabetes. Metabolism. 1986;35:814-7.

68. Samal KC, Das S, Parija CR, et al. C-peptide responses to glycaemic stimuli. J Assoc Physicians India. 1987;37:362-4.

69. Workshop Report: Consensus statement from the International Workshop on type of diabetes peculiar to tropics. Acta Diabetologia. 1996;33:62-4.

70. Hoet JJ, Tripathy BB, Rao RH, Yajnik CS. Malnutrition and diabetes in the tropics. Diabetes Care. 1996;19:1014-7.

71. Kar BC. Observations on clinical pattern of diabetes mellitus in Orissa. Bihar University; 1963.

72. Tripathy BB, Kar BC. Observations on clinical patterns of diabetes mellitus in India. Diabetes.s 1965;14:404-12.

73. Tripathy BB, Samal KC. Protein-deficient diabetes mellitus (PDDM) in India. Int J Diab Dev Countries. 1993;13:3 -13.

74. Khan AKA, Barik NG, Mahatabh. Malnutrition related diabetes in Bangladesh. In Roflom J, Coluell JA, Taylor L (Eds): Diabetes 1991. Amsterdam: Exerpta Medica; 1997. pp. 944-9.

75. Panda NC, Tripathy BB, Parija CR, et al. Observations on endocrine function in adults with chronic malnutrition. In Rastogi GK (Ed): Proceedings of V Asia Oceans in Congress on Endocrinology. Chandigarh: Endocrine Society of India. 1971;1:305.

76. Hazra DK, Singh R, Singh B, et al. Autoantibodies in tropical ketosis resistant but insulin dependent diabetes mellitus. In Bajaj JS (Ed): Diabetes Mellitus in Developing Countries. New Delhi: Interprint; 1984. pp. 165-7.

77. Fajans SS, Conn JW. An approach to the prediction of diabetes mellitus by modification of the glucose tolerance test with cortisone. Diabetes 1954;3:296-304.

78. Rimn E, Manson J, Stamfer M, et al. Oral contraceptive use and the risk of type 2 diabetes in a large population of women. Diabetologia. 1992;35:967-72.

79. Whitehead MI, Lobo RA. Progestogen use in post menopausal women. Lancet. 1988;ii:1243-4.

80. Sonksen PH, Greenwood FC, Ellis JP, et al. Change in carbohydrate tolerance in acromegaly with progress of the disease and in response to treatment. J Clin Endocrinol Metab 1967;27:1418.

81. Bowes SB, Benn JJ, Scobie IN, et al. Glucose metabolism in patients with Cushing's syndrome. Clin Endocrinol. 1991;34:311.

82. Gifford RW, Manger WM, Bravo EL. Pheochromocytoma. Endocrino Metab Clin North Am 1994;23:387-90.

83. McGarran MH, Linger RH, Recant L, et al. A glucagon secreting alpha-cell carcinoma of the pancreas. N Engl J Med. 1996;274:1408-13.

84. Shoelson S, Haneda M, Blix P, et al. Three mutant insulins in man. Nature. 1983; 302:540-3.

85. Steiner DF, Tager HS, Chan SJ, et al. Lessons learned from molecular biology of insulin gene mutation. Diabetes Care. 1990;13:600-9.

86. Ioan D, Dumitriu I, Belengeanu V, Bistriceanu M, Maximilian C. Leprechaunism report of two cases and review. Endocrinology. 1988;26:205-9.

87. Elders MJ, Schedewie HK, Olesfsky J, et al. Endocrine metabolic relationship in patients with leprechaunism. J Natl Med Assoc. 1982;74:1195-210.

88. Berardinelli W. An undiagnosed endocrine metabolic syndrome: report of 2 cases. J Clin Endocrine Metab. 1954;14: 193-204.

Chapter 79

DIABETES IN ELDERLY

Radha Reddy, SS Rastogi, KM Prasanna Kumar

CHAPTER OUTLINE

- Introduction
- Demographics of Diabetes in the Elderly
- Carbohydrate Metabolism in the Elderly
- Screening and Diagnosis of Diabetes
- Manifestations of Diabetes in the Elderly
- Common Geriatric Syndromes associated with Diabetes
- Acute Complications of Diabetes in the Elderly
- Chronic Complications of Diabetes in the Elderly
- Treatment of Diabetes in the Elderly
- Management of the Elderly Diabetic in Special Situations
- Conclusion

INTRODUCTION

The elderly, i.e. men and women over 65 years, are the most rapidly growing segment of the world's population and are expected to exceed 20% of the population by 2040.[1] Diabetes is a disease of aging, affecting nearly 10% of people between the ages of 65 to 74[2] and 20% of people over age 80 years.[2] The incidence declines among the very old.[3] It is estimated that one half of elderly are undiagnosed.[4] An additional 25% of older people have impaired glucose tolerance that increases their risk for macrovascular disease similar to overt diabetes.[4,5] Diabetes *per se* is a frequent cause for hospitalization and a poorer quality of life compared to those with undiagnosed diabetes, impaired glucose tolerance or normal glucose tolerance.[4-7]

There are several important differences between diabetes in the young and elderly that need to be addressed on an individual basis. Firstly, screening for diabetes in the elderly should be done carefully, as most of these people remain asymptomatic, secondly, as microvascular disease is related to the duration of diabetes, the longer the lifespan, the more *likely for these* patients will develop such a complication. Thirdly, a careful watch needs to be kept for macrovascular complications, for which the elderly are at increased risk. Fourthly, the elderly have multiple chronic diseases for which they are on polypharmacy that may interfere with their diabetes, insulin response and tolerability to hypoglycemia. Fifthly, the elderly diabetics are at increased risk for common geriatric syndromes like cognitive impairment, depression, urinary incontinence, falls and persistent pain. Finally, economic, social, functional and physiological issues may make adequate diabetes management difficult.[8-10]

DEMOGRAPHICS OF DIABETES IN THE ELDERLY

The prevalence of diabetes is increasing steadily with increase in the number of the aged and as people grow heavier. The overall prevalence for diagnosed cases of type 2 diabetes rises from 1.4% among individuals aged 25 to 44 years to 3.6% between ages of 45 to 54 years,

7.8% *between of 55 to 64 years and* over 10% over the age of 65.[2] Majority of these patients have type 2 diabetes, although 10 to 15% of people over age 70 years have type 1 diabetes or latent autoimmune diabetes of adulthood.[11] Diabetes also tends to be slightly more frequent in women with advancing age.[12]

Data from individual countries and worldwide demographics of diabetes in the elderly is lacking. Currently in India, there are 60 million people over the age of 60, and this number is expected to rise to 225 million by 2025. Surveys by Ramachandran et al in 1989 and in 1995, of urban Indian subjects, showed that the age-standardized prevalence of diabetes has increased from 8.2 to 11.6% and impaired glucose tolerance (IGT) from 8.7 to 9.1%, over a span of six years.[13] In another study, age, body mass index, waist hip ratio and urbanization were found to be the best predictors of type 2 diabetes in the Indian population.[14] The prevalence of type 2 diabetes and IGT tends to increase significantly with age (p<0.001), markedly so in the urban people compared to rural.

The prevalence of diabetes in India study (PODIS) random multistage cross-sectional population survey involving 41,270 subjects in 108 centers across India showed the prevalence of diabetes in the elderly (>60 years) to be 4.6% (5.4% urban vs 3.1% rural).[15] In this study, the prevalence of impaired fasting glucose (FBG—100–109 mg/dl) was 5.3% (5.8% in urban vs 4.3% in rural) elderly population.

CARBOHYDRATE METABOLISM IN THE ELDERLY

In 1920, Spence was the first to note that the prevalence of both impaired glucose tolerance and type 2 diabetes increased with advancing age.[16] The pathophysiology of type 2 diabetes in both young adults and elderly individuals is the same. But physiological changes with aging produce glucose intolerance even in healthy older individuals. This glucose intolerance is primarily manifested by increase in postprandial glucose (PPBG) response which may increase by as much as 15 mg/dl per decade after age 30.[17] Age-related fasting blood glucose increases are minimal 1 to 2 mg/dl per decade after age 30.[17,18] The increase in PPBG may be greater in men than women. Although the complete pathophysiology of glucose intolerance with aging is not well understood, many mechanisms may be involved. Increase in peripheral insulin resistance (IR) with postreceptor defects in insulin action may play a major role.[19] Leptin levels relate to insulin resistance in older

people and amylin secretion is associated with delayed return of glucose to baseline. Changes in tumor necrosis factor-alpha (TNF-α) and nitric oxide are also thought to play a role in the pathogenesis of age related insulin resistance.[20]

Other lesser contributory mechanisms for glucose intolerance with aging include impaired insulin secretion with lack of pancreatic β-cell compensation for IR, reduction in both early and late phase insulin release, increase proinsulin to insulin molar ratio and impaired hepatic glucose suppression by insulin.[21] The Baltimore Longitudinal Study has shown that decreased glucose tolerance in the elderly is independent of percent of body fat, distribution of fat and fitness of the individual.[22] In addition to the above, intrinsic factors leading to glucose intolerance of aging, a major contribution also comes from extrinsic factors including diet, physical activity, medications, chronic illness and stress, all of which cause changes in body composition or change in other organ mass or function with resultant glucose intolerance. Both the decline in lean body mass and increase in body fat that accompany aging, may contribute to insulin resistance.[23]

The clinical significance of glucose intolerance is due to the increased risk for cardiovascular disease and development of overt diabetes. The risk for development of diabetes among those over age 70 who are glucose intolerant is 2% per year, as compared to 0.04% per year for those older individuals with normal glucose tolerance.

SCREENING AND DIAGNOSIS OF DIABETES

Neither the World Health Organization (WHO) criteria nor the guidelines for diagnosis of diabetes issued by the Expert Committee on Diagnosis and Classification of Diabetes Mellitus adjust glycemic criteria for age.[24] This is due to the fact that even mild hyperglycemia in younger individuals is associated with a poor outcome. Therefore, the usual criteria for diagnosis of diabetes (ADA, 1997) apply, i.e.

- Fasting plasma glucose (FPG) >126 mg/dl, on two separate occasions.
- Random plasma glucose (RPG) >200 mg/dl with symptoms of diabetes such as polyuria, polydipsia, polyphagia and weight loss.
- Two-hour plasma glucose (PG) >200 mg/dl on 75 gm oral glucose tolerance test (OGTT).

The ADA is also recommending that all individuals be tested at age 45 and three yearly thereafter. The best screening test for diabetes mellitus in older adults is a determination of FPG.[1] OGTT is considered to be cumbersome, has poor reproducibility, uses a nonphysiological stimulus and is affected by a variety of factors including diet, drugs, illness, etc. Glycosylated hemoglobin has been proposed as a screening tool for diabetes, but has a low sensitivity and specificity. Its levels tend to increase with older age.[25] Data on serum fructosamine in the elderly are limited; initial data suggests it may be a useful tool to monitor diabetes in the elderly.[11,26]

MANIFESTATIONS OF DIABETES IN THE ELDERLY

Presentation of diabetes in the elderly can be quite variable. As patients may be totally asymptomatic, routine blood glucose screening is recommended. *Symptoms pertaining to other organ systems that are more prevalent in the elderly, weight loss and weakness that may be thought to be due to malignancy. Weight loss is usually multifactorial and may be due to poorly controlled diabetes, anorexia or certain neurological syndromes such as diabetic naturopathic cachexia.[21] Orthostatic, unsteadiness and confusion secondary to dehydration are typical manifestations of diabetes in the elderly, as their thirst perception is decreased and polydipsia may not occur.[27,28]* The nursing home or home/bed-bound patients may present with failure to thrive, increasing or new onset urinary incontinence, slowly resolving soft tissue infections or changes in levels of consciousness.

Several syndromes are specific to the diabetic elderly.[29] These include painful shoulder periarthrosis that occurs in 10% of the elderly diabetics, and is associated with moderate-to-severe limitation at the glenohumeral joint. Others include diabetic amyotrophy and diabetic neuropathic cachexia, which are almost exclusively seen in elderly diabetic men.[30] Diabetics over 70 years old may develop diabetic dermatopathy with intraepidermal bullae of the feet, which resolve spontaneously. Elderly diabetics are also more susceptible to hypothermia. Renal papillary necrosis is also more common in the elderly and frequently presents without flank pain or fever. Older diabetics, especially those in nursing homes are highly prone for tuberculosis. Also, the elderly are unable to mount a fever in response to infections, leading to delay in diagnosis of serious infections such as malignant otitis externa due to *Pseudomonas aeruginosa*, or polymicrobial necrotizing fasciitis.

COMMON GERIATRIC SYNDROMES ASSOCIATED WITH DIABETES

Diabetes is associated with increased risk of dementia and many older patients remain undiagnosed in the early stages. Cognitive function should be assessed in the elderly, whenever, there is noncompliance with therapy, frequent hypoglycemia or deterioration in glycemic control without obvious explanation. Depression occurs at a higher rate in older diabetics than age-matched controls and is frequently undiagnosed and under treated in this high-risk population.[31] Depression has been associated with poor glycemic control and accelerated rates of coronary heart disease in diabetic patients.[32] Early identification and treatment may achieve better glycemic control. Use of multiple drugs is common in the elderly in managing their diabetes and associated risk factors. Side effects may exacerbate comorbidities; therefore medication list should be kept current. Falls are also more common in this population due to neuropathy, muscle weakness, disability, loss of vision, polypharmacy, osteoarthritis and mild hypoglycemia. Exercise may reduce risk of falls. Diabetic women are more prone to urinary incontinence due to recurrent urinary tract infections, vaginal infections, neurogenic bladder and polyuria. Treatment of incontinence will improve quality of life.

ACUTE COMPLICATIONS OF DIABETES IN THE ELDERLY

Hyperglycemic Hyperosmolar Nonketotic State and Diabetic Ketoacidosis

The most serious acute complications of diabetes mellitus are diabetic ketoacidosis (DKA) and hyperglycemic hyperosmolar nonketotic coma (HHNC). Both DKA and HHNC state represent two ends of a continuum and are seen in patients with either type 1 or type 2 diabetes.[33,34] In one retrospective analysis of 600 hospitalized elderly patients, about one-third have an overlap syndrome of mixed DKA and HHNS.[33] But, HHNS is more associated with the elderly. One-third of all HHNS occur in patients with no prior history of diabetes. The predilection of the elderly to HHNS may be secondary to age-related impaired maintenance of serum osmolality, decreased thirst sensation or decreased cognitive function interfering with fluid intake.[35] In many elderly diabetic patients, the occurrence of DKA does not necessarily indicate that insulin therapy will be required for life.

An acute infection is the most frequent predisposing factor (40–60% of patients), with pneumonia being the most common illness. Other precipitating factors include stroke, myocardial infarction, renal failure, drugs such as glucocorticoids, stress, dehydration or even intravenous dextrose in water administered to hospitalized patients.

Mortality in HHNS can be as high as 35%.[36] Hyperosmolarity and dehydration are the principal cause for coma and death. Correcting the water deficit and hyperglycemia with fluids, and insulin corrects hyperosmolarity. The underlying cause should be treated and any electrolyte imbalance corrected. Caution should be exerted in the elderly with decreased cardiac reserve, with strict monitoring of cardiac and renal parameters. Ultimately, at the time of discharge, majority of patients with HHNS can be managed without insulin, and treated with diet and oral hypoglycemic agents.

Hypoglycemia

Usually hypoglycemia is a complication of insulin treatment or sulfonylureas. Although defined as plasma glucose less than 45 mg/dl, symptoms of hypoglycemia can occur at higher plasma glucose levels and correlate with rapidity of fall in glucose levels.[37] Risk of hypoglycemia, which may lead to impaired cognition and function, is substantially increased in the elderly. Even mild hypoglycemia can lead to falls and fractures in the elderly.

In older diabetic individuals, neuroglycopenic symptoms (dizziness, weakness, delirium) predominate compared to adrenergic symptoms (tremors, sweating, palpitations) and hypoglycemic unawareness can occur without history of tight control or repeat episodes of hypoglycemia. Recovery from hypoglycemia may be slower in the elderly. Hypoglycemia also occurs more frequently in the elderly as near-euglycemia is achieved. Secretagogues and polypharmacy are also more frequently associated with asymptomatic daytime hypoglycemia in the elderly.[38-41] Furthermore, elderly diabetics who become hypoglycemic are at a greater risk for myocardial infarction or cerebrovascular accidents.

Therefore, as the potential risks of hypoglycemia are more in the elderly diabetic, avoidance and careful monitoring for hypoglycemia, are key to management in this subset of the population.

CHRONIC COMPLICATIONS OF DIABETES IN THE ELDERLY

The chronic complications of diabetes add to its morbidity, associated with aging. Despite the United Kingdom Diabetes Prospective Study (UKPDS) and other studies having demonstrated that with good glycemic control, there is a decline in lifetime risk of developing blindness from diabetic retinopathy or end stage renal disease from diabetic nephropathy, with advancing age of onset of type 2 diabetes, appropriate yearly screening and prevention of long-term complications is advocated.[42] Hyperglycemia, along with the normal aging process and coexisting morbidity can hasten the onset and course of long-term complications of diabetes. Both micro- and macrovascular complications of diabetes develop faster in the elderly with poor glycemic control.[43] Cardiovascular and peripheral vascular disease are the most prevalent complications in elderly patients with diabetes, with the incidence of hypertension and cardiovascular disease continuing to increase in the diabetic elderly compared to the nondiabetics of this age group.

Diabetic Retinopathy

Prevalence of retinopathy increases progressively with increasing duration of diabetes. The natural history of retinopathy may differ in older patients. In one study, only 21% over the age of 70 years had any form of retinopathy and only 3.5% had poor vision due to diabetes.[44] Despite this, yearly eye examinations are important in elderly diabetics because poor vision can lead to social isolation, increased risk of accidents, inability to check blood glucose or draw up insulin. Also, cataracts are twice as common in people over the age of 65 with diabetes, compared to normal subjects, while glaucoma is three times more common.[45]

Diabetic Nephropathy

The prevalence of diabetic nephropathy increases with duration of diabetes and age.[46,47] There is a 20 to 30% progressive decline in renal mass and volume from the third to eight decade of normal individuals, causing a progressive decline in renal function. In addition to above, the older diabetic patient is at risk for other cause of renal insufficiency such as arteriosclerosis, hypertension, chronic heart failure (CHF), drug-induced renal problems.

Prevention and treatment of diabetic nephropathy in the elderly is similar to the younger diabetic.

Microalbuminuria testing should be done routinely, yearly. Adequate control of blood glucose and aggressive treatment of hypertension are required although, the elderly are particularly prone to side effects of antihypertensives, such as orthostatic hypotension. Low protein diet may be used after careful evaluation of their nutritional status. Angiotensin-converting enzyme (ACE) inhibitors and angiotensin II receptor blockers are underused in the elderly.[48] They may be used in normotensive as well as hypertensive diabetic patients.[49] Nephrotoxic drugs and dyes should be avoided. Dialysis and renal transplant are still options *in the elderly otherwise healthy diabetics*. The outcome of these patients is poor with the majority of these patients dying of cardiovascular causes.[50, 51]

Diabetic Neuropathy

Diabetic neuropathy also increases with age and duration of diabetes as shown in a study of 6487 diabetic patients.[52] The prevalence of neuropathy increased from 5% in the 20 to 29 year age group to 44.2% in the >65 year old age group. Also, 36.8% of patients who had diabetes >10 years had neuropathy.

Several specific syndromes are described in the elderly diabetics, which usually resolve spontaneously. Diabetic amyotrophy is characterized by asymmetric weakness, pain, wasting of pelvic girdle and thigh muscles, with minimal sensory changes, most often in elderly diabetic men. The condition is usually difficult to manage but it usually resolves spontaneously by one year.[53] Diabetic neuropathic cachexia also affects older diabetic men. It presents with peripheral painful neuropathy, depression and dramatic weight loss suggestive of malignancy. This condition usually recovers spontaneously in a year with good prognosis.

Peripheral neuropathy may be the presenting symptom of diabetes in the elderly patient and may also precede overt hyperglycemia. In general, the symptoms and signs of peripheral and autonomic neuropathy are similar in the elderly as in the young. But the presence of other comorbid conditions such as arthritis and cataracts make daily foot examinations difficult. This puts them at increased risk for foot ulcers, infections and amputations. Medical treatments for neuropathy are also less tolerated in the elderly. For instance, the side effects, of tricyclic antidepressants such as orthostatic hypotension and depression of mentation are less tolerated by the elderly.

Diabetic Cheiropathy

Carpal-Tunnel syndrome, Dupuytren's contracture, trigger finger and limited joint motility are all more frequent in the diabetic than the nondiabetic persons.[54] These rheumatological complications of diabetes are a cause of functional impairment in the older diabetic and hence can reduce quality of life. The pathogenesis of these disorders is thought to involve glycosylation of collagen with secondary inflammation and fibrosis. Most of these disorders are amenable to surgical release procedures.

Macrovascular Disease

Both diabetes and age are major risk factors for coronary heart disease. Coronary heart disease is the leading cause of death in elderly patients with diabetes and the effect of most interventions is more pronounced in them. In elderly diabetics, 50 to 70% of deaths are due to macrovascular disease, coronary artery disease (CAD), cerebrovascular disease (CVD) and peripheral vascular disease (PVD).[55]

The morbidity and mortality associated with macrovascular events far outweigh the microvascular complications in elderly people with diabetes. In the United Kingdom Prospective Diabetes Study (UKPDS), 9% of type 2 diabetic patients developed microvascular complications after nine years of follow-up compared to 20% for macrovascular complications.[56] Older people with diabetes should be treated as aggressively for diabetes and cardiovascular risk factor as in nondiabetic people with known CAD.[57]

Older patients with type 2 diabetes are at an increased risk for cerebrovascular disease than younger patients with type 1 diabetes or nondiabetic controls. A given stroke episode has higher morbidity and mortality in older diabetic patients. Poor glycemic control is thought to contribute to increased stroke severity and delayed recovery.[58,59]

Peripheral vascular disease is two to four folds more prevalent in the diabetic and is an important cause of morbidity and mortality. Diabetics have a 22-fold increased amputation rate compared to nondiabetic subjects. Amputations in the elderly diabetics are associated with considerable mortality and deterioration of functional status.

Cardiac risk reduction should focus on the following areas:
- *Smoking cessation:* Smoking is an independent risk factor for all cause mortality, due largely to cardiovascular disease, and has to be addressed.

- *Treatment of hypertension:* This is clearly beneficial in the elderly, even up to the age of 84.
- *Treatment of dyslipidemia:* Clinical benefits of lipid lowering are seen as early as six months.[60] CARE and Heart Protection Study showed similar benefits of LDL reduction in the elderly and young.[61,62]
- *Aspirin:* A meta-analysis of several secondary prevention trials has shown the greatest benefits of aspirin therapy in those over 65 years of age with diabetes and diastolic hypertension.[63]

TREATMENT OF DIABETES IN THE ELDERLY

General Treatment

The initial approach to an older adult with diabetes mellitus should include careful assessment of patient's current medical status and consideration of remaining life- expectancy. The optimal range for glycemic control in the elderly diabetic is unknown. The recent Canadian Consensus Conference recommended keeping: (1) HbA_{1c} less than 1% above upper limit of normal; (2) FPG of up to 140 mg/dl and (3) PPBG less than 180 mg/dl, in elderly diabetics with a life-expectancy greater than 5 years.[64] The American Geriatric Society (AGS) recommends as a treatment goal an HbA_{1c} value of 8% for selected older patients who are unable to achieve this goal or less likely to benefit from it.[9,65]

Geriatric assessment or functional assessment includes assessment of patient's capabilities for self care, basic and instrumental (feeding, bathing, housework, etc.). It also evaluates the amount of assistance required by the patient, financial status and the social support system available to the patient. There are a variety of age-related changes that can alter a patient's ability to perform the skills necessary to treat diabetes.[66,67] As with any age group, diabetes education is useful in the elderly.

The initial step in treating a patient with diabetes is to determine whether or not the patient has type 1 or type 2 diabetes. Only 5 to 10% of elderly patients presents with classic type 1 diabetes and need insulin till the end. For the type 2 diabetic patients, diet, exercise, and oral hypoglycemic agents (OHA) may suffice. After a period of time, however, a significant percentage of older type patients require insulin. A cut-off C-peptide value of 0.68 nmol after 100 gm glucose challenge administered orally can reliably predict a successful withdrawal from insulin therapy in insulin treated type 2 diabetic patients.[64]

Diet Management

Diet therapy is fundamental to management of diabetes. There is no age related change in dietary guidelines for the elderly. There are several factors unique to the elderly that limit the effectiveness of dietary therapy. These include, limited mobility, which restrict exercise, requiring substantial calorie restriction to achieve weight loss. This may put a patient at a risk for nutrient deficiency and is therefore not advisable. Thus, many recommend a noncalorie-restricted, low fat (<30% of calories), high carbohydrate (>50% of calories) diet.[68,69] Diet supplement may be required for the frail weight-losing elderly patients with diabetes.

Anorexia is also a major problem in the elderly. In nursing homes, 21% of patient's with diabetes were under their ideal body weight, while only 8.5% were overweight.[70] Factors predisposing to anorexia include visceral neuropathy, poorly fitting dentures and drugs.[71] Weight loss is associated with increased morbidity and mortality in the elderly.[72]

Exercise

Exercise benefits individuals of all ages, and should be used as an adjunct. Even moderate leisure activity is associated with reduced risk of developing diabetes. Appropriate precautions should be taken towards prevention of hypoglycemia. Duration, frequency and type of exercise should be tailored to individual needs.

Exercise is beneficial to help maintain physical function, reduce cardiac risk, and improve insulin sensitivity in patients with diabetes. In older adults, exercise also improves body composition and arthritic pain, reduces falls and depression, increases strength and balance, enhances the quality of life and improves survival.[73,74] Studies of frail elderly people have shown that weight training should be included in addition to aerobic exercises.[75]

Oral Hypoglycemic Agents

The type 2 diabetic patient, whose glucose levels remains consistently above 200 mg/dl despite diet and exercise, is a candidate for oral hypoglycemic agents (OHA). The five classes of OHA available for use include—sulfonylureas, biguanides, meglitinides, 5- alpha glucosidase inhibitors and thiazolidinediones. In all type 1 patients and in those type 2 diabetics who fail to respond to OHA, insulin may be initiated. Now, amylin analogs (types 1 and 2) and incretin mimetics, exanetide (type 2) are also available for use.[66]

Over time, most patients need multiple drug combinations. No consistent data demonstrates superiority of any particular drug over another in elderly patients.[76] *Start slow and go slow* is a good principle for the elderly. All classes of antidiabetic drugs can reasonably be used as first line therapy, since most demonstrate equivalent efficacy in reducing HbA_{1c} level. The glucose lowering effect of the second agent is additive but not synergistic.

Sulfonylureas

Sulfonylureas (SU) are the most widely used drugs in the elderly population. Although one-third of all patients with type 2 diabetes are being treated with these drugs, 70% of the prescriptions are for individuals over the age of 60.[77] SU may be the drugs of first choice in most elderly patients with if diet and exercise fail to achieve optimum center.

The sulfonylureas are insulin secretagogues. The major risk for older adults treated with sulfonylureas is hypoglycemia and weight gain.[78,79] Age alone has been shown to be a major risk factor for hypoglycemia in patients treated with OHA. The age-associated factors that increase risk for hypoglycemia include decline in hepatic and renal functions, impairment in autonomic nervous system and reduction in β-adrenergic receptor function. Frequently used drugs in the elderly that increase risk for hypoglycemia include beta-blockers, salicylates, warfarin, sulfonamides and alcohol.

The newer generation sulfonylureas, i.e. glibenclamide, glipizide, gliclazide and glimeperide are clearly preferred over the older generation sulfonylureas, owing to fewer interactions and favorable safety profile. Chlorpropamide, in particular, is known for its prolonged hypoglycemia and hyponatremia (antidiuretic hormone like action), both of which are more so in the elderly. Usually, half maximal dose is adequate for maximal glycemic control. All sulfonylureas are hepatically metabolized and should be used cautiously in cases with liver disease. Glibenclamide's liver metabolites have delayed action. For this reason, glipizide and gliclazide, which have a shorter half-life and generate few or no active hepatic metabolites, are the preferred sulfonylureas in elderly diabetic patients.[80] The long-acting formulations of glipizide with the osmotic gastrointestinal therapeutic delivery system and glimeperide may be the least likely sulfonylureas to be associated with hypoglycemia.

Biguanides

Metformin decreases hepatic glucose output and may increase muscle glucose uptake.[81] Its advantages over sulfonylureas, particularly in the elderly, include lack of hypoglycemia as it does not stimulate insulin secretion. In addition, metformin therapy is associated with weight loss or weight stabilization. Metformin therapy has modest benefits on lipid panel, lowering coronary risk, which is an important cause of morbidity and mortality in the elderly.[82] Metformin has the same efficacy in the elderly as in the young adults.

Metformin should not be used in conditions that are associated with increased production of lactate or its clearance, such as liver or renal failure, alcoholism, severe congestive heart failure, severe peripheral vascular disease, severe infection and severe chronic obstructive pulmonary disease.[83,84] Metformin should be used with caution in the frail elderly in whom lactic acidosis tends to occur, even though rare. In persons over the age of 80, creatinine clearance should be calculated to ensure renal sufficiency as serum creatinine may be deceptively normal due to reduced muscle mass. Metformin should be avoided in elderly with creatinine clearance less than 60 ml/min. Metformin therapy should be temporarily discontinued during radiographic studies using iodinated contrast, acute illness or hospitalization.

As long as renal function is reasonably intact, metformin may be the preferred initial agent in overweight elderly patient with type 2 diabetes.

Meglitinides

Repaglinide and nateglinide are the prototype. They stimulate insulin secretion by acting at a different site compared to sulfonylureas and do not stimulate direct insulin exocytosis. Repaglinide and nateglinide differ significantly from sulfonylureas in that they are primarily excreted by the liver rather than the kidney and have a short half-life of one hour. Therefore, potential for hypoglycemia due to a delayed or skipped meal or decreased excretion is much less and postprandial regulation is better.[85,86] Meglitinides may be given 0 to 15 minutes before a meal. It exerts its effect on the meal and carry little effects over to the next meal, therefore, making it a useful drug in the elderly. It may be used as monotherapy or as combination with metformin for type 2 diabetes. They are also a useful alternative for sulfa allergy.

5-alpha Glucosidase Inhibitors

Inhibition of α-glucosidase enzyme in the intestinal brush border retards digestion of complex carbohydrates and disaccharides to monosaccharides. This results in decreased postprandial glucose with reduction of HbA_{1c}.[87] Few reports have appeared in the elderly, but lack of hypoglycemia suggests an advantage in this section of the population. Acarbose has been shown to increase insulin sensitivity but not insulin release in elderly patients with diabetes. It commonly causes mild abdominal discomfort and flatulence. Its effect on HbA_{1c}, is modest, but its use is appropriate in early diabetes when the ability to secrete insulin in response to a meal is mildly impaired. Miglitol, is another relatively safe option in elderly diabetics.[88] It is more potent with less gastrointestinal side effects compared to acarbose.

Thiazolidinediones

Rosiglitazone and pioglitazone are the drugs of its class. They are insulin sensitizers, improving hyperglycemia in type 2 diabetics by improving insulin sensitivity in muscle and adipocytes.[89] These do not cause hypoglycemia and can be given to older patients with impaired renal function. However, fluid retention, congestive heart failure and liver dysfunction may limit their use.

New Antidiabetic Agents

Pramlintide and exanetide have only recently become available. Pramlintide, an amylin analog, lowers postprandial blood glucose by suppressing glucagon release, delaying gastric emptying and enhancing satiety. Therefore, it causes some weight loss and has been approved for use with insulin. It is unlikely to be favored in the elderly due to three injections per day dosage schedule and marginal glucose reduction.[66]

Exanetide activates glucagon like peptide 1 receptor and enhances glucose- dependent insulin secretion from the β-cells. Rest of its effects is similar to pramlintide-suppression of glucagon, delayed gastric emptying and increased satiety. It does not cause hypoglycemia and results in modest weight loss. It reduces HbA_{1c} by 1%. Its main side effect is nausea. It has been shown to be an effective option in elderly type 2 diabetics.[90]

Insulin

Insulin is essential for all patients with type 1 diabetes. It should also be used in those patients with type 2 diabetes wherein diet, exercise and OHA's have not been effective in meeting the treatment goals. Although the oral regimen can be maintained by simply adding insulin, the usual practice is to combine insulin with insulin sensitizers but to discontinue any secretagogues.[91] No specific form or insulin regimen has been identified as being more or less efficacious in older people. The choice of insulin must be individualized.

A single dose of insulin may be adequate to prevent symptomatic hyperglycemia, if this is the goal. For many elderly patients, use of intermediate or long-acting insulin at bedtime with daytime oral agent may improve their symptoms and diabetic control.[92,93] Another approach is to use premixed formulations of rapid and intermediate-acting insulins once or twice daily before meals. In those elderly, whose diabetes is difficult to control, the use of newer insulin analogs like lispro/aspart/glulisine may enable tighter plasma glucose control with minimal increased risk of hypoglycemia. The other advantages of use of insulin analogs in the elderly diabetic patients are improved predictability of response, greater flexibility in the more frail elderly patients such as those with variable oral intake or compromised renal function.[94] The newer pen devices and premixed insulins also enhance compliance of insulin use in the elderly due to their simplicity and ease of administration. More accurate dosing is associated with the use of these pens ensuring better long-term outcome. Inhaled insulin is better tolerated, with comparable glycemic control and less hypoglycemia.[64]

Studies show that elderly patients >60 years of age can perform self-monitoring of blood glucose (SMBG), and also benefit from intensive insulin treatment program to improve glycemic control. Intensive insulin treatment does lead to increased frequency of hypoglycemia and should be used with caution in the elderly.

Insulin therapy in the elderly requires some special considerations. Aging, as well as complications of diabetes, may impair vision and fine motor skills necessary for insulin self-administration or monitoring of blood glucose. Hyperglycemia and poor diabetes control may be associated with subtle impairments of cognitive function in older adults. This affects the ability of the individual to adhere to a complicated insulin regimen. Financial constraints also exist in this section of the population. Hypoglycemia in the elderly is associated with psychomotor retardation and altered counter-regulatory hormone responses inhibiting hypoglycemic awareness. Also, elderly who live alone and do not have family or support services are at risk for serious sequelae of hypoglycemia from insulin administration, as often, there is delay in recognition and institution of treatment.[95]

MANAGEMENT OF THE ELDERLY DIABETIC IN SPECIAL SITUATIONS

Hospitalized Elderly Patient with Diabetes

The rate of hospitalization among elderly patients with diabetes is 1.7 times the rate among elderly people without diabetes.[1] These include hospitalizations for diabetes and other reasons. The goals of glycemic control should be individualized.

Hypoglycemia is an important problem in the hospitalized elderly and is usually due to inadequate intake or inappropriate changes in insulin dose. It can be prevented by frequent glucose monitoring, changing insulin dose according to changes in the medical condition of the patient, and maintaining optimal in-hospital glycemic goals. Reasonable in-hospital glycemic goal would be plasma glucose of less than 200 mg/dl.

General measures include strict decubitus precautions, restriction of use of indwelling catheter and judicious use of psychoactive drugs. Early mobility and physical therapy should be encouraged. Discharge planning should be coordinated with the social worker from the time of admission, to ensure adequate family versus social support postdischarge.

Nursing Home or House-bound Patient

In India, only a minority of the elderly are in the nursing homes or old-age homes, but this concept is fast catching on. A good majority are still cared for at home, even if they are bedridden. The prevalence of diabetes in this population is twice that of the general population. Furthermore, this section of the population is more likely to have disease associated with diabetes such as CAD, PVD, amputations and immobility. Urinary tract and skin infections, chronic renal failure, retinopathy, neuropathy are also more common in diabetic compared to nondiabetic patients of this same age group. Furthermore, the care of these patients at nursing homes is at best, marginal.

The life-expectancy of the elderly home or nursing home-bound diabetic patient is markedly reduced. The functional status of the patient rather than diabetes per se is a predictor of outcome. Hence, goals for glycemic control should be individualized. Tight glycemic control will be inappropriate in those whose life-expectancy is reduced.[96] The basic approach should be to control hyperglycemia and prevent acute complications. Diet and OHA is the mainstay of treatment. A good number of these patients are underweight and some even malnourished. Therefore, these patients should be assessed by dietitians and calories adjusted to include factors like level of activity, wounds, infections, etc. Exercise and physical therapy should be encouraged.

OHA should be selected based on the guidelines in the section above. If ineffective or glycemic control is very brittle, then insulin may be necessary. Frequent monitoring of blood glucose should be encouraged. Glucose control may be more easily obtained in the elderly home-bound/nursing home diabetic, if meals and medications are provided on time.[97] Routine preventive medicine for diabetes should be continued including regular ophthalmologist, dental and foot check-ups.

CONCLUSION

Diabetes mellitus is a common disorder in the elderly, and often undiagnosed. Several features are unique to the presentation and management of diabetes in the elderly, even though the same fundamental principles apply. Diabetes and its complications, both macrovascular and microvascular are a major cause of mortality and morbidity, more so in the elderly, as they have other coexisting debilitating conditions. The lack of financial resources as well as social or emotional support makes treatment of diabetes in this section of the elderly population a challenging experience.

REFERENCES

1. Morrow LA, Halter JB. Treatment of the elderly with diabetes. In Kahn CR, Weir GC (Eds): Joslin's Diabetes Mellitus, 13th edn. Philadelphia: Malvern PA, Lea and Febiger, 1994.
2. Kenny SJ, Aubert RE, Geiss LS. Prevalence and incidence of NIDDM. In Diabetes in America, 2nd edn. Harris MI (Ed): NIH Publication. 1995;95-1468:47-67.
3. Rockwood K, Awalt E, MacKnight C, McDowell I. Incidence and outcomes of diabetes mellitus in elderly people: report from the Canadian Study of Health and Aging. CMAJ. 2000;162(6):769-72.
4. Harris MI. Epidemiology of diabetes mellitus among the elderly in the United States. Clin Geriatr Med. 1990;6:703-19.
5. Hiltunen L, Kuukinen H, Koski K, et al. Prevalence of diabetes mellitus in an elderly Finnish population. Diabet Med. 1994;11:241-9.
6. Damasguard EM. Why do elderly diabetics burden the health care system more than nondiabetics? Dan Med Bull. 1989;36:89-92.
7. Hiltunen L, Keinanen-Kinkaanniemi S. Does glucose tolerance affect quality of life in our elderly population? Diab Res Clin Pract. 1999;46(2):161-7.
8. Peters AL, Davidson MB. Treatment of the elderly with diabetes. In Alberti KGMM, Zimeet P, Dfronzo RA (Eds):

international textbook of diabetes mellitus, 2nd edn. Wiley 1997. pp 1151-77.

9. Brown AF, Mangione CM, Saliba D, et al. California Health Care Foundation/ American Geriatric Society Panel on Improving Care for Elders with Diabetes. Guidelines for improving the care of the older person with diabetes. J Am Geriartr Soc. 2003;51(5 Suppl guidelines):S265-80.

10. McCulloch DK, Munshi M. Treatment of diabetes mellitus in the elderly. UpToDate. 2005. p. 13.3.

11. Morley JE, Kaiser FE. Unique aspects of diabetes mellitus in the elderly. Clin Geriatr Med. 1990;6:693-702.

12. Meneilly GS, Tessier D. Diabetes in Elderly. Diabet Med. 1995;12:949-60.

13. Ramachandran A, Vishwanathan M, et al. Rising prevalence of NIDDM in an urban population in India. Diabetologia. 1997;40(2):232-7.

14. Ramachandran A, Vishwanathan M, et al. Prevalence of glucose intolerance in Asian Indians. Diabetes Care. 1992;15(10):1348-55.

15. Sadikot SM , Nigam A, Das S, Zarger AH, Prasanna Kumar KM, Sosale A, Munichoodappa C, et al. The burden of Diabetes and impaired fasting glucose in India using the ADA 1997 criteria: prevalence of diabetes in India study (PODIS). Diabetes Research and Clinical Practice. 2004;66:293-300.

16. Spence JC. Some observations on sugar tolerance, with special reference to variations found at different ages. Quart J Med. 1920-21;14:314-26.

17. Gumbiner B, Fink RI, et al. Effects of aging on insulin secretion. Diabetes. 1989;38:1549-56.

18. Jackson RA. Mechanisms of age-related glucose intolerance. Diabetes Care. 1990;13(suppl 2):9-19.

19. Meneilly GS, Rowe JW, et al. Insulin action in aging man: evidence for tissue specific differences at low physiologic insulin levels. J Gerontol. 1987;42:196-201.

20. Morley JE. An overview of diabetes medicine in older persons. Clin Ger Med. 1999;15(2):211-24.

21. Samos LF, Roos BA. Prevention and treatment of diabetes and its complications: diabetes mellitus in older persons. Med Clin North Am. 1998;82:791-803.

22. Garcia GV, Supiano MA, et al. Glucose metabolism in older adults: a study including subjects more than 80 years of age. J Am Geriatr Soc. 1997;45:813-7.

23. Shimokata H, Andres R, et al. Age as an independent determinant of glucose tolerance. Diabetes. 1991;40:44-51.

24. Expert Committee on the Diagnosis and Classification of Diabetes Mellitus. Report of the Expert Committee on the Diagnosis and Classification of Diabetes Mellitus. Diabetes Care. 1997;20:1183-97.

25. Arnetz BB, Theorell T, et al. The influence of aging on HbA$_{1c}$. J Gerontology. 1982;37:648-50.

26. Cefalu WT, Bell-Farrow AD, et al. Serum fructosamine as a screening test for diabetes in the elderly: A pilot study. J Am Geriatr Soc. 1993;41:1090-4.

27. Hiltunen L, Laara E, et al. Self-perceived health and symptoms of elderly persons with diabetes and impaired glucose tolerance. Age Ageing. 1996;25:59-66.

28. Hogikyan RV, Halter JB. In Porte D Jr, Sherwin RS (Eds): Ellenberg and Rifkins Diabetes Mellitus, 5th edn. Stanford, CT, Appleton and Lange. 1997.

29. Gregg EW, Engelgau MM, Narayan V. Complications of diabetes in elderly people. BMJ. 2002;325(7370):916-7.

30. Morley JE, Mooradian AD, Rosenthal MJ, et al. Diabetes mellitus in elderly patients: is it different? Am J Med. 1987;83:533-54.

31. Anderson RJ, Freedland KE, Clouse RE, Lustman PJ. The prevalence of comorbid depression in adults with diabetes: a meta-analysis. Diabetes Care. 2001;24:1069.

32. Lustman PJ, Clouse RE. Treatment of depression in diabetics: impact on mood and medical outcome. J Psychosom Res. 2002;53:917.

33. Siperstein MD. Diabetic ketoacidosis and hyperosmolar coma. Endocrinol Metab Clin North Am. 1992;21:415-33.

34. Wachtel TJ, Goldman DL, et al. Hyperosmolarity and acidosis in diabetes mellitus. J Gen Int Med. 1991;6:497-502.

35. Singh I, Marshall MC. Diabetes Mellitus in the elderly. Endo Clin North Am. 1995;24:255-72.

36. Umpierrez GE, Khajavi M, Kitabchi AE. Review: diabetic ketoacidosis and hyperglycemic hyperosmolar nonketotic syndrome. Am Med Sci. 1996;225-33.

37. Walter RM Jr. Hypoglycemia: still a risk in the elderly. Geriatrics. 1990;45:69-75.

38. Brodows RG. Benefits and risks with glyburide and glipizide in elderly NIDDM patients. Diabetes Care. 1992;15:75-80.

39. Matyka K, Evans M, Lomas J, et al. Altered hierarchy of protective responses against severe hypoglycemia in normal aging in healthy men. Diabetes Care. 1997;20:135.

40. Greco D, Angileri G. Drug induced severe hypoglycemia in Type 2 diabetic patients aged 80 years or older. Diabetes Nutr Metab. 2004;17(1):23-6.

41. Chelliah A, Burge MR. Hypoglycemia in elderly patients with diabetes mellitus: causes and strategies for prevention. Drugs Aging. 2004;21(8):511-30.

42. United Kingdom Prospective Diabetes Study (UKPDS) Group. Intensive blood glucose control with sulfonylurea or insulin compared to conventional treatment and risk of complications in patients with type 2 diabetes (UKPDS 33). Lancet. 1998;352:837-53.

43. Mooradian AD. Diabetes in the elderly: studies dispel common misconceptions. Cleve Clin J Med. 1996;68:5-7.

44. Hirvela H, Laatikainen L. Diabetic retinopathy in people aged 70 years or older. Br J Ophthalmol. 1997;81:214.

45. Klein R, Klein BE. Vision disorders in diabetes. In Diabetes in America, 2nd edn. Harris MI (Ed): NIH Publication. 1995;95-1468.

46. Herman WH. Eye disease and nephropathy in NIDDM. Diabetes Care. 1990;13 (Suppl 2):24-9.

47. Wingard DL, McPhillips JB, et al. Prevalence of cardiovascular and renal complications in older adults with normal or impaired glucose tolerance or NIDDM. Diabetes Care. 1993;16:1022-5.

48. Winkelmayer WC, Fischer MA, Schneeweiss S, Wang PS, Levin R, Avorn J. Underuse of ACE inhibitors and angiotensin II receptor blockers in elderly patients with diabetes. Am J Kidney Dis. 2005;46(6):1080-7.

49. Molitch ME. ACE inhibitors and diabetic nephropathy. Diabetes Care. 1994;17: 756-60.

50. Khan MA. Diabetes in the elderly population. Adv Renal Replace Ther. 2000;7(1):32-51.

51. Corsenello A, Pedone C, Incalzi RA, et al. Concealed renal failure and adverse drug reactions in older patients with type 2 diabetes mellitus. J Gerontol A Biol Sci Med Sci. 2005;60(9):1147-51.

52. Young MJ, Sonksen PH, et al. A multicenter study of the prevalence of diabetic peripheral neuropathy in the UK hospital clinic population. Diabetologica. 1993;36:150-4.

53. Thomas PK, Ward JD, Watkins PJ. Diabetic neuropathy. In Keen H, Jarett J (Eds): complications of diabetes, 2nd edn. London: Edward Arnold 1982. pp 117-8.

54. Spanheimer RG. Skeletal and rheumatological complications of diabetes. In Mazzefferri EL, Bar RS, Kreisberg RA (Eds): advances in endocrinology and metabolism. St Louis: Mosby Year Book. 1993 p. 4.

55. Panzram G. Mortality and survival in type 2 diabetes mellitus. Diabetologia. 1987;30:123-31.

56. Turner R, Cull C, Holman R. United Kingdom Prospective Diabetes Study (UKPDS 17): a 9 year update of a randomized controlled trial on the effect of impaired metabolic control on complications in NIDDM. Ann Intern Med. 1996;124:136-45.

57. Haffner SM, Laaska M, et al. Mortality from coronary heart disease in subject with and without prior MI. N Engl J Med. 1998;339:229-34.

58. Olsson T, Hagg E, et al. Prognosis after stroke in diabetic elderly patients: a controlled prospective study. Diabetologia. 1990;33:244-9.

59. Monkovsky BN, Molitch ME, et al. Cerebrovascular disorders inpatients with diabetes mellitus. J Diabetes Complications. 1996;10:228-42.

60. Scandinavian Simvastatin Survival Study. Randomized trial of cholesterol lowering in 4444 patients with coronary heart disease. Lancet. 1994;344:1383.

61. Scaks FM, Tonkin AM, Craven T, et al. Coronary heart disease in patients with low LDL cholesterol: benefit of pravastatin in diabetics and enhanced role for HDL cholesterol and triglycerides as risk factors. Circulation. 2002:105:1424.

62. MRC/BHF Heart Protection Study of cholesterol lowering with simvastatinin 20,536 high-risk individuals: a randomised placebo-controlled trial. Lancet. 2002:360:7.

63. Collaborative overview of randomized trials of antiplatelet therapy I: Prevention of death, myocardial infarction, and stroke by prolonged antiplatelet therapy in various categories of patients. Antiplatelet Trialists' Collaboration. BMJ. 1994;308:1540.

64. Lee A. Management of elderly diabetics in sub-acute care setting. Clinics in Geriatric Medicine. 2000;16(4):833-52.

65. American Diabetes Association. Standards of medical care in diabetes. Diabetes Care. 2005;(28 suppl 1):S4-36.

66. Sakharova OV, Inzucchi SE. Treatment of diabetes in the elderly. Postgraduate Medicine. 2005;118(5):19-29.

67. Gilden JL, Singh SP, et al. Support groups improve health care in older diabetic patients. J Am Geriatar Soc. 1992;40:147-50.

68. Wallace IJ. Management of diabetes in the elderly. Clinical Diabetes. 1999;17(1).

69. American Diabetes Association. Translation of diabetes nutrition recommendations for health care institutions: position statement. J Am Diet Assoc. 1997;36:391.

70. Morley JE, Silver AJ, et al. Nutrition in the elderly. Ann Intern Med. 1988;109: 890-904.

71. Couslton AM, Mandelbaum D, Reaven GM. Dietary management of nursing home residents with NIDDM. Am J Clin Nutr. 1990;51:67-71.

72. Wedick NM, Barrett-Connor E, Knoke JD, Wingard DL. The relationship between weight loss and all cause mortality in older men and women with and without diabetes mellitus: the Rancho Bernardo Study. J Am Geriatr Soc. 2002;50:1810.

73. Christmas C, Andersen RA. Exercise and older patients: guidelines for the clinician. J Am Geriatr Soc. 2000;48:318.

74. Morey MC, Pieper CF, Crowley GM, et al. Exercise adherence and 10-year mortality in chronically ill older adults. J Am Geriatr Soc. 2002;50:1929.

75. Fiatarone MA, O'Neill EF, Ryan ND, et al. Exercise training and nutritional supplementation for physical frailty in very elderly people. N Engl J Med. 1994;330: 1769.

76. Kimmel B, Inzuchi SE. Oral agents for type 2 diabetes: an update. Clin Diabetes. 2005;23:64-76.

77. Bloomgaden ZT. New and traditional treatment of glycemia in NIDDM. Diabetes Care. 1996;19:295-9.

78. Shorr RI, Ray WA, Daugherty JR, et al. Incidence and risk factors for serious hypoglycemia in older persons using insulin or sulfonylureas. Arch Int Med. 1997;157:1681.

79 Burge MR, Schmitz-Fiorentino K, Fischette C, et al. A prospective trial of risk factors for sulfonylurea-induced hypoglycemia in type 2 diabetes. JAMA. 1998; 279:137.

80. Graal MB. The use of sulfonylureas in the elderly. Drug and Aging. 1999;15(6): 471-84.

81. Davidson MB, Peters AL. An overview of Metformin in the treatment of type 2 diabetes mellitus. Am J Med. 1997;102:99-110.

82. United Kingdom Prospective Diabetes Study (UKPDS) Group. Effect of intensive blood glucose control with Metformin on complications in overweight patients with type 2 diabetes (UKPDS 34). Lancet. 1998;352:854-65.

83. Sulkin TV, Bosnian D, Krentz AJ. Contraindications to metformin therapy in patients with NIDDM. Diabetes Care. 1997;20:925-8.

84. Lalau JD, Hary L, et al. Type 2 diabetes in the elderly: an assessment of metformin (metformin in the elderly). Int J Clin Pharmacol Ther Toxicol. 1990;28:329-32.

85. Replaglinide for type 2 diabetes mellitus. Medical Letter 1998;40:55-6.

86. Hatorp V, Huang WC, Strange P. Pharmacokinetic profiles of Repaglinide in elderly subjects with type 2 diabetes. JCEM. 1999;84(4):1475-8.

87. Josse RG, Meneilly GS, et al. Acarbose in the treatment of elderly patients with type 2 diabetes. Diab Res Clin Pract. 2003;59(1):37-42.

88. Johnston PS, Munera CL, et al. Advantages of alpha-glucosidase inhibition as monotherapy in elderly type 2 diabetic patients. JCEM. 1998;83(5):151-2.

89. Yki-Jarvinen H. Thiazolindinediones. N Eng J Med. 2004; 351(11):1106-18.

90. Thearle M, Brillantes AM. Unique characteristics of the geriatric diabetic population and the role for therapeutic strategies that enhance glucagon like peptide-1 activity. Curr Opin Clin Nutr Metab Care. 2005;8(1):9-16.

91. Dailey GE III. Early insulin: an important therapeutic strategy. Diabetes Care. 2005;28(1);220-1.

92. Saudek CD. Feasibility and outcomes of insulin therapy in elderly patients with diabetes mellitus. Drugs and Aging. 1999;14(5):375-85.

93. Riddle MC, Rosenstock J, Gerich J. Insulin Glargine 4002 study investigators. The treat to target trial: randomized addition of glargine or human NPH insulin to oral therapy of type 2 diabetic patients. Diabetes Care. 2003;26(11):3080-6.

94. Barnett AH, Owens DR. Insulin Analogues. Lancet. 1997;349:47-51.

95. Bruce DG, Davis WA, Davis TME. Glycemic control in older subjects with type 2 DM in Fremantle Diabetes Study. J Am Geriatric Society. 2000;48(11):1449-53.

96. Tonino RP. Diabetes education: What should health care providers in long-term nursing care facilities know about diabetes? Diabetes Care. 1990;13 (Suppl 2):55.

97. Bernbaum M, McGinnis J, et al. The reliability of self blood glucose monitoring in elderly diabetic patients. J Am Geriatr Soc. 1994;42:79-81.

Chapter 80

DIABETES AND PREGNANCY (GESTATIONAL DIABETES)

V Seshiah, V Balaji

CHAPTER OUTLINE

- Introduction
- Fuel Metabolism in Normal Pregnancy
- Pathogenesis of Glucose Intolerance Developing during Pregnancy
- Fuel Metabolism in Diabetic Pregnancy
- Consequences of Diabetes on the Pregnant Mother

- Pregestational Diabetes
- Gestational Diabetes Mellitus (GDM)
- Screening for GDM
- Management
- Follow-up of GDM
- Summary

INTRODUCTION

A new structure arises *de novo* during pregnancy, develops and matures till it is expelled at the completion of the gestational period. The metabolic adaptations that occur during pregnancy are to accommodate a rapidly growing tissue transplant, i.e. the conceptus. For its own normal growth and development, the conceptus brings about alterations in maternal fuel metabolism and hormones. The placenta facilitates embryogenesis, growth, maturation and survival of the fetus. It has the capacity to synthesize steroid and peptide hormones and to modulate and transport maternal fuel to the fetus. Association of diabetes and pregnancy can occur in two different situations: (i) pregestational diabetes persons becoming pregnant and (ii) gestational diabetes GDM when diabetes or glucose intolerance is detected during gestation.

FUEL METABOLISM IN NORMAL PREGNANCY

The fuel metabolism during normal (nondiabetic) pregnancy is characterized by facilitated insulin action during the first half of pregnancy and diabetogenic stress during the second half of pregnancy. In the early weeks of gestation, fasting insulin concentrations rise as does glucose stimulated insulin release reaching a peak at the 18th to 20th weeks.[1] Serum levels of estrogen and progesterone rise and induce beta cell hyperplasia resulting in increased elaboration and secretion of insulin (hyperinsulinemia) and heightened sensitivity to insulin. Insulin, being an anabolic and anticatabolic hormone, favors tissue glycogen storage, prevents production of glucose from the liver and increases peripheral glucose utilization. The net effect of these anabolic changes is a decrease in fasting blood glucose by 10% compared to nonpregnancy fasting value. The other reason for the decrease in the fasting plasma glucose with advancing gestation is due to increase in plasma volume in early gestation and the increase in fetoplacental glucose utilization later in the late gestation.

During the later half of pregnancy, the facilitated insulin action continues, and at the same time, there is increased elaboration of placental chorionic

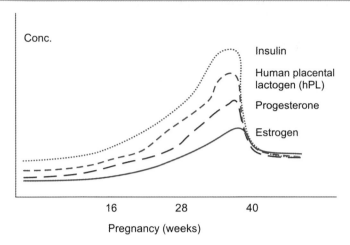

Figure 80.1 Hormonal changes during normal pregnancy

TABLE 80.1	Hormonal and metabolic changes in late pregnancy	
Hormonal	*Effect*	*Metabolic change*
↑ hCS	"Diabetogenic" ↓ Glucose tolerance	Facilitated anabolism during feeding
↑ Prolactin	Insulin resistance	Accelerated starvation during fasting
↑ Bound and free cortisol	↓ Hepatic glycogen stores	↓
	↑ Hepatic glucose production	Ensure glucose and AA to fetus

somatomammotropin (human placental lactogen, hPL), prolactin and cortisol. Hormonal profile and their effect on glucose metabolism is given in **Figure 80.1**.

These surges in counter regulatory hormones result in insulin resistance and stress on the carbohydrate metabolism (diabetogenic stress) and maternal insulin sensitivity is reduced approximately by 50%.[2] Extrainsulin compensates for the 50% reduction in the responsiveness of peripheral tissues to insulin action. In normal glucose tolerant women, first and second phases insulin response increases approximately by three-fold by the third trimester of pregnancy[3] and is associated with maternal B cell hypertrophy and hyperplasia.[4] Overall, the metabolic alterations under the influence of insulin and counterhormones facilitate anabolism during feeding and catabolism during fasting. As the pregnancy advances, the plasma glucose during fasting continues to be low, due to constant removal of glucose by the fetus since the fetus is a continually feeding boarder in an intermittently eating host, i.e. the mother. The lower level of FPG is also attributed to a fall in circulating amino acids particularly alanine needed for gluconeogenesis, a situation of "substrate deficiency syndrome." The conceptus removes both glucose and amino acids from the maternal circulation, the former by facilitated diffusion and the latter by active transport. Hence, during pregnancy, maternal nitrogen is conserved (for fetal use) by sparing protein and relying as little as possible on proteins and carbohydrates as substrate, the maternal metabolism necessarily shifts rapidly to catabolism when exogenous fuel is not available, using fat as the fuel source. Placental hormones help in this metabolic

shift by producing ketogenesis and a state of "accelerated starvation." The metabolic changes which should normally occur after 72 hours of food deprivation in a nonpregnant state occur within 18 hours during pregnancy **(Table 80.1)**.

During fed state, the levels of insulin and glucose are higher and more prolonged. Following a glucose load, glucagon is more readily suppressed during pregnancy than in the nonpregnant state. Though glucose suppresses the alpha cell, the aminogenic stimulation of glucagon is preserved. The combination of enhanced beta cell response to glucose and preserved alpha cell response to amino acids could 'facilitate anabolism' from 'mixed meals' as follows: The "extra" insulin could blunt the gluconeogenic potential of glucagon during the immediate postprandial hyperglycemic period and so "spare" ingested amino acids for both maternal and fetal anabolic utility. Contrarily, after disposal of the ingested carbohydrates, the responsiveness of the alpha cell to the persistent hyperaminoacidemia could initiate enough gluconeogenesis to prevent reactive hypoglycemia in the mother.[5]

In short, facilitated anabolism in the fed state and accelerated starvation in the fasted state characterize the maternal fuel adaptations during pregnancy. These hormonal and metabolic changes are geared towards facilitated anabolism under the actions of insulin throughout pregnancy. However, in the second half of the pregnancy, insulin resistance and diabetogenic stress due to placental hormones necessitate compensatory increased insulin secretion. Changes in maternal metabolism is given in **Table 80.2**.

Hence, the clinical expression of gestational diabetes occurs, where this compensation is inadequate, usually during the second half of pregnancy.

TABLE 80.2	Changes in maternal metabolism during later half of normal pregnancy

- Decreased fasting plasma glucose level
- Relative increase in postprandial plasma glucose level
- Increased fasting and postprandial plasma insulin levels
- β-cell hypertrophy and hyperplasia
- Decreased insulin sensitivity
- Enhanced lipolysis

PATHOGENESIS OF GLUCOSE INTOLERANCE DEVELOPING DURING PREGNANCY

Genetic Factors

The relative importance of genetic factors, are yet to be elucidated while increasing maternal age and obesity are significant contributing and compounding factors.

Gestational Factors

Islet Secretion

In gestational diabetes, during OGTT, the early insulin release is sluggish **(Figure 80.2)**. They have significantly lower insulin response at 30 and 60 minutes after oral glucose, compared to glucose tolerant controls. As pregnancy progresses, the time to reach the maximum glucose concentration also increases. The peak plasma glucose level is attained by 55 minutes at 38 weeks of gestation compared to the nonpregnant value of 34 minutes. [1] There is relative diminution in the biologic activity of circulating immunoreactive insulin while the alpha cell function in gestational diabetes remains normal.

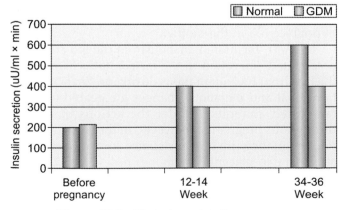

Figure 80.2 First phase insulin response
(*Courtesy*: Dr Patrick Catalano)

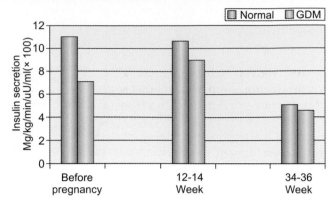

Figure 80.3 Insulin sensibility during gestation
(*Courtesy*: Dr Patrick Catalano)

Insulin Resistance and Hormones of Gestation

In about 20% with gestational diabetes, the sluggish early insulin secretion cannot be demonstrated. It may be that in these individuals, there is an increased elaboration of insulin in response to heightened sensitivity to one or more of the gestational counter hormones (like human placental lactogen, (hPL) leading to decreased insulin sensitivity **(Figure 80.3)**. The postreceptor defects in the insulin signaling cascade appears to be a cause for the decreased insulin sensitivity in both pregnant women with normal glucose tolerance and gestational diabetes[6] compared to weight matched nonpregnant controls. Insulin receptor substrate (IRS-1) expression is decreased in all pregnant women compared to controls. The down regulation of IRS-1 protein parallels the decreased ability of insulin in inducing further steps in insulin signaling cascade. The factors affecting IRS-1 function in the signaling cascade is due to cytokine tumor necrosis factor (TNF).[7] In other words, the pathophysiology of gestational diabetes has been related to excessive insulin antagonism by the pregnancy generated contrainsulin factors. When maternal insulinogenic compensation is inadequate to offset these factors, gestational diabetes supervenes. Further, when gestational diabetics that had reverted to normal glucose tolerance following delivery and women with normal glucose tolerance during last pregnancy were given prednisolone or hPL in the postpartum period and challenged with oral glucose load (OGTT), the former failed to increase plasma insulin levels similar those in the later despite greater hyperglycemia. Thus, the relatively decreased â cell function that occurs in GDM women may be the indication for the future susceptibility to diabetes.[8,9]

FUEL METABOLISM IN DIABETIC PREGNANCY

The effect of diabetic pregnancy on fuel metabolism is one of maternal underutilization of exogenous fuels in the fed state (facilitated anabolism reduced) and overproduction from endogenous sources in the fasted state ('hyper' accelerated starvation). The first sign of pregnancy in a diabetic subject (particularly pregnancy in type-1 DM) as early as the first week of gestation, even before nausea or vomiting sets in, may be early morning fasting ketonuria. This should not be construed as ketoacidosis.

Consequences of the Changes in Fuel Metabolism during Pregnancy on the Fetal Development

Consequences of the changes in fuel metabolism during pregnancy on the fetal development revolve around 'maternal hyperglycemia and fetal hyperinsulinemia' (**Figure 80.4**). Pregnancy is considered as a tissue culture experiment[10] implicating that placenta and fetus develop in an incubation medium that is totally derived

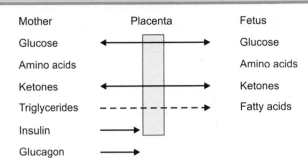

Figure 80.5 Schematic representation of maternal-fetal nutrient transport in humans

from maternal fuels[11] consisting of glucose, amino acids and lipids. The fuels travel the placenta by facilitated diffusion and active transport and enter the fetal circulation (**Figure 80.5**). The recent concept is that the placental glucose transport is dependent on the glucose transporter (GLUT) family and GLUT 1 is the principal transporter which is located in the syncytiotrophoblast.[12] GLUT 1 is present both on the microvilli and basal membranes. With the advancing gestation there is a two- to three-fold increase in the expression of syncytiotrophoblast glucose transportors.[13] The role of GLUT 3 and GLUT 4 remains speculative. Amino acids are actively transported against the concentration gradient from the mother to both placenta and fetus via energy requiring amino acid transporters. These processes are regulated by insulin and hence any disturbance in the secretion and action of insulin would influence the composition of nutrient to which fetus is exposed and may lead to fetal hyperinsulinemia. The abnormal mixture of maternal nutrients gain access to the developing fetus and modify phenotype gene expression in newly forming cells and thereby causing permanent short- and long-term effects upon the offsprings. Accordingly, the fetal and neonatal complications occur when the fetus is exposed to the abnormal fuel mixture during different periods of gestation (**Table 80.3**).

In the first trimester, the exposure to abnormal mixed nutrients during organogenesis (first 6–8 weeks of gestation) may cause spontaneous miscarriage, intrauterine growth retardation and malformations (**Table 80.4**). Most evidence from human pregnancies point to the maternal metabolic abnormalities as the most important cause for the increased risk of malformations in diabetic pregnancies. The mechanism suggested for the teratogenic effect due to disturbances in the early postimplantation stage of the embryo which are as follow:

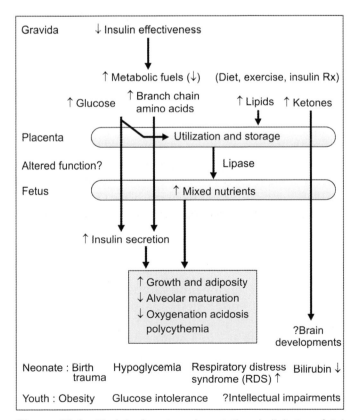

Figure 80.4 Model of maternal gestational diabetes, fetal hyperinsulinemia and infant outcome (Modified from Pedersen hypothesis)

TABLE 80.3	Fetal problems associated with maternal hyperglycemia by trimester wise		
First trimester	*Second trimester*	*Third trimester*	
Malformations	Hypertrophic	Hypoglycemia	
Growth Retardation	Cardiomyopathy	Hypocalcemia	
Fetal wastage	Polyhydramnios	Hyperbilirubinemia	
	Erythema	Respiratory	
	Placental	distress syndrome	
	insufficiency	Macrosomia	
	Pre-eclampsia	Hypomagnesemia	
	Fetal loss	Intrauterine death	
	Low IQ		

TABLE 80.4	Types and timing of malformation in infants of diabetic mothers	
Types of anomaly	*Timing of lesions (Weeks postconception)*	
Skeletal		
Caudal regression	3	
Spina bifida	6	
Neural		
Anencephaly	4	
Myelocele	4	
Hydrocephalus	5	
Cardiovascular		
Dextrocardia	4	
Conus arteriosus defects	5	
Ventricular septal defects	6	
Renal		
Renal agenesis/hypoplasia	6	

a. Disruption of normal functioning of the yolk sac which regulates nutrient transport from maternal plasma to embryo during early neural tube development.
b. Diffusion of intracellular myoinositol with resultant disruption of arachidonic acid and prostaglandin metabolism.
c. Oxidative metabolism and generation of free oxygen radicals that may be toxic to the embryos.
d. Glucose-induced mutations in embryonic DNA.

If this fuel mediated teratogenesis is to be avoided, then excellent control of maternal metabolism must commence before conception and must be maintained during the first eight weeks, a critical period when many women may not be aware that they are pregnant. Preventive medicine necessarily starts before conception reflecting the importance of prepregnancy counseling. Supplementation with folic acid dose (0.4 mg),

myoinositol and antioxidants may play a role in the prevention of malformations and lower the ratio from 7.5 to 0.8%.[14]

Hyperglycemia, during the second trimester when the formation and the development of brain cells takes place, alters the behavioral, intellectual and psychological pattern in childhood.[15,16] Insulin is detectable in the fetal pancreas as early as 9th week after conception. cell growth and replication are regulated by nutritional insulin secretagogues, such as glucose, mannose and essential amino acids.[17] Human studies have shown an increase in pancreatic fetal cell mass and insulin secretion in fetuses of poorly controlled diabetic women of 16th week of gestation and both abnormalities increase throughout second trimester until 26th week of gestation.[18] This priming of cell in mid gestation may account for the persistence of fetal hyperinsulinemia throughout the pregnancy and the risk of accelerated fetal growth even when mother achieves a good metabolic control later in pregnancy.[19]

Maternal hyperglycemia in the third trimester causes proliferation of fetal adipocytes, muscle cells and pancreatic beta cells and neuroendocrine systems. These form the basis for macrosomia and adiposity along with propensity for IGT and type 2 diabetes in later life.[20] Stillbirth in diabetic pregnancies is still unexplained, although both maternal hyperglycemia and fetal macrosomia are usually associated. Mechanisms implicated are fetal hypoxia, acidosis, hyperkalemia leading to dysrhythmias, placental dysfunction and competition for essential nutrients.[21] In an unexplained stillbirth, the possibility of undiagnosed GDM must be considered. At autopsy, the fetus may have islet cell hyperplasia (in the absence of rhesus problem) and increased interstitial tissue in the testis or luteinization of the theca interna of the ovary.

Neonatal Complications

Hypoglycemia

Because of the endogenous hyperinsulinemia and suppression of endogenous glucose production, the infant of the diabetic mother (IDM) is at increased risk of hypoglycemia at 1 to 3 hours after birth. About 50% of the hypoglycemic babies may remain asymptomatic. Twitching of the limbs, hypotonia, tachypnea and rarely seizures in severe hypoglycemia are the clinical presentations. Hypoglycemia is defined as blood sugar level less than 30 mg/dl in any infant regardless of gestational age. Once hypoglycemia is confirmed, IV glucose as an initial bolus at 200 mg/kg must be given and is followed by a continuous glucose infusion at 8 mg/kg/min. The factor mainly protective against fetal hypoglycemia is the optimal control of maternal hyperglycemia, especially during the third trimester and during labor. It has been shown that a mean maternal plasma glucose >105 mg/dl during the last four hours of labor in a diabetic mother leads to a higher incidence of neonatal hypoglycemia.

Hypocalcemia

About 25% of the IDMs may present with serum calcium of <7 mg/dl and this may remain mostly asymptomatic and is usually detectable during the 2nd or 3rd day of the birth. Asphyxia and prematurity, operating through elevated cortisol, induces vitamin D antagonism. Respiratory distress and fetal metabolic acidosis may result in calcium being shifted from intracellular to extracellular pools and reversal of this shift during correction of the acidotic event may produce hypocalcemia. Hypomagnesemia may coexist and may require correction.

Respiratory Distress Syndrome

Respiratory distress syndrome (RDS) observed in about 5% of infants of diabetic mothers. *In vitro* studies indicate that insulin antagonizes the stimulatory effects of cortisol on fibroblasts to induce the synthesis of fibroblast-pneumocyte factor (FPF), which in turn inhibits type II cells and phosphatidylcholine production. Measurement of phosphatidylglycerol alone or in combination with the lecithin phosphatidylcholine may be a more reliable indicator of lung maturity in diabetic pregnancies than the lecithin: sphingomyelin ratio alone. Prophylactic steroids to accelerate the lung maturity may be indicated, if the L:S ratio is less than 2:1. Such obstetric situations, requiring steroids or beta sympathomimetic drugs (e.g. salbutamol) may worsen the diabetes control and calls for frequent monitoring of blood glucose and correction with soluble insulin.

Polycythemia

Relatively common in infants of diabetic mothers (IDM). This is mostly due to the hypoxic stimulus by the placental insufficiency and elevated glycohemoglobin. Overtransfusion from the large placenta of diabetic pregnancy may also contribute. The resultant hyperviscosity may induce congestive heart failure and vascular thrombosis accounting for the increased risk of renal vein thrombosis in these infants.

Hyperbilirubinemia

This common abnormality is due to increased bilirubin production and decreased life span of the RBCs with glycosylated cell membranes. Hepatic conjugation of bilirubin may be impaired due to immaturity of the liver.

Macrosomia

Neonates weighing more than 4 kg are considered to be macrosomic. The Indian consensus is that newborn baby's weight >3.5 kg should be considered as macrosomia.[22] Macrosomic babies have considerable greater shoulder/head and chest/head differences and are prone to shoulder dystocia. Fetal hyperinsulinemia *per se* is accompanied by excessive transfer of nutrients to the fetus and external somatic growth. This phenomenon usually manifests around 28th week of gestation. The fetal insulin has a central role in fetal growth and development approximately around the last 10 weeks of gestation. Meticulous control of maternal metabolism (substrate concentration) tends to normalize the fetal growth to a certain extent. The reduction in size at birth is partly attributed to reduced amount of adipose tissue, which normally accumulates during the last 8 to 10 weeks of gestation.

Two types of macrosomic infants can be identified: (i) constitutional macrosomia, which represents the genetic drive to growth—this infant is LGA (>90th percentile) already in the second trimester and will continue to grow on its own growth curve during pregnancy; and (ii) metabolic macrosomia, which represents diabetic fetopathy as a result of abnormal glucose metabolism—this infant is characterized by increased liver and spleen size (greater abdominal circumference) and normal head size (head circumference). In addition, this infant suffers from an enlarged heart and increased subcutaneous fat.[23]

CONSEQUENCES OF DIABETES ON THE PREGNANT MOTHER

Complications of diabetes in pregnancy occur almost exclusively in pre-gestational diabetic women.

Hypoglycemia

Hypoglycemia may occur in the first trimester of the pregnancy. This is due to combination of physiological adaptation, attempt for strict control and the nausea of early pregnancy.

Diabetic Ketoacidosis

As pregnancy has some features of starvation state, ketoacidosis is a real hazard. DKA has deleterious effect on the fetus.

Retinopathy

Background diabetic retinopathy (BDR) can develop or worsen during pregnancy. It is not a risk for vision and usually regresses postpartum. If BDR is already present, may progress to proliferative diabetic retinopathy (PDR). It is essential to perform periodic ophthalmic examination and in a few photocoagulations may be necessary. The pregnant women in poor glycemic control and with hypertension are at an increased risk of developing PDR. These risks can be minimized by instituting preconception control of diabetes and hypertension

Nephropathy

The risk of worsening diabetic nephropathy depends on baseline renal function and the degree of hypertension. Diabetic women with microalbuminuria may develop albuminuria during pregnancy with regression postpartum. Some among them are likely to develop preeclamptic symptoms. If the initial renal function is impaired in pregnancy, almost 50% of them are likely to show further decline in renal function.

Hypertension

The safe and effective antihypertensive drug during pregnancy is methyldopa. The other alternate drugs are diltiazem, clonidine and prazosin. Better to avoid beta-blockers due to possible association with fetal growth retardation. Angiotensin inhibitors should never be used due to potential damage to the fetal kidneys.

Diabetic Gastropathy

This condition severely exacerbates nausea and vomiting. The drug such as cisapride or mosapride may give relief.

Polyhydramnios

This occurs in poorly controlled diabetic mothers attributed to increased glucose content in the amniotic fluid, creating an osmotic pressure that equilibrates in the presence of an increased volume of amniotic fluid.

TABLE 80.5	White's classification of diabetes in pregnancy
Diabetes Class	Description
A	Euglycemia maintained by diet alone; diabetes may be of any duration and onset may have occurred at any age
B	Onset at age 20 years or older and duration of less than 10 years
C	Onset during age 10–19 years or duration of 10–19 years
D	Onset at age below 10 years, duration of over 20 years, background retinopathy or hypertension (not preeclampsia)
F	Nephropathy with proteinuria exceeding 500 mg/day
R	Proliferative retinopathy or vitreous hemorrhage
RF	Criteria for classes R and F coexist
H	Atherosclerotic heart disease clinically evident
T	Prior to renal transplantation

PREGESTATIONAL DIABETES

This term denotes an already established diabetic marching through pregnancy. The accepted White's classification of diabetes in pregnancy is based on the patient's condition before pregnancy, the duration of diabetes, age of onset, and the complication **(Table 80.5)**.

GESTATIONAL DIABETES MELLITUS

Gestational diabetes mellitus (GDM) is defined as carbohydrate intolerance of variable severity with onset or first recognition during the present pregnancy. The definition applies irrespective of whether or not insulin is used for treatment or the condition persists after pregnancy. It does not exclude the possibility that glucose intolerance may have antedated the present pregnancy. GDM results from sluggish first phase insulin release and in addition to excessive resistance to action of insulin on glucose utilization due to placental hormones (placental lactogen, progestin, prolactin and cortisol). The insulin secretion pattern in nonpregnant women and in GDM is given in **Table 80.6**. They have significantly lower insulin response at 30 and 60 minutes after oral glucose compared to glucose tolerance in controls.[24] A pregnant woman who is not able to increase her insulin secretion to overcome insulin resistance that occurs during nondiabetic pregnancy develops gestational diabetes. The etiology and possible

TABLE 80.6	Insulin secretion in pregnancy

- Insulin secretion is considerably increased in both pregnant women with NGT and women with GDM
- Glucose-stimulated insulin secretion is increased more in normal pregnant women than in women with GDM
- Peak plasma insulin during an OGTT occurs later in women with GDM than in women with NGT
- First phase insulin response to intravenous glucose increases more during pregnancy in women with NGT than in women with GDM
- Increases in second phase insulin responses are of similar magnitude in women with NGT and those with GDM

TABLE 80.7	Etiology and pathogenesis of GDM: possible explanations

- Autoimmune destruction of pancreatic β cells
- Impaired β-cell function genetic, environmental, idiopathic
- Increased insulin degradation (unused)
- Decreased tissue sensitivity to insulin
  - Impaired insulin—insulin receptor binding
  - Impaired intracellular insulin signaling

pathogenesis is given in **Table 80.7**. A considerable proportion about 30% of women with GDM will progress to type 2 DM in the 2 to 20 years after pregnancy.

The risk factors for progression areas follows:
a. Low grade of glucose tolerance during and after pregnancy.
b. Elevated fasting plasma glucose >105 mg.
c. Need for insulin therapy during pregnancy.
d. Obesity.
e. Prior use of contraceptive and IUD.

Abnormal glucose tolerance during pregnancy is not only associated with increasing pregnancy related and perinatal morbidity but also increases the likelihood of subsequent diabetes in the mother. Maternal hyperglycemia has a direct effect on the development of fetal beta cell mass and is associated with increased susceptibility to the development of obesity and diabetes in the offspring **(Figure 80.6)**. This effect on the offspring is independent of other genetic factors. As such GDM has implications beyond the index pregnancy, identifying two generations (mother and her offspring) at risk greater of future diabetes.[25] The recognition of glucose intolerance during pregnancy is more relevant in the Indian context as; Indian women have 11-fold increased risk of developing GDM compared to White women.[25] It is important to detect these GDM cases because, if unrecognized, pregnancy may end in perinatal morbidity.

Effect of Maternal Fuels on Fetal Development

The hyperglycemia-hyperinsulinism hypothesis of Pedersen has been modified to include contributions of other maternal fuels besides glucose that are also responsive to maternal insulin. All of these can influence the growth of the fetus and the maturation of fetal insulin secretion. Within this formulation, growth will be disparately greater in insulin-sensitive than in insulin-insensitive tissues in the fetus.

SCREENING FOR GDM

Methods

Urine Glucose

Glucosuria is still practiced as a screening test for the detection of glucose intolerance. During pregnancy, the renal threshold for glucose is often lowered, due partly to an eight-fold increase in glomerular filtration of

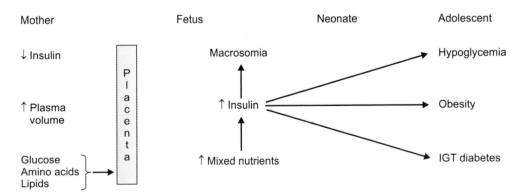

Figure 80.6 Pedersen/Freinkel hypothesis

glucose, and partly, to an intermittent tubular defect in glucose reabsorption. Since glucosuria occurs when the tubular maximum for glucose is exceeded, in some gravid women glucose is found in the urine at lower blood glucose levels than in the nongravid state. Pregnant women with diabetes will find more sugar in the urine even with the similar or better control of their disease. Low renal threshold for glucose during pregnancy renders glucosuria less specific for detection of GDM and must not be used as a diagnostic test.

Blood Glucose

The normally lower blood glucose levels during pregnancy make the nonpregnant blood glucose criteria unsuitable for extrapolation to pregnancy. Oral glucose tolerance test, carried out during each trimester of every pregnancy, is the ideal procedure. This unfortunately is not practicable especially in centers with high birth rates.

Practically, all the pregnant women should undergo screening for glucose intolerance particularly for high-risk population and ethnic groups with higher tendency to develop GDM **(Table 80.8)**. The usual recommendation for screening is between 24 and 28 weeks of gestation. The recent concept is to screen for glucose intolerance in the first trimester itself. If negative, repeated around 24th to 28th weeks and finally around 32nd to 34th weeks.[26]

Spot Test

The simplest practical screening procedures, which can be followed is the 'spot test' based on the study in Madras by Seshiah et al. Consecutive 971 pregnant women at various stages of gestation attending the antenatal clinic at the Institute of Obstetrics and Gynecology and Hospital for Women, Madras, were screened with the spot test. Venous blood sample was obtained at the time of consultation after ascertaining

the time at which the subject last had anything to eat. Interval between the time of last meal and the time of collection of blood sample was corrected to the nearest 30 minutes. Interval of over 3 hours was interpreted as fasting (zero hour) sample. Whole blood glucose was estimated by O-toluidine method. The spot test mean blood glucose values of mean at 0, 30, 60, 90, 120, 150 and 180 minutes with reference to their last meal in the pregnant women studied were 60.5 + 11.0, 68.4 + 13.8, 71.7 + 16.5, 73.0 + 15.2 and 67.1 + 11.4 mg/dl, respectively. The + 2 SD figure of the spot test blood glucose (corrected to nearest 5 mg) was 85 mg/dl at fasting and 105 mg/dl at nonfasting[27] state. The approximate round up plasma glucose values came to be around 90 mg/dl and 120 mg/dl, respectively. In reference pregnant women, the fasting and nonfasting glucose in spot tests did not exceed the above figures. Hence, any pregnant woman whose plasma glucose value exceeds these cutoff points should be subjected to an oral glucose tolerance test.

O'Sullivan's Screening Test

The screening test recommended by O'Sullivan and Mahan[28] was determination of blood glucose one hour after a 50 g oral glucose load. If plasma glucose measures more than 140 mg/dl an oral GTT is ordered. This procedure requires 50 g of glucose and the subject has to remain for only one additional one hour in the clinic.

O'Sullivan and Mahan Diagnostic Criteria

A three-hour oral glucose tolerance test is performed with 100 g of glucose **(Table 80.9)**. If any two of the values meet or exceed the cutoff levels, the test is positive for GDM. If the test is negative, it is repeated during subsequent trimester, particularly in those who gain excessive weight, or show by clinical examination or ultrasound evidence of macrosomia.

TABLE 80.8	Indications for screening
High risk for GDM	*Low risk for GDM*
• Family history of diabetes • Glucose in second fasting urine sample • History of unexplained perinatal loss • History of large for gestational age infant with a low prevalence of GDM • History of congenitally malformed infant • Maternal obesity	• Age <25 years • Weight normal before pregnancy • Member of an ethnic group • No known diabetes in first-degree relatives • No history of abnormal glucose intolerance • No history of poor obstetric outcome

GDM: Gestational diabetes mellitus

TABLE 80.9	O'Sullivan and Mahan diagnostic criteria	
	Blood glucose (mg/dl)	Plasma glucose (mg/dl)
Fasting	90	105
1 hr	165	190
2 hr	145	165
3 hr	125	145

ADA Recommends Two-step Approaches[29]

1. *One Step Approach*—Diagnostic: 100 g oral glucose tolerance test (No prior plasma or serum glucose screening).
2. *Two-step Approach:* An initial screening by measuring plasma glucose one hour after 50 g oral glucose load (glucose challenge test, GCT) and perform a diagnostic OGTT on that subset of women exceeding the glucose threshold value on the GCT. When the two-step approach is employed, a glucose threshold value > 140 mg/dl (7.8 mmol/L) identifies approximately 80% of women with GDM, and the yield is further increased to 90% by using a cutoff of >130 mg/dl (7.2 mmol/L).

Carpenter and Coustan Diagnostic Criteria

The American Diabetes Association has adopted Carpenter and Coustan criteria given in **Table 80.10**.

TABLE 80.10	Diagnosis of GDM	
	100 g OGTT	75 g OGTT
Fasting	95 mg/dl (5.3 mmol/L)	95 mg/dl
1 hr	180 mg/dl (10 mmol/L)	180 mg/dl
2 hr	155 mg/dl (8.6 mmol/L)	155 mg/dl
3 hr	140 mg/dl (7.8 mmol/L)	—

GDM: Gestational diabetes mellitus; OGTT: Oral glucose tolerance test
Two or more of the venous plasma concentrations must be met or exceeded for a positive diagnosis.

WHO Criteria

A Standard OGTT should be performed after over night fasting by giving 75 g of glucose. Plasma glucose is measured at fasting and after two hours. Pregnant women who meet WHO criteria for IGT (2 hr PG > 140 mg/dl are classified as having gestational diabetes mellitus (GDM)[30] **(Table 80.11)**.

If the screening has fasting plasma glucose more than 126 mg and/or 2 hr post glucose more than 200 mg/dl probably she has been having undetected diabetes prior

TABLE 80.11	WHO criteria (plasma glucose)	
	FPG (mg/dl)	2 hr PG (mg/dl)
IGT	<126	140–200
Diabetes	>126	>200

to conception (pre-gestational diabetes) that can be confirmed by A_{1c} estimation.

Glycosylated hemoglobin (A_{1c}): A_{1c} is not suitable for screening for gestational diabetes, since it yields false-positive results in 41% and false-negative in 26%. A_{1c} estimation is useful in pregestational diabetes to know the retrospective blood glucose control at the time of conception if performed in the early first trimester. A_{1c} is also useful in monitoring the control during pregnancy but not for day-to-day management.

Serum fructosamine: Like A_{1c}, serum fructosamine is not a useful screening test for gestational diabetes. This test is useful to assess the short-term state of maternal glucose control during the past two weeks.

Recommendations

American Diabetes Association suggests selective screening for GDM **(Table 80.12)**. Selective screening is applicable for women belonging to ethnic groups with the low prevalence of GDM, whereas ethnically Indian women are more prone to develop glucose intolerance during pregnancy and have eleven-fold increased risk compared to White Caucasians necessitating universal screening during pregnancy.[25]

Disadvantages of Selective Screening

a. Screening for abnormal glucose tolerance (AGT) during pregnancy based on historical risk factors

TABLE 80.12	Indications for screening

- Age >25 years
- Family history of diabetes
- Obesity (Prepregnancy BMI >25)
- BOH - previous history of
  - Unexplained perinatal loss
  - IUD
  - Large for gestational age infant
  - Congenitally malformed infant
  - Polyhydramnios
  - Preeclampsia
- Glucose in second fasting urine sample.

alone leaves 45.4% of the pregnant women unscreened. Among the unscreened 35% had abnormal glucose tolerance.[31]

b. Compared with selective screening, universal screening for GDM detects more cases and improves maternal and offspring prognosis.[32]

The hyperglycemia and adverse pregnancy outcome (HAPO) study was initiated on April 1, 1999. The objective of the study is to clarify unanswered questions on associations of maternal glycemia, less severe than overt diabetes mellitus, with risks of adverse pregnancy outcome. The glucose tolerance is assessed by a 75 g OGTT at 24 to 32 weeks of gestation. The primary outcomes to be assessed in relation to maternal glycemia are cesarian delivery, increased fetal size (macrosomia/LGA/obesity), neonatal morbidity (hypoglycemia), and fetal hyperinsulinism. The study is for five years duration.[33] Till the results of this study are available, a uniform policy of adopting WHO screening and diagnostic criteria is recommended for the following reasons:

1. GDM diagnosis based on two hour 75 g OGTT defined by either WHO or ADA criteria predicts adverse pregnancy outcome.[34]
2. The criteria recommended by WHO are simple and cost-effective and is practiced in many centers. [35,36]
3. Further assuming that effective treatment is available, WHO criteria of 2 hr post Glucose PG >140 mg/dl identifying a large number of cases may have a greater potential for prevention.[37]
4. One step procedure of WHO serves dual purpose of both screening and diagnosis.

Impaired Gestational Glucose Tolerance (IGGT)/Isolated Abnormal Plasma Glucose (IAPG)

Woman with only one abnormal glucose value in 100 g GTT particularly two-hour value >120 mg/dl (IGGT) do have adverse fetal outcome. Maternal and fetal morbidity increases in women with only a single abnormal value in glucose tolerance test during pregnancy.[37] Another study also supports this view, as minor elevations of maternal glucose levels which are insufficient to significantly rise A_{1c} levels are sufficient to produce neonatal macrosomia.[38] Further patients with any glucose value above the upper limit of normal while not necessarily diabetes showed increased placental growth and perinatal mortality. An elegant study using innovative computer based technology indicate patients with one elevated blood glucose value

during formal glucose tolerance testing have higher blood glucose values under ambulatory conditions. Furthermore, these elevated ambulatory glucose values were significantly correlated with fetal macrosomia.[39]

MANAGEMENT

The important predictor of fetal outcome either in pregestational or gestational diabetes is the glycemic control attained immediately before and during pregnancy. The plasma glucose level of normal pregnant women is less than 90 and 120 mg%, respectively during fasting and nonfasting states.[40] Hence, the best fetal outcome can be expected by maintaining the mean plasma glucose level around 105 mg in a pregnant diabetic woman.

Management of Diabetes in Pregnancy
(*Pregestational Type 1 and Type 2 Diabetic Women*)

The congenital malformation remains the leading cause of mortality and serious morbidity in infants of mother with type 1 or type 2 diabetes, in spite of advancement in understanding pregnancy metabolism and treatment. Studies have established association between elevated maternal glucose during embryogenesis and high rates of spontaneous abortions and major malformations in newborn. Clinical trials also have established preconception care to achieve tight glycemic control and during first trimester have resulted in striking reductions in malformations. Unfortunately, unplanned pregnancy occurs in a considerable number of women with diabetes resulting in fetal mortality and morbidity.

The perinatal morbidity attributable to conditions, such as macrosomia and metabolic disorders remain relatively high in women who develop glucose intolerance of any degree with onset or first recognized during pregnancy [Gestational Diabetes Mellitus (GDM)]. Yet, another observation was that in pregnant women with one elevated blood glucose during formal glucose tolerance test have abnormality in glucose values under continuous ambulatory glucose monitoring.[39] These elevated ambulatory glucose values were significantly correlated with fetal macrosomia. Thus, the fetus of pregestational diabetic women, gestational diabetic women or women with any degree of abnormal glucose tolerance during pregnancy is at risk of developing either congenital malformation or morbidity in the form of macrosomia.

To minimize the occurrence of lethal malformations, pregestational counseling is essential. The pregnant women with diabetes need standard care throughout pregnancy. The goal for glycemic management in the preconception period and during the first trimester should be to obtain the lowest A_{lc} test level possible without undue risk of hypoglycemia in the, would be mother. Practical self-management skills are essential for attaining good glycemic control in preparation for pregnancy and during pregnancy.

- Use of appropriate meal plan
- Self monitoring of blood glucose
- Self-administration of insulin and adjustment of insulin doses
- Treatment of hypoglycemia (patient and family members)
- Incorporate safe physical activity
- Development of techniques to reduce stress and cope with the denial.

All these measures are applicable in women with gestational diabetes also.

Insulin Requirement in Pre-GDM

If appropriate prepregnancy counseling has occurred and near euglycemia had been achieved before conception and, if the prepregnancy insulin regimen incorporates two or more insulin injections a day, it may be suitable to achieve the near euglycemia necessary for a successful outcome of the pregnancy. A split/mixed regimen (NPH and regular or lispro or aspart) given in the morning and evening is ideal. NPH insulin given before supper has the likelihood of producing overnight hypoglycemia if the dose is increased to control the next morning's fasting value (even though the patient eats a bedtime snack). This happens because the peak action of the intermediate-acting insulin occurs during the middle of the night. Moving the injection of the evening NPH insulin to bedtime shifts the time of peak action towards early morning and minimizes the possibility of overnight hypoglycemia. Injecting NPH insulin in the morning, however, limits a patient's flexibility in regard to eating and exercise patterns. Unanticipated changes are more difficult to deal with because once the intermediate-acting insulin is given, it exerts its preordained effect for many hours. Using three injections of regular human insulin or rapid acting insulin analogs (Humalog/Novorapid) before each meal gives a patient more flexibility with regard to eating and exercise. Preprandial regular or rapid acting insulin analogs can be particularly helpful during the first trimester, when nausea and anorexia (morning sickness) are common. Controlling the fasting plasma glucose concentration requires evening NPH insulin.

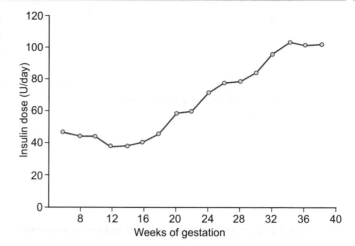

Figure 80.7 Usual changes in insulin requirement in a patient with type 1 DM

Regular insulin is usually given half hour before a meal, because it does not start to work until approximately 30 minutes after injection. On the other hand, the new rapid-acting insulin analogs start to act within 10 to 15 minutes, hence they are much more effective in controlling the postprandial peaks.

Adjusting insulin doses is simpler with self-monitoring of blood glucose (SMBG) administrating of each regular insulin four times a day, because dose of each regular insulin injection affects only one SMBG value. Monitoring before breakfast and 1 to 2 hours postprandial is recommended routinely. Most high-risk and precious pregnancies may require frequent monitoring of blood glucose to find out the fluctuations in levels and adjustment of the dose of insulin. Continuous glucose monitoring system (CGMS) and glucowatch can be more useful in this regard.

In a pregestational type 1 diabetic woman, the requirement of insulin may fall during the early part of first trimester due to increased insulin sensitivity. Insulin requirement increases during later half of pregnancy because of the increased concentration of circulating contrainsulin hormones. Constant adjustment of insulin dosage is necessary to keep up with the increasing insulin requirement of pregnancy **(Figure 80.7).** The insulin dose is increased from 0.7 U / kg/day in the first trimester to 0.8 U/kg/day at week 18, 0.9 U/kg/day at week 26 and 1.0 U/kg/day at week 36 in women who maintain within 15% of ideal body weight. The insulin doses vary from person to person even when weight is almost the same. In a study of 11 patients who were markedly obese at the start of pregnancy, 6 required 1.2 U/kg/day, 3 required 2U/kg/day and 2

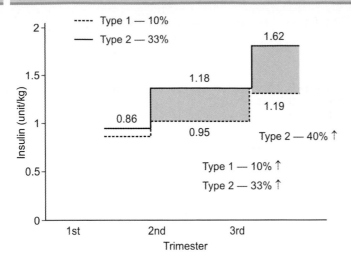

Figure 80.8 Increase in insulin requirement during 2nd and 3rd trimesters in types 1 and 2 diabetes (Adapted from Langer O)

required 3U/kg/day at term. Further type 2 DM patients may require significantly higher dose of insulin during each trimester compared to type 1 DM. During first trimester, no difference was found between type 1 and type 2 subjects. During the second trimester, a significant increase in insulin requirement was observed (10 percent for patients with type 1 compared with 33 percent for those with type 2 DM). In the third trimester a 40% increase has been observed in a group of women with type 2 DM **(Figure 80.8)**. This has been attributed to increased body mass and heightened insulin resistance in type 2 diabetic women with pregnancy.[41] Rarely, a pregestational type 2 diabetic women may require a very high dose of insulin even up to 200 units/day given in divided dose. It is appropriate to use the dose needed to achieve near normal glycemic level without undue concern about giving too much insulin to the patient. The main concern should be blood glucose results rather than the dose of insulin.[42] Failure to increase in the demand for increased insulin dose as pregnancy advances reflects poor placental growth, intrauterine growth retardation and impending intra-uterine death. This situation requires close coordination with obstetrician. A few pregnant women may require less insulin in the last week of pregnancy attributed to fetal handling of maternal glucose due to hypertrophic fetal β cells. At approximately 36 weeks, placental growth stops and contrainsulin hormone production plateaus. Thus, insulin requirement may decline.

Management of GDM

Medical Nutrition Therapy (MNT)

All women with GDM should receive nutritional counseling. The meal pattern should provide adequate calories and nutrients to meet the needs of pregnancy. The expected weight gain during pregnancy is 300 to 400 gm/week and a total weight gain is 10 to 12 kg by term. Hence, the meal plan aims to maintain euglycemia and to provide sufficient calories to sustain adequate nutrition for the mother and fetus and to avoid excess weight gain and postprandial hyperglycemia. Calorie requirement depends on age, activity, prepregnancy weight and stage of pregnancy. Approximately, 30 to 40 kcal/kg ideal body weight or an increment of 300 kcal/day above the basal requirement is needed **(Table 80.13)**. Pregnancy is not the ideal time for obesity correction. Underweight subjects or those not gaining weight as expected, particularly in the third trimester, require admission to ensure adequate nutrition to prevent low birth weight infants.

As a part of the medical nutrition therapy, pregnant diabetic woman are advised to wisely distribute their calorie consumption, especially the breakfast. This implies splitting the usual breakfast portion into two equal halves and consumption of the portions with a two hours gap inbetween. By this the undue peak in plasma glucose levels after ingestion of the total quantity of breakfast at one time is avoided. For example, if 4 slices of bread is suitable for consumption by

TABLE 80.13	Dietary allowances for women 25 to 50 years of age		
Constituent	Non pregnant	Pregnant	Increase
Protein (g)	50	60	10
Average kcal	2,200	2,500	300
Vitamin C (mg)	60	70	10
Vitamin B$_6$ (mg)	1.6	2.2	0.6
Folate (μg)	180	400	220
Calcium (mg)	800	1,200	400
Magnesium (mg)	280	320	40
Iron (mg)	15	30	15
Zinc (mg)	12	15	3

Additional calories are needed during the second and third trimesters only

subjects with DM (applies to all type of breakfast menu) is taken for breakfast at 8 am and two hours plasma glucose at 10 am is 140 mg: the same quantity divided into two portions, i.e. two slices at 8 am and remaining two slices after 10 am, the two hours post-prandial plasma glucose at 10.00 am falls by 20 to 30 mg.

This advice has distinct scientific basis as the peaking of plasma glucose is high with breakfast (due to Dawn phenomenon) compound to lunch and dinner. Further in a normal person, insulin secretion is also high with breakfast than with lunch or dinner.[43] Since GDM mothers have deficiency in first phase insulin secretion and to match this insulin deficiency the challenge of glycemic load at one time should also be less.

Insulin Treatment (Human Insulin)

Insulin is essential, if medical nutrition therapy fails to achieve euglycemia. The treatment of GDM with insulin requires several decisions. In a normal (nondiabetic) pregnancy, the fasting plasma glucose (FPG) concentration ranges between 55 and 70 mg/dl, the 1 hour postprandial glucose level is <120 mg/ dl.[40]

Various criteria have been proposed for the initiation of insulin therapy **(Table 80.14)**. To interpret these values, one must take into account the relationship between plasma and whole blood glucose concentrations, the site of sampling and whether the value is a fasting or a postprandial one. It is enough to realize that a plasma value is approximately 12% higher than a whole blood value. A finger stick yields arterialized blood, which does not influence the fasting glucose concentration because in the fasting state there is little glucose uptake by muscle tissue. After eating, however, muscle glucose utilization becomes a factor. Measurement of glucose concentrations in blood samples obtained by a finger stick yields higher values than if a venous sample had been obtained. This is because the arterialized blood in the sample has not yet traversed muscle and glucose removal by this tissue has not occurred.

If the FPG concentration on the OGTT is >120 mg/ dl, the patient is started on insulin immediately. Others are seen within 3 days and are also taught self monitoring of blood glucose (SMBG) to be performed before breakfast and 2 hours after each meal. Insulin is started within 1 to 2 weeks if the majority (i.e. at least four of seven per week) of fasting BG values exceed 95 mg/dl. Similarly, if the majority of postprandial values after a particular meal exceed 120 mg/dl, insulin is started. Pen injectors are very useful and the patients acceptance is excellent. The initial dose of NPH insulin could be as low as 4 units and adjusting the dose of insulin on follow-up. A few GDM patients may require combination of short-acting insulin and intermediate-acting insulin in the morning and evening. If a patient has elevated prelunch blood sugar, regular insulin is usually necessary in the morning to handle the post-breakfast hyperglycemia, because of the lag period before the intermediate-acting insulin begins to work. The above regimen of regular and intermediate-acting insulin in the morning controls hyperglycemia in most cases.

If the post-dinner blood sugar is high a small dose of regular insulin is necessary before dinner in addition to the regular and intermediate-acting insulin given in the morning. Combination of regular and intermediate-acting insulin before dinner may be necessary if fasting blood sugar is high. This combination of short and intermediate acting insulin in the morning and as well as in the evening is known as mixed and split dose of insulin regimen. In this regimen, two-thirds of the total daily dose of insulin is given in the morning and one-third in the evening. For each combination one-third dose should be regular insulin and two-thirds intermediate-acting insulin. With this regimen, if the patient continues to have fasting hyperglycemia, the intermediate acting insulin has to be given at bedtime instead of before dinner.

TABLE 80.14	Criteria recommended for the initiation of insulin therapy in women with gestational diabetes	
Fasting[a]	Postprandial	Reference
>80	1 hour >140	Jovanovic-Peterson and Peterson
105[b]	None	Metzger
>95	2 hour >120	Langer et al
>100	1 hour >130	Ramus and Kitzmiller
>90	1 hour >120	Jovanovic-Peterson

[a]Glucose concentrations (mg/dl) measured in finger-stick whole blood samples unless designated otherwise
[b]Venous plasma sample
Adapted from American Diabetes Association. Nutritional management during pregnancy in preexisting diabetes. In Jovanovic-Peterson L (Ed): Medical Management of Pregnancy Complicated by Diabetes. American Diabetes Association, Alexandria, VA; 1993. pp. 47-56.

TABLE 80.15	Mean glucose level perinatal mortality
>150 mg%	24%
100 to 150 mg%	15%
<100 mg%	4%

Ultrasound Fetal Measurement

GDM management based on fetal growth combined with glycemic criteria provides outcomes equivalent to management based on strict glycemic criteria alone. Inclusion of fetal growth might provide the opportunity to reduce glucose testing in low-risk pregnancies.[44]

Target Blood Glucose Levels

Maintenance of mean blood glucose level around 105 mg% is ideal for good fetal outcome.[45] A study by Karlson and Kjellman from Sweden showed that perinatal mortality is proportional to maternal blood glucose level during the last weeks of pregnancy[46] (Table 80.15).

The maintenance of mean plasma glucose around 105 mg% would protect the newborn from hypoglycemia (Fasting 80 to 90 mg% and 2 hour postmeal 110 to 120 mg%). The recent concept is to maintain 1 hr postprandial plasma glucose < 120 mg/dl. Excess glucose crosses the placenta and stresses the fetal β-cells which respond by increased elaboration of insulin. As long as fetus is in the uterine compartment, it has enough fuel to maintain its blood glucose level. When the fetus is expelled at the termination of pregnancy, the super charged β-cells of the neonate continue to secrete insulin but there is no fuel supply from the maternal compartment and the newborn develops hypoglycemia. On the contrary, if plasma glucose of the mother had been maintained at the acceptable level with diet and insulin, an excess flow of glucose from maternal to fetal compartment cannot occur to stimulate fetal β-cells and the newborn of this mother would not develop hypoglycemia. The fact that maternal hypoglycemia does not jeopardize fetal outcome, is very well brought out by a study done in Düsseldorf, Germany. Out of seventy-seven pregnant women with type 1 DM, 32 had 94 episodes of severe hypoglycemia with loss of consciousness requiring hospital admission in some. There was no difference in fetal outcome between those mothers who had severe hypoglycemia and those who did not. Nevertheless, all efforts should be taken to avoid hypoglycemia in the pregnant mother.

Species of Insulin

It is ideal to use highly purified porcine or human insulin which are least immunogenic. Though insulin does not cross the placenta, the anti-insulin antibodies due to bovine insulin can cross the placenta, and stress the fetal beta cell, increase insulin production and induce macrosomia. Rapid acting insulin analogs (Humalog/Novorapid) have been found to be safe during pregnancy.[47]

Oral Antidiabetic Drugs

Sometimes, an undiagnosed type 2 diabetic woman may progress through the early weeks of gestation at the risk of malformation in her offspring, or a known type 2 diabetic woman who is already on oral hypoglycemic agent may present to antenatal clinic after conception and at times in second or third trimester of pregnancy. The best course at this juncture is to withdraw oral hypoglycemic agents and introduce insulin. Though oral antidiabetic drugs are not recommended, the outcome in diabetic women who have conceived and continued to be on oral antidiabetic drugs is not gloomy, since many workers have used these drugs successfully in pregnant diabetics.[48] Recently, it has been reported good fetal outcome in GDM who were on glyburide (micronised form of glibenclamide). Oral glucose lowering agents have generally not been recommended during pregnancy. However, one randomized unblinded clinical trial compared the use of insulin and glyburide in women with GDM who were not able to meet glycemic goals on meal plan. Treatment with either agent resulted in similar perinatal outcomes. All these patients were beyond the first trimester of pregnancy at the initiation of therapy.[49]

A few more studies are required before routinely recommending glyburide during pregnancy. Metformin has been found to be useful in women with polycystic ovarian disease (PCOD) who failed to conceive. Continuing this drug after conception is still in controversy. But there are a few studies favoring continuation of metformin throughout pregnancy.[50]

Obstetric Considerations

About a decade ago sudden intrauterine fetal demise in the third trimester of diabetic pregnancy was not uncommon. To avoid this risk, preterm delivery was instituted but with this the incidence of respiratory distress syndrome (RDS) increased. In the event of

TABLE 80.16	Obstetrical management procedures		
Procedures	Risk based on glycemic control, vascular disease		
	Low-risk	High-risk	
Dating ultrasound	8–12 weeks	8–12 weeks	
Prenatal genetic diagnosis	As needed	As needed	
Targeted perinatal ultrasound: fetal echocardiography	18–22 weeks	18–22 weeks	
Fetal kick counts	28 weeks	28 weeks	
Ultrasound for fetal growth	28 and 37 weeks*	Monthly	
Antepartum fetal heart rate (FHR) monitoring, back up with biophysical profile	36 weeks, weekly	27 weeks, 1–3/week	
Amniocentesis for lung maturity	—	35–38 weeks	
Induction of labor	41 weeks**	35–38 weeks	

*Not needed in normoglycemic, diet-treated women with GDM.
**Earlier for obstetrical reasons or for impending fetal macrosomia

administering steroids for lung maturity or β adreno-receptor agonist to inhibit premature uterine contraction is likely to induce adverse metabolic effects due to their glycolytic and glycogenolytic and lipolytic effects and extrainsulin may be required to maintain euglycemia. Rarely, fetal demise can occur due to preeclampsia, which can produce fetal hypoxia via decreased utero-placental perfusion. The recent advances in techniques for detecting fetal well-being are given in **Table 80.16**. Unless maternal or fetal complications arise the goal for timing of delivery should be 39 to 40 weeks. Having a neonatologist support at the time of delivery is advisable. This applies particularly to subjects with good glycemic control throughout the 3rd trimester of pregnancy.

Fetal Evaluation

An ultrasound scan has to be performed around 18 to 20 weeks of gestation focusing on structures namely the spine, skull, kidney and heart. Fetal echocardiography has to be done around 20 to 24 weeks which allows to view all the four chambers of the heart. From 26th week onwards, fetal growth and liquor volume has to be monitored every 2 to 3 weeks. Fetal abdominal circumference provides baseline for further serial measurements, which gives growth acceleration or restriction. Fetal movements are monitored from 20 weeks onwards. Screening for chromosomal anomalies is necessary in pre-GDM. Screening should be done for Down syndrome, alpha fetoprotein for neural defects and human chorionic gonadotrophin to identify any chromosomal abnormalities.

Mid pregnancy (16–20 wk) to detect fetal anomalies
- Maternal serum alpha fetoprotein
- Screening for chromosomal anomalies
- Ultrasonography
- Fetal echocardiography.

Late Pregnancy (28 wk to delivery) to assess fetal well-being
- Maternal assessment of fetal activity (< 4/hr indicate fetal jeopardy)
- Nonstress test
- Contraction stress test
- Fetal biophysical profile
- Ultrasonography
- Lecithin-to-sphingomyelin (L/S) ratio (>3.0), lung profile.

Intrapartum Diabetic Management

Metabolic studies of nondiabetic pregnant women during labor revealed that glucose turnover increased four-fold with little change in insulin levels.[51] This strongly suggests that muscle contractions (probably both uterine and skeletal) independent of insulin are the predominant determinant of glucose utilization during labor. During active labor, the insulin requirement was zero while glucose requirements were relatively constant at 2.6 mg/kg/min or approximately 10 g/h in a 60 kg woman.[52]

The following approach is suggested for treating an insulin-requiring woman with pregestational diabetes, as she progresses through labor and delivery. If labor is to be induced, induction should start in the morning. The usual dose of evening NPH insulin is taken, but no morning insulin is given. The goal is to maintain the

TABLE 80.17	Plasma glucose and insulin IV fluid
Plasma glucose	Insulin/IV fluids
60–90 mg/dl	5% DNS-100 ml/hr
90–120 mg/dl	NS-100 ml/hr
120–140 mg/dl	NS-100 ml/hr *plus* 4 units of Reg. insulin added with IV fluid
140–180 mg/dl	NS-100 ml/hr *plus* 6 units of Reg. insulin added with IV fluid
>180 mg/dl	NS-100 ml/hr *plus* 8 units of Reg. insulin added with IV fluid

glucose concentration between 70 and 100 mg/dl. Most labor and delivery units have the ability to measure finger-stick glucose concentrations, and this should be done every hour. If labor is to be induced, intravenous saline is infused until active labor begins. If the initial glucose concentration is <70 mg/dl, 5% dextrose is infused at 100 ml/hr until the glucose level is in the appropriate range. The IV fluids, insulin dose to be given on monitoring the blood glucose level is given in **Table 80.17**.

When active labor begins, the same insulin infusion rate described earlier is used, depending on the glucose concentration at this time as well. In contrast, a woman with GDM does not require insulin once labor begins. If labor is to be induced in GDM, the usual evening NPH insulin should be taken the night before, but no subcutaneous insulin is given the following morning when induction begins and to follow the guidelines given in **Table 80.17**.

In a gestational diabetic subject the requirement of insulin is likely to fall precipitously and no insulin may be required immediately after expulsion of placenta. In a known diabetic the dose of insulin has to be adjusted by monitoring blood glucose.

FOLLOW-UP OF GDM

GDM may be viewed as:
- An unidentified preexisting disease, or
- The unmasking of a compensated metabolic abnormality by the added stress of pregnancy, or
- A direct consequence of the altered maternal metabolism stemming from the changing hormonal milieu.

Gestational diabetic women require follow-up and glucose tolerance test is repeated after 6 weeks and, if necessary, after 6 months to determine whether the glucose tolerance has returned to normal. A small proportion of gestational diabetic women may continue to have glucose intolerance.

GDM recurs approximately in 50% of subsequent pregnancies. The future risk of developing diabetes for a gestational diabetic is two-fold, if she becomes overweight but maintaining ideal weight approximately halves the risk. The requirement of insulin in addition to diet to maintain euglycemia during the index pregnancy is also predictive of future diabetes.

In conclusion, the scope of diabetes and pregnancy encompasses not only a known patient of diabetes marching through pregnancy (pregestational diabetes mellitus) but also any form of abnormal glucose tolerance developing during gestation. A known diabetic subject marching through pregnancy represents only the tip of the diabetic pregnancy iceberg. Abnormal glucose tolerance of any etiology, during pregnancy, is associated with a high-risk of a poor outcome like miscarriage, stillbirth, and neonates with heavy birth weight, hypotrophic infants and small for dates, children with lethal or handicapping congenital malformations which can be morally and socially demanding. The pregnant mothers may also develop hydramnios, toxemia and recurrent urinary tract infections. The maternal health and fetal outcome depends upon the care by the committed team of diabetologists, obstetricians and neonatologists. A short-term intensive care gives a long-term pay off in the primary prevention of obesity, IGT and diabetes, as the preventive medicine starts before birth.

SUMMARY

The fuel metabolism during normal (nondiabetic) pregnancy is characterized by facilitated insulin action during the first half of pregnancy and diabetogenic stress during the second half of pregnancy. In the early weeks of gestation, fasting insulin concentrations rise as does glucose stimulated insulin release reaching a peak at the 18th to 20th week.

During the later half of pregnancy, the basic facilitated insulin action continues and at the same time there is increased elaboration of placental chorionic somatomammotropin (human placental lactogen, hPL), prolactin and cortisol.

Facilitated anabolism in the fed state and accelerated starvation in the fasted state characterize the maternal fuel adaptations during pregnancy. Insulin secretion is considerably increased in both pregnant women with normal glucose tolerance and women with GDM. Peak plasma insulin during an OGTT occurs later in women with GDM than in women with normal glucose tolerance. However, in the second half of the pregnancy, insulin resistance and diabetogenic stress due to placental hormones necessitate compensatory increased insulin secretion. The clinical expression of gestational diabetes occurs, where this compensation is inadequate.

Consequences of the changes in fuel metabolism during pregnancy on the fetal development revolve around 'maternal hyperglycemia and fetal hyper-insulinemia.' Pregnancy is considered as tissue culture experiment implicating that placenta and fetus develop in an incubation medium that is totally derived from maternal fuels consisting of glucose, amino acids and lipids. The fuels travel the placenta by facilitated diffusion and active transport and enter the fetal circulation.

In the first trimester, the exposure to abnormal mixed nutrients during organogenesis (first 6–8 weeks of gestation) may cause spontaneous miscarriage, intra-uterine growth retardation, and malformations.

Hyperglycemia, during the second trimester when the formation and the development of brain cells takes place, alters the behavioral, intellectual and psychological pattern in childhood.

Maternal hyperglycemia in the third trimester causes proliferation of fetal adipocytes, muscle cells and pancreatic β-cells and neuroendocrine systems. These account for macrosomia and the development of obesity, IGT and type 2 diabetes in later life.

Complications of diabetes in pregnancy occur almost exclusively in pregestational diabetic women. Complications that are likely to be inducted or aggravated are hypoglycemia, diabetic ketoacidosis, retinopathy, nephropathy, hypertension, diabetic gastropathy and polyhydramnios. Neonatal complications are hypoglycemia, hypocalcemia, respiratory distress syndrome, polycythemia, hyperbilirubinemia and macrosomia.

Practically, all pregnant women should undergo screening for glucose intolerance while it is imperative for high-risk patients likely to develop GDM. Universal screening is recommended in population ethnically more prone to develop glucose intolerance during pregnancy.

The important predictor of fetal outcome either in pregestational or gestational diabetes is the glycemic control attained immediately before and during pregnancy. The plasma glucose level of normal pregnant women is less than 90 and 120 mg%, respectively during fasting and nonfasting states.

Congenital malformation remains the leading cause of mortality and serious morbidity in infants of mother with type 1 or type 2 diabetes. To minimize the occurrence of lethal malformations, pregestational counseling is essential.

If appropriate prepregnancy counseling has taken place and near euglycemia had been achieved before conception, and if, the prepregnancy insulin regimen incorporates two or more insulin injections a day, it may be suitable to achieve the near euglycemia necessary for a successful outcome of the pregnancy.

In a pregestational type 1 diabetic woman the requirement of insulin may fall during the early part of first trimester. Insulin requirement increases during later half of pregnancy because of the increased concentration of circulating contra insulin hormones. Constant insulin adjustment is necessary to keep up with the increasing insulin requirement of pregnancy.

All women with GDM should receive nutritional counseling. The meal pattern should provide adequate calories and nutrients to meet the needs of pregnancy. Insulin is essential, if medical nutrition therapy fails to achieve euglycemia. Maintenance of mean blood glucose level around 105 mg% is ideal for good fetal outcome.

Oral glucose lowering agents have generally not been recommended during pregnancy. However, one randomized unblinded clinical trial compared the use of insulin and glyburide in women with GDM who were not able to meet glycemic goals on meal plan. Treatment with either agent resulted in similar perinatal outcomes. All these patients were beyond the first trimester of pregnancy at the initiation of therapy. Metformin has been used in women with PCOS with successful fetal outcome.

Unless maternal or fetal complications arise the goal for timing of delivery should be 39 to 40 weeks. An ultrasound scan has to be performed around 18 to 20 weeks of gestation focusing on structures, namely the spine, skull, kidney and heart. Fetal echocardiography has to be done around 20 to 24 weeks which allows to view all the four chambers of the heart.

During intrapartum management of diabetes, the goal is to maintain the glucose concentration between 70 and 100 mg/dl. A woman with GDM does not require insulin once labor begins. In a gestational diabetic, the requirement of insulin is likely to fall precipitously and no insulin may be required immediately after expulsion of placenta. In a known diabetic, the dose of insulin has to be adjusted by monitoring blood glucose.

The future risk of developing diabetes for a gestational diabetic is over two-fold, if she becomes overweight; but maintaining ideal weight approximately halves the risk.

The maternal health and fetal outcome depends upon the care by the committed team of diabetologists, obstetricians and neonatologists.

A short-term intensive care gives a long-term pay off in the primary prevention of obesity, IGT and diabetes, as the preventive medicine starts before birth.

REFERENCES

1. Lind T, Billewicz WZ, Brown G. A serial study of changes occurring in the oral glucose tolerance test during pregnancy. J Obstet Gynaecol Br Commonw 1973;80:1033-9.
2. Buchanan TA, Metzger BE, Frienkel N, Bergman RN. Insulin sensitivity and cell responsiveness to glucose during late pregnancy in lean and moderately obese women with normal glucose tolerance or mild gestational diabetes. Am J Obstet Gynecol 1990;162:1008-114.
3. Catalano PM, Huston L, Amini SB, Kalhan SC. Longitudinal changes in glucose metabolism during pregnancy in obese women with normal glucose tolerance and gestational diabetes mellitus. Am J Obstet Gynecol 1999;180:903-16.
4. Van Assche FA, Aerts L, De Prins F. A morphological study of the endocrine pancreas in human pregnancy. Br J Obstet Gynaecol 1978;85:818-20.
5. Metzger BE, Unger RG, Frienkel N. Carbohydrate metabolism in pregnancy.XIV. Relationships between circulating glucagons, insulin, glucose, and amino acids in response to 'mixed meal' in late pregnancy. Metabolism 1977;26:151-6.
6. Friedman JE, Ishizuka T, Shao J, et al. Impaired glucose transport and insulin receptor tyrosine phosphorylation in skeletal muscle from obese women with gestational diabetes. Diabetes 1999;48:1807-14.
7. Catalano P, Highway T, Huston L, Friedman J. Relationship between reproductive hormones/TNF a and longitudinal changes in insulin sensitivity during gestation. Diabetes 1996;45:175A.
8. Buchanan TA, Xiang A, Kjos SL, et al. Gestational diabetes: antepartum characteristics that predict postpartum glucose intolerance and type 2 diabetes in Latino women. Diabetes 1998;47:1302-10.
9. Buchanan TA, Xiang AH, Peters RK, et al. Response of pancreatic cells to improved insulin sensitivity in women at high risk for type 2 diabetes. Diabetes 2000;49:782-8.
10. Frienkel N. Of pregnancy and progeny. Diabetes 1980;29:1023-35.
11. Pederson J. Foetal mortality in the pregnant diabetic and her newborn. Baltimore: Williams S Wilkins; 1967. pp 108-27.
12. Barros LF, Yudilevich DL, Jarvis SM, et al. Quantitation and immunolocalization of glucose transporters in the human placenta. Placenta 1995;16:623-33.
13. Jansson T, Wennergren M, Illsley NP. Glucose transporter expression and distribution in the human placenta throughout gestation and in intrauterine growth retardation. J Clin Endocrinol Metab 1993;77:1554-62.
14. Hod M. Clinical and experimental advances in diabetic embryopathy. Diabetes Reviews International 1997;6:10-4.
15. Philips AF, Porte PJ, Stabinsky S, Risenkrantz TS, Raye JR. Effects of chronic fetal hyperglycemia upon oxygen consumption in the bovine uterus and conceptus. J Clin Invest 1984;74:279-86.
16. Rizzo T, Metzger BE, Burns WJ, Burns K. Correlation between antipartum maternal metabolism and intelligence of offspring. N Engl J Med 1991;325:911-6.
17. Swenne I. Pancreatic beta-cell growth and diabetes mellitus. Diabetologia 1992;35:193-201.
18. Reiher H, Fuhramann K, Noack S, et al. Age dependent insulin secretion of the endocrine pancreas in vitro from fetuses of diabetic and non diabetic patients. Diabetes Care 1983;6:446-51.
19. Carpenter MW, Canick JA, Hogan JW, et al. Amniotic fluid insulin at 14-20 weeks gestation: associated with later maternal glucose intolerance and birth macrosomia. Diabetes Care 2001;24:1259-63.
20. Silverman BL, Metzger BE, Cho NM, Loeb CA. Impaired glucose tolerance in adolescent offspring of diabetic mothers: relationship to foetal hyperinsulinism. Diabetes Care 1995;18:611.
21. Salafia CM. The foetal, placental and neonatal pathology associated with maternal diabetes. In Reece EA, Coustan BR (Eds): Diabetes Mellitus in Pregnancy: Principles and Practice. NewYork: Churchill Livingston; 1988. pp. 143-81.
22. Vinod K Paul, Ashok K Deorari, Meharban Singh. Management of low birth weight babies. In Parthasarathy A (Ed): IAP Textbook of Pediatrics, 2nd edition. New delhi: Jaypee Brothers; 2002. p. 60.
23. Langer O, Kagan-Hallet K. Diabetic vs. non-diabetic infants: a quantitative morphological study. Proceedings of the 38th Annual Meeting of the Society for Gynaecologic Investigation, San Antonio, Texas, 1992.
24. Nicholls JSD, Chan SP, Ali K, Beard RW, Dornhorst A. Insulin secretion and sensitivity in women fulfilling WHO criteria for gestational diabetes. Diabet Med 1993;10:278-81.
25. Dornhost A, Paterson CM, Nicholls JS, Wadsworth J, Chiu DC, Elkeles RS, Johnston DG, Beard RW. High prevalence of GDM in women from ethnic minority groups. Diabetic Med 1992;9(9):820-2.
26. Nahum GG, Wilson SB, Stanislaw H. Early-pregnancy glucose screening for gestational diabetes mellitus. J Reprod Med 2002;47(8):656-62.
27. Seshiah V, Ramanakumar T.K, Sundaram A, Hariharan R.S, Anjalakshi A, Seshasainam M, Janakiram C, Sam GPMoses. The Antiseptic 1982;78:52-61.
28. O'Sullivan JM, Mahan CM. Criteria for the oral glucose tolerance test in pregnancy. Diabetes 1964;13:278-85.
29. ADA: Clinical practice recommendations 2002. Diabetes Care 2002;25: (Suppl 1).
30. WHO study group prevention of diabetes mellitus. Geneva. World Health org. 1994 (Tech Report series 844).
31. Anjalakshi Chandrasekhar, PhD thesis submitted to Dr. MGR. Medical University, 2002. Evaluation of diagnostic criteria for abnormal glucose tolerance AGT in south Indian pregnant women.
32. Cosson E, et al. Screening and insulin sensitivity in gestational diabetes. Abstract volume of the 40th Annual Meeting of the EASD, September 2004, A 350.

33. HAPO Study Co-operative Research Group. Special communication: the hyperglycemia and adverse pregnancy outcome (HAPO) study. Intern J Gynae Obstet 2002;78:69-77.

34. Schmidt MI, Duncan BB, Reichelt AJ, Branchtein L, Matos MC, Costa e Forti A, Spichler ER, Pousada JM DC, Teixeira MM, Yamashita T for the Brazilian Gestational Diabetes Study Group. Gestational diabetes mellitus diagnosed with a 2 h 75 g oral glucose tolerance test and adverse pregnancy outcomes. Diabetes Care 2001;24(7):1151-5.

35. Pettitt DJ, Bennett PH, Hanson RL, Venkat Narayanan KM, Knowler WC. Comparison of World Health Organization and National Diabetes Data Group procedures to detect abnormalities of glucose tolerance during pregnancy. Diabetes Care 1994;17:1264-8.

36. Moses RG. Is it time to modify the GTT for the diagnosis of gestational diabetes? (Letter) Diabetes Care 1995;18:886.

37. Lindsay MK, Graves W, Klein L. The relationship of one abnormal glucose tolerance test value and pregnancy complications. Obstet Gynecol 1989;73(1):103-6.

38. Jovanovic-Peterson L, Bevier W, Peterson CM. The Santa Barbara County Health Care Services Program: birth weight change concomitant with screening for and treatment of glucose intolerance of pregnancy: a potential cost-effective intervention? Am J Perinatol 1997;14(4):221-8.

39. Oded Langer. Scientific rational for management of diabetes in pregnancy. Recent approaches with innovative computer based technology. Diabetes Care 1988;11(Suppl. 1):67-72.

40. Jovanovic-Peterson L. The diagnosis and management of gestational diabetes mellitus. Clin Diabetes 1995;13:32.

41. Langer O, Anyaegbunam A, Brustman L, et al. Pregestational diabetes: insulin requirements throughout pregnancy. Am J Obstet Gynaecol 1988;159:616.

42. Oded Langer. Maternal glycemic criteria for insulin therapy in gestational diabetes mellitus. Diabetes Care 1998;21(suppl 2):B91-8.

43. Polonsky KS, Given BD, van Cauter E. Twenty-four- hour profiles and pulsatile patterns of insulin secretion in normal and obese subjects. J Clin Invest 1988;81:442-8.

44. Ute M. Schaefer-Graf, et al. A randomized trial evaluating a predominately fetal growth-based strategy to guide management of gestational diabetes in Caucasian women. 2004;27(2):297-302.

45. Langer O, Levy J, Brustman L, Anyaegubunam A, Merkatz R, Divon MY. Glycemic control in gestational diabetes mellitus: how tight is tight enough: small for gestational age versus large for gestational age? Am J Obstet Gynecol 1989;161:646-53.

46. Karlsson K, Kjellman I. The outcome of diabetic pregnancies in relationship to the mother's blood sugar level. Am J obstet Gynaecol 1972;112:213-20.

47. Patmore JE, Mason EA, Brash PD, Boxter M, Caldwell G, Gallen J, Price PA, Vice PA, Walker J, Lindow SW. Maternal outcome in type 2 diabetic pregnancy treated with insulin lispro. Abstract 2275 PO, the 61st Scientific sessions, American Diabetes Association, Philadelphia PA. 2001; June 22-26.

48. Coetzee EJ, Jackson WPU. The management of non-insulin dependent diabetes during pregnancy. Diabetes Res Clin Pract 1986;1:281.

49. Langer L, Conway DL, Berkus MD, et al. A comparison of glyburide and insulin in women with gestational diabetes mellitus. N Engl J Med 2000;343:1134-8.

50. Jakubowicz DJ, Iuorno MJ, Jakubowicz S, Roberts KA, Nestler JE. Effects of metformin on early pregnancy loss in the polycystic ovary syndrome. J Clin Endocrinol Metab 2002;87(2):524-9.

51. Maheux PC, Bonin B, Dizazo A, et al. Glucose homeostasis during spontaneous labor in normal human pregnancy. J Clin Endocrinol Metab 1996;81:209.

52. Ogata ES. Perinatal morbidity in offspring of diabetic mothers. Diabetes Rev 1995;3:652.

Chapter 81

SURGERY AND DIABETES

KM Prasanna Kumar, Geetha K Bhat

CHAPTER OUTLINE

- Introduction
- Metabolic Issues
- Effect of Surgery on Diabetes
- Morbidity and Mortality
- Preoperative Evaluation
- Preoperative Recommendation for Type 2 Diabetics on Oral Hypoglycemic Agents
- Type 2 Diabetics on Insulin
- Surgery in Type 1 Diabetic
- Moderate Control of Diabetes

- Postoperative Management
- Infections
- Anesthesia in a Diabetic Patient
- General Anesthesia
- Special Situation
- Open Heart Surgery
- Emergency Surgery in a Diabetic with Ketoacidosis
- Laparoscopic Surgery
- Cesarian Section
- Summary

INTRODUCTION

The last two decades has seen steady rise of prevalence of diabetes worldwide. Because of increasing longevity of people with diabetes, the likelihood of their undergoing surgery is increasing. One of the estimates in 1960 showed that diabetic patients have 50% chance of undergoing surgery at sometime during their lifetime.[1] With advances in various fields of surgery and anesthesia diabetics today, have much higher chances of undergoing surgery. A diabetic patient spends 30 to 50% more time in the hospital than a nondiabetic following major surgery, even if the surgery proceeds without an incident. In 1980, 11.3% of all surgeries were performed on diabetic patients, compared to 4.3% in nondiabetics. About 5.5% of ophthalmologic procedures involved diabetic patients compared with 3.3% in

persons without diabetes. Diabetes is the leading cause of lower extremity amputation. *In 1990, there were 54,000 hospital discharges listing this diagnosis.[2] Cataract surgery with intraocular implants, vitrectomy, renal transplant, penile prosthesis implantation, diabetic foot surgery, vascular reconstructions for peripheral vascular disease and coronary artery bypass surgery, are some of the surgeries commonly performed in the diabetics. Appendicectomy, cesareans, gall bladder surgery and surgery for malignancy are some of the surgeries, which are performed in diabetic patients.*

Perioperative care of diabetes involves a multi-speciality approach with participation of diabetologist, physician, anesthesiologist and surgeon. Clinicians should be familiar with the treatment of diabetes during the preoperative period, during which patients are vulnerable to metabolic crises.[3] The ultimate aim of perioperative care of diabetic patient undergoing surgery is a safe and effective outcome without complications.[43]

Surgery in diabetes should be discussed under two different situations namely type 1 and type 2 diabetics. The preoperative, postoperative and the intraoperative management also vary depending on whether the patient undergoing surgery is on insulin or oral hypoglycemic drugs preoperatively. Individuals with type 1 diabetes are at a greater risk for metabolic complications, if diabetes is not adequately managed preoperatively. They are particularly at greater risk for infections, metabolic, electrolyte, renal and cardiac complications during and after surgery.[4-7]

METABOLIC ISSUES

Surgery and general anesthesia stimulate a neuro-endocrine stress response with the release of cortico-tropin (ACTH), growth hormone, catecholamines,[40,44] and to varying degrees, glucagons. The magnitude of the counter-regulatory response is related to the severity of surgery and any complications which may develop, such as sepsis. In contrast to general anesthesia, epidural anesthesia has minimal effects on glucose metabolism. Indeed, splanchnic sympathetic outflow is abolished and epinephrine secretion is reduced, resulting in decreased hepatic glucose production. Thus, insulin resistance is not generally changed, and there may be a greater risk for hypoglycemia, especially in the absence of sufficient blood glucose monitoring.

To minimize the adverse consequences of these metabolic effects, detailed attention to metabolic control is required. The clinician should always recall that a major surgery with general anesthesia will cause a larger metabolic stress than a minor procedure with local anesthesia, and that individuals with type I diabetes with absolute insulin deficiency are at greater risk for a metabolic catastrophe, if little attention is provided to diabetes management.

EFFECT OF SURGERY ON DIABETES

Surgery like any trauma induces a complex series of hormonal and metabolic changes in a diabetic under-going surgery.[4] Counter regulatory hormones like catecholamines, cortisol, which are secreted in increased amount, suppresses the insulin secretion and its effectiveness as well. Decreased insulin secretion causes a loss of anti-catabolic effects of insulin. Thus, it leads to a catabolic state and increased hepatic glucose production and breakdown of protein and fat. These changes though of minor consequence in an otherwise healthy patient, can have serious consequences like ketosis in a type 2 diabetic, where there is absolute deficiency of insulin. Thus, the metabolic consequences are more pronounced in a type 1 diabetic compared to type 2 diabetic. The physician should take adequate precautions before certifying the diabetic for surgery and take preventive measures to prevent metabolic emergencies in the preoperative period.

MORBIDITY AND MORTALITY

There are several studies to show that that mortality is higher in diabetics compared to nondiabetics during surgery.[8-10] In the 1960s, surgery in diabetics was associated with 4 to 13% mortality.[11,12]

The best possible means of minimizing morbidity and mortality in diabetic patients undergoing surgery is to mimic normal metabolism, as closely as possible by avoiding hypoglycemia, excessive hyperglycemia, lipolysis, ketogenesis, protein catabolism and electrolyte disturbances. Adequate insulin infusion pre- and postoperatively with glucose infusion prevents the catabolic state.

Insulin is necessary in the early stages of inflam-matory response but seems to have no effect on collagen formation after the first 10 days. Healing epithelial wounds have minimal leukocyte infiltration and unlike deep wounds, are not dependent on collagen synthesis for the integrity of the tissue. Simple epithelial repair is not inhibited in the diabetic patient, whereas the repair of deeper wounds is impaired[13] with respect to collagen formation and defense against bacterial growth.

A major surgery with general anesthesia will cause a larger metabolic stress than a minor procedure with local anesthesia. Apart from hyperglycemia, neuropathy, atherosclerosis and small vessel disease may contribute to delayed wound healing.[14,15] However, some studies suggest that diabetes *per se* may be as important to the outcome as its end organ effects.[16]

The major risk factors for diabetics undergoing surgery are the associated end organ involvement like cardiovascular dysfunction, renal insufficiency, joint-collagen tissue abnormalities (limitations of head extension, poor wound healing), inadequate granulocyte function and neuropathies. If the patient has both diabetes and hypertension, it is associated with poor prognosis and increased risk of autonomic neuropathy.[16]

Carefully-managed diabetes does not add signi-ficantly to surgical risk. Most often, it is poor glycemic

TABLE 81.1	Current perioperative recommendations for diabetics

- History and clinical examination to review end organ function, focusing on signs and symptoms of associated autonomic dysfunction, cardiac disease (CAD, CHF, diastolic dysfunction), renal damage and retinal involvement
- Laboratory investigations: Fasting and postprandial plasma glucose, glycated hemoglobin, blood urea or serum creatinine, electrolytes, urinary albumin/micro-albuminuria estimation
- Chest X-ray, electrocardiogram, echocardiogram/dobutamine echocardiogram to assess the cardiac status
- Standard ASA monitoring supplemented by judicious use of central venous pressure (CVP), pulmonary artery catheter (PAC) or arterial monitoring
- Application of appropriate techniques to facilitate intubation and patient positioning to avoid nerve or soft tissue injury
- Glucose control: The tighter the control of preoperative glucose, the more frequent is the monitoring required
- Continuous infusion of glucose and insulin or frequent IV boluses to maintain the plasma glucose between 100 to 200 mg/dl would be the ideal approach

CAD: Coronary artery disease; CHF: Congestive heart failure

control, inefficient monitoring facilities, pre-existing unrecognized sepsis and most importantly advanced diabetic complications, which contribute to the adverse outcome. Insulin infusion is the most rational and physiological method available today for perioperative management of blood sugars in diabetic individuals. With the use of modern management protocols and the sophisticated monitoring facilities available, the mortality and morbidity of surgery are now comparable in diabetic and nondiabetic patients **(Table 81.1)**.

PREOPERATIVE EVALUATION

Assessment and treatment of the potential end organ effects of diabetes is as important as the assessment of the metabolic status of the individual. There is universal consensus regarding the preoperative evaluation of diabetic complications, especially cardiovascular, autonomic dysfunction and diabetic nephropathy and the need for frequent metabolic monitoring. However, there is no consensus pertaining to preoperative insulin administration.

History

A detailed history regarding the duration of diabetes control, end organ effects, dietary intake, therapeutic and exercise regimens should be recorded. Associated diseases and medications taken should be noted. History of previous surgeries, anesthetic response and drug allergies are to be recorded.

A complete physical examination including cardiac, renal, respiratory system examination and fundoscopy should be performed. Assessment of airway, joint mobility, identification of the *stiff man syndrome*, cervical instability and risk of aspiration should be done.

Laboratory Evaluation

This includes fasting plasma glucose, postprandial plasma glucose, electrolytes, blood urea and serum creatinine estimation, glycated hemoglobin, electrolytes, urinary albumin excretion, lipid profile, chest X-ray and electrocardiogram.

PREOPERATIVE RECOMMENDATION FOR TYPE 2 DIABETICS ON ORAL HYPOGLYCEMIC AGENTS (OHA)

One of the most important things in the preoperative management of diabetes is to set the targets for control and frequently monitor the plasma glucose to achieve the goal. Thus, there is a need for frequent metabolic monitoring specially plasma glucose, avoiding hypoglycemia, excess hyperglycemia, ketosis and electrolyte disturbance.[14,15,17,18]

The target for control in patients undergoing elective surgery should be postprandial plasma glucose of 120 to 180 mg/dl in the preoperative period.[19] A glycated hemoglobin of < 7% is desirable.

Patients on OHA who are well-controlled can continue the same medication preoperatively for minor surgeries except during special situations like infection, nonhealing of wound, hyperglycemia or inability to take oral medication where he may need insulin therapy. About 93% of the patients with type 2 diabetes can achieve acceptable blood glucose control without insulin.[20]

Chlorpropamide should be stopped at least five days before surgery, substituting a shorter acting sulfonylurea if necessary. Long acting sulfonylureas increases the potential hazard of hyperglycemia. Metformin should be discontinued 48 hours prior to and 48 hrs subsequent to the procedure and reinstituted only after renal function has been re-evaluated and found to be normal.[21] Metformin does cause hyperlactatemia and renal function may deteriorate during anesthesia.[14] There is a theoretical increased risk during the period of potential hypotension and increased anerobic metabolism.[22] Sulfonylureas are generally stopped on the morning of surgery and then withheld until after surgery when the patient resumes eating.[14] Glibenclamide can cause hypoglycemia in the elderly, who are the majority of diabetics undergoing surgery and hence it is preferable not to give glibenclamide on the day of surgery.

If the diabetes is poorly-controlled preoperatively, it is advisable to switch over to purified insulins. To achieve euglycemia faster, it is advisable to manage the patient with short-acting insulins three times a day given subcutaneously with each meal along with basal insulin, if required at night to control fasting hyperglycemia.

TYPE 2 DIABETICS ON INSULIN

There is no need to change the insulin regimen before surgery if the diabetes is well-controlled. Patients receiving bedtime insulin do well taking the normal dose of insulin at that time. If the patient is diagnosed preoperatively or needs emergency surgery, he will need to be started on insulin. In such situations, purified insulins are preferable, as the patient may not require insulin in the follow-up period. This prevents the development of insulin antibody in the susceptible individuals who are exposed to insulin for short periods of time.

Regimens of Insulin in Type 2 Diabetes Undergoing Surgery under General Anesthesia (GA)

Insulin may be used subcutaneously (SC) or through intravenous route (IV) during GA. The subcutaneous route of insulin administration is usually given in practice while the IV insulin is reserved for special situations like shock, diabetic ketoacidosis (DKA), pregnancy, high dose glucocorticoids, sepsis, transplantation and coronary artery bypass graft (CABG). However, the effect of subcutaneous insulin is unpredictable. As blood pressure variations and fluid shifts are common during surgery and subcutaneous route of administration is dependent on changes in peripheral blood flow, insulin absorption will be variable. In view of the above facts, most of the physicians prefer either a variable rate of IV insulin infusions or a glucose–insulin–potassium (GIK) infusion for diabetics undergoing surgery under general anesthesia. Type 2 diabetic patients undergoing major surgery that requires prolonged fasting are best managed using continuous glucose and insulin delivery.

TABLE 81.2	Perioperative management of diabetes in type 1 diabetics undergoing elective surgery

- Frequent home blood glucose monitoring before admission to hospital
- Preoperative assessment of metabolic, renal and cardiac status
- Patients with plasma glucose above 250 mg/dl should get arterial blood gas estimation done
- Regular monitoring of glucose level during insulin infusion

Regimens of insulin in type 2 diabetes undergoing surgery under LA: The metabolic changes in the non-insulin dependent diabetic undergoing minor surgery are minimal[23] and there is no advantage of GIK versus no insulin.[24]

SURGERY IN TYPE 1 DIABETIC

Surgical stress suppresses insulin release and stimulates counter-regulatory hormone secretion. This favors catabolic state, which may lead to hyperglycemia and ketosis in type 1 diabetic. The regimen of Watts et al[25] of variable insulin by separate infusion is the best for type 1 diabetics undergoing surgery under general anesthesia **(Table 81.2)**.

Elective Surgery and Preoperative Diabetes Control

Though there are various regimens of insulin administration during the preoperative period, simplicity of insulin regimen is essential. Junior doctors who might not have acquired specialized skills in the management of diabetes most often undertake the preoperative bedside management in our country. It is better to plan the insulin regimen suitable for the diabetic patient undergoing surgery day before surgery and attach the protocol to patient's chart before surgery. This will help the junior doctors to follow instructions regarding the regimen of insulin and appropriate monitoring of metabolic parameters during perioperative period.

Table 81.3 shows guidelines for minor surgery and invasive diagnostic procedures in patients with diabetes mellitus.

Management of Diabetes on the Day of Surgery

Timing of surgery: Starting the surgery in a diabetic early in the day avoids prolonging the catabolic state and minimizes the risk of hypoglycemia.

TABLE 81.3	Guidelines for minor surgery and invasive diagnostic procedures in patients with diabetes mellitus

Insulin treated	Oral hypoglycemic agents
• Type 1 and Type 2: Use insulin drip or combined insulin glucose infusion. Check blood glucose (BG) every 2–4 hrs	• Hold morning OHA • Check BG pre-and postsurgery • Give evening OHA
• Type 2 (< 50 U/day) HOLD morning NPH/Lente; treat with regular insulin as shown:	• Insulin rarely needed; if necessary treat with regular insulin as shown:

Insulin Regimens in Diabetics Undergoing Surgery

Tight control of Diabetes: Treatment regimens should not aim for near normoglycemia, as this doesn't improve the outcome of surgery but only increases the risk of hypoglycemia, which may be a major hazard during surgery. The aim of such a regimen is to keep plasma glucose levels between 100 mg/dl and 200 mg/dl, which may help in preventing postoperative infection and accelerate wound healing.

In the past, many regimens like bolus insulin,[26] low insulin infusion[27] rates like 0.5 to 1.0 Units/hour accompanied by a glucose infusion was used. These low dose insulin infusions are not preferred these days because it is accompanied by higher risk of metabolic decompensation during surgery. Recently higher rates of insulin delivery 2 to 4 Units/hour is given along with 5 to 10 grams of glucose per hour. This higher dose of insulin along with glucose provides a wider safely margin and greater flexibility for dose adjustment to achieve better glycemic control.

Continue nondextrose, nonlactate infusions on the day of surgery to maintain intraoperative fluids and electrolytes. During the surgery, measure the plasma glucose level hourly from the beginning of the surgery till the next 24 hours and adjust the insulin infusion rates. In case of hypoglycemia keep 25% or 50% glucose handy to tackle hypoglycemia and stop the insulin infusion and administer 25% glucose in case the plasma glucose falls below 50 mg/dl **(Table 81.4)**.

Glucose-insulin-potassium Regimen (GIK)

The GIK regimen has gained widespread acceptance because of its simplicity and effectiveness. In the GIK by supplying glucose, the need for protein catabolism to meet gluconeogenic needs in the diabetic patient is

TABLE 81.4	Guidelines for perioperative diabetes management with combined insulin-glucose infusion
Treatment (<50 U/day)	Diet, oral agents, or insulin (<50 U/day) Fasting blood glucose (FBG) 120-180 mg/dl: Add 10 U regular (human) insulin to 1000 mL of 5% dextrose plus 20 mEq KCl Blood glucose (BG) > 180 mg/dl: Increase insulin by 5 U BG < 120 mg/dl: Decrease insulin by 5 U Check BG hourly infuse at 100 mL/hour (1.0 U/hour)
Treatment (>50 U/day)	Insulin (>50 U/day) FBG 120-180 mg/dl: Add 15 U regular (human) insulin to 1000 mL of 5% dextrose plus 20 mEq KCl BG > 180 mg/dl: Increase insulin by 5 U BG <120 mg/dl: Decrease insulin by 5 U Check BG hourly infuse at 100 mL/hour BG <80 mg/dl: Stop infusion and administer intravenous bolus of 50% dextrose in water (25 mL). Once BG >80, restart insulin infusion Insulin needs increase for obesity, sepsis, steroid therapy, renal transplant, and coronary artery bypass

reduced and a less negative nitrogen balance results.[20] Three bags of 10% IV glucose (500 ml bags) are taken and numbered 1, 2 and 3; 10 millimols of potassium chloride are added to each bottle. To the first bottle 10 units of regular purified or human insulin, to the second bottle 15 units and to the third bottle 20 units of insulin is added. This glucose, insulin and potassium mixture is infused over a period of 5 hours at the rate of 100 ml per hour. This regimen is simple and can be used in peripheral hospitals also, as it does not require an infusion pump. The infusion rate is not so critical in a regimen where insulin and glucose are infused separately. When the three bags are prepared in GIK infusion set, it is imperative that the bags are labeled clearly with the dosages of glucose, potassium and insulin in the bag. The plasma glucose should be monitored hourly (with a glucometer) while infusing GIK mixture **(Tables 81.5 and 81.6)**. In case glucometer is not available, visual method of blood glucose measurement using glucose strips may be used. This is essential till the insulin requirements are stabilized. It is also advisable to measure the serum electrolytes once in three hours during GIK infusion and to adjust the potassium levels, if necessary. Start GIK infusion with bag number 1 (containing 10 units Insulin), and after

TABLE 81.5 Glucose-Insulin-Potassium (GIK)

GIK mixture

Bag 1: 10% dextrose solution + 10 units of regular insulin + 10 mmol KCl

Bag 2: 10% dextrose solution + 15 units of regular insulin + 10 mmol KCl

Bag 3: 10% dextrose solution 20 units of regular insulin + 10 mmol KCl

TABLE 81.6 GIK infusion during surgery

Plasma glucose 100–200 mg/dl IV GIK Bag 1

Plasma glucose 200–250 mg/dl IV GIK Bag 2

Plasma glucose > 200 mg/dl IV GIK Bag 3

GIK: Glucose-insulin-potassium regimen

infusion, if the plasma glucose is above 200 mg/dl change over to second bottle or if still higher to bag 3. In the same way if the plasma glucose is lower (below 100 mg/dl) during infusion, switch over to the bag with lower insulin content. Dilutional hyponatremia may occur if the GIK infusion is prolonged. In case, there is likelihood of fluid overload in a particular patient, the GIK infusion bags may be prepared with 20% dextrose with appropriate adjustment in insulin and potassium.

GIK Infusion with Separate Infusion Lines

The GIK infusion may be given in separate lines, insulin through infusion pump and glucose and potassium mixture in a bag. The advantage of this infusion is greater flexibility in the infusion, where depending on the plasma glucose either the insulin pump rate or glucose infusion may be modified. This separate GIK infusion system obviates the need of three bags and confusion that can arise in such a situation. The disadvantages of separate infusion lines are, pump malfunction, glucose infusion running out or blocking of intravenous cannula, which can lead to problems during infusion.

Insulin Infusion Pump

There are two types of insulin infusion pump available for use during surgery. The portable insulin infusion pump and the bigger insulin infusion pump that is a 100 ml electrically driven syringe, which is not portable. The portable insulin pump has the advantage of greater flexibility and wide range of insulin delivery dosage 1/20th of unit insulin per hour to 10 unit insulin per hour. Even postoperatively, the portable insulin pump can be used for several days, and switched over to subcutaneous insulin infusion. Use of a portable pump can cut short the stay in the hospital of a patient, before and after surgery, as it is useful in quicker diabetes control during preoperative period. The limitations of portable insulin pumps in our country are the high cost of the pump, lack of trained personnel to handle using the pump, nonavailability of local trained technicians to repair or service the insulin pump. With the introduction of miniature sophisticated programmable insulin pumps, the preoperative management of diabetes will be much easier than what it was before.

MODERATE CONTROL OF DIABETES

The aim of this nontight regimen is to prevent ketoacidosis and hyperosmolar states before and during surgery.

The patient is advised not to take any solids for 24 hours preceding surgery and nil by mouth after midnight. On the day of surgery, give half of usual morning dose of insulin and start IV 5% glucose infusion at the rate of 125 ml/h/70 kg in the morning. Continue 5% dextrose infusion preoperative and postoperatively. Monitor the plasma glucose in every 1 to 2 hours postoperatively and adjust the insulin infusion accordingly.

POSTOPERATIVE MANAGEMENT

The postoperative management depends on the type of surgery performed, the anesthesia and how soon the oral feeding is started. In most of the cases within 48 hours after surgery the patient will be allowed to take solid feeds. If the patient is unlikely to be on oral feeds for prolonged time, as in the case of major abdominal surgery, it is better to continue IV insulin regimen. In case the patient is on parenteral nutrition adjust the dose of insulin accordingly.

The insulin infusion should be continued till the patient starts taking solid foods. The plasma glucose is measured in every two to three hours and depending on the plasma glucose IV regular insulin is given intermittently, so as to keep the plasma glucose between 100 mg/dl and 200 mg/dl. Once the patient starts taking solid food, he is advised to take his usual dose of subcutaneous (SC) insulin. The intravenous insulin may be discontinued 30 minutes after the first subcutaneous insulin is given, as the subcutaneous dose is effective by that time **(Table 81.7)**.

TABLE 81.7	Patient is on Ryle's tube (RT) feeds

Give basal insulin approximately 24 units (if type 1 DM) spread over 24 hours or insulin requiring type 2
- Each alternate RT feed preceded by regular insulin
- If caloric content of RT feed known regular insulin/short acting insulin can be given almost accurately (bolus dose) one unit of insulin-decreases blood glucose by 50 mg/dl

INFECTIONS

Infections account for two-thirds of postoperative complications and about 20% of preoperative deaths in diabetic patients. Unfortunately, there are no controlled prospective studies directly comparing different levels of preoperative glycemia with rates of wound infection or breakdown. Alterations in leukocyte function, decreased chemotaxis, impaired phagocytic activity of granulocytes and reduce intracellular killing of pneumococci and staphylococci are noted during hyperglycemia in animal experiments and when diabetes is controlled and blood sugars are brought below 250 mg/dl most of these leukocyte dysfunctions are restored to near normal levels. Phagocyte dysfunction is believed to occur with blood glucose of more than 200mg/dl. Both plasma glucose levels above 200 mg/dl and high serum ketones provide a permissive milieu for the development of infectious complications.[28,29]

Nosocomial infection rates can probably be decreased without patient surgeries.[42] Those diabetics at higher risk for complications during surgery need tight control of diabetes and/or intensive postoperative reduce the rate of complications. Though the rate of infection in clean incision was higher (10.7%) in the diabetics compared to the nondiabetics (1.8%), when age is accounted for, the differences in the wound infection in diabetic and nondiabetics were not statistically significant Danish study of 224 diabetic and 224 matched nondiabetic subjects reported wound infection rates of 5.8 and 5.4% respectively in these groups.[9]

ANESTHESIA IN A DIABETIC PATIENT

In a diabetic undergoing surgery, the anesthetist, surgeon and the treating physician should critically evaluate the patient and decide as to which type of anesthesia is the best for the particular patient. The decision depends on the metabolic status of the patient, type of surgery, associated complications and the effect of surgery on the glycemic control.

GENERAL ANESTHESIA

Surgery and general anesthesia stimulate a neuroendocrine stress response with the release of ACTH, growth hormone, catecholamines and glucagon.[30,31] The magnitude of the counter-regulatory response is related to the severity of surgery and any complications, which may envelop like sepsis. In the early days of anesthetic use agents like ether causes hyperglycemia, insulin resistance and increased blood levels of lactate and ketone bodies. Modern general anaesthetics have little effect on plasma glucose, so that the choice of agent should be determined by the type and duration of operation rather than by diabetes. Hypoglycemia has been reported after epidural anesthesia and after infiltration of large amounts of lidocaine.[32] Anesthetic agents like halothane and enflurane can be safely used in diabetics. The most controversial aspect of insulin treatment during general anesthesia is the regimen and the type of insulin that is to be used. There is uniform opinion among all physicians that tight control of diabetes is essential during general anesthesia. Though various regimens of insulin therapy, routes of administration has been discussed with its advantages as well as limitations, every hospital and the diabetes management team should decide a particular regimen depending on the local situation, the facilities and expertise available in their set-up. A simple and convenient protocol should be drawn up and agreed upon by those involved in patient care-physicians, surgeons and anesthetist. It is better to evolve a *diabetes care team* to take care of the patient during preoperative period so that in the long-term uniform and quality medical care is delivered to the patient with diabetes undergoing surgery.

Hypertension, cardiomegaly, diffuse hypokinesia and previous myocardial infarctions are more likely in diabetics compared to nondiabetics, and thus may result in poorer outcome in diabetics. Type 1 diabetics with coronary artery disease appear to have stiffer ventricles with greater elevation to left ventricular end-diastolic pressure than do matched nondiabetic controls. Poorer diastolic function and decreased peripheral autonomic responses result in poorer pre-load control. Surgical mortality can be a high as 10 to 15% in diabetics with poor ventricular function undergoing coronary bypass surgery.

SPECIAL SITUATION

Autonomic Neuropathy

Diabetics with long-duration of the disease and type 1 diabetics are likely to have autonomic neuropathy. Preoperative assessment of these patients should include tests for autonomic neuropathy like electrocardiogram recording during inspiration and expiration, postural hypotension. Patients with autonomic neuropathy are at an increased risk of gastroparesis, cardiorespiratory arrest and aspiration at postoperative period. Current autonomic function tests however, do not assess cardiac sympathetic neuropathy. Use of 10 mg of metoclopramide pre-operatively facilitates gastric emptying of solids. Patients with advanced autonomic neuropathy warrant close, continuous cardiac and respiratory monitoring for 24 hours postoperatively. Forces that tend to perturb cardiovascular homeostasis abound in the postoperative period, when narcotics are frequently used, ventilation to perfusion ratio abnormality may lead to hypoxia and anesthetics depress both circulation and respiration.[33]

OPEN HEART SURGERY

Patients undergoing open-heart surgery require higher rates of insulin delivery[34] because of the glucose rich solutions, effects of induced hypothermia, which hampers the insulin action and interpose used during cardiopulmonary bypass, as well as the metabolic effects of hypothermia.[35] As a result of these factors, the usual GIK infusion system may not be very effective in tight control of diabetes during cardiopulmonary bypass and a separate line for insulin administration or an insulin pump may be used for effective control. Often IV insulin in the dose of 0.06 units/kg body weight/hour is needed to achieve good glycemic control. Such situations need more frequent plasma glucose monitoring and frequent adjustment of insulin infusion.

A study of 340 diabetics and 2522 nondiabetics undergoing CABG surgery showed marginal increase in operative mortality in diabetics (1.8%) compared to non-diabetics (0.6%).[36,37] In the post bypass phase, patients with diabetes required inotropic therapy and intra-aortic balloon pump support five times more frequently than nondiabetics. Diabetics with angina are more likely to have extensive coronary artery disease than nondiabetics. With improved care and better monitoring facilities the overall results of open-heart surgery is now similar in diabetics and nondiabetics.[38,39]

EMERGENCY SURGERY IN A DIABETIC WITH KETOACIDOSIS

In a type 1 or type 2 diabetic with ketoacidosis emergency, surgery may be contemplated either for trauma or infection. Diabetic patient who needs emergency surgery should be assessed fully both clinically and biochemically as the surgery may lead to metabolic decompensation. In such a situation very little time is available for stabilization of the patient and only few hours may be sufficient. The most important aspect of management in such a situation is to correct fluid and electrolyte imbalance and try to achieve near normal euglycemia. It is futile to delay surgery in such situations to eliminate ketoacidosis completely as the underlying surgical condition may lead to further metabolic deterioration. If the volume depletion and hypokalemia are partially corrected before surgery it is sufficient to prevent intraoperative cardiac arrhythmias and hypotension. It is better to use two separate IV lines for fluid and insulin infusion as it gives flexibility in managing hyperglycemia and correct the metabolic decompensation effectively. Use of portable or bedside insulin pump in these situations is very helpful. Start with 10 units of IV regular insulin followed by continuous insulin infusion. The insulin infusion rate should vary depending on the blood glucose response and individual insulin sensitivity. The actual amount of insulin administered is less important than regular monitoring of glucose, potassium and pH. The insulin infusion may be given through an insulin infusion pump or IV infusion set depending on the availability. The advantage of using an insulin pump is that it maintains a steady state plasma insulin level and if the pump rate and IV fluids infusion rate may be separately regulated. Rapid decline in serum potassium levels occur reaching a nadir within 2 to 4 hours after starting IV insulin infusion as the potassium moves into the intracellular space along with insulin when ketosis is corrected. About 3 to 10 mEq/kg body weight of potassium may be lost during treatment of ketoacidosis, which has to be replaced. Plasma phosphate levels should be measured and if it falls below 1.0 mg/dl to be replaced at a rate of 1 mmol/kg body weight.

Once the plasma glucose reaches 250 mg/dl, 5% glucose is added to the IV regimen to prevent hypoglycemia during surgery and insulin dosage or infusion is accordingly adjusted to maintain plasma glucose levels between 200 to 250 mg/dl.

LAPAROSCOPIC SURGERY

The laparoscopic or *key hole surgery* is gaining popularity among both surgeons and the patients. With the availability of laparoscopic surgery in many centers in our country, the number of patients undergoing laparoscopic surgery is bound to go up. Surgeries like appendicectomy, cholecystectomy and hysterectomy in a diabetic may be performed by laparoscopic surgery. Though there are few reports of laparoscopic surgery in diabetics, in future the data regarding such surgery in diabetics will help in choosing either laparoscopic or conventional surgery by surgeon or the patient. Theoretically, laparoscopic surgery should involve less of surgical trauma, preferable in diabetics because of least metabolic disturbance. One of the reports comparing conventional surgery and laproscopic surgery in diabetics has shown that the degree of metabolic disturbance and the severity of insulin resistance induced appear to be comparable.[40]

CESAREAN SECTION

Both type 1 patients and type 2 patients who are on insulin may have a situation where cesarean section may be necessary. If the cesarean section is an elective surgery, GIK regimen described previously may be used effectively to achieve euglycemia. When a diabetic woman goes into labor, start two separate IV lines with glucose infusion and insulin infusion. If emergency cesarean section is necessary IV insulin is continued and IV fluids to maintain the fluid and electrolyte balance. Use of beta-adrenergic agonist agents to delay the labor and dexamethasone to improve fetal lung maturity may increase insulin requirement during cesarean section. With the delivery of the placenta, the insulin requirement falls significantly. If the patient is getting GIK infusion, the insulin infusion rate may be reduced or stopped. Once patient is taking oral feeds, subcutaneous insulin is resumed.

SUMMARY

The key to success in diabetic patient undergoing surgery is not the choice of a specific regimen but the frequent monitoring of the patients metabolic status and appropriate responses to the metabolic state.[41]

With the advances in anesthesia, better and frequent monitoring of the metabolic status of a diabetic patient undergoing surgery, the surgery in a diabetic in well-equipped hospitals and with team approach, is as safe as in nondiabetic patient.

REFERENCES

1. Root HF. Perioperative care of the diabetic patient. Postgrad Med.1966;40:439-43.
2. Center for disease control and prevention. Diabetes surveillance 1993. Atlanta GA.US department of health and human services, public health services, 1993.
3. Irl B Hirsch, Douglas S Paauw. Diabetes management in special situations.Endocrinal Metab Clin North Am.1997;26:631-44.
4. Elliot MI, Alberti KGMM. Carbohydrate metabolism effects of pre-operative starvation and trauma. Clin Anaesthesiol. 1983;1:527-50
5. David S. Schade. Surgery and diabetes, Med Clin N Am. 1988;72:6,1531-43.
6. Robert L Schiff, Gail A Welsh. Perioperative evaluation and management of the patient with endocrine dysfunction. Med Clin N Am. 2003;87:175-92.
7. Hirsch IB, McGill JB. Role of insulin in management of surgical patients with diabetes mellitus. Diabetes Care 1990;13:980-91.
8. Fowkes FGR, Lunn JH, Farrow SC, Robertson IB, Samuel P. Epidemiology in anaesthesia III. Mortality risk in patients with coexisting physical disease. Br J Anaesth. 1982;54:819-24.
9. Hjortrup A, Sorenson C, Dyremose E, Hjortso NC, Kehlet H. Influence of diabetes mellitus on operative risk. Br J Surg. 1985;72:785-7.
10. Farrow SC, Fowkes FGR. Epidemiology in anaesthesia: a method for predicting hospital mortality. Eur J Anaesthisiolo.1983;1:77-84,.
11. Galloway JA Shuman Cr. AM J Med. 1963;34:177-191.
12. Alberti KGMM, Marshall SM. In Alberty KGMM, Krall LP(Eds): The Diabetic Annual 4. Elsevier, Amsterdam. 1988,p.248-71.
13. Mc Murry JF. Wound healing with diabetes mellitus. Surg Clin N Am. 1984;64:769-78.
14. Alberti KGMM. Editorial Views. Diabetes and Surgery. Anesthesiology. 1991;74:209-11.
15. Conill AM, Horowitz DA, Braunstein S. The surgical patient with diabetes mellitus. In Goldman DR, Brown FH, Guarnieri DM(Eds): Perioperative medicine. McGraw-Hill, New York.1994, p.243.
16. Michael F Roizen. Perioperative management of the diabetic patient, Annual Refresher course Lectures Oct 9-13,1993, Washington D.C.American Society of Anaesthesiologist. 1993;164:1-6.
17. Iri B Hirsch, Janet B Mcgill, Philip E Cryer and Paul F White. PRE-OPERATIVE management of surgical patients with diabetes mellitus. Medical intelligence article. In Julien F Biebuyck (Eds): Anesthesiology. 74;pp.346-59.
18. Gavin LA. Perioperative management of the diabetic patient. Endocrinol Metab Clin North Am 1992;21:457,.
19. Alberti KGMM. Diabetes and surgery. Ellenberg and Rifkin's Diabetes Mellitus: theory and practice. 4th edn. In Rifkin H, Porte D(Eds): Elsevier, New York. 1990;pp.626-33.
20. Husband DJ, Thai AC, Albertii KGMM. Management of diabetes during surgery with glucose-insulin potassium infusion. Diabet Med. 1986;3:69.
21. Glucophage (Metformin hydrochloride tablets) package insert. Bristol-Myers Squibb company.
22. Bailey CJ Turner RC. Drug therapy. Metformin. N Engl J Med. 1996;9:574.
23. Malling B, Knudsen L, Christiansen CL, Schurizek BA, Albrti KGMM, Hermansen K. Insulin treatment in non-insulin dependent diabetic patients undergoing minor surgery. Diabetes, nutrition and metabolism 1989;2:125-31.

24. Thompson J, Husband DJ, Thai AC, Alberty KGMM. Metabolic changes in the non-insulin dependent diabetic undergoing minor surgery. Effects of glucose-insulin -potassium infusion. Br J Surg. 1986;73:301-4.

25. Watts NB, Gebhart SP, Clark RV, Philips LS. Perioperative management of diabetes mellitus: steady state glucose control with bedside algorithm for insulin adjustment. Diabetes care 1986;9:40-5.

26. Hall GM. Insulin administration in diabetic patients-return of the bolus? Br J Anaesth. 1994;72:1-2.

27. Goldberg NJ, Wingert TD, Levin SR, Wilson SE, Villjoen JF. Insulin therapy in the diabetic surgical patient: metabolic and hormone response to low dose insulin infusion. Diabetes care.1981;4:279-84.

28. Hostetter MK. Handicaps to host defense: effects of hyperglycaemia on C3 and *Candida albicans*. Diabetes. 1990; 39:271.

29. Marhoffer W, Stern M, Maeser W, et al. Impairment of polymorphonuclear leukocyte function and metabolic control of diabetes. Diabetes care. ,1992;15:256.

30. Kennedy DJ, Butterworth JF. Endocrine function during and after cardiopulmonary bypass: recent observations. J Clin Endocrinol Metab. 1994;997.

31. Palmisano JJ. Surgery and siabetes. In Kahn CR, Weir GC (Eds): Joslin's Diabetes Mellitus ed 13. Malvern PA Lea and Febiger.1994,p.955.

32. Romano E, Gullo A. anesthesia. 1980;35:1084-6

33. Edwin DJ, Martin CN, Young RJ, Clark BF. The value for cardiovascular autonomic function tests. 10 years experience in diabetics. Diabetes care. 1985;8:491-8.

34. Gill GV, Sherif IH, Alberti KGMM. Management of diabetes during open heart surgery. Br J Surg.1981;68:171-2.

35. Crock PA, Ley CJ, Martin IK, Alford FP, Best JD. Hormonal and metabolic changes during hypothermic coronary bypass heart surgery in diabetic and nondiabetic subjects. Diabet Med. 1988;5:47-52.

36. Devineni R, Mckinzie FN. Surgery for coronary artery disease in patients with diabetic mellitus. Can J Surg 1985;28:367-70.

37. Lawrie GM, Morris GC. Glaeser DH. Influence of diabetes mellitus on the result of coronary bypass surgery. JAMA. 1986;256:1967-71.

38. Douglas JS, King SB, Craver JM,et al. Factors influencing risk and benefit of coronary bypass surgery in patients with diabetes mellitus. Chest. 1981;80:369.

39. Frater RWM,Oka Y,Kadish A, et al. Diabetes and coronary artery surgery. Mt Sinai J Med. 1982;49:237.

40. Hawthorne GC, Ashworth L, Alberti KGMM. The effect of laproscopic cholecystectomy in insulin sensitivity. Horm Metab Res. 1994;26:474-7.

41. Furnary AP, Zerr KJ, Grunkemeier GL. Continuous intravenous insulin infusion reduces the incidence of deep sternal wound infection in diabetic patients after cardiac surgical procedures. Ann Thorac Surg 1999;67:352-62.

42. Pomposelli JJ,Baxter JK,Babineau TJ, et al Early postoperative glucose control predicts nosocomial infection rate in diabetic patients. Journal of parenteral and enteral nutrition. 1998:22:77-81.

43. Scherpereel PA, Tavernier B. Perioperative care of diabetic patients. Eur J anaesthesiol. 2001;18:277-94

44. Hirsch IB, Janet B Mcgill, Philip E Cryer And Paul F White. Perioperative management of surgical patients with diabetes mellitus. Medical Intelligence Article. In: Julien F Biebuyck (Eds): Anesthesiology. 1991;74:346-59.

Section 12

LIVING WITH DIABETES

Chapter 82

PSYCHOSOCIAL ASPECTS OF DIABETES

GR Sridhar

CHAPTER OUTLINE

- Introduction
- Psychology and Diabetes—A Historical Perspective
- Diabetes-care Providers
- Lifestyle and Behavior, Perception of Life
- Biopsychosocial Model of Diabetes Management
- Studies in Children with Type I Diabetes Mellitus
- Studies in Parents of Children with Type I Diabetes
- Studies in Type 2 Diabetes
- Psychological Factors in Childhood Diabetes
- Model for Living Effectively with Diabetes
- Summary

INTRODUCTION

Diabetes mellitus is a lifestyle disorder that requires synergistic interaction among the patient, the family and the health care team. Being *nonurgent* or silent, diabetes and its complications are often allowed to go uncontrolled.[1] To prevent the disease and its complications, efforts are needed for a broad-based management plan, in which the patient, the family and society are integral parts. Crucial as medical interventions may be, lifestyle changes are equally important in treatment. A nationwide study in the USA has shown that most people with chronic diseases are neither old nor disabled.[2] Attention is now being paid to the importance of the perspective of the patient in health care.[3] Kravis suggested the physician's job description must change 'from a focus on patients' bodies to a focus on their lives.

Diabetes mellitus, which is projected to affect Asian Indians most among all others in the world by 2025,[4] has been described as the *most complex and demanding* of any common chronic disease to manage. It requires a combination of one or all of the following:

modification of dietary practices, weight management, exercise, biochemical, monitoring of body fluids (blood, urine), foot care, use of drugs, learning new technical skills such as home blood glucose monitoring.

The need for these may set in suddenly and without warning, or may be presaged by an apprehensive wait for the condition to be diagnosed. There is now increasing evidence that psychological stress may result in diabetes mellitus,[5] which is a component of metabolic syndrome (insulin resistance hyperglycemia, hypertension, truncal obesity, dyslipidemia). In addition, psychological issues are crucial in adhering to treatment.

Problems can occur in adhering to treatment, in attempting to prevent complications and in adjustment to complications if and when they occur. It is therefore difficult to adhere to such a complex management protocol 'to forestall some far-off poorly perceived danger particularly when they are made uncomfortable in the process'.

To paraphrase the American Declaration of Independence, the objective of treatment of diabetes is Life, Liberty and the Pursuit of happiness. *Life* can be interpreted as normalizing blood glucose to reduce disability and death; *Liberty* from oppression of associated risk factors such as hypertension, dyslipidemia, obesity, smoking and target organ damage; *Pursuit of happiness* is acceptability and quality of life profile. Like most ideals they are not often met.

It is the purpose of this chapter to define the hurdles in managing diabetes and to suggest ways to overcome them.

PSYCHOLOGY AND DIABETES—A HISTORICAL PERSPECTIVE

In the 17th century, diabetes was believed to be precipitated by sorrow. Attempts were then made to identify a *diabetic personality*, which predisposes such individuals to diabetes. The search was understandably unfruitful. There are no personality characters specific for a diabetic that can precipitate diabetes, but only those common to all chronic diseases. The circle is nearly turning around, with psychological stress being shown to elevate concentrations of interleukin-6 (IL-6), which could in turn have a role in pathogenesis of insulin resistance and glucose intolerance.[6] Presently, social psychology is applied to study psychological aspects of coping with diabetes and how to improve these for better management of diabetes.[7] These include the role of psychological factors in promoting and maintaining health, and identifying correlates of health and illness. Information gleaned from these studies leads to developing techniques to modify unhealthy behavior.[7] The concept of mental well-being as an integral component of *Ayurvedic* System of Medicine: '... the mental type of morbidity may be quieted by spiritual knowledge, philosophy, fortitude, remembrance and concentration'. Similarly, the emphasis has shifted from illness-centered medicine to patient-centered medicine.

DIABETES-CARE PROVIDERS

In tune with the need for multifaceted management, many professionals including the physician, dietician, lab personnel, diabetes educator, as well as the family and society around the individual provide diabetes care, directly or indirectly.

Unlike in the West, individuals in developing countries tend to place more emphasis on how they feel and on their ability to maintain their way of life rather than on a physiological state measured by a laboratory test.[8] In addition, there is a strong preference to maintain

asymptomatic or mildly symptomatic conditions in diabetes.[9]

A pilot study in India showed that although individuals with diabetes are fairly ignorant about the disease, they do not have many negative ideas about their disease.[10] Therefore, management by health care professionals can be built on this neutral base. A recent qualitative study on the health beliefs on diabetes mellitus among emigrant *Bangladeshis* (Bangladesh) evaluated the purported cause and nature of diabetes, food classification and knowledge of complications.[11]

One can tailor health promoting education programs that build on beliefs, attitudes and behavior already existing in culture, aiming at good diabetes control, preventing complications and improving quality of life.

LIFESTYLE AND BEHAVIOR, PERCEPTION OF LIFE

Adult lifestyles are laid down in childhood and adolescence. It is difficult to change social patterns encompassing diet, physical activity and risk taking behavior like smoking, and alcohol consumption. Passive entertainment exemplified by television viewing and computer games, along with intake of meals being isolated rather than social events all contribute to disorders of lifestyle.[12] Modern man prefers to rely more on pills than lifestyle changes in order to manage his health. These human tendencies must be considered in planning future health maintaining strategies.

Viewed from a wider perspective, the objectives of health policy, i.e. health, healthy lifestyle and risk-taking behavior depend on what the public perceives as the most acceptable pattern of life. It is essentially a political decision to which doctors make small, if any contribution.[13]

There is a little purpose in detecting the disease, stratifying the risk and attempting to promote change in behavior, if ultimately medical advice is not followed. It is essential that the doctor, who knows more about the clinical situation, should communicate with the patient, in order to allow him/her a reasonable choice of participating in treatment. Ultimately, implementing prevention and treatment measures need sustained confidence of the public and the individual patients.

The management approach to diabetes must be from a proactive public health perspective, rather than a reactive, traditional medical perspective.[14] Using the social cognitive theory, it is possible to identify risk factors, how people acquire and maintain behavioral patterns, and intervention models that preclude the need for costly pharmacological and medical intervention.[15]

BIOPSYCHOSOCIAL MODEL OF DIABETES MANAGEMENT

Managing diabetes is influenced not only by factors in each individual, but by the system that surrounds the individual. The biopsychosocial model is a new paradigm that recognizes that disease and behavior are functions and results from the interaction among biological, psychosocial, developmental, sociocultural and ecological factors.[16]

Several resources buffer the stress of managing a chronic illness in the family, family esteem and communication, sense of mastery, financial well-being and extended family support system. Anticipatory coping would help in families having diabetic children. It consists of gaining knowledge about what may happen in the near future, preparing themselves attitudinally and emotionally, gaining skills and ultimately being confident that the family can successfully cope with the disease and treatment, if necessary from outside social support.

In summary, the biomedical model emphasizes individual influences on diabetes management (physiological and physical). Equally, important are environmental contexts, because of their influence on preventive and management behaviors. Three social contexts—the family, the health care system and the community—have considerable impact on persons with diabetes throughout their lives.

Stress and Diabetes

Emotions and Psychological Stress

Advanced development of brain in the humans allows awareness of subtle social cues that can affect self-esteem. Social interactions with others are often necessary to maintain optimum functioning. Threats to self-esteem and fear of losing control over ones' environment also elicit a stress response. The balance between the stress and resilience determines an individual's vulnerability to stress.[17]

Vulnerability to stress depends on both genetic influences and early life experiences. Genetic polymorphisms alter gene expression that regulates stress system. Early life and later lives events may activate the stress response inappropriately.

Metabolic Syndrome and Hypothalamic— Pituitary Adrenal Axis (HPA)

Obesity and cortisol are closely associated. In obesity, circulating cortisol levels may be either normal or low.[18] Environmental stress was also shown to contribute to obesity along with other factors including perinatal influences and programming of HPA.

Bjorntop postulated that stress could activate the sympathetic nervous system and result in the metabolic syndrome through dysregulation of hormones. Psychosocial stress may trigger the onset of visceral obesity and other components of the metabolic syndrome. Difference in response among individuals to the same stimuli may be responsible for the stress being perceived as *distress* or *eustress*.[19]

HPA has been shown to be more active in centrally obese men and in the premenopausal centrally obese women.[20] Central android obesity and peripheral gynecoid obesity may be associated with differential regulation of HPA,[21] besides being targeted to metabolically important tissues such as liver and visceral fat.

Preferential deposition of fat in the abdomen may be due to activity of enzymes that metabolize glucocorticoids. The enzyme 11 β-HSD exists in two isoforms: Type 1 (11 β-HSD1) and type 2 (11 β-HSD2). The type 2 isoform irreversibly inactivates cortisol and corticosterone, oxidising their 11 β-hydroxy groups to metabolites which bind only weakly to hormone receptors.[22] The type 1 isoform catalyzes both the inactivating and activating reactions, which is principally seen in the liver. Stress-related metabolic response via glucocorticoids may be modulated by the different isoforms of the enzyme. The 11 β-HSD oxoreductase activity in subcutaneous abdominal fat tissue is increased in obese individuals,[23] which may activate local glucocorticoid receptors,[24] promoting obesity. There is also evidence suggesting that 11 β-HSD activity in the placenta may be responsible for active forms of stress hormones passing through the placenta and resulting in adverse effects *in utero*.[25]

Intrauterine exposure to stress may activate the HPA axis. In populations undergoing health transition metabolic syndrome and low birth weight may be linked through activation of HPA.[26] Experimental animals, when prenatally exposed to the corticosteroid dexamethasone, had lower birth weight, permanent elevation of blood pressure and hyperinsulinism. A resetting of neuroendocrine pathways may be responsible for this constellation of changes. Therefore along with maternal undernutrition, maternal exposure to stress may also contribute to later components of the metabolic syndrome.

In the Hoorn Study, chronic psychological stress was correlated with prevalence of type 2 diabetes mellitus and with visceral adiposity.[27] More than 2000 adults aged 50 to 74 years without a history of diabetes mellitus were studied for the number of major stressful events during the preceding five years. An oral glucose tolerance test was given after the history taking. The number of stressful events was positively associated with the prevalence of newly diagnosed diabetes.[27]

Stress is defined as a 'stimulus event of sufficient severity to produce disequilibrium in the homeostasis of physiological systems'.[28] Stressor is the stimulus that evokes a stress response. It is perceived as stressful depending on the meaning the individuals ascribes to the stimulus and which in turn results in a sensory or metabolic process which is inherently stressful. Therefore, the definition of stress and stressor depends on the person's perception of the stimulus as being stressful.

An Overview of Coping with Stress

Coping has been defined as 'constantly changing cognitive and behavioral efforts to manage specific external and/or internal demands that are taxing or exceeding the resource of the person'.[29] In other words, coping is an attempt to manage the situation effectively and consists not of one single act, but a process that allows one to deal with various stressors. The process can focus either on the emotional effects of the stressors or on solving the problems of stressors.

Emotion Focussed Strategies of Coping with Stress

These are emotional or cognitive changes that shape ones views on stressful situations, rather than adopting strategies to change the situations themselves. Defense mechanisms are one example, which are employed to avoid anxiety by distorting reality. Although these may alleviate feelings of anxiety and guilt, they may be harmful in the long run. People often use rationalization when they are frustrated in attaining goals, such as concluding that ones blood sugar is not under control because the spouse is not taking enough care about the diet, or that one does not have enough money to buy the 'best insulin'. Denial or refusing to acknowledge that the stress exists is another mechanism. Defense or denial can sometimes lead to dangerous results. For example, when a diabetic subject refuses to accept on upsetting fact, the result is precarious.

Anxiety and depression occur in persons with diabetes more frequently than in the general population.[30] In addition other problems that are also common include fear of the future, restriction of leisure activities and depression partly as a result of physical disability.[31]

As in other chronic incurable conditions over which one does not have control, the following psychological reactions can occur.[32]

Denial: This reaction can occur when the diagnosis is first made. As a defensive measure, one may believe that someone else's report has been mistakenly given. Denial is avoiding some situations that are restricting or uncomfortable, or something one does not want to do. It is a normal reaction, but it can keep one from following precautions to maintain ones health. The physician can deal with denial by asking the patient: What does diabetes mean to the patient? How does he/she reach if they have trouble accepting the diabetes? Is the patient avoiding the treatment plan? Is the patient avoiding telling others he/she has diabetes? What the patients propose to do if they have problems living with diabetes? Can the patients talk it out with someone else?

By thinking about these questions one may have made the initial steps toward adjusting to diabetes and can be considered positive steps.

Anger: Anger is normal and healthy when there are major changes in ones life, especially when those are unexpected, unwanted or uncontrollable, such as when diabetes is first diagnosed. Expressing anger should not be hurting, but should be done in less harmful ways. When anger is exhibited by the patient the physician should ask (or make the patient ask himself). Why is the patient angry? Is it due to diabetes or something else? Do the same circumstances make the patient angry all the time? What does the patient do when he/she is angry? Does the patient shout at the spouse or children? Does the patient stop taking care of diabetes? What could the patients do when they are angry? Can the patient do something to express anger without hurting others or themselves, such as talking it over with family, friends, or perhaps yelling in an empty room?

These questions help the patients identify the reasons for their anger and the way they are expressing it.

Guilt: This reaction occurs when the patient feels responsible for something wrong happening. Feelings of guilt may be realistic or unrealistic. When guilty, one can ask oneself: Why is the patient feeling guilty? Is it something the patient did which affected his/her diabetes or is it something beyond their control? Is the guilt realistic? What does the patient do when he/she feels guilty? Do they worry too much? Do they try to make positive changes?

Feeling guilty about events under ones control may help to change ones habits.

Depression: This psychological reaction can occur when faced with an unpleasant situation that one cannot change, or can be due to fear of the unknown. Withdrawal increases loneliness and adds to depression. Depression is a normal response to diabetes and the lifestyle changes it brings. However, it should not become overwhelming or last too long. When depressed, the patients can ask themselves (or the physician can ask the patients). Why does the patient feel depressed? Is it because they have diabetes or is it due to some other reason? How are they reacting because of their depression? Are they withdrawing from activities, sleeping less or more, eating less or more, or frequently complaining about little aches and pains?

Depression can be tackled by talking over ones feelings or becoming involved in a special enjoyable activity or finally by making changes one at a time. If it persists one should seek professional help.

Emotion-focussed forms of coping can be successful as positive coping strategies when they are accurate reappraisals of stressful situations. It is often necessary and more effective to confront the stressor directly, rather than the emotions evoked by the stressor.

Problem-focussed Strategies of Coping with Stress

These involve putting problem-solving skills to work. Problem-focussed forms of coping are ways to deal directly with the situation that will eventually decrease or eliminate the stress. In general, they are the same as problem-solving strategies and the better a person is at solving problems, the more likely it is that he or she develops effective coping strategies. The strategies consist of identifying the stressful problem, generating possible solutions, selecting the appropriate solution and applying the solution to the problem to eliminate stress.

Problem-focused strategies involve the overt behavioral response to the stressor. They are aimed at making the patient accept his/her disease. Acceptance means that one feels good about oneself as a person with diabetes. It can take time and patience, along with help from others. Resolution and acceptance may take up to a year after diagnosis of diabetes. It requires full understanding of why diabetes sets in, its metabolic

basis and is consolidated, when successful glycemic control is established within the parameters of one's lifestyle.[33]

Psychosocial Barriers

The general psychosocial barriers experienced by patients with diabetes are low levels of self-efficacy (fueled by the chronic nature of the disease) and the emphasis on self-care (necessitated by the treatment regimen). Some of the other barriers relate to the patients themselves and their physicians.

Family members and friends can inadvertently undermine a patient's efforts to adhere to dietary changes, exercise regimens or medications, if they do not provide the necessary support for the changes. They may also assume too many responsibilities for an ill relative, contributing to inactivity and loss of self-confidence.

Physicians: Physicians generally expect patients to assume a passive role, whereas remaining active and independent are high priorities for most people with diabetes. The doctors respond to symptoms and discussion focused on laboratory findings. As a result, visits to the doctor remain focused on clinical and laboratory results and on medical treatments, even when controlling symptoms and finding ways to remain active may be more important, both to the patient and to the ultimate outcome. Further, the physicians rarely ask chronically ill patients to share their understanding of their illness or to identify their goals.[1,2] Consequently, neither the health care provider nor the patient clarifies what objectives are most important. Finally, physicians often do not ask about illness-related problems at work or at home. When these problems are discussed, many doctors are reluctant to talk about how to adapt because they believe they must either solve the problem (which they may feel unprepared to do) or sanction disability (which they may feel is not in the patient's best interest).

In all circumstances, it is necessary for the patients and the physicians to work together to facilitate the former in adhering to the regimen of management.

Collaboration between Physicians and Patients

The collaboration between the physicians and the patients is best achieved by discussing on the definition of the problem, the goals to be achieved and planning for an active and sustained follow-up.

Definition of Problem: Patients and their physicians need to work together in defining what problems are most important. Physicians typically define problems related to diagnosis, poor compliance with treatment regimens or continuing unhealthy behaviors, such as smoking or lack of exercise. Patients, however, are more likely to define problems of pain and other symptoms, their inability to function as they once did, emotional distress, difficulty carrying out prescribed regimens or lifestyle changes or fear of unpredictable consequences of the illness. The question that immediately comes to mind is; which is more important compliance, unhealthy behaviors or fears of decreased ability or unpredictable consequences? A possible answer to this would require physicians to ask patients to identify their biggest problem. This would help to harmonize the two perspectives and decide on strategies to manage diabetes.

Goal setting and planning: Patients and physicians typically try to initiate many different changes at once. Too many goals can lead to discouragement and difficulty in following treatment regimens. Instead, patients and physicians should focus on a limited number of solvable problems, based both on the significance of the problems and on the patient's motivation and readiness to tackle them. Once targeted, having a clear goal and an action plan to achieve the goal allows both the patient and the doctor to check progress, which in turn promotes confidence and willingness to comply with regimens.

Interaction with patients: Physicians should encourage patients to stay in charge of the illness and its management, as it would facilitate self-care. They should also talk to the patients about their daily problems. The physicians should be ready to accept the patients' feelings and reframe them only when possible. They need to enquire about normal emotional responses and normalize their anger by pointing out that people with chronic illnesses do get angry at times. At the same time, it is advisable not to cheer up the patient.

Interaction with the family: Physicians should encourage the family to talk about the disease and give them all the information after prior sanction from the patients. The family members should be asked to support the patient to become self-confident. The feelings of the family members are equally important and signs of dysfunction in the caring family should be keenly observed. The treatment supporter in the family should be encouraged to develop skills (syringe driver skills). The services of a professional psychologist should be sought when the doctor feels constrained either due to lack of skills or time.

Active and sustained follow-up: Patients benefit most when contact with doctors is planned and sustained over time. By contacting patients at specified intervals, doctors can collect information on the medical and functional status of the patient. They can also identify potential complications early, check progress in implementing the care plan, make necessary adjustments and reinforce patients' efforts. All this can be done by scheduled return visits, or by such simple steps as telephone contacts.

An individual's adaptation or maladaptation to persistent stress such as having diabetes mellitus makes the difference between ability and inability to manage the stress.

Additional Resources for Coping with Stress

An ability to cope depends on the nature of the stress and also on resources available for 'background support' to the individual. Several major coping resources have been identified including:

Health and energy: The stronger and healthier people are, the longer they can cope with stress without exhaustion.

Positive beliefs: A positive self-image and a positive attitude are especially significant coping resources. Such positive belief can come from a belief in oneself, in others (e.g. doctors who can help) or in a just and helpful God. People who feel they have an internal locus of control, i.e. a feeling they have significant control over the events in their lives, tend to cope better than those who feel they have no control.[34]

Social skills: The better one's social skills, the less the stress. Social skills also help in communicating ones need, to enlist help and to decrease hostility.

Social support is an important coping resource, be it from families, friends or social organizations such as diabetes self-care groups. The findings from a study of 245 patients highlighted the interdependence of the persons with diabetes and the family in living with the disease. Asian Indians with diabetes mellitus tend to be more independent in self-care, i.e. exercising and taking medication, but seek and receive significant social and emotional support from their spouses. The results of the longitudinal analysis reiterate the role of the spouse in assisting the patient in living with diabetes. Gender differences show that female patients require more social support in coping with the disease and enhancing their sense of well-being and quality of life.[35]

Diabetes education programs, which are now more informal and interactive, offer forum for interaction. Courses developed to combine education with counseling and psychological intervention.[36]

Material resources are invaluable in coping with stress, although the adage goes *money is not everything*; it is something when one has to purchase medicines, blood glucose meters, and sticks or undergo other tests in managing diabetes. In facing minor or major stresses, people with money who can use it effectively generally fare better and experience less stress than those without money.

Other Sources of Stress

- **Restriction of daily life patterns:** Regimentation in lifestyle, fear of hypoglycemia and dependency induces anxiety. Close follow-up by diabetes care team, education and reinforcement help in normalizing attitude towards daily care. Understanding the rationale and acquiring skills can buffer the psychological effects.
- **Sexual dysfunction as an expression of stress:** Besides vascular and neural disorders leading to sexual dysfunction in men, stress can also result in reversible sexual dysfunction. Misconceptions abound regarding sexual function in diabetes.[37] It has been recently shown that erectile dysfunction is common among persons with type 2 diabetes, and is associated with a poorer quality of life.[38] A comprehensive approach is imperative in managing the situation.
- Sleep disturbances are four times common in diabetes mellitus compared to controls.[39] The stress of having the disease, along with physical symptoms, psychosocial factors including shift work may all contribute to sleep disturbances. Sleep problems in chronic diseases such as diabetes mellitus go hand-in-hand with poor work productivity, work quality and greater use of health services.[40] A recent study has suggested that individuals with short sleep had reduced leptin and elevated ghrelin. These differences in leptin and ghrelin could increase appetite, and lead to obesity and insulin resistance.[41]
- **Apprehension of complications and likely disability:** Onset of complications brings on extra-psychosocial problems. The single deciding factor is the degree of handicap resulting from complications, and how well the individual can cope with the resulting limitation. The health care team along with the individual's family and significant others form the major source of support in coping.

Psychological Instruments in Diabetes Mellitus

The outcome of treatment in acute conditions such as infectious diseases is measured by duration of illness and recovery. Diabetes mellitus cannot be evaluated similarly. The traditional measure of signs, symptoms and biochemical investigations form the doctors' *preoccupation with the disease process*.[42] Patients are encouraged to participate actively in their health promoting activities, including the decision on which mode of treatment and the degree of control that is required. All these call for new paradigms in adopting objective measures such as quality of life questionnaire,[43] including the recent ADDQOL questionnaire,[44] well-being[45] and diabetes treatment satisfaction.[46]

- Quality of life questionnaire (Diabetes quality of life questionnaire; DQOL) was originally developed for use in DCCT to evaluate the discomfort of intensive insulin therapy with conventional therapy. It was assumed that additional demands in intensive therapy including re-education, multiple daily insulin injections or pump, frequent blood glucose monitoring, greater need for adjustment of food exercise and insulin could affect the quality of life, and could affect the willingness to follow intensive treatment. The questionnaire evaluates the satisfaction, impact and worries associated with diabetes treatment. It can be used in both type 1 and type 2 diabetic patients using insulin, or diet and oral hypoglycemic agents.[43] It is acceptable and easy-to-use that is not difficult to understand. The newly developed ADDQOL instrument is sensitive to effects of diabetes, including treatment and complications. It was devised on the basis of schedule for the evaluation of individual quality of life, in which an individual is asked to generate aspects of life that are important, and to evaluate how good or bad each aspect is currently felt to be, and indicate the importance of each for quality of life.[44]
- **Well-being questionnaire:** The well-being questionnaire was originally designed to provide a measure of depressed mood, anxiety and also aspects of positive well-being in a WHO study evaluating new treatments for managing diabetes.[45] This questionnaire was specifically designed and scored so that diabetes related symptoms (such as tiredness, loss of appetite and libido) are not mistakenly attributed to depressed mood. Even though the original questionnaire was developed for adults with insulin-treated diabetes, it can probably be suitably used for people treated with diet alone.[45] It is now called the World Health Organization (WHO) (Bradley)

well-being questionnaire. It includes each of four subscales—depression, anxiety, energy and positive well-being. The scale is useful in determining the incremental benefits to well-being of new treatments designed to improve quality of life rather than just blood glucose control.

- **Diabetes treatment satisfaction questionnaire (DTSQ)** was specifically designed to measure satisfaction with diabetes treatment regimens in people with diabetes.[46] It is intended to measure satisfaction with treatment and is not designed to measure satisfaction with other aspects of the diabetes care service. It is a measure of psychological outcome to measure benefits of new treatments that can improve patients' quality of life rather than just the blood glucose control. This scale is claimed to be useful in individuals who are treated with diet and exercise alone. However, DTSQ scores should not be interpreted in isolation, but should be corroborated with other measures of metabolic control. Or else patients are likely to desire a treatment regimen that is easy to follow, but which does not achieve metabolic control.

Other Scales[17]

ATT[39] (Psychological adjustment to diabetes): This measures the psychological adjustment to diabetes.[47] It is sensitive to the psychological process unique to diabetes. The rationale for this is, blood glucose levels are affected both by stress-related neurohormonal perturbations as well as indirectly by compliance to treatment. It is a 39 item self-report measure with *attitudinal statements* related to patient's perception of disease and treatment. The psychological adjustment instrument measures how far diabetes is integrated into the patient's lifestyle and personality.

Diabetes specific health beliefs: The purpose of this scale is to measure beliefs about diabetes and its complications.[48] It evaluates the psychological processes rather than outcome and can be used to understand how the patients beliefs are associated with their behavior. Four belief factors are determined—perceptions of severity of disorder, vulnerability to disorder, benefits of treatment and barriers to treatments. The health belief measure gives a framework for conceptualizing the beliefs.

Perceived control of diabetes: Measures of perceived control of diabetes provide understanding of patients' preferences for treatment options.[49] Perceptions of patients and health care professionals may be discordant. The use of this instrument is to try to bridge the dichotomy. Three subscales are employed—personal control, medical and situational control. It measures psychological processes rather than outcomes.

Barriers to self-care: This evaluates the social-environmental factors in diabetes, and seeks to improve compliance.[50] It identifies environmental and cognitive factors that interfere with diabetes self-care. Thirty-one item statements are given to the subjects. The scale produces an overall barriers score. The current scale has been validated on adults with type 2 diabetes mellitus.

Other scales are being developed such as the diabetes distress scale, to assess diabetes-related emotional distress.[51]

Quality of life, well-being, social support and coping in diabetes mellitus.

When quality of life was assessed in individuals with diabetes mellitus and with impaired glucose tolerance[30] more subjects with impaired glucose tolerance rated their general perceived health as being excellent to good (72.23% with diabetes mellitus, 83.49% with impaired glucose tolerance).

Considering that diagnosis of chronic diseases such as diabetes mellitus may have a negative impact on the individual's perception of well-being, a study was carried out to determine the effect of being newly diagnosed with diabetes.[52] Using the medical outcomes study short form-36 (SF-36) instrument in 1,253 outpatients, screening for diabetes was shown to have minimal *labeling effect*. Similarly, education about primary prevention in offspring of persons with type 2 diabetes resulted in improved awareness about personal risk, but did not cause psychological harm.[53]

STUDIES IN CHILDREN WITH TYPE 1 DIABETES MELLITUS

A study of the impact of diabetes on overall quality of life (QOL) identified four major themes—restrictions, being different from others, negative emotion and adaptation. Adolescents were most bothered about dietary restrictions, and were worried the most about the future, specifically diabetic complications. Older adolescents, however, had lower worry and had better quality of life. A multicentric multinational study from 17 countries involving 2101 adolescents between the ages of 10 and 18 showed that lower glycosylated hemoglobin (i.e. better medium term glycemic control) was associated with fewer worries, greater satisfaction and better health perception.[54] Both the parents and the health care team perceived the burden of disease as being lesser in adolescence than in the younger age.

Personal models of diabetes could be proximal determinants of self-care in diabetes. Adolescent's beliefs about diabetes and its treatment were important in influencing self-care, emotional well-being and glycemic control.[55] Similarly, both friends and family were important sources of support to adolescents with diabetes.[56,57] Family support predicted good self-management.[26] Acceptance of the disease and a sense of coherence correlated with educational level.[27]

STUDIES IN PARENTS OF CHILDREN WITH TYPE 1 DIABETES

In type 1 diabetes mellitus, the parents and immediate family members face physical, psychological and social stress, especially in the very young.[58] Having a child with diabetes mellitus most affected the parental life satisfaction.[59] The event with the greatest impact was the frequency of telling others about the child's diabetes. The greatest worry was the possible development of diabetes complications. Parents of school-aged children manage to derive than parents of adolescents.

Parents employed various coping strategies such as planned problem solving, positive reappraisal and social support seeking.[60] Fathers were more likely to use distancing independent of whether the child was a boy or girl, in contrast to mothers who used all coping strategies when the child was a girl.

STUDIES IN TYPE 2 DIABETES

Quality of life in type 2 diabetes mellitus is an important health outcome measure.[61] In addition to medical treatment, social support, health education and psychological care are also required.[62]

A judicious blend of generic as well as disease-specific psychological instruments is required to measure quality of life and well-being. Scales have been designed encompassing cognitive and disease-specific dimensions, while accounting for cultural beliefs and specific norms.

In the United Kingdom Prospective Diabetes Study (UKPDS), complications of the disease were shown to affect the quality of life (QOL), whereas the treatment measures (intensive versus aggressive) did not affect QOL.[63] This is consistent with an earlier study, which showed that poor metabolic control and comorbid conditions were related to poor QOL.[64,65] Over time, insulin therapy was eventually related to poorer QOL.[66]

QOL was compared with metabolic control in 94 outpatients with type 2 diabetes who were referred for insulin therapy.[67] QOL improved in the total group with a reduction of mean blood glucose.

In contrast to this report, another study followed up 461 persons randomized into standard care or group with monitoring with diabetes nurse specialist.[68] The group that was monitored reported better mood, independent of glycemic control. Monitoring and discussing psychological well-being had favorable effects on the moods, even though metabolic control did not improve. This is similar to our study on a smaller group who were followed up by a psychological research scientist,[69,70] where improved well-being occurred independent of glycemic control.

It is therefore important that the balance between metabolic control and QOL be considered. Care must be taken not to sacrifice metabolic control with exclusive focus on well-being aspects, and vice versa. The purpose of QOL assessment is to improve patient satisfaction *pari passu* with metabolic control.

Quality of Life (QOL) and Complications of Diabetes

It may seem intuitive that QOL is adversely affected by complications by diabetes, but few formal studies were carried out. Aside from the substudy in the UKPDS referred to above,[63] complications were evaluated separately. Involvement of the foot had a negative impact on the QOL.[46] Currently, active foot ulcers and amputation resulted in a poorer QOL than those with healed ulcers, without amputation.[71,72] Lower limb ulcers had a negative impact not only on the patients but also on the caregivers.[73] Therefore prevention and management of foot involvement in diabetes must pay attention to improving mobility, and by to offer appropriate counseling.[74]

Symptomatic diabetic neuropathy was associated with impaired QOL,[75] on the following scores—emotional reaction, pain, physical mobility and sleep. In a recent report, sleep problems were directly associated with health-related QOL.[40] These are particularly relevant to India, where we have shown that both sleep disturbances[39] and symptomatic peripheral neuropathy[39] were common. There is also preliminary evidence that sleep deprivation may activate the hypothalamopituitary adrenal axis[76] and lead to the metabolic syndrome.

QOL Studies in Fine Tuning Management Strategies

Studies on well-being and QOL may be useful to fine tune management plan to improve well-being and compliance. Continuity of care in the diabetes clinic was associated with better well-being.[77] These measures can be implemented with little extra financial burden. On the contrary, there should be a consideration of how the physician perceives and is comfortable with the management relation with the patient. Not only can health care givers be affected by the burden of treating persons with chronic unrelenting diseases,[78] but it may dictate the doctor-patient relationship in achieving better glycemic control and QOL.[79]

Even in primary prevention of diabetes, inappropriate hope must not be offered. Whereas offspring of type 2 diabetes mellitus perceived greater threat of developing diabetes and hypertension themselves, they also adopted in health care behaviors to lower the risk.[80] On the contrary, first degree relatives with type 1 diabetes wrongly assumed that lifestyle changes can minimize the risk of developing diabetes.[81]

In the same way, inappropriate use of self-home blood glucose monitoring in type 2 diabetes persons who are not using insulin was counterproductive and led to greater distress.[82]

Social support contributes to physical and psychological well-being.[83] Individuals with type 2 diabetes mellitus tended to create stories of meaning of their diabetes *by linking their current management strategies* with past history.[84] Similarly, impaired access to specific positive memories was associated with poor adjustment to type 1 diabetes mellitus.[85] Other aspects such as spirituality[86] and personal transformation were related to well-being and positive outcomes.

Empowerment—the Concept

Empowerment enables the individual, the family and society to perceive the need for healthy lifestyle and the need for adherence to medical management. It can therefore be considered to have a broader sweep and include compliance as one of its end points. It refers to different components in various contexts. In the field of diabetes management, empowerment addresses not just disease management, but other components including emotional, spiritual, social and cognitive aspects.[87-89] Tailored education forms part of the empowerment pathway, incorporating it into the context of the individual's life.[90] Structured self-education led to empowerment and improved perception of self-efficacy.[91]

The Diabetes Empowerment Scale was developed to measure psychosocial self-efficacy.[92] The psychometric analyses resulted in a 28-item diabetes empowerment scale, with three subscales—managing the psychosocial aspects of diabetes, assessing dissatisfaction and readiness to change, and setting and achieving diabetes goals.

The goal is to improve outcome in the management of diabetes, by combining the efforts of the physician, educator, nutritionist, psychologist, with the individual and the family.[93] Ideally empowerment allows one to analyze data, identify patterns and solve them. It improves treatment outcomes and reduces diabetes-treatment frustration. Psychosocial barriers are identified and energy diverting family issues resolved.[94]

Diabetes Translational Research in Real-World Settings

The evidence-base of diabetes management is now mature. Poor outcomes in disease management are not due to lack of evidence, but mainly due to the inability to put principles into practice. Attention is now focussed on translating research in real world settings.[95] The following key priority areas were identified, external validity and applicability of programs and results in different settings, identifying and understanding barriers and facilitators to diabetes translation in different settings, moving from an acute-care paradigm to a multifaceted chronic-care model that is population-based, proactive, and patient-centered, and community-based participatory translational efforts involving partnerships among researchers, community members and governmental/private agencies. Such translational research outcomes are crucial in containing the diabetes epidemic in India.[95]

PSYCHOLOGICAL FACTORS IN CHILDHOOD DIABETES

Childhood diabetes forms a small percentage of the diabetic population reported from our country.[96,97] However, to those affected it entails considerable stress in management—the child, the family and the health care team. Medical skills and psychosocial support are nowhere more crucial than in the management of the very young child with diabetes.[58] Where trained manpower in supportive fields such as social work, psychology and nutrition is not available, the treating physician must often take on the additional role of providing psychosocial support for the child and the family. The extended family structure, which is still common in our country, offers additional family members in sharing the burden. However, managing the young child with diabetes requires empathy, tact, understanding and ingenuity.

Cognitive Function in Childhood Diabetes

Diabetes mellitus is known to be associated with neuro-behavioral and neuropsychological changes, involving learning, memory, mental speed and eye-hand coordination.[98]

Frequency of Cognitive Dysfunction

Children with diabetes were shown to have greater psychological disability compared to children with other chronic disorders.[99] Cognitive dysfunction identified by electrophysiological tests may antedate abnormal psychometric tests.[100] Lower performances on IQ scores were demonstrated one year after onset of childhood diabetes when associated with ketonuria and hospitalizations,[101] along with other mild neuropsychological dysfunction, such as information processing speed, acquisition of new knowledge and conceptual reasoning.[102] Similarly, there was an inability to express emotions verbally -alexithymia, as a form of emotional suppression.[103]

Studies in India

There are few published Indian studies except for the report from Chennai, Tamil Nadu, India.[104] Children with diabetes scored less compared to controls on all scores, Wechsler's coding, digit span test and Raven's colored progressive matrices. However, there was no correlation with duration of diabetes or early onset of diabetes. It was concluded that the lower scores were due to psychosocial factors in addition to metabolic control. In a study at our center, it was shown that cognitive function was poorer compared to control children on reaction time and memory. Sixteen children with diabetes (8 boys, 8 girls) aged 8 to 16 were compared to 32 age and sex-matched controls. Diabetic children had longer reaction times than controls.[105] Similarly, they scored poorly on memory scales including memory span, logical memory and associated learning.[106] However, there was no statistically significant difference in intelligence quotient between children with diabetes and controls.[107]

Cause and Course

A variety of causes were implicated in cognitive dysfunction including central nervous system vascular or metabolic dysfunction, emotional influence of the chronic illness on the intellectual and educational development or a central neuropathy (analogous to peripheral neuropathy).[108,109] There is strong evidence for recurrent hypoglycemic episodes being responsible for this disability in cognitive function.[110-112] Hyperglycemia has also been implicated for cognitive dysfunction.[113] Other associated factors include duration of illness, age of onset, episodes of ketonuria, ketoacidosis and hospitalization.[98] The role of social impact of the disorder must not be lost sight of.[114]

Significance of Cognitive Impairment

Children with diabetes missed school more often, performed more slowly and obtained lower scores than controls.[115] Cognitive impairment is associated with increased risk of learning problems.[116] This underscores the necessity for ascertaining educational skills in diabetic children when planning diabetic treatment regimens, especially with early onset long duration diabetes, who may be especially vulnerable.[117]

Diabetes and Child Development

It is always a struggle to balance the need for parental guidance in diabetes mellitus and allowing the child with diabetes to develop independence. The difficulties in coping can be categorized into the following empirical stages:

They may benefit from contact with other families with young children with type 1 diabetes as part of diabetes education programs.[118] There is no ideal way of management, which must be ultimately a balance of the ideal with the practical and realistic.

MODEL FOR LIVING EFFECTIVELY WITH DIABETES

Based on a detailed psychosocial analysis of more than 200 persons with diabetes mellitus,[35] a model was proposed for living effectively with diabetes.

- The model rests on the fundamental issue that metabolic control is essential to live effectively with diabetes. Even isolated instances of high or low blood glucose levels can affect the emotional well-being. Depression, anxiety, coping abilities, stress and host of other responses can be affected.
- Gender differences become crucial when one has to learn to live effectively with diabetes. Women need to develop a positive attitude towards the disease and its management. This is crucial especially in those responsible for household tasks, which may render it difficult for them to follow their own diets, medication and eating schedules. They need to realize that the disease can be controlled and it is they themselves who have to do so, undoubtedly, with support from others such as their physicians and family members.

- The age of the individual with diabetes is also important. Older people need to reconcile themselves to the fact that diabetes would not go away but that it could be managed satisfactorily with a disciplined lifestyle. They should be careful not to allow depression and anxiety arising out of age to overwhelm their psychological well-being. They must learn to consider diabetes as another problem, which needs to be carefully handled.

- Adoption of a positive approach in the management of the disease can enhance the effectiveness of living with diabetes. In many cases, especially type 2 diabetes, the patients themselves will be responsible for management of their illness.

Consistent with the above conclusion, a network of psychological variables in diabetes revealed that subjects who had 'strong beliefs in their self-efficacy and with an optimistic outlook on life were more likely to be satisfied with their doctor-patient relationships'. They also showed 'more active coping behavior' and had a better quality of life.[119]

SUMMARY

Diabetes mellitus being a lifestyle-related disorder, the role of psychosocial factors is closely interwoven in its management. Historically, efforts were made to identify *diabetes prone personality*. This was followed by using psychological skills to improve health-related behavior. Currently, psychological factors are studied in relation to the cause and prevention of metabolic syndrome, insulin resistance phenotype.

The biopsychosocial model recognizes the central role of the individual, the family and thereby society to perceive and act upon evidence in the management of lifestyle disorders such as type 2 diabetes mellitus. Rather than focus solely on biological factors, the model lays increasing emphasis on psychological and social factors to deal with diabetes mellitus.

Stress acts at many levels—individual, environment, genetic, hypothalamo-pituitary-adrenal—modulation of the stress response balances vulnerability and resilience to diseases, including diabetes mellitus. The exposure and resultant expression can occur from the intrauterine life through to birth and the entire lifespan. Coping strategies in stress are learned experiences and may be emotion focussed, or cognitive changes in how one views stress, rather than changing the stressful situation; or problem focussed, in which the stressful conditions are themselves changed. A combination of both strategies is necessary in different situations. Psycho-

social barriers must be broken among the family, the physician and significant others. Positive beliefs, social skills, social support and support groups, and material help all form additional resources for coping.

A variety of psychological instruments are available to quantify and follow-up various facets specifically to diabetes—quality of life, well-being, treatment satisfaction, psychological adjustment to diabetes, diabetes specific health beliefs, barriers to self-care and diabetes distress scale. Careful attention is paid to the construction, use and interpretation of psychological tools, as with any other clinical or laboratory measurement. These have been used and found to be useful in children with type 1 diabetes, in their parents, as well as in type 2 diabetes mellitus; in the latter, various facets were studied including complications, in fine tuning management plans and in identifying other aspects of conception. However, one should be careful in balancing psychological well-being and glycemic-metabolic control. As the aim is to improve treatment outcome, one should not take precedence over the other.

Ultimately evidence from research (DCCT, UKPDS) must be applied to clinical practice. This translational research is gaining importance, so that the individual with diabetes and the family is empowered, i.e. they are informed, educated and convinced of the rationale and outcomes of treatment, so that they form active partners in diabetes management.

Children with diabetes have to cope not only with the disease, but with various other developmental aspects to reach adulthood. Similarly cognitive function is another vital component.

The role and goal of psychosocial issues in diabetes spread both broad and deep. They are being utilized to improve diabetes care and outcome.

REFERENCES

1. Chang JC, Ng MC, Critchley JA, Lee SC, Cockram CS. Diabetes mellitus—a special medical challenge from a Chinese perspective. Diabetes Res Clin Pract. 2001;54 (Suppl 1):S19-27.
2. Huffman C, Rice K, Sung HY. Persons with chronic conditions—their prevalence and costs. JAMA. 1996;276:1473-9.
3. Lari MA, Tamburini M, Gray D. Patients' needs, satisfaction, and health-related quality of life: towards a comprehensive model. Health and Quality of Life Outcomes 2004;2:32. URL: http://www.hqlo.com/content/2/1/32).
4. King H, Aubert RE. Global burden of diabetes, 1995-2025: prevalence, numerical estimates, and projections. Diabetes Care. 1998;21:1414-31.
5. Sridhar GR, Madhu K. Stress in the cause and course of diabetes. Int J Diab Dev Countries. 2001;21:112-20.

6. Yudkin JS, Yajnik CS, Ali VM, Bulmer K. High levels of circulating proinflammatory cytokines and leptin in urban, but not rural, Indians. Diabetes Care. 1999;22:363.

7. Bradley C. Psychological aspects of diabetes. In Alberti KGMM, Krall LP (Eds): the Diabetes Annual I. Amsterdam: Elsevier Sci Pub.1985. pp. 374-88.

8. Hopper SV. Meeting the needs of the economically deprived diabetic. Nurs Clin North Am. 1983;18:813-25.

9. Testa MA, Simonson DC, Turner RR. Valuing quality of life and improvements in glycemic control in people with type 2 diabetes. Diabetes Care. 1998;21(Suppl 3):44-52.

10. Kapur A, Shishoo S, Ahuja MMS, Sen V, Mankame K. Diabetes care in India – patients perceptions, attitudes and practices. Intl J Diab Dev Countries. 1997;17:5-17.

11. Greenhalgh T, Helman C, Chowdhury AM. Health beliefs and fold models of diabetes in British Bangladeshis: a qualitative study. BMJ. 1998;316:978-83.

12. Peckhan C. Fetal and child development. In Marinker M, Peckham M (Eds): clinical futures. Chapter 7; BMJ Books. 1998.

13. Sridhar GR. Complementary and mainstream medicine: friend or foe? Curr Science. 2002;83:211-3.

14. Roman SH, Harris MI. Management of diabetes mellitus from a public health perspective. Endocrinol Metab Clin North Am. 1997;26:443-74.

15. Mobley CC. Health promotion and diabetes risk factors in children. Diabetes Care.1999;22:189-90.

16. Madhu K, Sridhar GR. Model for coping with diabetes. Intl J Diab Dev Countries. 2001;21:103-11.

17. Sridhar GR, Madhu K. Psychosocial and cultural issues in diabetes mellitus. Curr Science. 2002;83:1556--64.

18. Bjorntorp P, Rosmond R. Obesity and cortisol. Nutrition. 2000;16:924-36.

19. Bjorntorp P. Visceral fat accumulation: the missing link between psychosocial factors and cardiovascular disease? J Intern Med. 1991;230:195-201.

20. Katz JR, Taylor NF, Perry L, Yudkin JS, Coppack SW. Increased response of cortisol and ACTH to corticotrophin releasing hormone in centrally obese men, but not in postmenopausal women. Int J Obes Related Metab Disord. 2000;23(Suppl 2): S138-9.

21. Duclos M, Corcuff JB, Etcheverry N, Rashedi M, Tabarin A, Roger P. Abdominal obesity increases overnight cortisol excretion. J Endocrinol Invest. 1999;22:465-71.

22. Sapolsky RM, Romero LM, Munck AU. How do glucocorticoids influence stress responses? Integrating permissive, suppressive, stimulatory, and preparative actions. Endocrine Reviews. 2000;21:55-89.

23. Katz JR, Mohammad Ali V, Wood PJ, Yudkin JS, Cuppack SW. An *in vivo* study of the cortisol-cortisone shuttle in subcutaneous abdominal adipose tissue. Clin Endocrinol (Oxford). 1999;50:63-8.

24. Livingstone DE, Jones GC, Smith K, Jamieson PM, Andrew R, Kenyon CJ, Walker BR. Understanding the role of glucocorticoids in obesity: tissue-specific alterations of corticosterone metabolism in obese Zucker rats. Endocrinology. 2000;141:560-3.

25. Smith GCS, Stenhouse EJ, Crossley SA, Aitken DA, Cameron AD, Connor JM. Development: early-pregnancy origins of low birth weight. Nature. 2002;417:916.

26. Naomi S Levitt, Estelle V Lambert, David Woods, C Nick Hales, Ruth Andrew, Jonathan R Seckl. Impaired glucose tolerance and elevated blood pressure in low birth weight, nonobese, young South African adults: early programming of cortisol axis. J Clin Endocrinol Metab. 2000;85:4611-8.

27. Mooy JM deVries H, Grootenhuis PA, Bouter LM, Heine RJ. Major stressful life events in relation to prevalence of undetected type 2 diabetes: the Hoorn Study. Diabetes Care. 2000;23:197-201.

28. Mehta S. Stress and coping. In Behavioural sciences in medical practice. India: Jaypee Brothers Medical Publishers, New Delhi; 1998. pp. 81-91.

29. Lazarus RS, Folkman. Stress, appraisal and coping. New York: Springer; 1984.

30. Peyrot M, Rubin RR. Levels and risks of depression and anxiety symptomatology among diabetic adults. Diabetes Care.1997;20:585-90.

31. Haupt E, Herrmann R, Benecke-Timp A, Vogl H, Haupt A, Walter C. The KID Study II: Socioeconomic baseline characteristics, psychosocial strain, standard of current medical care and education of the Federal Insurance for Salaried Employees' Institution (BfA) diabetic patients in inpatient rehabilitation. Kissingen Diabetes Intervention Study. Exp Clin Endocrinol Diabetes. 1996;104:378-86.

32. Piotrowski M, Sochalski JA. Learning to live with diabetes. Michigan Diabetes Research and Training Center. University of Michigan; 1980.

33. Priti Chandra. Psychological aspects of diabetes. Intl J Diab Dev Countries. 1997;17:111-2.

34. Strickland BR. Internal-external expectancies and health related behaviours. J Consulting Clin Psychol. 1978;46:1192-211.

35. Veena S, Madhu K, Veena S. Gender differences in coping with type 2 diabetes mellitus. Intl J Diab Dev Countries. 2001;21:97-102.

36. Shobhana R. The existing model and future directions in diabetes patient-education. Intl J Diab Dev Countries. 1997;17:113-6.

37. Sridhar GR. Contribution of psychosocial and physical factors in diabetic sexual dysfunction. Social Science International. 1992;8:1-4.

38. De Berardis G, Franciosi M, Belfiglio M, et al. Erectile dysfunction and quality of life in type 2 diabetic patients: a serious problem too often overlooked. Diabetes Care. 2002;25:284-91.

39. Sridhar GR, Madhu K. Prevalence of sleep disturbances in diabetes mellitus. Diab Res Clin Pract. 1994;23:183-6.

40. Manocchia M, Keller S, Ware JE. Sleep problems, health-related quality of life, work functioning and health care utilization among the chronically ill. Qual Life Res. 2001;10:331-45.

41. Taheri S, Lin L, Austin D, Young T, Mignot E. Short sleep duration is associated with reduced leptin, elevated ghrelin, and increased body mass index. PLoS Med. 2004; 1(3):e62

42. Torres TT. Measuring health-related quality of life: an idea whose time has come. Natl Med J India. 1998;11:155-7.

43. Jacobson AM. The Diabetes control and complications trial research group. The diabetes quality of life measure. In Bradley C (Ed): handbook of psychology and diabetes. Switzerland: Hardwood Acad Pub; 1994. pp. 65-87.

44. Bradley C, Speight J. Patient perceptions of diabetes and diabetes therapy: assessing quality of life. Diabetes/Metabolism Res Reviews. 2002;18:S64-9.

45. Bradley C. The well-being questionnaire. In Bradley C (Ed): handbook of psychology and diabetes. Switzerland: Hardwood Acad Pub; 1994. pp. 89-109.

46. Bradley C. Diabetes treatment satisfaction questionnaire (DTSQ). In Bradley C (Ed): handbook of psychology and diabetes. Switzerland: Hardwood Acad Pub; 1994. pp. 111-32.

47. Welch G, Dunn SM, Beeney LJ. The ATT39: A measure of psychological adjustment to diabetes. In Bradley C (Ed): handbook of psychology and diabetes. Switzerland: Hardwood Acad Pub; 1994. pp. 223-45.

48. Lewis KS, Bradley C. Measures of diabetes-specific health beliefs. In Bradley C (ed): handbook of psychology and diabetes. Switzerland: Hardwood Acad Pub; 1994. pp. 247-89.

49. Bradley C. Measures of perceived control of diabetes. In Bradley C (Ed): handbook of psychology and diabetes. Switzerland: Hardwood Acad Pub; 1994. pp. 291-331.

50. Glasgow RE. Social environmental factors in diabetes: barriers to diabetes self-care. In Bradley C (Ed): handbook of psychology and diabetes. Switzerland: Hardwood Acad Pub; 1994. pp. 335-49.

51. Polonsky WH, Fisher L, Earler J, Dudl RJ, Lees J, Mullan J, Jackson RA. Assessing psychosocial distress in diabetes. Diabetes Care. 2005;28:626-31.

52. David Edelman, Maren K Olsen, Tara K Dudley, Amy C Harris, Eugene Z Oddone. Impact of diabetes screening on quality of life. Diabetes Care. 2002;25:1022-6

53. Pierce M, Ridout D, Harding D, Keen H, Bradley C. More good than harm: a randomised controlled trial of the effect of education about familial risk of diabetes on psychological outcomes. Br J Gen Pract. 2000;50:867-71.

54. Hilary Hoey, Henk-Jan Aanstoot, Francesco Chiarelli, Denis Daneman, Thomas Danne, Harry Dorchy, et al. Good metabolic control is associated with better quality of life in 2101 adolescents with type 1 diabetes. Diabetes Care. 2001;24:1923-8.

55. Chas Skinner, Sarah E Hampson. Personal models of diabetes in relation to self-care, well-being, and glycemic control: a prospective study in adolescence. Diabetes Care. 2001;24:828-33.

56. Skinner TC, John M, Hampson SE. Social support and personal models of diabetes as predictors of self-care and well-being: a longitudinal study of adolescents with diabetes. J Pediatr Psychol. 2000;25:257-67.

57. Skinner TC, Hampson SE. Social support and personal models of diabetes in relation to self-care and well-being in adolescents with type I diabetes mellitus. J Adolesc. 1998;21:703-15.

58. Sridhar GR. Diabetes mellitus in children below the age of five. Indian J Endocrinol Metab. 1997;1:13-5.

59. Faulkner MS, Clark FS. Quality of life for parents of children and adolescents with type 1 diabetes. Diabetes Educ. 1998;24:721-7.

60. Azar R, Solomon CR. Coping strategies of parents facing child diabetes mellitus. J Pediatr Nurs. 2001;16:418-28.

61. Rubin RR, Peyrot M. Quality of life and diabetes. Diabetes Metab Res Rev. 1999;15:205-18.

62. Shobhana R, Rama Rao P, Lavanya A, Padma C, Vijay V, Ramachandran A. Quality of life and diabetes integration among subjects with type 2 diabetes. J Assoc Physicians India. 2003;51:363-5.

63. United Kingdom Prospective Diabetes Study (UKPDS) Group. Quality of life in type 2 diabetic patients is affected by complications but not by intensive policies to improve blood glucose or blood pressure control (UKPDS 37). Diabetes Care. 1999;22:1125-36.

64. Larsson D, Lager I, Nilsson PM. Socio-economic characteristics and quality of life in diabetes mellitus—relation to metabolic control. Scand J Public Health. 1999;27:101-5.

65. Lloyd CE, Orchard TJ. Physical and psychological well-being in adults with Type 1 diabetes. Diabetes Res Clin Pract. 1999;44:9-19.

66. Davis TM, Clifford RM, Davis WA. Effect of insulin therapy on quality of life in type 2 diabetes mellitus: the Fremantle Diabetes Study. Diabetes Res Clin Pract. 2001;52:63-71.

67. Goddijn PP, Bilo HJ, Feskens EJ, Groeniert KH, van der Zee KI, Meyboom-de Jong B. Longitudinal study on glycaemic control and quality of life in patients with type 2 diabetes mellitus referred for intensified control. Diabet Med. 1999;16:23-30.

68. François Pouwer, Frank J Snoek, Henk M, van der Ploeg, Herman J Adèr, Robert J Heine. Monitoring of psychological well-being in outpatients with diabetes: effects on mood HbA$_{1c}$, and the patient's evaluation of the quality of diabetes care: a randomized controlled trial. Diabetes Care. 2001;24:1929-35.

69. Sridhar GR, Madhu K, Radha Madhavi P, Mattoo V. Psychological parameters of Asian South Indian persons using insulin—one year follow-up. Diabetes. 2000 (Supplement to ADA 60th meeting): Abstract no 1887.

70. Gumpeny RS, Kosuri M, Paravastu RM, Pedamallu AB, Bhaduri J. One year follow-up of psychological status among Asian Indians with type 2 diabetes mellitus. 11th International Congress of Endocrinology, Sydney, Oct-Nov 2000. p. 557.

71. Vileikyte L. Diabetic foot ulcers: a quality of life issue. Diabetes Metab Res Rev. 2001;17:246-9.

72. Ragnarson TG, Apelqvist J. Health-related quality of life in patients with diabetes mellitus and foot ulcers. J Diabetes Complications. 2000;14:235-41.

73. Brod M. Quality of life issues in patients with diabetes and lower extremity ulcers: patients and care givers. Qual Life Res. 1998;7:365-72.

74. Meijer JW, Trip J, Jaegers SM, Links TP, Smits AJ, Groothoff JW, Eisma WH. Quality of life in patients with diabetic foot ulcers. Disabil Rehabil. 2001;23:336-40.

75. Behbow SJ, Wallymahmed ME, MacFarlane IA. Diabetic peripheral neuropathy and quality of life. QJM. 1998;91(11):733-7.

76. Sridhar GR. Painful diabetic neuropathy. Intl J Diab Dev Countries. 1999;19:172-6.

77. Hanninen J, Takala J, Keinanen-Kiukaanniemi S. Good continuity of care may improve quality of life in Type 2 diabetes. Diabetes Res Clin Pract. 2001;51:21-7.

78. Charman D. Burnout and diabetes: reflections from working with educators and patients. J Clin Psychol. 2000;56:607-17.

79. Auerbach SM, Clore JN, Kiesler DJ, Orr T, Pegg PO, Quick BG, Wagner CJ. Relation of diabetic patients' health-related control appraisals and physician-patient interpersonal impacts to patients' metabolic control and satisfaction with treatment. J Behav Med. 2002;25:17-31.

80. Forsyth LH, Goetsch VL. Perceived threat of illness and health protective behaviors in offspring of adults with non-insulin-dependent diabetes mellitus. Behav Med. 1997;23:112-21.

81. Hendrieckx C, De Smet F, Kristoffersen I, Bradley C. Risk assessment for developing type 1 diabetes: intentions of behavioural changes prior to risk notification. Diabetes Metab Res Rev. 2002;18(1):36-42.

82. Monica Franciosi, Fabio Pellegrini, Giorgia De Berardis, Maurizio Belfiglio, Donatella Cavaliere, Barbara Di Nardo, Sheldon Greenfield, Sherrie H Kaplan, Michele Sacco, Gianni Tognoni, Miriam Valentini, Antonio Nicolucci. The Impact of blood glucose self-monitoring on metabolic control and quality of life in type 2 diabetic patients: an urgent need for better educational strategies. Diabetes Care. 2001;24:1870-7.

83. Zink MR. Social support and knowledge level of the older adult home-bound person with diabetes. Public Health Nurs. 1996;13:253-62.

84. Schoenberg NE, Amey CH, Coward RT. Spirituality and well-being: an exploratory study of the patient perspective. Soc Sci Med. 2001;53:1503-11.

85. Leung P, Bryant RA. Autobiographical memory in diabetes mellitus patients. J Psychosom Res. 2000;49:435-8.

86. Daaleman TP, Kuckelman Cobb A, Frey BB. Spirituality and well-being: an exploratory study of the patient perspective. Soc Sci Med. 2001;53:1503-11.

87. Mark F Peyrot. Theory in behavioral diabetes research. Diabetes Care. 2001;24:1703-5.

88. Arnold MSM, Busler PM, Anderson RM, Fummell MM, Feste C. Guidelines for facilitating a patient empowerment program. Diabetes Educ. 1995;21:308-12.

89. Anderson RM, Fummell MM, Butler PM, Arnold MS, Fitzgerald JT, Feste CC. Patient empowerment: results of a randomized controlled trial. Diabetes Care. 1995;18:943-9.

90. Brown F. Patient empowerment through education. Prof Nurs. 1997;13 (Suppl 3):S4-6.

91. Howarka K, Pumpria J, Wagner-Nosiska D, Grillmayr H, Schlusche C, Schabamam A. Empowering diabetes outpatients with structured education: short-term and long-term effects of functional insulin treatment on perceived control of diabetes. J Psychosom Res. 2000;48:37-44.

92. Anderson RM, Funnell MM, Fitzgerald JT, Marero DG. The Diabetes Empowerment Scale: a measure of psychosocial self-efficacy. Diabetes Care. 2000;23:739-43.

93. Sridhar GR, Anderson RM. Compliance or empowerment in diabetes mellitus? In Kelkar SK, Srishya MV, Joshi JK (Eds): Novo Nordisk Diabetes Update Proc. Mumbai: Business Network Inc; 2003. pp. 128-34.

94. Brink SJ, Miller M, Moitz KC. Education and multidisciplinary team care concepts for pediatric and adolescent diabetes mellitus. J Pediatr Endocrinol Metab. 2002;15:1113-30.

95. Sridhar GR. Containing the diabetes epidemic. Natl Med J India. 2003;16:57-60.

96. Sridhar GR. Gender differences in childhood diabetes. Intl J Diab Dev Countries.1996;16:108-13.

97. Ramachandran A, Snehalatha C, Joseph TA, Vijay V, Viswanathan M. Delayed onset of diabetes in children of low economic stratum—a study from Southern India. Diab Res Clin Pract. 1994;22:171-4.

98. Ryan CM. Neurobehavioral complications of type 1 diabetes. Examination of possible risk factors. Diabetes Care. 1998;11:86-93.

99. Cernele D, Hafner G, Kos S, Cenlec P. Comparative study of social and psychological analyses in asthmatic, rheumatic and diabetic children. Allerg Immunol (Leipz). 1977;23:214-20.

100. Pozzessere G, Valle E, de Crignis S, Cordischi VM, et al. Abnormalities of cognitive functions in IDDM revealed by P300 event-related potential analysis. Comparison with short-latency evoked potentials and psychometric tests. Diabetes. 1991;40:952-8.

101. Rovet JF, Ehrlich RM, Czuchta D. Intellectual characteristics of diabetic children at diagnosis and one year later. J Pediatr Psychol. 1990;15:775-88.

102. Northam EA, Anderson PJ, Werther GA, Warne GL, Adler RG, Andrewes D. Neuropsychological complications of IDDM in children 2 years after disease onset. Diabetes Care. 1998;21:379-84.

103. Abramson L, McClelland DC, Brown D, Kelner S Jr. Alexithymic characteristics and metabolic control in diabetic and healthy adults. J Nerv Ment Dis. 1991;179:490-4.

104. Jyothi K, Susheela S, Kodali VR, Balakrishnan S, Seshaiah V. Poor cognitive task performance of insulin-dependent diabetic children (6–12 years) in India. Diabetes Res Clin Pract. 1993;20:209-13.

105. Sangeeta B. A study on reaction time and sleep patterns among children with diabetes mellitus. Dissertation submitted for MPhil in Psychology to Andhra University, Andhra Pradesh, India; 1997.

106. Hymavathi B. A study on memory among diabetic and non-diabetic children. Dissertation submitted for MPhil in Psychology to Andhra University, Andhra Pradesh, India; 1997.

107. Radha Madhavi P. A study on intelligence among children with diabetes mellitus. Dissertation submitted for MPhil in Psychology to Andhra University, Andhra Pradesh, India; 1997.

108. Franceschi M, Ceechetto R, Minicucci R, Smizne S, Baio G, Canal N. Cognitive processes in insulin-dependent diabetes. Diabetes Care. 1984;7:228-31.

109. Ryan CM, Williams TM, Orchard TJ, Finegold DN. Psychomotor slowing is associated with distal symmetrical polyneuropathy in adults with diabetes mellitus. Diabetes. 1992;41:107-13.

110. Skenazy JA, Bigler ED. Neuropsychological findings in diabetes mellitus. J Clin Psychol. 1984;40:246-58.

111. Rovet JF, Ehrlich RM, Hoppe M. Specific intellectual deficits in children with early onset diabetes mellitus. Child Dev. 1988;59:226-34.

112. Lincoln NB, Faleiro RM, Kelly C, Kirk BA, Jeffocate WJ. Effect of long-term glycemic control on cognitive function. Diabetes. Care. 1996;19:656-8.

113. Davis EA, Soong SA, Byrne GC, Jones TW. Acute hyperglycaemia impairs cognitive function in children with IDDM. J Pediatr Endocrinol Metab. 1996;9:455-61.

114. Deary IJ, Crawford JR, Hepburn DA, Langan SJ, Blackmore LM, Frier BM. Severe hypoglycemia and intelligence in adult patients with insulin-treated diabetes. Diabetes. 1993;42:341-4.

115. Ryan C, Longstreet C, Morrow L. The effects of diabetes mellitus on the school attendance and school achievement of adolescents. Child Care Health Dev. 1985;11:229-40.

116. Holmes CS, Dunlap WP, Chen RS, Cornwell JM. Gender differences in the learning status of diabetic children. J Consult Clin Psychol. 1992;60:698-704.

117. Wolfdorf JI, Anderson BJ, Pasquerello C. Treatment of the child with diabetes. In Joslin's diabetes mellitus (Eds): Kahn CR, Weit GC. Lea and Febiger, Philadelphia; 1994. pp. 530-51.

118. Pontious SL. Diabetes mellitus and the preschool child. In Joshu DH (Ed): management of diabetes mellitus. St Louis: Mosby; 1996. pp. 579-634.

119. Rose M, Fliege H, Hildebrandt M, Schirop T, Klapp BF. The network of psychological variables in patients with diabetes and their importance for quality of life and metabolic control. Diabetes Care. 2002;25:35-42.

Chapter 83

PSYCHIATRIC PROBLEMS IN DIABETES

MV Muraleedharan, GR Sridhar

CHAPTER OUTLINE

- Introduction
- Coexistence of Diabetes and Psychiatric Illness
- Psychological Distress Caused by Screening and Diagnosis
- Management of Common Mental Problems
- Psychiatric Comorbidity in Type 1 Diabetes
- Conclusion

INTRODUCTION

While it is recognized that diabetes is common in India,[1-3] it is often not realized that psychiatric diseases are also common and are likely to coexist with diabetes mellitus. In addition, some drugs used for management of psychiatric conditions may initiate or worsen metabolic changes of diabetes mellitus.[4]

Neuropsychiatric disorders account for 12.7% of the global burden of disease.[5] A recent population-based study of 4319 individuals in USA[6] has shown that nearly a third had mental disorders. In another large New York City study, serious psychological distress (depression, anxiety and other disorders) was reported by 10.4% of persons with diabetes (80/857).[7]

Morbidity due to mental disorders in India is comparable to global rates.[8] In an epidemiological study from rural north India, psychiatric morbidity was higher in the elderly (43.32%) compared to those below the age of 60.[9] Another survey in a rural community, when repeated after 20 years[10] has shown that the prevalence of psychiatric morbidity did not change significantly, although the pattern of morbidity differed from the earlier study. In AIIMS, New Delhi, nearly one-third of 209 subjects above the age of 60 had a psychiatric illness.[11]

Despite comparable prevalence of psychiatric diseases, attitudes and concepts may vary across cultures.[12] In United Kingdom, the rate of common mental disorders were as common in women of Indian origin compared to others; lower frequency of medical consultation was a result of differences in conceptualizations of the disease.[13]

Given that both diabetes and psychiatric morbidity are common, they are likely to coexist, while one may worsen the other.[14]

COEXISTENCE OF DIABETES AND PSYCHIATRIC ILLNESS

There is little published data from the Indian subcontinent on the coexistence of diabetes and psychiatric illness. At Dhaka, 27.88% (n:29) subjects with newly diagnosed diabetes had depressive illness as assessed by Hamilton Rating Scale for Depression.[15] Patients with mental disorders are likely to receive even less intensive medical care for diabetes.[16,17]

Stress from natural calamities has been shown to be associated with higher prevalence of new cases of diabetes and impaired glucose tolerance.[18]

In diabetes, lesser degrees of psychological aberration not amounting to psychiatric morbidity is more common.[19] Women with type 2 diabetes mellitus reported poorer quality of life compared to men. Persons aged below 40 years reported better satisfaction with management, and had better quality of life. Gender differences were apparent in sense of well-being, men reported better adjustment, particularly in coping with and integration of the illness.

Counseling for psychological distress and treatment of depressive disorder would improve the well-being and/or metabolic control in diabetes mellitus.[19,20]

A recent study suggested that maternal pre- and perinatal depression can adversely impact the health of their infants, leading to poorer growth.[21]

People with schizophrenia have greater mortality than controls.[22] Among 370 patients with schizophrenia followed for 13 years, standardized mortality ratio (SMR) was above that for the general population. The SMR from diabetes was also increased (996; 95% confidence interval 205-2911).[23] Lifestyle factors such as smoking and poor compliance to treatment may have contributed to the mortality. In addition, antipsychotic medications also cause obesity, metabolic syndrome and type 2 diabetes mellitus.

PSYCHOLOGICAL DISTRESS CAUSED BY SCREENING AND DIAGNOSIS

As either both type 1 and type 2 diabetes is pronounced one must keep in mind the impact, it may impose on those who are screened. It is imperative that the resultant anxiety be properly managed. When screening leads to high stress among those with a positive result, or false reassurance in those with a negative result, the subjects are less likely to take appropriate corrective action.[24] Similarly, one must realize that lifestyle changes can minimize the risk of developing type 1 diabetes mellitus.[19]

A variety of psychological distress can occur when diabetes mellitus is first diagnosed: Denial, anger, guilt, reactive depression and finally acceptance. Physicians must be aware of these reactions which are anticipated with most chronic conditions. They must be trained to manage these[25] reactions which may take months to resolve.

MANAGEMENT OF COMMON MENTAL PROBLEMS

Common mental disorders include states of anxiety and depression; these were previously termed neuroses. Patel et al have shown that patient models of common mental disorders may evolve from somatic to psychological as the illness becomes chronic and severe.[26] When mental disorders confront the doctor on the face of heavy outpatient load, he may find it difficult to manage. In a teaching general hospital, physicians and surgeons tend to underestimate the occurrence of psychiatric morbidity in clinical practice.[27] Even with high degree of awareness that patients with physical disorders may psychological morbidity, doctors feel it *impractical for them to assess and treat emotional problems.*[28]

An interesting saving feature is that in developing countries, people with schizophrenia fare better due to the *healing power of social interventions.*[29]

Central Obesity, Hypothalamopituitary Axis (HPA) and Stress

Cortisol and obesity may be linked by stress. Other contributing factors could include conversion of cortisol to its metabolites, and the programming of the HPA axis. Central obesity has been called the Cushing's disease of the omentum as constant exposure to raised glucocorticoids specifically of the adipose tissue in the omentum may be responsible for central obesity. Bjorntop postulated that stress could be responsible for sympathetic nervous system activation, hormone abnormalities and obesity. Different persons may show *eustress* and *distress* responses to the same stimulus.[30]

HPA Activation and Obesity

HPA axis is more active in centrally obese men; central obesity in women was associated with differential cortisol secretary response to meal. Fat may also be preferentially deposited in the abdomen due to activity of enzymes that metabolize glucocorticoids. The level of activity of 11-β-HSD activity was highly related to body fat distribution and with central obesity.

Depression and Diabetes

Depression as a Cause of Diabetes

Depression could double the risk of developing type 2 diabetes mellitus,[31] and may be considered a risk factor for its development.[32] The Hoorn study evaluated, if psychological stress was positively associated with, among others, prevalence of diabetes mellitus.[33] The number of stressful life events during the preceding five years was assessed in 2,262 adults aged 50 to 74 years without known diabetes. A glucose tolerance test was done after the stressful-event questionnaire was answered. The events included death of a loved one, retirement, moving from a house and ending an intense relationship. Five percent (n : 112) had previously undiagnosed diabetes. Among single stressful events unrelated to work, death of a partner or moving from a house was related to greater percentage of undetected diabetes (10.6% and 6.9%). Similarly, more the number of stressful events reported, the greater the prevalence of undetected diabetes. This study suggests that stressful life events could lead to the onset of diabetes mellitus.

In a recent paper on the diabetes prevention program, it was examined whether depression markers (using the Beck Depression Inventory) altered during intervention among the three arms of the study (*viz* intensive lifestyle, metformin and placebo). Overall, participation in the program was not associated with changes in levels of depression. Any elevation of depression score was likely to be transient that did not require specific treatment. In a subgroup analysis, elevated symptoms score were found to be less likely in men, and in those with better education.[34]

The causal roles are unclear, although impaired central nervous system glucose metabolism, sedentary lifestyle, diet and smoking may all contribute.[35] Recently leptin, originally studied in relation to adipose tissue has been found to have receptors in the limbic system and thus a potential role in emotional processes. Increasing the brain leptin signal could be used as a new approach to treat depressive disorders.[36]

Depression in the Course of Diabetes

In 2001, a meta-analysis of studies on the prevalence of comorbid depression in adults with diabetes was published.[37] Medline and Psyclnfo search engines were used to identify studies that measured point prevalence or lifetime prevalence or both, of depression in adults with diabetes;[39] studies were included, with a total of 20218 subjects. The principal conclusion was that diabetes doubled the odds of depression,[37] i.e. persons with diabetes were twice as likely to have depression compared to those without diabetes. The odds of depression occurring in women were higher than in men.

Depression may be related to complexities in management of diabetes, or to neurohormonal abnormalities.[38]

In clinical practice, identification of depression in diabetes is often overlooked for a variety of reasons: Societal disapproval of depression, complicity between physicians and patients not to discuss depressive symptoms, and wrongly considering depression as a *normal consequence of difficult physical illness*.[43] The potential benefits of treatment are thereby missed. It may be suspected by history of depression, mental health treatment, family history of depression, symptoms out of proportion to medical explanation, persistent focus on bodily complaints, innocuous medical symptoms not responding to reassurance, sexual dysfunction or chronic pain as a dominant complaint.[39]

Management of Depression

Once diagnosed, depression can be managed by cognitive behavior therapy, antidepressant medications or electroconvulsive therapy. In cognitive behavior therapy, patients are reinvolved in pleasurable social and physical activities; stressful circumstances are resolved and cognitive techniques are used to identify distorted patterns; they are replaced with adaptive and useful ways of thinking.[39]

Before starting formal therapy, depressive symptoms must be reassessed after hyperglycemia is corrected. However, depressive attitude and affective symptoms (e.g. pessimism or crying spells) are unlikely to be only due to poorly controlled diabetes.[38]

Use of antidepressant medications can disturb glycemic control: Tricyclic antidepressants stimulate appetite; selective serotonin reuptake inhibitors suppress appetite, enhance insulin sensitivity and lead to hypoglycemia if diet is not regulated. Once depression is treated eating habits exercise and drug compliance may change, leading to unstable metabolic control. In the presence of autonomic neuropathy, tricyclic antidepressants may worsen orthostatic hypotension, and induce constipation and urinary retention.[38]

Diabetes and Dementia

Dementia and diabetes both increase with age, with one predisposing to the other.[40] Cerebral vascular atherosclerosis in diabetes reduces blood supply to the brain, in addition to formation of advanced glycation end product, oxidative stress and amyloid deposition due to diabetes. The association is pronounced in carriers of the APOE 4 allele.[41] Depleted neuronal insulin receptors mimic some features of Alzheimer's disease, which suggests that neuronal insulin resistance may be partly responsible. Such common pathological changes may occur in both type 2 diabetes and Alzheimer's disease.[42]

Loss of memory is not part of normal aging. Administering mini-mental state examinations questionnaire, along with clock-drawing test may be used as annual screening tests.[43]

Psychotic Disorders and Metabolic Syndrome

Even before neuroleptic drugs were introduced, schizophrenia was believed to be a predisposing factor to diabetes. Diabetes was considered to be an integral part of the disease.[44]

Currently used antipsychotic drugs lead to obesity, diabetes, insulin resistance and metabolic syndrome. One must integrate the role of metabolic factors, medications and lifestyle factors in its pathogenesis; newer evidence indicates that there could be an interaction of orexin peptides and dopamine systems in the prefrontal cortex.[45] Even after antipsychotic drugs were stopped, insulin resistance and hyperleptinemia may persist.[46]

Patients with severe mental illness had higher prevalence of metabolic syndrome;[39,47] similarly, outpatients with bipolar disorder had greater severity of illness with increasing number of comorbid conditions including diabetes mellitus.[48] Remission from borderline personality disorder was poor when associated with chronic physical conditions such as obesity or diabetes mellitus.[49]

Antipsychotic Drugs and Metabolic Changes

Antipsychotic drugs are used in the management of schizophrenia, bipolar disorders, dementia and delirium and other conditions.[50] Earlier agents (e.g. chlorpromazine, thioridazine, haloperidol) were called *typical or conventional*; though they were effective, they commonly induced neurological adverse effects and hyperprolactinemia. More recently introduced agents, called *atypical*, include clozapine, risperidone, olanzapine, ziprasidone and others; they have fewer neurological side effects and better relief of negative symptoms of schizophrenia.[50-51] Relapses are less common.

Metabolic Effects of Atypical Antipsychotic Drugs

Atypical antipsychotic drugs induce weight gain in the following order: Clozapine>olanzapine>thioridazine>quetiapine>chlorpromazine>risperidone>haloperidol>fluphenazine> ziprasidone.[50] The average short-term weight gain varies from a mean of 0.43 to 4.45 kg, with its attendant effects on carbohydrate and lipid metabolism. Clozapine and olanzapine, with a greater propensity to induce weight gain seem to be frequently associated with type 2 diabetes mellitus.[50] A similar hierarchy exists for hyperlipidemia, high for clozapine and olanzapine; low for risperidone. However, a recent study from India which compared the use of otanzapine

and haloperidol/ trifluoperazine for 12 weeks did not find a change in glycemic status, weight or body mass index among the three drugs.[51]

Mechanism of Action

Weight gain: The atypical antipsychotic agents can increase body weight by either the direct stimulation of appetite via feeding areas of the brain, or indirectly by endocrine effects such as hyperprolactinemia, decreased gonadal levels and hypercortisolism.[50] Environmental factors also contribute.[52] Neurotransmitter system changes, *viz* histamine receptor blockage was implicated in changed body weight. In animal studies, blockage of serotonin receptor 5-HT2C led to increased appetite and obesity. Similarly, anticholinergic activity (muscarinic M_3 receptor) may contribute to the development of diabetes.[24]

Using a candidate gene approach, polymorphisms of genes controlling weight regulation pathway can be identified; functional imaging studies of the brain could also give leads into the pathogenesis of weight gain.[52] Polymorphisms of histamine H_1 receptors and dopamine D_2 receptors, polymorphisms in β-adrenergic receptor genes were studied. Leptin and ghrelin levels are also being evaluated, though definite conclusions cannot yet be drawn.[52]

Effect on β-cells and insulin sensitivity: The adverse metabolic effects may be induced in other ways, such as,[46] induction of insulin resistance, either directly or by stimulation of cytokine production, and interference with glucose transport across membranes.

Recently, the effects of clozapine and of haloperidol on electrical and secretory activity of pancreatic β-cells were studied: While at lower glucose concentrations, clozapine in low doses had little effect on membrane potential, at higher doses, it led to marked depolarization of the membrane potential, despite differing glucose concentrations.[53] Similarly, both drugs increased basal insulin release, in contrast to conventional antipsychotics.[54] They produced hyperglycemia. hyperlipidemia and hyperleptinemia.[55] Studies in dogs showed that olanzapine caused weight gain, truncal obesity and insulin resistance.[56] In a prospective analysis, it was shown that olanzapine and risperidone negatively affected pancreatic β-cell function even in the absence of underlying disease. Both led to weight gain, which was greater and consistent with olanzapine. Food intake alone did not account for positive energy balance, but seemed to be related to both caloric intake and energy expenditure. Increased fat mass was reflected in body weight. An impairment of β-cell compensation for insulin resistance was attributed to impedance of neural regulation.[56]

Clinical Implications: In view of the epidemiological and biochemical association of adverse metabolic effects, one must be careful in choosing the antipsychotic agent- efficacy, side in effects and patient profile must all be considered.[57] Weight gain at three to six weeks is a robust clinical indicator for predicting total weight gain: Gain is rapid in the first month and stays constant after several months.[58] Other risk factors are activity level, family history of obesity/diabetes and ethnicity.[59]

In a review on the effects of atypical antipsychotic agents in schizophrenia, the author concluded that olanzapine and clozapine were associated with largest mean weight gain; all atypical antipsychotic drugs increase weight in some patients and weight gain is more in randomized clinical trials. Factors predicting weight gain included low BMI, better clinical response, increased appetite, early weight gain and first onset psychosis.[60]

The consensus statement published in 2004[51] suggested nondiabetic patients on atypical antipsychotic medications be monitored as follows: Body mass index be monitored at each visit, personal and family history and weight circumference be checked at baseline and every annual visit, blood pressure, fasting plasma glucose and lipid profile at baseline, at 12 weeks and annually thereafter.

Management of obesity does not differ in principle from obesity due to other causes: Calorie restriction in diet, physical exercise to induce negative calorie balance, cognitive-behavior therapy, and where necessary, use of drugs to reduce weight (appetite suppressant, lipase blockers).[61]

It should be emphasized that psychiatric disease must not let clinicians be lax in correcting metabolic abnormalities. In a 52-week trial, nutrition, exercise and behavior therapy in schizophrenia was effective in improving metabolic outcomes.[62] Similarly, correction of mental illness can improve insight into medical illness and in adherence to treatment.

PSYCHIATRIC COMORBIDITY IN TYPE 1 DIABETES

Even though childhood diabetes comprises of a small percentage of reported diabetic population in India, it is stressful for the child, the family and the health care team.[63,64] Nearly, a third of children develop psychologi-

cal aberration, such as transient adjustment disorder. It is a normal response to a debilitating chronic illness. Parents also experience adjustment problem, parti- cularly mothers. Anxiety and depression may also occur. Such reactions in the father predict poor glycemic control in children. Adolescents have the capacity to cope better and are often confident in self-management of the disease.

Cognitive Dysfunction

Diabetes mellitus can affect learning, memory, mental speed and eye-hand coordination.[65] Electrophysiological tests can identify cognitive dysfunction even earlier. There are few published Indian studies except for the report of Seshiah et al and our observations.[66,67] Children with diabetes scored less compared to controls (Wechsler's coding, digit span test and Raven's colored progressive matrices). Lower scores were attributed to both metabolic control and psychosocial factors.[66] Sangeeta, Hymavathi and Radha Madhavi have shown that cognitive function was poorer, reaction time longer, memory scale poorer, although intelligence quotient was comparable with control children.[67] Cognitive dysfunction may result from vascular or metabolic dysfunction, emotional influence of the chronic illness or a central neuropathy (analogous to peripheral neuropathy). Children tend to miss school more often, and obtain lower grades.[68] Therefore, when planning diabetes treatment regimens, one must take educational skills in children into account.

Diabetes and Child Development

Development in childhood diabetes may be compro- mised at different stages: Infancy and toddlers. The difficulties arise from irregular meal schedule, poor conception to understand the need for injections and testing, and finally conflict with other siblings who may resent unequal sharing of parental attention. Parents may need psychosocial support along with medical advice.[67] Diabetes care groups may offer fellowship and advice.

School-age child between the ages of 6 and 11, the child must master diabetes care regimen, modify the diet while completing common developmental tasks. Children with normal psychosocial development cope with diabetes well. Stunted growth, hepatomegaly and delay in sexual maturation (Mauriac syndrome) may occur in case of inadequate insulinization and poor control of glycemia.

Behavioral Problems

Even after resolution of initial adjustment disorder, depression is more common in children and adolescents with diabetes. Some continue to show internalizing symptoms (Somatic complaints, sleep disturbances, anxiety, antisocial behavior) and externalizing symptoms (aggressive behavior). Externalizing symptoms are commoner in boys. Multiple stressful events and family conflict adversely influence these problems. Severe symptoms of depression and anxiety foretell poor metabolic control. They also show increased suicidal ideation compared to controls.

Eating Disorders in Type 1 Diabetes

In western countries, eating disorders are being increasingly recognized in type 1 diabetes.[69-73] They may be associated with insulin misuse for control of hyperglycemia and resultant metabolic complications. In a small study where 36 subjects with eating disorder were reassessed after two years, 13.9% (n : 5) showed full remission for at least 12 weeks, 61.6% (n : 22) showed no change and the remaining shifted from subclinical to clinical eating disorder.[74] An increasing body mass index may be associated with ineffective dietary restraint, especially among girls.[75]

Eating disorders should be suspected when, despite efforts to prevent, diabetic ketoacidosis or poor glycemic control continue to occur[76] particularly among those with family dysfunction.[72] However, eating disorder may not be specific to diabetes, but may be due to living with chronic diseases (e.g. phenylketonuria) where dietary management/restriction are mandated.[77]

Intervention should be seriously attempted, for the risk of death may be increased.[78] Psychoeducation program in a group of young women with type 1 diabetes and disordered attitude reduced eating disturbance, but did not improve metabolic control.[79]

Coping with Stress

Coping with stress can be approached either by focussing on the emotional effects of stress or solving the problems of stress or both.[28] In *emotion focused coping* with stressful situations are viewed as being less stressful, i.e. the situations are unchanged, only the emotional response to stress may be maximized. In problem-focused coping, one learns problem-solving skills to directly deal with and change the stressor. A variety of resources can be used to cope with stress, *viz* positive beliefs, social skills, social support and finally on material resources.[80]

Individual psychotherapy involves counseling at clinic visits and is useful in children and adolescents with significant psychological stress.

Group therapy is usually problem oriented. Group leader is a mental health worker. It is best used in the setting of a complication and distress. About 10 participants from the group meet in multiple sessions spread over a year or more.

Cognitive behavior treatment can be used in depression. The individual is encouraged to replace distorted beliefs with accurate and adaptive thoughts to enable management of the disease and reduce its impact on the mental state.

CONCLUSION

The consensus meeting on antipsychotic drugs and obesity and diabetes[51] recommended that research focus on:

- Accurate measurement of body fat using MRI, CT and DEXA
- Contribution of HPA axis activation in altered body composition, contrasting the effects of acute and chronic stress
- Altered insulin sensitivity measurement using euglycemic-hyperinsulinemic clamp with labeled glucose, β-cell function by frequently sampled tVGTT and lipid metabolism using tracer infusions
- Identification of predictive factors for adverse metabolic effects
- Genetic markers as predictors of metabolic disturbances.

Both diabetes and psychiatric disorders are frequent; the two may worsen one another. It is important that they are first identified and the causative factors eliminated. A biopsychosocial approach of diabetes and psychiatric diseases[60] can leverage the social strengths. Application of drugs addition to broad and deep social networks in developing countries is both feasible and effective.[81,82]

REFERENCES

1. Ramachandran A, Snehalatha C, Kapur A, Vijay V, Mohan V, Das AK, et al. Diabetes Epidemiology Study Group in India (DESI). High prevalence of diabetes and impaired glucose tolerance in India: National Urban Diabetes Survey. Diabetologia. 2001;44:1094.
2. Sridhar GR, Rao PV. Prevalence of diabetes among rural Indians. In Das S (Ed): Medicine Update. Mumbai: Association of Physicians of India. 2003;13:370-3.
3. Sadikot SM, Nigam A, Das S, Bajaj S, Zargar AH, Prasannakumar KM, et al. The burden of diabetes and

impaired glucose tolerance in India using the WHO 1999 criteria: prevalence of diabetes in India study (PODIS). Diabetes Res Clin Pract. 2004:66:301-7.

4. Sridhar GR. Psychiatric co-morbidity & diabetes. Ind J Med Res 2007;125:311-20.

5. Weiss MG, Isaac M, Parkar SR, Chowdhury AN, Raguram R. Global, national, and local approaches to mental health: examples from India. Trop Med Int Health. 2001; 6:4-23.

6. Kessler RC, Dernier O, Frank RG, Olfson M, Pincus HA, Waiters EE, et al. Prevalence and treatment of mental disorders 1990-2003. N Engl J Med. 2005;352:2515-23.

7. McVeigh KH, Mostashari F, Thorpe LE. Serious Psychological Distress among Persons with Diabetes—New York City, 2003. MMWR. 2004:53:1089-92. Reported in JAMA. 2005;293:419-20.

8. Khandelwal SK, Jhingan HP, Ramesh S, Gupta RK, Srivastava VK. India mental health country profile. Intl Rev Psychiatry. 2004;16:126-41.

9. Tiwari SC. Geriatric psychiatric morbidity in rural northern India: implications for the future. Intl Psychogeriatr. 2000;12:35-48.

10. Nandi DN, Banerjee G, Mukherjee SP, Ghosh A, Nandi PS, Nandi S. Psychiatric morbidity of a rural Indian community. Change over a 20-year interval. Br J Psychiatry. 2000;176:351-6.

11. Dey AB, Soneja S, Nagarkar KM, Jhingan HP. Evaluation of the health and functional status of older Indians as a prelude to the development of a health programme. Natl Med J India. 2001;14:135-8.

12. Patel V, Andrade C. Pharmacological treatment of severe psychiatric disorders in the developing world: lessons from India. CNS Drugs. 2003;17:1071-80.

13. Jacob KS, Bhugra D, Lloyd KR, Mann AH. Common mental disorders, explanatory models and consultation behavior among Indian women living in the UK. J R Soc Med. 1998;91:66-71.

14. Aanth A, Kolli S, Gunatitake S, Brown S. Atypical antipsychotic drugs, diabetes and ethnicity. Expert Opinion on Drug Safety. 2005;4:1111-24.

15. Begum A, Mahtab H, Khan AKA. Psychiatric morbidity in recently diagnosed diabetic subjects. Bangladesh: J Diab Assoc. 1991;19:16-21.

16. Desai MM, Rosenheck RA, Druss B, Perlin JB. Mental disorders and quality of diabetes care in the Veterans Health Administration. Am J Psychiatry. 2002;159:1584-90.

17. Frayne SM, Hatanych JH, Miller DR, Wang F, Lin H, Pogach L, et al. Disparities in diabetes care: impact of mental illness. Arch Intern Med. 2005;165:2631-8.

18. Ramachandran A, Snehalatha C, Yamuna A, Bhaskar AD, Mary Simon, Vijay V, Shobhana R. Stress and undetected hyperglycemia in southern Indian coastal population affected by tsunami. J Assoc Physicians India. 2006;54:109-12.

19. Sridhar GR, Madhu K. Psychosocial and cultural issues in diabetes mellitus. Current Science. 2002;83:1556-64.

20. Katon W, Cantrell CR, Sokol MC, Chiao E, Gdovin JM. Impact of antidepressant drug adherence on comorbid medication use and resource utilization. Arch Intern Med. 2005;165:2497-503.

21. Rahman A, Iqbal Z, Bunn J. Lovel H, Harrington R. Impact of maternal depression on infant nutritional status and illness: a cohort study. Arch Gen Psychiatry. 2004;61:946-52.

22. Brown S. Excess mortality of schizophrenia: a meta-analysis. Br J Psychiatry. 1997;171:502-8.

23. Brown S, Inskip H, Barraclough B. Causes of the excess mortality of schizophrenia. Br J Psychiatry. 2000;177:212-7.

24. Marteau TM. Understanding and avoiding the adverse psychological effects of screening: a commentary. In Williams R, Herman W, Kinmonth L, Wareham NJ (Eds): the evidence base for diabetes care. John Wiley and Sons, West Sussex; 2002. pp. 235-41.

25. Madhu K, Sridhar GR. Stress management in diabetes mellitus. Intl J Diab Dev Countries. 2005;25:7-11.

26. Patel V, Pereira J, Mann AH. Somatic and psychological models of common mental disorder in primary care in India. Psychological Medicine. 1998;28:135-43.

27. Chadda RK. Psychiatry in non-psychiatric setting: a comparative study of physicians and surgeons. J Indian Mod Assoc. 2001;99:24,26-7,62.

28. Farooq S, Akhter J, Anwar E, Hussain I, Jadoon IH, Khan SA. The attitude and perception of hospital doctors about the management of psychiatric disorders. JCPSP. 2005;15:552-5.

29. Miller G. A spoonful of medicine and a steady diet of normality. Science. 2006;311:464-5.

30. Sridhar GR, Madhu K. Stress in the cause and course of diabetes. Intl J Diab Dev Countries. 2001;21:112-20.

31. Eaton WW, Armenian H, Gallo J, Pratt L, Ford DE. Depression and risk for onset of type 2 diabetes. A prospective population-based study. Diabetes Care. 1996;19:1097-102.

32. Freedland KE. Depression is a risk factor for the development of type 2 diabetes. Diabetes Spectrum. 2004;17:150-2.

33. Mooy JM, deVries H, Grootenhuis PA, Bouter LM, Heine RJ. Major stressful life events in relation to prevalence of undetected type 2 diabetes. Diabetes Care. 2000; 23:197-201.

34. The Diabetes Prevention Program Research Group. Depression symptoms and antidepressant medicine use in diabetes prevention program participants. Diabetes Care. 2005;28:830-7.

35. Haupt D, Newcomer J. Depression is associated with hyperglycemia and other metabolic abnormalities. Diabetes Spectrum. 2004;17:154-5.

36. Lu XY, Kim CS, Frazer A, Zhang W. Leptin: a potential novel antidepressant. Proc Natl Acad Sci. 2006;103:1593-8.

37. Anderson RJ, Freedland KE, Clouse RE, Listman PJ. The prevalence of comorbid depression in adults with diabetes. Diabetes Care. 2001;24:1069-78.

38. Sridhar GR, Madhu K. Depression and psychosocial stress in diabetes mellitus. In Kapur A, Joshi JK (Eds): Novo Nordisk Diabetes Update Proc. Mumbai: Business Network Inc; 2002. pp. 87-92.

39. Lustman PJ, Clouse RE. Practical considerations in the management of depression in diabetes. Diabetes Spectrum. 2004;17:160-6.

40. Llorente MD, Urrutia V. Diabetes, psychiatric disorders, and the metabolic effects of antipsychotic medications. Clin Diabetes. 2006;24:18-24.

41. Peila R, Rodriguez BL, Launer LJ. Type 2 diabetes, APOE gene, and the risk for dementia and related pathologies. Diabetes. 2002:51:1256-62.

42. Janson J, Laedtke T, Parisi JE. Brien PO, Petersen RC, Butler PC. Increased risk of type 2 diabetes in Alzheimer's disease. Diabetes. 2004;53:474-81.

43. Stahelin H, Monsch AU, Spiegel R. Early diagnosis of dementia via a two-step screening and diagnostic procedure. Int Psychogehatr. 1997;9:123-30.

44. Kohen D. Diabetes mellitus and schizophrenia: historical perspective. Br J Psychiatry Suppl. 2004;47:864-6.

45. Fadel J, Bubser M, Deutch A. Differential activation of orexin neurons by antipsychotic drugs associated with weight gain. J Neuroscience. 2002;22:137-41.

46. Arranz B, Rosel P, Ramirez N, Duenas R, Fernandez P, Sanchez JM, et al. Insulin resistance and increased leptin concentrations in noncompliant schizophrenia patients but not in antipsychotic-naïve first-episode schizophrenia patients. J Clin Psychiatry. 2004;65:1335-42.

47. Toalson P, Ahmed S, Hardy T, Kabinoff G. The metabolic syndrome in patients with severe mental illness. Prim Care Companion J Clin Psychiatry. 2004;6:152-8.

48. Beyer J, Kuchibhatla M, Gersing K, Krishnan KR. Medical comorbidity in a bipolar outpatient clinical population. Neuropsychopharmacology. 2005;30:401-4.

49. Frankernburg FR, Zanarini MC. The association between borderline personality disorder and chronic medical illness, poor health-related lifestyle choices, and costly forms of health care utilization. J Clin Psychiatry. 2004;65:1660-5.

50. Baptista T, DeMendoza S, Beaulieu S, Bermudez A, Martinez M. The metabolic syndrome during atypical antipsychotic drug treatment: mechanisms and management. Metabolic Syndrome and Rel Dis. 2004;2:290-307.

51. Consensus Development Conference on Antipsychotic Drugs and Obesity and Diabetes. Diabetes Care. 2004;27:596-601.

52. Guha P, Roy K, Sanyal D, Dasgupta T, Bhattacharya K. Olanzapine-induced obesity and diabetes in Indian patients: a prospective trial comparing olanzapine with typical antipsychotics. J Indian Med Assoc. 2005;103:660-4.

53. Tighe S, Dinan T. An overview of the central control of weight regulation and the effect of antipsychotic medication. J Psychopharmacology. 2005;19(Suppl):36-46.

54. Best L, Yates AP, Reynolds GP. Actions of antipsychotic drugs on pancreatic β-cell function: contrasting effects of clozapine and haloperidol. J Psychopharmacology. 2005;19:597-601.

55. Melkersson K. Clozapine and olanzapine, but not conventional antipsychotics, increase insulin release *in vitro*. Eur Neuropsychopharmacology. 2004;14:115-9.

56. Melkersson KL, Dahl ML. Relationship between levels of insulin or triglycerides and serum concentrations of the atypical antipsychotics clozapine and olanzapine in patients on treatment with therapeutic doses. Psychopharmacology (Berl). 2003;170(2):157-66.

57. Ader M, Kim SP, Catalano KJ, Ionut V, Hucking K, Richey JM, et al. Metabolic dysregulation with atypical antipsychotics occurs in the absence of underlying disease. A placebo-controlled study of olanzapine and risperidone in dogs. Diabetes. 2005;54:862-71.

58. Davis JM. The choice of drugs for schizophrenia. N Engl J Med. 2006;354:518-20.

59. Citrome LL, Jaffe AB. Relationship of atypical antipsychotics with development of diabetes mellitus. Ann Pharmacotherap. 2003;37:1849-57.

60. Haddad P. Weight change with atypical antipsychotics in the treatment of schizophrenia. J Psychopharmacology. 2005; 19(Suppl):16-27.

61. Schwartz TL, Nihalani N, Virk S, Jindal S, Chilton M. Psychiatric medication-induced obesity: treatment options. Obesity Reviews. 2004;5:233-8.

62. Menza M, Vreeland , Minsky S, Gara M, Radler DR, Sakowitz M. Managing atypical antipsychotic-associated weight gain: 12 month data on a multimodal weight control program. J Clin Psychiatry. 2004;65:471-7.

63. Sridhar GR. Gender differences in childhood diabetes. Intl J Diab Dev Countries. 1996;16:108-13.

64. Sridhar GR. Diabetes mellitus in children below the age of five. Indian J Endocrinol Metab. 1997;1:13-5.

65. Ryan CM. Neurobehavioral complications of type I diabetes. Examination of possible risk factors. Diabetes Care. 1998;11:86-93.

66. Jyothi K, Susheela S, Kodali VR, Balakrishnan S, Seshaiah V. Poor cognitive task performance of insulin-dependent diabetic children (6–12 years) in India. Diabetes Res Clin Pract. 1993;20:209-13.

67. Sridhar GR, Madhu K. Psychosocial aspects of diabetes. In Ahuja MMS. Tripathy BB, Moses SGP, Chandalia HB, Das AK, Rao PV, et al (Eds): RSSDI Textbook of Diabetes. Hyderabad: RSSDI; 2002. pp. 737-55.

68. Ryan C, Longstreet C, Morrow L. Child Care Health Dev. 1985; 11:229-40.

69. Peveler RC, Bryden KS, Neil HA, Fairburn CG, Mayou RA, Dunger DB, et al. The relationship of disordered eating habits and attitudes to clinical outcomes in young adult females with type 1 diabetes. Diabetes Care. 2005;28:84-8.

70. Cotton P, Olmsted M, Daneman D, Rydall AC, Rodin GM. Disturbed eating behavior and eating disorders in preteen and early teenage girls with type 1 diabetes: a case-controlled study. Diabetes Care. 2004;27:1654-9.

71. Maharaj SI, Rodin GM, Olmsted MP, Connolly JA, Daneman D. Eating disturbances in girls with diabetes: the contribution of adolescent self-concept, maternal weight and shape concerns and mother-daughter relationships. Psychol Med. 2003;33:525-39.

72. Rodin G, Olmsted MP, Rydall AC, Maharaj SI, Colton PA, Jones JM, et al. Eating disorders in young women with type 1 diabetes mellitus. J Psychosom Res. 2002;53:943-9.

73. Affenito SG, Adams CH. Are eating disorders more prevalent in females with type 1 diabetes mellitus when impact of insulin omission is considered? Nutr Rev. 2001;59:179-82.

74. Herpertz S, Albus C, Kielmann R, Hagemann-Patt H, Lichtblau K, Kohle K, et al. Comorbidity of diabetes mellitus and eating disorders: a follow-up study. J Psychosom Res. 2001;51:673-8.

75. Bryden KS, Neil A, Mayou RA, Peveler RC, Fairburn CG, Dunger DB. Eating habits, body weight, and insulin misuse: a longitudinal study of teenagers and young adults with type 1 diabetes. Diabetes Care. 1999;22:1956-60.

76. Hoffman RP. Eating disorders in adolescents with type 1 diabetes. A closer look at a complicated condition. Postgrad Med. 2001;109:67-9, 73-4.

77. Antisdel JE, Chrisler JC. Comparison of eating attitudes and behaviors among adolescent and young women with type 1 diabetes mellitus and phenylketonuria. J Dev Behav Pediatr. 2000;21:81-6.

78. Nielsen S, Emborg C, Molbak AG. Mortality in concurrent type 1 diabetes and anorexia nervosa. Diabetes Care. 2002;25:309-12.

79. Olmsted MP, Daneman D, Rydall AC, Lawson ML, Rodin G. The effects of psychoeducation on disturbed eating attitudes and behavior in young women with type 1 diabetes mellitus. Intl J Eat Disord. 2002;32:230-9.

80. Madhu K, Sridhar GR. Model for coping with diabetes. Intl J Diab Dev Countries. 2001;21:103-11.

81. Bolton P, Bass J, Neugebauer R, Verdeli H, Clougherty KF, Wickramaratne P, Speelman L, et al. Group Interpersonal Psychotherapy for Depression in Rural Uganda: a randomized controlled trial. JAMA. 2003;289:3117-24.

82. Sridhar GR. Containing the diabetes epidemic. Natl Med J India. 2003;16:57-60.

Chapter 84

ECONOMIC ASPECTS, INSURANCE, DRIVING AND EMPLOYMENT PROBLEMS IN DIABETICS

DK Hazra, S Sarin

CHAPTER OUTLINE

- Introduction
- Diabetes and Life Insurance
- Diabetes and Personal Insurance
- Medical Infirmities and Driving Restrictions Under Insurance Policies
- Summary and Conclusion

INTRODUCTION

The diabetic patient and his treating physician need to consider the insurance aspects in relation to four sectors:

1. Life insurance
2. Health insurance
3. Personal accident insurance
4. Driving insurance.

Apart from the treating physician, the doctor may be asked to give an expert opinion in the capacity of a medical examiner appointed by the insurance company.

It is also pertinent to consider driving in relation to disability as well as employment. An extension of this is the involvement of diabetics in air traffic as pilots, air traffic controllers or crew.

The protection available to diabetics under antidiscrimination laws and the social net provided by various organizations is also worth considering.

This chapter will primarily focus on the Indian scene but we will refer to the situation in the west particularly because our laws and regulations are often modeled on such systems.

DIABETES AND LIFE INSURANCE

The attitude of the life insurance to the diabetic is somewhat different from that of the health and driving general insurer. The life insurer ordinarily makes a detailed assessment of an individual before insuring his life and then either declines the risk (refuses to insure) or agrees to insure. This agreement may be at the usual premium rates or it may be at enhanced rates. This applies to everyone but for the diabetic in particular the following need mention.

Life insurance of diabetics is possible in cases where the patients are under continuous medical supervision. The following factors are considered while deciding the insurability of a proposal:

Proposer: The proposer should be resident in a city/town where round the clock medical care is available. His or her financial status should be such that he/she can reasonably bear the cost of medical treatment. His/her occupation should be one that makes the proposal acceptable, e.g. doctor, chemist, lawyer, professor, etc.

Proposals from traveling salesmen, etc. where it is not possible to maintain regulated diet are high-risk proposals which may or may not be accepted.

Age of the proposer: Ordinarily proposals from diabetics between the ages of 25 to 55 only are accepted.

Waiting period: Proposals from diabetics are considered only after lapse of sufficient time after the diagnosis of the disease so that fasting and feasting sugar levels are known at which the disease is stabilized. Stabilization is confirmed when there is no fluctuation in the proposer's weight, diet and antidiabetic medication dosage are fixed, and there has been no episode of diabetes induced coma in the recent past.

Ordinarily, in cases of diabetics up to the age 35, life insurance cover is granted after a waiting period of one year from the date of detection of the disease, or more until the diabetes has stabilized.

Medical care: It is necessary that such a proposer takes regular professional medical care. For this, a certificate from the attending doctor is taken to this effect. Regular professional medical care would mean at least one visit to the doctor every year.

Associated impairments: If the proposer suffers from any other serious infirmities or diseases in addition to diabetes, normally such proposals constitute very high-risk and are declined. It is necessary to determine whether heart, kidneys, circulatory system is affected in any way since diabetes normally causes the impairment of their functions.

Due to the increased probability of diabetics contracting tuberculosis, the weight of such proposers is a notable factor in the decision to accept the proposal. If there is any family history of cardiovascular/renal diseases, it goes against the proposer.

A standard questionnaire for diabetics: One declaratory, i.e. to be answered by the proposer and the other to be filled up by the attending medical practitioner is required to be submitted for taking life insurance. Specific medical reports are called for to determine the acceptability of such proposals on a case-to-case basis.

If a proposal is found to be acceptable for granting life insurance, it is specially rated to commensurate with risk. Accordingly, premium rates are quoted and proposer willing, the policy is issued.

Concealment: Since all insurance contracts are contracts of utmost good faith any concealment or misrepresentation by the proposer/patient or his physician would entitle the insurer to avoid the contract.

It is pertinent to remember that findings such as advanced diabetic retinopathy or left ventricular hypertrophy during a hospital admission can often strongly indicate the long duration of diabetes, hypertension or ischemic heart disease and help to prove that the patient's declaration of absolute good health made a short while before was false. A doctor should never therefore be a party to such concealment because in such circumstances his fellow brethren in the capacity of the insurance company's medical expert will be forced to point out such inconsistencies.

However, with due exposition of the facts, since diabetics in general have an adverse life course as compared to the nondiabetic, every diabetic should be urged to get his life insured as early as possible. With many policies if subsequent major illness causes the premium payments to be interrupted the policies may continue in force.

DIABETES AND PERSONAL INSURANCE

Commonly available personal insurance sold by Indian General Insurance Companies are either:
• Personal accident policies
• Health insurance policies
• A combination of the two.

Personal accident policies provide compensation in the event of accidental injury or death. Since the factum of accident is in itself a *fortuitous* event, these policies contain no stipulation regarding the health of the insured person.

Health insurance policies provide for reimbursement or medical expenses incurred for treatment of illness or accidental injuries, principally in a hospital or nursing home. However, in cases of medical treatment for a period exceeding 3 days which in the normal course, would require treatment at a hospital/nursing home but is actually taken whilst confined at home either because:
• The condition of the patient is such that he/she cannot be removed to the hospital/nursing home, or
• The patient cannot be removed to the hospital/ nursing home for lack of accommodation therein.

These policies provide for reimbursement of such domiciliary hospitalization expenses up to reduced limits.

But this domiciliary hospitalization benefit does not cover diseases like asthma, bronchitis, diabetes mellitus and insipidus, hypertension, etc.

Pre-existing disease: All health insurance policies specifically exclude pre-existing diseases, i.e. diseases which have been in existence at the time of proposing for the policy. Pre-existing condition means any sickness or its symptoms which existed prior to the date of the policy whether or not the insured person had knowledge that the symptoms were related to the sickness.

In the context of diabetes, this means that if symptoms related to diabetes existed at the time of insurance the policy will not cover diabetes mellitus. However, if symptoms of diabetes arise after the date of insurance, it would be covered.

However, as health insurance is aimed at covering extraordinary expenses such as would necessitate hospitalization; the domiciliary treatment of diabetes is not covered even if it arises after the date of proposal.

This is quite unlike most other conditions where domiciliary treatment is covered. This means that the diabetic cannot claim for investigations or treatment of diabetes at home, even if this is a new illness.

Complications of diabetes: In general, complications arising from pre-existing diseases are considered part of the pre-existing illness. Therefore, for a person in whom the symptoms of diabetes *per se* had existed at the time of proposal, not only will diabetes be excluded but also subsequently arising complications such as retinopathy, nephropathy or heart disease. However, since certain diseases can arise both in diabetics as well as nondiabetics, for example, coronary artery disease, it can be a moot point as to whether coronary disease was a complication of diabetes or arose independent of it.

It must be emphasized, however, that a diabetic can take health insurance for all the other illnesses which are unrelated to diabetics, e.g. cancer.

MEDICAL INFIRMITIES AND DRIVING RESTRICTIONS UNDER INSURANCE POLICIES

Insurance companies in India offer two types of motor insurance policies to vehicle owners:
1. The *A* or the *Act* policy
2. The *B* or the comprehensive policy

The *Act* policy popularly known as the *Third Party* policy covers a vehicle owner "against any liability which may be incurred by him in respect of the death of or bodily injury to any person or damages to any property of a third party caused by or arising out of the use of the vehicle in a public place".

The *comprehensive* policy in addition to the above covers a vehicle owner against loss of or damage to the insured motor vehicle itself, by specified causes. Terms and conditions of both policies in so far as they pertain to the coverage of third party risks are closely regulated by statute. Only such driving restrictions on medically infirm persons as are not ultravires the statute, are therefore permissible under these policies.

The Motor Vehicles Act, 1939 with its subsequent amendments lays down the law relating to inter alia the operation, use and compulsory insurance of motor vehicles in India. It:
- Lays down the requirements and procedure for obtaining a driving license
- Makes mandatory the insurance of vehicles against third party risks
- Binds insurance companies to satisfy judgments of tribunals awarding compensation for third party injury, death or property damage in case of an accident
- Carves out certain exceptions to this duty.

One such exception is where the vehicle at the time of accident is being driven "by any person who is not duly licensed or by any person who has been disqualified for holding or obtaining a driving license during the period of disqualification", and insurance company may defend the action before the Tribunal.

Motor insurance policies accordingly carry a clause embodying the aforesaid exception of the Act. In so far, as the law stipulates a requirement of physical fitness for obtaining or holding a driving license, and bars persons suffering from specified medical infirmities from holding or obtaining a driving license, a positive covenant takes the place of negative restrictions on medically infirm persons driving.

Under Section 7 of the Act of 1939:
  i. Every application for a driving license to the appropriate authority has to be made in a specified *form A*. Part III of this form is a declaration by the applicant of physical fitness (Appendix I).
  ii. Where the application is for a driving license to drive as a paid employee or to drive a transport vehicle, or, where in any other case the licensing authority for reasons to be stated in writing so requires, the application shall be accompanied by a medical certificate in *form C* signed by a registered medical practitioner (Appendix II).

If from the application or from the medical certificate it appears that the applicant is suffering from any disease or disability as specified in the Second Schedule (Appendix III) of the Act or any other disease or disability which is likely to cause the driving by him of a motor vehicle to be a source of danger to the public or the passengers, the licensing authority shall refuse to issue the driving license.

Section 11 of the Act prescribes the same conditions for renewal of a driving license while Section 12 of the Act provides for revocation of driving license on grounds of disease or disability if the licensing authority has reasonable grounds to believe that the holder of the driving license is by virtue of any disease of disability, unfit to drive a motor vehicle.

The consensus of opinion of State Governments had been that medical certificates should be obligatory for all drivers other than owner drivers and that even for owner drivers the licensing authority should be empowered to demand a medical certificate if the authority is not satisfied as to the applicant's general appearance of fitness. This would infuse some life in the declaratory health requirement, otherwise a dead letter provision in practice, in a country where:

- Majority of the applicants being illiterate are not aware of the significance of the declaration.
- Licensing offices are over-run with touts working merely for a fee for each approved application.
- A license means a ticket to employment for many and therefore must be obtained.

The above position prevailed until enactment of the Motor Vehicles Act, 1988. A working group was constituted in 1984 to review the Act of 1939. An important modification suggested related to concern for improved road safety standards and the Bill provided for stricter procedures relating to grant of driving licenses and period of validity thereof.

The new law made it compulsory to first obtain a learner's license before applying for a driving license. Every application for learner's license would have to be accompanied by:

- A declaration of sound health by the applicant
- A medical certificate from a notified medical officer.

If from the application or from the medical certificate, it appeared that the applicant was suffering from any disease or disability to cause the driving by him of a motor vehicle to be a source of danger to the public or the passengers, the licensing authority would refuse to issue the learner's license. Similarly, a medical certificate is a must for renewal of driving license and the provision for revocation of driving license on grounds of disease or disability continued.

The Motor Vehicle Act 1988 with these laudable road safety measures came into force on July 1st, 1989. Government received a number of representations from transport operators, etc. regarding the inconvenience faced by them because of the operation of some of the provisions of the Act. A review committee was therefore constituted within 10 months to examine and review the Act. Its recommendations were placed before the Transport Development Council which made important suggestions on account of inter alia concern for road safety standards.

Act 54 of 1994 amended the Motor Vehicles Act, 1988. The requirement of medical certificate while applying for a driving license has been dropped except for applications for licenses to drive transport vehicles.

The list of specified medical infirmities discussed above does not include diabetes (Appendix III). However, whether by reason of diabetes or independent of it, if a person is suffering from epilepsy, sudden attacks of disability, giddiness or fainting, impairment of vision which prevents reading of a number plate at 25 meters, or defective movement control or muscle power of either arm or leg, he may be refused a license. Since such conditions may arise in persons prone to recurrent hypoglycemia or severe diabetic retinopathy or following cerebrovascular accidents in a diabetic, such individuals could be barred from driving.

In addition under the Act as presently amended a Medical Certificate of health is required for drivers of transport vehicles (trucks, buses, cabs, etc.) and therefore the doctor issuing such a certificate should take care in a diabetic that he does not suffer from epilepsy, vertigo, defects of vision, heart or lung disorder, or deformity which would interfere with the performance of his duties as driver.

Needless to say, this is in the best interests of the passengers, the public at large and the driver himself.

It would appear therefore that except for the existence of disabilities as mentioned above, a diabetic is legally entitled to obtain a driving license and also to obtain motor driving insurance.

Medical Studies on Diabetics as Drivers

Since insulin therapy can cause hypoglycemia which in turn can cause fainting and epilepsy, it is natural to be concerned about the safety of diabetics as drivers. Joslin's diabetes book has quoted a number of studies (Quickel, 1994) some of which show increased and other decreased frequencies of traffic violations and accidents among diabetics as compared to nondiabetics the ratios varying from 0.76 to 1.78. However, in one study only 5.2% of accidents among juvenile diabetics were due to low blood sugar.

There is an interesting study comparing the frequency of accidents among siblings with or without diabetes (Songer, 1988). Diabetic siblings had more accidents but this was not statistically significant.

The physician must use common sense in advising a particular patient as to whether he can or should drive. Assessment of visual disability is a must. Secondly, one should look at his hypoglycemia record. How often has he had hypoglycemia episodes? Does he monitor his blood and urine glucose regularly? Does he suffer from hypoglycemia unawareness? Is he literate or not? Is he, in general, a predictable patient or one prone to depression, *rebellion*, or erratic behavior. Finally is he alcoholic? The risks of alcohol are much greater in a diabetic. Further, the symptoms of hypoglycemia in a diabetic driving home can often be confused with those of alcohol intoxication.

In some diabetics with heart disease, it may be prudent to prohibit driving under stressful conditions which can exacerbate heart disease.

Driving, Employment and the Alcoholic

Apart from driving as a job, i.e. driving transport vehicles, in many countries driving is the only convenient way of reaching a place of work or performing a job. For such subjects, prohibition of driving may mean inability to hold several jobs.

In the USA, the American Diabetes Association until 1977 did not advise diabetics requiring insulin to drive in interstate commerce because such professional drivers often drove for very long periods with unpredictable meal stops and often were subjected to the physical work of loading and unloading. Later the ADA adopted a more liberal approach and requested the Federal Highway Administration to permit insulin requiring diabetics to drive provided, they had been free of severe hypoglycemia and strictly followed glucose monitoring and record-keeping, with provision for annual re-examination and re-certification.

Similar concerns arise for airline pilots, air-traffic controllers (ATCs) and flight crew. In general, diabetics are not permitted to fly airplanes as pilots even though they are on oral drugs rather than insulin. As regards air-traffic controllers, in 1990 an ATC had severe hypoglycemia on duty and all ATCs taking insulin was taken off duty. In 1992, they were permitted to return to duty provided they are under intensive medical supervision. The policies regarding flight attendants vary from airline to airline.

SUMMARY AND CONCLUSION

The legal aspects of insurance for a diabetic in India have been outlined in relation to:
- Life insurance
- Health insurance
- Personal accident insurance
- Driving insurance.

The health considerations in relation to hypoglycemia have been described. The individual physician using common sense can readily decide whether a particular diabetic should be allowed to drive. If he is unfit to drive safely, then he is also unfit to obtain driving insurance.

APPENDIX I: FORM A-III

Declaration as to physical fitness of applicant and knowledge of driving regulation and traffic signs.

The applicant is required to answer "Yes" or "No" in the space provided opposite each question:

a. Do you suffer from epilepsy, or from sudden attacks of disability, giddiness or fainting?
b. Are you able to distinguish with each eye at a distance of 25 meters in good daylight (with glasses, if worn) a motorcar number plate containing seven letters and figures?
c. Have you lost either hand or foot or are you suffering from any defect in movement, control or muscular power of either arm or leg?
d. Can you readily distinguish the pigmentary colours red and green?
e. Do you suffer from night blindness?
f. Are you so deaf as to be unable to hear the ordinary sound signals?
g. Do you suffer from any other disease or disability likely to cause your driving of a motor vehicle to be a source of danger to the public?

I declare that the best of my knowledge and belief the particulars give in Section II and the declaration made in Section III hereof are true.

Note 1: An applicant who answers "Yes" to any of the question (a), (c), (e), (f) and (g) or "No" to either of the questions (b) and (d) should amplify his answer with full particulars, and may be required, to give further information relating thereto.

Note 2: An applicant who answers "Yes" to question (b) and (d) in the declaration and "No" to the other questions may claim to be subjected to a test as to his competency to drive vehicles of a specified class or classes.

Date

Signature or thumb-impression of applicant

APPENDIX II: FORM C

Form of medical certificate in respect of an applicant for a license to drive any transport vehicle or to drive any vehicle as a paid employee:

(To be filled up by a registered medical practitioner)
1. What is the applicant's apparent age?
2. Is the applicant, to the best of your judgement subject to epilepsy, vertigo or any mental ailment likely to affect his efficiency?
3. Does the applicant suffer from any heart or lung disorder which might interfere with the performance of his duties as a driver?
4. a. Is there any defect of vision? If so, has it been corrected by suitable spectacles?
   b. Can the applicant readily distinguish the pigmentary colour red and green?
   c. Does the applicant suffer from night blindness?
   d. Does the applicant suffer from a degree of deafness which would prevent his hearing ordinary sound signals?
5. Has the applicant any deformity or loss of members which would interfere with the efficient performance of his duties a driver?
6. Does he show any evidence of being addicted to the excessive use of alcohol, tobacco or drugs?
7. Is he, in your opinion, generally fit as regards (a) bodily health, and (b) eyesight?
8. Mark of identification.

I certify that to the best of my knowledge and belief the applicant……..is the person herein above described and that the attached photograph is a reasonably/correct likeness.

(Signature)…………..…………

Name……….......................

Space of Photograph

Designation…….................

Note: Special attention should be directed to distant vision and to the condition of the arms and hands and the joints of both extremities.

APPENDIX III: THE SECOND SCHEDULE

I. Diseases and disabilities absolutely disqualifying a person for obtaining a license to drive a motor vehicle:
   1. Epilepsy
   2. Lunacy
   3. Heart disease likely to produce sudden attacks of giddiness or fainting.
   4. Inability to distinguish with each eye at a distance of twenty-five meters in good daylight (with the aid of glasses, if worn) a series of seven letters and figures in white on a black background of the same size and arrangement as those of the registration mark of a motorcar.
   5. A degree of deafness which prevents the applicant from hearing the ordinary sound signals.
   6. Inability to readily distinguish the pigmentary colours and red and green
   7. Night-blindness.
II. Diseases and disabilities absolutely disqualifying a person for obtaining a license to drive a public service vehicle.
   1. Leprosy.

Section 13

HEALTH CARE DELIVERY

Chapter 85

ORGANIZING A DIABETES CLINIC

Anant Nigam, SV Madhu

CHAPTER OUTLINE

- Introduction
- Rationale of Organized Diabetes Care
- Components of a Diabetes Clinic
- Improved Diabetes Care in Practice—the Organization Process
- How Does Organized Diabetes Care Become Effective?
- Follow Evidence-based Clinical Guidelines

- Guideline Implementation
- Patient Self-management Program
- Advantages of Organized Diabetes Care
- Impact of Organized Diabetes Clinic Care on Various Health Care Practices
- A Day at the Diabetes Clinic
- Conclusion
- Summary

INTRODUCTION

Diabetes mellitus is a disease-complex involving multiple systems of the body. Diabetes is the fifth most common cause of return visits in office-based practice with only hypertension, pregnancy, otitis and well-child where visits may be required more frequently.[1] It is a chronic disease requiring lifelong management on the part of the patient and the physician. The management of diabetes requires patience, commitment and has to be focused and individualized. Continuity of care and being able to provide education along with specific therapy is extremely important.

Chronic disease management requires an entire system of care, a team of providers to supply the necessary range of expertise, a system of information to track care and risk factors, and a system to provide patient education to encourage self-management. Many providers underestimate the time and expertise involved in building this systematic approach.

Much of the difficulty of providing good care is a *system problem*, not a *person problem*.[2,3] Diabetes care should be organized to be practical, cost-effective, flexible and individualized. Updated and repetitive information helps improve care.

The impact of organized diabetes care can be measured on various health care practices like improved rates of glycated hemoglobin estimation, foot inspection, low-density lipoprotein cholesterol control and decreased rates of hospitalization because of foot infections and smoking.

RATIONALE OF ORGANIZED DIABETES CARE

The goal of diabetes care is to reduce complications and provide a good quality of life.

Zgibor et al in a clinic-based study showed better process outcome in patients followed by specialists as compared with nonspecialist care.[4] Similar results were published in another report by Hellman et al in a private practice endocrinology setting in which longitudinal data were available over a 14-year follow-up.[5] Additionally, Zgibor et al pointed out that many studies in Europe, have reported lower rates of proliferative retinopathy, other long-term clinical complications, and mortality in patients who receive care in specialized diabetes centers. A long-term follow-up from the Pittsburgh Epidemiology of Diabetes Complications Study also showed that specialist physicians and clinics contribute to better outcome for patients with type 1 diabetes.

Thus diabetes care should be a comprehensive and coordinated effort to improve the outcomes which could be measured as health status, clinical status, patient satisfaction, and cost of therapy of all diabetic patients seen at an *Organized Diabetes Clinic*.

COMPONENTS OF A DIABETES CLINIC

Patient Database (Registry)

The patient database **(Table 85.1)** forms one of the most important components of a diabetes clinic organization. It provides useful information about the complete profile of the patient.

When and where possible computerized patient records help to organize medical data into a coherent flow sheet for rapid review. The computerized patient database can also be programmed to provide related useful information such as: (a) Number of patients with different types of diabetes; (b) Association of a particular type of diabetes with each type of diabetes-related complication. Each new patient receives a specific *Diabetes Clinic Registration Number*. The data in the computer is programmed in such a way that by punching the registration number, the last name or first name, or the city from which he comes, one is able to retrieve his complete profile.

How can the Diabetes Registry be Useful?

The registry helps the practice of diabetes to be interactive and helps the doctor and his patients to manage their diabetes, its related complications and their key clinical measures better. An updated registry may, for example, remind the diabetologist which patients need HbA_{1c} monitoring.

The diabetes registry also helps in analyzing data which then answers questions about whether the patients are deriving benefit in clinical outcome.

Diabetes Specific Laboratory Services

The laboratory needs to be standardized, accurate and reasonably priced. Investigations which need to be done

TABLE 85.1	The database sheet of each patient (manual and computerized record) has the following essential details
Personal details	Name, age, sex, husband's/father's name, complete address, phone numbers, email ID, name of referring doctor, occupation *Diet*: Vegetarian/nonvegetarian, history of smoking/alcohol
Family history	Yes (in grandparents, parents, siblings, children/others) No
Past medical history	Hypertension, cardiovascular disease, stroke, renal or hepatic disease, diabetes in pregnancy, abortions, stillbirths, neonatal death
Age of onset diabetes	
Symptoms of diabetes	
Clinical examination	*Anthropometric details*: Height, weight, BMI, waist circumference *Blood pressure*: Lying/sitting cardiovascular, central nervous system, gastrointestinal, foot examination, retinal examination
Laboratory investigations	Blood sugars, HbA_{1c}, renal functions (blood urea, serum creatinine, urinary protein, microalbuminuria), lipid profile
	Other investigations: ECG, chest skiagram, thyroid profile
Clinical diagnosis (coded)	Type 1 diabetes/type 2 diabetes/gestational diabetes/other types
Complications	All coded

BMI: Body mass index; ECG: Electrocardiogram

on a regular basis include blood sugars, blood urea, serum creatinine, urine protein, microalbumin, lipid profile, liver enzymes, thyroid functions, and glycated hemoglobin. An electrocardiogram (ECG) is also required. Chest skiagram and other relevant examinations are arranged.

Patient Education Material

Patient education forms the cornerstone of treatment of chronic diseases such as diabetes mellitus. Amongst the important components of the diabetes clinic environment are *patient educational posters* on the walls of the waiting area. These need to be in the vernacular language. The posters should have material directed to all aspects of diabetes care. They must be changed periodically to avoid monotony.

Audiovisual education is of value for people in the waiting area. New patients are grouped and educated together. Question-answer session after a lecture helps to improve learning. Patients receive education for diet, investigations related to diabetes treatment, complications of diabetes, podiatry care and for prevention of diabetes in other members of the family.

Diabetes Educator/Diabetes Nurse Specialist

The diabetes educator could give advice about foot care, review of insulin injection techniques or discuss self-monitoring, eye examination, measurement of U-glycosylated hemoglobin, microalbuminuria and the importance of control of blood pressure and lipid levels. Complications of diabetes and sick-day care are other issues which could be discussed.

Dietary Advice Service

This is an important component of any diabetes clinic. A dietician in consultation with the diabetologist should provide dietary advice to the patient, which is practical and useful.

Referral Advice

Referring the patient at the appropriate time for foot care, a retinal examination or a cardiac work-up is an important component of *organized diabetes care.* The ophthalmologist then may advise fluorescein fundus angiography or laser photocoagulation. Similarly, a patient needs referral advice for a cardiac evaluation or a podiatric check-up.

IMPROVED DIABETES CARE IN PRACTICE—THE ORGANIZATION PROCESS

The *organization process* requires that one pays attention to the following to improve diabetes care in practice.

Update Oneself and Know What to do?

Several standards, guidelines and consensus statements have been developed by many organizations. They should set and modify these according to patient needs and requirements and try to stick to them to provide comprehensive care.

Do not Forget Targets

Make a list of what has to be done. Flow charts can help as important reminders, at all desks in the clinic.

Remember What to do?

Simple paper charts help providers remember that care for patients has several components and each one needs attention. This information can also be formatted as a flow sheet to track recommended screening procedures. Brightly colored stickers can be used to indicate high-risk conditions, such as a high-risk foot.

Plan a Preventive Care Visit

One can have effective preventive care if the visit is scheduled for that. Patients need to know what they would be learning about a particular complication on their next visit in addition to their routine investigations.

Since complications related to diabetes are initially a symptomatic, a visit designated for example for foot care could be more productive.

Distribution of Tasks

Office staff must be given materials for various tests or services needed periodically. For example, different staff members could be made responsible for scheduling investigations like a glycated hemoglobin, a cholesterol test or a timely eye referral or a foot examination. The staff can also direct the patient for education service in a particular area. For example, foot examinations are more likely to occur, if nurses have patients remove their shoes before the doctor arrives in the examination room.[6]

Empower Patients

In any chronic disease management, patients should be active participants in taking care of their disease.

Patients can serve as powerful reminders and collaborators in their own care.

HOW DOES ORGANIZED DIABETES CARE BECOME EFFECTIVE?

Organized diabetes care improves both short-term and long-term outcomes. Organized diabetes care is helpful in the following ways:

Better and Updated Information

The diabetologist and his team have updated scientific information which is transformed into clinical practice for the patient's benefit.

Continuity of Care and Delivery of Frequent Repetitive Information

Continuity of care can improve care for persons with diabetes mellitus.[7] The provider would be more likely to know when tests are needed and treatment changes are indicated. Continuity might, therefore, have even greater benefits for persons with diabetes than it does for the general population.[8] Frequent and repetitive information has a better retention value. For example, when a patient on each visit hears about the importance of better blood pressure control or sees a poster about the benefits of foot care, he or she gets the message better and the retention of information is long lasting. A more recent study suggested that higher provider continuity might lead to better glucose control.[9]

Monitoring of Medical Compliance

Compliance of therapy is the essence of any good treatment protocol. An organized diabetes clinic improves when staff is trained in monitoring. Thus, compliance is increased.

Ongoing Teaching and Patient-Diabetes Team Interaction

This allows the patient to continually reassess his/ her treatment and make appropriate adjustments. A periodical interaction between the patient and the diabetes-team serves as an excellent platform for monitoring of the disease, change therapy to improve short-term goals and thereby prevent complications. It also helps in early detection complications and timely intervention. For productive interactions to occur, practice systems must ensure that provider teams have requisite expertise, appropriate patient information,

organized clinical practice support and, that patients have ready access to self-management support resources.

Familiar Personnel

The patient on arrival in the clinic feels comfortable with the same staff and this has an overall advantage.

FOLLOW EVIDENCE-BASED CLINICAL GUIDELINES

The outcome at the diabetes clinic can be improved significantly if the staff is trained to follow evidence-based clinical guidelines for various parameters.

Retinal Screening

All patients with type 2 diabetes at diagnosis or at presentation to the center and all patients with type 1 diabetes beginning five years after diagnosis are subjected to annual dilated eye-examination performed by a retinal specialist. The staff at the center checks the reminder sheet and plans the examination. Having realized the importance of retinal examination over a period of time, patients themselves volunteer for the eye test.[10]

Foot Care

The purpose of this examination is to identify persons at high-risk for developing foot ulcers in the next few years because of neuropathy, deformities, or peripheral vascular disease.[11,12]

All patients with type 2 diabetes have foot screening examination annually from the time of diagnosis, and all patients with type 1 diabetes should have this examination annually beginning 5 years after diagnosis.

Screening for Microalbuminuria

All patients undergo a screening for microalbumin on an annual basis, since it is an important marker for cardiovascular disease.[13]

Advice for Blood Pressure Control

Control of blood pressure is as important as good glycemic control. Organized diabetes care helps in ensuring that this becomes a regular check index when assessing a patient in follow-up. New Targets of blood pressure control and its importance need to be communicated to the patients as well and should be applied to nonpregnant adults with either type 1 or type 2 diabetes.[14]

Advice on Cardiac Risk Reduction

Since diabetes carries a great cardiovascular risk and is responsible for majority of diabetes-related hospitalization and premature death, it becomes imperative for the diabetologist and his team to pay special attention to factors which will eventually reduce cardiac risk.[15]

Glycemic Management To Target HbA$_{1c}$ less than 7%

A guideline suggesting how and when to use diet, exercise, oral hypoglycemic agents, and insulin are discussed in detail with the patients with the aim of reducing HbA$_{1c}$ to less than 7%.[16]

Pregnancy and Glycemic Control

It is of paramount importance to have special clinic personnel dedicated for the care of women with pregestational type 1 and type 2 diabetes or gestational diabetes. These patients will require specific nutritional instructions and also very strict glycemic control for a good fetal outcome.

Counseling about Smoking Cessation

A sincere and persistent effort should be made by the diabetologist and his team to motivate his patient to discontinue smoking because of the markedly increased cardiovascular risk that it carries.[17]

GUIDELINE IMPLEMENTATION

Guidelines can be implemented in several ways:

Continuing Medical Education

Continuing medical education programs are useful to implement guidelines. This includes lectures and workshop on several aspects of diabetes care like retinal screening, foot care, screening of microalbuminuria and glycemic management. Active participation of the patients improves compliance and ultimately clinical outcomes.

Patient-Specific Decision Support

Specific patient education materials exist for each guideline requiring patient self-management activities. For example, a small pamphlet containing information on protective foot care, importance of self-monitoring of blood glucose are distributed to patients and then discussed on subsequent visits.

Measure Guideline Implementation

As providers of diabetes care, it becomes imperative to assess how one is doing and are various guidelines being implemented and with what success. These are helpful in improving care in the future (*details www.diabetes.org/ada/prpqa.htm*).

PATIENT SELF-MANAGEMENT PROGRAM

Practice and implementation of self-management behavior plays an important role in the control of disease. For example, a detailed plan is drawn up for a patient ready to actively participate in self-monitoring of blood glucose. With proper education, more patients come forward for self-management programs.

Evaluation of the Impact of the Program

This is assessed by an annual survey of randomly sampled patients. They are asked to answer questions in a proforma, for example on screening for microalbuminuria or retinal screening or foot care.

ADVANTAGES OF ORGANIZED DIABETES CARE

Observational studies have indicated that endocrinologists in private practice and in institutional settings are able to provide process outcomes significantly different than those of generalists,[18] and are comparable to those achieved in the diabetes control and complications trial.[19]

Improvement in Short-term Clinical Outcomes

Studies have demonstrated that the involvement of diabetes-specialist clinics and diabetes team management have a significant impact on such short-term, clinically significant outcomes as cost for diabetic ketoacidosis,[20] length of hospital stay,[21] emergency room visits and hospitalizations,[22] hypoglycemia,[23] and foot infections.[24]

In the Medical Outcomes Study report by Greenfield et al[24] in 1996, endocrinologists fared better than family physicians in the mean summary clinical outcomes index, which includes [HbA$_{1c}$], foot ulcers, foot infections, albumin excretion, systolic and diastolic blood pressure, visual acuity, vibration sense, and serum creatinine.

Improvement in Long-term Clinical Outcomes

In the study by Hellman et al in a private endocrinology setting, doctors intensively followed 209 people and reported that they developed significantly less end-stage renal disease, had fewer cardiac events and had lower overall mortality rates compared with 571 patients who had been followed by standard community care.[5] Attention to this model of service would provide long-term benefits in a number of practice settings.

IMPACT OF ORGANIZED DIABETES CLINIC CARE ON VARIOUS HEALTH CARE PRACTICES

The Nigam Diabetes Center Experience

In our practice, we have found that over the years, *organized diabetes care* has made a significant difference on various health practices. Specific intermediate-targeted outcomes include increased rates of retinal screening, increased performance and documentation of foot inspection and risk-related education, increased testing for microalbuminuria, increased testing for HbA_{1c}, reduced HbA_{1c} levels, and improved patient satisfaction. More patients realized the importance of regular follow visits and, therefore, more patients underwent diabetes education. **Figure 85.1** shows the effect of *organized diabetes care* on HbA_{1c}, to assess diabetes control.

Between the years 1987 and 1992, the rate of foot infection did increase from 20.4 to 33.4% but the rate of hospitalization due to foot infection continued to increase from 30.6 to 38.6%.

This made us change our strategy at our centre and we made efforts to include a larger number of people for foot inspection. Between the period 1992 and 2002,

therefore, as the rate of foot inspection increased at our centre from 33.4 to 81.5%, the percentage of patients admitted for foot infection/amputation fell from 38.6 to 25.5%.

The percentage of people performing self-monitoring of blood glucose increases from 12.5% in 1987 to 51.5% in 2002 with better and repetitive education at the diabetes center.

Low-density lipoprotein cholesterol and blood pressure targets were also better achieved. With education, percentage of patients who smoked decreased from 29 in 1987 to 14.5 in 2002.

Similarly, percentage of patients who were referred for retinal examination increased significantly from 30.6 in 1987 to 91 in 2002.

A DAY AT THE DIABETES CLINIC

Registration/Appointments

All patients should be seen with an appointment to provide best care.

Patients being given an appointment are: (a) Requested to report at the registration desk after about 10 hours of fast and (b) Get all previous medical record, and up-to-date prescription and present medication. Registration desk fills up details including address and phone numbers.

Measurements

The outpatient clinic nurse records height, weight and waist circumference.

Meeting the Diabetes Doctor

This is a critical part of the patient. On the first visit, it is a detailed history taking and clinical examination which includes blood pressure recording, examination of feet, inspection of insulin injection sites (in a patient already on insulin), and arranging for eye examination.

The Doctor will then advise blood examination, see what medication the patient is taking. He then advises consultation with other members of the diabetes team, the dietician and the diabetes educator.

Blood Samples

Blood sample is taken by one of the clinic nurses for various investigations.

The Diabetes Dietician

The Diabetes Dietician discusses diet with the patient. The dietician advises about healthy eating, weight loss

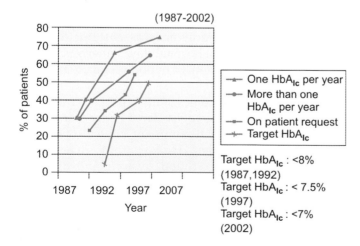

Figure 85.1 Rates of HbA_{1c} estimation and glycemic control (*Source*: Nigam Diabetes Centre, Jaipur, Rajasthan, India)

and adjusting insulin doses in accordance with the patient's food intake.

The Diabetes Educator

The diabetes educator plays a very important complimentary role to the diabetes doctor. He or she can guide the patient about various aspects of diabetes management.

The Next Appointment

The reception desk then gives the next appointment for the patient to be seen by the doctor when the reports are ready and then medication has to be planned.

CONCLUSION

Organized diabetes care demands that the health care provider is to be dedicated, updated and follows one of the consensus guidelines best suited for the patients. It is important to distribute tasks amongst various members of the diabetes care team.

Consensus among the community of health care professionals, scientists, providers on a single set of measures could provide a powerful tool for focusing on key components of care as a basis for quality improvement. It would also allow for valid comparison of care delivered within and across health care settings.

Consensus on these guidelines and quality standards by managed care organizations could simplify reporting quality comparisons. Development of consensus guidelines must be based on evidence supporting each recommendation and must allow flexibility to accommodate unique clinical settings. Consensus on evaluation standards must be based on the validity of the measures, the importance of the care practice to overall outcome, and the cost involved in obtaining these measures.

Finally, better techniques to assist providers in their efforts to provide quality diabetes care are needed. These include educational efforts, organizational changes, and informational support.

SUMMARY

Organized care, with its enforcement of information on each visit, improves clinical outcomes in the management of diabetes mellitus.

Among the many components of an *organized diabetes clinic*, the patient database is the most important. It provides patient information and can be designed to be interactive for reminders about periodic investigations and data analysis. Diabetes-specific laboratory investigations, patient education material, services of a diabetes educator and a dietician, and proper referral for foot care or a retinal examination are the other important components of an organized diabetes clinic.

There should be a constant effort to improve quality of care and much of this is achieved by properly distributing various tasks among staff members of the diabetes clinic. Empowering patients is also helpful.

Updated information, delivery of the same information repetitively, a better adherence to clinical guidelines, ongoing teaching programs which include patient-diabetes team interaction and an overall dedicated and committed staff help in achieving this goal.

Guidelines should be followed properly and methods to measure guideline implementation should be adopted.

Organized diabetes care improves both short-term and long-term clinical outcomes. Short-term clinical outcomes like length of hospital stay, emergency room visits, and attacks of hypoglycemia are lessened. Long-term clinical outcomes show improvement in the form of significantly less end-stage renal disease, fewer cardiac events and lower overall mortality rates.

Organized diabetes care over years can make a significant difference on various health practices. Specific intermediate-targeted outcomes include increased rates of retinal screening, increased performance and documentation of foot inspection and risk-related education, increased testing for microalbuminuria, increased testing for HbA_{1c}, reduced HbA_{1c} levels, and improved patient satisfaction.

REFERENCES

1. Janes GR. Ambulatory medical care for diabetes. In National Diabetes Data Group (Eds): Diabetes in America, 2nd edn. Washington DC: National Institutes of Health 1995, pp 541-5 (NIH pub No 95-1468).
2. General Accounting Office. Medicare: Most beneficiaries with diabetes do not receive recommended monitoring services. Report to the Chairman, Subcommittee on Health and Environment, Committee on Commerce, House of Representatives. Washington DC, General Accounting Office, 1997.
3. Oxman AD, Thomson MA, Davis DA, Haynes RB. No magic bullets: a systematic review of 102 trials of interventions to improve professional practice. Can Med Assoc J. 1995;153:1423-31.
4. Zgibor JC, Songer TJ, Kelsey SF, Weissfeld J, Drash AL, Becker D, Orchard TJ. The association of diabetes specialist care with health care practices and glycemic control in patients with

type 1 diabetes: a cross-sectional analysis from the Pittsburgh Epidemiology of Diabetes Complications Study. Diabetes Care. 2000;23:472-6.

5. Hellman R, Regan H, Rosen H. Effect of intensive treatment of diabetes of the risk of death or renal failure in NIDDM and IDDM. Diabetes Care. 1997;20:258-64.

6. Cohen SJ. Potential barriers to diabetes care. Diabetes Care. 1983;6:499-500.

7. Diabetes requires considerable medical management. American Diabetes Association. Standards of medical care for patients with diabetes mellitus. Diabetes Care. 2001;24:S33-43.

8. Wagner EH. Managed care and chronic illness: health services research needs. Health Serv Res. 1997;32:702--14.

9. Parchman ML, Pugh JA, Noel PH, Larme AC. Continuity of care, self-management behaviors, and glucose control in patients with type 2 diabetes. Med Care. 2002;40:137-44.

10. Aiello LP, Gardner TW, King GL, Blackenship G, Cavallerano JD, Ferris FL III, Klein R. Diabetic Retinopathy (Technical Review). Diabetes Care. 1998;21:143-56.

11. McNeely MJ, Boyko EJ, Ahroni JH, et al. The independent contributions of diabetic neuropathy and vasculopathy in ulceration. How great are the risks? Diabetes Care. 1995;18:216-21.

12. Rith-Najarian SJ, Stolusky T, Gohdes DM. Identifying diabetic patients at high risk for lower-extremity amputation in a primary health care setting: a prospective evaluation of simple screening criteria. Diabetes Care. 1992;15:1386-9.

13. Earle KA, Mishra M, Morocutti A, et al. Microalbuminuria as a marker of silent myocardial ischaemia in IDDM patients. Diabetologia. 1996;39:854--6.

14. Arauz-Pacheco C, Parrott MA, Raskin P. The treatment of hypertension in adults with diabetes (Technical Review). Diabetes Care. 2002;25:134-47.

15. Uusitupa MI, Niskanen LK, Siitonen O, Voutilainen E, Pyörälä K. Ten-year cardiovascular mortality in relation to risk factors and abnormalities in lipoprotein composition in type 2 non-insulin- dependent) diabetic and non-diabetic subjects. Diabetologia. 1993;36:1175-84.

16. Goldstein DE, Little RR, Lorenz RA, Malone JI, Nathan D, Paterson CM. Tests of glycemia in diabetes (Technical Review) Diabetes Care 1995; 18:896-909.

17. Harie-Joshi D, Glasgow RE, Tibbs TL. Smoking and diabetes (Technical Review). Diabetes Care 1999; 22:1887-1898.

18. Ho M, Marger M, Beart J, Yip I, Shekelle P. Is the quality of diabetes care better in a diabetes clinic or in a general medicine clinic? Diabetes Care. 1997;20:472-5.

19. Miller CD, Philips LS, Tate MK, Porwoll JM, Rossman SD, Cronmiller N, Gebhart SS. Meeting American Diabetes Association Guidelines in endocrinologist practice. Diabetes Care. 2000;23:444-8.

20. Levetan CS, Passaro MD, Jablonski KA, Ratner RE. Effect of physician specialty on outcomes in diabetic ketoacidosis. Diabetes Care. 1999;22:1790-5.

21. Levetan CS, Salas JR, Wilets IF, Zumoff B. Impact of endocrine and diabetes team consultation on hospital length of stay for patients with diabetes. Am J Med. 1995;99:22-8.

22. Laffel LM, Brackett J, Ho J, Anderson BJ. Changing the process of diabetes care improves metabolic outcomes and reduces hospitalization. Qual Manag Health Care. 1998;6:53-62.

23. Ho J, Anderson BJ. Changing the process of diabetes care improves metabolic outcomes and reduces hospitalization. Qual Manag Health Care. 1998;6:53--62.

24. Greenfield S, Rogers W, Mangotich M, Carney ME, Tarlov AR. Outcomes of patients with hypertension and non-insulin dependent diabetes mellitus treated by different systems and specialties: results from the Medical Outcomes Study. JAMA. 1995;274:1436-44.

Chapter 86

COMPUTERS IN DIABETES MANAGEMENT

GR Sridhar, PV Rao

CHAPTER OUTLINE

- Introduction
- Electronic Medical Records
- Linking Electronic Medical Records to Hospital Information System
- Scope and Limitations of Electronic Medical Records and Hospital Information System
- Accessing Medical Information
- Bioinformatics

INTRODUCTION

The use of computers in clinical medicine has become ubiquitous and the computer as it was known even a decade earlier is now a metaphor for information technology, which it represents.

Information technology has a broad sweep:[1] It is defined in the *Oxford Dictionary* as '...*technology involved in the recording, storage and dissemination of information, especially using computers, telecommunications, etc.*' In this chapter, use of computers will be discussed in the following areas: (a) Electronic medical records (EMRs); (b) Networking of EMR with hospital information systems; (c) Accessing information from Internet, especially the PubMed database; and (d) Bioinformatics as related to clinical practice and research in diabetes.

ELECTRONIC MEDICAL RECORDS

Essentially, there is nothing very new about electronic medical records (EMRs), except for *electronic*—the records exist in electronic format, instead of paper. The main purpose of clinical care and research is to discern patterns and modify treatment according to changing parameters, be they weight, blood pressure, plasma glucose or serum lipids.[1] EMR supports clinical processes and provides quality health care. It also permits individual health care targets to be set, not only by the physicians but also by the health care team and also enables faster consultations.[2]

Strengths and Weaknesses of Paper Records

Undoubtedly, records on paper have their advantages: They are familiar, mobile and are flexible, allowing one to record subjective data. Besides they can be scanned and browsed easily.[3] Yet, they have their limitations: Data may not be recorded in a uniform fashion, papers may be lost, misplaced or become complex and unmanageable; multiple problem assessment is difficult, sorting according to relevance is not easy, and they cannot be accessed across different locations.

Medical Software for Use in EMR

Electronic medical records (EMRs) have advantages in several of the above areas, but they have flaws as well: Entry of data is nonintuitive and physicians often have to learn to enter data in EMRs. The ideal EMR should fit in the work habits of a physician so that it does not impede work flow, should improve quality of care by

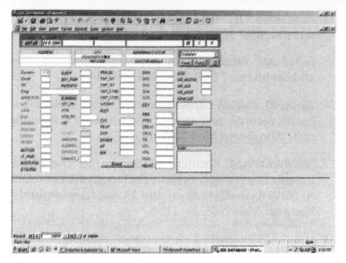

Figure 86.1 Screenshot of EMR for data entry at first visit

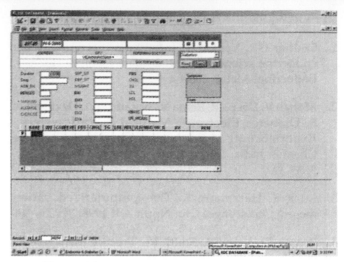

Figure 86.2 Screenshot of EMR for data entry at follow-up visit(s)

work audit and transparently accomplish tasks traditionally provided by other staff, besides being an aid in practice management tools.[1,4] Such as ideal has not yet been met.

The most important practical difficulty in implementing EMRs is an inability to replicate the non-structured capture of data in the physician-patient interaction, which depends on face-to-face interview.[5] Software can be developed consisting of a structured database incorporating a detailed symptoms or signs checklist; but it needs feedback from the clinician in dovetailing what and how much data to collect. The interaction between these two is the usual bottleneck. Besides, to think in a structured format and not lose social and emotional contact with patients requires a new set of skills. Therefore, physicians who plan to use EMRs must first carefully analyze and plan what can be captured: The kind of data, the order and the details, without losing focus of the patient in the interview **(Figures 86.1 and 86.2)**. A discussion with the software developer must be followed by user feedback.

Despite drawbacks, EMRs have undeniable advantages over paper records, viz complete and comprehensive flexibility in storage and retrieval of data, which can be used for publication, presentation and research.[6] Computerized guidelines can provide evidence-based recommendations by allowing access to references, showing errors and sending reminders.[7] Besides, interactive telemedicine support is possible **(Figure 86.3)**. However, all practical questions must be answered before they can be put into application: How and when would the data be entered—self or assisted? What are

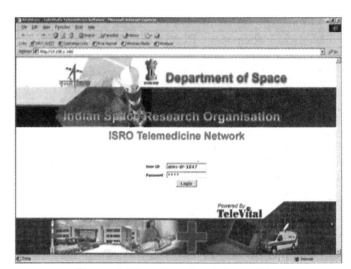

Figure 86.3 Interactive telemedicine

the levels of computer skills and typing skills needed? Are there programs available for the purpose? Solutions to these problems must be found for implementing EMRs.

Readymade Programs

Readymade programs (EMRs), employing a standard format for diabetes, are available in varying degrees of complexity. They are useful for a wide variety of uses besides EMR: Pharmacy data, prescription generation, accounts and billing. Such a comprehensive, standardized and naturally expensive programs may not be relevant to individual practitioners but may be useful for group practice and for hospitals.

Software Programs Records—Made by Doctors

In contrast, programs developed by individual physicians may provide only the basic functions, without harnessing the full potential of programs made by experts. However, the leanness and flexibility may be all that is needed for individual practice where the focus is to store patient data.

This is a situation where the clinician provides the software experts who then create the program. It is tested initially in dummy-record entry and trouble-shooted prior to live operation of the program. This often provides best of both worlds, provided the requirements can be decided and conveyed clearly and comprehensively.[1] The further assistance of a software professional is also needed to solve problem which are expected to occur when having live operation of the software in clinical setting.[6]

Hardware Needs

With the rapid expansion of powerful processors, insufficient hardware is usually not a problem; a recent version hardware which can support office application programs, pictures, videos and sound are necessary. Output devices like printers for prescription, referrals and reports are also available. One should be in a position to be networked if in a hospital or group practice, and as a practical point, there should be support including standby machine provision in case of breakdown.[6] A regular and systematic back-up of all data is imperative to guard against machine failure.

What Information or Data can be Stored?

It is possible to record and store all patient information, laboratory details including X-rays and imaging data, as well as patient photographs when relevant **(Figure 86.4)**.

Utilization of Information

When one is interested in presentation or research, the program should have capability of statistical operation, including facility for creation of graphs or ability to export the data to a program when graphs can be created and imported back.

Caveats in Going for EMRs

Despite all the potential advantages, one should consider the problems that may crop-up in terms of software and hardware support, the time as well as cost needed to familiarize with software for routine data

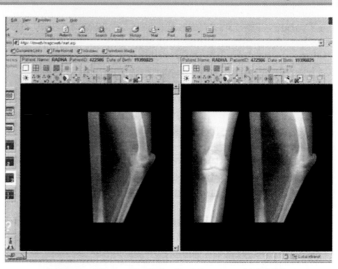

Figure 86.4   Radiological images in EMR

entry, and more importantly the possibility of data loss and how to avoid it, besides security and legal issues.[6] They must be balanced against the advantages of enhanced speed, efficiency, ease of data retrieval, applicability for purposes other than patient care including planning of services, and in the follow-up program for diabetes—when to call a patient back for check-up. All these translate into improved patient care.

Legal Aspects and Ownership of Information

Information laws of the country can be expected to consider EMR as a legal document. They may be electronically signed and must be permanent. An identifier must be attached to any further modifications.[8] Similarly, the question of ownership may arise because electronic information is much more easily transferable. Privacy issues are rampant in the developed countries; we must be aware of such issues cropping up and must plan accordingly.[1]

LINKING ELECTRONIC MEDICAL RECORDS TO HOSPITAL INFORMATION SYSTEM

Hospital Information System (HIS)

Information technology and computerization have been in use for administrative purposes for a long time in medical organizations for a variety of purposes, e.g. financial iInformation systems (FIS), management information systems (MIS), ward-related nursing information systems (NIS), radiology information systems (RIS) and pharmacy information systems (PIS)[6] **(Figure 86.5)**.

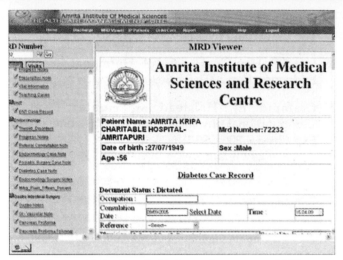

Figure 86.5 Hospital information system (HIS)

The HIS has traditionally included a broad sweep: In-patient administration, outpatient administration, patient care, tests and results, pharmacy control, purchase department, patient billing, financial accounting, human resources management and medical insurance policies.

The online activities include entering the patient profile into database for subsequent retrieval/analysis, reservation for inpatients, transfer of patients from one bed to another, pending discharges, displaying specified physicians patients, displaying patient details by name inquiry and displaying bed availability by nursing station.[6] In addition, offline activities can also be performed such as reservation list, daily inpatient report, list of patients admitted, transferred or discharged, bed census report indicating bed availability, and monthly maternity and death report.

Why Link EMR with HIS?

The purpose and strength of EMRs is to make available information independent of time and space. Therefore linking EMRs with HIS is a crucial, if difficult decision. The key issue is the integration of digital data so that authorized personnel can retrieve the necessary information anywhere and at any time they need it.

Data can be of different variety. Physician may have to look into radiographic images, listen to voice, hear live signals from intensive care and read the notes of other physicians. Such integration is only possible by linking EMR to HIS.

Local Area Networking (LAN) and HIS

Such linking of EMR and HIS is possible by local area networking (LAN), which is a data communication system interconnecting large mainframe system to peripheral computer terminals. It allows a large number of devices to share organizational resources like storage devices, printers, programs and data files. A server on the network provides a specific service like storage, access facility, printing, etc. for all terminals connected to LAN.

Advantages of EMR-HIS

A confluence of EMR-HIS results in improved quality of care, boost in patient safety, reduced length of hospital stay, and increased efficiency and timeliness of care. In health care, benefits are usually found in cost avoidance, rather than in revenue enhancement. Return of investment analysis is not an easily calculated with clinical and decision support applications—add value to patient encounter rather than add revenue.[6]

Automation results in fewer preventable medical errors; misinterpretation of doctors orders resulting from poor physician handwriting, pharmacists trying to clarify prescription and medication doses can all be overcome by HIS, besides cost reduction from decreased staffing, improved billing practices and charge capture. Besides, clinical outcomes can be improved by ensuring better adherence to clinical protocols. Real-time alerts reduce medical errors, drug interaction prevention. Finally, there is also organization value: Decreased waiting time, increased provider satisfaction. Nurses' time saved from documentation to caregiver role.[6]

Disadvantages of EMR-HIS

As in implementing any new technology, in the first few months following implementation, physician may find it difficult to learn new skills in the effort required to create the chart, cost may be high for some of these technologies, and privacy is an issue.

Security

Security can be controlled in a variety of ways:

Authentication: Verification of the identity of the person who is using the service: Username/password, smartcard or token, fingerprint or retinal scan.

Authorization: If the identified person is authorized to use the services requested—list of registered users and their access rights and privacy: Encrypt the message into

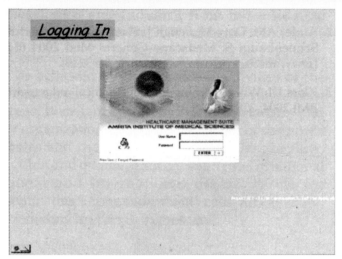

Figure 86.6 Log-in screen to hospital information system

mathematical formula, e.g. 128-bit encryption **(Figure 86.6)**.

Clinical Database Networking

Over time, clinical database networking across institutions offers advantages such as pattern recognition from a much larger database than a single institution or individual can possess; secondly patients may be allowed access to their health records.[9,10] Such access helps them to communicate with their physicians, in seeking appointments and other administrative matters. Eventually, context-related information can be accessed or sent to individuals (e.g. to stop smoking or to start exercise). They can also develop a patient database of experiences, analogous to peer-reviewed medical journals (e.g. database of individual patients experience of illness).[9] Technical advances in computation and matched human-machine interaction should make this possible.

SCOPE AND LIMITATIONS OF ELECTRONIC MEDICAL RECORDS AND HOSPITAL INFORMATION SYSTEM

Alluring as the scope of information technology in clinical practice, is, how does it translate in real life? A recent survey in USA has shown that adoption of information technology tools was slow; important barriers to use were cost to set-up and lack of time to learn new skills.[11]

One should not confuse knowledge with judgment in clinical interactions. A combination of new technology and human interaction is needed.[12] Development of interface is crucial, as a factor in being implemented to improve life.[13] One must also consider the effect on quality of life of physicians by the use of new technologies.[14] Ultimately, change in practice management is likely to be the one stumbling block to implement a new system such as electronic medical records.[15]

ACCESSING MEDICAL INFORMATION

Internet, Pubmed and Other Open Access Sources

Internet, which has become ubiquitous for many in today's world is a global information system that is linked together by a globally unique address space, which can support communications using standard protocols.[1] It is at once a worldwide broadcasting capability for information dissemination and a medium for collaboration independent of geography.

The Internet helps in putting together data that already exists, on a *just in time* basis. However, caution must be exercised in using information from the Internet just as from any other source.

Literacy in information technology for physicians is no longer a choice but a necessity.[1] Among 880 adult outpatients at a tertiary care private hospital in Mumbai, Maharastra, India, nearly a third were accessing the Internet; 75% of those who surfed accessed health-related information.[16] Simultaneous availability of information to both physicians and patients is likely to change the equation between them.[17] Nevertheless, the information must be interpreted by the physician to guide on either the diagnosis or management.[1]

Similarly, the physician has a wide variety of websites to educate oneself.[17] Beside scientific journal both specific to diabetes, endocrinology and metabolism, a variety of other general medical journal are also available (See Appendix). In addition, professional societies and dedicated sites to diabetes/endocrinology exist both from other countries and in India (e.g. *www.rssdi.org, www.diabetes-india.com, www.diabetesindia. com, www.endocrine-india.com, www. endocrineindia.com*).[18]

Specifically, PubMed (*http://www.ncbi.nlm.nih.gov/ entrez/query.fcgi? DB=pubmed*) is an invaluable resource, which has now been joined recently by *www.scholar. google.com.*

PubMed gives access to more than 15 million citations from biomedical literature and is available via NCBI Entrez retrieval system. Entrez is a text-based search and retrieval system; the others have data from nucleotides, protein, protein structures and genomes.

Search Techniques and Search Field Descriptions in PubMed

A detailed description of search field descriptions is available online at the URL *http://www.nlm.nih.gov/ bsd/ pubmed_tutorial/m7001.html*.

Searching with title words is a good way to find a specific citation.
- Enter significant terms and/or numbers from the title of an article
- Follow each term with the **[ti]** tag
- Use the **AND** connector between the words.

To search for an article, the title of which is *Chocolate: food or drug?*, type **chocolate[ti] AND food[ti] AND drug[ti]** into the query box and click on **Go**.

Author Searching [AU]

PubMed recognizes the format last name plus initials as an author search. PubMed will automatically truncate the author's name to account for varying initials.

To search for articles authored by J O'Brien, regardless of middle initials, type **o'brien j[au]** and click on **Go** to review the displayed citations. Notice the author values in the illustration include O'Brien JJ, and O'Brien JT.

To turn off automatic truncation of an author's name, surround the name with double quotes and use the **[au]** tag.
- *Example:* **o'brien j[au]** The citations returned will be restricted to O'Brien, J. If you are searching a last name only (no initials), be sure to use the **[au]** tag.
- *Example:* **o'brien[au]**.

Journal Title [TA]

Use the **[ta]** tag with the journal title abbreviation, full journal name, or ISSN (International Standard Serial Number).
- *Examples:*
  J Biol Chem [ta] Journal of Biological Chemistry [ta]0021-9258 [ta] [Show Me]
  If the journal name contains parentheses or brackets, enter the name without the special characters.
- *Example:* Occup Med (Lond) should be searched as **Occup Med Lond [ta] "**

Scholar Google (www.scholar.google.com)

Google Scholar (scholar.google.com), like PubMed in that it is a search engine that focuses on academic

papers, bringing many results from PubMed. However, there are differences: It is more comprehensive, indexing all academic fields, including nonbiomedical ones. In the case of Google Scholar, links are citations from different papers. Google Scholar does not have the precise searching of PubMed, and does not easily show up new papers, because they would not have been cited often enough.[19]

Open Access and Commercial Conflict

Information technology has the potential to narrow disparities in access to scientific information and literature. Most biomedical information is now controlled and distributed by publishers, whereby access is generally purchased by the reader (either online or as a hard copy journal). A number of journals are, however, available free of charge online in developing countries such as India. Yet a new business model is put forward, where authors pay for publication in open-access journals, which are available free of charge to readers (e.g. Plo S Biology, Plo S Medicine, published by the Public Library of Science, and other journals published by BioMed Central).[20]

BIOINFORMATICS

Computer scientists call bioinformatics '… a bright new field, and is defined as a science of developing computer databases and algorithms for the purpose of speeding up and enhancing biological research'.[21] Similarly, it is the '…study of how information technologies are used to solve problems in biology.'[22] It refers to application of *computational and analytical methods to biological problems… specifically.. the search for and use of patterns and inherent structure in biological data….*[23] Computational biology on the other hand refers to *physical and mathematical simulation of biological processes* although the distinction between bioinformatics and computational biology is not watertight.

Overview of Bioinformatics

In general, three major types of information are studied: (a) One-dimensional structural data from DNA and genes, (b) Three-dimensional structure of proteins and (c) Complete biological systems.[23] Put it another way, the three categories can be considered as *application of principles of physics and chemistry to the modeling of biological systems at the atomic and molecular level; dynamical systems modeling…; and pattern analysis, the process of searching for patterns in sequences of genes or proteins to gain insight into how a biosystem works.*[24]

Especially, after the availability of nucleotide sequences from the human genome project, the major focus is now on identification of genes that code for peptides/proteins, phylogenetic relation over evolution and as mentioned earlier, an integrated view of 'sequence, mRNA and protein expression, as well as cellular and organismal function for a limited number of genes'.[25]

Concept of Systems Biology and Computational Physiology

Research was focussed on a reductionistic scale, with studies progressively looking down from organs to tissues to cells to subcellular structures and to genes. Now attempts are made to integrate all this information into a comprehensive system: The *Physiome Project* aims to quantitatively describe *physiological dynamics and functional behavior of the intact organism*.[26] Distinguishing the genetic role on cell and organ function requires integration provided by computational science. The future challenge lies in quantitatively predicting *physiological outcomes from genome knowledge*.[26]

Application of Bioinformatics Research in Diabetes Mellitus

Ultimately, bioinformatics involves a new set of tools to integrate computational technology, mathematics, statistics and molecular biology; it offers a comprehensive view of physiological processes. This approach in turn could be used in understanding and thereby preventing pathological changes. It is also applicable for treatment and prognostication. Concepts obtained from each could be examined iteratively by wet-lab processes, and the results in turn would be analyzed *in silico*.

REFERENCES

1. Sridhar GR, Venkat Y. Information technology and endocrine sciences in the new millennium. Indian J Endocrinol Metab. 2000;4:70-80.
2. Mohan V, Deepa R, Rema M, Natarajan A, Devanathan S. Diabetes Electronic Medical Record system—Experience at MV Diabetes Specialities Centre, Chennai, India. International Diabetes Monitor. 2000;5:35-9.
3. Lusk R, Herrmann K. The computerized patient record. Otolaryngol Clin North Am. 1998;31:289-300.
4. Brooks RJ, Kahn JA, Smith RL. Practice management, health maintenance, and the use of computers in today's medical office. Medical Clin North Am. 1996;80:279-97.
5. Sridhar GR, Venkat Y. Computers and information technology in diabetes mellitus. In Shah S (Ed): Diabetes Update North Eastern Diabetes Society, Guwahati, Assam, India. 2001;.pp 82-4.
6. Sridhar GR, Appa Rao A, Muraleedharan MV, Jaya Kumar RV, Yarabati V. Electronic medical records and hospital management systems for management of diabetes. Diab Metab Syndr Clin ResRev. 2009;3:55-9.
7. Sullivan F, Wyatt JC. How decision support tools help define clinical problems? BMJ. 2005;331:831-3.
8. Bolling JP. Implementing a comprehensive computerized patient record. Ophthalmol Clin North Am. 2000; 13: June (from the Internet)
9. Sridhar GR, Rao YSV. Clinical database network. Curr Sci. 2000;79:549-50.
10. Sullivan F, Wyatt JC. How computers help make efficient use of consultations? BMJ. 2005;331:1010-2.
11. Audet AM, Doty M, Peugh J, Shamasdin J, Zapert K, Schoenbaum S. Medscape General Med. 2004;6(4) [www.medscape.com/viewarticle/493210]
12. Klass DJ. Will e-learning improve clinical judgement? BMJ. 2004;328:1147-8.
13. Gustafson DH. Evaluation of e-health systems and services. BMJ. 2004;328:1150-1.
14. Jadad AR. What next for electronic communication and health care? BMJ. 2004; 328:1143-4.
15. Baron RJ, Fabens EL, Schiffman M, Wolf E. Electronic health records: just around the corner? Or over the cliff? Ann Intern Med. 2005;143:222-6.
16. Shashank AM, Kanitkar M, Bichile LS. Use of the Internet as a resource of health information by patients: a clinic-based study in the Indian population. J Postgrad Med. 2005;51:116-8.
17. Jadad AR. Promoting partnerships: challenges for the Internet age. BMJ. 1999;319:761-4.
18. Hariom Y, Shalini J, Suman K, Prasad GBKS. Internet resources for diabetes. Indian J Med Sci. 2005;59:32-42.
19. Al-Ubaydli M. Using Search Engines to Find Online Medical Information. PLoS Med. 2005;2(9):e228.
20. Arunachalam S. Open access and the developing world. Natl Med J India. 2004;17:289-91.
21. Mayumi Kato, Chia-Tien Dan Lo. Growing adaptation of computer science in Bioinfomatics. ACM International Conference Proceeding Series; Vol. 90; Proceedings of the 2004 international symposium on Information and communication technologies; URL: http://portal.acm.org/citation.cfm?id=1071509.1071553)
22. Altman RB. Bioinformatics in support of molecular medicine. Proc AMIA Symp. 1998; http://www-smi.stanford.edu/pubs/SMI_Reports/SMI-980731.pdf
23. Yu U, Lee SH, Kim YJ, Kim S. Bioinformatics in the post-genome era. J Biochem Mol Biol. 2004;37:75-82.
24. Ouellette J. Bioinformatics moves into the mainstream. The Industrial Physicist. 2003; Oct/Nov 14-18
25. Leo CP, Hsu SY, Hsueh JW. Hormonal Genomics. Endocrine Rev. 2002;23:369-81.
26. Crampin EJ, Halstead M, Hunter P, et al. Computational physiology and the physiome project. Exp Physiol. 2004;89.1:1-26.

Chapter 87

ORGANIZATION OF HEALTH CARE FOR PERSONS WITH DIABETES

Vijay Panikar

CHAPTER OUTLINE

- Introduction
- The Saint Vincent Declaration
- Diabetes Patient Education
- Problems in India
- Proposed Approach to Diabetes Care in India

INTRODUCTION

Diabetes mellitus has been recognized for centuries. However, its heterogeneity of cause, course and outcome has been fully appreciated only relatively recently. The discovery of insulin in 1920 was a great advance in the treatment of diabetes. This advance also demanded organization of diabetes care to provide to the patients with the apparatus, techniques and knowledge for its effective use. The increasing number of diabetics[1,2] with their attendant burden of complications, both short-term and long-term, demands an organization for optimizing diabetes care.

Many measures, which are well documented and evidence-based are now available for minimizing the acute metabolic complications and preventing or minimizing the late complications of diabetes. It is the recognition that these feasible and achievable measures are not being adequately implemented that has reinforced the demand for better organization of diabetes care. Primary prevention of diabetes is high on the agenda. Whether this is pursued on a whole population or directed towards "high-risk" groups or both, it has major organizational implications at scientific, public health and economic level.[3]

Organization of diabetes care involves not only medical treatment but also extends to broader aspects of a healthy way of living with diabetes, taking care of the emotional, social and economic impact of the disease. It should also help eradicate the myths, prejudices and unfounded restrictions, which the diagnosis may impose on life, work and social relationships.

The first international attempt at organizing proper diabetes care was the St. Vincent initiative in 1989.[4]

THE SAINT VINCENT DECLARATION

The need to identify and mobilize resources for improving health and quality of life for people with diabetes was mainspring of the St. Vincent initiates.[4] It was convened jointly by the European region, WHO and IDF. Representatives of patients' organizations, government health politicians, healthcare professionals and industry from more than 30 European nations met in St. Vincent in 1989.

General goals and five-year targets listed below can be achieved by the organized activities of the medical services in active partnership with diabetic citizens, their families, friends and workmates and their organizations; in the management of their own diabetes and the education for it; in the planning, provision and quality audit of health care; in national regional and international organizations for disseminating information about health maintenance; in promoting and applying research.

General Goals for People (Children and Adults) with Diabetes

- Sustained improvement in health experience and a life approaching normal expectation in quality and quantity.
- Prevention and cure of diabetes and of its complications by intensifying research effort.

Five-year Targets

- Elaborate, initiate and evaluate comprehensive programs of detection and control of diabetes and of its complications with self-care and community support as major components.
- Raise awareness in the population and among health care professionals of the present opportunities and the future needs for prevention of the complications of diabetes and of diabetes itself.
- Organize training and teaching in diabetes management and care for people of all ages with diabetes, for their families, friends and working associates and for the health care team.
- Ensure that care for children with diabetes is provided by individuals and teams specialized both in the management of diabetes and of children, and that families with a diabetic child get the necessary social economic and emotional support.
- Reinforce existing centers of excellence in diabetes care, education and research. Create new centers where the need and potential exist.
- Promote independence, equity and self-sufficiency for all people with diabetes—children, adolescents, those in the working years of life and the elderly.
- Remove hindrances to the fullest possible integration of the diabetic citizen into society.
- Implement effective measures for the prevention of costly complications.
- Reduce new blindness due to diabetes by one third or more.
- Reduce number of people entering end-stage diabetic renal failure by at least one-third.
- Reduce by one-half the rate of limb amputations for diabetic gangrene.

- Cut morbidity and mortality from coronary heart disease in the diabetic by vigorous programs of risk factor reduction.
- Achieve pregnancy outcome in the diabetic women that approximates that of the nondiabetic women.
- Establish monitoring and control systems using state of the art information technology for quality assurance of diabetes health care provision and for laboratory and technical procedures in diabetes diagnosis, treatment and self-management.
- Promote European and international collaboration in programs of diabetes research and development through national, regional and WHO agencies and in active partnership with diabetes patients' organizations.
- Take urgent action in the spirit of the WHO program, "Health for All" to establish joint machinery between WHO and IDF, European region, to initiate, accelerate and facilitate the implementation of these recommendations.

At the conclusion of the St. Vincent meeting, all those attending formally pledged themselves to strong and decisive action in seeking implementation of the recommendations on their return home.

The WHO has suggested the following six assumptions as the foundation for diabetes program development at the local, national and global level:[5]

1. Diabetes is a heterogeneous disease requiring detection, prevention and control measures in individuals and communities which are tailored at local, cultural and practical considerations.
2. A substantial part of diabetes care is patient self-care. Thus, patients must be educated before being delegated the responsibility for daily management of their condition.
3. Optimal diabetes care by the patient and provider can prevent or delay the development of complications.
4. Properly designed and integrated diabetes care programs may result in sizeable reductions in morbidity, disability and mortality.
5. Diabetes health care costs may be reduced using a variety of cost-containment strategies.
6. Diabetes control programs do not work in isolation. Their function is enhanced with intersectoral training/planning and integration of service at all levels in the healthcare system. Close linkage is encouraged with other chronic disease prevention and treatment programs.

Intervention Strategies

The most important intervention methods in diabetes control programs are health education of the public, patient education and organization of primary health care. Community analysis should be designed in such a way that these control issues are satisfactorily covered. The review of existing data from earlier studies statistics and other sources in invaluable.

Epidemiological knowledge about diabetes and its complications in the target population provide the essential basis for the program—prevalence, incidence, mortality and their distribution within and between different population groups; the factors influencing the natural course of diabetes, and their prevalence.[6] It is also important to understand the social and cultural features of the populations and the country. Information about health behavior related to diabetes and its risk factors, about factors in the community influencing these behavior complexes, and about community leadership and social interaction, are essential for program development and implementation. Much of the success of any community program depends on the support of the population. For this reason information on how people and their official representatives see the problems and how they feel about the possibilities of solving them, should be part of the community analysis. Because the program would also depends heavily on their cooperation, the knowledge, attitudes and therapeutic practices of the health personnel should be surveyed too. The main objectives of a program are usually set by the perceived health needs of the community.

There is much evidence of the feasibility and effectiveness of primary and secondary prevention of major noncommunicable diseases (NCD). Primary prevention has been defined as all measures designed to reduce the incidence of a disease in a population by reducing its onset. Secondary prevention includes measures designed to reduce the prevalence of a disease in a population, by shortening its course and duration. Both types of prevention are necessary to achieve effective control of major NCDs, including type 2 diabetes, in the community. Knowledge about the natural history of the disease, effective intervention methods, occurrence of the disease and the quality of the existing health care system will dictate the priorities between different types of intervention used in the health program. Ideally, primary prevention should take precedence, because intervention after the clinical stage of a disease have been reached will have only a limited impact on the epidemic of type 2 diabetes and other major NCDs experience in developed countries and in many developing countries today.

Unfortunately, we cannot claim that such a priority setting actually obtains with regard to diabetes care **(Figure 87.1)**.

In the development of methods for modern community health programs, diabetes-related activities might even serve as a model for more general NCD prevention and control in some countries.

Diabetes care has several important components that can be effectively incorporated into primary health care services. These include the following at the very least:

1. Health education of the public.
2. Guided patient self-care .
3. Continuous education of patients .
4. Training of health personnel and lay workers.
5. Community participation.
6. Organizing and maintenance of primary diabetes health care supported by specialist consultations.
7. Attempts to improve the environment.
8. Social support.
9. Development of diabetes registers or other relevant information systems.

To identify and mobilize all community resources, it is necessary to work closely with both official and voluntary organizations.

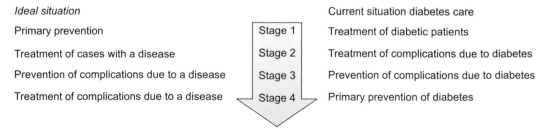

Priority of the activities of community health programs

Ideal situation		Current situation diabetes care
Primary prevention	Stage 1	Treatment of diabetic patients
Treatment of cases with a disease	Stage 2	Treatment of complications due to diabetes
Prevention of complications due to a disease	Stage 3	Prevention of complications due to diabetes
Treatment of complications due to a disease	Stage 4	Primary prevention of diabetes

Figure 87.1 Priority order of different intervention strategies in community health programs with special reference to diabetes care

The following groups of program activities need to be considered and developed:

1. Media-related and general educational activities.
2. Training of local health personnel and other active groups.
3. Organizations of health services—primary health care services, specialized supportive services, etc.
4. Community activities for the modification of the environment.
5. Information services for monitoring the development of the program and for providing feedback.

An evaluation component is required for any efficient diabetes prevention and control program in order to carry out the following strategic actions:

1. Add to the knowledge of disease etiology.
2. Evaluate the feasibility and effects of primary, secondary and tertiary prevention action.
3. Evaluate the effectiveness of secondary prevention activities.
4. Devise and test new intervention strategies for disease prevention.

Media-related and General Educational Activities

Numerous mass media activities on diabetes especially those related symptoms, diet, treatment and prevention of complications are regularly seen in many countries in the west. However, little attention has been paid to the primary prevention of diabetes, which was advocated as early as the 1920s.[7]

DIABETES PATIENT EDUCATION

Diabetes education has become an essential part of any modern diabetes control program. The philosophy of self-care and health education for an improved long-term quality of life is probably best illustrated in diabetes.[8]

Traditional strategies to reduce the burden of diabetes have focused primarily on the patient and the one-to-one relationship between doctor and patient. In today's world, we need to have a much wider perspective of diabetes as a whole. The burden of diabetes in India is likely to be huge, and keeping this in mind we need to have a specific public health approach to its management. Organization of diabetes care in India will be a mammoth task and should comprise the following:

a. Define the nature, extent and cause of the increase in diabetes, i.e. surveillance.

b. Develop innovative population-based strategies to reduce this burden.
c. Implement these 'environmental strategies' throughout the country through the central and state health departments.
d. These government efforts should be coordinated with all agencies involved in diabetes care, e.g. private doctors, corporate, diabetic associations, academic forums, etc.

PROBLEMS IN INDIA

Magnitude of the Problem

The incidence of diabetes is on the rise in India. Recent surveys in India have shown a high prevalence of diabetes in the urban population 8% to 12%. It is estimated that 31.7 million adults in India have diabetes, and this figure is likely to cross 79.4 million by the year 2030,[10] giving India the dubious distinction of having the largest diabetic population in the world. Organization of diabetes care in India is practically nonexistent, except in a few metro cities.

The problems of diabetes care in India are as diverse and mammoth as India itself.

Manpower Resources

India as an agricultural nation with 80% of its population living in rural areas. The physician to population ratio is 1:2100 as per official statistics. Unfortunately, this is not so in reality. Almost 75% of medical practitioners cater to the 20% urban population and barely 25% serve the remaining 80% rural population, giving a 1:20000 ratio in the rural areas.

Manpower Resources

One doctor per 2100 population
One (Nurse + Midwife) per 2238 population

Health Care Delivery Structure in India

Subcenters   : Total 1,30,336 (1 for 5000 population)
Each center   : 1 Medical health worker
                     1 Auxiliary nurse midwife
                     2-3 Village health guides
PHC (Primary : Total 21024 (1 for 30,000 population)
health centre)
Each center   : 1 doctor and 1 female health assistant
CHC   : Total 2293 (1 for 100,000 population)
(Community
health center)

Each center	: Physician, surgeon, obstetrics and gynecology nurse, health educator
District level	: Civil Hospital
State level	: Referral centers and medical colleges.

Literacy

Literacy levels are still alarmingly low. The problem of the use of different languages and dialects in different parts of the country can compound the problem for effective implementation of healthcare delivery programs.

Education Programs

Education programs for diabetics have a major impact on the management of diabetes.[11,12] Such programs are available only in very few institutions in India. Thus, today millions of our diabetics are not exposed to any kind of formal education at all.

Communication and Transport

Most of India lives in the villages which have inadequate infrastructure, poor roads, lack of electricity, telephone and transport facilities. These inadequacies are major impediments to deliver healthcare.

Religious Beliefs and Taboos

India is a land of diversity. There are all possible religious groups, castes and subcastes that one can think of. Add to these, the age old customs, rituals, beliefs and taboos. The practice of ancients systems of medicines like Ayurveda, Unani, Siddha, homeopathy and not to mention the local village medicine man or bhagat all together can confuse and misguide the populace. They contribute and strengthen misconceptions about diabetes and its treatment, which are quite deep rooted in the minds of the people. One such misconception is that rice is to be avoided in diabetic. In India, diet is mainly cereal based which is cheap.

Financial Resources

The financial resources to meet the challenges for providing health care are dismal. The government spending on health is very meager. This is not likely to improve in the population in the near future.

PROPOSED APPROACH TO DIABETES CARE IN INDIA

In various countries, different models of health care have been operative. In Sweden, the primary care physician 'has' been utilized as a 'key personnel' in diabetes care. The Chinese and Croatian model (Vuk Vrhovac Institute) consists of primary, secondary and tertiary care centers. In India, too, we have similar system established since independence and it may be possible to integrate diabetes care with the existing healthcare delivery system.[13] The current thrust of these services is towards the treatment and prevention of communicable disease. This needs to be reviewed and an added impetus towards preventing and treating noncommunicable diseases is the need of the hour. To be cost-effective, diabetes health care should be linked with health care to control risk factors like hypertension, hyperlipidemia, tobacco and alcohol abuse, etc. For this purpose, the health care professional should receive additional training and this can yield rich dividends at a low cost. As our financial resources are scarce, the main emphasis should be an education and empowerment of the patients and general populace at large. Education and information about the disease can also correct the attitude of the people towards the disease.

REFERENCES

1. King H, Rewers M. Global estimates for prevalence of diabetes mellitus and impaired glucose tolerance in adults. Diabetes Care 1993;16:157-77.
2. Zimmet PZ. Challenges in diabetes pidemiology—from west to the rest. Diabetes Care 1992;15:232-52.
3. World Health Organization Study Group Report. Prevention of diabetes mellitus. Technical Report Series No. 844. WHO, Geneva 1994.
4. Home P, Hallet L. The St. Vincent Declaration initiative: a movement for people with diabetes. IDF Bulletin 1996; 41(2):6-9.
5. Reiber G, King H (Eds). Guidelines for the development of a national programme for diabetes mellitus. Geneva: World Health Organization; 1991.
6. Herman WH, Sinnock P, Brenner E, et al. An epidemiologic model for diabetes mellitus: incidence, prevalence and mortality. Diabetes Care 1998;7:367.
7. Elliot PJ. The prevention of diabetes mellitus. JAMA 1921;76:79-84.
8. Mazzuca SA, Moorman NH, Wheeler ML, et al. The diabetes education study: a controlled trial of the effects of diabetes patient education. Diabetes Care 1986;9:1-10.
9. Ramachandran A, Snehalatha C. NIDDM in India and Indians: Is it increasing? IDF Bulletin 1995;40: 277-9.
10. Wild S,Roglic G, Green A, Sicree R,King H. Global prevalence of diabetes: Estimates for the year 2030. Diab care 2004; 27:1047-53.
11. Beggan MP, Cregan D, Drury MI. Assessment of the outcome of an educational program of diabetes self care. Diabetologia 1982;23:246-51.
12. Chandalia HB, Bagrodia J. Effect of nutritional counselling on the blood glucose and nutritional knowledge of diabetic subjects. Diabetes Care 1979; 2:353-6.
13. Chandalia HB. Health care delivery in diabetes: the Indian scene. In Kapur A (Ed): Novo Nordisk Diabetes Update. Proceedings, Health Care Communications 1996;65-9.

Chapter 88

ROLE OF PRIMARY CARE PHYSICIANS

GS Sainani, Rajesh G Sainani

CHAPTER OUTLINE

- Introduction
- Recommended Standards of Medical Care for Diabetic Patients
- Role of Dietitian
- Self Management

- Patient Education
- Lacunae in Medical Care
- Primary Care-based Models
- Primary Care Setting

INTRODUCTION

Recently attention has been paid on the organizational and economic aspects of medical care for diabetics.[1,2] The diabetes control and complications trial (DCCT) results[3] have heightened interest in the metabolic control of diabetes and its implication for healthcare policy.[4] We have now available the results of several studies conducted on representative section of diabetic patients. These results underline the importance of role of primary care physician and paramedical personnel (diabetes nurse or diabetes educator) in the management of diabetes mellitus. Patient's knowledge and methods used for glycemic control seem to be inadequate to achieve a tight glycemic control that will delay or prevent diabetic complications. Furthermore, majority of diabetic patients have associated hyperlipidemia, hypertension that contribute to the morbidity and mortality in diabetes. Achieving tight glycemic, lipid and blood pressure control would need support and motivation from primary care physician and paramedical personnel.

The load of diabetic patients (20 million diabetics, the majority of them having type 2 diabetes) in our country is tremendous and the problem is on the increase in view of the epidemic like situation. The numbers of diabetologists, endocrinologists and specialists are very few and they may be able to handle only 10% of the diabetic population. Hence, large majority of diabetic patients, particularly in rural and semiurban areas, have to be guided by primary care physician and/or diabetes educator. Providing such a level of management to all diabetic patients would require major changes in health care system.

The primary care physician has to appreciate that the management of diabetes is a labor-intensive process as it involves many metabolic abnormalities. Practically, every organ in the body can be affected. Hence, patient should be aware of the standards of medical care, which have been recommended for primary care.[1] These are mentioned below. These guidelines incorporate recommendations of National Cholesterol Education Program (NCEP), High Blood Pressure Education Program, expert committees of the American Diabetes

Association (ADA) and finding from the DCCT in which type 1 DM patients experienced marked lowering of the incidence of microvascular complications in patients with tight glycemic control.[4,5]

RECOMMENDED STANDARDS OF MEDICAL CARE FOR DIABETIC PATIENTS[1]

1. Plasma glucose (treatment goals): Fasting 80-110 mg/dl; Postprandial 120-140 mg/dl; Bedtime glucose 100-140 mg/dl; Hemoglobin A_{1c} <7% (normal range 4-7%).
2. Lipids: Total cholesterol <200 mg/dl; LDL cholesterol <130 mg/dl (<100 mg/dl for those with known CHD); Fasting triglycerides <200 mg/dl.
3. Blood pressure (treatment goal): Systolic <130 mm Hg; Diastolic <85 mm Hg.
4. Urine albumin <30 mg/24 hours.

The primary care physician is responsible to advise insulin, oral antidiabetic drugs, diet and exercise program to patients to achieve target blood glucose levels while minimizing risk of hypoglycemia. The primary care physician and/or paramedical personnel should aim at patient education, nutrition education for self management and teach patients for self monitoring of blood glucose and for self insulin injections.

Regular visits to primary care physician are essential (at least quarterly for insulin treated patients and atleast semi-annually for all other patients until achievement of all treatment goals) for medical history, physical examination, laboratory tests, assessment and alteration of management plan as and when required. Blood pressure measurement and foot examination must be done at every visit. Detailed examination of eyes after dilatation must be done annually. Paramedical personnel (diabetic nurse and/or diabetic educator) should examine and guide the patients more often (say every 4-6 weeks) and refer the patients to primary care physician when in doubt or difficulty. Thus, with help of paramedical personnel and primary care physicians, patients should be educated for self management.[5]

ROLE OF DIETITIAN

Dietitian or nutritionist plays a vital role in the management of diabetes. Patients managed in hospitals whether attending outpatients or diabetic clinics or as indoor patients have an easy access to dietitian of the diabetic clinic of hospital. However, patients getting treated from primary care physicians, learn about diet from their family physician. Epidemiologic survey reported by Harris[6] revealed that only 20% of diabetic adults in the survey had seen a dietitian in the past year. Approximately 64% of adult patients indicated that they followed a diet for diabetes, although 90% believed that such a diet is important for proper control of diabetes mellitus.

SELF MANAGEMENT

Approximately 26% of insulin treated patients with type 2 DM reported that they test their blood glucose at least once a day. But for type 2 DM, only 5.3% patients were self monitoring blood glucose.[7] The proportion who self monitored at least once a day declined markedly with increasing age.[7] The majority of patients examined their feet at least once per week. All self care practices were more frequent among patients who were insulin treated in comparison with those treated with oral agents or diet alone.

PATIENT EDUCATION

It is well known that patient education can result in increase in self management skills but only 35% of diabetic persons in USA have ever attended an education program. Approximately 40% of insulin treated type 2 DM and 24% of oral drug treated type 2 DM patients have received patient education. Almost all patients surveyed have obtained information from some source with a physician being by far the most common source (86% of patients). Other major sources include diabetes nurse or other diabetic patients.[8]

LACUNAE IN MEDICAL CARE

In the DCCT, glycemic control was achieved by the coordinated efforts of physicians, diabetes educators, dietitians, and behavioral specialists. However, in practice, such a team is usually not available for financial and logistic reasons. Large majority of diabetic patients receive primary care guidance from internist and family practitioner. Less than 10% of all office-based visits are made to diabetologists, endocrinologist. A small number of patients receive care from ophthalmologists and dietitians or nutritionists. The overwhelming majority of patients with diabetes are cared for by primary care practitioners.

PRIMARY CARE-BASED MODELS

As type 2 DM is a complex disease with multisystem complications, the current focus is on the primary care in various countries. In this model, the role of primary care physician incorporating into the primary case setting is very vital. The characteristics of the successful practice parameters of the DCCT include patient education to enhance and support patient self management, expert opinion for therapeutic management and the ensured delivery of effective intervention for treatment and screening. Models of care should support early diagnosis of diabetes and early detection and treatment of complications, as they improve glycemic control and empower patients to improve self care practices. In some situations, comanagement by primary care physician and diabetologist has been recommended.[9] In this model, the overall care of patients remains the responsibility of the primary care physician, and patients are seen by the diabetes specialist and diabetes team at regular intervals to review overall diabetes status. Here, recommendations concerning a plan of care including goals of management and requirements of nutritional counseling are addressed, screening and management of complications are carried out. The degree of involvement of diabetologist varies depending on the severity of diabetes as well as the skills and interest of the primary care physician. Comanagement model provides the support of a diabetic specialist for primary care physicians to implement patient education for self management, optimization of glycemic control, and prevention and management of complications. Most patients would benefit from intermittent access to diabetic team during the course of the disease. Success of such a model would be dependent upon ease of access to the diabetes specialist team and the rapport between the diabetes team and the primary care physician.[5]

It is important to establish target set goals. Health care goals are relatively easy to measure. The measurement of HbA_{1c}, blood pressure, urinary protein and regular eye and foot examinations are examples of care processes that can be related to quality diabetes management.

If HbA_{1c}, blood pressure measurement and urinary protein or microalbumin levels are not determined periodically, interventions to improve glycemic control reduce hypertension and delay the progression of nephropathy.

1. *HbA_{1c} Testing:* HbA_{1c} is a measure of the average level of blood glucose during the previous three months. The DCCT,[3] the Kumamoto trial[10] and the UKPDS[11] have established a relationship between the HbA_{1c} level and the development of complications. Hence, one can rationally use HbA_{1c} as a surrogate for future complications risk and a measure of recent glycemia. It is recommended that HbA_{1c} should be measured every 3 months for insulin treated diabetic patients and every 6 to 12 months for diabetic patients on oral medications who are in good control.

2. *Blood pressure measurements:* Regular blood pressure measurements should be carried out and the recommended goal of blood pressure for diabetic patients is less than 130/85 mm Hg.

3. *Lipid profile:* As per ADA recommendation, lipid profile should be carried out at least once a year.

4. *Monitoring for early diabetic nephropathy:* Screening diabetic patients for proteinuria once a year is recommended. Proteinuria exceeding 300 mg/daily usually progresses to renal insufficiency. In absence of proteinuria, test for microalbuminuria should be carried out.

5. *Eye examination:* Detailed eye examination after dilatation is carried out at the time of diagnosis of diabetes mellitus and subsequently at least once a year.

6. *Foot examination:* Diabetes is the leading cause of non-traumatic lower extremity amputations. Foot examination preferably at every office visit should be carried out but one documented foot examination once a year is a must.

PRIMARY CARE SETTING

The role of primary care physician shifts from providing direct medical care to facilitating self management of the disease by patients and relatives. Many primary care physicians use team approach and delegate the educational and skills-building components by referring patients to a diabetes team comprising of diabetes nurse, dietitian, exercise physiologist and a social worker.

The setting of goals and targets for both primary care physicians and patients stresses the fact that diabetes is a serious condition requiring regular screening and adjustments of therapy from time to time. Periodic monitoring of hemoglobin HbA_{1c} seems the most logical choice to serve as the designated-outcome marker because it integrates overall glucose control. The awareness of both the public and physicians concerning hemoglobin HbA_{1c} levels should be increased. Also hemoglobin HbA_{1c} level target should be given wide publicity as that would improve early detection and result in fewer undiagnosed cases of diabetes mellitus.[5] In the management of diabetes, goals can be achieved when patients appreciate and cooperate in the management skills, problem solving interventions and get goals for behavioral changes. Patients have to be motivated by primary care physicians and diabetic educators for diet, lifestyle changes, regular exercise, cessation of smoking and learning skills such as home glucose monitoring.[3] Primary care physicians and diabetic educators have also to address some of the psychosocial demands of implementing lifestyle modifications and diabetic treatment. Home-based educational material regarding diabetic diet, virtues of regular exercise may be of help in many educated homogenous populations but this may not be useful in populations with high rates of illiteracy or in ethnically diverse populations. Use of lay persons in the community (after having had orientation course) for guiding diabetic patients has been shown to be useful in ethnic communities.[12,13] However, in educated group, computer-based instructions in self management either at home or at practice site may be helpful. Audio and video presentation in groups at diabetic clinics has tremendous potential of patient education. Apart from diabetes nurse and diabetes educators, training of allied health professionals at the practice site or diabetic clinic to deliver the information to patients is also useful.[5]

Paramedical personnel should also emphasize on preventive care. They should observe a planned and scheduled follow-up, which should include periodic foot examination, screening for microalbuminuria, fundus examination after proper dilatation. Primary care physicians have to supervise adjustment of antidiabetic treatment (insulin, drugs), antihypertensive drugs and timely use of lipid lowering drugs for achieving reduction of complications. Preventive screening is expected of the primary physician and patient so as to detect and treat complications well in time.[5]

One may conclude that in view of the enormous diabetes load in our country, it is impossible for diabetologists and endocrinologists (being very few in number) to handle education and management of diabetic patients. Therefore, the role of primary care physician, diabetes nurse, diabetes educators is very vital and we should train an army of paramedical personnel to educate patients and supervise their management. In case of problems or severe complication, advice of diabetes specialist should be sought.

With such a health care delivery system, one would achieve improved patient adherence to medical regimens, enhanced patient confidence, improved utilization of effective treatments with proper glycemic control, reduction of ischemic heart disease, decreased progression to blindness, decreased progression to renal failure and less number of lower extremity amputations. This would also cause a shift in overall health utilization from high cost complication related hospitalizations to low cost preventive services. Hence, we should make a serious attempt to change the pattern of healthcare delivery to a proactive public health approach, if we wish to improve overall the health of diabetes patients.

REFERENCES

1. American Diabetes Association. Clinical practice recommendations, 1997. Position statement-standards of medical care for patients with diabetes mellitus. Diabetes Care 1997;20(Suppl):S1-S70.
2. Harris MI. Epidemiological correlates of diabetes in Hispanics, Whites, and Blacks in the US population. Diabetes Care 1999;(Suppl. 3):639.
3. The Diabetes Control and Complications Trial Research Group. The effect of intensive treatment of diabetes on the development and progression of long-term complications in insulin-dependent diabetes mellitus. N Engl J Med 1993;329:977.
4. American Diabetes Association. Position statement: implications of the diabetes control and complications trial. Diabetes 1993;42:1555.
5. Roman SH, Harris MI. Management of diabetes mellitus from a public health perspective. Endocrinol Metab Clin North Am 1997;26:443-74.
6. Harris MI. Medical care for patients with diabetes: epidemiologic aspects. Ann Intern Med 1996; 124(1pt2):117.
7. Harris MI, Cowie CC, Eastman R. Health insurance coverage for adult with diabetes in US population. Diabetes Care 1993;16:116.
8. Cowie CC, Harris MI. Ambulatory medical care for non-Hispanic whites, African Americans, and Mexican Americans with NIDDM in the US. Diabetes Care 1997;20:142.
9. Hiss RG, Greenfied S. Forum Three: Changes in the US health care system that would facilitate improved care for non-insulin dependent diabetes mellitus. Ann Intern Med 1996;124:180.
10. Ohkubo Y, Kishikawa H, Araki E et al. Intensive insulin therapy prevents the progression of diabetic microvascular complications in Japanese patients with non-insulin-dependent diabetes mellitus: A randomized prospective 6-year study. Diabetes Res Clin Pract 1995;28:103. (abstract) .
11. UKPDS Group. Intensive blood glucose control with sulfonylureas or insulin compared with conventional treatment and risk of omplications in patients with type 2 diabetes (UKPDS 33) (Abstract). Lancet 1998;352:837.
12. American Diabetes Association. National standards for diabetes self-management education programs. Diabetes Care 1985;8:391.
13. Corkery E, Palmer C, Foley ME et al: Effect of a bicultural community health worker on completion of diabetes education in a Hispanic population. Diabetes Care 1997;20:254.

Chapter 89

ROLE OF PARAMEDICAL PERSONNEL

SV Madhu

INTRODUCTION

Diabetes mellitus is a lifetime chronic condition with a need for coordinated management of the diabetic state as well as a number of comorbid conditions and complications. In addition, several other educational, emotional, psychological and behavioral needs of the diabetic patients have to be addressed. A team approach is crucial in providing such an integrated care and requires close cooperation of medical and paramedical personnel. A diabetes care team the fundamental unit in diabetes care as envisaged by WHO, consisting of a physician and a diabetes educator can be set-up at primary, secondary or tertiary levels of health care delivery depending on available resources of a country.

There is an increasing recognition that the diabetes patient should be an active part of his management and not merely a passive receiver of treatment and that he should be made an independent and responsible for most of his management. This would require effective empowerment of the patient with diabetes-related knowledge and skills (therapeutic patient education) and it is here that the role of paramedical personnel like diabetes educators, dietitians nursing personnel and behavior specialists become critical. The beneficial effects of patient education in preventing complications of diabetes particularly acute metabolic complications and amputations has been well documented although its role in achieving better glycemic control is not as clear. Suitable training and upgradation of knowledge and skills of paramedical personnel is essential for optimal use in diabetes care that can yield highly successful outcome.

Diabetes is a chronic condition requiring collaboration between patients and the care providers for most efficient management. The use of a team approach has been shown to improve health outcomes in diabetes management. The optimum use of paramedical personnel in diabetes care helps facilitate better patient participation in his own management and closer cooperation between the patient and the treating physicians. All these would improve outcome in diabetes care.

NEEDS OF PEOPLE WITH DIABETES

Diabetes patients have several kinds of needs, all of which have to be addressed in the management program. The quality of diabetes care provided depends to a large extent on the efficiency with which each of these needs are met and by implication the extent of use of paramedical personnel in delivering care. These needs include[1]:

Basic Needs

People with diabetes have a right to the best possible quality of life and must be helped to achieve it. They also have a right to information concerning the status and progress of their condition. In this regard, it must be understood that type 2 DM is no less difficult to manage than type 1 DM.

Medical Needs

This includes measures to manage glycemia as well as related comorbidities, efforts for early detection of complications and access to comprehensive diabetes care.

Educational Needs

Acquiring knowledge and skills in instituting diet, exercise, medication and self-monitoring is critical to a successful management program for diabetes patients. This would not only require a reasonable professional wisdom but also involves adequate patient education to empower the diabetic patient to manage his own condition.

In a study[2] evaluating the education needs of diabetic patients with low socioeconomic and literacy levels by our institution, 100 patients with diagnosed diabetes were interviewed for assessment of their knowledge of diabetes. Overall diabetes awareness (ODA) for the group was poor (mean score 34%) while their knowledge of self-monitoring was very poor (23.7%). ODA correlated with socioeconomic status and education level but not with age and duration of diabetes. However, knowledge of complications and self-monitoring improved with increasing duration of diabetes. Patients were not aware of food exchange (89%), glucometer (88%) and benefits of exercise (81%). Females had uniformly lower scores than males for all aspects of diabetes studied. The study highlighted the inadequacy of existing diabetes education methods and pointed to the difficulties in educating low socio-economic, low-literacy, and multilingual patient groups particularly women. This again emphasized the critical role of paramedical personnel in diabetes care.

Chennai Urban Rural Epidemiology Study (CURES-9)[3], a population-based study also assessed the level of awareness of diabetes in the population of Urban Chennai and concluded that awareness and knowledge regarding diabetes is still grossly inadequate in India and that there was an urgent need for massive diabetes education programs in our country. Only 25% of Chennai population were aware of a condition called diabetes. Knowledge of role of obesity and physical activity in genesis of diabetes was very low (11.9%). Even among the self-reported diabetic subjects, only 40.6% were aware that diabetes could produce a lot of complications.

Another study[4,5] reported that more than half the diabetic patients attending a hospital did not know whether good long-term control of diabetes prevented complications. Knowledge regarding individual complications was equally poor. A study[6] of the knowledge, beliefs and practices of diabetic patients showed a large gap between knowledge and action and reinforced the need for increased efforts towards patient education regarding diabetes. Viswanathan et al[7] found that awareness of general foot care principles and basic facts about foot complications were poor. In a study, carried out to assess oral health education among diabetic patients,[8] it has been reported that a majority of them did not know the factors in diabetes that can contribute to oral ill health including the need for good glycemic control.

All the above-mentioned studies underscore the need for an urgent, focused and targeted education program for diabetic patients as well as the general public and emphasize the need for team approach and active involvement of paramedical personnel in diabetes care.

Emotional Needs

Diabetes patients even long after they are diagnosed can feel isolated and depressed. This requires appropriate psychological and emotional support. Children with type 1 diabetes and adolescents have specific needs for psychological guidance.

PARAMEDICAL PERSONNEL AND STRICT GLYCEMIC CONTROL

The Diabetes Controls and Complications Trials (DCCT)[9] clearly demonstrated the benefits of coordinated efforts in achieving glycemic control. The strict glycemic goals achieved in this study was made possible only through close cooperation between the physicians and a number of other paramedical personnel, viz diabetes educators, dietitians and behavioral specialists. In a practical clinical care setting, however, this may not always be possible. At the same time, it can be said that the success in achieving strict glycemic control would depend to a great extent on the level of involvement of paramedical personnel.

CONCEPT OF SELF CARE AND SELF-MANAGEMENT

The concept of self care and self-management is being increasingly emphasized in the management of chronic conditions such as diabetes mellitus. It is now being appreciated that any state of illness, especially chronic illness, can cause psychosocial destabilization of the patient and by helping the patient gradually to adapt to his state of health and illness and by empowering him to deal with the illness, paramedical personnel play an important role in reducing the chances of occurrence of complications.[10] Providing the necessary competence to patients to adapt their treatment to the variations of daily life make them architects of their own treatment and not mere treatment receivers. The concept of self care management is fast becoming crucial in the health care delivery system particularly in the field of diabetes care. In one center in USA, diabetes self management education (DSME) aims at making the diabetic patient responsible for 99% of his day-to-day management. The process of DSME includes individualized assessment, goal-oriented plan, educational interventions and evaluation.

DIABETES HEALTH CARE TEAMS

Diabetes team is the fundamental unit[11] that has to be constituted at one or the other level of health care delivery regardless of whether the resources available are minimal, desirable or optional. If the resources are minimal, then diabetes team is placed only at the tertiary care centers. If they are at desirable levels, then diabetes team can be in place at secondary care centers also, and if optimal they should start functioning right from primary care settings **(Figure 89.1)**. In developing countries, diabetes care may be provided by paramedical staff, health workers, other lay workers, health extension officers or trained volunteers working at rural health centers. These individuals would be based at primary care settings and would require basic training for skills in diagnosis and in use of essential drugs while the physician would be managing diabetes and its complications at secondary health care settings.

A diabetes team, as envisaged by WHO, comprises of a physician and a professional diabetes educator.[11] This is the fundamental unit that is thought to be essential for providing quality diabetes care and education. The physician who is the leader of the team that provides diabetes treatment and care should have specific interest in diabetes. The educator should have knowledge and proficiency to educate diabetic patients and may be anyone of the following codes, viz nurse, dietitian, health educator or pharmacist. A diabetes unit is comprised of a diabetologist/endocrinologist or an internist with especial training in diabetes, a diabetes educator, and other health personnel such as a behavior specialist, podiatrist, dietitian and nephrologist. In India, podiatry is still not an established specialty and services of a surgeon may be needed for the purpose.

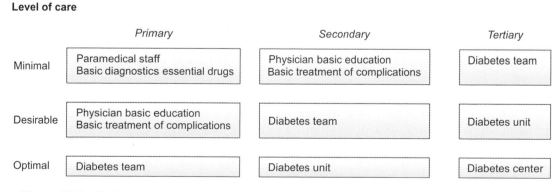

Figure 89.1 Options for level of diabetes care given the level of development and resource

It has to be realized paramedical personnel particularly diabetes educators are an integral part of any diabetes care team that can be expected to deliver diabetes care effectively. Several studies over the last 2 to 3 decades have demonstrated the need for tight control of glycemia for preventing or delaying long-term complications of diabetes mellitus.[9,12] However, this requires a high level of motivation on the part of the patient and a deeper understanding by him of the disease, its complications as well as the risks and benefits of its treatment. Also, the importance of various comorbid conditions such as dyslipidemia, hypertension, and coronary artery disease needs to be realized. All these requires constant support, education and motivation from dedicated paramedical personnel such as diabetic educator in addition to the efforts of primary physicians.

ROLE OF DIABETES EDUCATOR IN DIABETES MANAGEMENT

According to WHO, *education is the cornerstone of diabetic therapy and vital to the diabetic in the society*. In view of the growing epidemic of diabetes and the fact that diabetes is a chronic lifelong disease, there is an urgent and constant need to educate and empower diabetic patients and their relatives to deal with all the tribulations of this disease.

The primary aim of diabetes education[13] is to change behavior of people and promote self management. Diabetes education consists of providing tools and necessary support to patients as they acquire the knowledge and skills to manage their disease. The ultimate goal of patient education is to achieve three levels of competency:

1. Intellectual—knowledge of the disease and its treatment.
2. Practical—skill in knowing how to monitor the disease and control it.
3. Adaptation—change of behavior or attitude to better apply knowledge and skill for better diabetes management.

General health education about the disease is inadequate for a chronic disorder like diabetes, since the patient needs to know and understand a lot in order to participate actively in the management of his problems. Especially because diabetes mellitus is a vacillating ongoing process requiring constant monitoring of the disease and its treatment lifelong.

The WHO has thus adopted the term, therapeutic patient education (TPE), which envisages a more patient-oriented and problem-oriented approach of educators designed to provide effective therapeutic intervention.[14] TPE can only be given by health care professionals unlike general health educators. The role of nursing professionals becomes central to this concept.

TPE is directed at those who are already afflicted with the aim to limit the progression of the illness in order to minimize advent of complications (secondary prevention) and to control the complications already present to avoid disability (tertiary preventions).[15] The expanded role of health care providers in therapeutic education, which goes beyond the hitherto mainstream role given to them includes:

- To enable patients to gain and maintain abilities that allows them an optimal management of life with their disease
- To be used as a continuous process in integrated health care
- To be patient oriented and to provide organized awareness, information, self-care learning and psychological support regarding disease, prescribed treatment and health status
- To help patients and their families to understand the disease and the treatment, cooperate with health care providers, live healthily and maintain or improve their quality of life.

The broad goals of a diabetes educator that emerge in such a strategy are:[14]

- To help the patients and his family accept the disease
- To educate the patient about the disease including its causes, diagnosis, clinical features and complications
- To stress the importance of diet control, benefits of exercise and the need for regular use of tablets/ insulin for glycemic control
- To make the patient realize the importance of self-monitoring of diabetes control and to impart necessary skills for the same
- To empower the patients sufficiently so as to make them independent and active participants in decision making regarding their management.

The role of the diabetes educator is thus central to the management of diabetes and can be particularly important for:

- Diet and lifestyle changes
- Behavior therapy and weight management
- Self-monitoring skills and interpretation including self monitoring of blood glucose (SMBG)

- Blood pressure measurement and appropriate referral for lipid management
- Basic foot care
- Adjustment of diabetes medications
- Initiation and technique of insulin injection
- Education of other health care professionals.

Paramedical personal should also emphasize on preventive care such as need for daily foot examination, need for regular dilated eye check-ups, need for urine albumin/microalbumin ratio estimations and pregnancy planning among other aspects of diabetes management.

Diabetes education programs have been shown to reduce the frequency of acute metabolic complications and have been particularly effective in decreasing hospital admissions due to diabetic ketoacidosis[16] and severe hypoglycemia[17] all of which are important components of diabetes care. However, the benefits of education on glycemic control among diabetic subjects are not as clear.[18-20]

The evidence that diabetes education *per se* leads to improved long-term glycemic outcomes is not particularly strong.[21-23] Only a 0.16% difference in HbA_{1c} levels was found after three years between an intervention group receiving diabetes self management education (DSME) and a control group receiving regular conventional care in the Japanese Complications Study.[23] On the basis of this JDC trial, they concluded that the moderate but significant improvement effected by DSME on glycemic control of adult patients with (Type 2 diabetes mellitus) is maintained in the long-term.[23] Norris et al[21] demonstrated a decrease of 0.76% in GHb levels in patients with (Type 2 diabetes mellitus) given DSME at an immediate follow-up, of 0.26% at one to three month follow-up and of 0.26% at 7.4 months of follow-up. Their meta-analysis revealed that while the short-term benefits of DSME on GHb were significant, the long-term effects still needed to be improved. Overall, so far the glycemic effects of diabetes education on glycemic control particularly in the long-term are equivocal.

In the context of chronic complications, diabetes education strategies have been most effective in reducing foot ulceration and preventing leg amputations[24,25] particularly in high-risk individuals. High-risk patients are those with neuropathy, peripheral vascular diseases, and those with other foot abnormalities, viz callosities or deformities. The risk of amputations has been shown to decrease by 45 to 85% and this protection can persist for up to 10 years.

A diabetes educator can provide support by encouraging patients to talk about their concerns or fears about diabetes. This can help patients to cope with different complications and setbacks. In short, diabetes educator can help patients live life with diabetes. A systematic review[26] of 36 studies to study the impact of intervention in the form of education self-management and psychological counseling for diabetes, it was concluded that improvements in depression especially followed psychological interventions, while improvement in quality of life were more following self management interventions.

Grey et al[27] showed that behavioral intervention to enhance coping skills in young and adolescents with diabetes mellitus achieved improved metabolic control and quality of life. A study from India concluded that behavioral intervention can be reckoned as an effective adjunct to routine medical care in the management of type 1 diabetes, more so far in the management of complications, better metabolic control, enhancement of knowledge and improvement in the quality of life.[28] In general, it has been observed that the competence and preferences in self-treatment are considered as the determining factors in reducing complications in diabetes. It is here that, the role of paramedical personnel like psychologists, behavioral therapists or nurses assume greater important. Litaker et al[29] studied the impact of physician-nurse team care vs physician alone care in diabetes patient and demonstrated the value of team approach in providing better metabolic and quality of life (QOL) outcomes. Similarly, an analysis of six trials followed up for up to a year,[30] revealed that there was a significant reduction in HbA_{1c} at six months in the presence of a diabetes specialist nurse/nursing care manager. One of the studies also showed reduction in hypoglycemic episodes.

Intensive educational approaches have been shown to improve knowledge, compliance and foot problems[31] in type 2 diabetes. They have also been shown to cast significant impact on favorable dietary changes in these patients.[32] It has also been shown that SMBG can become a more effective tool in diabetes management, provided it is part of a wider educational strategy that aims at promoting patient autonomy.[33] Here also, paramedical personnel have a key role to play.

ROLE OF THE DIETITIAN IN DIABETES MANAGEMENT

A dietitian or a nutritionist plays a vital role in the management of diabetes. Dietitians are available and are generally part of diabetes management teams in most hospital care settings. Diet has always been the key to the success of any diabetes treatment regimen and hence the role of a dietitian in planning and monitoring the diet of diabetic patients is of crucial importance. In one survey, only 20% of patients reported visiting a dietitian over the past year[34] and we need to work seriously to improve this figure. The dietitian is an invaluable in guiding the patient to make the right food choices. The dietitian can contribute significantly by making a thorough assessment of the patient which would include anthropometric and current dietary assessments, and then evaluate risk and accordingly provide counseling on diet and lifestyle.[35] Dietary assessment should include, besides nutrient intake, a detailed account of food preferences and habits, which should help construct a comprehensive diet plan with a high likelihood of compliance. This is an essential component of any successful dietary management and would therefore determine the success of diabetes management overall.

In addition to planning and advising the patient on the details of dietary choices and providing diet charts the patient can follow, the dietitian should also make every effort to provide nutrition education to the patient on various facets of diabetic diet and lifestyle as well as the need to closely adhere to the same. Frequent follow-up to monitor the implementation and compliance of dietary advice also needs to be undertaken by the dietitian from time-to-time. Chandalia et al[36] demonstrated that patient's nutritional knowledge improved significantly after nutritional counseling and this improved control of diabetes significantly.

ROLE OF THE NURSING PERSONNEL IN DIABETES MANAGEMENT

Health care providers other than doctors constitute the largest professional group in the health sector. The nursing personnel is the most important segment in this group. Their role in health care delivery is one of a facilitator in carrying out the prescribed treatment and here they act as a link between the doctor and the patient. By having a continuous interaction with the patient, they are uniquely placed to gain insight into the psychosocial factors operating in his case and thus are most suited to provide TPE as a successful and effective intervention.[37]

TPE is a lifelong process and so is the association of the health care provider with the diabetic patient. The interaction starts from the day the diagnosis of diabetes

is made and begins with an assessment of the patients knowledge of diabetes and lifestyle preferences that help the nurse in planning and providing effective patient education and counseling. Nurses must teach the patient to balance a number of factors life diet, exercise, stress and medications for him to be able to achieve tight glycemic control and delay long-term complications.[30]

Nursing personnel can also be trained to be actively involved in the administration of medications, adjustments of antidiabetic agents particularly oral agents and in recording any adverse effects to treatments. This would need only a minor upgradation of their skills. These nurses could then function as diabetes management nurses and their services may prove invaluable in dealing with the huge load of diabetes patients that need to be seen. Also, primary care physicians need to see diabetic patients regularly, to monitor complications and glycemic control every few months. Paramedical personnel, particularly nurses can examine and guide the diabetic patients more often, e.g. every 4 to 6 weeks and refer the patients to primary care physicians when in doubt or difficulty.[38]

It can be concluded that in a disease like diabetes mellitus the availability of a skilled and highly motivated nursing care is absolutely essential. This would facilitate effective management of diabetes by motivating the patient, inculcating a positive thinking in him and by promoting his self-management skills. The nursing personnel can act not only as a caregiver but also as a counselor and an educator that are crucial to successful diabetes outcome.

EMPOWERING THE PARAMEDICAL PERSONNEL

While paramedical personnel form an important section of the diabetes care team, all efforts must be made to initially empower and orient these workers suitably so that they can optimally carry out their roles. In a recent pilot study from South India,[39] which was conducted to determine awareness and practices relating to diabetic retinopathy among paramedical personnel, it was reported that a significant proportion (75%) of them had inadequate levels of awareness of diabetic retinopathy. The study reinforces the need for considerable effort in improving awareness of diabetes and diabetes-related complications among paramedical personnel so that their services can be utilized effectively while providing diabetes care. Optimally empowered paramedical personnel are the key to successful diabetes management and successful outcome in diabetes mellitus.

REFERENCES

1. Roman SH, Harris MI. Management of diabetes mellitus from a public health perspective. Endocrinol Metab Clin North America. 1997;26:443-4.
2. Madhu SV, Lalitha K. Education needs of diabetic patients with low socioeconomic and literacy levels. 15th International Diabetes Federation (IDF) Congress, Kobe, Japan 1994; Scientific Supplement. pp 137 (Abstract # 10C3OP1804).
3. Mohan D, Raj D, Shanthirani CS, Datta M, Unwin NC, Kapur A, Mohan V. Awareness and knowledge of diabetes in Chennai—the Chennai Urban Rural Epidemiology Study (CURES-9). J Assoc Physicians India. 2005;53:283.
4. Bajaj S, Melhotra R, Singh K, Kumar D. Assessment of knowledge regarding metabolic control in diabetes. J Assoc Physicians India. 2001;49:296
5. Malhotra R, Bajaj S, Kumar D, Singh KG. Influence of education and occupation on knowledge about diabetes control. Natl Med J India. 2000;13:293
6. Sivagnanam G, Namasivayam K, Rajasekaran M, Thirumalaikolundusubramanian P, Ravindranath C. A Comparative Study of the knowledge, beliefs, and practices of diabetic patients cared for at a Teaching Hospital (Free Service) and those cared for by private practitioners (Paid Service). Ann NY Acad Sci. 2002;958:416-9.
7. Viswanathan V, Shobhana R, Snehalatha C, Seena R, Ramachandran A. Need for education on footcare in diabetic patients in India. J Assoc Physicians India. 1999 ;47:1083-5.
8. Taiwo JO. Oral health education needs of diabetic patients in Ibadan. African Journal of Medicine Med Sci. 2000;29:269-74.
9. The Diabetes Controls and Complications Trials (DCCT) Research Group. The Effect of intensive treatment of diabetes on the development and progression of long-term complications in insulin-dependent diabetes mellitus. N Engl J Med. 1993; 329:977.
10. Polit D, Hungler BP. Nursing Research Principles and Methods, 5th edn, Philadelphia: Lippincott.1995.
11. Rorber GE, King H. WHO guidelines for the development of a national programme for diabetes mellitus. 1991. pp 22-5.
12. United Kingdom Prospective Diabetes Study (UKPDS) Group. Intensive blood glucose control with sulfonylureas or insulin compared with conventional treatment and risk of complications in patients with type 2 diabetes (UKPDS 33). Lancet. 1998;352:837-53.
13. Soundarya M, Asha A, Mohan V. Role of a diabetes educator in the management of diabetes. Intl J Diab Dev Countries. 2004;24:65-8.
14. Report of WHO working group on *Therapeutic Patient Education*, Copenhagen, Denmark: WHO EURO. 1998 ESBN 92-890,1288-9.
15. Assal JP, Dayer-Metroz MD. Follow-up, therapeutic education and pharmacological treatment of patients with type 2 diabetes mellitus: Various critical views. Rev Med Suisse Romande. 2002;122:231-5.
16. Faich GA, Fishbein HA, Ellis SE. The epidemiology of diabetic acidosis: a population based study. Am J Epidemiol. 1983;117:551-8.
17. Goldgewciht C, Papol A, Tchobroutsky G. Hypoglycemic reactions in 172 type 1 diabetic patients. Diabetologia. 1983;24:95-9.
18. Deweend I, Visser AP, Kokg J, Deweerdt O, Vanderveen EA. Randomised controlled multicenter evaluation of an education programme for insulin-treated diabetic patient effects on metabolic control quality of life and costs of therapy. Diabetic Med. 1991;8:338-45.
19. Mazucca SA, Morrman NH, Wheeler ML. The diabetes education study: a controlled trial of the effects of diabetes patient education. Diabetes Care. 1986;9:1-10.
20. Brown SA. Studies of educational intervention and outcomes in diabetic adults: a meta-analysis revisited. Patient Educ Couns. 1990;16:189-215.
21. Norris SL, Lan J, Smith SJ, Schmid CH, Engelgau MM. Self-management education for adults with type 2 diabetes: a meta-analysis of the effect on glycemic control. Diabetes Care. 2002;25:1159-72.
22. Clement S. Diabetes self-management education. Diabetes Care. 1995;18:1204-14.
23. Sone H, Ito H, Yamashita H, Ishibashi S, Katayama S, Abe R, Ohashi Y, Akanuma Y, Yamada N. The Japan Diabetes Complication Study Group: the long-term effects of self-management education for patients with type 2 diabetes on glycemic control. Diabetes Care. 2002;25:2115.
24. Malone JM, Synde M, Anderson G. Prevention of amputation by diabetic education. Am J Surg. 1989;158:52-3.
25. Viswanathan V, Madhavan S, Rajasekhar S, Chamukuttu S, Ambady R. Amputation prevention initiative in South India: positive impact of foot care education. Diabetes Care. 2005;28:1019-21.
26. Steed L, Cooke D, Newman S. A systematic review of psychosocial outcomes following education, self-management and psychological interventions in diabetes mellitus. Patient Education Couns. 2003;51:5-15.
27. Grey M, Boland EA, et al. Coping skills training for youth with diabetes mellitus has long-lasting effects on metabolic control and quality of life. Journal of Pediatrics. 2000;37:107-13.
28. Matam P, Kumaraiah V, Munichoodappa C, Kumar KM, Aravind S. Behavioral Intervention in the management of compliance in young type-I diabetes. J Assoc Physicians India. 2000;48:967-71.
29. Litaker D, Mion L, Planavsky L, Kippes C, Mehta N, Frolkis J. Physician-nurse practitioner teams in chronic disease management: the impact on costs, clinical effectiveness, and patients' perception of care. J Interprof Care. 2003;17:223-37.
30. Loveman E, Royle P, et al. Specialist nurses in diabetes mellitus. Cochrane Database Syst Rev. 2003;CD003286.
31. Barth R, Campbell LV, Allen S, Jupp JJ, Chisholm DJ, et al. Intensive education improves knowledge, compliance, and foot problems in type 2 diabetes. Diabet Med. 1991;8:111-7.

32. Campbell LV, Barth R, Gosper JK, Jupp JJ, Simons LA, Chisholm DJ, et al. Impact of intensive educational approach to dietary change in NIDDM. Diabetes Care. 1990; 16:841-7.

33. Franciosi M, Pellegrini F, De Berardis G, Belfiglio M, Cavaliere D, Di Nardo B, Greenfield S, Kaplan SH, Sacco M, Tognoni G, Valentini M, Nicolucci A. The impact of blood glucose self-monitoring on metabolic control and quality of life in type 2 diabetic patients: an urgent need for better educational strategies. Diabetes Care. 2001;24:1870-7.

34. Harris MI. Medical care for patients with diabetes: epidemiological aspects. Ann Intern Med. 1996;124:117-22.

35. Worth JM, Vyas A: Diabetes Dietitian Or Diabetes Educator? Practical Diabetes International 2002; 19:180-1.

36. Chandalia HB, Bagrodia J. Effect of nutritional counseling on the blood glucose and nutritional knowledge of diabetic subjects. Diabetes Care. 1979;2:353-6.

37. Brunner SB , Suddarth DS. Medical surgical nursing. Philadelphia: JB Lippincott Company, 7th edn 1991. pp 41-2.

38. The place of nurses in management of diabetes (editorial). Lancet. 1982;1:145-8.

39. Namperumalsamy P, Kim R, Kallaperumal K, Sekar A, Karthika A, Nirmalan PK, et al. A pilot studies an awareness of diabetic retinopathy among nonmedical persons in south India: the challenge for eye care programmes in the region. Indian J Ophthalmol. 2004;52:247-51.

Section 14

PREVENTION

Chapter 90

PREDICTION AND PREVENTION OF TYPE 1 DIABETES

CB Sanjeevi

INTRODUCTION

Type 1 diabetes (Type 1 diabetes mellitus) is an autoimmune disease where the autoimmunity is mediated by T-helper cells in a genetically susceptible individual. Several studies have been done in both the mouse model (NOD)[1] and the rat (BB) model[2-5] of autoimmune diabetes to understand the mechanism of destruction mediated by the immune system on the β-cells. T1DM is most common in Sweden and it is third most frequent in the world, next to Finland and Sardinia.[6-9] The incidence increases approximately 20% every 10 years. The incidence of T1DM in Asian countries like India,[10-12] China and Japan is very low (1 in 250,000) when compared to Sweden where the incidence rate is very high (1 in 400). A recent estimate suggests that 1% of all children born in Sweden may develop T1DM during their lifetime.

There are several genes implicated in the etiology of T1DM. They are called IDDM genes and 18 of them are known till now.[13] (For details of these genetic markers, Chapter 24 titled *Immunogenetics of Type 1 Diabetes*). The major susceptibility and protection loci are in the short arm of chromosome 6 in the major histocompatibility gene complex (MHC). This group of MHC genes is categorized to Class I, Class II and Class III. HLA-DR and DQ genes are located in the HLA-class II region.[14] HLA-DR4/DQ8 and DR3/DQ2 are the susceptibility genes and DQ6 is the protective gene.[15-20] In Swedish children with T1DM, only 89% of the newly diagnosed patients can be accounted for by the high-risk susceptibility markers especially HLA-DQ8 and DQ2. The remaining 11% develop diabetes without the high-risk HLA. In addition, environmental factors play a major role in the etiology of the disease. This is evident from the studies on monozygotic twins where only 33 to 50% concordances is observed **(Table 90.1)**.[21-24] It is likely that environmental factors operate very early in life. Infection during pregnancy and nutrition have also been attributed as likely environmental trigger.[25-28]

For prevention strategy to be effective, there should be an efficient prediction strategy. The immune and genetic markers are used in the prediction strategies. The markers used in the prediction strategies are being evaluated and their limitations are discussed below before the prevention is discussed in detail.

TABLE 90.1	Lifetime risk for the development of T1DM in relatives of patients compared to general population

Sample	Risk
General population	0.7–1.5%
Offspring of type 1 diabetes mother	2–3%
Offspring of type 1 diabetes father	5–6%
Siblings of type 1 diabetes patients	5–6%
HLA identical siblings	10–16%
Monozygotic twins	33–50%

IMMUNE AND GENETIC MARKERS USED IN PREDICTION OF TYPE 1 DIABETES

The major autoantigens in T1DM are Insulin,[29] glutamic acid decarboxylase-isoform 65 (GAD65)[30-31] and protein tyrosine phosphatase. Antibodies to insulin (IAA), GAD65 and protein tyrosine phosphatase (ICA512 or IA-2)[32] are markers for the disease and they are not responsible for the causation of the disease. Their presence in the serum denotes the underlying β-cell autoimmunity. They are formed well before the development of clinical diabetes and their presence in the serum of nondiabetic individuals may indicate impending diabetes development. Therefore these autoantibody markers along with the high-risk genetic markers (e.g. HLA-DR and DQ gene) have been used in the strategies for the prediction of T1DM. Additional markers are being added to improve the prediction approach.

PREDICTION OF TYPE 1 DIABETES

In order to prevent T1DM, there is need for identifying susceptible subjects by applications of good prediction strategies.

Many studies are in progress to address this issue. Data on two important factors contribute to the prediction of T1DM. They are genetic and immunological markers. Currently, studies aimed at prediction of T1DM have largely been performed in relatives of individuals with T1DM rather than in the general population. However, 90% of patients with T1DM do not have a close relative with the disease and therefore prediction in the general population must be considered in order to design prevention trials on a public health scale. The newborn screening studies and subsequent prevention in the high-risk children are done in Finland called diabetes prediction and prevention project

(DPPP). The details of these projects are available at the website: *http://research.utu.fi/dipp/*. Similar studies are on in Sweden on the prediction strategies but intervention for prediction is not permitted thus far. All newborn babies in six countries in south-east Sweden are followed up since 1998. The details of this study are available on the website: *http://www.liu.se/hu/ihm/abis/index.htm*. Similarly, another study in southern Sweden addresses questions in a similar way and the details of this study are available at another website: *www.dipis.info*. In USA newborn studies are carried out in the University of Colorado at the Barbara Davis Center for Childhood Diabetes (*www.uchsc.edu/daisy/*).

The single most useful test for the prediction of T1DM had been the assay of ICA by immunohistochemistry.[33-35] However, the ICA assay is semiquantitative and remains difficult to standardize, despite improvements resulting from standardization workshop.[36] In contrast, radioimmunoassays utilizing a 96-well plate format and 96-well plate b counter are highly sensitive, reproducible and readily lend themselves to mass screening of populations.[37-38] The autoantibodies to the three different antigens insulin (IAA), GAD65 and protein tyrosine A2 phosphates (IA2) assort independently in prediabetic individuals and new-onset patients with T1DM. Approximately 80% of patients with new-onset diabetes[39] and prediabetes express at least two of the above autoantibodies and around 45% of all three autoantibodies while antibodies to insulin, GAD65 and ICA512/IA2 were each positive in 1% or less when tested in 200 healthy control subjects. Moreover none of the control subjects was positive for more than one of these autoantibodies, indicating that the presence of two or more of autoantibodies such as IAA, GAD65 and ICA512/IA2 is highly specific.[40]

In the University of Florida study on nondiabetic relatives of T1DM probands, 5-year risk for developing T1DM was calculated depending on the number of autoantibody positivity. The results are shown in the **Table 90.2**.

For first-degree relatives of patients with T1DM with two or more of these autoantibodies the risk of diabetes within 3 years is 39% and the risk within 5 years is 68%. For relatives with all three of these autoantibodies, the estimated risk within 5 years approaches 100%. When relatives of T1DM patients are stratified by the number of autoantibodies (as measured by radioimmunoassay), the additional presence of ICA does not increase the risk for T1DM.[40]

Another useful and widely used predictive marker is determination of first phase insulin release (FPIR)

TABLE 90.2	University of Florida Study of nondiabetic relatives of T1DM probands[41]
Islet autoantibody status	*5-year risk of developing T1DM*
ICA-negative	3.2%
ICA alone positive	5.3%
IAA alone positive	9.1%
Any two islets autoantibody positive	28.2%
ICA-positive and one other islets autoantibody positive	50.3%
IAA-positive and one other islets autoantibody positive	55.7%
Any three or four islets autoantibody positive	66.2%

with intravenous glucose tolerance test (IVGTT). This measures the ability of β-cells for prompt acute secretion of insulin in response to IV glucose. The FPIR is usually impaired variably predicts before the clinical onset of T1DM. The rate of fall of FPIR predicts the time of onset of overt diabetes in ICA and/or IAA positive relatives of patients with T1DM and other susceptible subjects. The presence of low FPIR increases the risk of diabetes in the subgroups positive for single autoantibody and the subgroup positive for multiple autoantibodies as measured by radioimmunoassay.[40]

RISK GROUPS LIKELY TO BENEFIT FROM PREVENTION APPROACH

The first degree relatives of patients with T1DM are more likely to develop T1DM than the general population as shown in **Table 90.1**. However, the **Table 90.3** gives additional list of groups who might from benefit intervention.

Women with gestational diabetes mellitus (GDM), from a special group who develop glucose intolerance during pregnancy because they already have initiated diabetes pathogenic process. Pregnancy in them appears as a window through which we can see the future

TABLE 90.3	Risk groups for prediction and prevention of T1DM

- First degree relatives of patients with T1DM
- Autoantibody positive offsprings gestational diabetes mellitus (GDM)
- Children born to older mothers
- General population.

development of full blown diabetes. Measuring autoantibodies in these patients have been shown to predict risk for the future development of T1DM. Di Mauricio and de Leiva's review give a glimpse of this problem in a lucid way.[42] The prevalence of ICA in GDM mothers in different populations vary widely 1.8% in one study compared to 38% in another population. However, when GAD65Ab was compared, the frequencies of 1.8% and 38% were the lowest and highest respectively.[42] In GDM mothers, ICA positivity gave a risk of 75% for development of T1DM in 11 years.[43,44] When GAD65, IA-2 or ICA was tested, the risk for the development of T1DM at 2 years postpartum was 17%, if one autoantibody was present, 61% if two autoantibodies were present and 84%, if three autoantibodies were present. Women with one or more pregnancies before the index pregnancy have 15% additional risk for the development of T1DM. If the risk for development of T1DM is calculated based on the presence of high-risk HLA markers, the risk at 2 years postpartum was, 22% if they are either DR3 or DR4 positive. If they are insulin treated, then the risk increases to 50%. Combined determination of DR3 or DR4 with islet autoantibody positivity increased the sensitivity of identifying T1DM up to 92%.[45]

Age of the mother at the time, she delivers the baby and the age of the biological father at the time, the T1DM child is conceived are also important risk factors for the development of T1DM in the offspring. A study by Bingley et al in the Bart-Oxford study group shows influence of maternal age and birth order on the risk of T1DM. In children born to mothers in the age group of 40 and above incidence of T1DM was three times higher than the children born to mothers in the age group of 20 to 25. The risk increased by 25% for each 5-year slab of maternal age.[46] The risk was highest in the first born and decreased progressively with increasing birth order. Paternal age was associated with 9% increase for each 5-year increase in paternal age.[46]

PREVENTION TRIALS

Two main large-scale prevention studies have been completed while others are in progress. European Nicotinamide Diabetes Intervention Trial (ENDIT)[47,48] and Diabetes Prevention Trial-1 (DPT-1) of North America[49] have been completed. Both studies recruited first degree relatives of patients with T1DM. The five-year ENDIT study was meant to prove whether oral nicotinamide[48,50] could prevent or postpone development of T1DM and the DPT-1 study was to show whether small doses of subcutaneous insulin administration could prevent T1DM development.

DPT-1 is a collaborative multicentered study performed in USA to test whether parenteral and/or oral insulin therapy can prevent or delay the onset of clinical type 1 diabetes. Using immunologic, genetic and metabolic testing, relatives of patients with type 1 diabetes were evaluated for risk of development of diabetes. High-risk relatives (risk of diabetes greater than 50% in five years) are eligible for the parenteral insulin trial and are randomized to active treatment vs a control group. Active treatment consists of four-day insulin infusion once per year and subcutaneous ultralente insulin twice per day for rest of the time. Intermediate risk relatives (risk of diabetes greater than 25% in five years) are eligible for the oral insulin trial and are randomized to oral insulin vs placebo daily. The parenteral insulin trial began in 1994 and the oral trial in 1996.

The results from both DPT-1 and ENDIT studies were found to be negative, at the dosage of insulin given and the route of administration chosen for the intervention in the first degree relative.[49] Similarly, nicotinamide oral orally at the dosage given was not effective in prevention of T1DM in the first degree relatives.[48]

VACCINE STRATEGIES FOR THE PREVENTION OF TYPE 1 DIABETES

The vaccine strategies currently tried can be broadly divided into five categories:
1. Induction of tolerance
2. Peptide-based vaccine strategy
3. DNA vaccine
4. Adjuvants as vaccines and others
5. Vaccine as adjuvants

Induction of Tolerance

Oral tolerance is a term used to describe the tolerance, which can be induced by the administration of exogenous antigen via the gut to activate immune system. It is meant to provide antigen driven peripheral tolerance and appears to involve two main mechanisms, which are in part dependent on antigen dose. The tolerance induced by lower doses of orally administered antigen appears to be mediated predominantly by active suppression whereas higher doses tend to induce clonal deletion. The active suppression of low doses of oral antigen appear to be mediated by the oral antigen

generating regulatory T-cells that migrate to lymphoid follows and to other tissues processing the ingested antigen in order to confer suppression of immune reaction via the secretion of downregulatory cytokines such as IL-4, IL-10 and TGF β. Such the type immune responses are preferentially generated by antigen presentation via the gut.

A method for induction of tolerance that is currently showing promise is administration of oral insulin conjugated to b-subunit of the cholera toxin (CTB).[51] It has been shown recently that oral administration of microgram amounts of antigen coupled CTB subunit, can effectively suppress systemic T-cell reactivity in native as well as in immune animals. Bergerot now reports that feeding small amounts (2-20 µg) of human insulin conjugated to CTB can effectively suppress β-cell destruction and clinical diabetes in adult nonobese diabetic (NOD) mice.[43] The protective effect could be transferred by T-cells from CTB-insulin-treated animals and was associated with reduced lesions of insulitis. Furthermore, adoptive cotransfer experiments involving injection of Thy-1, 2 recipients with diabetogenic T-cells from syngenic mice and T-cells from congenic Thy-1, 1 mice fed with CTB-insulin demonstrated a selective recruitment of Thy-1, 1 donor cells in the peripancreatic lymph nodes concomitant with reduced islet cell infiltration. These results suggest that protection against autoimmune diabetes can be achieved by feeding minute amounts of a pancreas islet cell autoantigen linked to CTB and appears to involve the selective migration and retention of protective T-cells into lymphoid tissues draining the vulnerable site of organ injury.

CTB subunit carries the insulin to the intestine and helps in the transfer of the insulin molecule across the intestinal barrier. The CTB conjugation also helps in the reduction of the dosage of insulin that can be administered orally without causing hypoglycemia. Further, this approach has also been tried successfully by intranasal administration. Both approaches have prevented the development of diabetes in the NOD mouse model of the autoimmune disease.

Peptide-based Vaccine Strategy

Peptide-based vaccine strategy has been successfully tried in the NOD mouse model with peptide derived from GAD65, by Dr Kaufman's group in University of California Los Angeles (UCLA).[52] This method has immense potential and is now being tried in the humans.

DiaPep277 Vaccine

One of the trials that has passed phase I and phase II is a peptide from 60 KDA Heat Shock Protein (HSP60). This is an immunomodulatory peptide called p277 (DiaPep277) which was tried successfully to prevent T1DM in NOD mice. In the phase II, clinical trial in latent autoimmune diabetes of adults (LADA) patients (n=35), 1 mg of p277 was given at entry, one month and 6 months or three placebos (n=17). The primary endpoint was glucagon-stimulated C-peptide production. Secondary end points were metabolic controls and T-cell autoimmunity to HSP60 and to p277. At the end of 10 months, the mean C-peptide had fallen in the placebo group but were maintained in the DiaPep 277 group (p<0.05). The need for exogenous insulin was higher in the placebo group compared to the DiaPep277 group (p<0.05). In both groups, T-cell reactivity to DiaPep277 enhanced T-helper 2 cytokine phenotype.[53] No adverse effect was noted. These findings were strengthened at the end of 24 months follow-up.

Diamyd GAD65 Vaccine

Studies in NOD mouse have shown that destruction of islet β-cells was associated with expressing T-cells recognizing GAD65. Studies by Kaufman show that GAD65 effectively prevent autoimmune β-cell destruction along with reduction and delay in the development of spontaneous diabetes.[52] Diamyd company of Sweden evaluated this by using alum-formulated human recombinant GAD65 in LADA patients. They selected diabetic patients of both sexes aged 30 to 70 years presenting as T2DM while positive for glutamic acid decarboxylase 65 antibodies (GAD65). These patients were either treated with diet or oral tablets. Only females of non-childbearing age were included. Thirty-four patients and 13 controls were treated with 4, 20, 100 and 500 μg doses, injected subcutaneously twice 4 weeks apart. No serious adverse effects were reported. Only GAD65 given at 500 μg dose produced GAD65 antibodies in one individual. In the follow-up, the C-peptide level (both fasting and stimulated) was significantly elevated only in those receiving 20 μg dose compared to placebo. Mean HBA_{1c} and glucose levels were significantly lowered in the 20 μg dose group compared to placebo. The Df+CD25+T-cells levels reflecting the increase of regulatory T-cells associated with nondestrucition of β-cell were elevated in the 20 μg dose group but not in others. All these findings were relevant even after a follow-up of 24 months (www.diamyd.com). It is construed that the prevention of β-cell destruction and β-cell recovery was due to shifting of immune response from destructive to nondestructive pathway which is mediated by the Diamyd GAD65 vaccine. The results of this study were presented in the ADA meeting in 2003 and published as abstract in the Diabetes 2005 Supplement 1.

DNA Vaccine

DNA vaccine is administering the GAD65 gene in a plasmid vector intramuscularly so that GAD65 protein is produced in the body that can induce tolerance.[54] The technique of DNA-based vaccination used to generate a T-cell-dependent antibody response to glutamic acid decarboxylase (GAD) in BALB/c, C57BL/6, and non-obese diabetic (NOD) mice. Plasmids expressing GAD65 (rGAD65) on the rat GAD67 (rGAD67) gene was constructed with the immediate early region promoter of the human cytomegalovirus (pCMV). This *naked* plasmid DNA was then injected into the regenerating muscles of the studied mice. In the vaccinated animals, antibody responses to GAD65 or to GAD67 were induced. Epitope recognition of GAD was studied by protein footprinting, a technique that makes use of a limited protcolysis of antibody-bound antigen. Diabetes incidence was unchanged in NOD mice, while no diabetes was observed in C57BL/6 and BALB/c mice, respectively. The data demonstrate that genetic immunization is a suitable novel tool to stimulate and to manipulate an immune response against the diabetes-associated protein glutamic acid decarboxylase. Interestingly, our results indicate that, by genetic vaccination, distinct β-cell epitopes were generated in the various studied mouse strains studied.

This approach has produced conflicting results. A group from San Francisco did not find this method useful in the NOD mouse model[55] but a Japanese group has showed that this method prevents the development of diabetes in the NOD mouse.

Adjuvants as Vaccine and Others

BCG vaccine has been tried in the prevention of T1DM both in the animal models and in humans.[56] The way this works is by shifting the T-cell response from destructive (Th1) to nondestructive (Th2). Several trials are being conducted to test the efficacy of this approach. In the mean time, a group headed by Dr Kevin Lafferty in Australia has tried Q fever vaccine in the prevention of T1DM in the animal models. This approach appears to be more efficient the prevention of T1DM than BCG. This is currently being evaluated in Australia with the help of a biotechnology organization.

Vaccine Delivery Systems

The vaccines that are developed have to be administered in a way that can deliver the substance of choice in an efficient manner for induction of tolerance. Several approaches are being tried. One is CTB as mentioned earlier.[57] The other novel approach is to clone human genes in plant products and consumption of these plant products would effectively induce tolerance. The plants that can be used easily for cloning human genes are tobacco.[58] GAD67 gene has been cloned into tobacco and when these were fed to diabetes prone NOD mice. These mice did not develop diabetes. Since tobacco is not fit for human consumption, GAD65 genes have been cloned into potatoes successfully and the animals fed with GAD-potato did not develop diabetes. However, good this might be one cannot consume raw potato and cooked potato may not have the GAD65 available in the right form for induction of tolerance. More recently carrots have been used successfully to clone GAD65 genes and are being currently evaluated for the prevention of diabetes in the mouse model.

These studies hopefully would give us a tool to prevent autoimmune diabetes in the humans and the experiments in the animal models look promising.

REFERENCES

1. Atkinson MA, Maclaren NK. Autoantibodies in nonobese diabetic mice immunoprecipitate 64,000-Mr islet antigen. Diabetes. 1988;37:1587-90.
2. Gotfredsen CF, Buschard K, Frandsen EK. Reduction of diabetes incidence of BB Wistar rats by early prophylactic insulin treatment of diabetes-prone animals. Diabetologia. 1985;28:933-5.
3. Like AA. Spontaneous diabetes in experimental animals. In Volk W (Ed): The diabetic pancreas. New York: Plenum Press; 1977. pp. 381-423.
4. Like AA, Weringer EJ, Holdash A, McGill P, Atkinson D, Rossini AA. Adoptive transfer of autoimmune diabetes mellitus in Biobreeding/Worcester (BB/W) inbred and hybrid rats. J Immunol. 1985;134:1583-6.
5. Baekkeskov S, Dyrberg T, Lernmark Å. Autoantibodies to a 64-kilodalton islet cell protein precede the onset of spontaneous diabetes in the BB rat. Science. 1984;224:1348-50.
6. Falorni A, Kockum I, Sanjeevi CB, Lernmark Å. Pathogenesis of insulin-dependent diabetes mellitus. Clinical Endocrinology and Metabolism. 1995;9(1):25-46.
7. Greenbaum C, Brooks-Worrel B, Palmer J, Larnmark Å: Autoimmunity and prediction of insulin-dependent diabetes mellitus. Diabetes Annual. 1994;8:21-52.
8. LaPorte RE, Tajima N, Åkerblom HK, Berlin N, Brosseau J, Christy M, Drash AL, Fishbein H, Green A, Hamman R, Harris M, King H, Laron Z, Neil A. Geographic differences in the risk of insulin-dependent diabetes mellitus: the importance of registries. Diabetes Care. 1985;8:101-7.
9. Karvonen M, Tuomilehto J, Libman I, LaPorte R, Group F. A review of the recent epidemiological data on incidence of type I diabetes mellitus worldwide. Diabetologia. 1993;36:883-92.
10. Menon P, Viramani A, Shah P, Raju R, Sethi A. Childhood onset diabetes in India: an overview. J Diab Dev Countries. 1990;10:11-6.
11. Asha Bai P, Krishnaswami CV, Chellamariappan M, Vijayakumar G, Subramanium J. Glycosuria and diabetes mellitus in children and adolescents in South India. Diab Res Clin Prac. 1991;13:131-6.
12. Ramachandran A, Snehalatha C, Krishnaswamy CV. Registry MI: incidence of IDDM in children in urban population in Southern India. Diab Res Clin Prac. 1996;34:79-82.
13. Pugliese A. Unravelling the genetics of insulin-dependent type 1A diabetes: the search must go on. Diabetes Reviews. 1999;7:39-54.
14. Bodmer J, Marsch S, Albert E, et al. Nomenclature for factors of the HLA system, 1996. Tissue Antigens. 1997;49:297-321.
15. Sanjeevi CB, Lybrand TP, Landin-Olsson M, Kockum I, Dahlquist G, Hagopian WA, Palmer JP, Lernmark Å. Analysis of antibody markers, DRB1, DRB5, DQA1 and DQB1 genes and modeling of DR2 molecules in DR2 positive patients with insulin-dependent diabetes mellitus. Tissue Antigens. 1994;44:110-9.
16. Sanjeevi CB, Lybrand T, DeWeese C, Landin-Olsson M, Kockum I, Dahlqvist G, Sundkvist G, Stenger D, Lernmark Å. Polymorphic amino acid variations in HLA-DQ are associated with systematic physical property changes and occurrence of insulin-dependent diabetes mellitus. Diabetes. 1995;44:125-31.
17. Sanjeevi CB, Landin-Olsson M, Kockum I, Dahlqvist G, Lernmark Å. Effects of the second haplotype on the association with childhood insulin-dependent diabetes mellitus. Tissue Antigens. 1995;45:148-52.
18. Sanjeevi CB, Kockum I, Lernmark Å. The role of major histocompatibility complex in insulin-dependent diabetes. Current Opinion in Endocrinology and Diabetes. 1995;2:3-11.
19. Sanjeevi CB, Höök P, Landin-Olsson M, Kockum I, Dahlquist G, Lybrand T, Lernmark Å. DR4 subtypes and their molecular properties in a population based study of Swedish childhood diabetes. Tissue Antigens. 1996;47:275-83.
20. Sanjeevi CB, DeWeese C, Landin-Olsson M, Kockum I, Dahlquist G, Lernmark Å, Lybrand T. Analysis of critical residues of HLA-DQ6 molecules in insulin-dependent diabetes mellitus. Tissue Antigens. 1997;50:61-5.
21. Deschamps I, Boitard C, Hors J, Busson M, Marcelli-Barge A, Mogenet A, Robert J-J. Life table analysis of the risk of type 1 diabetes in siblings according to islet-cell antibodies and HLA markers. An 8-year prospective study. Diabetologia. 1992;35:951-7.
22. Olmos P, Aherne R, Heaton DA, Millward BA, Risley D, Pyke DA. Significance of concordance rates in identical twins of insulin dependent diabetics. Diabetologia. 1988;31:747-50.
23. Kaprio J, Tuomilehto J, Koskenvuo M, Romanov K, Reunanen A, Eriksson J, Stengård J, Kesäniemi YA. Concordance for type 1 (insulin-dependent) and type 2 (non-insulin-dependent) diabetes mellitus in a population-based cohort of twins in Finland. Diabetologia. 1992;35:1060-7.
24. Verge CF, Gianani R, Yu L, Pietropaolo M, Smith T, Jackson RA, Soeldner JS, Eisenbarth GS. Late progression to diabetes

and evidence for chronic beta-cell autoimmunity in identical twins of patients with type I diabetes [see comments]. Diabetes. 1995;44(10):1176-9.

25. Menser MA, Forrest JM, Bransby RD. Rubella infection and diabetes mellitus. Lancet. 1978;i:57-60.

26. Rubinstein P, Walker ME, Fedun B, Witt ME, Cooper LZ, Ginsburg-Fellner F. The HLA system in congenital rubella patients with and without diabetes. Diabetes. 1982;31:1088-91.

27. Yoon J-W, Kim CJ, Pak CY, McArthur RG. Effects of environmental factors on the development of insulin-dependent diabetes mellitus. Clin Invest Med. 1987;10:457-69.

28. Tuvemo T, Dahlquist G, Frisk G, Blom L, Friman G, Landin-Olsson M, Diderholm H. The Swedish childhood diabetes study III: IgM against coxsackie B viruses in newly diagnosed type 1 (insulin-dependent) diabetic children—no evidence of increased antibody frequency. Diabetologia. 1989;32:745-7.

29. Palmer JP, Asplin CM, Clemons P, Lyen K, Tatpati O, Raghu PK, Paguette TL. Insulin antibodies in insulin-dependent diabetics before insulin treatment. Science. 1983;222:1337-9.

30. Lernmark Å, Freedman ZR, Hofmann C, Rubenstein AH, Steiner DF, Jackson RL, Winter RJ, Traisman HS. Islet-cell-surface antibodies in juvenile diabetes mellitus. N Engl J Med. 1978;299:375-80.

31. Baekkeskov S, Nielsen JH, Marner B, Bilde T, Ludvigsson J, Lernmark Å. Autoantibodies in newly diagnosed diabetic children immunoprecipitate human pancreatic islet cell proteins. Nature. 1982;298:167-9.

32. Gianani R, Rabin DU, Verge CF, Yu L, Babu SR, Pietropaolo M, Eisenbarth GS. ICA512 autoantibody radioassay. Diabetes. 1995;44(11):1340-4.

33. Bottazzo GF, Florin-Christensen A, Doniach D. Islet-cell antibodies in diabetes mellitus with autoimmune polyendocrine deficiencies. Lancet. 1974;304:1279-83.

34. Bonifacio E, Bingley PJ, Shattock M, Dean BM, Dunger D, Gale EAM, Bottazzo GF. Quantitative islet cell antibody measurement assists in the prediction of insulin dependent diabetes. Lancet. 1990;335:147-9.

35. Schatz D, Krisher J, Horne G, Riley W, Spillar R, Silverstein J, Winter W, Muir A, Derovanesian D, Shah S, Malone J, Maclaren N. Islet cell antibodies predict IDDM in United States school age children as powerfully as unaffected relatives. J Clin Invest. 1994;93:2403-7.

36. Landin-Olsson M. Precision of the islet cell antibody assay depends on the pancreas. J Clin Lab Anal. 1990;4:289-94.

37. Falorni A, Grubin C, Takei I, Shimada A, Kasuga A, Murayama T, Ozawa Y, Kasatani T, Saruta T, Li L, Lernmark Å. Radio-immunoassay detects the frequent occurrence of autoanti-bodies to the Mr 65,000 isoform of glutamic acid decarboxylase in Japanese insulin-dependent diabetes. Autoimmunity. 1994;19:113-25.

38. Falorni A, Örtqvist E, Persson B, Lernmark Å. Radio-immunoassays for glutamic acid decarboxylase and GAD65 antibodies using 35S or 3H recombinant human ligands. J Immunol Methods. 1995;186:89-99.

39. Hagopian WA, Michelsen B, Karlsen AE, Larsen F, Moody A, Grubin CE, Rowe R, Petersen J, McEvoy R, Lernmark Å.

Autoantibodies in IDDM primarily recognize the 65,000 Mr rather than the 67,000 Mr isoform of glutamic acid decarboxylase. Diabetes. 1993;42:631-6.

40. Verge CF, Gianani R, Kawasaki E, et al. Prediction of type I diabetes in first degree relatives using a combination of insulin, GAD and ICA512bdc/IA-2 autoantibodies. Diabetes 1996;45(7):926-33.

41. Winter WE, Harris N, Schatz C. Clinical Diabetes. 2002;4:183.

42. Di Mauricio, A de Leiva. Diabetes Metabolism Research and Reviews. 2001;17:422-8.

43. Damm P, et al. Diabetic Medicine. 1994;11:558-63.

44. Fuchtenbusch M, et al. Diabetes. 1997;46:1459-67.

45. Ferber KM, et al. Journal of Clinical Endocrinology and Metabolism. 1999;84:2342-8.

46. Bingley PJ, et al. British Medical Journal. 2000;321:420-4.

47. Bingley P, Christie M, Bonifacio E, et al. Combined analysis of autoantibodies improves prediction of IDDM in islet cell antibodies positive relatives. Diabetes. 1994;43:1304-10.

48. European Nicotinamide Diabetes Intervention Trial (ENDIT): a randomized controlled trial of intervention before the onset of T1DM. Lancet. 2004;363:925-31.

49. Diabetes Prevention Trial Type 1 Diabetes Study Group. New Engl J Med. 2002;346:1685-91.

50. Uchigata Y, Yamamoto H, Nagai H, Okamoto H. Effect of poly (ADP-ribose) synthetase inhibitor administration to rats before and after injection of alloxan and streptozotocin on islet proinsulin synthesis. Diabetes. 1983;32(4):316-8.

51. Bergerot I, Ploix C, Petersen J, Moulin V, Rask C, Fabien N, Lindblad M, Mayer A, Czerkinsky C, Holmgren J, Thivolet C. A cholera toxoid-insulin conjugate as an oral vaccine against spontaneous autoimmune diabetes. Proc Natl Acad Sci USA. 1997;94(9):4610-4.

52. Kaufman D, Clare-Salzar M, et al. Spontaneous loss of T-cell tolerance to glutamic acid decarboxylase in murine insulin-dependent diabetes. Nature. 1993;366:69-72.

53. Raz I, Elias D, Avron A, et al. Beta cell function in new-onset T1DM and immunomodulation with heat-shock protein peptide (DiaPep277): a randomized, double-blind, phase II trial. Lancet. 2001;358:1749-53.

54. Wiest-Ladenburger U, Fortnagel A, Richter W, Reimann J, Boehm **BO**. DNA vaccination with glutamic acid decarboxy-lase (GAD) generates a strong humoral immune response in BALB/c, C57BL/6, and in diabetes-prone NOD mice. Horm Metab Res. 1998;30(10):605-9.

55. Coon B, An L, Whitton J, von Herrath M. DNA immunization to prevent autoimmune diabetes. J Clin Invest. 1999;104(2):189-94.

56. Sadelain MWJ, Oin HY, Lauzon J, Singh B. Prevention of type 1 diabetes in NOD mice by adjuvant immunotherapy. Diabetes. 1990;39:583-9.

57. Czerkinsky C, Sun J, Holmgren J. Oral tolerance and anti-pathological vaccines. Curr Top Microbiol Immunol. 1999;236:79-91.

58. Ma S, Zhao D, Mukherjee R, Singh B, Qin H, Stiller C, Jevnicker A. Transgenic plants expressing autoantigens fed to mice to induce oral tolerance. Nature Medicine. 1997;3:793-6.

Chapter 91

PREVENTION OF TYPE 2 DIABETES

Hemraj B Chandalia

CHAPTER OUTLINE

- Introduction
- Target Population
- Diabetes Prevention Studies

- Lessons from Epidemiology
- Preferred Strategy for Prevention
- Summary

INTRODUCTION

Prevention of any disease is a laudable goal. When this is applied to type 2 diabetes mellitus, it gains further importance, because of the fact that diabetes is gaining epidemic proportions. Furthermore, the cost of treatment, more so the cost of treatment of complications of diabetes is staggeringly high for even an advanced economy in the western world to sustain. There is no question that developing world should allocate its scarce resources in the health care segment for prevention than treatment. The last decade has witnessed immense activity in this field leading towards the testing of the possible strategies. Each of these strategies now needs further research to evaluate its suitability and applicability to the large populations inhabiting the diabetes-prone regions of the world. Research is also needed on the socioeconomic factors, cultural mores, food and exercise habits of diverse populations so as to devise population-specific preventive strategies.

TARGET POPULATION

Preventive strategies must define the target population. In countries passing through an explosive epidemic, it may be advisable to target the whole population. This is probably true of a population like Pima Indians. The prevalence of diabetes among adult Pima Indians is as high as 50%.[1] This epidemic is now catching up with the young Pima Indians; 5.1% of the 15 to 19 years old subjects suffer from type 2 diabetes, a six-fold increase over the last 20 years.[2] Apart from such exceptions it is indeed difficult to apply any intensive preventive strategy to the whole population for simple logistic and cost considerations. Hence, more practicable strategies have to be thought of such as general education towards healthy lifestyle, healthy town planning; invoking help from food industries for marketing of healthy foods. Such global methods may not necessarily be effective or may only have a marginal effect. These have not been studied systematically anywhere. Most frequently advocated approach at present is application of the interventional strategy to highly susceptible groups. These groups can be identified by the presence of risk factors for the development of diabetes **(Table 91.1)**.

DIABETES PREVENTION STUDIES

Lifestyle Intervention

Prevention of type 2 diabetes by changes in lifestyle among subjects with impaired glucose tolerance (IGT)

TABLE 91.1	Groups at high-risk for the development of type 2 diabetes mellitus

- *Family history of type 2 diabetes:* Risk can be graded depending upon the history of diabetes in one sibling or parent; one sibling and a parent; both parents
- *Obesity:* Mild (BMI >23), moderate (BMI 25-30) or severe obesity (BMI >30). There is considerable work on Asian Indians indicating that BMI >22 is also a risk factor in this population[3]
- Gestational diabetes
- Stress hyperglycemia
- Common endocrine diseases like polycystic ovarian syndrome
- *Drug therapy:* Corticosteroid therapy, diuretics and oral contraceptives

was studied by Tuomilehto and his colleagues from Finland.[4] They studied 522 subjects with IGT, mean age 55 years, mean BMI 31 for a mean duration of 3.2 years. The subjects were divided into intervention and control groups. The intervention group received individualized counseling aimed at reducing weight and total and saturated fat intake; and increasing intake of fiber and physical activity. The weight loss at 1 year, weight loss at 2 years and cumulative incidence of diabetes in intervention group were 4.2-3.7 kg, 3.5-5.5 kg and 11% while in the control group the respective parameters were: 0.8 ± 3.7 kg, 0.8 ± 4.4 kg and 23%, respectively. Thus, the risk of diabetes was reduced by 58% (P<0.001) in the intervention group.

The most revealing study in the prevention of type 2 diabetes is the diabetes prevention program[5] where 3234 subjects with IGT, mean age 51 years, mean BMI 34 were randomized to placebo, metformin (850 mg twice a day) or a lifestyle-modification program aimed at 7% or more weight loss and 150 minutes of physical activity per week. The incidence of diabetes on follow-up (average 2.8 years) was 11.0, 7.8 and 4.8 cases per 100 person-years on placebo, metformin and lifestyle groups, respectively. Thus, compared to control group progress to type 2 diabetes mellitus was reduced by 58% in the lifestyle modification group and 31% in the metformin group. The study was monumental in its size, design and execution. The lifestyle intervention group was followed so intensively, that to match it in a large section of population is indeed a very difficult proposition.

The Da Qing study[6] was reported much earlier than the above two. In that study, 577 patients of impaired glucose tolerance (IGT) were recruited for the three study arms, diet alone, exercise alone and diet plus exercise. A control group was also followed up without any intervention. The cumulative incidence of diabetes at 6 years was 67.7% in the control group as compared to 43.8% in the diet group, and 41.1% in the diet plus exercise group. When adjusted for baseline differences in BMI and fasting glucose, the diet, exercise and diet plus exercise interventions were associated with 31%, 46% and 42% reductions in risk of developing diabetes respectively.

Manipulating dietary fat can result in weight loss and prevention of type 2 DM. A 5-year study of reduced fat intake induced by monthly discussion sessions for a year was reported by Swinburn and colleagues.[7] During the active phase of interaction for one year, the treatment group (reduced diet fat) had significantly more weight loss (3.3 kg) as compared to controls and lower emergence of type 2 diabetes (reduced fat diet vs controls: 47% vs 67%). However, these differences gradually disappeared over a 5 year follow-up. This brings out the fact that continuous reinforcement is needed to produce results in the long-run.

Role of dietary fat was evaluated by studying the fat intake in a group of 35988 Iowa women by a food frequency questionnaire.[8] Dietary PUFA, vegetable fat and n-3 fatty acids were negatively associated while transfatty acids, cholesterol and high keys score (higher score means more saturated fat and cholesterol intake) were positively associated with the prevalence of diabetes. The findings in this study are at variance to those in the Nurses Health Study, where intake of transfatty acids was associated with an increased incidence and w-3 or n-3 fatty acids a decreased incidence of diabetes. In another study, feasibility and effectiveness of educational methods to induce a reduction in dietary fat was proven on a short-term basis.[9]

Pharmacological Intervention

Diabetes prevention program evaluated the effect of metformin in dosage of 850 mg twice a day. This produced a 31% reduction in the emergence of type 2 diabetes as compared to a 58% reduction produced by intensive lifestyle intervention. Acarbose was used in the STOP-Noninsulin-dependent diabetes mellitus (STOP-**NIDDM**) trial.[10] A total of 1418 subjects diagnosed to have IGT were randomized in this double blind study to either acarbose 100 mg tid or placebo. At the end of the study, a reduction of 25% was noted in the cumulative incidence of diabetes.

A study of troglitazone in the prevention of diabetes (TRIPOD) was conducted on a group of 266 Hispanic women previously known to have suffered from gestational diabetes.[11] Troglitazone was administered in this double-blind study to 133 women randomized to the treatment group and compared with 133 women on the placebo. A few important conclusions emerged from this study. Troglitazone protected, these subjects from the development of diabetes (annual diabetes incidence rate 12.1 in placebo group vs 5.4% in troglitazone group). Those responding to troglitazone by increased insulin sensitivity benefited more compared to those not responding in terms of this parameter. Although troglitazone had to be discontinued quite early because of its potential hepatotoxicity, a follow-up at 8 months of discontinuation showed that the protective effect of troglitazone continued till that period. Other thiazolidinediones, namely pioglitazone and rosiglitazone are much safer drugs and are being currently evaluated for prevention of diabetes.

Analysis of Heart Outcomes Prevention Evaluation (HOPE) study revealed protective effect of angiotensin-converting-enzyme inhibitor, rampiril on the development of diabetes.[12] Ramipril suppressed fibrosis of islets in an animal model of type 2 diabetes.[13] In the West of Scotland Coronary Prevention Study, pravastatin reduced the development of diabetes by 30%.[14] Pravastatin retarded the progression of glucose intolerance in an animal model.[15] Similar observations have been documented in two more recent studies involving perindopril.

LESSONS FROM EPIDEMIOLOGY

The epidemiological studies reported from India[16,17] and elsewhere raise a few very important issues. Based on two-point determinations of prevalence, a number of projections have been made. The alarming increase in prevalence so predicted assumes that the escalation in the prevalence of the disease will continue in a linear fashion over the next two to three decades. However, such presumptions are likely to be affected by a variety of environmental factors. For example, increasing rate of urbanization, increasing obesity, diminishing physical inactivity and increasing fat intake will escalate the prevalence of diabetes. On the other hand, education promoting a healthy lifestyle, planned urban development leading to increased exercise opportunities, an enlightened food industry making low fat and high fiber foods available can decrease the prevalence of diabetes. The dynamics of these sociocultural and economic

factors is expected to influence the prevalence of diabetes. Although a polygenic disease, the frequency of these susceptibility genes may remain fairly constant if social practices continue to be the same. Hence, the effect of the onslaught of environmental factors is likely to wear off, as increasing numbers of susceptible individuals convert into IGT or overt diabetes. The residual population may be genetically at low risk. Hence, on an optimistic note, the incidence of type 2 diabetes may decline as we go along. On the other hand, the population of India will consist of increasing number of older people in the course of next two to three decades, which would lead to an increased incidence of diabetes. Suffice to say that dynamics of these equations needs to be appreciated and if possible, the influence of these forces to be quantified in order to arrive at more realistic estimates.

PREFERRED STRATEGY FOR PREVENTION

The prevention studies have pointed out clearly that the preferred modality for prevention appears to be lifestyle intervention. These modalities have not yet been applied to study hard endpoints like myocardial infarction and death. It is possible that a modality like lifestyle intervention has more secular, all pervasive effects on other cardiovascular risk factors like hypertension or dyslipidemia and hence, influences the endpoints in addition to those thus far studied. Besides lifestyle intervention, search is on to recognize the pleiotropic effect of drugs like statins and ACE inhibitors. Further research may give us molecules that have more profound pleiotropic effects, like retinoid receptor agonists and would therefore tend to correct both the dyslipidemias and dysglycemias.

As a preventive measure, a treatment modality is applied to an asymptomatic population. Hence, it should be virtually nontoxic, must have been documented to be effective and must be economical. Considering these facts, presently the lifestyle interventions come out as clear winners in the prevention of type 2 diabetes.

Assessment of applicability of preventive methods to large populations is dependent upon the knowledge of sociocultural-economic factors which has not yet been studied for different populations. The method used will at times need to be population-specific. This type of translational research[18] is sorely needed before large scale prevention can be undertaken. In the Indian context, indigenous drugs may have a role in the prevention. The Indian Council of Medical Research has recognized this fact and has made an initiative in this direction by studying scientifically a herbal remedy, *Vijaysar*.[19] The herbal indigenous drugs probably meet the criteria of low toxicity, low cost and easy acceptability and hence, are worth studying.

SUMMARY

Prevention of type 2 diabetes is an important public health measure. The target population has to be defined for this purpose. Obese individuals and those with family history of diabetes are important target groups.

Some landmark prevention studies published over the past five years have brought out the importance of lifestyle intervention. Weight loss by a low fat, high fiber diet and drugs such as glitazone, metformin and acarbose are likely to be effective. ACE inhibitors, and statins also may offer some protection.

Epidemiological studies have projected a very grim picture regarding the increasing prevalence of type 2 diabetes in the next two decades. However, interplay of sociocultural, economic and other environmental factors are likely to alter the prevalence of type 2 diabetes. Debate continues regarding the preferred modality of prevention. Applicability of these modalities to the society at large and outcome thereof requires further studies.

REFERENCES

1. Knowler WC, Bennett DH, Hamman RF, Miller M. Diabetes incidence and prevalence in Pima Indians: a 19-fold greater incidence than in Rochester, Minnesota. Am J Epidemiol. 1978;108:497-505.
2. Harwell TS, Mc Dowall JM, Moorek, et al. Establishing surveillance for diabetes in American Indian youth. Diabetes Care. 2001;24:1029-32.
3. Banerji MA, Faridi N, Atluri R, Chaiken RL, Lebovitz HE. Body composition, visceral fat, leptin and insulin resistance in Asian Indian Men. J Clin Endocr Metab. 1999;84:137-44.
4. Tuomilehto J, Lindstrom J, Eriksson JG, et al. Prevention of type 2 diabetes mellitus by changes in lifestyle among subjects with impaired glucose tolerance(Finnish Diabetes Prevention Study Group). New Engl J Med. 2001;344:1343-50.
5. Diabetes Prevention Program Research Group. Reduction in the incidence of type 2 diabetes with lifestyle intervention or metformin. New Engl J Med. 2002;346:393-403.
6. Panxiao-Ben, Liguang-Wei, Hu Ying-Hua, et al. Effects of diet and exercise in preventing NIDDM in people with impaired glucose tolerance (The Da Qiang IGT and Diabetes Study). Diabetes Care. 1997;20:537-44.
7. Swinburn BA, Metcalf P, Ley SJ. Long-term (5 years) effects of a reduced fat diet intervention in individuals with glucose intolerance. Diabetes Care. 2001;24:619-4.
8. Meyer KA, Kushi LH, Jacobs DR, Folsom AR. Dietary fat and incidence of type 2 diabetes in older Iowa women. Diabetes Care. 2001;24:1528-35.
9. Auseander W, Hairi-Jorhu D, Houston C, et al. A controlled evaluation of staging dietary patterns to reduce the risk of diabetes in African-American Women. Diabetes Care. 2002;25:809-14.
10. Chiasson JL, Jose RG, Gomis R, et al. Acarbose for prevention of type 2 diabetes mellitus. The STOP-NIDDM randomized trial. Lancet. 2002;359:2072-7.
11. Buchanan AB, Xiang AH, Peters RK, et al. Preservation of pancreatic beta cell function and prevention of type 2 diabetes by pharmacological treatment of insulin resistance in high-risk Hispanic women. Diabetes. 2002;51:2796-803.
12. The Heart Outcomes Prevention Evaluation Study Investigators. Effects of an angiotensin-converting-enzyme inhibitor, ramipril, on cardiovascular events in high-risk patients. New Engl J Med. 2000;342:145-53.
13. Ko SH, Kwon HS, Kim SR, et al. Ramipril treatment suppresses islet fibrosis in Otsuka Long-Evans Tokushima fatty rats. Biochem Biophys Res Commun. 2004;316:14-22.
14. Freeman DJ, Norrie J, Sattar N, et al. Pravastatin and the development of diabetes mellitus: evidence for a protective treatment effect in the West of Scotland Coronary Prevention Study. Circulation. 2001;103:357-62.
15. Yu Y, Ohmori K, Chen Y, et al. Effects of pravastatin on progression of glucose intolerance and cardiovascular remodeling in a type 2 diabetes model. J Am Coll Cardiol. 2004;44:904-13.
16. Ramachandran A, Jali MV, Mohan V, Snehlatha C, Vishwanathan M. High prevalence of diabetes in an urban population in South India. Br Med J. 1988;297:587-90.
17. Ramachandran A, Snehlatha C, Latha E, Vijay V, Vishwanathan M. Rising prevalence of NIDDM in an urban population in India. Diabetologia. 1997;40:232-7.
18. Engelgau MM, Venkat Narayan KM. Translation search for improving diabetes care: a perspective for India. Intl J Diab Dev Countries. 2004; 24:7-10.
19. Indian Council of Medical Research (ICMR) Collaborating Centers. Flexible dose open trial of *Vijaysar* in cases of newly diagnosed non-insulin dependent diabetes mellitus. Indian J Med Res. 1988;108:24-9.

Chapter 92

PREVENTION OF DIABETES—INDIAN ANGLE

A Ramachandran

CHAPTER OUTLINE

- Introduction
- Primary Prevention of Diabetes
- Impaired Glucose Tolerance (IGT) and Impaired Fasting Glucose (IFG)

- Secondary Prevention
- Conclusion
- Summary

INTRODUCTION

The prevalence of type 2 diabetes mellitus is increasing all over the world, especially in the developing countries.[1,2] According to the recent WHO report, by the year 2025, there will be 84 to 224 million diabetes subjects in the developing countries and the highest number would be in India (57 million), China and the US. Studies from different parts of India showed an increasing trend in the prevalence of diabetes **(Table 92.1)**. A series of epidemiological studies carried out by the Diabetes Research Centre, Chennai, Tamil Nadu, India, showed that the prevalence of diabetes had steadily increased among urban Indian adults from 5.0% in 1984 to 13.9% in 2000 **(Figure 92.1)**.[3] A national urban diabetes study conducted in six major Indian cities covering many regions in the country showed that the average prevalence of diabetes in urban Indian adults is 12.1%, the rates ranging from 9.3 to 16.6% **(Table 92.2)**.[4] Concomitantly, there has been a high prevalence of impaired glucose tolerance (IGT) also. Considering the magnitude of the population, the number likely to suffer from morbidity due to the disorder would be very high. Therefore, prevention is

TABLE 92.1	Studies showing a rising trend in the prevalence of type 2 diabetes in urban India		
Year	Author	Place	Prevalence %
1971	Tripathy et al	Cuttack	1.2
1972	Ahuja et al	New Delhi	2.3
1979	Gupta et al	Multicenter	3.0
1984	Murthy et al	Tenali	4.7
1986	Patel	Bhadran	3.8
1988	Ramachandran et al	Kudremukh	5.0
1991	Ahuja et al	New Delhi	6.7
1992	Ramachandran et al	Chennai	8.2
1997	Ramachandran et al	Chennai	11.6
2000	Ramankutty et al	Kerala	12.4
2001	Ramachandran et al (DESI)	National	12.1
2001	Misra et al	New Delhi	10.3
2001	Mohan et al	Chennai	12.1
2001	Kutty et al	Kerala	12.4

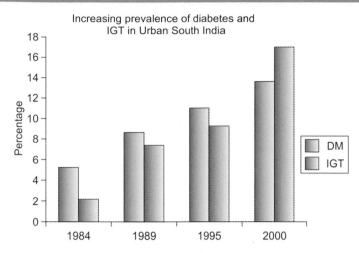

Figure 92.1 The temporary change in prevalence of diabetes mellitus (DM) and impaired glucose tolerance (IGT) in urban South India, Chennai, Tamil Nadu, India is shown. In the year 2000, IGT for diabetes ratio is >1

the most important factor in the crusade against the disorder. Prevention of type 2 diabetes is a possibility with changes in lifestyle.[5-7]

There are three main levels for the prevention of type 2 diabetes:
1. *Primary prevention* refers to the prevention of the onset of the disease.
2. *Secondary prevention* refers to the early diagnosis and treatment of the disease so as to prevent complications.
3. *Tertiary prevention* refers to limiting physical disability resulting from the complications and institution of rehabilitation measures.

Among these, it is imperative that presently more stress should be laid on primary prevention of diabetes. It includes genetic counseling, health promotion and specific protection. Genetic and environmental factors are of equal importance in the causation of diabetes. Details on secondary and tertiary preventions are discussed in Chapters on Management.

PRIMARY PREVENTION OF DIABETES

For implementation of primary prevention of diabetes, two major strategies are involved—the population-based approach and the high-risk approach. Both have relevance in community-based programs. In a country like India, where the prevalence and the risk of type 2 diabetes are high, both approaches have to be implemented.

Population-based Approaches

The benefits of a population-based approach would be far reaching as it not only prevents the conversion of high-risk group to type 2 diabetes but also prevents conversion of low-risk individuals to high-risk group.[8] In addition, it also has collateral benefits such as reduction of risks of coronary heart diseases, hypertension and several other noncommunicable diseases. However, implementation of such programs is beset with several hurdles. Firstly, in a large country like India with social, cultural and economic disparities and no comprehensive national health programs for diabetes or other noncommunicable disease, a population-based prevention program is rather an insurmountable task. It is gratifying to note that some positive steps are now

TABLE 92.2	Age and gender standardized prevalence of diabetes and IGT In different Indian cities, urban Indian population was used as standard					
	1 *Chennai*	*2* *Bengaluru*	*3* *Hyderabad*	*4* *Kolkata*	*5* *Mumbai*	*6* *New Delhi*
N	1668	1359	1427	2378	2084	2300
M:F	708:960	638:721	685:742	1163:1215	987:1097	107:1193
DM%	13.5 (11.8-15.2)	12.4[b] (10.5-14.3)	16.6 (14.6-18.6)	11.7[a,b] (10.4-13.0)	9.3[a,b,c] (7.7-10.1)	11.6[a,b] (10.3-12.9)
IGT%	16.8[b,f] (14.6-19.0)	14.9[b,f] (12.8-16.9)	29.8[f] (26.9-32.8)	10.0[a,b,d] (8.7-11.4)	10.8[a,b,d] (9.3-12.2)	8.6[a,b,d,e,f] (7.4-9.7)

95% confidence interval are shown in brackets
P<0.001
A vs Chennai, b vs Hyderabad, c vs New Delhi,
D vs Bengaluru, e vs Kolkata , f vs Mumbai

being initiated at national level to create awareness about the disease among the public.

Genetic Counseling

Though genetic counseling is one of the accepted methods for prevention of any hereditary disorder, it has not got into practice in the case of diabetes because the exact genetic mechanisms are unknown. In the light of the evidence already present, it is known that the stronger the family history, the higher the incidence of diabetes.[9,10] Hence, marriages between two diabetic subjects are not advisable in view of greater hazard for the offsprings.

Identification of High-risk Groups

Various epidemiological studies have shown that people with positive family history, obesity/central adiposity, insulin resistance and early biochemical abnormalities form a high-risk group for diabetes. Subjects undergoing rapid urbanization experience lifestyle changes which cooperates with the genetic tendency for diabetes in the evolution of the disease.

Familial Aggregation

Asian Indians possibly have stronger familial aggregation of diabetes with more frequent occurrence of diabetes among the first degree relatives and vertical transmission through 2 or more generations. It was found that 45% of the Indians compared to 38% of the Europeans have positive family history of diabetes. Among the type 2 diabetic subjects attending the Diabetes Research Centre, Chennai, Tamil Nadu, India, 54% of the probands had a parent with known diabetes and an additional 22.8% of siblings had diabetes.[10] The prevalence of diabetes increased with stronger family history of diabetes. The offsprings of diabetic parents developed the disease at least a decade earlier than their parents. In a survey in a South Indian population, it was noted that 43% of the diabetic patients had first degree family history of diabetes. Individuals at a high-risk of developing diabetes can be identified from a detailed analysis of their family history. Uncovering hidden diabetes becomes extremely successful if families are screened periodically for diabetes.

Detection of Early Biochemical Abnormalities

In its natural history, diabetes passes through some preclinical phases before it manifests as clinical diabetes

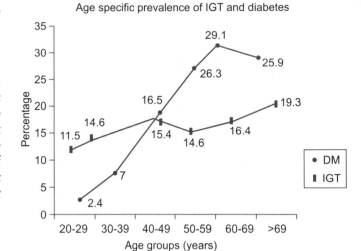

Figure 92.2 Age specific prevalence of impaired glucose tolerance (IGT) and diabetes for the urban Indian population is shown. The National Urban Diabetes Survey (2000) data was used for the analysis. Prevalence of impaired glucose tolerance is higher than diabetes in the group with <40 years of age

(Figure 92.2). Definite abnormalities of glucose tolerance and hormonal secretion and action, especially of insulin, have been detected in genetic prediabetic individuals, several years before clinical diabetes is detected.[11,12]

The identifiable biochemical markers in type 2 diabetes are:
- Elevated plasma insulin with normoglycemia
- Mean fasting and GTT derived area of glucose in the upper limit of normal-higher than control subjects
- Low insulin to glucose ratio at 2 hours in IGT
- Low incremental insulin to glucose ratio at 30 minutes (insulinogenic index).

More recently adiponectin, protective hormone secreted by the adipose tissue has been found to be playing key roles in controlling energy metabolism. A low blood adiponectin value has been documented to be predictive of future diabetes. A prospective study at our center showed that subjects who developed diabetes had low baseline adiponectin values.[13] Although it is a research tool, at present, it indicates availability of early indicators of future diabetes.

By proper screening procedures, these abnormalities can be detected early and corrective measures can be instituted. These measures help to improve insulin sensitivity.

Correction of Environmental (Diabetogenic) Factors

Having identified the high-risk group, the next step is to avoid or minimize the influence of the environmental factors. While genetic wing is not amenable for correction, the environmental factors can definitely be influenced to an appreciable extent. Several factors are known to predispose to diabetes in a susceptible population. These factors are: (1) Obesity, (2) Excessive intake of calories, fat and free sugar, (3) Lack of physical activity.

Modernization has led to consumption of excess calories, refined carbohydrates and fats and also need for minimal physical activity has resulted in adverse conditions result in obesity and high insulin resistance. Thus, the energy balance has tilted towards conservation of energy as depot fat, which is hardly needed to be utilized. High carbohydrate diet, as several studies have shown, produces high insulin sensitivity. However, this occurs mostly with complex carbohydrates and soluble food fiber. The western diet rich in energy and low in fiber promotes weight gain and insulin resistance, even in the low-risk populations such as the ethnic Europeans. The mechanisms responsible for this might operate more strongly in high-risk populations, who already have insulin resistance. A program involving alteration in lifestyle, complemented by pharmacological intervention with metformin, especially in those having impaired glucose tolerance and/or strong family history of diabetes has to be implemented to arrest the exploding epidemic of diabetes mellitus.

A study by Prof Viswanathan at the Diabetes Research Centre, Chennai, Tamil Nadu, India, conducted on 262 nondiabetic offsprings of noninsulin-dependent diabetic patients registered under the prevention program showed that rate of development of diabetes was greater in those who gained body weight in comparison with those who lost weight or showed no change.[14] Reduction in body weight, even in non-obese individuals helps to prevent the onset of diabetes. Although the rate and degree of obesity is less among Indians, it has been observed in several earlier studies that even a minor increase in body mass index increases the risk of diabetes. Recent studies have demonstrated that the healthy BMI for Asian Indians is less than 23 kg/m[2].[15,16]

The threshold of waist circumference for risk of diabetes is also lower. The cutoff values for normal waist girth are 85 cm (men) and 80 cm (women).[15] For a given BMI, Indians have higher central obesity and higher fat mass also. Results of another analysis of the data showed that lack of exercise, presence of mental stress and high 2-hour plasma glucose were the factors associated with development of diabetes.[17] Therefore, it was inferred that prevention strategies such as weight control by proper diet and exercise helps greatly in the crusade against diabetes.

Age at Development of Diabetes

Indians develop diabetes at a younger age than the western population. The risk is higher in those with parental history of diabetes. The offsprings develop diabetes at least a decade earlier than their parents. Therefore, it is necessary to screen for early changes in glucose tolerance at a young age (<30 years), in subjects with a high-risk for diabetes.

Prevalence of Overweight among Children

Overweight in childhood is a forerunner of obesity/overweight in adulthood. The association of obesity with metabolic syndrome such as diabetes and cardiovascular diseases is well known. Reports of increasing occurrence of type 2 diabetes among children in urban India[18] indicate that the epidemic of diabetes could become worse with the increasing epidemic of obesity now seen even among children. In a study in urban southern India, the prevalence of overweight was 17.8% among boys and 15.8% among girls aged 14-19 years.[19] There was a strong association of overweight with lack of physical activity and higher socioeconomic status.

IMPAIRED GLUCOSE TOLERANCE (IGT) AND IMPAIRED FASTING GLUCOSE (IFG)

Impaired glucose tolerance (IGT) and impaired fasting glucose (IFG) represent distinct stages in the natural history of diabetes **(Figure 92.3)**. Both conditions have a high-risk of conversion to diabetes. Approximately 40% of subjects with IGT progress to diabetes over a period of 5 to 10 years. The recently defined category of IFG also indicates an exaggerated predisposition to diabetes.[20] It is well known that IGT is associated with cardiovascular risk factors and as such is considered to be a proatherogenic condition. Recent studies have shown that incidence of the metabolic syndrome occurs frequently in association with IGT and IFG.[21] In India, IGT (8.1%) and IFG (8.7%) are prevalent in similar proportions and overlap in 3.5% of subjects.[22] Both conditions are associated with a high degree of insulin resistance. In the National Urban Diabetes Survey, the overall prevalence of diabetes was 12.1% and IGT 14%.

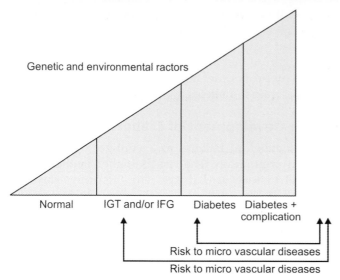

IGT: Impaired glucose tolerance
IFG: Impaired fasting glucose

Figure 92.3 Natural history of diabetes. It also shows the stages associated with the risk of complications

In most cities, the IGT: diabetes ratio was more than 1.0. This was an indicator of a high potential for a further rise in prevalence of diabetes due to conversion of IGT to diabetes. Another important observation made in the survey was that IGT was as common in younger age groups (<40 years of age) as in older subjects.[22]

An important observation made in the Madras Diabetes Survey, Chennai, Tamil Nadu, India, in 1992 was that although the prevalence of diabetes was 4 times lower in the rural population, the prevalence of IGT was almost similar in both urban and rural populations (8.7% and 7.8% in the urban and rural areas, respectively).[23] Recently, a survey conducted in rural areas of Chennai, Tamil Nadu, India, revealed several important demographic changes taking place in rural India.[24] Due to socioeconomic developments, lifestyle pattern in rural South India had changed considerably and the prevalence of type 2 diabetes had risen to 6.3%. Prevalence of IGT remained at the same level (7.3%). Probably a larger number of the susceptible IGT subjects are progressing to develop diabetes while the pool of IGT continues to be replenished. IGT can be easily identified by oral GTT and individuals with IGT should be advised preventive measures, as it has been shown to be a reversible condition.

Lifestyle Modification and Pharmacotherapy

In the pathophysiology of diabetes, an interaction between genetic predisposition and lifestyle factors such as obesity, sedentary behavior and unhealthy diet habits has been consistently demonstrated in many epidemiological studies. Increasing baseline BMI had been associated with increasing prevalence of diabetes in the Nurses Health Study.[25] The risk increases by 20-fold with a BMI of 30 to 35, in comparison with a BMI of 23 kg/m². Recently, three large, randomized, controlled long-term studies, the Da Qing study from China,[8] the Finnish Diabetes Prevention Program (DFS)[7] and the Diabetes Prevention Program (DPP), United States of America,[6] have unequivocally shown that lifestyle modifications reduced the risk of conversion of IGT to diabetes by up to 58%. The DPP study had shown that metformin could also be useful in preventing the conversion to IGT. In the study to prevent noninsulin-dependent diabetes mellitus (STOP-NIDDM)[26] trial proved that Acarbose—an α-glucosidase inhibitor produced a reduction by 24.8% in conversion of IGT to diabetes, and also increased the reversal to normal glucose tolerance **(Table 92.3)**.

The troglitazone in prevention of diabetes (TRIPOD) study[27] involving Hispanic women with history of gestational diabetes showed that troglitazone (now withdrawn) could reduce the progression to diabetes by 56% over a median follow-up period of 30 months. More recently results from the DREAM trial reveals that 8 mg of rosiglitazone/day can prevent progression of IGT to diabetes in around 60% of 2306 subjects as compared to placebo[28] while metformin is known to be effective in 31% only.

Education

Regular follow-up and constant motivation are required to ensure that the preventive measures are put into practice over a number of years. Education regarding diabetes has to be imparted not only to diabetic patients but also to their families and the community in general. It has been stressed that by not instituting these remedial

TABLE 92.3	Prevention of type 2 diabetes—completed trials in impaired glucose tolerance	
Trial reduction	*Description*	*Risk*
Da Qing Study 1997	Diet and/or	31–46
Diabetes Prevention Study (DPS) 2001	Intensive lifestyle	58
Diabetes Prevention Program (DPP) 2002	Metformin Lifestyle	31 58
STOP–NIDDM Study	Acarbose	24.8

measures one loses the chance of a lifetime to prevent the disease.

SECONDARY PREVENTION

Prevention of Complications

The landmark studies, the United Kingdom Prospective Diabetes Study (UKPDS)[29] in type 2 diabetes and diabetes control and complication trial[30] in type 1 diabetes (DCCT) highlighted the definite benefits of tight control of glycemia and blood pressure on development of vascular complications. However, it must be noted that in the UKPDS study, the glucose control deteriorated over a period of time suggesting that intervention prior to the onset of diabetes may be the best strategy to prevent the onslaught of the debilitating complications.

CONCLUSION

A few population-based prospective studies have been initiated in India to study the feasibility and efficacy of preventive strategies in Indians. Indians develop diabetes at younger age, with a relatively low body mass but high rates of insulin resistance. Suitable preventive strategies have to be worked out to combat the onslaught of the disease, which is imposing the gravest burden on this continent.

An inexplicable inertia exists today in accepting diabetes as a preventable disease though many other chronic diseases has been submitted to effective preventive regimen. The need of the hour is a drastic change in our approach with more emphasis on the preventive aspects of diabetes for the benefit of the community.

SUMMARY

India has the highest number of diabetic subjects in the world. The risk factors include high racial and genetic tendency to low-risk threshold for age and overweight and commonly present insulin resistance. Primary prevention of diabetes is possible for imparting preventive measures in the high-risk group such as offsprings of diabetic parents, obese—especially centrally obese, insulin resistant as well as subjects with impaired glucose tolerance (IGT) or impaired fasting glucose (IGF). Efficacy of lifestyle modification is proved in several prospective prevention trials. Pharmacological agents such as metformin and glitazones may also have a role in primary prevention of diabetes. Tight control of glycemia and blood pressure significantly reduces the risk of diabetes complications.

REFERENCES

1. King H, Aubert RE, Herman WH. Global burden of diabetes 1995-2025: prevalence, numerical estimates, and projection. Diabetes Care. 1998;21:1414-31.
2. Zimmet PZ. Challenges in diabetes epidemiology—Form west to the rest. Diabetes Care. 1992;15:232-52.
3. Ramachandran A, Snehalatha C, Vijay V. Temporal changes in prevalence of type 2 diabetes and impaired glucose tolerance in urban southern India. Diab Res Clin Prac. 2002;58:55-60.
4. Ramachandran A, Snehalatha C, Kapur A, et al. For the Diabetes Epidemiology Study Group in India (DESI) high prevalence of diabetes and impaired glucose tolerance in India: National Urban Diabetes Survey. Diabetologia. 2001;44:1094-101.
5. Viswanathan M. Prevention in diabetes. J Assn Phy Ind. 1981;29:251-61.
6. Knowler WE, Barrett-connor E, Fowler Se, et al. Reduction in the incidence of type 2 diabetes with lifestyle intervention or metformin. N Engl J Med. 2002;346:393-403.
7. Tuomilehto J, Lindstrom J, Eriksson JH, et al. Prevention of type 2 diabetes mellitus by changes in lifestyle among subjects with impaired glucose tolerance. N Engl J Med. 2001;344:1343-50.
8. Pan X, Li G, IIu Y, Wang J, An Z, et al. Effects of diet and exercise in preventing NIDDIM in people with impaired glucose tolerance: the Da Qing IGT Diabetes Study. Diabetes Care. 1997;20:537-44.
9. Ramachandran A, Mohan V, Snehalatha C, Viswanathan M. Prevalence of non-insulin-dependent diabetes mellitus in Asian Indian families with single diabetic parent. Diab Res Clin Prac. 1988;4:241-5.
10. Viswanathan M, McCarthy MI, Snehalatha C, Hitman GA, Ramachandran A. Familial aggregation of type 2 (noninsulin-dependent) diabetes mellitus in south India: absence of excess maternal transmission. Diabetec Medicine. 1996;13:232-7.
11. Ramachandran A., Snehalatha C, Mohan V, Viswanathan M. Development of carbohydrate intolerance in offspring of Asian Indian conjugal type 2 diabetic parents. Diab Res Clin Prac. 1990;8:269-73.
12. Snehalatha C, Ramachandran A, Satyavani K, et al. Study of genetic prediabetic south Indian subjects: importance of hyperinsulinemia and B-cell dysfunction. Diabetes Care. 1998;21:76-9.
13. Snehalatha C, Ramachandran A, Mukesh B, Mary Simon, Vijay V, Haffner SM. Plasma adiponectin is an independent predictor of type 2 diabetes in Asian Indians. Diabetes Care. 2003;26:3226-9.
14. Viswanathan M, Snehalatha C, Vijay V, Vidyavathi P, Indu J, Ramachandran A. Reduction in body weight helps to delay the onset of diabetes even in nonobese with strong family history of the disease. Diab Res Clin Prac. 1997;35:107-12.
15. Snehalatha C, Vijay V, Ramachandran A. Cut-off values of normal anthropometric variables in Asian Indian adults. Diabetes Care. 2003;26:1380-4.
16. World Health Organization (WHO) Recommendations. Obesity: preventing and managing the global epidemic.

Geneva: World Health Organization (Tech Rep. Series) 2000; p. 894.

17. Ramachandran A, Snehalatha C, Shobana R, Vidyavathi P, Vijay V. Influence of lifestyle factors in development of diabetes in Indians. J Assn Phy Ind. 1999;47:764-6.

18. Ramachndran A, Snehalatha C, Satyavani K, Sivasankari S, Vijay V. Type 2 diabetes in Asian—Indian Urban Children Diabetes Care. 2003;26:1022-5.

19. Ramachandran A, Vinitha R, Megha Thayyil, et al. Prevalence of overweight in urban Indian adolescent school children. Diab Res Clin Prac. 2002;57:158-90.

20. Shaw JW, Zimmet PZ, De Courten M. Impaired fasting glucose or impaired glucose tolerance. What best predicts future diabetes in Mauritius? Diabetes Care.1999;22:399-402.

21. Snehalatha C, Ramachandran A, Satyavani K, Sivasankari S, Vijay V. Clustering of cardiovascular risk factors in impaired fasting glucose and impaired glucose tolerance. Int J Diab Dev Count. 2003;23:58-60.

22. Ramachandran A, Snehalatha C, Satyavani K, Vijay V. Impaired fasting glucose and impaired glucoe tolerance in urban population in India. Diabetic Medicine. 2003;20: 220-4.

23. Ramachandran A, Snehalatha C, Daisy D, et al. Prevalence of glucose tolerance in Asian Indians: urban rural difference and significance of upper body adiposity. Diabetes Care. 1992;15:1-7.

24. Ramachandran A, Snehalatha C, Baskar ADS, et al. Temporal changes in prevalence of diabetes and impaired glucose tolerance associated with lifestyle transition occurring in rural population in India. Diabetologia. 2004;47:860-5.

25. Hu FB, Manson JE, Josse RG, Gomis R, Hanefeld M, Karasik A, Laakso M. Acarbose for prevention of type 2 diabetes mellitus in women. N Engl Med. 2001;345:790-7.

26. Chiasson JL, Josse RG, Gomis R, Hanefeld M, Karasik A, Laakso M. Acarbose for prevention of type 2 diabetes mellitus: the STOP-NIDDM randomized trial. Lancet. 2002;359:2072-2777.

27. Buchanan TA, Xiang AH, Peters RK, Kjos SL, Marroquin A, Goico J, Ocha C, Tan S, Berkowitz K, Hodis HN, Azen SP. Preservation of pancreatic B-cell function and prevention of type 2 diabetes by pharmacological treatment of insulin resistance in high-risk Hispanic women. Diabetes. 2002;51: 2796-2803.

28. The Diabetes Reduction Assessment with Ramipril and Rosiglitazone medication (DREAM) Trial Investigators. Effect of rosiglitazone on the pregnancy of diabetes in patients with impaired glucose tolerance or impaired fasting glucose: randomised control trial. Lancet. 2006; 368:1096-1105.

29. United Kingdom Prospective Diabetes Study (UKPDS) Group. Intensive blood-glucose control with sulfonylureas or insulin compared with conventional treatment and risk of complications in patients with type 2 diabetes (UKPDS 33). Lancet. 1998;352:837-53.

30. Diabetes Control and Complication Trial (DCCT) Research Group. The effect of intensive treatment of diabetes on the development and progression of long-term complications insulin- dependent diabetes mellitus. N Engl J Med. 1993;329:977-86.

Chapter 93

YOUTH-ONSET DIABETES IN INDIA: NATURE OF DIABETES AND USE OF BOVINE INSULIN IN THEIR TREATMENT

N Kochupillai, R Goswami

CHAPTER OUTLINE

- Introduction
- Subtypes of Youth-onset Diabetes in Northern India
- Insulin Antibody Response to Bovine Insulin Therapy and its Functional Significance Among Insulin Requiring Young Diabetics in India

---

INTRODUCTION

Around 10% of diabetics in India have onset below 30 years of age. Youth-onset diabetes in developing countries is a heterogeneous set of disorders. Till recently, information on occurrence, clinicopathological and biochemical features as well as etiology of youth onset diabetes in India were not coherent. Though in 1985, a WHO group of experts classified youth-onset diabetes in developing countries into different categories, that classification has recently been questioned and is now under review. Meanwhile type 1 diabetes as seen in the west being more clearly defined immunologically subcategories are emerging on the basis of natural history and immune markers.

At the All India Institute of Medical Sciences (AIIMS), India, we operate a *Diabetes in the Young* clinic. Patients with age of onset of diabetes <30 years are registered in this clinic and provided state-of-the-art diabetic care free of cost. The clinic has registry of 1033 with an average of 110 fresh patients registered each year. Catchment area of the clinic spreads beyond confinement of Delhi, India and includes States like Uttar Pradesh, Rajasthan, Haryana, Bihar, Jammu and Kashmir, West Bengal, Assam and Orissa. A recent analysis of the patients attending clinic showed that 60%

of them were socioeconomically poor with monthly income of parents up to Rs. 2,000. In our clinic, it is common to have patients with type 1 diabetes mellitus presenting with ketoacidosis as a result of interrupted insulin therapy due to financial constraints. Young patients with ketosis-resistant diabetes present in states of extreme wasting due to chronically poor glycemic control.

SUBTYPES OF YOUTH-ONSET DIABETES IN NORTHERN INDIA

The study subjects comprised of 132 consecutive patients with diagnosis of diabetes under 30 years of age who attended the *Diabetes in the Young* clinic on the All India Institute of Medical Sciences (AIIMS), India, during the two year period spanning 1995 to 1997. The mean age was 25 ± 8.0 and mean duration 5.5 ± 6.0 years. Forty-nine patients were females while 83 were males. Clinical characteristics, insulin requirement, ketosis proneness on insulin withdrawal, family history of diabetes, nutritional status and radiological and ultrasonographical evidences of pancreatic calculi were assessed. C-peptide was measured at 0 and 6 m postglucagon (1 mg IV). The daily insulin dose requirements were assessed by close monitoring of blood glucose with administration of purified insulin before the three principal meals to achieve ideal glycemic status throughout the day (fasting blood glucose <120 mg% and postmeal <140 mg%). The patients were categorized as type 1, type 2 and fibrocalculous pancreatopathy diabetes (FCPD). Type 1 diabetes was diagnosed, if ketosis developed on insulin withdrawal. Fibrocalculous pancreatopathy was diagnosed on the basis of pancreatic calculi on plain X-ray abdomen or ultrasonography. Diagnosis of type 2 diabetes was made, if subjects achieved glycemic control without insulin and with normal or above normal body mass indices (BMI). Diabetes as part of an autoimmune polyglandular syndrome was considered, if there was a coexisting clinically overt autoimmune thyroid disorder. No other organ specific autoimmune disorder coexisted with the present group of youth-onset diabetic individuals. Additionally, an entity designated as *ketosis resistant type* was categorized. These were insulin requiring youth-onset diabetic individuals, who were resistant to ketosis on insulin withdrawal and who has low BMI with other features of malnutrition. More recently, an International Workshop (1995)[1] named this entity *malnutrition modulated diabetes mellitus (MMDM)*. They did not have pancreatic calculi or coexisting thyroid autoimmunity.

Immunological markers for islet cell autoimmunity were assessed by determining autoantibodies against recombinant human glutamic acid decarboxylase (GAD65) and tyrosine phosphatase (IA-2) on blinded sample from the patients as well as a group of age-matched nondiabetic controls (n=20) with no family history of diabetes. Autoantibodies against thyroid

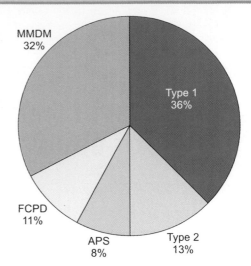

Figure 93.1 Distribution of clinical types among youth-onset diabetes in North India
MMDM: Malnutrition modulated diabetes mellitus
FCPD: Fibrocalculous pancreatic diabetes mellitus
APS: Autoimmune polyglandular syndrome

microsomal antigen (TMA) were assayed by hemagglutination method using commercial kits.

Briefly, five types of diabetes were delineated type 1 (37%) (ketosis in 32%), type 2 (13%), fibrocalculous pancreatopathy (11%), autoimmune polyglandular syndrome (7%) and ketosis-resistant young diabetes (32%). The last category corresponds to malnutrition modulated diabetes mellitus (MMDM) **(Figure 93.1, Table 93.1)**.

TABLE 93.1	Clinical characteristics and C-peptide in youth-onset diabetes				
Variable n (%) Gender	Type 1 49 (37%) M = 27, F = 22	Ketosis resistant type (MMDM)[42] M =32, F = 10	Fibrocalculous Pancreatopathy diabetes (FCPD) 14 (11%) M = 11, F = 3	Autoimmune polyglandular syndrome (APS) 10 (7%) M = 3, F = 7	Type 2 17 (13%) M = 10, F = 7
Age at onset of diabetes (years)	16.7 ± 7.4	20.5 ± 5.6	20.4 ± 5.3	22.4 ± 5.7	22.4 ± 6.3
Family history of diabetes (years)	29	28	25	33	82
Duration of diabetes (years)	5.9 ± 6.0	4.8 ± 6.3	4.5 ± 4.9	5.2 ± 5.1	6.8 ± 6.8
BMI (kg/m^2)	17 ± 2.8	16.6 ± 3.4	16.8 ± 2.6	21.5 ± 4.6	24.8 ± 6.1
C-peptide basal (ng/ml)	*0.27 ± 0.29	*0.66 ± 0.78	—	0.48 ± 0.47	—
C-peptide post-glucagon (ng/ml)	*0.31 ± 0.37	*0.79 ± 0.79	—	0.89 ± 0.81	—

*$p < 0.5$
MMDM: Malnutrition modulated diabetes mellitus; BMI: Body mass index

A total of 22.4% of type 1 and 30% of autoimmune polyglandular syndrome patients showed both GAD65 plus IA-2 autoantibody positivity, significantly more than 4.7% of the ketosis-resistant type. However, GAD65 antibody positivity alone was seen in 38% of resistant subjects which was significantly more than the 14.2% and 10% positivity seen in type 1 and autoimmune polyglandular groups, respectively. The fibrocalculous pancreatopathy group showed GAD65 plus IA-2 autoantibody positivity in 14.2% and lone GAD65 autoantibody positivity in 7.1%. Twenty-six percent and 60% respectively of the type 1 and autoimmune polyglandular syndrome groups had thyroid microsomal autoantibody positivity. Type 1 showed significantly less C-peptide response to glucagons when compared to the ketosis-resistant and autoimmune polyglandular syndrome groups. The controls and type 2 diabetic individuals tested negative for islet cell autoimmunity markers.

Thus, the largest group among youth-onset diabetes in north India can be categorized as type 1 diabetes.

The ketosis-resistant group was the second most prevalent type. The unique features of the entity brought forward by the present study include:
- High frequency of GAD65 positivity (38%)
- Relatively low frequency of combined GAD65 and IA-2 autoantibody positivity.
- Better basal and glucagons stimulated C-peptide response when compared to type 1 diabetic individuals.

The fibrocalculous pancreatopathy related diabetes is another well-recognized group of youth-onset diabetic individuals. Three of fourteen such patients had either GAD65 and/or IA-2A positivity with an overall, islet cell autoimmunity marker positivity of 21.3%. These observations suggest that diabetes causation in this syndrome may also involve autoimmune islet cell damage presumably triggered by islet cell destruction in pancreatitis. Overall the results of the present study, thus, indicate a dominant role of islet cell autoimmunity in the pathogenesis of most types of youth onset diabetes in northern India.

INSULIN ANTIBODY RESPONSE TO BOVINE INSULIN THERAPY AND ITS FUNCTIONAL SIGNIFICANCE AMONG INSULIN REQUIRING YOUNG DIABETICS IN INDIA

Seventy patients (43 males and 27 females), mean (SD) age 17.9 ± 6.1 years, mean duration of Bovine insulin therapy 5.1 ± 5.4 years, were studied.

Radiobinding assays for specific insulin binding were carried out by using a ^{125}I tracer of human insulin prepared in our laboratory using chloramine-T technique. The mean and specific binding of 100 healthy subjects without any family history of diabetes or other autoimmune disease was 0.9 ± 1.1%. The insulin antibody titers observed in patients was expressed in the assay precision unit, SD score.

Briefly, all the patients treated with bovine insulin showed high titers of insulin antibodies with SD score ranging from 5.1 to 42. No significant difference was observed in the mean SD score of insulin antibodies in the three diabetic groups. Insulin antibodies SD score and its affinity did not show significant relationship with daily insulin dose and HbA$_{1c}$ at admission. Only 27±7% variations in daily insulin dose requirement were accounted for by total insulin binding power. There was a significant inverse relationship between insulin antibody SD score and duration of insulin therapy (r = –0, 4172, p <0.0004).[2]

There was no relationship between insulin antibody titers and daily insulin dose requirement. In fact despite presence of high insulin antibody titers, daily insulin dose requirement remained within physiological range in all three types of diabetics studied. The major variation in insulin dose requirement is thus governed by factors other than insulin antibody.

Overall, these results indicate that bovine insulin-related antibody response does not result in any clinically significant impact in terms of daily insulin requirement for diabetes control.

REFERENCES

1. Tripathy BB, Samal KC. Overview and consensus statement on diabetes in tropical areas. Diabetes Metabol Rev. 1997;13:63-76.
2. Goswami R, Jaleel A, Kochupillai N. Insulin antibody response to bovine insulin therapy: functional significance among insulin requiring young diabetics in India. Diabetes Research and Clinical Practice. 2000;49:7-15.

Chapter 94

PREVENTION OF COMPLICATIONS OF DIABETES

V Mohan, R Deepa

CHAPTER OUTLINE

- Introduction
- Prevalence of Microvascular Complications in Indian Population
- Prevalence of Macrovascular Complications in Indian Population

- Diabetes Complications—Economic Burden
- Prevention of Complications
- Future Perspectives
- Summary

INTRODUCTION

Diabetes, a potentially life-threatening disorder, is considered as *an apparent epidemic which is strongly related to lifestyle and economic change* by the World Health Organization (WHO).[1] Lifestyle and economic drift along with increase in life-expectancy has markedly increased the diabetes epidemic in India by affecting more than 32 million people presently.[2] This metabolic disorder causes profound alterations in both the micro- and macrosections of the vascular tree affecting nearly every organ in the body.[3,4] Diabetes magnifies the risk for vascular diseases several fold and is thus one of the major causes of morbidity and mortality worldwide.[5,6] Surprisingly, in spite of the enormous growth in the field of diabetology, measures taken to prevent these dangerous complications of diabetes are woefully inadequate.

Among the several categories of diabetes, the most common is type 2 affecting more than 85% of the total diabetic population, the next common being type 1, accounting for around 5 to 10% worldwide. Although the pathophysiology of type 1 and type 2 diabetes are different, the pathological sequence of complications appears to be similar in both these types of diabetes.[7] Hence, they are considered together in this Chapter. The micro- and macrovascular complications of diabetes are indicated in **Figure 94.1**.

PREVALENCE OF MICROVASCULAR COMPLICATIONS IN INDIAN POPULATION

The most specific complications of diabetes are microvascular complications (retinopathy and nephropathy) of which diabetic retinopathy is considered as the hallmark of diabetes. Diabetic retinopathy is the most common cause of blindness in the working age group in developed countries.[8] Prevalence of this disorder among type 2 diabetic subjects in Indians has been reported to range from 7.3 to 4.1%.[9-12] Diabetic neuropathy may affect around 50% of all diabetic subjects and is considered to be a main cause for morbidity. Prevalence of peripheral neuropathy in type 2 diabetic subjects has been reported to be 17.5 to 19.1% in India,[13,14] while autonomic neuropathy is prevalent in 35.7%.[15] Diabetic nephropathy is the leading cause of

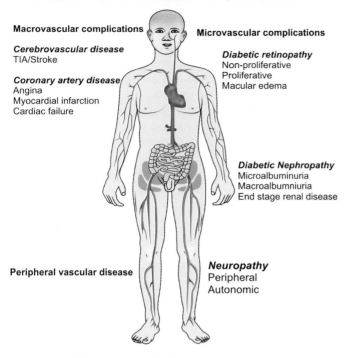

Figure 94.1 Diabetes complications

end-stage renal disease worldwide[16] and accounts for more than one-third of all cases of end-stage renal disease. The stage of microalbuminuria, which is reversible, precedes overt proteinuria, which is indicative of definitive or irreversible diabetic nephropathy. The prevalence of microalbuminuria was reported to be 36.3% at a major referral center in South India.[17]

PREVALENCE OF MACROVASCULAR COMPLICATIONS IN INDIAN POPULATION

Compared to type 1 diabetes, type 2 diabetes has a higher risk for cardiovascular disease, which is estimated to be 2 to 4-fold higher compared to nondiabetic subjects.[18] This is because type 2 diabetes is a component of the metabolic cluster, which is associated with other risk factors like insulin resistance, dyslipidemia, hypertension, abdominal obesity and prothrombotic state.[19] Cardiovascular disease includes peripheral vascular disease, cerebrovascular disease and coronary artery disease all of which are atherosclerotic in origin. Prevalence of coronary artery disease is also increasing at an alarming proportion in India. The present prevalence of this disease among Indians ranges from 9 to 14%.[20,21] Prevalence of CAD among diabetic subjects is reported to be 17 to 21%.[20,22] The prevalence of peripheral vascular disease (PVD) is several fold

higher in diabetic patients compared to nondiabetic subjects but the prevalence of PVD appears to be relatively lower in Indians.[23] In the Chennai Urban Population Study (CUPS), the prevalence of PVD was 3.2% among nondiabetic subjects while among diabetic subjects, it was 6.3%.[23]

DIABETES COMPLICATIONS— ECONOMIC BURDEN

Diabetes is an expensive disease.[24-26] Most of the expenses incurred could be attributed to the morbid complications. Treatment of diabetic complications constitutes the highest cost. The expenses include both direct cost of treatment and indirect cost due to man-hours lost in loss of productivity. Medical expenditure for a diabetic is estimated to be two to five times more than a nondiabetic subject.[24] This imposes a heavy burden both at the individual and at the societal level, which underscores the need for prevention of complications of diabetes.

PREVENTION OF COMPLICATIONS

The natural history of type 2 diabetes provides chances for prevention at three transition points **(Flow chart 94.1)**. Primary prevention targets prevention of diabetes itself by early diagnosis through screening programs, which conclude that presently there are very few drugs targeting the complications directly. Preventive approaches to diabetes complications can be categorized into three levels—first the early approach where early detection and appropriate treatment are the cornerstones for delaying the onset of the diabetic complications. Once some complication sets in, preventing progression of the same would form the second approach or the intermediate approach by introducing specific drugs and lifestyle intervention for combating complications. Third would be the late approach where complications have reached a very critical stage and

Flow chart 94.1 Stages of prevention of diabetes

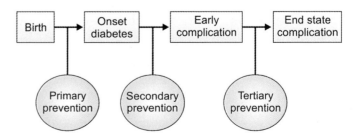

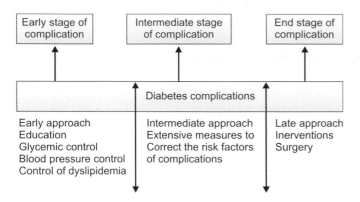

Flow chart 94.2 Strategies to protect target organ damage in diabetic subjects

interventional procedures like surgery are required to ameliorate progression to end-stages of the complications **(Flow chart 94.2)**.

Early Detection of Diabetes Complications (Screening)

Early detection of diabetes complications by routine screening is an important aspect in prevention of diabetes complications. Screening is beneficial in diseases, which impose a significant burden on the society, where the natural history is known and intervention in early stages can prevent further

progression of the disease. Diabetes satisfies all these criteria. Several studies have clearly demonstrated that intervention at an early stage can help in preventing morbidity and mortality.[27-31] The American Diabetes Association (ADA) in its clinical practice recommendations[32] has indicated the frequency of screening for various complications of diabetes.

Diabetic Retinopathy

Even if visual symptoms are absent, initial retinal screening is recommended at the time of diagnosis for type 2 diabetic subjects and for type 1 diabetic subjects, within 3 to 5 years after diagnosis of diabetes when patient age is 10 years or older. Thereafter, an annual screening is recommended for all diabetic subjects regardless of the type of diabetes **(Table 94.1)**. Since retinal screening involves pupil dilatation, then a detailed eye examination by an ophthalmologist is advisable. In patients with any degree of retinopathy, more frequent examinations are indicated. In diabetes complicating pregnancy, a comprehensive eye examination at the first trimester and a close follow-up throughout pregnancy is recommended by the ADA.[32] Retinal color photography helps to document early retinal lesions while fundus fluorescein angiography (FFA) helps to document diabetic macular edema and subtle new vessels in the retina.

TABLE 94.1	Screening schedule for diabetic complications		
Complications	*Test to be done*	*First screening—when?*	*Monitoring*
Macrovascular complications			
Peripheral vascular disease	Examine pedal pulses, auscultate for bruits, Peripheral Doppler—ankle brachial index	At diagnosis for type 2 diabetes As clinically appropriate for type 1 diabetes At diagnosis for type 2 diabetes	Annually
Coronary artery disease	12-lead electrocardiography	As clinically appropriate for type 1 diabetes	Annually
Microvascular complications			
Diabetic retinopathy	Retinal screening—ophthalmoscopy/fundal photography Visual acuity	At diagnosis for type 2 diabetes 3 to 5 years after diagnosis for type 1 diabetes	Annually
Diabetic nephropathy	Microalbuminuria—spot urine	At diagnosis for type 2 diabetes 3 to 5 years after diagnosis for type 1 diabetes	Annually
Peripheral neuropathy	Foot examination Assess protective sensation in feet (Semmes-Weinstein 10G monofilament), Biothesiometry Plantar pressure measurement	At diagnosis for type 2 diabetes As clinically appropriate for type 1 diabetes	Annually

Diabetic Nephropathy

In the natural history of diabetic nephropathy, excretion of low but abnormal levels of albumin in the urine is considered as the initial stage and is referred as microalbuminuria which is also regarded as incipient nephropathy. Detection at this stage is helpful, as sufficient evidence has accumulated to show that intervention at this stage prevents progression of the disease and indeed sometimes even reverses to normo-albuminuria stage.[33-35] In addition to hyperglycemia, hypertension is also a contributing factor for diabetic nephropathy which could also be controlled using adequate measures. Thus detection of microalbuminuria in diabetic subjects is crucial to prevention of overt diabetic nephropathy. According to the ADA clinical practice recommendations, annual screening of microalbuminuria is recommended in type 1 and type 2 diabetic subjects **(Table 94.1)**. The easiest method as suggested by ADA for diagnosis of microalbuminuria is measurement of the albumin to creatinine ratio (ACR) in a random spot collection. Microalbuminuria is diagnosed, if ACR is >30 mg/mg of creatinine while ACR >300 mg/mg of creatinine is categorized as clinical albuminuria. Care should be taken while diagnosing microalbuminuria because conditions like exercise, urinary tract infection, marked hypertension, heart failure and acute febrile illness can cause a transient increase in excretion of albumin in the urine. As day-to-day variability has been observed in albumin excretion, at least two to three collection within a time span of 3 to 6 months is required for diagnosis of micro-albuminuria.

Diabetic Neuropathy

Though neuropathic pain is one of the important causes of morbidity in diabetic subjects,[36] unlike micro-albuminuria, there is no direct measure for screening of peripheral neuropathy. Several tests may be necessary to designate a subject as having diabetic neuropathy. To determine the small fiber function, protective sensation in the feet, temperature discrimination threshold and skin integrity tests could be used. For large myelinated fibers, vibration perception threshold (VPT) using biothesiometry has been shown to be a good predictor of foot ulceration.[37] Though not used for routine purposes, motor and sensory conduction velocities gives an assessment of function of large myelinated fibers. Wasting, weakness and ankle reflexes would indicate alterations in motor nerve function. For detecting sensory nerve dysfunction, vibration using tuning fork, sensitiveness to monofilament and pin-prick should be useful. Annual screening for peripheral neuropathy is recommended using measures suggested in **Table 94.1**.

Macrovascular Disease

A common cause of foot amputations in diabetic subjects is peripheral vascular disease (PVD). As lower limb amputations are preventable, detection at an earlier stage is advisable. Most of the diabetic subjects are symptom-free for PVD. Subjects with asymptomatic PVD not only have a higher risk for frank PVD but also an increased risk for cardiovascular deaths.[38] One of the easiest measures for detecting PVD is ankle brachial index (<0.9) measured by peripheral Doppler. This has been shown to have a sensitivity of 70 to 97% and specificity of 89 to 97%.[39,40] In addition, studies have shown ankle brachial pressure index to be a good predictor of subsequent cardiovascular events.[41,42] Sophisticated measures for assessing PVD include Duplex Doppler studies and angiography.

Coronary artery disease (CAD) can often be asymptomatic and early screening is therefore advantageous in preventing major events. Since diabetes is considered as a risk equivalent[43] for CAD routine screening for CAD in these patients is justified. The recommended initial test for routine screening for CAD is resting electrocardiography (ECG). This provides evidence of previous silent myocardial infarctions and silent or inducible myocardial ischemia. Cardiac stress test (Treadmill) is useful in detecting latent CAD but the test has a substantial false positive and false negative rates. Thallium-201 scintigraphy, exercise echocardiography, and ambulatory ECG are less commonly used for screening purposes. Another test, which is gaining importance in the field of cardiology, is measurement of carotid intimal medial thickness (IMT). Several studies have indicated IMT to be a strong predictor for cardiovascular events.[44,45] IMT has been clearly shown to be higher among diabetic subjects compared to nondiabetic subjects.[46-48] IMT has also shown to be a good predictor for cerebrovascular disease.[49,50] However, this measurement requires a high resolution ultrasound. Recently, functional changes in the artery, which can be assessed by determining the endothelial dysfunction and arterial stiffness, have been shown to be indicative of future cardiovascular events.[47] These measurements also require sophisticated instruments like high resolution B mode ultrasonography system or Sphygmocor apparatus.

Prevention of Metabolic Complications

The metabolic consequences of diabetes include hyperglycemia, hypertension and dyslipidemia. Landmark trials and intervention studies have clearly documented the beneficial effects of glycemic control, blood pressure control and lipid control in delaying the onset of complications.

Glycemic Control

Hyperglycemia is responsible for many functional vascular changes, which include endothelial dysfunction, impairment of blood flow, increased leukocyte, monocytes adhesion, etc. It also has many indirect metabolic effects that alter lipid patterns resulting in dyslipidemia. Evidence from various studies suggests a continuous relationship of hyperglycemia with microvascular complications (retinopathy and nephropathy) and neuropathy.[51-53] It has been shown that for every 1% decrease in glycosylated hemoglobin (HbA$_{1c}$), there is dramatic decrease in prevalence of complications **(Figure 94.2)**. However, the effect of glycemia on macrovascular disease is not so clear.

Glycemic Control and Prevention of Microvascular Complications

Three landmark studies on glycemic control in diabetes namely the Diabetes Complications and Control Trial (DCCT), the United Kingdom Prospective Diabetes Study (UKPDS) and Kumamoto study[27,28,54] have clearly

TABLE 94.2	Glycemic control and risk reduction of microangiopathy in intervention studies		
	DCCT[27] (Type 1 diabetes)	UKPDS[28] (Type 2 diabetes)	Kumamoto[54] (Type 2 diabetes)
Number studied	n = 1441	n = 5102	n = 110
Duration of follow-up	9 years	10 years	6 years
Retinopathy	76%	21%	69%
Albuminuria	56%	33%	70%
Neuropathy	60%	—	57%

documented the beneficial effects of glycemic control in preventing microvascular complications **(Table 94.2)**.

The DCCT,[27] a multicentric prospective study conducted by the National Institute of Diabetes and Digestive and Kidney Diseases (NIDDK) involved 1441 type 1 diabetic subjects in the age range 13 to 39 from 29 centers in the United States and Canada. Seven hundred and twenty-six patients who had no retinopathy formed the primary prevention cohort and 715 subjects with mild-to-moderate retinopathy formed the secondary prevention cohort. These subjects were then randomized to either a conventional (710 patients) or an intensive (726 patients) regimen of therapy and were followed for 3.5 to 9.0 years. A difference in glycosylated hemoglobin (HbA$_{1c}$) by 0.9% between the conventional and intensive therapy groups reduced retinopathy by 76%, albuminuria by 54% and neuropathy by 60%. The DCCT study subjects were followed four years later in the epidemiology of diabetes and its complications (EDIC) study after their intensive interventions were stopped, while the conventional therapy continued.[55] This study showed that although the HbA$_{1c}$ of the two groups had become equal, those who were in the intensive group in the DCCT continued to do better with respect to complications. The Stockholm diabetes intervention study (SDIS) on type 1 diabetic subjects based on a ten-year follow-up showed a similar reduction in diabetic retinopathy with the intensive group having lower frequency of retinopathy compared to the conventional group.[56]

Two long-term studies on the type 2 diabetic subjects, the United Kingdom Prospective Diabetes Study (UKPDS) and the Kumamoto study showed clearly that intensive therapy decreased the risk of retinopathy compared to conventional therapy. The UKPDS[28] recruited 5102 patients with newly diagnosed

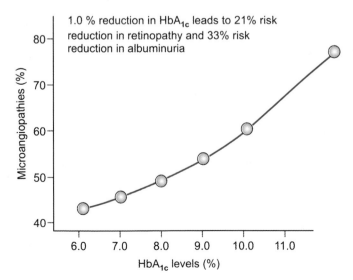

Figure 94.2 Relation of glycemic control with microvascular complications

type 2 diabetes in 23 centers in the United Kingdom. The intensive therapy yielded 0.9% decrease in HbA_{1c} level compared to the conventional. This decrease led to a risk reduction of 21% for retinopathy and 33% for albuminuria. The Kumamoto study[54] done on 110 Japanese type 2 diabetic subjects had two arms—the multiple insulin injection therapy (MIT) group (intensive group), who were administered three or more daily insulin injections or conventional insulin injection therapy (CIT). This study concluded that the glycemic threshold to prevent the onset and progression of diabetic microvascular complications as $HbA_{1c} < 6.5\%$, fasting plasma glucose concentration <110 mg/dl, and 2 hour postprandial plasma glucose concentration <180 mg/dl.

The importance of continuous infusion of insulin to reduce symptomatic neuropathy was assessed in a four-month follow-up study which revealed achieving near normoglycemia in patients with symptomatic neuropathy achieved symptomatic and objective benefit.[36]

A meta-analysis by Wang et al[57] on 16 randomized trials estimated the impact of glycemic control over progression of microvascular complications. It summarized that *long-term intensive blood glucose control significantly reduced the risk of diabetic retinopathy and nephropathy.*

Glycemic Control and Prevention of Macrovascular Complication

Earlier studies in the western population like the Whitehall study, Honolulu Study, PADY study and several others have shown that hyperglycemia contributes to cardiovascular disease.[58-61] Indian studies have shown that the risk for CAD increases with increase in plasma glucose.[62-64] Hyperglycemia increases glycation of proteins resulting in advanced glycation end products (AGE). AGE *per se* can trigger the atherosclerotic process, in addition, as the arterial wall components also get glycated, this leads to arterial stiffness and thence to vascular disorders. It could be postulated that glycemic control reduces nonenzymatic glycation, which in-turn could reduce the occurrence of cardiovascular events. Several studies on antidiabetic agents, particularly thiazolidinediones have shown beneficial reduction in cardiovascular risk factors like LDL, fibrinogen, inflammatory markers and preclinical atherosclerotic markers.[65-67] A randomized double blind multicentric study conducted on over 3000 patients showed that pioglitazone effectively decreased triglycerides and increased HDL-cholesterol both when used as monotherapy or in combination with metformin.[68] Further studies have also shown differential effects on lipid parameters with regard to glitazones, pioglitazones beneficially reduces triglycerides and particle concentration of LDL and increases HDL-cholesterol compared to rosiglitazone.[69] In addition, the recent Prospective Pioglitazone Clinical Trial in Macrovascular Events (PROACTIVE) study suggested that pioglitazone reduced main secondary endpoint of life-threatening events, the risk of heart attacks, strokes and death by 16% (p = 0.027).[70] However, it reduced the primary endpoint of all cause mortality by only 10% which did not reach statistical significance by study end (p=0.095). However, in the UKPDS study, by glycemic control alone, the risk reduction of myocardial infarction was reduced by 16% but this just missed statistical significance (p=0.052) leading to the conclusion that by glucose control alone, macrovascular complications cannot be prevented.[28] Some of the reasons for this could be that the study was underpowered for macrovascular events, tight enough glycemic control was not established or that drugs like sensitizers were not used.[71] Though the DIGAMI[72] trial showed that 24-hour intensive treatment with intravenous insulin, glucose, and potassium followed by tight blood sugar control with insulin significantly reduced mortality, this study has several flaws and recent studies have not been able to confirm these findings.[73]

Though hyperglycemia plays a major role in complications, the consensus today is that to prevent macrovascular complications in diabetic patients tight control of factors like hypertension and dyslipidemia are equally important and these are described below. **Table 94.3** summarizes the current evidence with respect of control of risk factors and prevention of diabetic complications.

Hypertension Control

Blood pressure is another key factor which can affect both micro- as well as macrovasculature. Over 50% of type 2 diabetic subjects may have hypertension. It has been hypothesized that both type 2 diabetes and hypertension have common pathogenic mechanisms. Controlling blood pressure is an important aspect in treating complications, as untreated hypertension results in declining renal function.[74] In the PROCAM study, the prevalence of CAD was several fold higher in diabetic hypertensives compared to diabetic normotensives.[75] The risk for CAD in males with hypertension was two-fold higher and in females four-fold higher

TABLE 94.3	Benefits of risk factor control on diabetes complications			
Risk factor	Retinopathy	Nephropathy	Neuropathy	Macrovascular diseases
Glucose control	Definite benefit	Definite benefit	Definite benefit	Possible benefit
Blood pressure control	Definite benefit	Definite benefit	Unknown value	Significant benefit
Lipid control benefit	Possible	Possible benefit	Possible benefit	Significant
Smoking control	Benefits unclear	Benefits unclear value	Unknown benefit	Significant

compared to normotensives.[75] Based on these and other studies, the goals recommended for blood pressure for diabetic subjects both by the ADA as well as the Joint National Committee on Prevention, Detection, Evaluation, and Treatment of High Blood Pressure (JNCP) are lower than those recommended for nondiabetic subjects.[76,77]

Hypertension Control and Microvascular Complication

Hypertension hastens the progression of diabetic retinopathy. Exudates were reported to be more among diabetic subjects with systolic blood pressure greater than 145 compared to those with less than 125 mm Hg.[78] The UKPDS study also addressed the issue of hypertension control in reducing microvascular complications. A reduction of 105 mm Hg blood pressure yielded a 34% reduction in risk of diabetic retinopathy.[79] The EUCLID study, which assessed the impact of lisinopril on microvascular complications in type 1 diabetic subjects, suggested a decrease in progression of retinopathy among the drug intervention arm compared to placebo (odds ratio: 0.50, p = 0.02).[80]

ACE inhibitors and angiotensin II receptor antagonists have been shown to have greater benefits in diabetic subjects in preventing progression of microalbuminuria to macroalbuminuria stage.[34,81-86] Further, ACE inhibition has been shown to be beneficial in diabetic subjects at all stages of nephropathy. In microalbuminuric patients, ACE inhibitors reduce the progression to macroalbuminuria and in macroalbuminuric patients, they reduce the decline in glomerular filtration rate [GFR].[81-86] Indeed ACE inhibitors slow down the progression of nephropathy independent of their effects on blood pressure.[86] In the Microalbuminuria, Cardiovascular, and Renal Outcomes-Heart Outcomes Prevention Evaluation (MICRO—HOPE) study, which is a substudy of HOPE, 3,577 subjects with diabetes received either ramipril (10 mg) or placebo. After a median follow-up period of 4.5 years, ramipril

treatment was associated with a decreased risk of development of overt nephropathy.[35] Overall, hypertension control seems to be beneficial in reducing both nephropathy and retinopathy in diabetic subjects.

Hypertension Control and Macrovascular Complication

Though the UKPDS study failed to show a significant reduction in macrovascular endpoints with glycemic control, hypertension control yielded impressive results in reducing cardiovascular endpoints. Each 10 mm Hg decreases in mean systolic blood pressure was associated with 11% reduction for myocardial infarction.[79] In the hypertension optimal treatment (HOT) trial , 51% reduction in major cardiovascular events was observed in the target group with diastolic blood pressure ≤ 80 mm Hg compared to the group with ≤ 90 mm Hg.[87] The prevention of events from macrovascular disease seems to be dose dependent as subjects with greater blood pressure control were the most benefited.[88] Lisinopril was shown to reduce mortality in diabetic subjects with acute myocardial infarction in the GISS-3 study.[89] The Captopril Prevention Project **(CAPP)** study showed that captopril reduces cardiovascular mortality in subjects with hypertension.[90] Calcium-channel antagonist like verapamil have also been shown to reduce reinfarction rates in diabetic subjects.[91] However, ACE inhibitors and β-blockers appeared to be more beneficial than calcium-channel blockers in reducing myocardial infarction.[71] The MICRO-HOPE study showed that ramipril reduced myocardial infarction by 22%, cardiovascular death by 37% and revascularization by 17%.[35] A summary of the studies, which have shown a remarkable reduction in cardiovascular mortality are depicted in **Table 94.4**.[86,92-95]

Dyslipidemia and Microvascular Disease

Dyslipidemia, particularly increased serum cholesterol and low-density lipoprotein (LDL) cholesterol have been shown to be associated with diabetic retinopathy

TABLE 94.4	Antihypertensive agents that reduce cardiovascular risk in patients with type 2 diabetes
Study	*Drugs*
Systolic hypertension in the elderly program (SHEP)[92]	*Diuretics:* Chlorthalidone *β-blocker:* Atenolol
Heart outcome prevention evaluation (HOPE)[86]	*ACE inhibitor:* Ramipril
United kingdom prospective diabetes study (UKPDS)[79]	*ACE inhibitor:* Captopril *β-blocker:* Atenolo
Appropriate blood pressure control in diabetes (ABCD)[93]	*ACE inhibitor:* Enalpril
Fosinopril versus amlodipine cardiovascular events randomized trials (FACET)[94]	*ACE inhibitor:* Fosinopril
Losartan intervention for endpoint reduction in hypertension study (LIFE)[95]	*Angiotensin receptor blocker:* Losartan

especially hard exudates in macula.[96-98] Abnormalities in serum lipid are hypothesized to alter the coagulation, fibrinolytic system, membrane permeability, endothelial dysfunction and thereby result in altered capillary blood flow leading to worsening of diabetic retinopathy and nephropathy. In addition, dyslipidemia also hastens the decline in glomerular filtration rate and progression of albuminuria to overt nephropathy.[99] A prospective study on 297 type 1 diabetic patients showed serum triglycerides to predict diabetic nephropathy and diabetic retinopathy.[100] Some intervention studies have shown lipid control could help prevent diabetic nephropathy,[101] but not many studies have assessed its role in diabetic retinopathy. Although studies have shown serum lipids to be associated with microvascular complications, the effect of intervention with lipid-lowering therapy has not been widely investigated.

Control of Dyslipidemia and Macrovascular Disease

Cross-sectional, prospective and interventional studies have consistently documented the association of dyslipidemia with cardiovascular disease.[102-104] Lipid control plays a major role on the course of than that of microvascular disease. Several intervention studies have very clearly demonstrated the positive benefits of lipid control in cardiovascular disease.[71]

More than 50 clinical trials have supported the clinical benefit of cholesterol management in prevention of cardiovascular disease.[105-108] The role of simvastatin in reducing mortality rates was shown in the Scandinavian Simvastatin Survival Study (4S) trial conducted on 4444 subjects.[105] Both the long-term intervention with pravastatin in ischemic disease **(LIPID)**

and cholesterol and recurrent events (CARE) studies demonstrated the effect of pravastatin and simvastatin in increasing survival.[106,107] In studies, such as the west of Scotland coronary prevention study (WOSCOPS) and the Air Force coronary atherosclerosis prevention study (AFCAPS) use of pravastatin in subjects without CVD showed a 25% reduction in CVD rates on follow-up.[108,109] Most of these studies had substudies on diabetic subjects, which indicated that diabetic subjects more markedly benefited by cholesterol reduction compared to the nondiabetic.[71] The data on risk reduction of cardiovascular events in diabetic subjects from various trials are presented in **Table 94.5**. The heart protection study included 5,963 adults aged 40 to 80 years with diabetic subjects of whom 90% were type 2 diabetic subjects. The mean LDL-cholesterol level was reduced from 125 to 86 mg/dl and this reduction yielded a 22% reduction of major cardiovascular events in the simvastatin group compared to the placebo-allocated group. There was also a 33% reduction in events among diabetic subjects without evident cardiovascular disease at baseline.[110]

Another class of drugs, the fibrates has been shown to markedly reduce triglycerides and moderately elevate high density lipoprotein (HDL) cholesterol and thereby reduce cardiovascular events.[108-111] In the veterans affairs high-density lipoprotein intervention trial **(VA-HIT)** study gemfibrozil significantly increased HDL levels resulting in remarkable decrease in the incidence of myocardial infarction.[111] The Helsinki heart study and bezafibrate infarction prevention trial and diabetes atherosclerosis intervention study (DAIS) are the other major trials which have shown fibrates to be protective **(Table 94.5)**.[112-114]

TABLE 94.5	Lipid lowering agents that reduce cardiovascular risk in patients with type 2 diabetes	
Study	Drug	Risk reduction
Statin trials		
Scandinavian simvastatin survival study [4S][105]	Simvastatin	55%
Long-term intervention with pravastatin in ischemic disease (LIPID)[106]	Pravastatin	19%
Cholesterol and recurrent events (CURE)[107]	Pravastatin	25%
Air Force/Texas coronary atherosclerosis prevention study (AFCAPS/TexCAPS)[109]	Lovastatin	43%
Heart protection study (HPS)[110]	Simvastatin	22%
Fibrate trials		
Veterans administration high density lipoprotein intervention trial (VA-HIT)[111]	Gemfibrozil	24%
Helsinki heart study (HHS)[112]	Gemfibrozil	68%
Bezafibrate infarction prevention study (BIP)[113]	Bezafibrates	42%
Diabetes atherosclerosis intervention study (DAIS)[114]	Fenofibrate	23%

Multifactorial Approaches to Prevention of Cardiovascular Disease (CVD) in Diabetics

Although in clinical practice, most diabetologists advice simultaneous control of blood glucose, blood pressure and lipids so as to take care of all the above mentioned risk factors, there were no studies on the effect of tackling all these risk factors on macrovascular complications until the recent Danish Steno 2 study.[115]

The Steno 2 study had two arms—the conventional and intensive groups with 80 type 2 diabetic individuals in each. The treatment regimen focused on glycemic control, hypertension control, lipid control and antiplatelet therapy, with the intensive group having a lower target than the conventional group. After a mean follow-up of 7.8 years, the outcomes, which included death from cardiovascular causes, nonfatal myocardial infarction, nonfatal stroke, revascularization, and amputation, were assessed. There was a significant decrease in the glycosylated hemoglobin values, systolic and diastolic blood pressure, serum cholesterol and triglyceride levels in the intensive group compared to conventional group. This decrease resulted in lower risk of cardiovascular disease, nephropathy, retinopathy, and autonomic neuropathy. The cardiovascular event rate in conventional-therapy group was 44% compared to 24% in the intensive group. Overall, in the intensive group, there was a significant reduction in cardiovascular disease (CVD) with a hazard ratio of 0.47 in 7.8 years of follow-up. This risk reduction was statistically significant even after adjusting for baseline duration of diabetes, age, sex, smoking status, and presence or absence of cardiovascular disease. The risk reduction in cardiovascular events observed in this study is higher than other studies, which have used single-factor intervention strategies, targeting glycemic control, hypertension control or lipid control.

Patients receiving intensive therapy also had a significant reduction in CVD (hazard ratio, 0.47; 95% confidence interval, 0.24 to 0.73), nephropathy (hazard ratio, 0.39; 95% confidence interval, 0.17 to 0.87), retinopathy (hazard ratio, 0.42; 95% confidence interval, 0.21 to 0.86), and autonomic neuropathy (hazard ratio, 0.37; 95% confidence interval, 0.18 to 0.79). Results from this study emphasized the need for a multifactorial approach to present cardiovascular disease in diabetic subjects.

Lifestyle Measures

Lifestyle changes like dietary modification, regular exercise and cessation of smoking has been suggested as measures to reduce cardiovascular disease.[116] One of the most important modifiable risk factor for prevalence of both PVD and CAD is cessation of smoking. One of the lifestyle intervention program which included smoking cessation showed clinical benefits for subjects with PVD.[117] Cessation of smoking has been constantly emphasized particularly in subjects with high-risk for vascular disease.[117,118]

Though dietary modification is always a challenge as the dietary patterns differ in different countries, there are a few strategies, which could be of benefit to everyone.

Type of fat: Substituting saturated fat and transfatty acids with nonhydrogenated mono- and polyunsaturated fats.

Improving quality of carbohydrate: Substitute high glycemic index (GI) foods with low GI ingredients and increase intake of cereals rich in fibers.

Reduce salt intake:[119] Physical activity has shown to have a strong relation with coronary artery disease.[116] A prospective study on 8302 Finnish men and 9139 women aged 25 to 64 years without a history of antihypertensive drug use, coronary heart disease, stroke, and heart failure at baseline showed that subjects with heavy grade of physical activity had low prevalence of hypertension.[116] Exercise helps in weight reduction and also reduces cholesterol levels which would prevent vascular disorders.

A multidrug approach coupled with lifestyle measures would be ideal to prevent the onset of complications. However, once complications set in, specific measures to tackle the consequences of the complications have to be incorporated into the patient's treatment regimen.

Intermediate Approach for Prevention of Diabetes Complications

These approaches are specific for diabetes-related complications as suggested in **Table 94.6**.

Diabetic Retinopathy

The Diabetic retinopathy study (DRS) assessed the effect of panretinal photocoagulation on the risk of vision loss from PDR. Photocoagulation significantly reduced visual loss and this effect persisted throughout the entire follow-up.[120] The early treatment diabetic retinopathy study (ETDRS) investigated the timing for initiating photocoagulation and suggested that scatter photocoagulation be deferred in eyes with mild-to-moderate nonproliferative diabetic retinopathy.[29] By timely screening for retinopathy and aggressive use of photocoagulation both the sight-threatening forms of retinopathy namely proliferative diabetic retinopathy and microaneurysms can be effectively tackled.

Diabetic Nephropathy

The measures taken for regressing the progression of diabetic nephropathy include tight blood pressure control, use of ACE inhibitors, and protein restriction in diet.[121] Protein restriction in type 1 diabetic subjects reduced the decline in glomerular filtration rate.[122] Similarly, creatinine clearance decreased more slowly in subjects with low protein diet compared to those on high protein diet.[122]

Diabetic Neuropathy

Nearly 5% of painful peripheral neuropathy in diabetic subjects could be due to nondiabetic causes. The management of symptomatic neuropathy is given in **Table 94.7**. For painful peripheral neuropathy, the drug recommended, is tricyclic antidepressant drugs, i.e. phenytoin, carbamazepine and topical capsaicin.[36] Nonsteroidal anti-inflammatory drugs **(NSAIDs)** should be used with caution could be of great risk in subjects with renal insufficiency. The new drugs in market like the gamma linolenic acid and α-lipoic acid and methylcobolamine have been reported to be of some benefits.

TABLE 94.6	Strategies for prevention of diabetes complications		
Complication	*Early approach*	*Intermediate approach*	*Late approach*
Diabetic retinopathy	Glycemic control Blood pressure control Lipid control	Photocoagulation	Vitreoretinal surgery
Diabetic nephropathy	Glycemic control Blood pressure control Lipid control	ACE inhibitors	Dialysis Transplantation
Peripheral neuropathy	Glycemic control Footwear	γ-linolenic acid α-lipoic acid Drugs for relief of pain	Prompt intervention (antibiotic, local surgery) Custom made footwear Corrective surgeries
Macrovascular disease	Glycemic control Blood pressure control Lipid control	Antiplatelet drugs	Revascularization Surgery

TABLE 94.7	Management of symptomatic neuropathy

Step	Action
1	Exclude nondiabetic causes
2	Explanation and education to the patient
3	Tight glycemic control
4	Consider symptomatic therapy

Drug class	Drug
Tricyclics	Amitriptyline
	Imipramine
Anticonvulsants	Gabapentin
	Lamotrigine
	Carbamazepine
Antiarrhythmics	Mexiletine
Other agents	Tramadol
Topical application	Capsaicin

Macrovascular Diseases

Drugs, which are considered to be of great use in preventing cardiovascular diseases, include aspirin and antiplatelet drugs like GP IIb/IIIa inhibitors. The CURE study on 12,562 patients with acute coronary syndrome using aspirin demonstrated that adding clopidogrel to aspirin effectively prevents the combined incidence of cardiovascular death, myocardial infarction, or stroke.[123] Indeed diabetic subjects had more benefit by using GP IIb/IIIa inhibitors compared to nondiabetic subjects according to a meta-analysis on six large studies which involved 23,072 patients without and 6,458 patients with diabetes admitted for non-ST-segment elevation myocardial infarction or unstable angina.[124]

Late Approach for Prevention of Diabetes Complications

This forms the last step and is used in the end stages of the diabetes complications. The late approaches have been sequenced in **Table 94.6**. Vitreoretinal surgery is used to regain sight in those with bleeding due to proliferative retinopathy and in cases of retinitis proliferans and retinal detachment. Dialysis and kidney transplantation are used in end-stage renal failure with good results. In macrovascular disease, intervention like angioplasty and bypass surgery has been used with varying degrees of success. New types of stents like the drug-eluting stents are considered to be major breakthroughs in preventing restenosis.[125] However, it can be appreciated that most of these are not curative but palliative therapies and it is better to try to prevent patients going into these late stages of complications.

FUTURE PERSPECTIVES

With rapid advances in the field of diabetology, newer drugs are now in the pipeline, which could specifically address the consequences of complications. For diabetic retinopathy, protein kinase C inhibitors and similar products may form the basis of future treatments for diabetic retinopathy.[126] Ruboxistaurin (LY333531), a compound that shows a high degree of specificity over the protein kinase C (PKC) gene family for inhibiting PKC β-isoforms is considered to be useful in preventing microvascular complications.[127] The potentials of aldose reductase inhibitors and antioxidant therapy in preventing complications are also under study.[36] For preventing cardiovascular and cerebrovascular diseases, new generation statins and fibrates may be more effective than at present.

Owing to the importance of multifactorial approach to drugs, poly pharmacy is the rule. An important task for the pharmaceutical industry is to try to develop combinations of drugs that are safe and effective thereby helping the diabetic patient to live an easier, longer and healthier life despite diabetic.

SUMMARY

- Both the economic burden and loss quality of life experienced by a diabetic individual could be attributed to its morbidity associated with microvascular and macrovascular complications.
- The natural history of type 2 diabetes provides chances for prevention at three transition points: Primary prevention of diabetes itself, secondary prevention—early detection to prevent onset of complications and tertiary prevention—retardation of progression of complications and prevention of disability.
- The early detection of diabetic complications by routine screening is an important aspect in prevention of diabetes complications. Annual screening is recommended for all diabetic patients for all complications. This includes retinal screening for detecting retinopathy, microalbuminuria for diabetic nephropathy, examination of pedal pulses and peripheral doppler for peripheral vascular disease, 12-lead electrocardiography for coronary artery disease and if indicated treadmill and echocardiography as well as a complete foot examination including monofilament testing and biothesiometry for diabetic neuropathy.

- The early approaches for prevention of complications should target glycemic control, hypertension control and control of dyslipidemia. Such a multifactorial approach is necessary to prevent complications, particularly macrovascular disease.

- Lifestyle measures to prevent complications should include dietary modification, which includes substituting: (i) Saturated fat, and transfatty acids with nonhydrogenated mono- and poly-unsaturated fats; (ii) High glycemic load items with low glycemic items, increasing fiber intake and reducing salt intake. Regular exercise and cessation of smoking would also help in preventing macrovascular complications.

- The intermediate approach should target prevention of progression of complications after the complications set in. This includes panretinal photocoagulation for reducing the risk of visual loss in subjects with retinopathy, tight blood pressure control and protein restriction in subjects with nephropathy and use of antiplatelet therapy for macrovascular disease.

- Late approach includes interventional procedures to prevent progression to end stage of the complications, like vitreoretinal surgery (proliferative retinopathy), dialysis and kidney transplantation (renal failure), angioplasty and bypass surgery (macrovascular disease).

REFERENCES

1. King H, Rewers M. Diabetes in adults is now a Third World problem. The WHO Ad Hoc Diabetes Reporting Group. Bull World Health Organ. 1991;69:643-8.

2. Bjork S, Kapur A, King H, Nair J, Ramachandran A. Global policy: aspects of diabetes in India. Health Policy. 2003;66:61-72.

3. Nathan DM. Long-term complications of diabetes mellitus. N Engl J Med. 1993;328:1676-85.

4. Songer TJ, Zimmet PZ. Epidemiology of type II diabetes: an international perspective. Pharmacoeconomics. 1995;8 (Suppl 1):1-11.

5. Zimmet PZ. Diabetes epidemiology as a tool to trigger diabetes research and care. Diabetologia. 1999;42:499-518.

6. King H, Aubert RE, Herman WH. Global burden of diabetes, 1995-2025: prevalence, numerical estimates and projections. Diabetes Care. 1998;21:1414-31.

7. Sheetz MJ, King GL. Molecular understanding of hyperglycemia's adverse effects for diabetic complications. JAMA. 2002;288:2579-88.

8. Harper CA. Treatment of diabetic retinopathy. Clin Exp Optom. 1999;82:98-101.

9. Rema M, Ponnaiya M, Mohan V. Prevalence of retinopathy in noninsulin-dependent diabetes mellitus at a diabetes centre in southern India. Diabetes Res Clin Pract. 1996;34:29-36.

10. Rema M, Shanthirani CS, Deepa R, Mohan V. Prevalence of diabetic retinopathy in a selected South Indian Population—the Chennai Urban Population Study (CUPS). Diabetes Res Clin Pract. 2000;50:S252.

11. Dandona L, Dandona R, Naduvilath TJ, McCarty CA, Rao GN. Population based assessment of diabetic retinopathy in an urban population in southern India. Br J Ophthalmol. 1999;83:937-40.

12. Rema M, Deepa R, Mohan V. Prevalence of retinopathy at diagnosis among type 2 diabetic patients attending a diabetic centre in South India. Br J Ophthalmol. 2000;84:1058-60.

13. Ashok S, Ramu M, Deepa R, Mohan V. Prevalence of neuropathy in type 2 diabetic patients attending a diabetes centre in South India. J Assoc Physicians India. 2002;50:546-50.

14. Ramu M, Premalatha G, Deepa R, Mohan V. Prevalence of neuropathy using biothesiometry in a selected South Indian Population—the Chennai Urban Population Study (CUPS). Diabetes Res Clin Pract. 2000;60:S270.

15. Mohan V, Sastry NG, Premalatha G. Autonomic dysfunction in non-insulin-dependent diabetes mellitus and fibrocalculous pancreatic diabetes in south India. Diabet Med. 1996;13:1038-43.

16. Locatelli F, Canaud B, Eckardt KU, Stenvinkel P, Wanner C, Zoccali C. The importance of diabetic nephropathy in current nephrological practice. Nephrol Dial Transplant. 2003;18:1716-25.

17. Varghese A, Deepa R, Rema M, Mohan V. Prevalence of microalbuminuria in type 2 diabetes mellitus at a diabetes centre in southern India. Postgrad Med J. 2001;77:399-402.

18. Haffner SM, Agostino RD Jr, Saad MF, et al. Carotid artery atherosclerosis in type 2 diabetic and nondiabetic subjects with and without symptomatic coronary artery disease (The Insulin Resistance Atherosclerosis Study). Am J Cardiol. 2000;85:1395-400.

19. Reaven GM. A syndrome of resistance to insulin stimulated uptake (Syndrome X). Definitions and implications. Cardiovasc Risk Factors. 1993;3:2-11.

20. Mohan V, Deepa R, Rani SS, Premalatha G. Prevalence of coronary artery disease and its relationship to lipids in a selected population in South India: the Chennai Urban Population Study (CUPS No. 5). J Am Coll Cardiol. 2001;38:682-7.

21. Gupta R, Gupta VP, Sarna M, et al. Prevalence of coronary heart disease and risk factors in an urban Indian population: Jaipur Heart Watch-2. Indian Heart J. 2002;54:59-66.

22. Mohan V, Premalatha G, Sastry NG. Ischaemic heart disease in South Indian NIDDM patients: a clinic-based study on 6597 NIDDM patients. Int J Diab Dev Countries. 1995;15:64-7.

23. Premalatha G, Shanthirani S, Deepa R, Markovitz J, Mohan V. Prevalence and risk factors of peripheral vascular disease in a selected South Indian population: the Chennai Urban Population Study. Diabetes Care. 2000;23:1295-300.

24. Ritchie LD, Ganapathy S, Woodward-Lopez G, Gerstein DE, Fleming SE. Prevention of type 2 diabetes in youth: etiology, promising interventions and recommendations. Pediatr Diabetes. 2003;4:174-209.

25. American Diabetes Association. Economic consequences of diabetes mellitus in the US in 1997. Diabetes Care. 1998;21:296-309.

26. The Economics of Diabetes and Diabetes Care. A Report of the Diabetes Health Economics Study Group, WHO and International Diabetes Federation, 1998. Diabetes Health Economics, International Diabetes Federation, 1999.

27. The Diabetes Control and Complications Trial Research Group. The effect of intensive treatment of diabetes on the development and progression of long-term complications in insulin-dependent diabetes mellitus. N Engl J Med. 1993;329:977-86.

28. United Kingdom Prospective Diabetes Study (UKPDS) Group. Intensive blood glucose control with sulphonylureas or insulin compared with conventional treatment and risk of complications in patients with type 2 diabetes (UKPDS 33). Lancet. 1998;352:837-53.

29. Early Treatment Diabetic Retinopathy Study Research Group. Photocoagulation for diabetic macular edema. Early Treatment Diabetic Retinopathy Study Report no 1. Arch Ophthalmol. 1985;103:1796-806.

30. Feldt-Rasmussen B, Mathiesen ER, Deckert T. Effect of two years of strict metabolic control on progression of incipient nephropathy in insulin-dependent diabetes. Lancet. 1986;2:1300-4.

31. American Diabetes Association. Clinical Practice Recommendations 2004. Nephropathy in Diabetes. Diabetes Care. 2004;27:S79-83.

32. American Diabetes Association. Clinical Practice Recommendations 2004. Retinopathy in Diabetes. Diabetes Care. 2004;27:S84-7.

33. Martins D, Norris K. Combating diabetic nephropathy with drug therapy. Curr Diab Rep. 2001;1:148-56.

34. Deferrari G, Ravera M, Berruti V. Treatment of diabetic nephropathy in its early stages. Diabetes Metab Res Rev. 2003;19:101-14.

35. Gerstein HC. Reduction of cardiovascular events and microvascular complications in diabetes with ACE inhibitor treatment: HOPE and MICRO-HOPE. Diabetes Metab Res Rev. 2002;18 (Suppl 3):S82-5.

36. Boulton AJ. Treatment of symptomatic diabetic neuropathy. Diabetes Metab Res Rev. 2003;19 (Suppl 1):S16-21.

37. Ward JD. Improving prognosis in type 2 diabetes—diabetic neuropathy is in trouble. Diabetes Care. 1999;22 (Suppl 2):B84-8.

38. Leng GC, Lee AJ, Fowkes FG, et al. Incidence, natural history and cardiovascular events in symptomatic and asymptomatic peripheral arterial disease in the general population. Int J Epidemiol. 1996;25:1172-81.

39. Premalatha G, Ravikumar R, Sanjay R, Deepa R, Mohan V. Comparison of colour duplex ultrasound and ankle-brachial pressure index measurements in peripheral vascular disease in type 2 diabetic patients with foot infections. J Assoc Physicians India. 2002;50:1240-4.

40. Ouriel K, McDonnell AE, Metz CE, Zarins CK. Critical evaluation of stress testing in the diagnosis of peripheral vascular disease. Surgery. 1982;91:686-93.

41. Leng GC, Fowkes FG, Lee AJ, Dunbar J, Housley E, Ruckley CV. Use of ankle-brachial pressure index to predict cardiovascular events and death: a cohort study. BMJ. 1996;313:1440-4.

42. Sikkink CJ, van Asten WN, van 't Hof MA, van Langen H, van der Vliet JA. Decreased ankle/ brachial indices in relation to morbidity and mortality in patients with peripheral arterial disease. Vasc Med. 1997;2:169-73.

43. Executive Summary of the Third Report of the National Cholesterol Education Program (NCEP). Expert Panel on Detection, Evaluation, and Treatment of High Blood Cholesterol in Adults (Adult Treatment Panel III). JAMA. 2001;285:2486-97.

44. O' Leary DH, Bryan FA, Goodison MW, et al. Measurement variability of carotid atherosclerosis: real-time (B-mode) ultrasonography and angiography. Stroke. 1987;18:1011-7.

45. Geroulakos G, O'Gorman D, Kalodiki E, Sheridan DJ, Nicolaides AN. The carotid intima media thickness as a marker of the presence of severe symptomatic coronary artery disease. Eur Heart J. 1994;15:781-5.

46. Mohan V, Ravikumar R, Shanthirani S, Deepa R. Intimal medial thickness of the carotid artery in south Indian diabetic and nondiabetic subjects: the Chennai Urban Population Study (CUPS). Diabetologia. 2000;43:494-9.

47. Ravikumar R, Deepa R, Shanthirani CS, Mohan V. Comparison of carotid intima-media thickness, arterial stiffness and brachial artery flow medicated dilatation in diabetic and nondiabetic subjects. The Chennai Urban Population Study (CUPS NO: 9). Am J Cardiol. 2002;90:702-7.

48. Kawamori R, Yamasaki Y, Matsushima H, et al. Prevalence of Carotid atherosclerosis in diabetic patients. Ultrasound high resolution B-mode imaging on carotid arteries. Diabetes Care. 1992;15:1290-4.

49. Simon A, Gariepy J, Chironi G, Megnien JL, Levenson J. Intima-media thickness: a new tool for diagnosis and treatment of cardiovascular risk. J Hypertens. 2002;20:159-69.

50. Kastelein JJ, Wiegman A, de Groot E. Surrogate markers of atherosclerosis: impact of statins. Atheroscler Suppl. 2003;4:31-6.

51. Duby JJ, Campbell RK, Setter SM, White JR, Rasmussen KA. Diabetic neuropathy: an intensive review. Am J Health Syst Pharm. 2004;61:160-73.

52. Nosadini R, Tonolo G. Blood glucose and lipid control as risk factors in the progression of renal damage in type 2 diabetes. J Nephrol. 2003;16 (Suppl 7):S42-7.

53. Speicher MA, Danis RP, Criswell M, Pratt L. Pharmacologic therapy for diabetic retinopathy. Expert Opin Emerg Drugs. 2003;8:239-50.

54. Shichiri M, Kishikawa H, Ohkubo Y, Wake N. Long-term results of the Kumamoto Study on optimal diabetes control in type 2 diabetic patients. Diabetes Care. 2000;23:B21-9.

55. Writing Team for the Diabetes Control and Complications Trial/Epidemiology of Diabetes Interventions and Complications Research Group. Sustained effect of intensive treatment of type 1 diabetes mellitus on development and progression of diabetic nephropathy: the Epidemiology of Diabetes Interventions and Complications (EDIC) study. JAMA. 2003;290:2159-67.

56. Reichard P, Pihl M, Rosenqvist U, Sule J. Complications in IDDM are caused by elevated blood glucose level: the Stockholm Diabetes Intervention Study (SDIS) at 10-year follow-up. Diabetologia. 1996;39:1483-8.

57. Wang PH, Lau J, Chalmers TC. Meta-analysis of the effects of intensive glycemic control on late complications of type I diabetes mellitus. Online J Curr Clin Trials. 1993;Doc No 60.

58. Klein R. Hyperglycemia and microvascular and macrovascular disease in diabetes. Diabetes Care. 1995;18:258-68.

59. Fuller JH, Shipley MJ, Rose G, Jarrett RJ, Keen H. Mortality from coronary heart disease and stroke in relation to degree of glycaemia: the Whitehall study. Br Med J. 1983;287:867-70.

60. Donahue, RP, Abbott RD, Reed DM, Yano K. Postchallenge glucose concentration and coronary heart disease in men of Japanese ancestry. Honolulu Heart Program. Diabetes. 1987;36:689-92.

61. McGill Jr HC, McMahan CA, Malcolm GT, Oalmann MC, Strong JP. Pathological Determinants of Atherosclerosis in Youth (PADY) Research Group. Relation of glycohaemoglobin and adiposity to atherosclerosis in youth. Arterioscler Thromb Vasc Biol. 1995;15:431-40.

62. Pais P, Pogue J, Gerstein H, et al. Risk factors for acute myocardial infarction in Indians: a case-control study. Lancet. 1996;348:358-63.

63. Deepa R, Arvind K, Mohan V. Diabetes and risk factors for coronary artery disease. Current Science. 2002;83:1497-505.

64. Arvind K, Pradeepa R, Deepa R, Mohan V. Diabetes and coronary artery disease. Indian J Med Res. 2002;116:163-76.

65. Buse JB, Tan MH, Prince MJ, Erickson PP. The effects of oral anti-hyperglycaemic medications on serum lipid profiles in patients with type 2 diabetes. Diabetes Obes Metab. 2004;6:133-56.

66. Sidhu JS, Cowan D, Kaski JC. The effects of rosiglitazone: a peroxisome proliferator-activated receptor-gamma agonist, on markers of endothelial cell activation, C-reactive protein, and fibrinogen levels in non-diabetic coronary artery disease patients. J Am Coll Cardiol. 2003;42:1757-63.

67. Sidhu JS, Kaposzta Z, Markus HS, Kaski JC. Effect of rosiglitazone on common carotid intima-media thickness progression in coronary artery disease patients without diabetes mellitus. Arterioscler Thromb Vasc Biol. 2004.

68. Rajagopalan R, Iyer S, Khan M. Effect of pioglitazone on metabolic syndrome risk factors: results of double-blind, multicenter, randomized clinical trials. Curr Med Res Opin. 2005;21:163-72.

69. Goldberg RB, Kendall DM, Deeg MA, Buse JB, Zagar AJ, Pinaire JA, Tan MH, Khan MA, Perez AT, Jacober SJ. GLAI Study Investigators: a comparison of lipid and glycemic effects of pioglitazone and rosiglitazone in patients with type 2 diabetes and dyslipidemia. Diabetes Care. 2005;28:1547-54.

70. Dormandy JA, Charbonnel B, Eckland DJ, Erdmann E, Massi-Benedetti M, Moules IK, et al. PROactive investigators. Secondary prevention of macrovascular events in patients with type 2 diabetes in the PROactive Study (PROspective pioglitazone Clinical Trial In macrovascular Events): a randomized controlled trial. Lancet. 2005;366:1279-89.

71. Zarich SW. Treating the diabetic patient: appropriate care for glycemic control and cardiovascular disease risk factors. Rev Cardiovasc Med. 2003;4(Suppl 6):S19-28.

72. Malmberg K, Ryden L, Efendic S, et al. Randomised trial of insulin-glucose infusion followed by subcutaneous insulin treatment in diabetic patients with acute myocardial infarction (DIGAMI study): effects on mortality at 1 year. J Am Coll Cardiol. 1995;26:57-65.

73. Mehta SR, Yusuf S, Diaz R, et al. CREATE-ECLA Trial Group Investigators. Effect of glucose-insulin- potassium infusion on mortality in patients with acute ST-segment elevation myocardial infarction: the CREATE-ECLA randomized controlled trial. JAMA. 2005;293:437-46.

74. National High Blood Pressure Education Program Working Group report on hypertension and chronic renal failure. Arch Intern Med. 1991;151:1280-7.

75. Assmann G, Schulte H. The Prospective Cardiovascular Munster (PROCAM) study: prevalence of hyperlipidemia in persons with hypertension and/or diabetes mellitus and the relationship to coronary heart disease. Am Heart J. 1988;116:1713-24.

76. American Diabetes Association. Treatment of hypertension in adults with diabetes. Diabetes Care. 2003; 26(Suppl 1):S80-2.

77. National High Blood Pressure Education Program. The seventh report of the Joint National Committee on Prevention, Detection, Evaluation, and Treatment of High Blood Pressure. JNC 7 Express. pp. 1-52.

78. Knowler WC, Bennett PH, Ballintine EJ. Increased incidence of retinopathy in diabetics with elevated blood pressure. A six-year follow-up study in Pima Indians. N Engl J Med. 1980;302:645-50.

79. United Kingdom Prospective Diabetes Study Group. Tight blood pressure control and risk of macrovascular and microvascular complications in type 2 diabetes. UKPDS 38. Br Med J. 1998;317:703-13.

80. Chaturvedi N, Sjolie AK, Stephenson JM, et al. Effect of lisinopril on progression of retinopathy in normotensive people with type 1 diabetes. The EUCLID Study Group. EURODIAB controlled trial of lisinopril in Insulin-dependent diabetes mellitus. Lancet. 1998;351:28-31.

81. Lewis EJ, Hunsicker LG, Bain RP, Rohde RD. The effect of angiotensin-converting-enzyme inhibition on diabetic nephropathy. The Collaborative Study Group. N Engl J Med. 1993;329:1456-62.

82. Laffel LM, McGill JB, Gans DJ. The beneficial effect of angiotensin-converting enzyme inhibition with captopril on diabetic nephropathy in normotensive IDDM patients with microalbuminuria. North American Microalbuminuria Study Group. Am J Med. 1995;99:497-504.

83. Parving HH, Lehnert H, Brochner-Mortensen J, Gomis R, Andersen S, Arner P. Irbesartan in Patients with Type 2 Diabetes and Microalbuminuria Study Group. The effect of irbesartan on the development of diabetic nephropathy in patients with type 2 diabetes. N Engl J Med. 2001;345:870-8.

84. Brenner BM, Cooper ME, de Zeeuw D, et al. RENAAL Study Investigators. Effects of losartan on renal and cardiovascular outcomes in patients with type 2 diabetes and nephropathy. N Engl J Med. 2001;345:861-9.

85. Lewis EJ, Hunsicker LG, Clarke WR, B, et al. Collaborative Study Group. Renoprotective effect of the angiotensin-receptor antagonist irbesartan in patients with nephropathy due to type 2 diabetes. N Engl J Med. 2001;345:851-60.

86. Heart Outcomes Prevention Evaluation Study Investigators. Effects of ramipril on cardiovascular and microvascular outcomes in people with diabetes mellitus: results of the HOPE study and MICRO-HOPE substudy. Lancet. 2000;355:253-9.

87. Hansson L, Zanchetti A, Carruthers SG, et al. Effects of intensive blood-pressure lowering and low-dose aspirin in patients with hypertension: principal results of the Hypertension Optimal Treatment (HOT) randomised trial. HOT Study Group. Lancet. 1998;351:1755-62.

88. Bakris GL. The importance of blood pressure control in the patient with diabetes. Am J Med. 2004;116(Suppl 5A):30-8S.

89. Zuanetti G, Latini R, Maggioni AP, Franzosi M, Santoro L, Tognoni G. Effect of the ACE inhibitor lisinopril on mortality in diabetic patients with acute myocardial infarction: data from the GISSI-3 study. Circulation. 1997;96:4239-45.

90. Hansson L, Lindholm LH, Niskanen L, et al. Effect of angiotensin-converting-enzyme inhibition compared with conventional therapy on cardiovascular morbidity and mortality in hypertension: the Captopril Prevention Project (CAPPP) randomised trial. Lancet. 1999;353:611-6.

91. The Danish Verapamil Infarction Trial II (DAVIT II). Effect of verapamil on mortality and major events after acute myocardial infarction Am J Cardiol. 1990;66:779-85.

92. The Systolic Hypertension in the Elderly Program Cooperative Research Group. Implications of the systolic hypertension in the elderly program. Hypertension. 1993;21:335-43.

93. Estacio RO, Jeffers BW, Hiatt WR, Biggerstaff SL, Gifford N, Schrier RW. The effect of nisoldipine as compared with enalapril on cardiovascular outcomes in patients with non-insulin-dependent diabetes and hypertension. N Engl J Med. 1998;338:645-52.

94. Tatti P, Pahor M, Byington RP, Di Mauro P, Guarisco R, Strollo G, Strollo F. Outcome results of the Fosinopril versus Amlodipine Cardiovascular Events Randomized Trial (FACET) in patients with hypertension and NIDDM. Diabetes Care. 1998;21:597-603.

95. Lindholm LH, Ibsen H, Dahlof B, et al. LIFE Study Group. Cardiovascular morbidity and mortality in patients with diabetes in the Losartan Intervention for Endpoint reduction in hypertension study (LIFE): a randomised trial against atenolol. Lancet. 2002;359:1004-10.

96. Klein BE, Moss SE, Klein R, Surawicz TS. The Wisconsin Epidemiologic Study of Diabetic Retinopathy XIII. Relationship of serum cholesterol to retinopathy and hard exudate. Ophthalmology. 1991;98:1261-5.

97. Chew EY, Klein ML, Ferris FL 3rd, et al. Association of elevated serum lipid levels with retinal hard exudate in diabetic retinopathy. Early Treatment Diabetic Retinopathy Study (ETDRS) Report 22. Arch Ophthalmol. 1996;114:1079-84.

98. Rema M, Mohan V, Susheela L, Ramachandran A, Viswanathan M. Increased LDL cholesterol in non-insulin-dependent diabetes with maculopathy. Acta Diabetologica Latina. 1984;21:85-9.

99. Misra A, Kumar S, Kishore Vikram N, Kumar A. The role of lipids in the development of diabetic microvascular complications: implications for therapy. Am J Cardiovasc Drugs. 2003;3:325-38.

100. Hadjadj S, Duly-Bouhanick B, Bekherraz A, et al. Serum triglycerides are a predictive factor for the development and the progression of renal and retinal complications in patients with type 1 diabetes. Diabetes Metab. 2004;30:43-51.

101. Battisti WP, Palmisano J, Keane WE. Dyslipidemia in patients with type 2 diabetes. relationships between lipids, kidney disease and cardiovascular disease. Clin Chem Lab Med. 2003;41:1174-81.

102. Durrington P. Dyslipidaemia. Lancet. 2003;362:717-31.

103. Nabel EG. Cardiovascular disease. N Engl J Med. 2003;349:60-72.

104. Gotto AM Jr. Triglyceride: the forgotten risk factor. Circulation. 1998;97:1027-8.

105. Scandinavian Simvastatin Survival Study (4S) Group. Randomised trial of cholesterol lowering in 4444 patients with coronary heart disease: the Scandinavian simvastatin survival study (4S). Lancet. 1994;344:1383-9.

106. The Long-term Intervention with Pravastatin in Ischaemic Disease (LIPID) Study Group. Prevention of cardiovascular events and death with pravastatin in patients with coronary heart disease and a broad range of initial cholesterol levels. N Engl J Med. 1998;339:1349-57.

107. Sacks FM, Pfeffer MA, Moye LA, et al. For the Cholesterol and Recurrent Events Trial Investigators: the effect of pravastatin on coronary events after myocardial infarction in patients with average cholesterol levels. N Engl J Med. 1996;335:1001-9.

108. West of Scotland Coronary Prevention Study Group. Influence of pravastatin and plasma lipids on clinical events in the West of Scotland Coronary Prevention Study (WOSCOPS). Circulation. 1998;97:1440-5.

109. Downs JR, Clearfield M, Weis S, et al. For the AFCAPS/TexCAPS Research Group, primary prevention of acute coronary events with lovastatin in men and women with average cholesterol levels: results of AFCAPS/TexCAPS. JAMA. 1998;279:1615-22.

110. Goldberg RB. Statin treatment in diabetic subjects: what the heart protection study shows—Landmark Study. Clinical diabetes. 2003;21:151-2.

111. Robins SJ, Collins D, Wittes JT, et al. Veterans Affairs High-Density Lipoprotein Intervention Trial (VAHIT) Study Group. Relation of gemfibrozil treatment and lipid levels with major coronary events. VA-HIT: a randomized controlled trial. JAMA. 2001;285:1585-91.

112. Manninen V, Tenkanen L, Koskinen P, et al. Joint effects of serum triglyceride and LDL cholesterol and HDL cholesterol concentrations on coronary heart disease risk in the Helsinki Heart Study: implications for treatment. Circulation. 1992;85:37-45.

113. Secondary prevention by raising HDL cholesterol and reducing triglycerides in patients with coronary artery disease: the Bezafibrate Infarction Prevention (BIP) study. Circulation. 2000;102:21-7.

114. Effect of fenofibrate on progression of coronary artery disease in type 2 diabetes—the Diabetes Atherosclerosis Intervention Study: a randomized study. Lancet. 2001;357:905-10.

115. Gaede P, Vedel P, Larsen N, Jensen GV, Parving HH, Pedersen O. Multifactorial intervention and cardiovascular disease in patients with type 2 diabetes. N Engl J Med. 2003;348:383-93.

116. Hu G, Barengo NC, Tuomilehto J, Lakka TA, Nissinen A, Jousilahti P. Relationship of physical activity and body mass index to the risk of hypertension: a prospective study in Finland. Hypertension. 2004;43:25-30.

117. Burns DM. Epidemiology of smoking-induced cardiovascular disease. Prog Cardiovasc Dis. 2003;46:11-29.

118. Hobbs SD, Bradbury AW. Smoking cessation strategies in patients with peripheral arterial disease: an evidence-based approach. Eur J Vasc Endovasc Surg. 2003;26:341-7.

119. Cernea S, Hancu N, Raz I. Diet and coronary heart disease in diabetes. Acta Diabetol. 2003;40(Suppl 2):S389-400.

120. Ferris FL 3rd, Podgor MJ, Davis MD. Macular edema in diabetic retinopathy study patients. Diabetic Retinopathy Study Report Number 12. Ophthalmology. 1987;94:754-60.

121. Walker JD, Bending JJ, Dodds RA, et al. Restriction of dietary protein and progression of renal failure in diabetic nephropathy. Lancet. 1989;2:1411-5.

122. Zeller K, Whittaker E, Sullivan L, Raskin P, Jacobson HR. Effect of restricting dietary protein on the progression of renal failure in patients with insulin-dependent diabetes mellitus. N Engl J Med. 1991;324:78-84.

123. Peters RJ, Mehta SR, Fox KA, et al. Clopidogrel in Unstable angina to prevent Recurrent Events (CURE) Trial Investigators. Effects of aspirin dose when used alone or in combination with clopidogrel in patients with acute coronary syndromes: observations from the Clopidogrel in unstable angina to prevent Recurrent Events (CURE) study. Circulation. 2003;108:1682-7.

124. Roffi M, Chew DP, Mukherjee D, et al. Platelet glycoprotein IIb/IIIa inhibitors reduce mortality in diabetic patients with non-ST-segment-elevation acute coronary syndromes. Circulation. 2001;104:2767-71.

125. Hodgson JM, Bottner RK, Klein LW, et al. Drug-eluting stent task force: Final report and recommendations of the working committees on cost-effectiveness/ economics, access to care, and medicolegal issues. Catheter Cardiovasc Interv. 2004;62:1-17.

126. Aiello LP, Cahill MT, Cavallerano JD. Growth factors and protein kinase C inhibitors as novel therapies for the medical management diabetic retinopathy. Eye. 2004;18:117-25.

127. Tuttle KR, Anderson PW. A novel potential therapy for diabetic nephropathy and vascular complications: protein kinase C beta inhibition. Am J Kidney Dis. 2003;42:456-65.

Chapter 95

GLIMPSE INTO THE FUTURE

Hemraj B Chandalia, Shaival H Chandalia

CHAPTER OUTLINE

- Introduction
- Etiopathogenesis
- Self-monitoring of Blood Glucose and Glucose Sensors
- Therapy of Diabetes
- Complications of Diabetes

INTRODUCTION

Diabetes mellitus is perhaps the most important non-infective epidemic to hit the globe in the present millennium. We in India, especially face an enormous problem. There were an estimated 84 million people with diabetes in the developing world in 1995. The Indian subcontinent accounted for nearly a quarter of these. This number is likely to increase three-fold to 226 million by the year 2025 and India shall continue to maintain the dubious distinction of having the maximum number of diabetics in the world.[1]

This chapter gives you a glimpse into the future. What will diabetics expect in the next two decades: a disease beset with more problems than before or a disease that is easily controlled and treated or a disease on the brink of eradication? Being optimists, we believe that easy control of most forms and eradication of a few select types is possible.

We shall review various areas to see what is happening at present and what direction it is likely to take in the near future.

ETIOPATHOGENESIS

Type 1 Diabetes Mellitus

The interlink between genetic susceptibility and environmental factors is now well established. It is a polygenic or an oligogenic disease with 30 to 70% of susceptibility explained by association with genes located on the major histocompatibility complex (MHC) on chromosome 6. The only known non-MHC association is in close proximity to the insulin gene on chromosome 11. The environmental factors include association with various viruses (Coxsackie Rota, Mumps, Rubella, and Cytomegalovirus), bovine milk and nitrosamines. However, the precise environmental trigger still remains enigmatic. What has proven to be more exciting is the unfolding of the sequence of events leading to β-cell damage and apoptosis in type 1 diabetes. This has led to remarkable advances in the ability to modify or halt the immunologically mediated β-cell damage and may lead to the ultimate goal of preventing type 1 diabetes through vaccination or some such other means.

Certain HLA types impart distinct genetic suscepti-bility to type 1 diabetes mellitus. Absence of aspartate at position 57 in the HLA-DQ β-chain strongly predis-poses to type 1 diabetes mellitus in Caucasians. Presence of an aspartate residue at this site exerts a potent protective effect. The differential binding of various gene products of HLA-DQ genes to various peptides determines the susceptibility towards autoimmunity and type 1 diabetes mellitus.[2] Another susceptibility gene is located in the variable number of tandem repeats (VNTR) in the 5'-position of the insulin gene or on the insulin gene itself. A large number of genetic loci predisposing to type 1 diabetes mellitus have been identified but the strength of their association is not certain.[3]

Environmental factors continue to receive attention because of the fact that concordance for type 1 diabetes mellitus in monozygotic twins averages only 50%. The most important environmental factor is viral infection, but toxins, dietary factors and stress have also been implicated. Most lessons on these environmental factors have emerged from animal models of diabetes mellitus.[4] Proteins contained in food can influence the expression of diabetes mellitus in NOD mice and BB rats. In animal studies, feeding natural chow has shown lower prevalence of diabetes mellitus than a semi-purified chow. Milk protein, especially of bovine origin, as an etiological factor continues to be controversial.[5]

The process of immunopathogenesis of type 1 diabetes mellitus is under extensive study. A few examples of inadvertent transfer of type 1 diabetes mellitus by allogenic bone marrow transplantation have been reported. This suggests that the genetic predis-position to type 1 diabetes mellitus may initially be expressed in stem cells.[6] Animal studies suggest that development of intrathymic cell population may be defective or predispose to production of autoreactive cell lines. Some studies suggest that autoimmune process is initiated by CD8+ cells and amplified by CD4+ cells.[7]

The β-cell and β-cell environment have been studied by a large number of investigators. Expression of a neoantigen or hyperexpression of self-antigen by β-cell is not the cause of autoimmunity. The production of cytokines IFN-γ, IL-2, TNF-α or TNF-β and their role in the induction of β-cell damage or immune tolerance has been described.[8]

Administration of autoantigens in animal studies has produced conflicting results. Insulin, oral or parenteral has been used in animal studies.[9] Administering maximal doses of insulin in BB rats can prevent diabetes mellitus. Such doses probably lead to concealment of immunological targets by producing complete β-cell rest. In BB rats, oral insulin does not prevent but may exacerbate production of diabetes mellitus. Answers to such conflicting evidence may emerge from diabetes mellitus prevention trials on humans. Diabetes Prevention Trial-1 (DPT-1) is testing both, oral and paren-teral insulin to produce a state of immune tolerance. The results were disappointing, as 60% of those receiving parenteral insulin as well as those not receiving any treatment developed diabetes over a 5-year follow-up.[10] Diabetes Prediction and Prevention Project (DIPP) is studying mucosal tolerance induction by administration of nasal insulin. Many other peptides, including β-chain of insulin and Heat Shock Protein-65 (HSP-65) are also being studied clinically.

Peri-insulinitis can be induced by a variety of agents but does not lead to β-cell damage unless it progresses to diffuse intra-insulinitis. If progression of insulinitis can be stopped at the peri-insulitis phase, salvation of β-cells maybe possible. IL-12, IL-18 and TNF-α have a distinct role in the progression of insulinitis, as evi-denced by studies on knockout and transgenic animal models, where receptors of these molecules are deleted.

Type 2 Diabetes Mellitus

Type 2 diabetes has remained more enigmatic. The defects in both the β-cell (insulin pulsatility, first phase insulin secretion, proinsulin and proinsulin split products, amylin) and peripheral insulin sensitivity are well recorded. The key to these defects and a unifying theory still eludes us.

There is a continuing controversy whether insulin resistance or insulin secretory defect is more important in the etiology of type 2 diabetes mellitus (DM) and whether one precedes the other. It is difficult to resolve such issues by any direct studies as insulin resistance affects insulin secretion and vice versa. Most studies thus far favor the hypothesis that insulin resistance precedes insulin deficiency. Obesity is another confusing factor and whether obesity is the cause or the effect of insulin resistance has been debated all along. In a group of obese subjects serum insulin levels continued to be elevated, when the estimations were obtained after three days of refeeding following an effective weight loss program. This supports the fact that insulin resistance is a primary event. Insulin resistance can be present with impaired glucose tolerance (IGT).[11] Alternatively, instead of assigning a cause and effect relationship, it is safe to visualize obesity and insulin resistance both as stemming from a combination of genetic and environmental factors.

In various phases of type 2 diabetes mellitus, insulin resistance or insulin deficiency may predominate, but they often coexist. Hyperglycemia induced by insulin deficiency itself begets hyperglycemia via production of insulin resistance.

Insulin resistance is usually considered important in skeletal muscle, liver and adipose tissue. However, two other sites are considered important at present: The vascular endothelium and smooth muscle. This can result into insulin secretory defect at the β-cell level and micro- and macrovascular complications at the endothelial site.[12,13]

The insulin signal transmission pathway has been a subject of intensive studies. The receptor activation leads to activation of its intrinsic tyrosine kinase activity, which in turn is essential for transmission of the insulin signal.[14] Insulin receptor mutations do occur, but are not considered significant in the etiology of type 2 diabetes mellitus. The signal transmission further occurs through a series of insulin receptor substrates (IRS 1,2,3,4, Shc and GAB1). These proteins dock with each other and transmit signal through a serine/threonine kinase system. Polymorphism of IRS-1 gene differs significantly between normals and subjects with type 2 diabetes mellitus (5.8% vs 10.7%), and may thus be an important molecular mechanism of insulin resistance. This is not so in case of IRS-2, while data for other IRS are yet scanty. The IRS proteins recruit PI-3 kinase, a key enzyme involved in producing the metabolic effects of insulin. Some degree of polymorphism in p85 regulatory subunit of PI-3 has been described, but this needs further evaluation.

Keeping aside the specific gene disorders, type 2 diabetes definitely has a stronger genetic predisposition than type 1 diabetes, as inferred from twin, family and population studies. Many monogenic subtypes of type 2 diabetes have now been identified. These include maturity onset diabetes of the young (MODY) or autosomal dominant diabetes of which six subtypes have all been found to be single gene disorders. The list of monogenic diabetes is likely to be enhanced as we go along, but is not likely to constitute more than 3 to 5% of all types of diabetes. Most patients of type 2 diabetes are definitely polygenic and considerable progress is being made in identifying this polygenic element. The number of genes implicated so far might also point to the heterogeneity of the disease. Some of these genes include apolipoprotein B, glucokinase, HLA (HLA-A2, Bw62, Bw61, Bw22, C4B2), insulin gene, insulin receptor, GLUT-1 and GLUT-2, glycogen synthase, adenosine deaminase and other apolipoprotein genes, C-fos promoter, mitochondrial RNA and locations on chromosomes 1, 4 and 6. Genetic polymorphism of PC-1 K121Q region is associated with insulin resistance in Asian Indians.[15] This has been further identified to be responsible for genetic susceptibility to type 2 diabetes in other ethnic groups, including Caucasians.[16] The importance of these findings lies in the fact that better understanding of the etiology can lead to development of effective preventive or interventional strategies.

Dysinsulinemia is an important biochemical feature of type 2 diabetes. Insulin is secreted in a pulsatile manner throughout the day. These are larger sustained pulses that last for approximately 1 to 2 hours, accompanied by smaller, rapid cycle of insulin secretion lasting 12 to 15 minutes. More pulses occur during the postprandial period than fasting periods. One of the earliest abnormalities in type 2 diabetes is an abnormality in both the timing and amplitude of pulsatile insulin secretion. Immediate postprandial pulses corresponding to the first phase insulin release seem to be the most affected. The loss of first phase insulin secretion is a well-known early change in both overt type 2 diabetes and IGT.[17,18] In addition to the insulin secretory defects, there is an associated rise in proinsulin and 32/33 split proinsulin products.[19] Together with peripheral insulin resistance, the profound alteration in insulin release contributes to the pathogenesis of type 2 diabetes.[20,21]

The cause and degree of β-cell dysfunction is unknown in most cases. Genetic factors play an important role,[22,23] although some insulin secretory disturbances seems to be acquired and at least partially reversible, because optimal glucose control can lead to a significant improvement in glucose-induced insulin release.[24] Several alterations secondary to relative insulin deficiency, such as hyperosmolarity, high concentrations of free fatty acids (FFA) and triglycerides (TG) and lack of postprandial suppression of glucagon, resulting in much lower insulin/glucagon ratio,[25,26] are frequently seen during hyperglycemia and can modify or suppress insulin release.[26] In addition high glucose concentration itself plays a key role in β-cell dysfunction. This phenomenon has been termed as glucotoxicity.[27,28]

Postprandial glucose homeostasis requires an abrupt insulin secretory response and normal tissue responses to the released insulin. The relative contribution of defective insulin secretion and peripheral insulin resistance to postprandial hyperglycemia is still a matter of debate. Importantly, the sluggish insulin response causes reduced suppression of hepatic glucose release after carbohydrate ingestion in type 2 diabetes,[29,30] but perhaps equally important is the peripheral glucose disposal, mainly in the skeletal muscle.[31]

Common to the β-cell and peripherally glucose sensitive tissues such as skeletal muscle, adipose tissue and the hepatocytes, are the glucose transporters. GLUT-2 is the predominant transporter at the β-cell and is closely linked to glucose uptake and subsequently insulin release by the β-cell.[32] The affinity of GLUT-2 transporter for glucose is low (K_m 20–66 mM)[33,34] and hence it has the ability to mediate cellular glucose uptake or release over a large range of physiological glucose concentration. Experimental studies in animal models have shown marked effect of glucose concentration on GLUT expression in β-cells. Prolonged hypoglycemia resulted in a complete loss of GLUT-2 mRNA expression in pancreatic islets, whereas prolonged hyperglycemia increased GLUT-2 mRNA levels by 46%.[35,36] It has also been demonstrated that loss of β-cell expression of GLUT-2 is reversible and can be induced by a diabetic environment.[37]

GLUT-1 transporter is found in all tissues, and has an important role to play in noninsulin sensitive tissues such as the brain. GLUT-4 on the other hand, is the predominant transporter for insulin sensitive tissues such as the skeletal muscle and the adipocyte.

GLUT-2 and GLUT-4 are potential candidates for involvement in the pathogenesis of defective glucose induced insulin secretion and impaired insulin action in glucose metabolism in type 2 diabetes. A few polymorphisms of GLUT genes have been detected, but they are not of great clinical significance.[32,38-42] As yet we are unable to clearly define the role of glucose transporters in the etiology of diabetes mellitus. However, studies have taught us that they undergo regulation at pre- and post-translation levels in a subtype and tissue specific manner. The regulatory factors include age, diet, exercise, hormones and metabolites. To gain further insight into this field, the intermediaries between such promoters and transacting elements need to be explored.[32]

SELF-MONITORING OF BLOOD GLUCOSE AND GLUCOSE SENSORS

To develop a nontraumatic glucose sensor has been a high priority. A large number of investigators are using different technologies to be able to achieve this aim. Noninvasive glucose sensing technologies currently being developed involve either radiation or fluid extraction. With radiation technology an energy beam is: (1) Applied to the body, (2) Modified proportionate to the amount of glucose in blood, and (3) Measured. The blood glucose concentration is then calculated. The most promising of these approaches are:

- Near-infrared light spectroscopy
- Far-infrared radiation spectroscopy
- Radiowave impedance
- Rotation of polarized light.

The fluid extraction technology employs the principle of extracting a body fluid containing glucose (from skin) either by reverse iontophoresis or by near noninvasive insertion of micro-cannula and the glucose is estimated in the transcutaneous intestinal fluid. The technologies involved are:

- Fluid extraction from skin (reverse iontophoresis)
- Interstitial fluid harvesting.

Currently, each method has features predictive of commercial viability as well as technical problems, which have yet to be overcome. A diabetes watch has already been developed by Cygnus therapeutic systems and is in wide use. In not so distant future invasive (capillary/finger prick) monitoring of blood sugar will be a thing of the past.[43-45] Till then, for brittle or labile diabetics and for those who are on insulin pumps a continuous glucose monitoring system (CGMS) can be used periodically to determine the cause of very high or very low blood glucose. A sensor is placed subcutaneously for this purpose; the sensor estimates the interstitial fluid glucose level continuously, in the form of an ionic charge. This is automatically calibrated to fine blood glucose values by feeding 4 to 6 blood glucose values determined by a blood glucose meter during the monitoring period. More recently, this system has been upgraded to give real-time blood glucose values. The real-time blood glucose system has been also linked to an open-loop insulin pump.

THERAPY OF DIABETES

Diet, exercise, oral hypoglycemic agents, insulin and patient education continue to remain the mainstay of treatment of diabetes. For nearly five to six decades sulfonylureas, biguanides and insulin remained the cornerstones of diabetic management. The nineties and especially the last decade has seen the emergence of new classes of drugs, ranging from the antihyperglycemics such as acarbose and thiazolidinediones to the hypoglycemic drugs like nonsulfonylurea β-cell

---

TABLE 95.1 | Fat replacers

Fat mimetics

Agents belonging to other macronutrient categories
- *Carbohydrates*: Starch, cellulose, gums, dextrins
- *Proteins*: Whey, zein, microparticulated egg, milk proteins

Low calorie fats (less than 9 kcal/gm)
- Medium chain triglycerides (8 kcal/gm)
- Caprenin (5 kcal/gm)
- Salatrim (5 kcal/gm)

Fat substitutes (nonabsorbable fats)
- Olestra
- Sorbestrin
- Esterified propoxylated glycerolesters (EPGs)

---

agonists (meglitinide group of drugs), designer insulins (Lispro, Aspart, Glargine and Detemir insulin) and inhaled insulin. Many more promising drugs are in the wings and are likely to be in commercial use very soon.

Diet Therapy

Reduction of dietary fat is the single most important tool in the control of obesity and diabetes. Today, we have a large number of fat mimetics, low calorie fats and fat substitutes **(Table 95.1)**. More are in the developmental stages. These substances will drastically reduce calories without sacrificing the organoleptic properties of foods.

Fat Replacers

These can be divided into three types:
1. Fat mimetics
2. Low calorie fats
3. Fat substitutes.

Fat mimetics are materials belonging to other macronutrient categories, i.e. carbohydrates or proteins, which replace the bulk, body and taste of fats. Examples include starch, cellulose, gums, and dextrins amongst carbohydrates, and whey, zein, microparticulated egg and milk proteins amongst proteins. These mimetics are digestible but are less energy dense than fats and as these are hydrated, the caloric reduction is even greater due to dilution. These are generally used for hydrated products such as desserts and spreads. They do not have adverse effects but suffer from sizeable sensory and functional limitations as general fat replacers and cannot be used as a frying media and finally have a short shelf-life.[46,47]

Low calorie fats include triglycerides that are chemically altered to become less energy dense, i.e. to provide fewer than 9 kcal/day. Examples are medium chain triglycerides (MCT), caprenin and salatrim. Medium chain triglycerides are made up of 8 to 12 carbon fatty acids that provide 8 kcal/g. They are rapidly absorbed from the portal bloodstream and provide a small caloric advantage, but a larger metabolic advantage.

Caprenin is a triglyceride in which two fatty acids are medium chain fatty acids (caprylic and capric) and the third is behenic acid. The latter is poorly absorbed and thus caprenin provides 5 kcal/kg. Salatrim is a randomized triglyceride containing short- and long-chain fatty acids. The short-chain fatty acids are acetic, propionic and butyric while the long-chain fatty acid is stearic. The stearic acid is poorly absorbed. The caloric value of salatrim is also 5 kcal/g.[46,47]

Fat substitutes are materials that have the properties of fats and oils, but are not absorbed or metabolized by the body. Examples include olestra, sorbestrin and esterified propoxylated glycerol esters (EPGs). Sucrose polyester or olestra is a mixture of hexa-, hepta- and octa-fatty acids of sucrose. The fatty acid distribution can range from 8 to 22 carbon fatty acids, either saturated or unsaturated. This allows for the formation of various sucrose polyesters ranging from a liquid to plastic to hard fat. Olestra is neither digested nor absorbed in the human body, thus its caloric value is close to zero. The other advantage is that it keeps its fat like qualities when heated and has a good flavor. Olestra reduces the absorption of fat-soluble vitamins and can cause malabsorption like syndrome. Studies have shown it to be efficacious in obesity and hyperlipidemia.[48,49] Sorbestrin, like olestra is indigestible. It is a hexa-fatty acid ester of sorbitol and does not provide any calories.

EPGs are made from naturally occurring fats with propylene oxide inserted between glycerol and fatty acids. Any fat can be altered to its EPG counterpart. These also have a zero caloric value and have the attendant problem of malabsorption of fat and fat-soluble vitamins.[46]

A dietary supplement containing soya protein with fiber and isoflavones reduced LDL-cholesterol, triglycerides and homocysteine and improved the LDL/HDL ratio.[50] Such dietary supplements can be used in lipid management in type 2 diabetes. Omega-3 fatty acid supplementation was demonstrated to have a cardioprotective effect as early as 4 months of therapy; hence, the mechanism seems to be antiarrhythmogenic.[51] A meta-analysis of randomized controlled trials of low glycemic-index diets revealed a small (lowering of HbA$_{1c}$ by 0.43%), yet clinically important influence on glycemic control.[52] The resting energy expenditure declines on hypocaloric diets, but to a less extent when a low glycemic index diet is used for weight reduction.[53] By using activity and nutrition control in obese patients, number of prescription indications was reduced and quality of life improved in 7 out of 9 domains.[54]

Exercise Therapy

Exercise continues to be recognized as an important aspect of obesity management. It promoted loss of body weight and fat in a group of obese postmenopausal women.[55] In morbidly obese subjects, exercise reduced the intramyocellular fat content, a factor responsible for enhanced insulin sensitivity.[56] Behavior modification is key to success in promoting diet adherence. Hence, increasing research will be conducted in this area in the near future.

With self-monitoring of blood glucose, safety of exercise therapy has increased considerably. The physiology of both aerobic and anaerobic exercise is now well understood. In future, indigenous exercise forms, like *Yoga* and *Pranayam* are going to be studied in detail in the management of the IGT and diabetes. The Research Society for the Study of Diabetes in India has mounted a collaborative study in the year 2006, where *Yoga* and fenugreek powder are the two study arms for prevention of type 2 diabetes. The results of this study will be of great importance towards the planning of preventive strategies in India. The behavior modification strategies are again very important in exercise adherence; hence new research in this area will be highly fruitful.

Oral Drugs and Insulin Therapy

Postprandial Glucose Regulation

Postprandial state (meals and postmeal periods) covers about 66% of the day's duration and is characterized by glucose and other nutrient influx into the blood. Postprandial hyperglycemia can be an early feature of glucose intolerance but can further deteriorate into fasting hyperglycemia and be associated with coagulation activation and/or lipid abnormalities, the latter being considered as cardiovascular risk factors, even in nondiabetic population. Thus, the need and search for effective postprandial glycemia regulators is now gaining paramount importance. Short-acting insulin analogs (Lispro and Aspart insulin), nonsulfonylurea prandial regulators such as repaglinide and nateglinide

and α-glucosidase inhibitors such as acarbose, miglitol and voglibose are already available for control of postprandial hyperglycemia. However, a search for more effective and specific regulators is ongoing.

Correction of Insulin Pulsatility and First Phase Insulin Secretion

Restoration of insulin pulsatility and the ultradian rhythm in type 2 diabetes and IGT would be an ideal method of regularizing postprandial hyperglycemia.[57-60] To date, no agents have been discovered which could restore these physiological phenomena. However, the loss of first phase insulin secretion (the hallmark of β-cell dysfunction in type 2 diabetes and IGT) could be to some extent replaced by usage of the fast-acting insulin analogs. Rapid progress has been made in this field and Lispro and Aspart insulins are already in commercial use. Aerosol insulin has undergone extensive trials and is now available for use in many countries.[61] This could be an effective agent for replacing first phase insulin secretion and could be useful for all types of diabetes.

A whole new vista has been opened with the development of nonsulfonylureas, benzoic acid derivatives and the meglitinide series. The first amongst these is repaglinide and many more analogs such as mitiglinide (KAO 122a) and senaglinide (A-4166) are undergoing clinical evaluation. These short acting, ultrafast, insulin secretagogues, cause rapid release of insulin from β-cells and thus help reduce postprandial hyperglycemia. A recently published study[62] reported that repaglinide amplifies insulin secretory burst mass and basal secretion, with no change in burst frequency. Perhaps we are now entering into the era of control over insulin pulsatility.

A-4166, 9N-trans-isopropyl (cyclohexyl-carbonyl-phenylalanine), a phenylalanine analog, stimulates meal-related insulin release and decreases post-prandial hyperglycemia. This agent shows promise as a postprandial glycemic regulator.[63]

Morphilinoguanidine compounds (BTS 67582) act on a site different form the sulfonylurea receptor at the β-cell. They may have a role in control of postprandial hyperglycemia.[63]

Reduction of Carbohydrate and Fat Absorption

More gradual and slow absorption of nutrients, especially carbohydrates will prevent postprandial glucose rise. A diet rich in complex carbohydrates and fiber will definitely help. However, in most cases, this measure is not adequate by itself. The α-glucosidase inhibitors effectively delay the absorption of complex carbohydrates and sucrose. Acarbose and miglitol are already in clinical use and voglibose is likely to be available shortly. These drugs also affect the energy expenditure, diet-induced thermogenesis and alter the respiratory quotient. However, the limiting factor is that this group of drugs has a minimal effect on HbA_{1c} in long-term users (approx 0.5%).[64]

Orlistat is a pancreatic lipase inhibitor, which produces a 30% reduction in fat absorption at a dose of 120 mg three times daily. This leads to a clinically significant weight loss in obese subjects during continuous treatment. Additionally, by interfering with fat absorption, it has a salutary effect on postprandial glucose concentrations by reducing the nutrient load.[65]

Insulin Biosynthesis and Secretion

Attempts are being made to treat the defects of glucose sensing mechanisms (GLUT-2) and proinsulin biosynthesis and processing by the β-cells by pharmacological means. But these are currently in a very preliminary stage of development. Succinate esters are potential agents.[63]

Potentiators of Insulin Secretion and Action through Enteroinsular Axis

The study of the enteroinsular axis and the incretins has gained importance in the search for postprandial glycemic control. Molecular targets now include the various hormones and peptides interacting with insulin synthesis and release, glucagon suppression or release, and hepatic glucose production.

Peptides affecting gastric emptying and interfering with glucose absorption have also gained prominence. Putative agents include glucagon-like peptide-1 (GLP-1), calcitonin gene-related peptide (CGRP), Glucose dependent insulinotropic polypeptide (GIP), pancreatic polypeptide (PP), gastrin, amylin, galanin, and somatostatin. **Table 95.2** lists the putative targets and drugs undergoing trials for containing postprandial hyperglycemia.[66-70]

A large number of agents are being developed which enhance nutrient-induced insulin secretion and these agents have several putative targets within the β-cell. The most prominent of these are glucagon-like peptide-1 (GLP-1) and its congeners. Additionally, drugs that inhibit destruction of GLP by dipeptidyl-peptidase (DPP inhibitors) are highly promising. Liraglutide—a GLP-analog and sitagliptin, saxagliptin or denagliptin

TABLE 95.2	Molecular targets for control of pre- and postprandial hyperglycemia

- A. *Insulin pulsatility, ultradian rhythm and first phase insulin secretion*
    Short-acting insulin analogs (Lispro, Aspart)
    Aerosol insulin
    Rapid-acting insulin secretagogues
        Meglitinides
            Repaglinide
            Nateglinide
            Senaglinide
            Morphilinoguanide
                BTS 67582
    B. *Insulin biosynthesis and secretion*
        Succinate ester
- Reduction of carbohydrate and fat absorption
    Ingestion of complex carbohydrate meals and fiber
    α-glucosidase inhibitors (Acarbose, miglitol, voglibose)
    Biguanides
    Orlistat (pancreatic lipase inhibitor)
- *Potentiators of insulin secretion and action through enteroinsular axis*
    GLP-1 and analogs
    Phosphodiesterase inhibitors
    Imidazoline derivatives PMS 812 (S21663)
    Amylin agonist (Pramlintide)
    Glucagon receptor antagonist BAY 27-9955
- *Reducing hepatic glucose output*
    Biguanides
    GLP-1
- Reduction of peripheral insulin resistance
    Insulinomimetic agents
        Vanadium salts
        IGF–1
        PPAR-γ agonists: Thiazolidinediones
            Troglitazone
            Rosiglitazone
            Pioglitazone
    PPAR-γ agonists: Nonthiazolidinediones
        G 1262570X[GG 570]
        D-chiro-inositol
    Retinoid X receptor agonists
    Biguanides
    Antiobesity drugs
        Orlistat
        Sibutramine

which are DPP inhibitors are undergoing phase IV trials and are about to be marketed for clinical use.

Glucagon-like peptide-1 (GLP-1) is a potent gut hormone, which stimulates meal-related insulin release from the β-cell. Additionally, it suppresses glucagon release, has insulinomimetic effects on gluconeogenesis in the liver and muscles and on lipogenesis in the adipose tissues. It further reduces postprandial hyperglycemia by delaying gastric emptying. Hence, GLP-1 is perhaps the most potent activator of first phase insulin secretion. It has further beneficial effects by suppression of hepatic neoglucogenesis and increased peripheral glucose disposal. It does not cause hypoglycemia, as the insulin release is glucose dependent. Due to its very short duration of action, various GLP-1 receptor agonists (Exendin 4), inhibitors of GLP-1 deactivation and its GLP-1 analogs are all under development, to find a suitable long-acting agent.[66,68,71-74]

Exendin-4, a long-acting agonist of GLP-1 receptor reduces fasting and postprandial glucose and reduces energy-intake in healthy volunteers.[75] GLP-1 enhances noninsulin mediated glucose uptake in elderly diabetics.[76] Another important incretin, glucose-dependent insulinotropic peptide (GIP) is also degraded by dipeptidyl-peptidase IV (DPP IV). Hence, inhibitors of DPP IV like valine-pyrrolidide enhanced the effectiveness of GIP.[77] Physiological doses of GLP-1 stimulate glucose-induced insulin secretion in a linear fashion.[78] Chronic inhibition of DPP IV delays the onset of diabetes in male Zucker fatty rats.[79] GLP-1 suppresses glucagons levels, yet there is no significant effect on glucose counter-regulation.[80] Impaired GLP-1 and gastric inhibitory polypeptide (GIP) response is associated with insulin resistance and maybe another biochemical feature of IGT.[81] GLP-1 inhibits cell apoptosis of isolated human islet cell and enhances their glucose responsiveness.[82] Chronic DPP-IV inhibition improves metabolic control in type 2 diabetes.[83] A combination of GLP-1 and pioglitazone produces an additional glucose lowering effect in type 2 diabetics.[84] Exenatide significantly decreases HbA_{1c} in diabetics not responding to maximal doses of sulfonylurea.[85] Based upon these studies, orally effective DPP-IV inhibitors, like sitagliptin or saxagliptin have been developed and are entering the therapeutics arena.

Phosphodiesterase inhibitors and imidazoline derivatives PMS 812 (S-21663) also enhance meal-related insulin secretion and are potential candidates for postprandial glycemic regulation.[63]

Amylin suppresses insulin secretion and action. An amylin antagonist (IAPP 8-37) has been developed and has been found to stimulate insulin secretion.[86,87] On the other hand amylin agonist, pramlintide slows gastric emptying and suppresses glucagon secretion. These too may have a role to play in achieving postprandial glycemic control.[88,89]

Potential incretins include CGRP, PP and GIP. CGRP[8-37] causes a dose dependent release of GLP-1. Galanin on the other hand inhibits its release. GIP is a potent insulin secretagogue.[70] Glucagon antagonists and receptor blockers are also under development. BAY 27-9955 is a nonpeptide glucagon receptor blocker and has shown promise in animal studies.[90] Researchers are targeting various agonists and antagonists of the hormones or their receptors as potential postprandial glucose regulators.

Biguanides have predominant action through suppression of hepatic glucose output and hepatic neoglucogenesis. They have a more pronounced effect on postprandial glucose concentrations than on fasting hyperglycemia. Thus, they too form a part of postprandial regulators.[24]

Suppression of Hepatic Glucose Output

The liver is a major player in the postprandial state and about 10 to 20% of ingested glucose is retained within the liver in the first pass.[91,92] Furthermore, it is the suppression of hepatic neoglucogenesis mediated by insulin, GLP-1 and some other incretins, which prevents the postprandial glucose surge. Suppression of glucagon is an important part of this phenomenon. If this were to be deficient, about 20 g of glucose load will be added at each meal. Potent suppressors of hepatic glucose release include the biguanides, BAY 27-995, a nonpeptide glucagon receptor inhibitor may have a similar action.[91]

Peripheral Insulin Resistance

Broadly, these can be grouped into insulinomimetic drugs and insulin sensitizers.

Vanadium salts such as orthovanadate, metavanadate and peroxovanadium, have been demonstrated to have insulinomimetic effects on adipocytes, hepatocytes and skeletal muscles. They produce hypoglycemia in both hyperinsulinemic and hypoinsulinemic models of diabetes. They act by a mechanism independent of insulin and near-euglycemia is achieved in animal models, in a couple of weeks. They act by increasing phosphorylation of insulin receptor sites (nitrogen-activated protein kinase and cytosolic insulin independent tyrosine kinase). Importantly, these salts are also effective in situations where the insulin signal transduction pathway is defective. These salts have an anorectic effect and thus an additional benefit is weight loss in type 2 diabetes. The major drawbacks are gastrointestinal intolerance and their mitogenic potential.

These compounds hold promise for the future and may be excellent postprandial regulators.[60,88,93]

Insulin-like growth factor-1 (IGF-1) is a member of the growth family and has a structural homology with proinsulin. In addition to its major function of mediating growth and mitogenic activities of growth hormone, it has insulinomimetic activities on the skeletal muscle and the adipocyte. These activities are mediated through the insulin and IGF-1 receptor, which have considerable homology in the quaternary structure and the amino acid sequences of their α- and β-subunits. IGF-1 is now readily available through recombinant technology and has the remarkable feature of reversing insulin resistance (observed especially in type A insulin resistance). It is effective in a single or twice a day dosage and has a good potential for treatment of type 2 diabetes. IGF-1 analogs are designed to annul the mitogenic and growth promoting activities of IGF-1. IGF-1 receptor agonists are also under development which maybe action-specific, have a prolonged duration of action and perhaps be used by the oral route.[60,88]

Insulin Sensitizers

All insulin sensitizers have a great potential for use as postprandial regulators. They can be broadly divided into the thiazolidinediones (rosiglitazone, pioglitazone, troglitazone) which are PPAR-γ receptor agonists, newer nonthiazolidinediones PPAR-γ receptor agonists such as G 1262570 X (GG 570) and D-chiro-inositol[60,88] and the retinoid X receptor agonists.[94] These drugs lower insulin resistance and have great potential for postprandial regulation. In experimental animal retinas, rosiglitazone inhibits retinal neovascularization by a mechanism that is mostly downstream of vascular endothelial growth factor expression.[95] Pioglitizone-induced weight gain is associated with an increase in the subcutaneous fat and a decrease in the visceral fat.[96] Thiazolidinediones increase the uptake of fatty acids in the skeletal muscle of type 2 diabetics.[97] Rosiglitazone entrains high frequency insulin pulsatability in β-cells of type 2 diabetics.[98] Pioglitizone can be combined with metformin in type 2 diabetes.[99] Rosiglitazone alone or in combination with insulin enhances adiponectin levels in obesity, which may account for its insulin sensitizing and anti-inflammatory properties.[100] Oral rosiglitazone is safe in post-transplant patients, as it does not alter serum creatinine, cyclosporin or tacrolimus levels and produces safe and effective blood glucose control.[101] Pioglitazone exerts a protective effect on the murine

pancreatic islet structure and secretory function, thus has a role in the prevention or progression of type 2 diabetes.[102] The newer generation drugs may be able to overcome the limitations of weight gain and have a more favorable impact on the lipid profile. Retinoid X receptor agonists hold this promise by their effect on both PPAR-α and PPAR-γ receptors. Ragaglitazar has a dual effect on PPAR-γ and PPAR-α receptors and has pronounced effect on both the blood glucose and lipids.[103]

Designer (Newer) Insulins

From the days of Banting and Best, insulin therapy held a lot of promise. For many decades, clinicians fretted with problems related to inadequate glycemic control, insulin allergy, lipoatrophy, lipohypertrophy, hyperinsulinemia, brittle diabetes, insulin resistance and the ever omnipresent, hypoglycemia. We are still not able to deliver insulin intraperitoneally, the physiological route. The ideal replacement for loss of first phase insulin secretion and the ideal basal insulin delivery has yet to be achieved. Human insulin has been with us for more than a decade, but it has yet not obviated many of our problems in achieving a good glycemic control.

It is in this setting that the designer insulins are coming to the fore. The advent of the fast-acting insulin analogs (Lispro and Aspart) has made first phase insulin replacement possible.[104-106] Use of Lispro and Aspart insulin in situations such as brittle diabetes, insulin resistance and its use in insulin pumps has already started and has shown good results. Although Lispro and Aspart insulin regulate postprandial glucose levels more effectively, the blood glucose rise before the next meal is exaggerated with their use. This is because of the fact that their peak effect is at 30 to 60 minutes and the effect wears off in about two hours. In order to obviate this problem, it is suggested that human NPH insulin be used in small dosage with each dose of Lispro or Aspart insulin. We will soon have *reverse split insulins* available with 70 to 80% of Lispro or Aspart and 20 to 30% of NPH insulin.

Numerous basal analogs have been developed, of which glargine insulin (Lantus) and detemir (Levemir) is already in commercial use. These insulins provide a smooth 24-hour basal effect without any sharp peak.[107-109] However, these analogs are required to be administered parenterally, in a separate injection. Glargine can be administered at any time of the day, unlike the original recommendation that it be administered at bedtime.[110] Glargine was compared to NPH insulin in a treat-to-target study.[111] In this study, fasting blood glucose goal of 100 mg/dl was pursued aggressively. The incidence of nocturnal hypoglycemia was much less in the glargine group as compared to NPH group.

Nonparenteral insulin delivery has always been a dream for the patient; perhaps the only barrier to insulin therapy is its parenteral mode of delivery. Pulmonary aerosol insulin delivery is now a reality. Only about 10 to 15% of it is absorbed, but it is effective. Inhaled insulin (Exubera) is administered either in tablet form or liquid after being aerosolized in a small, mechanically powered inhaler. It has been shown to have similar time action profile as Lispro or Aspart insulin.[61] A head-on comparison of inhaled insulin with SC injected insulin showed same degree of metabolic control and frequency of hypoglycemia. The coefficient of variation of insulin action is same or slightly better with inhaled insulin as compared to the subcutaneously injected insulin. Inhaled insulin is well tolerated and does not significantly alter pulmonary function tests, spirometry, lung volumes and diffusion capacity.[112] However, lung functions need to be monitored and those demonstrating unusual reduction in lung function after 1 to 3 months of inhaled insulin use should be switched back to subcutaneous insulin. Thus, inhaled insulin in multiple doses combined with a single injection of glargine or detemir insulin may constitute the most convenient form of insulin therapy in the near future. Insulin delivery by other routes, such as ophthalmic, nasal, rectal, and skin has not been very successful so far. The development of hexyl-insulin, which can be taken orally, has shown some promise. With unlimited amounts of human insulin now available through recombinant biological techniques, insulin supply is no more a problem. Hence, even if absorption is limited to less than 15 to 20%, nonparenteral insulin delivery is likely to be commercially viable.

Insulin therapy has been shown to be highly beneficial in critically ill patients.[113] Maintaining blood glucose at or below 110 mg/dl reduced morbidity and mortality (8% with conventional therapy, 4.6% with intensive therapy) in critically ill patients. Intensive insulin therapy helped maximally in patients with multiple organ failure with septic shock. It also reduced bloodstream infections by 46%, acute renal failure by 41% and critical care polyneuropathy by 44%.

Insulin Pumps

The currently available insulin pumps are the open loop system where after blood glucose values are sensed, the patient or his/her doctor, orders the delivery of the required amount of insulin. These pumps were plagued by problems of pump failure and pump runaway, but the modern day pumps are free of such problems.

The newer closed loop systems under development obviate the need of patient/doctor intervention. These devices are termed as implanted insulin pumps (IIP) and are implanted subcutaneously. The catheter is placed intraperitoneally to provide a continuous intraperitoneal insulin delivery. After the initial programming, an implantable (permanent) glucose sensor detects the concurrent blood glucose values, the information is sent to the computer (teleradiometry), which then decides the insulin dosage to be delivered automatically and completes the function by directing the pump to deliver the insulin. The major limitation in this system has been to find a reliable glucose sensor, which can function within the body systems for at least a couple of years. Sensors under development, use technologies such as enzymatic, optical, intravenous placement, reverse iontophoresis and microdialysis. Currently, the life of implanted glucose sensor measures only in weeks and months due to many technological problems such as inflammatory response and fibrous tissue formation. With ongoing advances in research and technology, the dream of having a permanent implanted device like the cardiac pacemaker, should only be a few years away. In the meanwhile, patients have to be content with an open loop, insulin pump coupled with a real-time blood glucose monitoring system (Medtronic Guardian). Patient well trained with insulin/food algorithms can utilize this system to achieve excellent metabolic control.

Pancreatic and Islet Transplants

Transplanting a healthy pancreas into a person with diabetes can restore normal blood sugar levels and prevent diabetic complications without the need for insulin injections. Yet transplanting the whole pancreas is a traumatic and complex procedure, so researchers are trying to just transplant the islets of Langerhans. Though a large number of islet transplants have been performed (including fetal islet transplants), problems continue to plague success, as potentially toxic immunosuppressive drugs have to be given to the patients to prevent the recipient's immune system from destroying the islets and their survival is usually for a short duration of months to a couple of years. Today most islet transplants are done in conjunction with renal transplants because these patients are on immuno-suppression anyway. In such instances, the survival of kidney takes the prime priority and the survival of islet cells assumes secondary importance. There is no reason to restrict the benefit of islet transplantation to patients with renal failure alone. Any patient with diabetes should be able to benefit from this procedure. Currently, researchers are focusing on solitary islet cell transplants. They also face the problem of immune rejection. It is already established that the immunosuppressive drugs used for renal transplant are not effective in suppressing the immune response against islets. Researchers are thus developing other safer immunotherapies.[114,115] Successful pancreatic transplant can improve macrovascular disease significantly. In a group of 25 type 1 diabetics successfully transplanted (HbA$_{1c}$ <6.5%, creatinine <2.4 mg/dl), the carotid intima media thickness (IMT) reduced significantly. The IMT compared with those diabetics having diabetes for six years or lesser duration.[116] Pancreatic transplant alone are not justified as compared to pancreas and kidney transplant undertaken simultaneously.[117]

Two experimental studies now head the list. The first is *mixed bone marrow chimerism*. This involves reconstituting the recipient's immune system using a bone marrow transplant partly from the recipient himself and partly from the organ donor. This appears not only to render the transplant recipient tolerant to tissue from an outside donor, but it also appears to overcome auto-immunity. This approach has been used successfully in animals for years. The other approach is *costimulatory blockade*, which stops the body's attack on its own β-cells. Antigens on the transplanted β-cells are taken up by antigen presenting cells in the bloodstream, which present these antigens to the T-cells in order to activate them or turn them on against the donor β-cells. This is not possible unless another step takes place. Other proteins on the antigen presenting cells have to interact with certain proteins on the T-cells, a process termed as *costimulation*. By blocking this interaction and by preventing the costimulation from occurring, the attack on the β-cell can be prevented.[114,115]

One of these, two approaches may come to the fore in the near future. However, there are about a dozen or more approaches under experimental study and we never know which one of these may prove to be more promising.

Genetically engineered β-cells offer a wide variety of approaches towards the β-cell transplantation. There are many kinds of genes, which when expressed, slowdown the immune response against the β-cells in type 1 diabetes. If β-cells were to be made invisible to the T-cells, an immune reaction would not occur and the β-cells would be safe from destruction. Class I antigens on the surface of β-cells attract the attention of the immune system. By inserting certain genes into the β-cells, one would regulate or decrease the expression of these class I antigens and make them less of a target.

Genetic manipulation would enable β-cells to send out *missiles* to modify or destroy the invading T-cells. Cells of the immune system communicate with each other by using *messenger proteins* called cytokines. Some cytokines promote inflammatory disease that destroys β-cells, while others appear to downregulate or slowdown the inflammatory process. β-cells could be genetically manipulated to produce these protective cytokines in order to slowdown the disease process.

Another type of missile would be a protein that blocks costimulation of the T-cells. Researchers have already been successful in manipulations rat β-cells to produce a costimulatory blocking protein CTL-4Ig, which greatly prolongs their survival when transplanted into mice. A third approach is to make the β-cells sturdier, scientists have now understood several important steps in the destruction of β-cells and have identified certain substances and genes that slowdown the process of destruction.[118-120] A different approach is, to block the costimulatory response by using special antibodies called anti-CD-40 ligand. Vaccination with either insulin or a protein called GAD65 has been shown to be successful in protecting the β-cells against type 1 diabetes in rodents.[121,122]

A critical limitation for islet or pancreatic transplant is that not nearly enough human islets are available for the prospective number of patients. Experimenters are now exploring the use of islets from other species (especially pigs), but again they have to surmount the problem of immune rejection. The rejection response in xenotransplantation (transplant from another species) is particularly severe.

To prevent this problem a technique known as *immunoisolation* is being developed.[123] Porcine (pig) islets are put into slabs of alginate, a semipermeable membrane derived from seaweed. This alginate membrane is designed to allow nutrients and oxygen to pass from the bloodstream into the islets and to allow insulin to flow from the islets to the bloodstream. At the same time, components of the immune system, such as T-cells are prevented from coming into contact with the porcine transplanted islets thus preventing an immune response against them.[124]

Surrogate β-cells, is another approach. Other cells in the body are altered by molecular biology to act as β-cells. The advantage of this approach is that there will be no immune reaction against such cells as they are from the patient himself. The goal is to alter them to act as much as possible like normal β-cells, sensing the blood sugar levels and responding by secreting appropriate amounts of insulin. One such cell line AtT-20-ins, has been made by altering pituitary cells by addition of genetic material for a molecule which produces GLUT-2 (a known glucose transporter). This cell line responds to glucose in blood by secreting more insulin. More attractive candidates maybe muscle and skin cells, but these cells are unable to package insulin into secretory granules. How to make these cells produce secretory granules is one of the current challenges.[124,125]

Perhaps the best surrogate cell would be the β-cell itself, if it could be induced to replicate and grow. Unfortunately, β-cells once removed from the body do not expand or grow. You can use them for transplant, but cannot be used to solve the problem of supplying cells for millions of people with diabetes. Yet β-cells can be transformed or *immortalized* so that they can constantly reproduce. This feat is accomplished by using oncogenes (genes causing cancer).[125] Recently, researchers began work on insulin producing cell line from rodents called RIN 1046-38. They have been able to place genes for human insulin, GLUT-2 and glucokinase (one of the glucose sensors) into RIN 1408-38 T-cells, so that they act similarly to human β-cells in several aspects. Unfortunately, even, if this cell line is made to behave more like human β-cells, still it will be a xenotransplant and face immune rejection as pig cells. Currently, there are no documented human β-cell lines, but recent investigations show a lot of promise .The status of islet cell transplantation has been comprehensively reviewed.[126]

Stem cells appear as the most promising source of islet cells. Besides the embryonic stem cells, the most exciting development has been the discovery of adult, differentiated cells, especially the pancreatic ductal cells which are capable of differentiating into β-cells. The ductal cells are functional precursor cells, which when stimulated by various growth factors, expand into cultivated human islet buds.[127] This can expand availability of islet cells and also make cultivation of islets from patients own ductal cells.

COMPLICATIONS OF DIABETES

Recent research has led to the discovery of many interlinking mechanisms, which lead to the manifestations of diabetic complications. The discovery of receptor for advanced glycation endproducts (RAGE) receptors and the macrophage receptors has given us an understanding about how glucotoxicity occurs. The many paracrine and endocrine factors that are a link to endothelial damage are being daily discovered. Similarly, better understanding of oxidative and carbonyl stress in diabetes, genesis of lipid abnormalities and the genetic predisposition along with vasoactive factors and hemodynamic factors, have been developed. These developments are bound to have far reaching therapeutic implications. RAGE blockers and AGE lytics are examples.[128-131] A study in normal twins has shown that the level of an advanced glycation end product (carboxymethyl lysine) is genetically determined and is independent of genes affecting fasting glucose or HbA_{1c}.[132] Similarly, the discovery that angiostatin is the endocrine mediator of the benefits of laser photocoagulation may lead to pharmacological prevention of retinopathy.[132] Better understanding of neuropathy has led to the development of nerve growth factor (NGF) as a possible therapeutic agent. Similarly, a lot of research has been centered on finding early markers for diabetic complications. Intimal medial thickness (IMT) and microalbuminuria are now universally accepted as markers of macroangiopathy. Na/Li countertransport dysfunction is a molecular marker. Interest is again been generated in using the skeletal muscle basement membrane as a marker. Homocysteine levels correlate with the glycemic control in type 2 diabetes, thus suggesting yet another mechanism by which poor glycemic control may produce vascular complications.[133] Analysis of DCCT date has shown that a biologic variation in HbA_{1c} level between individual patients, which is distinct from the variation attributable to mean blood glucose level, was a strong predictor of vascular complications.[134] The control of risk factors and comorbidities is important for the prevention of vascular complications but the real-life situation shows that much needs to be done in this regards.[135] Increased oxidative stress is an important mechanism of vascular complications, but antioxidant supplements have been disappointing while antioxidants in natural form in vegetables, fruits and whole grains are effective.[136] Control of cardiovascular risk factors and comorbid conditions has a huge impact on the cardiovascular complications. Our ability to control hypertension is improving continuously and achieving target values without producing distressing postural hypotension is possible. Control of obesity improves glycemia almost pari passu with weight reduction. We do not yet have very effective antiobesity drugs, but this situation will improve soon. Besides sibutramine and xenical, cannabinoides hold a great promise. Control of hyperlipidemia has improved considerably; the combination of a statin with a newer fibric acid derivative like fenofibrate has been approved. This is required in many diabetics with dyslipidemia, because both high LDL-cholesterol and high triglycerides, more commonly the latter, is the commonest form of dyslipidemia seen in diabetics. Raising HDL-cholesterol is as yet a difficult proposition, but nicotinic acid has shown some efficacy in this regard. Hyperhomocysteinemia is not seen frequently, but is eminently treatable. In females, postmenopausal women, hormone replacement therapy should not be considered for the prevention of ischemic heart disease. It has been proven amply by Women's Health Initiate Study that it is not a good option.[137]

Ischemic Heart Disease

This is the commonest clinical manifestation of macrovascular disease. Physical activity can reduce the risk for cardiovascular events in diabetic women.[138] Relative risk for cardiovascular events was 0.52 in those women who engaged in 7 hours/week of moderate to vigorous physical activity.[138] Coronary artery calcification scores are higher in diabetics as compared to nondiabetic controls.[139] Contrary to the often quoted study of Haffner,[140] a study from Scotland[141] showed that the nondiabetics with previous myocardial infarction had a 3-fold risk of repeat myocardial infarction as compared to diabetics without previous myocardial infarction. The differences between Haffner's study and the Scottish study probably arose out of different selection criteria and duration of diabetes in these studies. Alcohol has been projected as a cardioprotective substance in the studies, one in women[142] and other in men.[143] Contrary to Women's Health Initiative and HERS Study, one study showed that estrogen therapy reduces risk of cardiovascular events among women with type 2 diabetes.[144] The results of this study maybe attributed to factors governing selection of patients, whereby women having health advantage tend to use preventive medications.

The beneficial effect of lipid lowering in diabetics has been further confirmed in two studies.[145,146] It is a fact that diabetics with near normal baseline LDL-cholesterol may also benefit from atorvastatin as primary prevention. It is difficult to draw National guidelines based upon these studies and probably some more studies will clarify the situation.

The question of silent myocardial ischemia in diabetics has been looked at again.[147] It is estimated that 1 in 16 patients have large perfusion abnormalities which can only be detected by detailed noninvasive testing such as stress myocardial perfusion. The prognosis of patients with silent myocardial ischemia is similar to that for patients without a history of IHD or Q waves.[148]

Rosiglitazone has been shown to prevent restenosis after coronary stent implantation. The rate of restenosis was significantly reduced in the Rosiglitazone group compared with the control group (17.6% vs 38.2%).[149] However, such beneficial effects have to be confirmed in the long-run by using hard endpoints like reinfarction or death.

Insulin has been shown to exert an anti-inflammatory and profibrinolytic effect in acute ST-segment elevation myocardial infarction.[150] Thus, indications of insulin therapy are expanding and all critically ill diabetics or those with vascular events will continue to receive intensified insulin therapy.

Atherosclerosis and Cardiomyopathy

Research has indicated that a molecule called advanced glycation endproduct (AGE) is responsible for the aggressive, severe form of atherosclerosis seen in diabetics. This molecule is found in all people, but it accumulates rapidly in the presence of high blood glucose. AGE molecules bind to the cells and trigger of an abnormal behavior in these cells, which in-turn creates havoc in the patient with diabetes. Researchers have isolated the possible link between AGE activity and diabetes. This is the cell surface receptor termed as RAGE. This receptor is found in very high numbers in patients with diabetes. Efforts were then initiated to prevent AGE from being attached to RAGE. They have succeeded in making a decoy molecule, which soaks up the RAGE receptors and prevents AGE from reacting with it.[130-131] The result is that in diabetic animals, atherosclerosis was drastically suppressed. At present, this molecule is too big and expensive to be given to humans, but it is very likely that a suitable molecule will be discovered soon.

In addition to disease of the blood vessels, diabetes directly affects the cardiac muscle leading to diabetic cardiomyopathy, a debilitating disease that also accounts for the lower survival rates in patients with diabetes with a heart attack. Protein kinase C (PKC) is an enzyme, which is elevated in diabetics and has already been linked to both diabetic retinopathy and nephropathy. One fraction of PKC, PKC-β is specifically found to be elevated in diabetics. Workers have found that mice with excess PKC-β bred into their hearts developed severe cardiomyopathy.[151] An inhibitor of PKC-β has already been developed and is being used in patients with diabetic retinopathy. Workers have already established that PKC-β inhibitors prevent development of cardiomyopathy in mice. This has exciting potential for use in humans.[151]

Diabetic Neuropathy

Diagnosis and follow-up of diabetic neuropathy has become more accurate by systematic clinical inquiry followed by quantitative sensory testing. Activating cutaneous sensory receptors by measurable physical stimuli and studying the evoked potentials gives quantitative somatosensory function. The results are modifiable by patient's attention and motivation, yet it is possible to standardize these tests.[152] The vibration perception threshold (VPT)) is measured by a biothesiometer. A VPT greater than 25V at the foot is associated with increased risk of foot ulceration. The thermal perception threshold (TPT) signifies the function of C-fibers. Pressure perception cutaneous threshold (PPCT) is easily measured by a Semmes-Weinstein monofilament. Absence of sensation with a 10 gm filament is associated with risk of foot ulceration.

Several new research techniques have been developed for assessing peripheral nerve function. A skin punch biopsy with immunostaining with specific antibodies to human protein gene product 9.5 Substance P and calcitonin gene product peptide is a new technique. This can replace the more traumatic technique of peripheral nerve biopsy.[153] Single fiber electromyography (EM) and macro-EM has been applied in diabetic neuropathy to demonstrate deficient innervation in diabetic neuropathy.[154]

For autonomic testing, three tests continue to be used most widely; beat-to-beat variation in heartbeat; heartbeat variation during deep breathing, lying-to-standing and the Valsalva maneuver; and blood pressure response to standing. It is possible to image the myocardial sympathetic innervation by measuring the uptake of ^{123}I-metaiodobenzylguanidine (MIBG) by postganglionic fibers. This isotope is an analog of noradrenaline and its concentration can be measured by single photon emission computed tomography (SPECT). These data provide an objective quantitation of diabetic dysautonomia.[155,156]

Good glucose control can make an important difference in progression of diabetic peripheral neuropathy.[157] High blood glucose speeds-up the programmed cell death of both nerve cells and their protective covering (Schwann cells). A new family of drugs known as neurotropins or NGF has been able to reverse damaged nerve cells in patients without diabetes (e.g. cancer) and should be able to do the same in diabetics. One such neurotropin, (IgF$_1$) shows exceptional promise in the laboratory. It protects both the neurons (nerve cells) and the Schwann cells even in the presence of high blood glucose.

In diabetic rodents, deficiency of γ-linolenic acid has been demonstrated. This leads to an imbalance between the lipo-oxygenase and cyclo-oxygenase systems and consequent deficient production of vasodilatory prostaglandins. Use of GLA supplements in diabetic neuropathy in humans has only been partially successful.[157] Although aldose reductase inhibitors were theoretically expected to produce some therapeutic benefits, the results with some earlier compounds such as Sorbinil have been disappointing. A series of new aldose reductase inhibitors are now under long-term clinical trials. Anti-oxidants are also expected to confer some benefits in peripheral neuropathy. In animal studies, α-tocopherol has proved beneficial, but there is no convincing human data in this regard. Alpha-lipoic acid is another antioxidant used in diabetic neuropathy. It has undergone extensive trials in Germany[160] with fair results, as confirmed in the Adult, Learning, Documentation and Information Network (ALADIN) study.[158]

In practice, relief of pain becomes extremely important in cases of painful diabetic neuropathy. Besides glycemic control and use of tricyclic antidepressants, anticonvulsant drugs like gabapentin in dosage of 900 to 3600 mg/day, and antiarrhythmic agents like mexiletine in dosage of 10 mg/kg in three divided doses have shown some promise. At times, an opioid like tramadol will also be required. Possibility of using transcutaneous electrical nerve stimulation (TENS) need to be evaluated in greater detail, as it holds promise as a nonpharmacological measure. A new technique, where monochromatic near-infrared photoenergy was administered by an Anodyne therapy system for 6 to 12 sittings demonstrated almost 50% improvement in peripheral sensation.[159] The duration of such studies has been short, but it holds good promise for a seemingly hopeless situation.

Diabetic Retinopathy

Retinopathy due to diabetes in one of the leading causes if blindness. Currently, the proven therapies include intensive insulin therapy and photocoagulation or laser surgery for advanced disease. Researchers are now focusing on what causes retinopathy and if that process could be nipped in the bud. Cells lining the retinal blood vessel walls abut each other in tight junctions, much like tiles on a wall. Normal concentration of a protein called occludin is needed to maintain the integrity of these tight junctions. In diabetic rodents, the amount of occludin is known to be decreased by 35%.[160] However, this is not confirmed in diabetic human retina, perhaps because of methodological problems.[161] The leakage from these junctions' results into macular edema, the type of retinopathy more commonly seen in type 2 diabetes mellitus and less amenable to laser treatment. Leakage from these tight junctions is perhaps mediated by histamine. Histamine is thought to inhibit occludin, a key protein that regulates junction permeability. Occludin is greatly reduced in retinas of diabetics. Furthermore, the nerve cells in retina (neurons and glial cells) also interact with the vascular cells. Glial cells (nerve cells with connective properties) become functionally impaired in diabetics at about the same rate that occludin reduces. An antihistamine *hismanal* is being currently tried to increase the levels of occludin in retina. Results should be out by early next year. This offers hope to salvaging eyesight in diabetics.

Besides disturbance of tight junctions, there are certain abnormalities of glial cells; more specifically the Müller cells. In diabetics, these cells are known to overexpress a protein called glial fibrillary acidic protein (GFAP), which is a hallmark of *reactive astrocytosis*.[162] Müller cells express GLUT-1 and thus are affected by hyperglycemia.

The proliferative retinopathy has its genesis from retinal ischemia, the first event probably being that of a capillary closure. The pericytes as well as endothelial cells have a role in this initial event. Closure of capillaries is caused by microthrombosis[163] and leukostasis.[164] Another pathology described is of accelerated apoptosis.[165] Present data brings out the complexity of this process and involvement of a variety of cells in the retina. It is possible that many of these mechanisms work simultaneously or sequentially to produce retinopathy. When properly understood, specific treatment modalities can be developed for prevention or treatment of retinopathy.

Diabetic Nephropathy

The prevalence of nephropathy was estimated to be 30 to 40% in type 1 diabetics. This has shown a downward trend recently probably because of improved glycemic control.[166] Only about 5 to 10% of type 2 diabetics develop nephropathy, but in absolute numbers they equal or exceed type 1 diabetics.[167] In all studies, probably a small number of patients with glomerulonephritis have been included as diabetic nephropathy. With decline in the prevalence of poststreptococcal glomerulonephritis, this component of mistaken diagnosis has also diminished. Renal insufficiency in the absence of albuminuria (micro or macro) and retinopathy could be due to interstitial nephritis. This situation is known to occur in 30% of patients of renal insufficiency in type 2 diabetes.[168]

On the other hand, microalbuminuric renal insufficiency in type 2 diabetes could be nothing but diabetic nephropathy.[169] These issues are expected to be resolved only when larger studies are done with renal biopsies.

The basic pathophysiology at the level of glomerular basement membrane (GBM) consists of thickening of the GBM and increased permeability. Thickening is caused by increased deposition of the collagen with abnormal crosslinking and porosity is caused by a reduction in the strong negative charge of the endothelial cells. The GBM collagen forms crosslinking with amino acid residues like lysine. The collagen is also glycated to yield advanced glycosylation end products; these are more resistant to degradation. The diminished negative change of the glomerular endothelium results in impaired repulsion and increased passage of negatively charged molecules like albumin.

Genetic Factors in Diabetic Nephropathy

Familial clustering of diabetic nephropathy is known; thus 45% siblings of diabetics with nephropathy have chronic renal failure and other 45% have overt proteinuria. In siblings of diabetics without nephropathy, only 10% have CRF or proteinuria.[170,171] The metabolic control of diabetes is also important as evidenced by the natural history of the disease and kidney transplants from diabetic animals to nondiabetics and vice versa. Studies like DCCT have further supported the facts that glycemia is important in the development of nephropathy. Probably what is inherited is a genetic protection of development of diabetic nephropathy, because 60% of type 1 diabetics do not develop nephropathy. A type 1 diabetic who has not developed retinopathy after 20 to 25 years of diabetes is highly unlikely to develop it later on. However, he does have a very low (1% per year) chance of developing the disease. The nature of this genetic protection has been a subject of intensive study and is likely to be elucidated further in the near future. An insight into the protective genes or gene products may make prevention of diabetic nephropathy a reality.[172]

Microalbuminuria, Hyperfiltration and Diabetic Nephropathy

The importance of microalbuminuria in predicting the future development of diabetic nephropathy is well established. In order to be of predictive value, micro-albuminuria needs to be estimated on a timed urine collection or correlated with creatinine excretion. Thus, more than 20 mg/min of albumin is labeled as microalbuminuria and more than 200 mg/min as macroalbuminuria. An albumin (mcg)/creatinine (mg) ratio of less than 30 is normal, 30 to 300 is indicative of microalbuminuria and more than 300 indicative of macroalbuminuria. The methods for estimation of urinary albumin are getting accurate and faster.

Microalbuminuria is now considered an indicator of generalized endothelial disease and hence correlates well with many macrovascular diseases, like ischemic heart disease, peripheral vascular disease and stroke.[173] In another study, both microalbuminuria and proteinuria were predictive of all cause mortality in patients with type 1 diabetes of more than 30 years duration.[174]

The natural history of diabetic nephropathy is well visualized at present, thanks to the pioneering work of Mogenson. However, the early hyperfiltration phase and its relationship to the development of diabetic nephropathy is controversial. While Mogenson has shown a close relationship between these two phases,[175] many investigators have not been able to document a link between this early phase and final nephropathy.[176] Regression of microalbuminuria occurs more frequently in type 1 diabetes as its progression.[138] This is an interesting facet of natural history of this disease and lends hope for interventional measures like meticulous control of hypertension and hyperglycemia.

Management of Diabetic Nephropathy

Management of hypertension: Control of hypertension gains precedence over metabolic control, once microalbuminuria has set in. However, glycemic control cannot be neglected and in fact, usually gets easier to manage as renal function gets compromised. Newer antihypertensive agents, mainly ACE inhibitors are metabolically neutral, or in fact have a favorable influence on insulin resistance. In addition, they have a definitive renoprotective effect, a benefit over and above accrued by the control of hypertension. Many other antihypertensive drugs may have similar effects; for example nonpyridine calcium-channel blockers (amlodipine, verapamil). As the prevalence of side effects like persistent dry cough is high with ACE inhibitors, the ACE receptor blockers are now in use for the same purpose. The drugs have shown the same beneficial affects in short-term studies on parameters like urinary albumin excretion rate and offer the same long-term protection of renal function. Irbesartan and losartan have both been documented to offer this benefit.[177-179] In several head-on trials with ACE inhibitors and angiotensin II receptor blockers, the renoprotective effect of both the groups of drugs was found to be similar.[180-183] However, these studied were not designed or powered to reveal differences in cardiovascular endpoints like myocardial infarction and death. ACE inhibitors have been shown to reduce all cause mortality by almost 20%, which remains to be proven for ARB drugs (Benedict Bergamo Nephrologic Diabetes Complications Trial Study). Trandolapril alone or with verapamil was shown to reduce microalbuminuria but verapamil alone failed to do so.

Protein restriction: The beneficial effect of protein restriction in renal disease of diverse etiology has been adequately documented. This has also been demons-trated in type 1 diabetes mellitus.[184] However, this has been questioned in a recent study,[185] where protein intake of 0.58 gm/kg was compared with an intake of 1.3 gm/kg. The beneficial effect of protein restriction was probably masked by the beneficial effect of ACE inhibition. Hence, when ACE inhibition is used, protein restriction can be very mild, while in the absence of ACE inhibition, moderate restriction can be used. The rate of decline of GFR is also less with the use of vege-table proteins rich in branch-chain amino acids.[185]

Role of Estrogens: Epidemiological data from United States Renal Data System (USRDS) reveal a strong relationship between estrogen deficiency and increased risk of diabetic nephropathy. The progression of diabetic nephropathy is rapid in postmenopausal women, as compared to premenopausal women. The human mesangial cells express estrogen receptor subtypes, ER-α and ER-β. Estrogens increase matrix metallo-proteinases in the mesangial cells, thus promoting removal of mesangial tissues. The role of estrogens in females with diabetic nephropathy needs to be explored.[186,187]

REFERENCES

1. Hillary K, Ronald EA, William HH. Global burden of diabetes (1995-2025): prevalence, numerical estimates and projections. Diabetes Care. 1998;21:1414-31.
2. Nepom GT, Keok WW. Molecular basis for HLA-DQ association with IDDM. Diabetes. 1998;47:1177-84.
3. Concannon P, Gogolin G, Wens K, Hind DA, et al. A second-generation screen of the human genome for susceptibility to IDDM. Nature Genet. 1998;19:292-6.
4. Yoon JW, Elliott RB. Discussion: environmental factors, viruses and diet. In Frontiers in Diabetes Research: lessons from animal diabetes III. Shafrir E (Ed). London. Smith Gordon. 1991. pp 198-203.
5. Scherzenmeir J, Jagla A. Milk and diabetes. J Am Coll Nutr. 2000;19:1765-905.
6. Sorli CH, Greiner Dl, Mordes JP, Rossini AA. Stem cell transplantation for treatment of autoimmune disease. Graft. 1998;1:71-81.
7. Graser RT, DiLorenzo PP, Wong FM, Christianson GJ, et al. Identification of a CD8 cell that can independently mediate autoimmune diabetes development in the complete absence of CD4 T-cell helper function. J Immune. 2000;164:3913-8.
8. Grewal IS, Flavell RA. New insights into insulin dependent diabetes mellitus from studies with transgenic mouse models. Lab Invest. 1997;76:3-10.
9. Atkinson M, Leiter EH. The NOD mouse model of insulin dependent diabetes mellitus. As good as it gets. Nature Med. 1999;5:601-4.
10. Effects of insulin in relatives of patients with type 1 diabetes mellitus. N Engl J Med. 2002;346:1685-91.
11. Boshell BR, Chandalia HB, Kreisberg RA, Roddam RF, Serum insulin in obesity and diabetes. Am Jour Cli Nutr. 1968;21:1419.
12. Kulkarni RN, et al. Tissue-specific knock out of the insulin receptor in the pancreatic β-cells creates an insulin secretory defect similar to that in type 2 diabetes mellitus. Cell. 1999;96:329-39.
13. Jiang ZY, et al. Characterization of selective resistance to insulin signaling in the vasculature of obese Zucker (fa/fa) rats. J Clin Invest. 1999;104:447-57.
14. Virkamaki A, et al. Protein-protein interaction in insulin signaling and the molecular mechanisms of insulin resistance. J Clin Invest. 1999;103:931-43.
15. Nicole A, Lucia C, Chandalia M, et al. Genetic polymorphism PC-1 K121Q and ethnic susceptibility to insulin resistance. J Clin Endocrinol Metab. 2003;88:5927-34.
16. Nicole A, Chandalia M, Pankaj S, et al. ENPP1/PC-1 K121Q polymorphism and genetic susceptibility to type 2 diabetes. Diabetes. 2005;54:1207-13.
17. Davies MJ, Rayman G, Grenfall A, et al. Loss of first phase insulin response to intravenous glucose in subjects with impaired glucose tolerance. Diabetic Med. 1994;11:432-6.
18. Cerasi E, Luft R, Efendic S. Decreased sensitivity of the pancreatic beta-cells to glucose in prediabetic and diabetic subjects. A glucose dose response study. Diabetes. 1972;21:224-34.
19. Davies MJ, Rayman G, Gray IP, Day JL, Hales CN. Insulin deficiency and increased plasma concentration of intact and 32/33 split proinsulin in subjects with impaired glucose tolerance. Diabetes Med. 1993;10:313-20.
20. Lerner PL, Porte D Jr. Acute and steady state insulin responses to glucose in nonobese diabetic subjects. J Clinical Invest. 1972;51:1629-31.
21. DeFronzo RA, Bonadonna RC, Ferrannini E. Pathogenesis of NIDDM: a balanced overview. Diabetes Care. 1992;15:318-68.
22. Leah JL. Beta-cell dysfunction in type II diabetes mellitus. Curr Opin Endocrinol Diabetes. 1995;2:300-6.
23. Matschinsky FM, Glaser B, Magnuson MA. Pancreatic beta-cell glucokinase: closing the gap between theoretical concepts and experimental realities. Diabetes. 1998;47:307-15.
24. Landraf R. Approaches to the management of postprandial hyperglycemia. Exp Clin Endocrinol Diab. 1999;107 (Suppl 4):S128-32.
25. Dinneen S, Alziad A, Turk D, Rizza R. Failure of glucagon suppression contributed to postprandial hyperglycemia in IDDM. Diabetologia. 1995;38:337-43.
26. McGarry JD, Dobbin RL. Fatty acids, lipotoxicity and insulin secretion. Diabetologia. 1999; 42:128-38.
27. Yki-Jarvinen H. Glucose toxicity. Endocrine Rev. 1992;13: 415-31.
28. Rossetti L, Giaccari A, DeFronzo RA. Glucose toxicity. Diabetes Care. 1990;13:610-30.
29. Luzi L, DeFronzo RA. Effect of loss of first phase insulin secretion on hepatic glucose production and tissue glucose disposal in humans. Am J Physiol. 1989;257:E241-6.
30. Bruce DG, Chisholm DJ, Storlein LH, Kraegen EW. Physiological importance of deficiency in early prandial insulin secretion in noninsulin-dependent diabetics. Diabetes. 1988;37:736-44.
31. Yki-Jarvinen H, Williams J. Insulin resistance in noninsulin-dependent diabetes mellitus. In Pickup J, Williams G (Eds): Textbook of Diabetes, 2nd edn. Blackwell Science Oxford; 1997. pp. 20.1-20.4
32. Pederson O. Glucose transporters and diabetes mellitus. In the Diabetes Annual: Marshall SH, Home PD, Alberti KGMM, Krall LP (Eds): Elsevier Science Publications; 1993. pp. 30-53.
33. Mueckler M. Family of glucose transporter genes. Implications for glucose homeostasis and diabetes. Diabetes Care. 1990;13:198-200.
34. Gould GW, Thomas HM, Jess TJ, Bell GI. Expression of human glucose transporters in xenopus oocytes. Kinetic characterization and substrate specificities of the erythrocyte, liver and brain isoforms. Biochemistry. 1991;30:S139-45.
35. Chen L, Alan T, Johnson JH, Hughes S, Newgard CB, Unger RH. Regulation of beta-cell glucose transporter gene expression. USA: Proc Natl Acad Sci. 1990;87:4088-92.
36. Orcii L, Ravazzola M, Baetens D, Inman L, et al. Evidence that downregulation of β-cell glucose transporter in noninsulin-dependent diabetes mellitus maybe the cause of diabetic hyperglycemia. USA: Proc Natl Acad Sci. 1990;87:9953-57.

37. Thorens B, Wu YJ, Leah JL, Weir GC. The loss of GLUT-2 expression by glucose unresponsive β-cells of db/db mice is reversible and is induced by the diabetic environment. J Clin Invest. 1992;90:77-85.

38. Li SR, Baroni MG, Oelbaun RS, Stock J, Galton DJ. Association of genetic variant of the glucose transporters with noninsulin-dependent diabetes mellitus. Lancet. 1988;2:368-70.

39. Cox NJ, Xiang KS, Bell GI, Karam JH. Glucose transporter gene and noninsulin-dependent diabetes mellitus. Lancet. 1988;2:793-4.

40. Kalu K, Metsutani A, Mireckler M, Permmut MA. Polymorphisms of Hep G2/erythrocyte glucose transporter gene. Linkage relationship and implications for genetic analysis of NIDDM. Diabetes. 1990;3:49-56.

41. Matsutani A, Korijani L, Cox N, Permmut MA. Polymorphisms of GLUT-2 and GLUT-4 genes: use in evaluation of genetic susceptibility in blacks. Diabetes. 1990;39:1534-42.

42. Bjorbaek C, Vestergaard H, Heding LG, Cohen P, Pedersen O. Analysis of genes encoding 3 key proteins in insulin resistant glucose utilization of skeletal muscle in type 2 diabetes. Diabetologia. 1992;35 (Suppl 1):A72.

43. Hoss UDO, Gessler R, Kalatz B, et al. Continuous online glucose monitoring using pattern recognition: the comparative microdialysis technique. Diabetes. 1999;48 (Suppl 1) Abs 0445:A103-4.

44. Heinemann L, Kraemer UWE, Kloetzer HM, et al. Non-invasive continuous glucose monitoring using physiological blood glucose changes in volunteers and diabetic patients. Diabetes. 1999;48 (Suppl 1) Abs 1573:A359.

45. Gabreily I, Wozniak R, Mevorach M, et al. Performance of a novel near-infrared (NIR) transcutaneous glucose monitor during hypoglycemia. Diabetes. 1999;48(Suppl 1) Abs 0426:A99.

46. Chandalia SH, Modi SV. Fat replacers and flat blockers. Int Jour Diabetes Dev Countries. 1999;19:139-43.

47. Mela DJ. Nutritional implications of fat substitutes. J Am Diet Assoc. 1992;92:412-6.

48. Mellies MJ, Jandaeck RJ, Taulber JD, et al. A double blind placebo controlled study of sucrose polyester in hypercholesterolemia outpatients. Am J Clin Nutr. 1993; 37:339-46.

49. Mellies MJ, Vitale C, Jandaeck RT, et al. The substitution of sucrose polyester for dietary fat in obese, hypercholesterolemia patients. Am J Clin Nutr. 1985;41:1-12.

50. Hermansen K, Søndergaard M, Høie L, et al. Beneficial effects of a soy-based dietary supplement on lipid levels and cardiovascular risk markers in type 2 diabetic subjects. Diabetes Care. 2001;24:228-33.

51. Marchioli R. For the GISSI-Prevenzione Investigators, early protection against sudden death by n-3 polyunsaturated fatty acids after myocardial infarction: time-course analysis of the results of the Gruppo Italiano per to Studio della Sopravvivenza nell'Infarto Miocardico (GISSI). Prevenzione. Circulation. 2002;105:1897-903.

52. Brand-Miller J, Hayne S, Petocz P, et al. Low-glycemic index diets in the management of diabetes: a meta-analysis of randomized controlled trials. Diabetes Care. 2003;26:2261-7.

53. Pereira MA, Swain J, Goldfine AB, et al. Effects of a low-glycemic load diet on resting energy expenditure and heart disease risk factors during weight loss. JAMA. 2004; 292:2482-90.

54. Wolf AM, Conaway MR, Crowther JQ, et al. Translating lifestyle intervention to practice in obese patients with type 2 diabetes: Improving Control with Activity and Nutrition (ICAN) Study. Diabetes Care. 2004;27:1570-6.

55. Irwin ML, Yasui Y, Ulrich CM, et al. Effect of exercise on total and intra-abdominal body fat in postmenopausal women: a randomized controlled trial. JAMA. 2003;289:323-30.

56. Gray RE, Tanner CJ, Pories WJ, et al. Effects of weight loss on muscle lipid content in morbidly obese subjects. Am J Physiol. 2003;284:E726-32.

57. O'Rahilly S, Turner RC, Mathew DR. Impaired pulsatile secretion of insulin in relatives of patients with noninsulin-dependent diabetes mellitus. N Eng J Med. 1988;318;1225-30.

58. Polonsky KS, Given BD, Hirsch LJ, et al. Abnormal patterns of insulin secretion in noninsulin-dependent diabetes mellitus. N Eng Med. 1988;318:1231-9.

59. Mathews DR. Insulin secretion, pulsatility and signaling attributes. In The Diabetes Annual: Marshall SM, Home PD, Alberti KGMM, Krall LP (Eds). Elsevier Science Publishers BV; 1993. pp. 18-29.

60. Chandalia HB, Lamba PS. Futuristic antidiabetic agents. The Indian Practitioner. 2000;53(1):37-45.

61. Weiss SR, Berger S, Cheng SL, et al. Adjunctive therapy with inhaled human insulin in type 2 diabetic patients failing oral agents: a multicentric phase II trial. Diabetes. 1999;48 (Suppl 1):A12.

62. Juhl CB, Pørksen N, Hollingdal M, Sturis J, et al. Repaglinide activity amplifies pulsatile insulin secretion by augmentation of burst mass with no effect on burst frequency. Diabetes Care. 2000;23:745-81.

63. Evans AJ, Krentz AJ. Recent developments and emerging therapies for type 2 diabetes mellitus. Drugs RD. 1999;2:75-94.

64. Manson JE, Faich GA. Pharmacotherapy of obesity—do the benefits to outweigh the risks? N Eng J Med. 1998; 335:659-60.

65. Sjostron L, Rissanen A, Anderson T, et al. Randomized placebo-controlled trial of orlistat for weight loss and prevention of weight regain in obese patients. Lancet. 1998;352:167-72.

66. Nauck MA. Glucagon like peptide-1. Curr Opin Endocrinol Diabetes. 1997;4:291-9.

67. Lam WF, Masclee AA, De Boer SY, Lamers CB. Hyperglycemia reduced gastrin-stimulated gastric acid secretion in humans. Eur J Clin Invest. 1998;10:826-30.

68. Rinke CH, McGregor CP, Goke B. Calcitonin gene related peptide potentially stimulates glucagon like peptide-1 release in the isolated perfused rat ileum. Peptides. 2000;3:431-7.

69. Meyer LV, Laedreirel L, Fulendroff J, Melaisse WJ. Stimulation of insulin and somatostatin release by two meglitinide analogs. Endocrine. 1997;3:311-7.

70. Ranganath L, Schaper F, Gama R, et al. The effect of glucagon on carbohydrate-mediated secretion of glucagon dependent insulinotropic polypeptide (GIP) and glucagon like peptide-1 (7-36 amide) (GLP-1). Diabetes Mellitus Res Rev. 1999;6:390-4.

71. Holst JJ, Wojdemann M, Andre W, Lars R. Potent enterogastrone action of the insulinotropic hormone, glucagon-like

peptide-1 (GLP-1): mechanism of action. Diabetes. 1999;48(Suppl 1):A21.

72. Gallawitz BJ, Ropiter T, Morys-Wortmann C, et al. Characterization of GLP-1 and analogs with n-terminal modifications in position-1. Diabetes. 1999;48(Suppl 1):A423.

73. Seidenstrucker A, Gallwitz B, Reinke-Ludtke A, et al. GLP-1 (7-36 amide) and biologically active analogs increase insulin secretion from pancreatic islets in cirrhotic rats. Diabetes. 1999;48 (Suppl 1):A424.

74. Maksond H, Barrow BA, Ayres A, et al. Glucagon like peptide (7-36 amide) stimulates insulin secretion in proportion to the underlying beta cell function to an equal extent in late onset type 1 and type 2 diabetes. Diabetes. 1999;48(Suppl 1):A425.

75. Edwards CMB, Stanley SA, Davis R, et al. Extendin reduces fasting and postprandial glucose and decreases energy intake in healthy volunteers. Am J Physiol. 2001;281:E155-61.

76. Meneilly GS, Gingerich R, McIntosh CHS, et al. Effect of glucagon-like peptide 1 on noninsulin-mediated glucose uptake in the elderly patient with diabetes. Diabetes Care. 2001;24:1951-6.

77. Deacon CF, Danielson P, Klarskov L, et al. Dipeptidyl pepetidase IV inhibition reduces the degradation and clearance of GIP and potentiates its insulin tropic and antihypertensive effects in anesthetized pigs. Diabetes. 2001;50:1588-97.

78. Brandt A, Katschinski M, Arnold R, et al. GLP-1-induced alterations in the glucose-stimulated insulin secretory dose-response curve. Am J Physiol. 2001;281:E242-7.

79. Sudre B, Broqua P, White RB, et al. Chronic inhibition of circulating dipeptidyl peptidase IV by FE 999011 delays the occurrence of diabetes in male Zuccker diabetic fatty rats. Diabetes. 2002;51:1461-9.

80. Nauck MA, Heimesaat MM, Behle K, et al. Effects of glucagon-like peptide-1 on counter regulatory hormone responses, cognitive functions, and insulin secretion during hyper-insulinemic, stepped hypoglycemic clamp experiments in health volunteers. J Clin Endocrinol Metab. 2002;87:1239-46.

81. Rask E, Seckl J, Olsson T, et al. Impaired incretin response after a mixed meal is associated with insulin resistance in nondiabetic men. Diabetes Care. 2001;24:1640-5.

82. Farilla L, Bulotta A, Hirshberg B, et al. Glucagon-like peptide 1 inhibits cell apoptosis and improves glucose responsiveness of freshly isolated human islets. Endocrinology. 2003; 144:5149-58.

83. Ahren B, Landin, Olsson M, Jansson PA, et al. Inhibition of dipeptidyl peptidase-4 reduces glycemia, sustains insulin levels and reduces glucagons levels in type 2 diabetes. J Clin Endocrinol Metab. 2004;89:2078-84.

84. Zander M, Christiansen A, Madsbad S, et al. Additive effects of glucagons-like peptide and pioglitazone in patients with type 2 diabetes. Diabetes Care. 2004;27:1910-4.

85. Buse JB. Effects of exenatide (Exendin-4) on glycemic control over 30 weeks in sulfonylurea-treated patients with type 2 diabetes. Diabetes Care. 2004;27:2628-35.

86. Ye J, Bonner VM, Lim-Fraser M, et al. An amylin antagonist has opposite effects to amylin on basal lipids and counteracts insulin resistance in high fat fed rats. Diabetes. 1999;48(Suppl 1):A273.

87. Bailey CJ. Novel compounds for NIDDM. Diabetes Reviews International. 1996;5:9-12.

88. Fineman M, Bahner A, Gottlieb A, Kolterman OG. Effect of six months administration of pramlintide as an adjunct to insulin therapy on metabolic control in people with type 1 diabetes. Diabetes. 1999;48 (Suppl 1):A113.

89. Muralidharan R, Dash RJ. Newer modes of therapy for NIDDM. Jour Assoc Physicians of India. 1998;46:8:716-23.

90. Livingston JW, Macdougall M, Landoucher G, Schoen W. BAY-27- 9955, a novel nonpeptide antagonist of the glucagon binds to the glucagon receptor. Diabetes. 1999;48(Suppl 1):A199.

91. Radzuick J, McDonald TJ, Rubenstein D, Dupre J. Initial splanchnic extraction of ingested glucose in normal man. Metabolism. 1978;27:657-79.

92. Ferrnanni E, Bjorkmann O, Reichard GA, et al. The disposal of an oral glucose load in healthy subjects: a quantitative study. Diabetes. 1985;34:580-8.

93. Malaber UH, Dryden S, McCarthy HD, Kilpatrick A, Williams G. Effects of chronic vandate administration in STZ-induced diabetic rats. Diabetes. 1994;43:9-15.

94. Ogilvie KM, Saladin R, Nagy TR, et al. Reduced adiposity in Zucker fatty rats treated with a retinoid X receptor agonist. Diabetes. 1999;48(Suppl 1):A6.

95. Murata T, Hata Y, Ishibashi T, et al. Response of experimental retinal neovascularization to thiazolidinediones. Arch Ophthalmol. 2001;119:709-17.

96. Miyazaki Y, Mahankali A, Matsuda M, et al. Effect of pioglitizone on abdominal fat distribution and insulin sensitivity in type 2 diabetic patients. J Clin Endocrinol Metab. 2002;87:2784-91.

97. Wilmsen HM, Ciraldi TP, Carter L, et al. Thiazolidinediones upregulate impaired fatty acid uptake in skeletal muscle of type 2 diabetic subjects. Am J Physiol. 2003;285:E354-62.

98. Juhl CB, Hollingdal M, Pørksen N, et al. Influence of rosiglitazone treatment on β-cell function in type 2 diabetes: evidence of an increased ability of glucose to entrain high-frequency insulin pulsatility. J Clin Endocrinol Metab. 2003;88:3794-800.

99. Pavo I, Jermendy G, Varkonyi TT, et al. Effect of pioglitizone compared with metformin on glycemic control and indices of insulin sensitivity in recently diagnosed patients with type 2 diabetes. J Clin Endocrinol Metab. 2003;88:1637-45.

100. Motoshima H, Wu X, Sinha MK, et al. Differential regulation of adiponectin secretion from cultured human omental and subcutaneous adipocytes: effects of insulin and rosiglitazone. J Clin Endocrino Metab. 2002;87:5662-7.

101. Baldwin D Jr, Duffin KE. Rosiglitazone treatment of diabetes mellitus after solid organ transplantation. Transplantation. 2004;77:1009-14.

102. Diani AR, Sawada G, Wyse B, et al. Pioglitazone preserves pancreatic islet structure and insulin secretory function in three Murine models of type 2 diabetes. Am J Physiol. 2004;286:E116-22.

103. Saad MF. Ragaglitazar improves glycemic control and lipid profile in type 2 diabetic subjects: a 12-week, double-blind, placebo-controlled dose ranging study with an open pioglitizone arm. Diabetes Care. 2004;27:1324-9.

104. Fineberg SE, Fineberg NS, Anderson JH, et al. Insulin immune respone to Lispro human insulin therapy in type 1 and type 2 diabetic patients. Diabetologia. 1995;38(Suppl 1):A4.

105. Howey DC, Bowsher R, Brunelle RL, et al. Lys (B28), Pro (B29) human insulin rapidly absorbed analogue of human insulin. Diabetes. 1994;43:396-402.

106. Uwe B, Ebraham S, Hirschberger S, et al. Effect of rapid acting insulin analogue, insulin Aspart on quality of life and

treatment satisfaction in type 1 diabetic patients. Diabetes. 1999;48(Suppl 1) Abs 0481;A112.

107. Dashora U, Dashora V. Insulin Glargine. Int J Diabetes Dev Countries. 2000;20(4):140-4.

108. Heinemann L, Linkeschova R, Rave K, et al. Time action profile of the long acting insulin analogue of insulin glargine (HOE 901) in comparison with those of NPH insulin and placebo. Diabetes Care. 2000;23:644-9.

109. Yki-Jarvinen H, Dessler A, Ziemen N. Study group-HOE 901/ 3002. Comparison of insulin glargine (HOE 901) vs NPH during one year of insulin therapy in type 2 diabetes. Diabetes. 2000;49(Suppl 1):A130.

110. Hamann A. A randomized clinical trial comparing breakfast, dinner, or bedtime administration of insulin glargine in patients with type 1 diabetes. Diabetes. 2003;26:1738-44.

111. Riddle MC. The treat-to-target trial: randomized addition of glargine or human NPH insulin to oral therapy of type 2 diabetic patients. Diabetes Care. 2003;26:3080-6.

112. Skyler JS. For the Inhaled Insulin Phase II Study Group. Efficacy of inhaled human insulin in type 1 diabetes mellitus: a randomized proof-of-concept study. Lancet. 2001;357:331-5.

113. Van den Berghe G, Wouters P, Weekers F, et al. Intensive insulin therapy in critically ill patients. N Engl J Med. 2002;345:1359-67.

114. Secchi A, Falqui L, Davalli A, Pozza G. New hope from organ and tissue transplantation in diabetic patients. In Diabetes in the New Millineum: Mario UD, Leonetti F, Pugliese G, Sbraccia P, Signore A (Eds). John Wiley and Sons; 2000. pp. 89-100.

115. Federlin K, Brendel M, Bretzel RG. Islet cell transplantation in type 1 diabetes. In Diabetes in the New Millinneum: Mario UD, Leonetti F, Pugliese G, Sbraccia P, Signore A (Eds). John Wiley and Sons; 2000. pp. 81-8.

116. Larsen JL, Colling CW, Ratanaswan T, et al. Pancreas transplantation improves vascular disease in patients with type 1 diabetes. Diabetes Care. 2004;27:1706-11.

117. Venstrom JM, McBride MA, Rother KI, et al. Survival after pancreas transplantation in patients with diabetes and preserved kidney function. JAMA. 2003;290:2817-23.

118. Abai AM, Hobart PM, Norman JA, et al. Gene therapy for type 1 diabetes: insulin delivery with plasmid DNA. Diabetes. 1999;48(Suppl 1):A12.

119. Bach JF. Restoring cell tolerance in diabetes. In Diabetes in the New Millennium. Mario UD, Leonetti F, Pugliese G, Sbraccia P, Signore A (Eds). John Wiley and Sons; 2000. pp. 39-46.

120. Pozilli P, Cavallo MG. Tolerance induction for prevention of type 1 diabetes. In Diabetes in the New Millennium: Mario UD, Leonetti F, Pugliese G, Sbraccia P, Signore A (Eds). John Wiley and Sons; 2000. pp. 47-54.

121. Giordano C, Bompiani GD, Galluzo A. Clinical trials in prediabetes: an overview. In Diabetes in the New Millennium: Mario UD, Leonetti F, Pugliese G, Sbraccia P, Signore A (Eds). John Wiley and Sons; 2000. pp. 55-64.

122. Shapiro AMJ, Lakey RJ, Ryan E, et al. Insulin independence after solitary islet transplantation in type 1 diabetic patients using steroid free immunosuppression. Transplantation. 2000;55:354-9.

123. Lanza RP, Sullivan CJ, Chick WC. Islet transplantation with immunoisolation. Diabetes. 1992;41:1503-10.

124. Newgard CB. Cellular engineering and gene therapy strategies for insulin replacement in diabetes. Diabetes. 1994;43:341-50.

125. Faradji R, Havari E, Mulligan RC, et al. Cellular engineering approaches to the treatment of IDDM. 60th Annual ADA Meeting 1999, San Deigo, California.

126. Robertson RP. Islet cell transplantation as a treatment for diabetes—a work in progress. N Engl J Med. 2004;350:694-705.

127. Bonner-Weir M, Taneja M, Weir GC, et al. In vitro cultivation of human islet cells from expanded ductal tissue. Proc Natl Arad Sc (USA). 2000;97:7999-8004.

128. Hamada Y, Araki N, Kahn N, Nakamura J, Horiuchi S, Holta N. Formation of advanced glycation end products by intermediate metabolites of glycolytic pathways and polyol pathway. Biochem Biophys Res Commun. 1998;228:539-43.

129. Valsarra H, Bucala R. Recent progress in advanced glycation and diabetes vascular disease. Role of advanced glycation end products. Diabetes. 1996;45 (Suppl 3):S65-6.

130. Baynes JW. Role of oxidative stress in development of complications of diabetes. Diabetes. 1991;40:405-12.

131. Oturai PS, Christensen M, Rolin B, et al. Effects of advanced glycation end products inhibition and protein crosslinked breaking in diabetic rats. Diabetes. 1999;48(Suppl 1): Abs151;A35.

132. Leslie RD, Beyan H, Sawtell P, et al. Level of an advanced glycated end product is genetically determined: a study of normal twins. Diabetes. 2003;52:2441-4.

133. Passaro A, Calzoni F, Valpato S, et al. Effect of metabolic control on homocysteine levels in type 2 diabetic patients: a 3-year follow-up. J Intern Med. 2003;254:264-71.

134. McCarter RJ, Hempe JM, Gomez R, et al. Biological variation in HbA$_{1c}$ predicts risk of retinopathy and nephropathy in type 1 diabetes. Diabetes Care. 2004;27:1259-64.

135. Arun CS, Stoddart J, Mackin P, et al. Significance of microalbuminuria in long-duration type 1 diabetes. Diabetes Care. 2002;26:2144-9.

136. Baynes JW, Thorpe SR. Role of oxidative stress in diabetic complications. A new perspective on an old paradigm. Diabetes. 1999;48:1-9.

137. Rossouw JE, et al. Risks and benefits of estrogen plus progestin in healthy postmenopausal women: principal results from the Women's Health Initiative Randomized Controlled Trial. JAMA. 2003;288:321-33.

138. Hu FB, Stampfer MJ, Solomon C, et al. Physical activity and risk for cardiovascular events in diabetic women. Ann Intern Med. 2001;134:96-105.

139. Schurgin S, Rich S, Mazzone T. Increased prevalence of significant coronary artery calcification in patients with diabetes. Diabetes Care. 2001;24:335-8.

140. Haffner SM, Lehtos, Ronmemaa T, et al. Mortality with coronary heart disease in subjects with type 2 diabetes in nondiabetic subjects with and without prior myocardial infarction. N Engl J Med. 1998;339:229-43.

141. Evan JMM, Wang J, Morris AD. Comparison of cardiovascular risk between patients with type 2 diabetes and those who had a myocardial infarction. BMJ. 2002;324:939-42.

142. Davies MJ, Baer DJ, Judd JT, et al. Effects of moderate alcohol intake on fasting insulin and glucose concentrations and insulin sensitivity in postmenopausal women: a Randomized Controlled Trial. JAMA. 2002;287:2559-62.

143. Tanasescu M, Hu FB, Willet WC, et al. Alcohol consumption and risk of coronary heart disease among men with type 2 diabetes mellitus. J Am Coll Cardiol. 2001;38:1836-42.

144. Newton KM, LaCroix AZ, Heckbert SR, et al. Estrogen therapy and risk of cardiovascular events among women with type 2 diabetes. Diabetes Care. 2003;26:2810-6.

145. Vijan S, Hayward RA. Pharmacologic lipid-lowering therapy in type 2 diabetes mellitus—Background Paper for the American College of Physicians. Ann Intern Med. 2004;140: 650-8.

146. Colhoun HM, et al. Primary Prevention of Cardiovascular Disease with Atorvastatin in Type 2 Diabetes in the Collaborative Atorvastatin Diabetes Study (CARDS): Multicenter Randomized Placebo-controlled Trial. Lancet. 2004;364:685-96.

147. Wackers FJT. Detection of Silent Myocardial Ischemia in Asymptomatic Diabetic subjects: the DIAD Study. Diabetes Care. 2004;27:195-61.

148. Davis TME, Fortun P, Mulder J, et al. Silent myocardial infarction and its prognosis in a community-based cohort of type 2 diabetic patients: the Fremantle Diabetes Study. Diabetologia. 2004;47:395-9.

149. Choi D, Kim SK, Choi SH, et al. Preventative effects of rosaglitazone on restenosis after coronary stent implantation in patients with type 2 diabetes. Diabêtes Care. 2004;27: 2654-60.

150. Chaudhuri A, Janicke D, Wilson MF, et al. Anti-inflammatory and profibronolytic effect of insulin in acute ST-segment-elevation myocardial infarction. Circulation. 2004;109:849-54.

151. Inoguchi T, Battan R, Handler E, et al. Preferential activation of protein kinase C isoform B II and diacylglycerol levels in aorta and heart of diabetic rats. USA: Proc Natl Acad Sci. 1992;89:11059-63.

152. Kahn R. Proceedings of a consensus development conference on standardized measures in diabetic neuropathy. Diabetes Care. 1992;15:1081-103.

153. Arezzo JC. New developments in diagnosis of diabetic neuropathy. Am J Med. 1999;107:9S-16S.

154. Andersen H. Motor function in diabetic neuropathy. Acta Neurol Scand. 1999;100:211-20.

155. Spallone V, Menzinger G. Diagnosis of cardiovascular autonomic neuropathy in diabetes. Diabetes. 1997;46 (Suppl 2):S67-S76.

156. Stevens MJ, Raffel DM, Allman KC, et al. Cardiac sympathetic dysinnervation in diabetes. Implications for enhanced cardiovascular risk. Circulation. 1998;98:961-8.

157. Ward JD. Improving prognosis in type 2 diabetes. Diabetes Care. 1999;22(Suppl 2):B84-8.

158. Ziegler D, Hanefeld M, Ruhnau KJ, et al. The ALADIN III study group: treatment of symptomatic diabetic polyneuropathy with α-lipoic acid. Diabetes Care. 1999;22:1296-301.

159. Leonard DR, Farooqi MH, Myers S. Restoration of sensation, reduced pain, and improved balance in subjects with diabetic peripheral neuropathy: a double-blind, randomised, placebo-controlled study with monochromatic near infrared treatment. Diabetes Care. 2004;27:168-72.

160. Antonetti DA, Alistair JB, Khin S, et al. Penn State Retina Research Group: vascular permeability in experimental diabetes is associated with reduced endothelial occludin content. Diabetes. 1998;47:1953-9.

161. Gerhardinger C, Podesta F, Lorenzi M. Retinal levels of occludin are increased in background diabetic retinopathy and are associated with over expression of glial fibrillar acidic protein. Diabetes.1999;48(Suppl 1):A20.

162. Eddleston M, Mucke L. Molecular profile of reactive astrocytes—implications for their role in neurologic disease. Neuroscience. 1993;54:15-36.

163. Sima AAF, Chakrabarti S, Garcia-Salinas R, Basu PK. The BB rat—an authentic model of human diabetic retinopathy. Curr Eye Res. 1985;4:1087-92.

164. Miyamoto K, Khosrof S, Bursell SE, et al. Prevention of leukostasis and vascular leakage in streptozotocin-induced diabetic retinopathy via intercellular adhesion molecule-1 inhibition. USA: Proc Natl Acad Sci. 1999;96:10836-41.

165. Mizutani M, Kern TS, Lorenzi M. Accelerated death of retinal microvascular cells in human and experimental retinopathy. J Clin Invest. 1996;97:2883-91.

166. Bojestig M, Arnqvist HJ, Hermansson G, et al. Declining incidence of nephropathy in insulin-dependent diabetes mellitus. N Engl J Med. 1994;330:15-8.

167. Fabre J, Balant LP, Dayer PG, et al. The kidney in maturity onset diabetes mellitus: a clinical study of 510 patients. Kidney Int. 1982;21:730-8.

168. Earle K, Viberti GC. Familial, hemodynamic and metabolic factors in the predisposition to diabetic kidney disease. Kidney Int. 1994;45:434-7.

169. Kramer HJ, Nguyen QD, Curhan G, et al. Renal insufficiency in the absence of albuminuria and retinopathy among adults with type 2 diabetes mellitus. JAMA. 2003;289:3273-7.

170. MacIsaac RJ, Tsalamandris C, Panagiotopoulos S, et al. Nonalbuminuria renal insufficiency in type 2 diabetes. Diabetes Care. 2004;27:195-200.

171. Krolewski AS, Canessa M, Warram JH, et al. Predisposition to hypertension and susceptibility to renal disease in insulin-dependent diabetes mellitus. N Engl J Med. 1988; 318:140-5.

172. Borch-Johnsen K, Norgaard K, Hommel E, et al. Is diabetic nephropathy a inherited complication? Kidney Int. 1992;41: 719-22.

173. Muir A, Schatz DA, Maclaren NK. The pathogenesis, prediction and prevention of diabetes mellitus. Endocrinol Metab Clin North Am. 1992; 21(2):199-219.

174. Valmadrid CT, Klein R, Moss SE, Klein BEK. A population based study of the risk of cardiovascular disease mortality associated with microalbuminuria and gross proteinuria in people with older onset diabetes. Diabetes. 1999;48(Suppl 1):Abs 0062;A15.

175. Mogensen CE, Christensen CK. Blood pressure changes and renal function in incipient and overt diabetic nephropathy. Hypertension. 1985;7(Suppl II):64-73.

176. Castellino P, Shohat J, DeFronzo RA. Hyperfiltration and diabetic nephropathy: is it the beginning? Or is it the end? Semin Nephrol. 1990;10:228-41.

177. Dasbach EJ, Shahinfar S, Santanello NC, et al. Quality of life in patients with NIDDM and nephropathy at baseline: the Losartan Renal Protection Study. Diabetes. 1999; 48(Suppl 1):A389.

178. KR, Whittaker E, Sullivan L et al. Effects of restricting dietary protein of renal failure in patients with insulin-dependent diabetes mellitus. N Engl J Med. 1991;324:78-84.

179. Perkins BA, Ficociello LH, Silva KH, et al. Regression of microalbuminuria in type 1 diabetes. N Engl J Med. 2003; 348:2285-93.

180. Parving HH. The effects of Irbesartan on the development of diabetic nephropathy in patients with type 2 diabetes. N Engl J Med. 2001;345:870-8.

181. Lewis EJ. Renoprotective effect of the angiotensin-receptor antagonist irbesartan in patients with nephropathy due to type 2 diabetes. N Engl J Med. 2001;345:851-60.

182. Brenner BM. Effects of losar on renal and cardiovascular outcomes in patients with type 2 diabetes and nephropathy. N Engl J Med. 2001;345:861-9.

183. Barenett AH. Angiotensin-receptor blockade versus converting-enzyme inhibition in type 2 diabetes and nephropathy. N Engl J Med. 2004;351:1952-61.

184. Jenkins DJA, Kendall CWC, Marchie A, et al. Effects of a dietary portfolio of cholesterol-lowering foods vs lovastatin in on serum lipids and C-reactive protein. JAMA. 2003; 290:502-10.

185. Viberti GC, Walker JD. Diabetic nephropathy: etiology and prevention. Diabetes Metab Rev. 1988;4:147-62.

186. Striker G, Poter M, Elliot SJ, et al. Pathophysiology of diabetic nephropathy: role of estrogens. In Diabetes in the New Millennium: Di Mario U, Leonetti F, Pugliese G, Sbracca P, Signo A (Eds). United Kingdom: John Wiley and Sons Ltd, West Sussex; 2000. pp. 297-310.

187. Wingrove CS, Garr E, Godsland IF, Stevenson JC. 17β estradiol enhances release of matrix metalloproteinases-2 from human vascular smooth muscle cells. Biochem Biophys Acta. 1998;1406(2):169-74.

APPENDIX

APPENDIX

Analyte	SI units	Conventional units
Activated clotting time	70–180 sec	70–180 sec
Albumin (Female)	41–53 g/L	4.1–5.3 g/dl
Albumin (Male)	40-50 g/L	4.0–5.0 g/dl
Aminotransferases		
AST (SGOT)	0–0.58 µkat/L	12–35 µ/L
ALT (SGPT)	0–0.58 µkat/L	7–35 µ/L
Ammonia	15–47 µmol/L	25–80 µgm/dl
Anion gap	7–16 mmol/L	7–16 mmol/L
Arterial blood gas (ABG)		
(HCO_3)	21–28 mmol/L	21–30 mEq/L
PCO_2	4.7–5.9 kPa	32–45 mm Hg
pH	7.38–7.44	7.35–7.45
PO_2	11–13 kPa	72–104 mm Hg
b_2-microglobulin (serum)	1.2–2.8 mg/L	1.2–2.8 mg/L
Bilirubin		
Total	5.1–17 µmol/L	1.2–2.8 mg/dl
Direct	1.7–5.1 µmol/L	0.1–0.3 mg/dl
Indirect	3.4–12 µmol/L	0.2–0.7 mg/dl
Bleeding time (adult)	2–9.5 min	2–9.5 min
Body fluids		
Total volume (lean) of body weight	50–70%	
Intracellular	0.3–0.4 of body weight	
Extracellular	0.2–0.3 of body weight	
Blood		
Male	69 ml/kg body weight	
Female	65 ml/kg body weight	
Plasma volume		
Male	39 ml/kg body weight	
Female	40 ml/kg body weight	
Calcium		
Ionized	1.1–1.4 mmol/L	4.5–5.6 mg/dl
Total	2.2–2.6 mmol/L	9–10.5 mg/dl
Ceruloplasmin	250–630 mg/L	25–63 mg/dl
Chloride	98–106 mol/L	98–106 ng/dl
Clot retraction time	0.5–1/2 hours	50–100%/2 hours
C–reactive proteins	0.08–3.1 mg/L	0.08–3.1 mg/L
Creatine kinase (Total)		
Female	0.67–2.5 µkat/L	39–238 µ/L
Male	1.00–6.6 µkat/L	51–294 µ/L
CK–MB	0–5.5 µg/L	0.0–5.5 ng/ml
Creatinine (Female)	44–80 µmol/L	0.5–0.9 ng/ml
(Male)	53–106 µmol/L	0.6–1.2 ng/ml

Contd...

Contd...

Analyte	SI units	Conventional units
Differential blood count		
Neutrophil	0.40–0.70	40–70%
Lymphocyte	0.20–0.50	20–50%
Monocyte	0.04–0.08	4–11%
Eosinophils	0.0–0.6	0–8%
Basophil	0.0–0.02	0–3%
Erythrocyte count		
Adult (Male)	$4.5–5.9 \times 10^{12}$/L	$4.5–5.9 \times 10^{6}$/mm^3
(Female)	$4.5–5.20 \times 10^{12}$/L	$4.5–5.2 \times 10^{6}$/mm^3
Lifespan	120 days	120 days
Erythropoietin		
Erythrocyte sedimentation rate (ESR)		
Female	0–20 mm/h	0–20 mm/hour
Male	0–15 mm/h	0–15 mm/hour
Ferritin		
Male	30–300 µg/L	30–300 ng/ml
Female	10–150 µg/L	10–150 ng/ml
Fibrinogen	2.33–4.96 g/L	233–496 mg/dl
Gamma-glutamyltransferase	1–94 µ/L	1–94 u/L
Hematocrit		
Male	0.41–0–0.53	41.0–53.0
Female	0.35–0.44 mmol/L	35.4–44.4 g/dl
Homocysteine	4.4–10.8 µmol/L	4.4–10.8 µmol/L
Iron	5.4–29.7 µmol/L	30–160 µg/dl
Lactate dehydrogenase	1.7–3.2 µkat/L	100–190 µ/L
Lipase	0.51–0.73 µkat/L	3–43 µ/L
Magnesium	0.62–0.95 mmol/L	1.5–2.3 mg/dl
MCHC	310–370 g/L	31–37 g/dl
MCH	26–34 pg/cell	26–34 pg/cell
Myoglobulin		
Male	19–92 µg/L	19–92 µg/L
Female	12–76 µg/L	12–76 µg/L
Osmolality (Plasma)	285–295 mmol/kg of serum water	
Phosphatases	275–295 mOsmol/kg of serum water	
Acid	0.9 µkat/L	0.5–5.0 U/L
Alkaline	0.52 µkat/L	30–120 U/L
Phosphorus (inorganic)	1.0–1.4 mmol/L	3–4.5 mg/dl
Plasminogen		
Antigen	84–140 mg/L	8–14 mg/dl
Platelet count	$150–350 \times 10^{9}$/L	$150–350 \times 10^{3}$/mm^3
Potassium	3.5–5.0 mmol/L	3.5–5.0 mEq/L
Proteins (total)	55–80 g/L	5.5–8.0 g/dl
Albumin	35–55 g/L	3.5–5.5 g/dl (50–60%)
Globulin	20–35 g/L	2.0–3.5 g/dl (40–50%)
α_1	2–4 g/L	0.2–0.4 g/dl (4.2–7.2%)
α_2	5–9 g/L	0.5–0.9 g/dl (6.8–12.0%)
β	6–11 g/L	0.6–1.1 g/dl (9.3–15.0%)
γ	7–15 g/L	0.7–1.7 g/dl (13–23%)

Contd...

Contd...

Analyte	SI units	Conventional units
Protein C and S		
Total antigen	0.70–1.4	70–140%
Functional	0.70–1.4	70–140%
PT	11.1–13.1 sec	11.1–13.1 sec
Red cell distribution width	0.115–0.145	11.5–14.5%
Reticulocyte count		0.5–2.5% of red cells
Sodium	136–145 mmol/L	136–145 mEq/L
Thrombin time	16–24 sec	16–24 sec
Troponin T	0–0.4 µg/L	0–0.4 ng/ml
Urea nitrogen	3.6–7.1 mmol/L	10–20 mg/dl
Uric acid		
Male	0.18–0.41 µmol/L	3.1–7.0 mg/dl
Female	0.15–0.33 µmol/L	2.5–5.6 mg/dl
Viscosity plasma	1.7–2.1	1.7–2.1
Vitamin B_{12}	206–735 pmol/L	279–996 pg/ml

mg/dl=mmol/L x atomic/molecular weight 10

DIABETES RELATED MEASUREMENTS

Analyte	SI units	Conventional units
ANTHROPOMETRY		
Body mass index	Wt (kg)/Ht(m^2)	
N	18.5–22.9	
Overweight	23–27.5	
Obese	>27.5	
Waist (central obesity present)		
Male	>90 cm	
Female	>80 cm	
W/H ratio		
Male	>0.9	
Female	>0.8	
Body fat standards (Asian standard)		
Male	24%	
Female	32%	
Ammonia	15–47 µmol/L	25–80 mg/dl
Amylase	0.8–3.2 µkat/L	60–180 µ/L
Acetones	negative	
Acetoacetate	<100 µmol/L	<1 mg/dl
B-hydroxybutyrate	<300 µmol/L	<3 mg/L
Glucose		60–96 mg/dl

Contd...

Contd...

Analyte	SI units	Conventional units
Growth hormone (resting)	0.1–5 ng/ml	0.5–17.0 ng/ml
Lactate P (arterial)	0.6–1.7 mmol/L	5–15 mg/L
Lactate P (venous)	0.6–1.7 mmol/L	5–15 mg/L
Osmolality (plasma)	285–295 mmol/kg of serum water	

HbA$_{1c}$ levels (glycosylated hemoglobin)

Normal	3.8–6.1%	
HbA$_{1c}$ values%	glycemic control	
<7.0	good	
7.0–8.0	fair	
>8.0	Poor	

75gm OGTT (8–12 hours fasting)

	Fasting plasma glucose (mg/dl)	Post challenge glucose (2 hours) (mg/dl)
NGT	<100	<140
Impaired glucose tolerance	>100	>139 to <200
Impaired fasting glucose	>99 to <126	<140
Diabetes mellitus	>125	>199
Diabetes (type 1) autoantibodies levels	Normal values	
IAA (nu/ml)	<42	
Glutamic Acid Decarboxylase (GAD)	<0.032	
ICAs 12 bdc AA (islet cell autoantibodies)	<0.071	
Basal C–peptide	0.9–4.0 ng/dl	
Glucagon stimulated C peptide	1.5–9.0 ng/dl	

Proinsulin levels

Normal	<0.20 ng.ml	
Suspicious for insulinoma	>0.20–0.30 ng/ml	
Insulinoma	>0.30 ng/ml	
Serum osmolality	$= 2 \times (Na^+ + K^+) + \dfrac{glucose}{18} + \dfrac{BUN}{2.6}$	

LIPID PROFILE

Analyte	SI units	Conventional units
APO A1	119–240 mg/dl	
APO B	52–163 mg/dl	
Cholesterol		
HDL		
Low	<1.03 mmol/L	<40 mg/dl
High	≥1.55 mmol/L	≥60 mg/dl
LDL		
Optimal	<2.59 mmol/L	<100 mg/dl
Near normal	2.59–3.34 mmol/L	100–129 mg/dl
Borderline high	3.36–4.11 mmol/L	130–159 mg/dl
High	4.14–4.89 mmol/L	160–189 mg/dl
Very high	≥4.91	>189 mg/dl
Total cholesterol		
Desirable	<5.17 mmol/L	<200 mg/dl
Borderline high	5.17–6.18 mmol/L	200–239 mg/dl
High	≥6.21 mmol/L	>240 mg/dl

Contd...

Contd...

Analyte	SI units	Conventional units
Triglycerides		
Normal		<150
Borderline high		150–199
High		200–499
Very high		>499
LDL (total cholesterol triglyceride/5) – HDL		
Free fatty acids	<0.28–0.89 mmol/L	8–25 mg/dl
Lipoprotein (a)	0.300 mg/L	0–30 mg/dl

RENAL FUNCTION TESTS

Analyte	SI units	Conventional units
Clearance corrected to 1.72 m^2 BSA		
Measures of GFR		
Insulin clearance		
Male	2.1±0.4 ml/s	124 ± 25.8 ml/min
Female	2.0±0.2 ml/s	119 ± 12.8 ml/min
Endogenous creatinine clearance	1.5–2.2 ml/s	91–130 ml/min
Specific gravity	1.002–1.028	1.002–1.028
Protein excretion	0.15 g/day	<150 mg/day

URINARY ANALYSIS

Analyte	SI units	Conventional units
Ammonia	30–50 mmol/dl	30–50 mEq/d
Calcium	<7.5 mmol/d	<300 mg/d
Creatine		
Female	<760 µmol/d	<100 mg/d
Male	<380 µmol/d	<50 mg/d
Creatinine	8.8–14 mmol/d	1.0–1.6 g/d
Glucose	0.3–1.7 mmol/d	50–300 mg/d
24 hours urine albumin (N)	<0.031 g/24 hours	<31 mg/24 hours
Microalbuminuria	0.03–0.30 g/d	30–300 mg/d
pH	5.0–9.0	5.0–9.0
Phosphate	12.9–42.0 mmol/d	400–1300 mg/d
Sodium	100–260 mmol/d	100–260 mEq/d
Potassium	25–100 mmol/d	25–100 mEq/d
Sp gravity	1.001–1.035	1.001–1.035
Urea nitrogen	214–607 mmol/d	6–17 g/d
Uric acid	1.49–4.76 mmol/d	250–800 mg/d
ENDOCRINE TESTS		
Adrenocorticotrophin (ACTH)	1.3–16.7 pmol/L	6.0–7.60 pg/ml
Androstenedione	1.75–8.73 nmol/L	50–250 ng/dl

Contd...

Contd...

Analyte	SI units	Conventional units
Cortisol		
Fasting 8 am–12 noon	138–690 nmol/L	5–25 µg/dl
12 noon–8 pm	138–414 nmol/L	5–15 µg/dl
8 pm–8 am	0–276 nmol/L	0–10 µg/dl
Deoxycorticosterone	61–576 nmol/L	2–19 ng/dl
11–Deoxycortisol	0.34–4.56 nmol/L	12–158 ng/dl
Dihydrotestosterone		
Male	1.03–2.92 nmol/L	30–85 ng/dl
Female	0.14–0.76 nmol/L	4–22 ng/dl
Epinephrine	0–109 nmol/day	0–20 µg/day
Fructosamine	<285 µmol/L	<285 µmol/L
Glucagon	20–100 ng/L	20–100 pg/ml
Growth hormone	0.5–17.0 µg/L	0.5–17.0 ng/ml
Insulin	14.35–143.5 pmol/L	2–20 µU/ml
PTH (parathyroid hormone)	8–51 ng/L	8–51 pg/ml
Parathyroid hormone related peptide	<1.3 pmol/L	<1.3 pmol/L
Progesterone (Female)		
Follicular	<3.18 nmol/L	<1.0 ng/ml
Midluteal	9.54–63.6 nmol/L	3–20 ng/ml
Male	<3.18 nmol/L	<1.0 ng/ml
Somatostatin	<25 ng/L	<25 pg/ml
Testosterone (total)		
Female	0.21–2.98 nmol/L	6–86 ng/dl
Male	9.36–37.10 nmol/L	270–1070 ng/dl
Thyroglobulin	0.5–5.3 µg/L	0.5–53 ng/ml
TSH	0.34–4.25 mIU/L	0.34–4.25 µIU/ml
T4	70–151 nmol/L	5.4–11.7 ug/dl
T3	1.2–2.1 nmol/L	77–135 ng/dl
fT4	10.3–21.9 pmol/L	0.8–1.7 ng/dl
fT3	3.7–6.5 pmol/L	2.4–4.2 pg/ml
Vasoactive intestinal polypeptide (VIP)	0–60 ng/L	0–60 pg/ml

INDEX

Page numbers with *f* and *t* indicate figure and table, respectively.